KEITH L. MOORE, PhD, FIAC, FRSM
Professor Emeritus of Anatomy and Cell Biology
Faculty of Medicine, University of Toronto
Toronto, Ontario, Canada

Professor of Human Anatomy and Cell Science
Department of Anatomy, Faculty of Medicine
University of Manitoba
Winnipeg, Manitoba, Canada

T.V.N. PERSAUD, MD, PhD, DSc, FRCPath (Lond.)
Professor and Former Head
Department of Human Anatomy and Cell Science
Professor of Pediatrics and Child Health
Professor of Obstetrics, Gynecology, and Reproductive Sciences
University of Manitoba, Faculty of Medicine

Consultant in Pathology and Clinical Genetics
Health Sciences Centre
Winnipeg, Manitoba, Canada

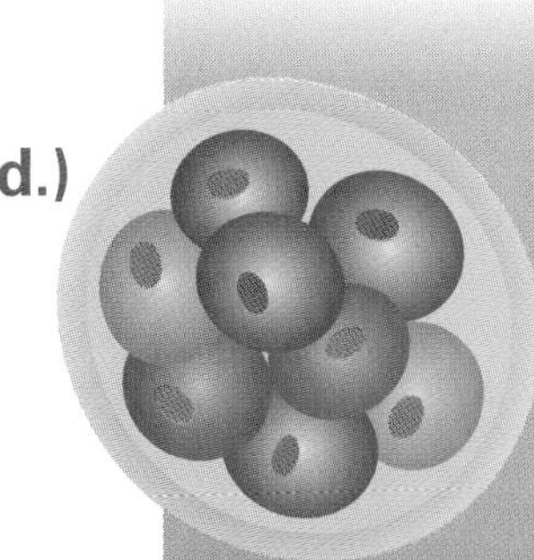

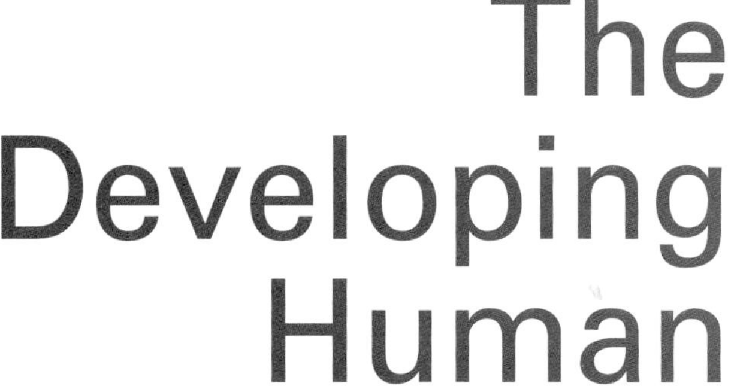

The Developing Human

Clinically Oriented Embryology

6th EDITION

W.B. SAUNDERS COMPANY
A Division of Harcourt Brace & Company
Philadelphia London Toronto Montreal Sydney Tokyo

W.B. SAUNDERS COMPANY
A Division of Harcourt Brace & Company

The Curtis Center
Independence Square West
Philadelphia, Pennsylvania 19106

Library of Congress Cataloging-in-Publication Data

Moore, Keith L.
The developing human: clinically oriented embryology / Keith L. Moore, T.V.N. Persaud.—6th ed.

p. cm.

Includes bibliographical references and index.

ISBN 0–7216–6974–3

1. Embryology, Human. 2. Abnormalities, Human. I. Persaud, T.V.N. II. Title. [DNLM: 1. Embryology. QS 604 M822d 1998]

QM601.M66 1998 612.6′4—dc21

DNLM/DLC 97–27844

THE DEVELOPING HUMAN: CLINICALLY ORIENTED EMBRYOLOGY ISBN 0-7216-6974-3

Printed in the United States of America.

Last digit is the print number: 9 8 7 6 5 4 3 2

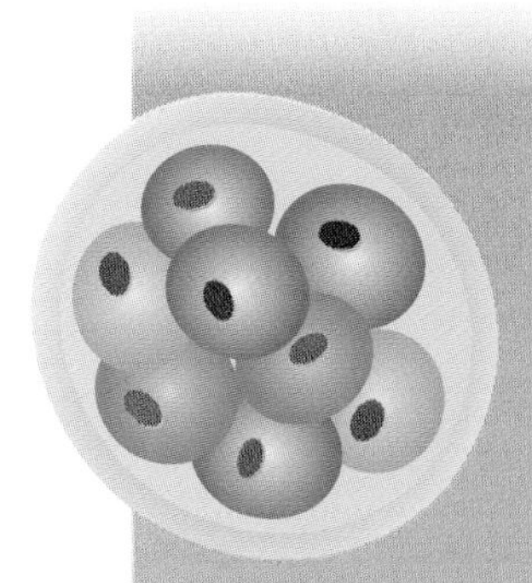

The Developing Human

Clinically Oriented Embryology

To our wives, Marion and Gisela, our children,
and our grandchildren — especially the two latest
grandchildren —
Courtney Michaella (KLM) and Brian (TVNP)

Preface

The sixth edition of *The Developing Human* contains more clinically oriented material than previous editions. These sections are highlighted in color to set them apart from the rest of the text. In addition to focusing on clinically relevant aspects of embryology, there are clinically oriented problems with brief answers and case studies that emphasize that embryology is an important part of medical practice.

This edition includes numerous new color photographs of embryos (normal and abnormal). Many of the illustrations have been improved using *three-dimensional renderings* and more effective use of colors. There are also additional diagnostic images (ultrasound and MRI) of embryos and fetuses, and more scanning electron micrographs have been incorporated to illustrate three-dimensional aspects of embryos.

The coverage of *teratology* has been increased because the study of abnormal development is helpful in understanding risk estimation, the causes of anomalies, and how malformations may be prevented. Recent advances in the molecular aspects of developmental biology have been highlighted throughout the book, especially in those areas that appear promising for clinical medicine or have the potential for making a significant impact on the direction of future research. National board examinations now require some knowledge of the molecular mechanisms that are involved in embryonic development.

We have continued our attempts to give an *easy-to-read account of human development before birth.* Every chapter has been thoroughly revised to reflect new findings in research and their clinical significance. The chapters are organized to present a systematic and logical approach that explains how embryos develop. The first chapter introduces the reader to the scope and importance of embryology, the historical background of the discipline, and the terms used to describe the stages of development. The next four chapters cover embryonic development, beginning with the formation of gametes and ending with the formation of basic organs and systems. The development of specific organs and systems is then described in a systematic manner, followed by chapters dealing with the highlights of the fetal period, the placenta and fetal membranes, and the causes of human congenital anomalies. At the end of each chapter are lists of references that contain classic works and the most recent research publications. This updating of references will be appreciated by serious students and those wishing to use the book as a reference text.

Many of our colleagues (listed alphabetically) have helped with the preparation of this edition. It is a pleasure to record our indebtedness to them: *Dr. Albert E. Chudley,* Professor of Pediatrics and Child Health, Director of Clinical Genetics, Health Sciences Centre, University of Manitoba, Winnipeg, Manitoba, Canada; *Dr. Angelika J. Dawson,* Director, Cytogenetics Laboratory, Health Sciences Centre and Department of Pediatrics and Child Care, University of Manitoba, Winnipeg, Manitoba, Canada; *Dr. Raymond Gasser,* Louisiana State University School of Medicine, New Orleans, Louisiana; *Dr. Christopher R. Harman,* Department of Obstetrics, Gynecology, and Reproductive Sciences, Women's Hospital and University of Manitoba, Winnipeg, Manitoba, Canada; *Dr. Elizabeth Hay,* Pfeifer Professor of Embryology, Department of Cell Biology, Harvard Medical School, Boston, Massachusetts; *Professor K. Hinrichsen,* Rühr-Universität, Medizinische Fakultät, Institut für Anatomie, Bochum, Germany; *Dr. Dagmar K. Kalousek,* Program Head, Cytogenetics/Embryopathology Laboratory and Professor of Pathology, University of British Columbia, Vancouver, British Columbia, Canada; *Dr. Peeyush K. Lala,* Professor of Anatomy and Cell Biology, Faculty of Medicine, University of Western Ontario, London, Ontario, Canada; *Dr. Bernard Liebgott,* Professor of Anatomy and Cell Biology, Faculty of Medicine and Department of Biological Sciences, Faculty of Dentistry, University of Toronto, Toronto, Ontario, Canada; *Dr. Edward A. Lyons,* Professor of Radiology and Obstetrics and Gynecology, Health Sciences Centre, University of Manitoba, Winnipeg, Manitoba, Canada; *Dr. Kohei Shiota,* Professor and Chairman of the Department of Anatomy and Developmental Biology and Director of the Congenital Anomaly Research Center, Faculty of Medicine, Kyoto University, Kyoto, Japan; *Dr.*

Gerald S. Smyser, Altru Health System, Grand Forks, North Dakota; and *Dr. Michael Wiley,* Associate Professor, Department of Anatomy and Cell Biology, Faculty of Medicine, University of Toronto, Toronto, Ontario, Canada.

Those who have contributed photographs are individually acknowledged in the figure legends. The new illustrations were prepared by Hans Neuhart, President of the Electronic Illustrators Group in Fountain Hills, Arizona. Marion Moore in Toronto did the word processing and helped with the review of the manuscript, as did Gisela Persaud in Winnipeg. William Schmitt, Medical Editor, Laurie Sander, Production Manager, and Agnes Byrne, Project Manager, W.B. Saunders Company, and their colleagues have been most helpful with our work. To all these people, we extend our sincere thanks. Last, but not least, we thank our wives, Marion and Gisela, for their continued understanding and support.

KEITH L. MOORE
T.V.N. PERSAUD

Contents

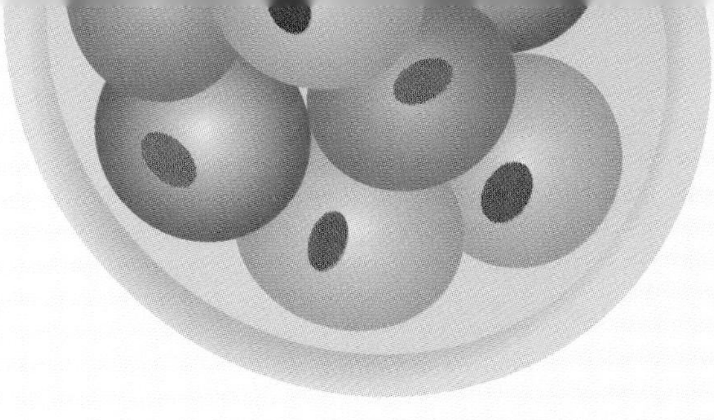

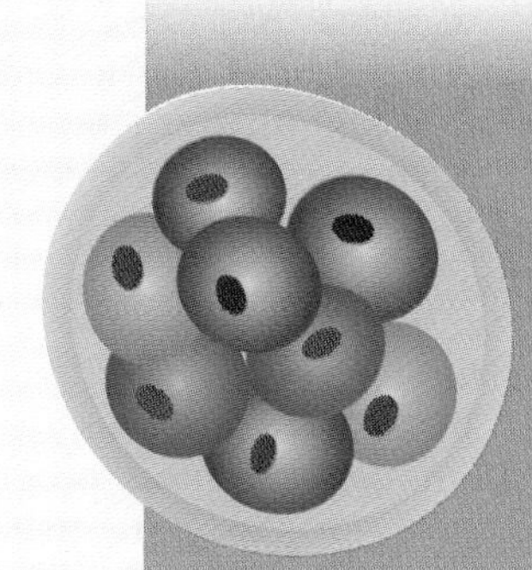

1

Introduction to the Developing Human

■ *Interest in human development before birth is widespread*, largely because of curiosity about our beginnings and the desire to improve the quality of life. The intricate processes by which a baby develops from a single cell are miraculous, and few events are more exciting than a mother's viewing of her embryo during an ultrasound examination. The adaptation of a newborn infant to its new environment is also exhilarating to witness.

Human development is a continuous process that begins when an **oocyte** (ovum) from a female is fertilized by a **sperm** (or spermatozoon) from a male. Cell division, cell migration, programmed cell death, differentiation, growth, and cell rearrangement transform the fertilized oocyte, a highly specialized, totipotent cell — a **zygote** — into a multicellular human being. Although most developmental changes occur during the embryonic and fetal periods, some important changes occur during later periods of development: infancy, childhood, adolescence, and adulthood.

DEVELOPMENTAL PERIODS

Although it is customary to divide human development into *prenatal* (before birth) and *postnatal* (after birth) periods, birth is merely a dramatic event during development resulting in a change in environment. *Development does not stop at birth*. Important changes, in addition to growth, occur after birth (e.g., development of teeth and female breasts). The brain triples in weight between birth and 16 years; most developmental changes are completed by the age of 25.

Prenatal Period

The main developmental changes occurring before birth are illustrated in the *Timetable of Human Prenatal Development* (Figs. 1-1 and 1-2). This developmental calendar is based on the examination of many embryos and fetuses by the authors, and on studies by Streeter (1942), Gasser (1975), Persaud et al. (1985), Butler and Juurlink (1987), Shiota (1991), O'Rahilly and Müller (1992), and Moore et al. (1994). Study of the *Timetable of Human Prenatal Development* reveals that the most visible advances occur during the third to eighth weeks of embryonic development, but the embryo begins to develop as soon as the oocyte is fertilized.

EMBRYOLOGICAL TERMINOLOGY

The following terms are commonly used in discussions of developing humans; several of these terms are used in the *Timetable of Human Prenatal Development*. Most embryological terms have Latin (L.) or Greek (Gr.) origins. Understanding the origin of embryological terms adds clarity and often serves as a memory key. The zygote, for example, is derived from the Greek word *zygōtus,* meaning yoked, which indicates that the sperm and oocyte unite to form a new cell, the zygote. Latin and Greek terms are given in this book for clarity and interest.

Oocyte (L. *ovum*, egg). This term refers to the female germ or sex cell produced in the *ovaries*. When mature, the oocyte is called a secondary oocyte or mature ovum. A *blighted ovum* refers to an early embryo whose development has ceased. Although the embryo is dead, the other products of conception, the chorionic (gestational) sac, for example, may survive for several weeks (Callen, 1994).

Sperm (Gr. *sperma*, seed). The term spermatozoon also has a Greek origin (*spermatos*, seed + *zōon*, animal). The sperm, or spermatozoon, refers to the male germ cell produced in the *testes* (testicles). Sperms (spermatozoa) are expelled from the male urethra during ejaculation.

Zygote (Gr. *zygōtos*, yoked). This cell results from the union of an oocyte and a sperm. A zygote is the beginning of a new human being (i.e., an embryo). The expression *fertilized ovum* refers to a secondary oocyte (ovum) that is impregnated by a sperm; when fertilization is complete, the oocyte becomes a zygote.

Fertilization or Conception Age. It is difficult to determine exactly when fertilization (conception) occurs because the process cannot be observed *in vivo* (within the living body). Physicians calculate the age of the embryo or fetus from the first day of the last normal menstrual period (LNMP). This is the *gestational age*, which is about two weeks longer than the *fertilization age* because the oocyte is not fertilized until about two weeks after the preceding menstruation (Fig. 1-1). Consequently, when a physician gives the age of an embryo or fetus, two weeks must be deducted to determine the actual or fertilization age of the developing human.

Cleavage. This term refers to *the series of mitotic cell divisions of the zygote* that result in the formation of the early embryonic cells, the *blastomeres*. The size of the early embryo remains unchanged because at each succeeding cleavage division, the blastomeres become smaller.

Morula (L. *morus*, mulberry). The blastomeres change their shape and tightly align themselves against each other to form a compact ball of cells. This phenomenon — **compaction** — is probably mediated by cell surface adhesion glycoproteins (Gilbert, 1997). When 12 or more blastomeres have formed, the spherical group of cells is called a morula. It was given this name because of its resemblance to the fruit of a mulberry tree. The morula stage occurs 3 to 4 days after fertilization, just as the developing human enters the uterus.

Blastocyst (Gr. *blastos*, germ + *kystis*, bladder). After the morula enters the uterus from the uterine tube (fallopian tube), a fluid-filled cavity — the *blastocyst cavity* — develops inside it. This change converts the morula into a blastocyst. Its centrally located cells —

the *inner cell mass* or embryoblast—are the primordium or beginning of the embryo.

Implantation. This is the process during which the blastocyst attaches to the *endometrium*—mucous membrane or lining of uterus—and subsequently embeds in it. The *preimplantation period of embryonic development* is the time between fertilization and the beginning of implantation—a period of about 6 days.

Gastrula (Gr. *gaster*, stomach). During gastrulation (transformation of a blastocyst into a gastrula), a three-layered or trilaminar embryonic disc forms (third week). The three germ layers of the gastrula (ectoderm, mesoderm, and endoderm) subsequently differentiate into the tissues and organs of the embryo (e.g., the stomach).

Neurula (Gr. *neuron*, nerve). During neurulation—formation of neural tube—the embryo in the fourth week is sometimes called a neurula. The neural tube is the primordium of the central nervous system (brain and spinal cord).

Embryo (Gr. *embryon*). This term refers to the developing human during its early stages of development. The *embryonic period* extends to the end of the eighth week, by which time the beginnings of all major structures are present. Only the heart and circulation are functioning. The *size of embryos* is given as crown-rump length (CRL), which is measured from the vertex of the skull (crown of the head) to the rump (buttocks).

Stages of Prenatal Development. Early embryonic development is described in stages because of the variable period it takes for embryos to develop certain morphological characteristics (Fig. 1-1). *Stage 1 of development* begins at fertilization and embryonic development ends at *stage 23*, which occurs on day 56. The *fetal period* begins on day 57 and ends when the fetus is completely outside the mother. The stages of embryonic development can be assessed by *ultrasonography* (Filly, 1994).

Conceptus (L. *conceptio*, the derivatives of a zygote). This term refers to the embryo and its adnexa (L., appendages or adjunct parts) or associated membranes (i.e., *the products of conception* or fertilization). The conceptus includes all structures that develop from the zygote, both embryonic and extraembryonic. Hence it includes the embryo as well as the embryonic part of the placenta and its associated membranes—amnion, chorionic (gestational) sac, and yolk sac (see Chapter 7).

Primordium (L. *primus*, first + *ordior*, to begin). This term refers to the beginning or first discernible indication for the earliest stage of development of an organ or structure. The terms *anlage* or *rudiment* have similar meanings. The primordium or anlage of the upper limb appears as a bud on day 26 (Fig. 1-1).

Fetus (L., unborn offspring). After the embryonic period (eight weeks), the developing human is called a fetus. During the *fetal period* (ninth week to birth), differentiation and growth of the tissues and organs formed during the embryonic period occur. Although developmental changes are not so dramatic as those happening during the embryonic period, they are very important because they make it possible for the tissues and organs to function. The rate of body growth is remarkable, especially during the third and fourth months (Fig. 1-2), and weight gain is phenomenal during the terminal months.

Abortion (L. *aboriri*, to miscarry). This term means a premature stoppage of development and refers to the premature expulsion of a conceptus from the uterus or expulsion of an embryo or fetus before it is *viable*—capable of living outside the uterus. There are different types of abortion:

- *Threatened abortion* (bleeding with the possibility of abortion) is a complication in about 25% of clinically apparent pregnancies. Despite every effort to prevent an abortion, about half these pregnancies ultimately abort (Filly, 1994).
- An *accidental abortion* is one that occurs because of an accident (e.g., during a fall down a stairs).
- A *spontaneous abortion* is one that occurs naturally and is most common during the third week after fertilization. About 15% of recognized pregnancies end in spontaneous abortion, usually during the first 12 weeks.
- A *habitual abortion* is the spontaneous expulsion of a dead or nonviable fetus in three or more consecutive pregnancies.
- An *induced abortion* is a birth that is induced before 20 weeks (i.e., before the fetus is viable). This type of abortion refers to the expulsion of an embryo or fetus that is brought on intentionally (e.g., by *vacuum curettage*—removal of the conceptus after dilatation by means of a hollow curette introduced into the uterus, through which suction is applied).
- A *complete abortion* is one in which all the products of conception are expelled from the uterus.
- A *criminal abortion* is one that is produced illegally.
- *Legally induced abortions*, elective, justifiable, or *therapeutic abortions* are usually produced by drugs or suction curettage. Some abortions are induced because of the mother's poor health (physical or mental), or to prevent the birth of a severely malformed child (e.g., one without most of its brain).
- A *missed abortion* is the retention of a conceptus in the uterus after death of the embryo or fetus.
- A *miscarriage* refers to the spontaneous abortion of a fetus and its membranes before the middle of the second trimester.
- An *abortus* refers to the products of an abortion (i.e., the embryo/fetus and its adnexa or membranes). An embryo or nonviable fetus and its ad-

Text continued on page 8

TIMETABLE OF HUMAN PRENATAL DEVELOPMENT
1 TO 6 WEEKS

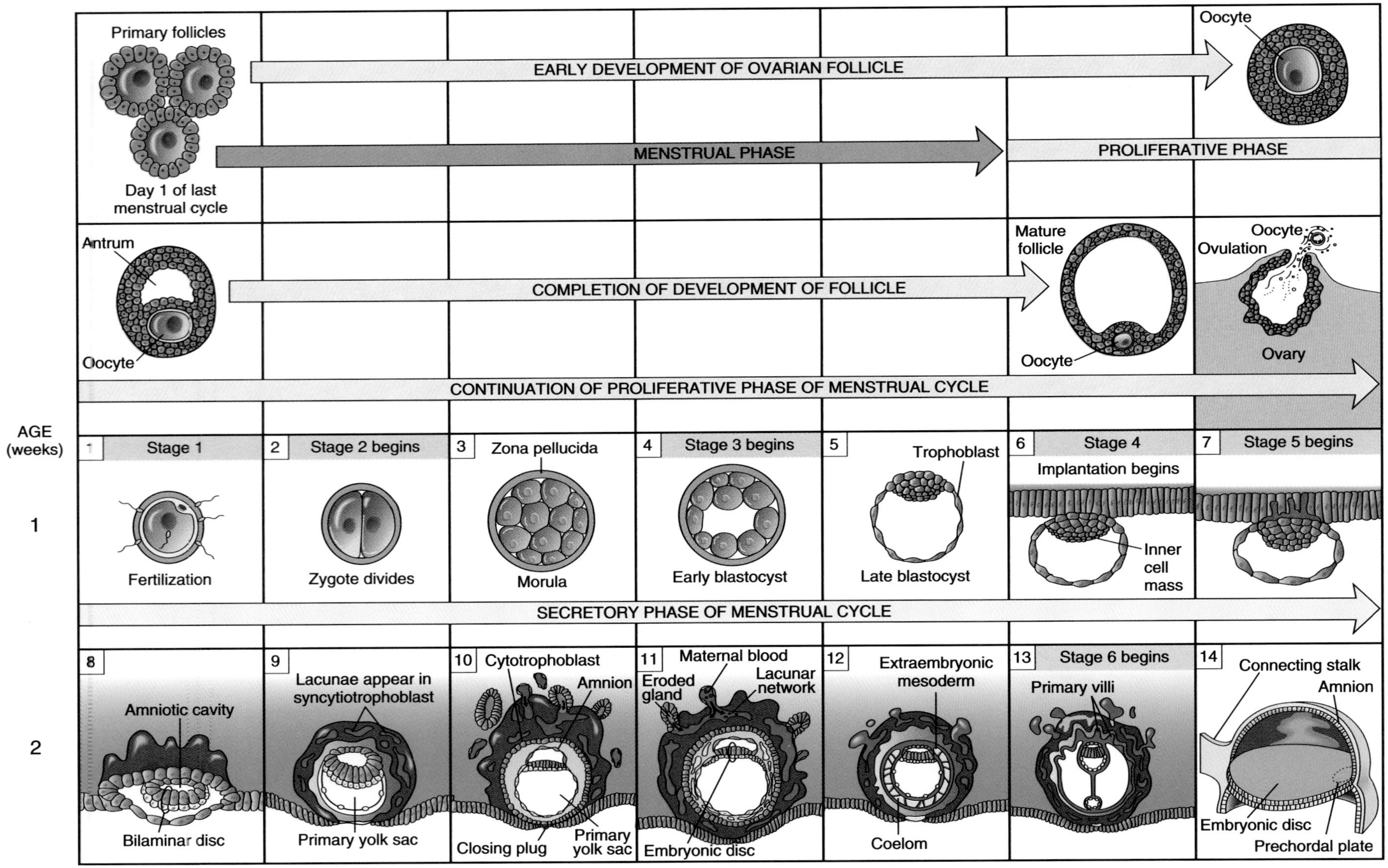

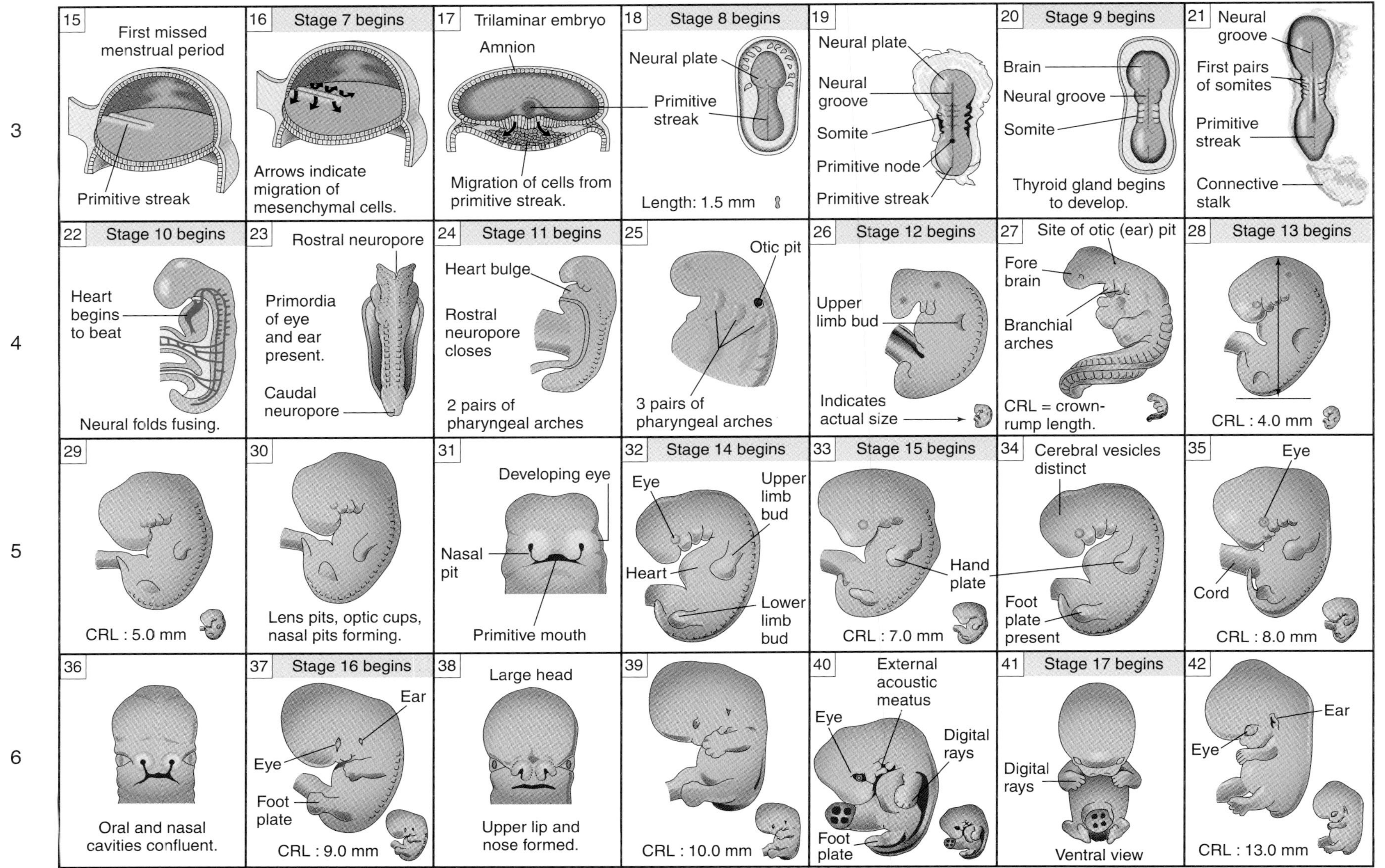

Figure 1–1. Early stages of development. Development of an ovarian follicle containing an oocyte, ovulation, and the phases of the menstrual cycle are illustrated. Human development begins at fertilization, about 14 days after the onset of the last menstruation. Cleavage of the zygote in the uterine tube, implantation of the blastocyst, and early development of the embryo are also shown. For a full discussion of embryonic development, see Chapter 5. Beginning students should make no attempt to memorize these tables or the stages (e.g., that Stage 3 begins on day 4 and Stage 5 on day 7).

TIMETABLE OF HUMAN PRENATAL DEVELOPMENT
7 to 38 weeks

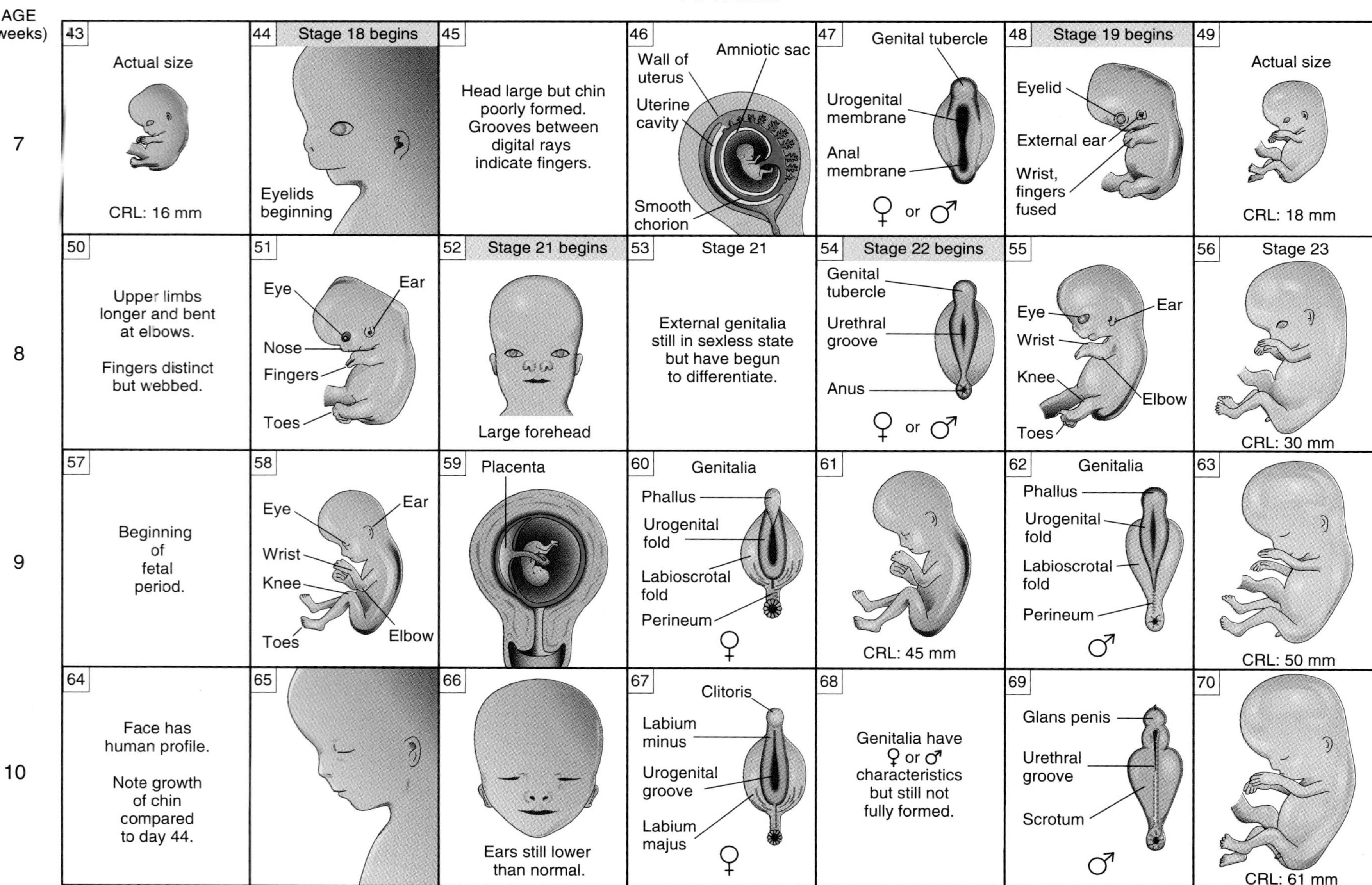

Eleventh Week to Full Term

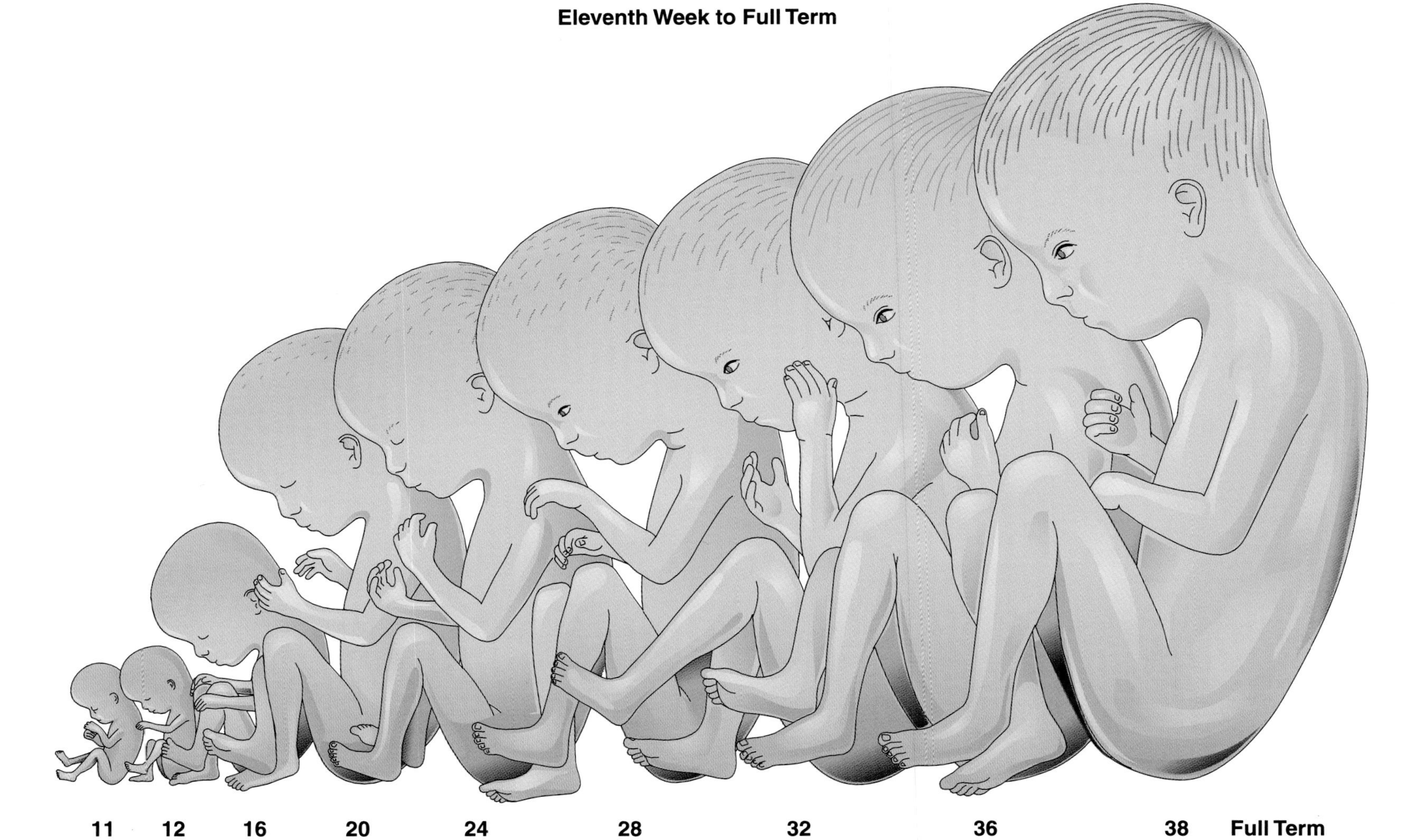

Figure 1–2. Conclusion of the embryonic period and features of the fetal period. The embryonic period terminates at the end of the eighth week; by this time, the beginnings of all essential structures are present. The fetal period, extending from the ninth week to birth, is characterized by growth and elaboration of structures. Sex is clearly distinguishable by 12 weeks. Fetuses are viable 22 weeks after fertilization, but their chances of survival are not good until they are several weeks older. The 11- to 38-week fetuses shown above are about half their actual sizes. For more information, see Chapter 6.

nexa weighing less than 500 gm that are expelled from the uterus is an abortus (aborted embryo or fetus).

Trimester. This is a period of *three calendar months* during a pregnancy. Obstetricians commonly divide the 9-month period of gestation (stages of intrauterine development) into three trimesters. The most critical stages of development occur during the first trimester (12 weeks) when embryonic and early fetal development is occurring.

Congenital Anomalies. Birth defects, or congenital malformations, are abnormalities of development that are present at birth (L. *congenitus*, born together or with); a cleft lip, for example. In some cases the anomalies are not detected until childhood or even adulthood; e.g., three kidneys instead of two. For a full discussion of birth defects and congenital anomalies (malformations), see Chapter 8.

Postnatal Period

The changes occurring after birth—the development of teeth and breasts, for example—are more or less familiar to most people. Explanations of frequently used developmental terms and periods follow.

INFANCY

Infancy refers to the earliest period of extrauterine life; roughly *the first year after birth*. The first 4 weeks are designated as the newborn or *neonatal period*. Transition from intrauterine to extrauterine existence requires many critical changes, especially in the cardiovascular and respiratory systems. If newborn infants, or *neonates*, survive the first crucial hours after birth, their chances of living are usually good. The body as a whole grows particularly rapidly during infancy; total length increases by about one-half and weight is usually trebled. By the age of 1 year, most children have six to eight teeth. For details of development during infancy, see Behrman et al. (1996).

CHILDHOOD

Childhood is the period from about 13 months until puberty (sexual maturity). The primary (deciduous) teeth continue to appear and are later replaced by the secondary (permanent) teeth. During early childhood there is active ossification (formation of bone), but as the child becomes older, the rate of body growth slows down. Just before puberty, however, growth accelerates during the *prepubertal growth spurt*.

PUBERTY

Puberty (L. *pubertas*, development of sex characteristics) is the period, usually between the ages of 12 and 15 years in girls and 13 and 16 years in boys, during which *secondary sexual characteristics develop* and the capability of sexual reproduction is attained. The stages of pubertal development follow a consistent pattern for individuals and are defined by the development of primary and secondary sexual characteristics (pubic hair development, breasts in females, and growth of external genitalia in males). Puberty ends in females with the first menstrual period or *menarche*, the beginning of the menstrual cycles or periods. Puberty ends in males when mature sperms are produced. The *legal age of presumptive puberty* is 12 years in girls and 14 years in boys.

ADOLESCENCE

Adolescence (L. *adolescentia*) is the period from about 11 to 19 years of age, which is characterized by rapid physical and sexual maturation. It extends from the earliest signs of sexual maturity—the appearance of pubes (pubic hairs) or *pubertal development*—until the attainment of physical, mental, and emotional maturity. *The ability to reproduce is achieved during adolescence*. The general growth rate decelerates as this period terminates, but growth of some structures accelerates (e.g., female breasts and male genitalia).

ADULTHOOD

Adulthood (L. *adultus*, grown up)—attainment of full growth and maturity—is generally reached between the ages of 18 and 21 years. Ossification and growth are virtually completed during early adulthood, 21 to 25 years. Thereafter, developmental changes occur very slowly.

SIGNIFICANCE OF EMBRYOLOGY

Literally, **embryology** means the study of embryos; however, the term generally refers to prenatal development—the study of embryos and fetuses. **Developmental anatomy** is the field of embryology concerned with the changes that cells, tissues, organs, and the body as a whole undergo from a germ cell of each parent to the resulting adult. Prenatal development is more rapid than postnatal development and results in more striking changes; however, the developmental mechanisms of the two periods are similar.

Teratology (Gr. *teratos*, monster) is the division of embryology and pathology that deals with abnormal development (anomalies, birth defects, congenital malformations). This *branch of embryology* is concerned with various genetic and/or environmental factors that disturb normal development and produce birth defects (see Chapter 8).

Embryology

- Bridges the gap between prenatal development and obstetrics, perinatal medicine, pediatrics, and clinical anatomy.
- Develops knowledge concerning the beginnings

of human life and the changes occurring during prenatal development.
- Is of practical value in helping to understand the causes of variations in human structure.
- Illuminates gross anatomy and explains how normal relations and abnormalities develop.

Knowledge that physicians have of normal development and of the causes of anomalies is necessary for giving the embryo and fetus the greatest possible chance of developing normally. Much of the modern practice of obstetrics involves what may be called **applied embryology**. Embryological topics of special interest to obstetricians are ovulation, oocyte and sperm transport, fertilization, implantation, fetal-maternal relations, fetal circulation, critical periods of development, and causes of birth defects. In addition to caring for the mother, physicians guard the health of the embryo and fetus. *The significance of embryology is readily apparent to pediatricians* because many of their patients have congenital anomalies resulting from maldevelopment, e.g., diaphragmatic hernia, spina bifida, and congenital heart disease.

Developmental anomalies cause most deaths during infancy. Knowledge of the development of structure and function is essential for understanding the physiological changes that occur during the newborn period and for helping fetuses and babies in distress. Progress in surgery, especially in the fetal, perinatal, and pediatric age groups, has made knowledge of human development even more clinically significant. *Surgical treatment of the fetus is now possible* (Harrison et al., 1991). The understanding and correction of most congenital anomalies depend upon knowledge of normal development and of the deviations that may occur. An understanding of common congenital anomalies and their causes also enables physicians, dentists, and others to explain the developmental basis of abnormalities, often dispelling parental guilt feelings.

Physicians and other health care professionals who are aware of common anomalies and their embryological bases approach unusual situations with confidence rather than surprise. For example, when it is realized that the renal artery represents only one of several vessels originally supplying the embryonic kidney, the frequent variations in number and arrangement of renal vessels are understandable and not unexpected.

HISTORICAL GLEANINGS

"If I have seen further, it is by standing on the shoulders of giants."

—SIR ISAAC NEWTON, ENGLISH MATHEMATICIAN, 1643–1727

This statement, made over 300 years ago, emphasizes that each new study of a problem rests on a base of knowledge established by earlier investigators. The theories of every age offer explanations based on the knowledge and experience of investigators of the period. Although we should not consider them final, we should appreciate rather than scorn their ideas. People have always been interested in knowing how they originated, developed, and were born, and why some people develop abnormally. Ancient people, filled with curiosity, developed many answers to these questions.

Ancient Views of Human Embryology

A brief *Sanskrit treatise* on ancient Indian embryology is thought to have been written in 1416 B.C. This scripture of the Hindus, called *Garbha Upanishad*, describes ancient ideas concerning the embryo. It states:

> From the conjugation of blood and semen the embryo comes into existence. During the period favorable for conception, after the sexual intercourse, (it) becomes a *Kalada* (one-day-old embryo). After remaining seven nights, it becomes a vesicle. After a fortnight it becomes a spherical mass. After a month it becomes a firm mass. After two months the head is formed. After three months the limb regions appear.

Greek scholars made many important contributions to the science of embryology (Persaud, 1984; Horder et al., 1986; Dunstan, 1990). The first recorded embryological studies are in the books of **Hippocrates of Cos** (Fig. 1-3), the famous Greek physician (circa 460-377 B.C.), the *Father of Medicine*. In order to understand how the human embryo develops, he recommended:

> Take twenty or more eggs and let them be incubated by two or more hens. Then each day from the second to that of hatching, remove an egg, break it, and examine it. You will find exactly as I say, for the nature of the bird can be likened to that of man.

Aristotle of Stagira (circa 384-322 B.C.), a Greek philosopher and scientist, wrote a treatise on embryology in which he described development of the chick and other embryos. Aristotle is regarded as the *Founder of Embryology*, despite the fact that he promoted the idea that the embryo developed from a formless mass, which he described as a "less fully

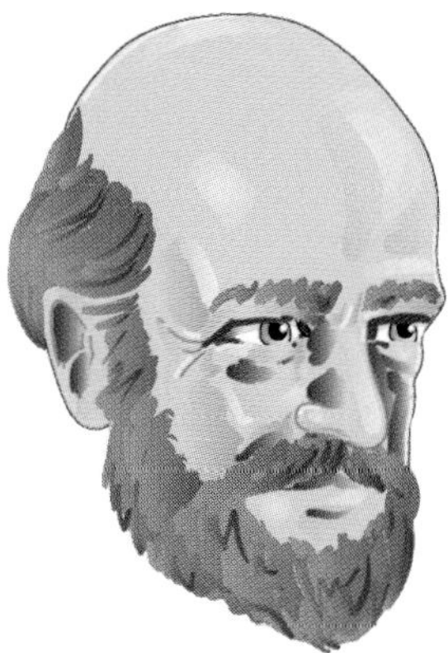

■ **Figure 1-3.** A drawing of Hippocrates, "the Father of Medicine" (460-377 B.C.). He placed medicine on a scientific foundation. In addition to the Hippocratic oath attributed to him, he wrote several books on anatomy, including one on embryology.

concocted seed with a nutritive soul and all bodily parts." This embryo, he thought, arose from menstrual blood after activation by male semen.

Claudius Galen (circa 130-201 A.D.), a Greek physician and medical scientist in Rome, wrote a book *On the Formation of the Foetus*, in which he described the development and nutrition of fetuses and the structures that we now call the allantois, amnion, and placenta.

Embryology in the Middle Ages

Growth of science was slow during the medieval period, and few high points of embryological investigation undertaken during this time are known to us. However, it is cited in the Qur'an (seventh century A.D.), the Holy Book of the Muslims, that human beings are produced from a mixture of secretions from the male and female. Several references are made to the creation of a human being from a *nutfa* (small drop). It also states that the resulting organism settles in the womb like a seed, 6 days after its beginning. Reference is also made to the leechlike appearance of the early embryo. Later the embryo is said to resemble a "chewed substance." For more information about embryological references in the Qur'an, see Musallam (1990).

Constantinus Africanus of Salerno (circa 1020-1087 A.D.) wrote a concise treatise entitled *De Humana Natura*. He gave the West many classical learnings in readable Latin through his many translations of Greek, Roman, and Arabic scholars. Africanus described the composition and sequential development of the embryo in relation to the planets and each month during pregnancy, a concept unknown in antiquity (Burnett, 1990).

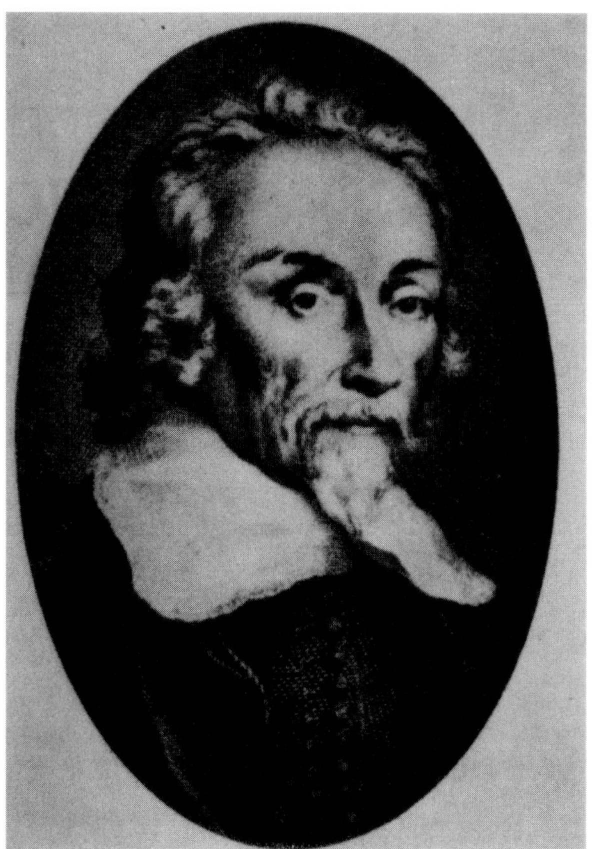

■ **Figure 1-5.** William Harvey (1578–1657). He discovered the circulation of blood and made many observations on the development of embryos. (From Sabiston BC, Jr, Lyerly HK: *Sabiston Essentials of Surgery,* 2nd ed. Philadelphia, WB Saunders, 1997, p 2.).

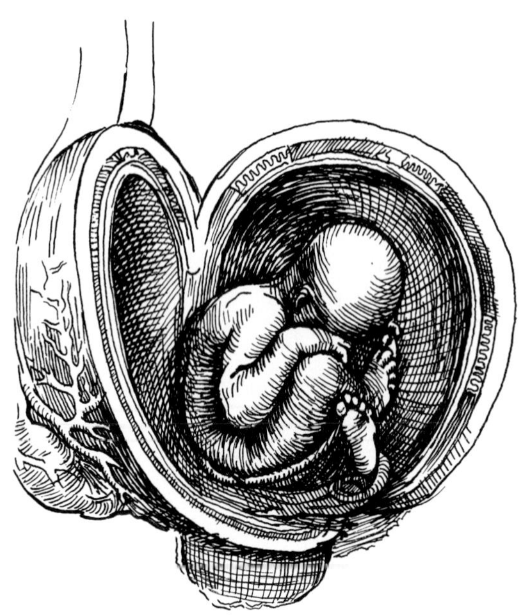

■ **Figure 1-4.** Reproduction of Leonardo da Vinci's drawing made in the fifteenth century A.D., showing a fetus in a uterus that has been incised and opened.

The Renaissance

Leonardo da Vinci (15th century A.D.) made accurate drawings of dissections of the pregnant uterus containing a fetus (Fig. 1-4). He introduced the quantitative approach to embryology by making measurements of prenatal growth.

According to Brockliss (1990), the embryological revolution began with the publication of Harvey's book, *De Generatione Animalium*, in 1651. He believed that the male seed or sperm, after entering the womb or uterus, became metamorphosed into an egg-like substance from which the embryo developed. **William Harvey** (1578-1657) was greatly influenced by one of his professors at the University of Padua, **Fabricius of Aquapendente**, an Italian anatomist and embryologist who was the first to study embryos from different species of animals. Harvey (Fig. 1-5) examined chick embryos with simple lenses and made many new observations. He also studied development of the fallow deer; however, when unable to observe early stages, concluded that embryos were secreted by the uterus. **Girolamo Fabricius** (1537-1619) wrote two major embryological treatises, including one entitled *De Formato Foetu* (The Formed Fetus), which contained many illustrations of embryos and fetuses at different stages of development.

Early microscopes were simple but they opened an exciting new field of observation. In 1672 **de Graaf** observed little chambers in the rabbit's uterus and concluded that they could not have been secreted by the uterus. He concluded that they must have come from organs that he called *ovaries*. Undoubtedly, the little chambers de Graaf described were blastocysts. He also described vesicular ovarian follicles, which are still sometimes called *graafian follicles* in his honor. **Marcello Malpighi,** studying what he believed were unfertilized hen's eggs in 1675, observed early embryos. As a result, he thought the egg contained a miniature chick. **Hamm** and **Leeuwenhoek**, using an improved microscope in 1677 (Fig. 1-6), first observed human sperms or spermatozoa (Gr. *sperma*, seed + *zōon*, animal). However, they misunderstood the sperm's role in fertilization. They thought the sperm contained a miniature preformed human being that enlarged when it was deposited in the female genital tract (Fig. 1-7).

Caspar Friedrich Wolff refuted both versions of the *preformation theory* in 1759, after observing parts of the embryo develop from "globules" (developing embryonic tissues). He examined unincubated eggs and could not see the embryos described by Malpighi. He proposed the *layer concept*, whereby division of what we call the zygote produces layers of cells (now called the embryonic disc) from which the embryo develops. His ideas formed the basis of the *theory of epigenesis*, which states that development results from growth and differentiation of specialized cells. These important discoveries first appeared in Wolff's doctoral dissertation, *Theoria Generationis*. He also observed embryological masses of tissues that partly contribute to the development of the urinary and genital systems—Wolffian bodies and Wolffian ducts—now called the mesonephros and mesonephric ducts, respectively (see Chapter 13).

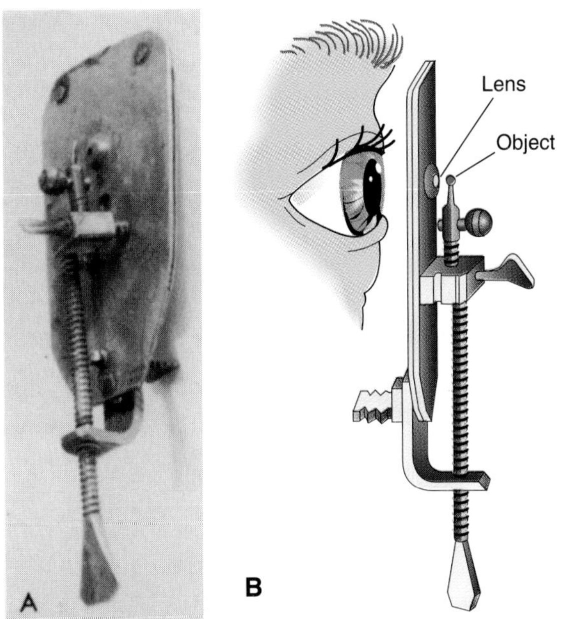

■ **Figure 1–6.** *A,* Photograph of a 1673 Leeuwenhoek microscope. *B,* Drawing of a lateral view illustrating the use of this primitive microscope. The object was held in front of the lens on the point of the short rod, and the screw arrangement was used to adjust the object under the lens.

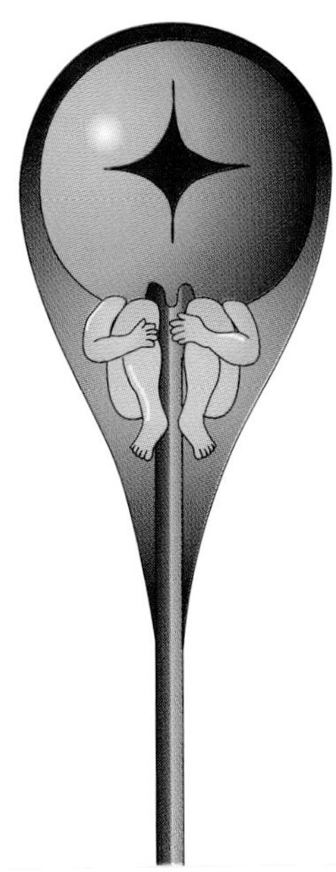

■ **Figure 1–7.** Copy of a seventeenth century drawing of a sperm by Hartsoeker. The miniature human being within it was thought to enlarge after the sperm entered an ovum. Other embryologists at this time thought the oocyte contained a miniature human being that enlarged when it was stimulated by a sperm.

Heinrich Christian Pander discovered the three germ layers of the embryo, which he named the *blastoderm*. He reported this discovery in 1817 in his doctoral dissertation. The preformation controversy ended in 1775 when **Spallanzani** showed that both the ovum and sperm were necessary for initiating the development of a new individual. From his experiments, including artificial insemination in dogs, he concluded that the sperm was the fertilizing agent that initiated the developmental processes.

Saint Hilaire and his son made the first significant studies of abnormal development in 1818. They performed experiments in animals that were designed to produce developmental abnormalities, initiating what we now know as the *science of teratology*.

Von Baer described the oocyte in the ovarian follicle of a dog in 1827, about 150 years after the discovery of the sperm. He also observed dividing zygotes in the uterine tube and blastocysts in the uterus. He contributed new knowledge about the origin of tissues and organs from the layers described earlier by Malpighi and Pander. *Von Baer formulated two important* *embryological concepts*: corresponding stages of embryonic development and that general characteristics precede specific ones. His significant and far-reaching contributions resulted in his later being regarded as the *Father of Modern Embryology*.

Schleiden and **Schwann** were responsible for great advances being made in embryology when they *formulated the cell theory* in 1839. This concept stated that the body is composed of cells and cell products. The cell theory soon led to the realization that the embryo developed from a single cell, the *zygote*, which underwent many cell divisions as the tissues and organs formed. **Wilhelm His** (1831-1904), a Swiss anatomist and embryologist, developed improved techniques for fixation, sectioning, and staining of tissues, and for reconstruction of embryos (O'Rahilly, 1988). His method of graphic reconstruction paved the way for producing current three-dimensional, stereoscopic, and computer-generated images of embryos.

Franklin P. Mall (1862-1917), inspired by the work of His, began to collect human embryos for scientific study. Mall's collection forms a part of the *Carnegie Collection* of embryos that is known throughout the world. It is now in the National Museum of Health and Medicine in the Armed Forces Institute of Pathology in Washington, DC.

Wilhelm Roux (1850-1924) pioneered analytical experimental studies on the physiology of development in amphibia, which was pursued further by **Hans Spemann** (1869-1941). For his discovery of the phenomenon of primary induction—how one tissue determines the fate of another (Allen, 1993)—*Spemann received the Nobel Prize in 1935*. Over the decades, scientists have been attempting to isolate the substances that are transmitted from one tissue to another, causing induction. Recent studies suggest that endogenous *retinoic acid*, a hydrophobic molecule that specifically binds to nuclear receptors, is a likely *morphogen*—a diffusible substance in embryonic tissue that influences morphogenesis, which is the evolution and development of form (Bard, 1992)—that induces the normal pattern of embryonic structures. Moreover, there is some evidence that *retinoic acid receptors* (RARs), as well as an *orphan receptor* (RXR), may be uniquely involved in the regulation of normal embryonic development (Eichele, 1989; Slack, 1991; Giguere, 1994).

Edwards and **Steptoe** pioneered one of the most revolutionary developments in the history of human reproduction—the technique of *in vitro fertilization*. These studies resulted in the birth of Louise Brown in 1978, the first "test tube baby". Since then, thousands of couples throughout the world who were considered infertile have experienced the miracle of birth because of this new reproductive technology.

Genetics and Human Development

In 1859 **Charles Darwin** (1809-1882), an English biologist and evolutionist, published the book *On the Origin of Species*, in which he emphasized the hereditary nature of variability among members of a species as an important factor in evolution. **Gregor Mendel**, an Austrian monk, developed the principles of heredity in 1865, but medical scientists and biologists did not understand the significance of these principles in the study of mammalian development for many years.

Flemming observed chromosomes in 1878 and suggested their probable role in fertilization. In 1883, **von Beneden** observed that mature germ cells have a reduced number of chromosomes. He also described some features of *meiosis*, the process whereby the chromosome number is reduced in germ cells.

Sutton and **Boveri** declared independently in 1902 that the behavior of chromosomes during germ cell formation and fertilization agreed with Mendel's principles of inheritance. In the same year, **Garrod** reported *alcaptonuria* as the first example of mendelian inheritance in human beings. Many consider Garrod to be the *Father of Medical Genetics*. It was soon realized that the zygote contains all the genetic information necessary for directing the development of a new human being.

Von Winiwarter reported the first observations on human chromosomes in 1912, stating that there were 47 chromosomes in body cells. **Painter** concluded in 1923 that 48 was the correct number, a conclusion that was widely accepted until 1956, when **Tjio** and **Levan** reported finding only 46 chromosomes in embryonic cells. Their descriptions and photomicrographs were so superior to those of previous workers that few cytologists doubted the accuracy of their chromosome counts.

Chromosome studies were soon used in medicine in a number of important ways, e.g., clinical diagnosis, chromosome mapping, and prenatal diagnosis (Thompson et al., 1991). Once the normal chromosomal pattern was firmly established, it soon became evident that some persons with congenital anomalies had an abnormal number of chromosomes. A new era in medical genetics resulted from the demonstration by **Lejeune and associates** in 1959 that infants with mongolism (now known as *Down syndrome*) have 47 chromosomes instead of the usual 46 in their body cells. It is now known that chromosomal aberrations are a significant cause of congenital anomalies and embryonic death (see Chapter 8).

Molecular Biology of Human Development

Advances in molecular biology have led to the development of sophisticated techniques for studying embryonic development. The application of *recombinant DNA technology*, chimeric models, and transgenic mice are now widely used in research laboratories to address such diverse problems as the genetic regulation of morphogenesis, the temporal and regional expression of specific genes, and how cells are committed to form various parts of the embryo. For the first time we are beginning to understand how, when, and

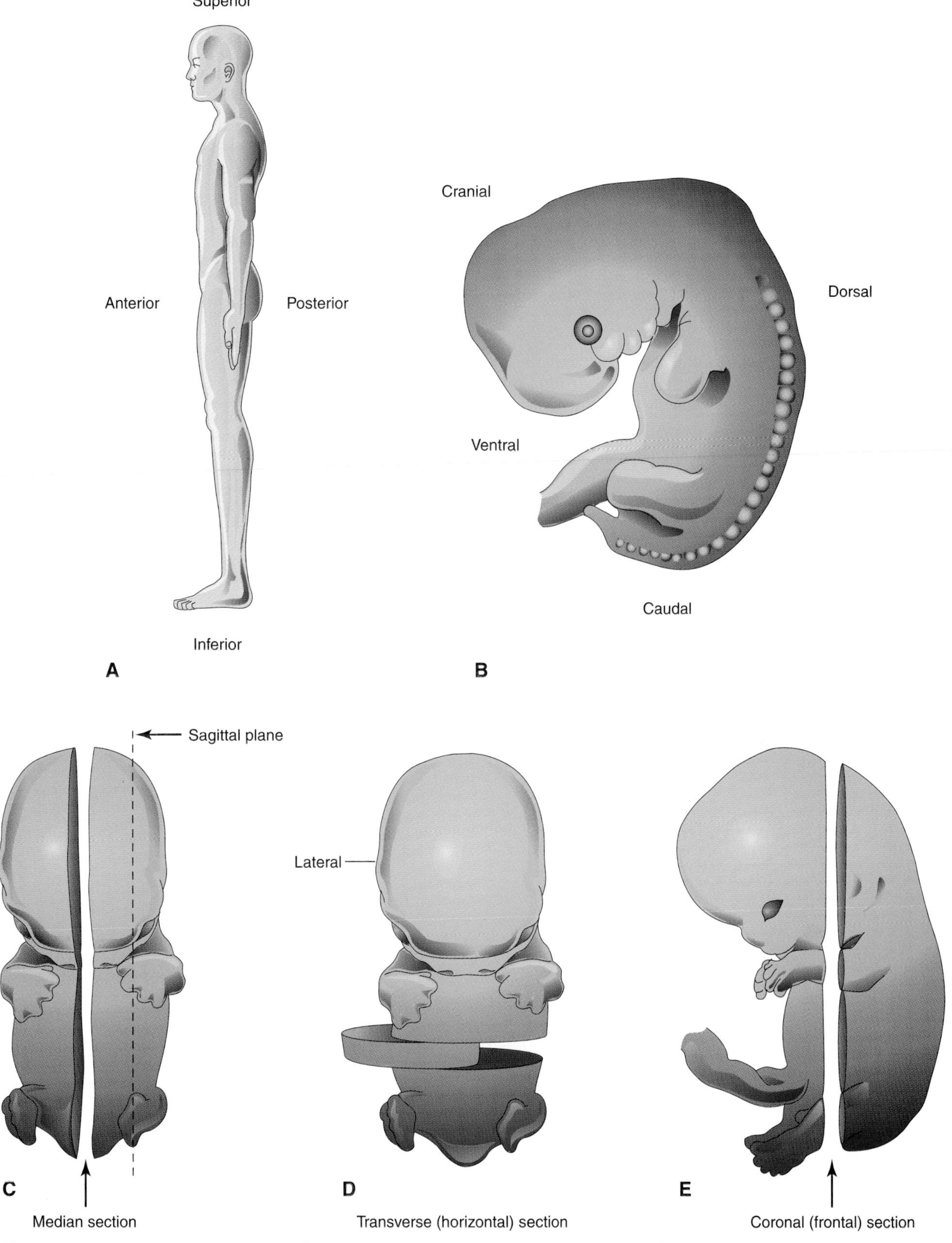

■ **Figure 1–8.** Drawings illustrating descriptive terms of position, direction, and planes of the body. *A,* Laterial view of an adult in the anatomical position. *B,* Lateral view of a five-week embryo. *C* and *D,* Ventral views of six-week embryos. *E,* Lateral view of a seven-week embryo. In describing development, it is necessary to use words denoting the position of one part to another, or to the body as a whole. For example, the vertebral column (backbone) develops in the dorsal part of the embryo, and the sternum (breast bone) develops ventral to it in the ventral part of the embryo.

where selected genes are activated and expressed in the embryo during normal and abnormal development (Goodwin, 1988; Rossant and Joyner, 1989; Rusconi, 1991; Smith, 1996). *Endogenous retinoic acid* has been identified as an important regulatory substance in embryonic development. Apparently, it acts as a transcriptional activator for specific genes that are involved in embryonic patterning (Eichele, 1989; Giguere, 1994).

Homeobox-containing (HOX) genes now appear to be important in controlling pattern formation during embryonic development (Muragaki et al., 1996). The Nobel prize for physiology or medicine was awarded to Edward B. **Lewis**, Christiane **Nüsslein-Volhard**, and Eric F. **Wieschaus** in 1995 for their discovery of genes that control embryonic development (Blum, 1995). Their findings are helping us to understand the causes of spontaneous abortion and congenital anomalies.

DESCRIPTIVE TERMS IN EMBRYOLOGY

Most terms used in this book are based on the third edition of *Nomina Embryologica*, which was published as part of the sixth edition of *Nomina Anatomica* (Warwick, 1989). The English equivalents of the standard Latin forms of anatomical terms are given in some cases, e.g., sperm (spermatozoon). Eponyms commonly used clinically appear in parentheses, such as uterine tube (fallopian tube).

In anatomy and embryology several terms relating to position and direction are used, and reference is made to various planes of the body. All descriptions of the adult are based on the assumption that the body is erect, with the upper limbs by the sides and the palms directed anteriorly (Fig. 1-8*A*). This is the **anatomical position**. The terms anterior or ventral and posterior or dorsal are used to describe the front or back of the body or limbs, and the relations of structures within the body to one another. When describing embryos, the terms dorsal and ventral are used (Fig. 1-8*B*). Superior and inferior are used to indicate the relative levels of different structures (Fig. 1-8*A*). For embryos, the terms cranial and caudal are used to denote relationships to the head and tail, respectively (Fig. 1-8*B*). Distances from the source or attachment of a structure are designated as proximal or distal. In the lower limb, for example, the knee is proximal to the ankle and the ankle is distal to the knee.

The *median plane* is an imaginary vertical plane of section that passes longitudinally through the body. Median sections divide the body into right and left halves (Fig. 1-8*C*). The terms *lateral* and *medial* refer to structures that are respectively farther from or nearer to the median plane of the body. A *sagittal plane* is any vertical plane passing through the body that is parallel to the median plane (Fig. 1-8*C*). The sagittal planes are named after the sagittal suture of the skull (see Chapter 15), to which they are parallel. A *transverse (horizontal)* plane refers to any plane that is at right angles to both the median and coronal planes (Fig. 1-8*D*). A *coronal (frontal) plane* is any vertical plane that intersects the median plane at a right angle (Fig. 1-8*E*) and divides the body into anterior or ventral and posterior or dorsal parts. The coronal planes are named after the coronal suture of the skull (see Chapter 15), to which they are parallel.

Clinically Oriented Problems

1. At what embryonic stage does a new human being start to develop? When do developmental stages end?
2. What is the human embryo called at the beginning of its development? Why is this an appropriate term? Could it be referred to as a conceptus?
3. How do the terms conceptus and abortus differ?
4. What sequence of events occurs during puberty? Are they the same in males and females? What are the respective ages of presumptive puberty in males and females?
5. How do the terms embryology and teratology differ? Are these studies applicable to clinical practice?

Discussion of these problems appears at the back of the book.

REFERENCES AND SUGGESTED READING*

Allen GE: Inducers and "organizers": Hans Spemann and experimental embryology. *Pubbl Stn Zool Napoli 15*:229, 1993.

Bard J: *Morphogenesis. The Cellular and Molecular Processes of Developmental Anatomy*. Cambridge, Cambridge University Press, 1992.

Behrman RE, Kliegman RM, Arvin AM (eds): *Nelson Textbook of Pediatrics*, 15th ed. Philadelphia, WB Saunders, 1996.

Beller FK, Zlatnik GP: The Beginning of Human Life. *J Assist Reprod Genet 12*:477, 1995.

Biggers JD: Arbitrary partitions of prenatal life. *Hum Reprod 5*:1, 1990.

Blum HE: Nobelpreis für Medizin 1995. *Dtsch Med Wochenschr 120*: 1797, 1995.

Brockliss LWB: The embryological revolution in the France of Louis XIV: The dominance of ideology. *In* Dunstan GR (ed): *The Human Embryo. Aristotle and the Arabic and European Traditions*. Exeter, University of Exeter Press, 1990.

Burnett CSF: The planets and the development of the embryo. *In* Dunstan GR (ed): *The Human Embryo. Aristotle and the Arabic and European Traditions*. Exeter, University of Exeter Press, 1990.

Butler H, Juurlink BHJ: *An Atlas for Staging Mammalian and Chick Embryos*. Boca Raton, CRC Press, Inc, 1987.

Callen PW: *Ultrasonography in Obstetrics and Gynecology*, 3rd ed. Philadelphia, WB Saunders, 1994.

Churchill FB: The rise of classical descriptive embryology. *Dev Biol (NY) 7*:1, 1991.

Cunningham BA: Cell adhesion molecules and the regulation of development. *Am J Obstet 164*:939, 1991.

De Pomerai D: *From Gene to Animal*, 2nd ed. New York, Cambridge University Press, 1991.

Dunstan GR (ed): *The Human Embryo. Aristotle and the Arabic*

*In this and other chapters, the references include not only those cited in the text, but ones that are classical (e.g., Streeter, 1942) and others that will be helpful to those wishing more details about embryology and related subjects.

and European Traditions. Exeter, University of Exeter Press, 1990.

Eichele G: Retinoids and vertebrate limb pattern formation. *Trends Genet 5*:246, 1989.

Filly RA: Ultrasound evaluation during the first trimester. *In* Callen PW (ed): *Ultrasonography in Obstetrics and Gynecology*. Philadelphia, WB Saunders, 1994.

Gasser R: *Atlas of Human Embryos*. Hagerstown, Harper & Row, 1975.

Giguere V: Retinoic acid receptors and cellular retinoid binding proteins: complex interplay in retinoid signaling. *Endocr Rev 15*:61, 1994.

Gilbert SF: *Developmental Biology*, 5th ed. Sunderland, Sinauer Associates, Inc., 1997.

Goodwin BC: Problems and prospects in morphogenesis. *Experientia 44*:633, 1988.

Hanson AE: *Paidopoiia*: Metaphors for conception, abortion, and gestation in the *Hippocratic Corpus. Clio Med 27*:291, 1995.

Harrison MR, Golbus MS, Filly RA: *The Unborn Patient: Prenatal Diagnosis and Treatment*, 2nd ed. Philadelphia, WB Saunders, 1991.

Hawkins J: *Gene Structure and Expression*, 2nd ed. New York, Cambridge University Press, 1991.

Horder TJ, Witkowski JA, Wylie CC (eds): *A History of Embryology*. Cambridge, Cambridge University Press, 1986.

Kalthoff K: *Analysis of Biological Development*. New York, McGraw/Hill, 1995.

Kohl F, von Baer KE: 1792-1876. Zum 200. Geburtstag des "Vaters der Embryologie." *Dtsch Med Wochenschr 117*:1976, 1992.

Longo LD: De formato foetu-Girolamo Fabrici. *Am J Obstet Gynecol 173*:1617, 1995.

Moore KL: A scientist's interpretation of references to embryology in the Qur'an. *JIMA 18*:15, 1986.

Moore KL, Persaud TVN, Shiota K: *Color Atlas of Clinical Embryology*. Philadelphia, WB Saunders, 1994.

Muragaki Y, Mundlos S, Upton J, Olsen BR: Altered growth and branching patterns in synpolydactyly caused by mutations of HOXD 13. *Science 272*:548, 1996.

Musallam B: The human embryo in arabic scientific and religious thought. *In* Dunstan GR (ed): *The Human Embryo: Aristotle and the Arabic and European Traditions*. Exeter, University of Exeter Press, 1990.

Nathanielsz PW: *Life Before Birth. The Challenges of Fetal Development*. New York, WH Freeman and Company, 1996.

Needham J: *A History of Embryology*, 2nd ed. Cambridge, Cambridge University Press, 1959.

O'Rahilly R: One hundred years of human embryology. *In* Kalter H (ed): *Issues and Reviews in Teratology*, vol 4. New York, Plenum Press, 1988.

O'Rahilly R, Müller F: *Developmental Stages in Human Embryos*. Washington, DC, Carnegie Institution of Washington, 1987.

O'Rahilly R, Müller F: *Human Embryology and Teratology*. New York, Wiley-Liss, 1992.

Persaud TVN: *Problems of Birth Defects: From Hippocrates to Thalidomide and After*. Baltimore, University Park Press, 1977.

Persaud TVN: *Early History of Human Anatomy*. Springfield, Charles C Thomas, 1984.

Persaud TVN: *A History of Anatomy: The Post-Vesalian Era*. Springfield, Charles C Thomas, 1997.

Persaud TVN, Chudley AE, Skalko RG: *Basic Concepts in Teratology*. New York, Alan R Liss, Inc, 1985.

Rossant J, Joyner AL: Towards a molecular-genetic analysis of mammalian development. *Trends in Genet 5*:277, 1989.

Roush W: "Smart" genes use many cues to set cell fate. *Science 272*: 652, 1996.

Rusconi S: Transgenic regulation in laboratory animals. *Experientia 47*:866, 1991.

Schumacher GH: *Monster und Dämonen*. Berlin, edition q Verlags-GmbH, 1993.

Shiota K: Development and intrauterine fate of normal and abnormal human conceptuses. *Cong Anomalies 31*:67, 1991.

Slack JMW: *From Egg to Embryo*, 2nd ed. New York, Cambridge University Press, 1991.

Smith J: How to tell a cell where it is. *Nature 381*:367, 1996.

Streeter GL: Developmental horizons in human embryos. Description of age group XI, 13 to 20 somites, and age group XII, 21 to 29 somites. *Contrib Embryol Carnegie Inst 30*:211, 1942.

Thompson MW, McInnes RR, Willard HF: *Thompson & Thompson's Genetics in Medicine*, 5th ed. Philadelphia, WB Saunders, 1991.

Warwick R: *Nomina Anatomica*, 6th ed. Edinburgh, Churchill Livingstone, 1989.

Wolpert L: *The Triumph of the Embryo*. Oxford, Oxford University Press, 1991.

Wolpert L: Positional information and pattern formation in development. *Dev Genet 15*:485, 1994.

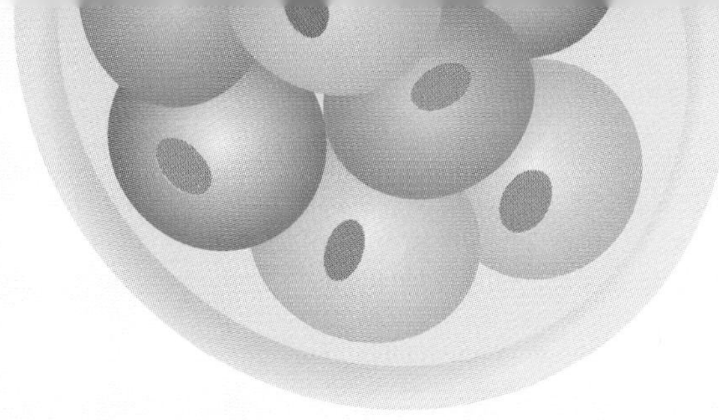

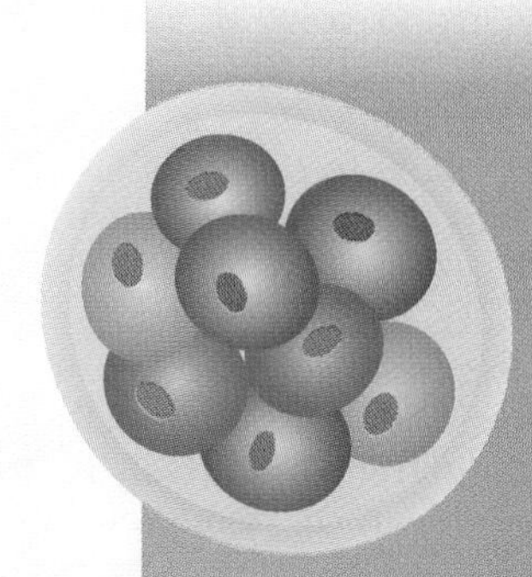

The Beginning of Human Development: The First Week

He who sees things grow from the beginning will have the finest view of them.

—ARISTOTLE, 384–322 B.C.

2

■ *Human development begins at fertilization,* the process during which a male gamete or sperm (spermatozoon) unites with a female gamete or oocyte (ovum) to form a single cell called a **zygote**. This highly specialized, totipotent cell marked the beginning of each of us as a unique individual. The zygote, just visible to the unaided eye as a tiny speck, contains chromosomes and genes (units of genetic information) that are derived from the mother and father. The unicellular organism, or zygote, divides many times and becomes progressively transformed into a multicellular human being through cell division, migration, growth, and differentiation (Gilbert, 1997).

Although development begins at fertilization, the stages and duration of pregnancy described in clinical medicine are calculated from the commencement of the mother's *last normal menstrual period* (LNMP), which is about 14 days before conception occurs (see Fig. 1-1). Although referred to as the *gestational age,* this method overestimates the actual gestational age by over 2 weeks because the embryo does not begin to implant in the uterus until about 20 days after the LNMP. However, gestational (menstrual) age is widely used in clinical practice because the onset of the LNMP is usually easy to establish.

Before describing the beginning of development, gametogenesis and the female reproductive system will be reviewed.

GAMETOGENESIS

The sperm and oocyte, the male and female gametes, are highly specialized sex cells. They contain half the number of chromosomes (haploid number) that is present in somatic (body) cells. The number of chromosomes is reduced during **meiosis**, a special type of cell division that occurs during gametogenesis. This maturation process is called **spermatogenesis** in males and **oogenesis** in females (Fig. 2-1). The history of male and female gamete formation is different, but the sequence is the same. It is the timing of events during meiosis that differs in the two sexes.

Gametogenesis (*gamete formation*) is the process of formation and development of specialized generative cells called **gametes** (Gr. *gamete,* wife; *gametes,* husband). This process, involving the chromosomes and cytoplasm of the gametes or germ cells, *prepares the sex cells for fertilization* (union of male and female gametes). During gametogenesis, the chromosome number is reduced by half and the shape of the cells is altered. A *chromosome* is defined by the presence of a *centromere* — the constricted part of a chromosome. Before DNA replication in the *S* phase of the cell cycle, chromosomes exist as *single chromatid chromosomes.* A chromatid consists of parallel DNA strands. After DNA replication, chromosomes exist as *double chromatid chromosomes.*

Meiosis

Meiosis is a special type of cell division that *involves two meiotic cell divisions*; it takes place in germ cells only (Fig. 2-2). Diploid germ cells give rise to haploid *gametes* (sperms and oocytes).

The **first meiotic division** is a *reduction division* because the chromosome member is reduced from diploid (Gr., double) to haploid (Gr., single) by pairing of homologous chromosome in prophase and their segregation at anaphase. *Homologous chromosomes* (one from each parent) pair during prophase and then separate during anaphase, with one representative of each pair going to each pole. Homologous chromosomes or homologs are pairs of chromosomes, one inherited from each parent. At this stage, they are *double chromatid chromosomes.* The X and Y chromosomes are not homologs but they have homologous segments at the tips of their short arms. They pair in these regions only. By the end of the first meiotic division, each new cell formed (secondary spermatocyte or secondary oocyte) has the *haploid chromosome number* (double chromatid chromosomes), i.e., half the number of chromosomes of the preceding cell (primary spermatocyte or primary oocyte). This separation or disjunction of paired homologous chromosomes is the *physical basis of segregation* — the separation of allelic genes during meiosis.

The **second meiotic division** follows the first division without a normal interphase (i.e., without an intervening step of DNA replication). Each chromosome divides and each half, or *chromatid,* is drawn to a different pole; thus, the haploid number of chromosomes (23) is retained and each daughter cell formed by meiosis has the reduced haploid number of chromosomes, with one representative of each chromosome pair (now a single chromatid chromosome). The second meiotic division is similar to an ordinary mitosis except that the chromosome number of the cell entering the second meiotic division is haploid. For more details about meiosis, see Thompson et al. (1991).

IMPORTANCE OF MEIOSIS

The significance of meiosis is that it:

- provides for *constancy of the chromosome number* from generation to generation by reducing the chromosome number from diploid to haploid, thereby producing haploid gametes.
- allows random *assortment of maternal and paternal chromosomes* between the gametes.
- relocates segments of maternal and paternal chromosomes by *crossing over of chromosome segments,* which "shuffles" the genes and produces a recombination of genetic material.

Abnormal Gametogenesis

Disturbances of meiosis during gametogenesis, e.g., **nondisjunction** (Fig. 2-3), result in the formation of *chromosomally abnormal gametes.* If involved in fertilization, these gametes with numerical chromosome abnormalities cause abnormal development such as occurs in infants with the *Down syndrome* (see Chapter 8).

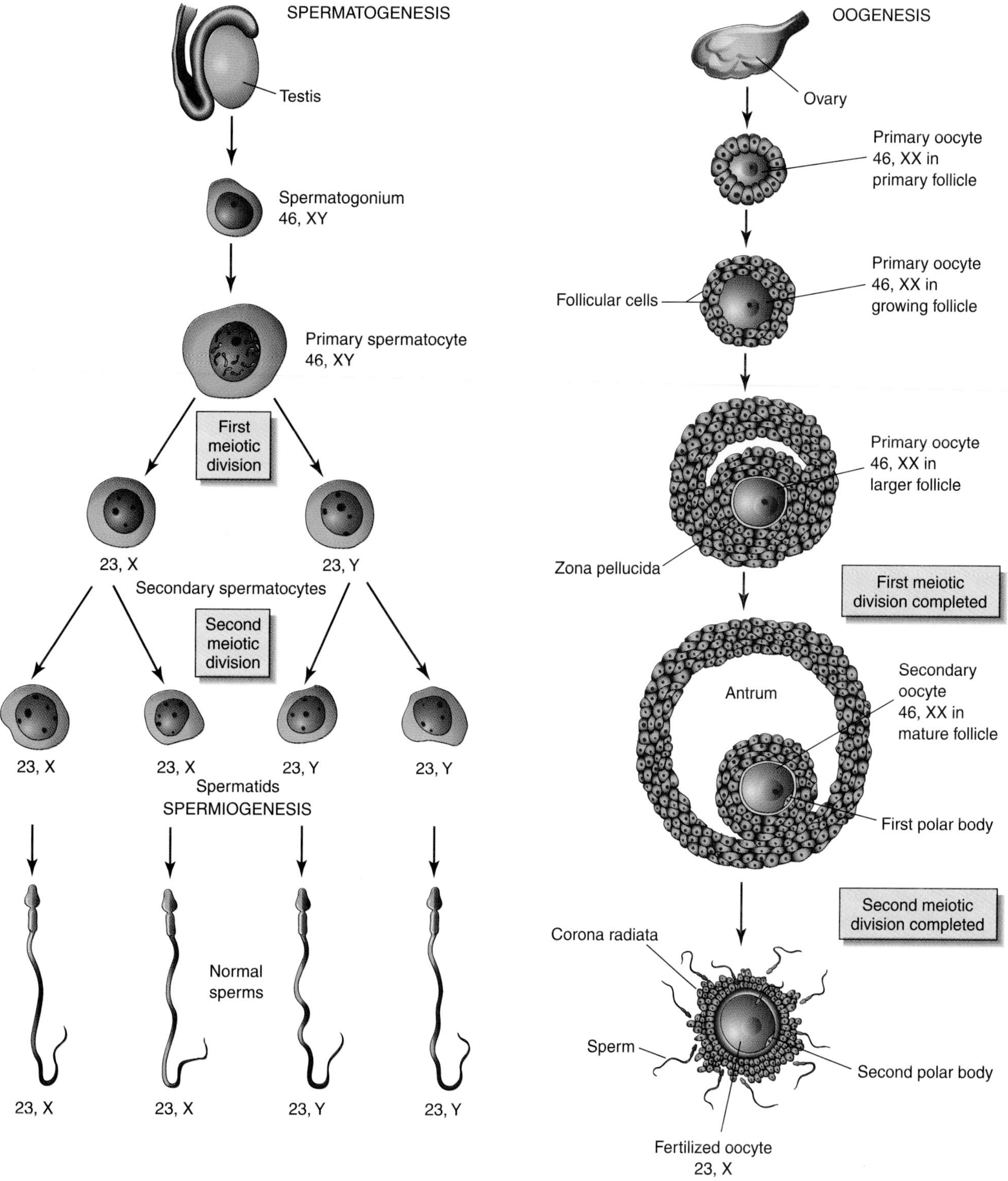

■ **Figure 2–1.** Gametogenesis—conversion of germ cells into gametes. The drawings compare spermatogenesis and oogenesis. Oogonia are not shown in this figure because they differentiate into primary oocytes before birth. The chromosome complement of the germ cells is shown at each stage. The number designates the total number of chromosomes, including the sex chromosome(s) shown after the comma. Note: (1) following the two meiotic divisions, the diploid number of chromosomes, 46, is reduced to the haploid number, 23; (2) four sperms form from one primary spermatocyte, whereas only one mature oocyte results from maturation of a primary oocyte; and (3) the cytoplasm is conserved during oogenesis to form one large cell, the mature oocyte or ovum. The polar bodies are small nonfunctional cells that eventually degenerate.

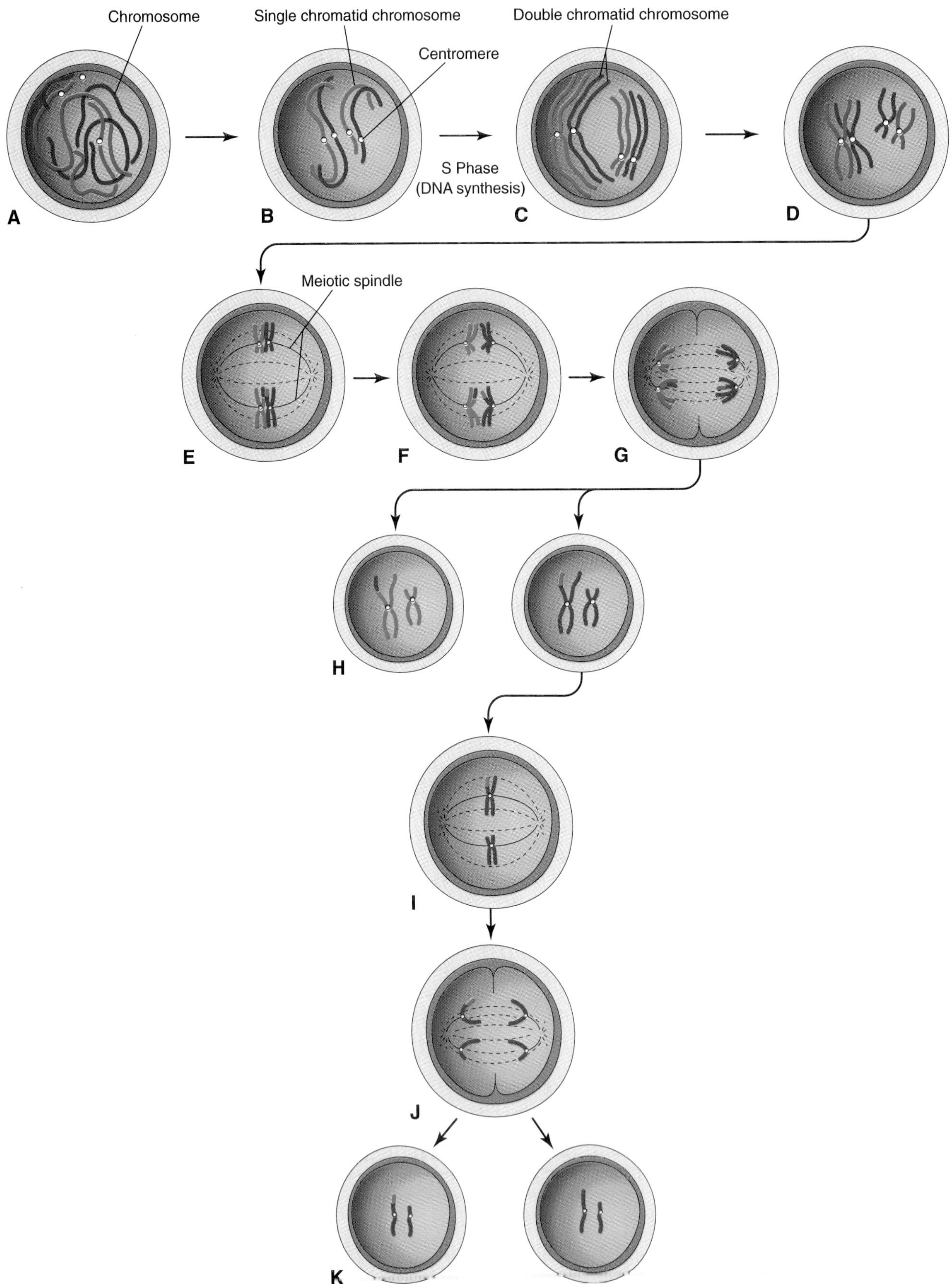

■ **Figure 2–2.** Diagrammatic representation of meiosis. Two chromosome pairs are shown. *A* to *D*, Stages of prophase of the first meiotic division. The homologous chromosomes approach each other and pair; each member of the pair consists of two chromatids. Observe the single crossover in one pair of chromosomes, resulting in the interchange of chromatid segments. *E*, Metaphase. The two members of each pair become oriented on the meiotic spindle. *F*, Anaphase. *G*, Telophase. The chromosomes migrate to opposite poles. *H*, Distribution of parental chromosome pairs at the end of the first meiotic division. *I* to *K*, Second meiotic division. It is similar to mitosis except that the cells are haploid.

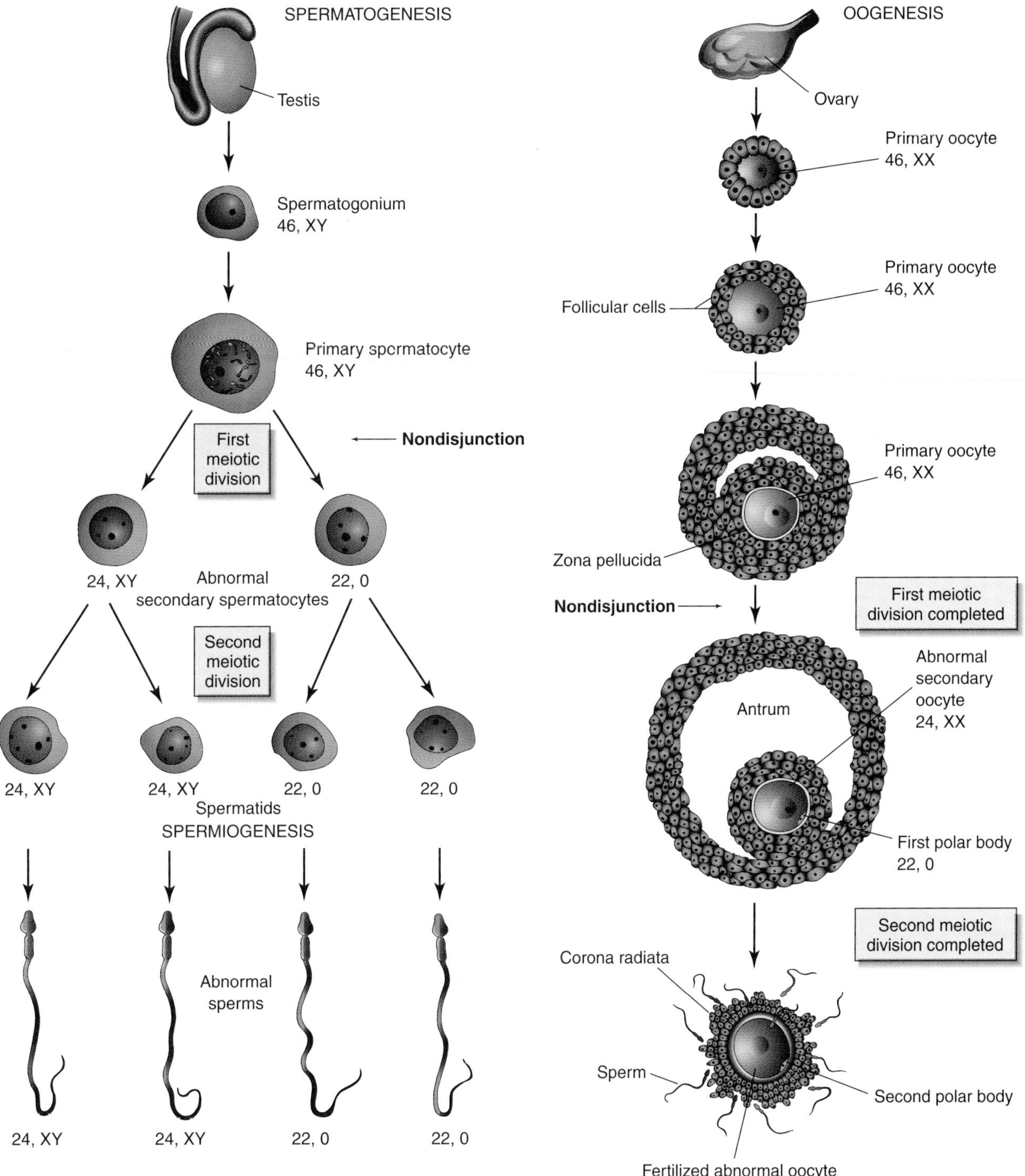

■ **Figure 2–3.** Abnormal gametogenesis. The drawings show how nondisjunction, an error in cell division, results in an abnormal chromosome distribution in germ cells. Although nondisjunction of sex chromosomes is illustrated, a similar defect may occur during the division of autosomes. When nondisjunction occurs during the first meiotic division of spermatogenesis, one secondary spermatocyte contains 22 autosomes plus an X and a Y chromosome, and the other one contains 22 autosomes and no sex chromosome. Similarly, nondisjunction during oogenesis may give rise to an oocyte with 22 autosomes and two X chromosomes (as shown) or may result in one with 22 autosomes and no sex chromosomes.

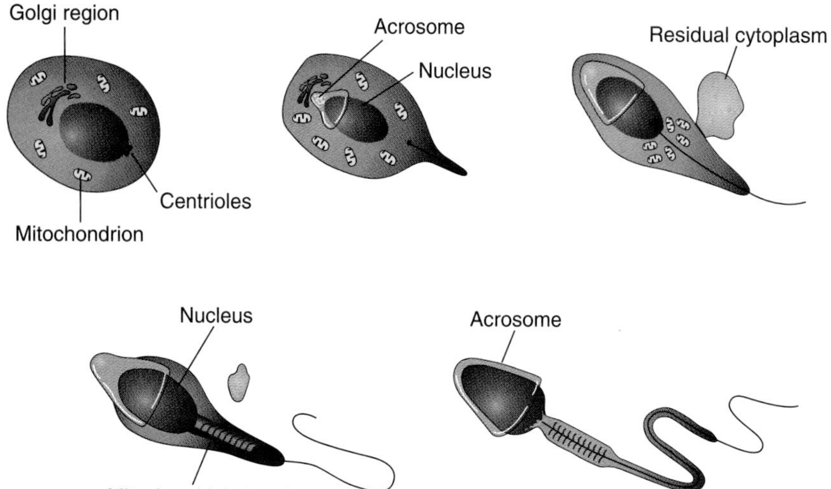

■ **Figure 2-4.** Drawings illustrating spermiogenesis, the last phase of spermatogenesis. During this process the rounded spermatid is transformed into elongated sperm. Note the loss of cytoplasm, development of the tail, and formation of the acrosome. The acrosome, derived from the Golgi region of the spermatid, contains enzymes that are released at the beginning of the fertilization process to assist the sperm in penetrating the corona radiata and zona pellucida surrounding the secondary oocyte. The mitochondria arrange themselves end-to-end in the form of a tight helix, forming a collarlike mitochondrial sheath. Note that excess cytoplasm is shed during spermiogenesis.

SPERMATOGENESIS

Spermatogenesis refers to the entire sequence of events by which primitive germ cells—*spermatogonia*—are transformed into sperms or spermatozoa. This maturation process of germ cells begins at puberty (13 to 16 years) and continues into old age. **Spermatogonia,** which have been dormant in the seminiferous tubules of the testes since the fetal period, begin to increase in number at puberty. After several mitotic divisions, the spermatogonia grow and undergo gradual changes that transform them into **primary spermatocytes,** the largest germ cells in the seminiferous tubules. Each primary spermatocyte subsequently undergoes a reduction division—*the first meiotic division*—to form two haploid **secondary spermatocytes**, which are about half the size of primary spermatocytes. Subsequently the secondary spermatocytes undergo a *second meiotic division* to form four haploid **spermatids**, which are about half the size of secondary spermatocytes. The spermatids are gradually transformed into four mature sperms by a differentiation process known as **spermiogenesis** (Fig. 2-4). The entire process of spermatogenesis, which includes spermiogenesis, takes about two months. When spermiogenesis is complete, the sperms enter the lumina of the seminiferous tubules.

Sertoli cells lining the seminiferous tubules support and nurture the germ cells, and may be involved in the regulation of spermatogenesis. Sperms are transported passively from the seminiferous tubules to the *epididymis*, where they are stored and become func-

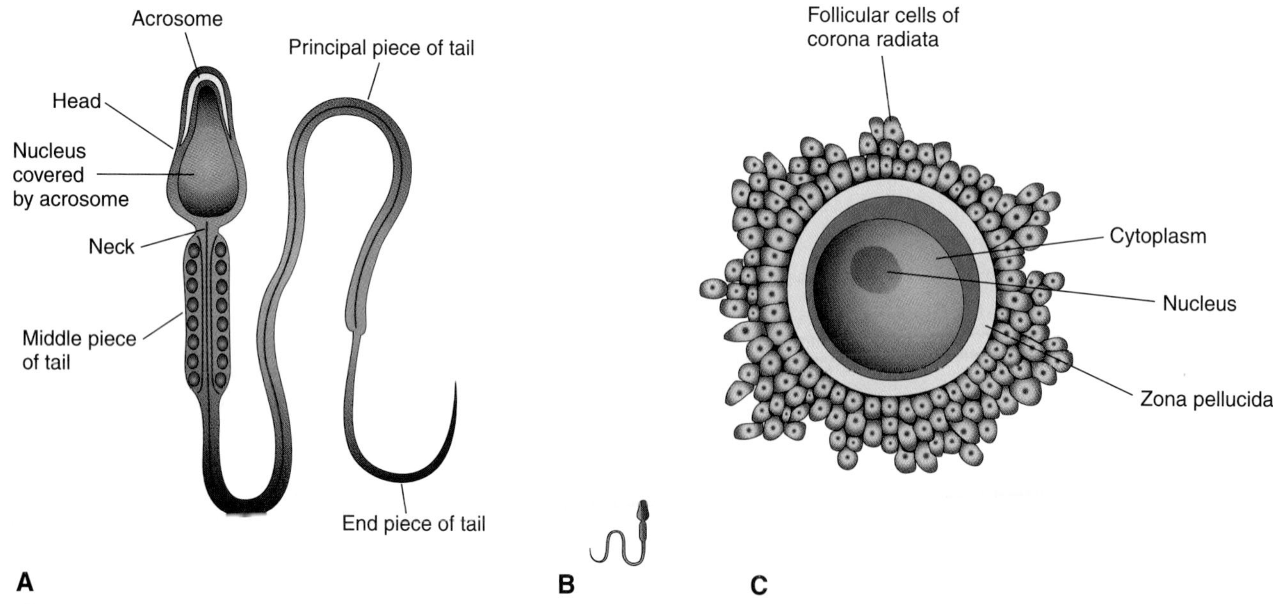

■ **Figure 2-5.** Male and female gametes (sex cells). *A*, Drawing showing the main parts of a human sperm (×1250). The head, composed mostly of the nucleus, is partly covered by the caplike acrosome, an organelle containing enzymes. The tail of the sperm consists of three regions: the middle piece, principal piece, and end piece. *B*, A sperm drawn to about the same scale as the oocyte. *C*, Drawing of a human secondary oocyte or ovum (×200), surrounded by the zona pellucida and corona radiata.

tionally mature. The epididymis is the elongated coiled duct along the posterior border of the testis (see Fig. 2-15). It is continuous with the *ductus deferens* (vas deferens), which transports the sperms to the urethra.

The **mature sperm** is a free-swimming, actively motile cell consisting of a head and a tail (Fig. 2-5*A*). The *neck of the sperm* is the junction between the head and tail. The **head of the sperm** forms most of the bulk of the sperm and contains the *haploid nucleus*. The anterior two-thirds of the nucleus is covered by the **acrosome**, a caplike saccular organelle containing several enzymes, including an important one called *acrosin*. When released, these enzymes facilitate sperm penetration of the corona radiata and zona pellucida during fertilization. The **tail of the sperm** consists of three segments: middle piece (midpiece), principal piece, and end piece (Fig. 2-5*A*). The tail provides the motility of the sperm that assists its transport to the site of fertilization. The *middle piece of the tail* contains mitochondria, which provide the adenosine triphosphate (ATP) necessary for activity. The **mitochondrial (fibrous) sheath** is believed to promote the lashing movements of the tail (Oura and Toshimori, 1990).

Recently, the cryopreservation of rat spermatogonial stem cells and their later implantation after thawing in mouse testis, has been reported. Because the donor cells generated new and functional sperms in the host, as well as new stem cells, the possibility of transplantation of spermatogonial stem cells across species (*xenogenic spermatogenesis*) has been discussed. The biological and medical implications of this are numerous (Clouthier et al., 1996).

OOGENESIS

Oogenesis (ovogenesis) refers to the sequence of events by which primitive germ cells called **oogonia** are transformed into **mature oocytes**. This maturation process begins before birth and is completed after sexual maturity (puberty) has been reached.

Prenatal Maturation of Oocytes. During early fetal life, oogonia proliferate by mitotic division. *Oogonia enlarge to form primary oocytes before birth*; for this reason, no oogonia are shown in Figures 2-1 and 2-3. As a **primary oocyte** forms, connective tissue cells (ovarian stromal cells) surround it and form a single layer of flattened, follicular epithelial cells. The primary oocyte enclosed by this layer of cells constitutes a *primordial follicle* (see Fig. 2-8*A*).

As the primary oocyte enlarges during puberty, the follicular epithelial cells become cuboidal in shape and then columnar, forming a **primary follicle** (Fig. 2-1). The primary oocyte soon becomes surrounded by a covering of amorphous acellular glycoprotein material called the **zona pellucida** (see Fig. 2-8*B*). Scanning electron microscopy of the surface of the zona pellucida reveals a regular meshlike appearance with intricate fenestrations, not unlike swiss cheese. When the primary follicle has more than one layer of cuboidal follicular cells, it is called a maturing or **secondary follicle**.

Primary oocytes begin the first meiotic division before birth, but completion of prophase does not occur until adolescence. The primary oocytes remain in suspended prophase (dictyotene) until sexual maturity and the reproductive cycles begin during puberty. The follicular cells surrounding the primary oocyte are believed to secrete a substance called the *oocyte maturation inhibitor* (OMI), which keeps the meiotic process of the oocyte arrested (Scott and Hodgen, 1990).

Postnatal Maturation of Oocytes. Beginning during puberty, usually one follicle matures each month and ovulation occurs, except when oral contraceptives (birth control pills) are used. The long duration of the first meiotic division (up to 45 years) may account in part for the relatively high frequency of meiotic errors, such as **nondisjunction** (failure of paired chromatids to dissociate), that occur with increasing maternal age. The primary oocytes in suspended prophase I (dictyotene) are vulnerable to environmental agents such as radiation.

No primary oocytes form after birth in females, in contrast to the continuous production of primary spermatocytes in males after puberty. The primary oocytes remain dormant in the ovarian follicles until puberty. As a follicle matures, the **primary oocyte** increases in size and, shortly before ovulation, completes the first meiotic division. Unlike the corresponding stage of spermatogenesis, however, the division of cytoplasm is unequal.

The **secondary oocyte** receives almost all the cytoplasm (Fig. 2-1), and the *first polar body* receives very little. The first polar body is a small, nonfunctional cell that soon degenerates. At ovulation, the nucleus of the secondary oocyte begins the second meiotic division, but progresses only to metaphase, when division is arrested. If a sperm penetrates the secondary oocyte, the second meiotic division is completed, and most cytoplasm is again retained by one cell, the **fertilized oocyte**, or mature ovum (Fig. 2-1). The other cell, the *second polar body*, is a small nonfunctional cell that soon degenerates. As soon as the second polar body is extruded, maturation of the oocyte is complete.

There are about two million primary oocytes in the ovaries of a newborn female infant, but many regress during childhood so that by adolescence no more than 40 thousand remain. Of these, only about 400 become secondary oocytes and are expelled at ovulation during the reproductive period. Few of these oocytes, if any, become mature (Scott and Hodgen, 1990). The number of oocytes that ovulate is greatly reduced in women who take contraceptive pills because the hormones in them prevent ovulation from occurring.

COMPARISON OF MALE AND FEMALE GAMETES

The sperm and secondary oocyte are dissimilar in several ways because of their adaptation for specialized roles in reproduction. The oocyte is a massive cell compared with the sperm and is immotile (Fig. 2-5), whereas the microscopic sperm is highly motile. The oocyte is surrounded by the zona pellucida and a layer of follicular cells called the *corona radiata* (Fig. 2-5*C*). The oocyte also has an abundance of cytoplasm containing yolk granules, which provide nutrition to the dividing zygote during the first week of development. The sperm bears little resemblance to an oocyte or any other cell because of its sparse cytoplasm and specialization for motility.

With respect to sex chromosome constitution, there are *two kinds of normal sperm:* 23, X and 23, Y, whereas there is only *one kind of normal ovum:* 23, X (Fig. 2-1). In the foregoing descriptions and illustrations, the numbers 23 and 46 indicate the total number of chromosomes in the complement, including the sex chromosomes. For example, the number 23 is followed by a comma and an X or Y to indicate the sex chromosome constitution; e.g., 23, X indicates that there are 23 chromosomes in the complement, consisting of 22 autosomes and 1 sex chromosome (an X in this case). *The difference in the sex chromosome complement of sperms forms the basis of primary sex determination.*

Abnormal Gametes

The ideal maternal age for reproduction is generally considered to be from 18 to 35 years of age. The likelihood of chromosomal abnormalities in the embryo increases significantly after the mother is 35. In older mothers, there is an appreciable risk of Down syndrome or some other form of trisomy in the infant (see Chapter 8). The likelihood of a fresh *gene mutation* (change in DNA) also increases with age. The older the parents are at the time of conception, the more likely they are to have accumulated mutations that the embryo might inherit. For fathers of children with fresh mutations, such as the one causing *achondroplasia*, this age relationship has continually been demonstrated (Stoll et al., 1982). This does not hold for all dominant mutations and is not an important consideration in older mothers. For a full discussion of *gene mutations*, see Thompson et al. (1991).

During meiosis, homologous chromosomes sometimes fail to separate and go to opposite poles of the germ cell. As a result of this error of cell division—**nondisjunction**—some gametes have 24 chromosomes and others only 22 (Fig. 2-3). If a gamete with 24 chromosomes unites with a normal one with 23 chromosomes during fertilization, a zygote with 47 chromosomes forms (see Fig. 8-1). This condition is called **trisomy** because of the presence of three representatives of a particular chromosome, instead of the usual two. If a gamete with only 22 chromosomes unites with a normal one, a zygote with 45 chromosomes forms. This condition is known as *monosomy* because only one representative of the particular chromosome pair is present. For a description of the clinical conditions associated with numerical disorders of chromosomes, see Chapter 8.

Up to 10% of sperms in an ejaculate may be grossly abnormal (e.g., with two heads), but it is generally believed that these abnormal sperms do not fertilize oocytes, due to their lack of normal motility. Most morphologically abnormal sperms are unable to pass through the mucus in the cervical canal. Measurement of forward progression is a subjective assessment of the quality of sperm movement. X-rays, severe allergic reactions, and certain antispermatogenic agents have been reported to increase the percentage of abnormally shaped sperms. Such sperms are not believed to affect fertility unless their number exceeds 20%.

Although some oocytes have two or three nuclei, these cells die before they reach maturity. Similarly some ovarian follicles contain two or more oocytes, but this phenomenon is infrequent. Although compound follicles could result in multiple births, it is believed that most of them never mature and expel the oocytes at ovulation.

UTERUS, UTERINE TUBES, AND OVARIES

A brief description of the structure of the uterus, uterine tubes (fallopian tubes, oviducts), and ovaries is presented as a basis for understanding reproductive cycles and implantation of the blastocyst.

Uterus

The uterus (L., womb) is a thick-walled, pear-shaped muscular organ that varies considerably in size (Moore, 1992). The uterus averages 7 to 8 cm in length, 5 to 7 cm in width at its superior part, and 2 to 3 cm in thickness. The uterus consists of two major parts (Fig. 2-6*A*):

- Body, the expanded superior two-thirds
- Cervix, the cylindrical inferior third

The **body** of the uterus narrows from the **fundus**—the rounded part of the body superior to the orifices of the uterine tubes—to the **isthmus**, the 1-cm long constricted region between the body and cervix (L., neck). The **cervix** of the uterus is its tapered vaginal end that is nearly cylindrical in shape. The lumen of the cervix, the **cervical canal**, has a constricted opening or *os* at each end. The **internal os** (ostium) communicates with the cavity of the uterine body and the **external os** communicates with the vagina.

The *walls of the body of the uterus* consist of three layers (Fig. 2-6*B*):

- perimetrium, the thin external layer
- myometrium, the thick smooth muscle layer
- endometrium, the thin internal layer

The *perimetrium* is a peritoneal layer that is firmly attached to the myometrium. At the peak of its development, the *endometrium* is 4 to 5 mm thick. During the secretory phase of the menstrual cycle, *three layers of the endometrium* can be distinguished microscopically (Fig. 2-6*C*):

- thin **compact layer** consisting of densely packed, connective tissue around the necks of the uterine glands

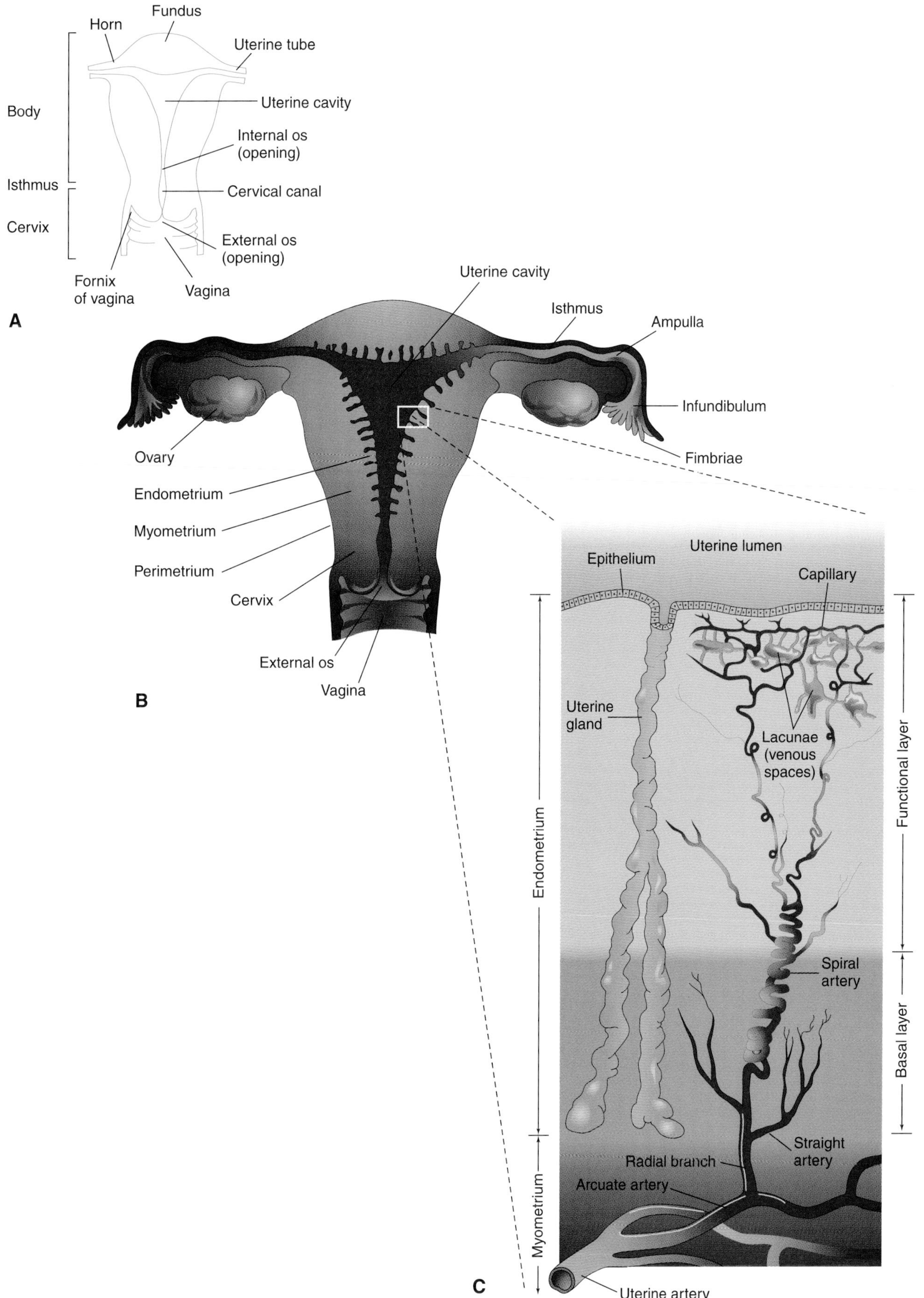

■ **Figure 2–6.** *A,* Parts of the uterus. *B,* Diagrammatic coronal section of the uterus, uterine tubes, and vagina. The ovaries are also shown. *C,* Enlargement of the area outlined in *B.* The functional layer of the endometrium is sloughed off during menstruation, the monthly endometrial shedding and discharge of bloody fluid from the uterus.

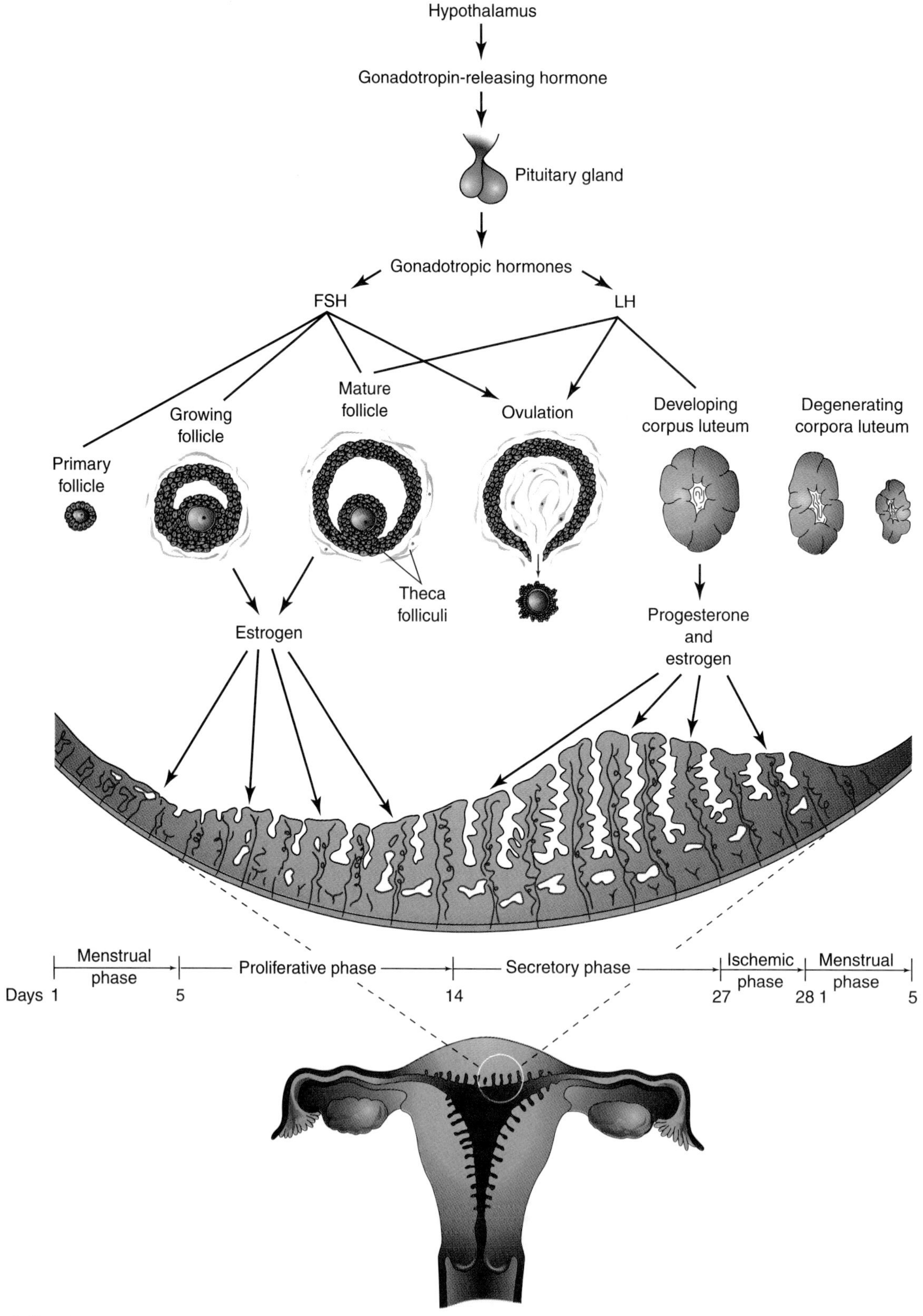

■ **Figure 2–7.** Schematic drawings illustrating the interrelations of the hypothalamus of the brain, pituitary gland, ovaries, and endometrium. One complete menstrual cycle and the beginning of another are shown. Changes in the ovaries, the ovarian cycle, are induced by the gonadotropic hormones (FSH and LH). Hormones from the ovaries (estrogens and progesterone) then promote cyclic changes in the structure and function of the endometrium, the menstrual cycle. Thus, the cyclical activity of the ovary is intimately linked with changes in the uterus. The ovarian cycles are under the rhythmic endocrine control of the adenohypophysis of the pituitary gland, which in turn is controlled by gonadotropin-releasing hormone (GnRH) produced by neurosecretory cells in the hypothalamus of the brain.

- thick **spongy layer** composed of edematous connective tissue containing the dilated, tortuous bodies of the uterine glands
- thin **basal layer** containing the blind ends of the uterine glands

The basal layer of the endometrium has its own blood supply and is not sloughed off during menstruation. The compact and spongy layers, known collectively as the *functional layer*, disintegrate and are shed during menstruation and after parturition (delivery of a baby).

Uterine Tubes

The uterine tubes, 10 to 12 cm long and 1 cm in diameter, extend laterally from the **horns** (L. *cornua*) of the uterus (Fig. 2-6*A*). The uterine tubes carry oocytes from the ovaries and sperms entering from the uterus to reach the fertilization site in the **ampulla of the uterine tube** (Fig. 2-6*B*). The uterine tube also conveys the dividing zygote to the uterine cavity. Each tube opens at its proximal end into the horn of the uterus and into the peritoneal cavity at its distal end. For descriptive purposes, *the uterine tube is divided into four parts*:

- infundibulum
- ampulla
- isthmus
- uterine part

Ovaries

The ovaries are almond-shaped reproductive glands located close to the lateral pelvic walls on each side of the uterus (Fig. 2-6*B*). The ovaries produce estrogen and progesterone, the hormones responsible for the development of secondary sex characteristics and regulation of pregnancy. The ovaries are also responsible for producing and maintaining oocytes.

FEMALE REPRODUCTIVE CYCLES

Commencing at puberty and normally continuing throughout the reproductive years, human females undergo monthly reproductive cycles (sexual cycles), involving activities of the **hypothalamus** of the brain, **pituitary gland** (L. *hypophysis cerebri*), **ovaries**, uterus, uterine tubes, vagina, and mammary glands (Fig. 2-7). These monthly cycles prepare the reproductive system for pregnancy.

A *gonadotropin-releasing hormone* (GnRH) is synthesized by neurosecretory cells in the hypothalamus and is carried by the *hypophyseal portal system* to the anterior lobe of the pituitary gland. **GnRH** stimulates the release of two hormones produced by this gland that act on the ovaries:

- *Follicle stimulating hormone* **(FSH)** stimulates the development of ovarian follicles and the production of **estrogen** by its follicular cells.

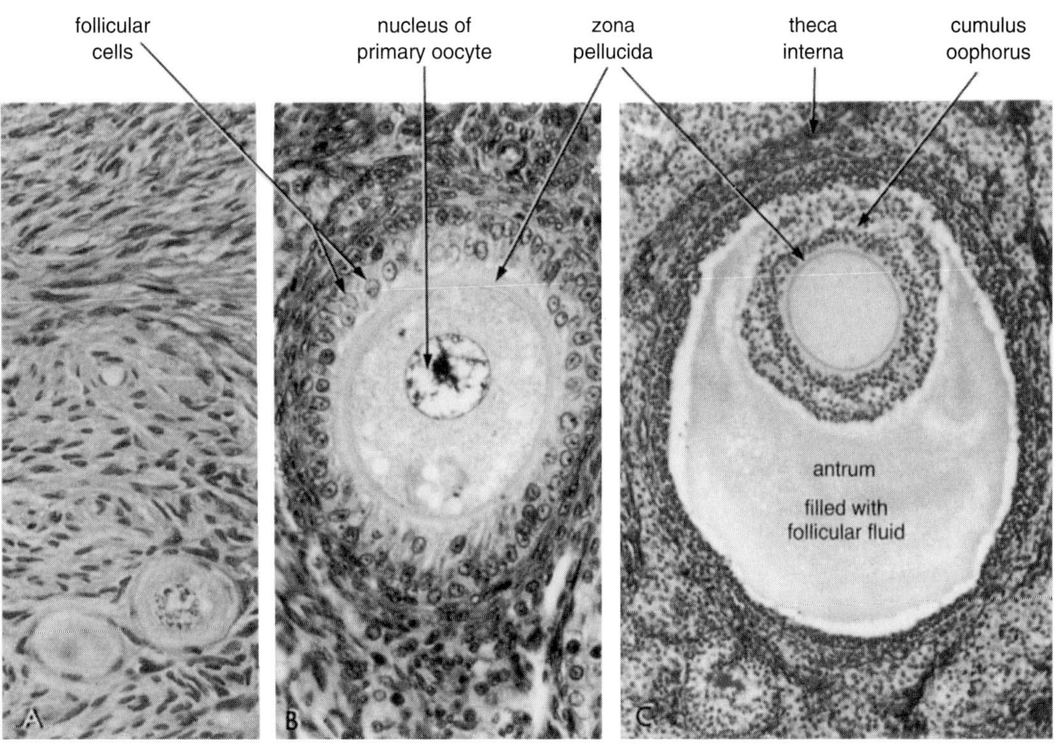

■ **Figure 2-8.** Photomicrographs of sections from adult human ovaries. *A*, Ovarian cortex showing two primordial follicles containing primary oocytes (×250). *B*, Growing follicle containing a primary oocyte, surrounded by the zona pellucida and a stratified layer of follicular cells (×250). *C*, An almost mature follicle with a large antrum. The oocyte, embedded in the cumulus oophorus, does not show a nucleus because it has been sectioned tangentially (×100). (From Lesson CR, Leeson TS: *Histology,* 3rd ed. Philadelphia, WB Saunders, 1976.)

- *Luteinizing hormone* (**LH**) serves as the "trigger" for ovulation (release of secondary oocyte) and stimulates the follicular cells and corpus luteum to produce **progesterone**.

These hormones also induce growth of the endometrium.

Ovarian Cycle

FSH and LH produce cyclic changes in the ovaries (development of follicles, ovulation, and corpus luteum formation) known as the ovarian cycle (Fig. 2-7). During each cycle, FSH promotes growth of several *primordial follicles* into primary follicles (Fig. 2-8*A*); however only one primary follicle usually develops into a mature follicle and ruptures through the surface of the ovary, expelling its oocyte (see Fig. 2-11). Hence, 4 to 11 follicles degenerate each month.

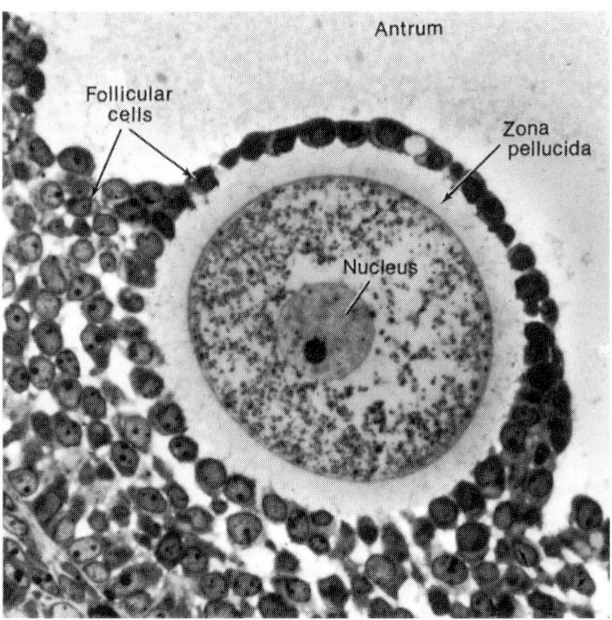

■ **Figure 2-9.** Photomicrograph of a human primary oocyte in a secondary follicle, surrounded by follicular cells. The whole mound of tissue, the cumulus oophorus, projects into the antrum. The zona pellucida is a refractile, deeply staining layer of uniform thickness. (From Bloom W, Fawcett DW: *A Textbook of Histology,* 10th ed. Philadelphia, WB Saunders, 1975. Courtesy of L. Zamboni.)

FOLLICULAR DEVELOPMENT

Development of an ovarian follicle (Figs. 2-8 to 2-10) is characterized by:

- growth and differentiation of a primary oocyte
- proliferation of follicular cells
- formation of the zona pellucida
- development of a connective tissue capsule, the theca folliculi (Gr. *theke*, box)

As the **primary follicle** increases in size, the adjacent stroma (connective tissue) organizes into a capsule, the **theca folliculi** (Fig. 2-7). The theca soon differentiates into two layers, an internal vascular and glandular layer—the *theca interna*—and a capsulelike layer, the *theca externa*. Thecal cells are thought to

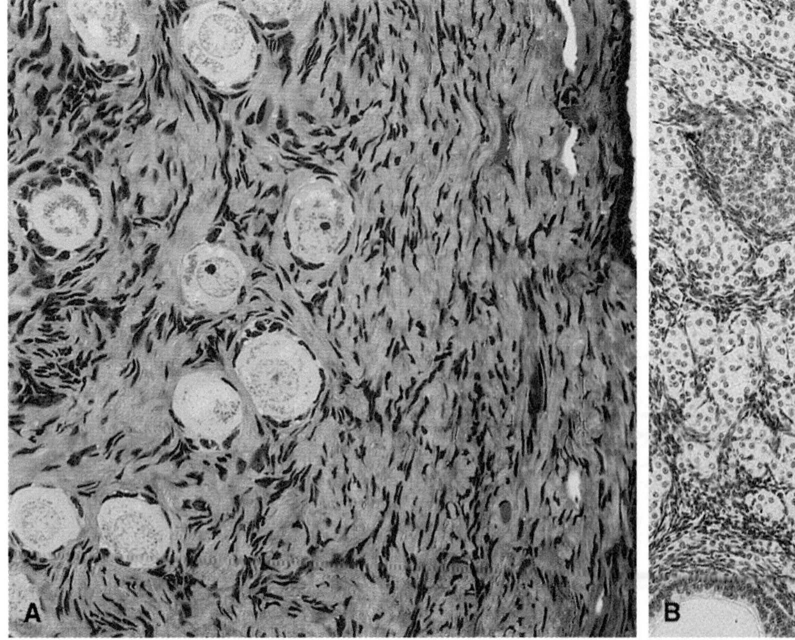

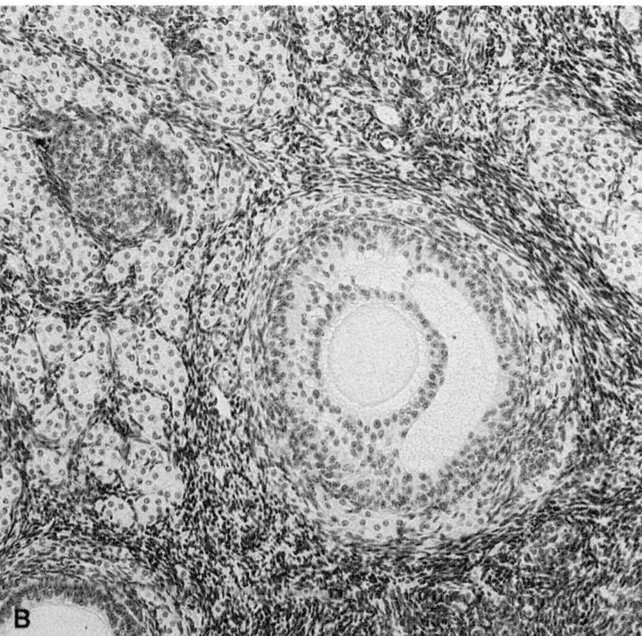

■ **Figure 2-10.** Light micrographs of ovarian cortex. *A*, Several primordial follicles are visible (×270). Observe that the primary oocytes are surrounded by follicular cells. *B*, Secondary ovarian follicle. The oocyte is surrounded by granulosa cells of the cumulus oophorus that project into the fluid-filled antrum (×132). (From Gartner LP, Hiatt JL: *Color Textbook of Histology.* Philadelphia, WB Saunders, 1997.)

produce an *angiogenesis factor* that promotes growth of blood vessels in the theca interna (Fig. 2-8*C*), which provide nutritive support for follicular development. The follicular cells divide actively, producing a stratified layer around the oocyte (Fig. 2-8*B*). The ovarian follicle soon becomes oval and the oocyte eccentric in position because proliferation of the follicular cells occurs more rapidly on one side. Subsequently, fluid-filled spaces appear around the cells, which coalesce to form a single large cavity, the **antrum**, which contains **follicular fluid** (Figs. 2-8*C*, 2-9, and 2-10*B*).

After the antrum forms, the ovarian follicle is called a vesicular or **secondary follicle**. The primary oocyte is pushed to one side of the follicle, where it is surrounded by a mound of follicular cells, the **cumulus oophorus**, that projects into the enlarged antrum (Figs. 2-8 and 2-9). The follicle continues to enlarge until it reaches maturity and forms a swelling on the surface of the ovary (Fig. 2-11*A*). It is now a **mature follicle** (graafian follicle).

The early development of ovarian follicles is induced by FSH, but final stages of maturation require LH as well. Growing follicles produce **estrogen**, a hormone that regulates development and function of the reproductive organs. The vascular *theca interna* produces follicular fluid and some estrogen. Its cells also secrete *androgens* that pass to the follicular cells in the **membrana granulosa** (Fig. 2-10), which convert them into estrogen. Some estrogen is also produced by widely scattered groups of stromal secretory cells, known collectively as the *interstitial gland of the ovary*.

Ovulation

Around midcycle (14 days in an "average" 28-day menstrual cycle) the ovarian follicle — under the influence of FSH and LH (Balasch et al., 1995) — undergoes a sudden *growth spurt*, producing a cystic swelling or bulge on the surface of the ovary. A small avascular spot, the **stigma**, soon appears on this swelling (Fig. 2-11*A*). Prior to ovulation, the secondary oocyte and some cells of the cumulus oophorus detach from the interior of the distended follicle (Fig. 2-11*B*).

Ovulation is triggered by a surge of LH production (Fig. 2-12). Ovulation usually follows the LH peak by 12 to 24 hours. The **LH surge**, elicited by the high estrogen level in the blood, appears to cause the stigma to balloon out, forming a vesicle (Fig. 2-11*A*). The stigma then ruptures, expelling the secondary oocyte with the follicular fluid (Fig. 2-11*B* to *D*). Expulsion of the oocyte is the result of intrafollicular pressure and possibly contraction of smooth muscle in the theca externa owing to stimulation by prostaglandins. *Enzymatic digestion of the follicular wall* seems to be one of the principal mechanisms leading to ovulation (Oehninger and Hodgen, 1993). The expelled secondary oocyte is surrounded by the zona pellucida and one or more layers of follicular cells, which are radially arranged as the **corona radiata** and a cumulus layer (Fig. 2-11*C*), forming the oocyte-cumulus complex (Talbot, 1985). The LH surge also seems to induce resumption of the first meiotic division of the primary oocyte. Hence, mature ovarian follicles contain secondary oocytes (Fig. 2-11*A* and *B*).

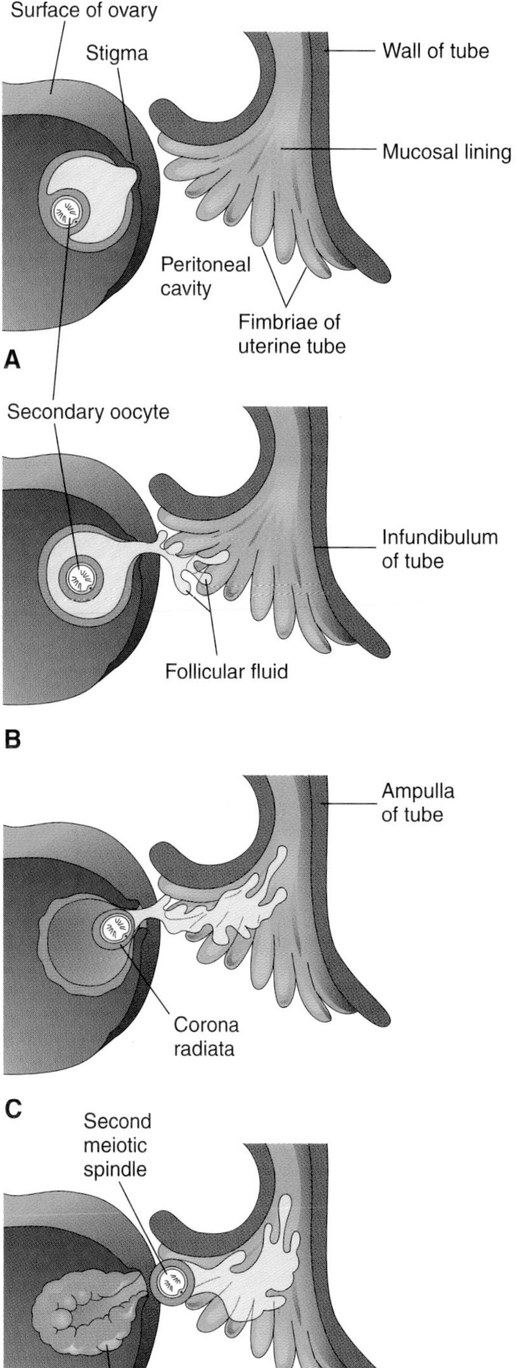

■ **Figure 2-11.** Diagrams (*A-D*) illustrating ovulation. The stigma ruptures and the secondary oocyte is expelled from the ovarian follicle with the follicular fluid. After ovulation the wall of the follicle collapses and is thrown into folds. The follicular wall is transformed into a glandular structure, the corpus luteum.

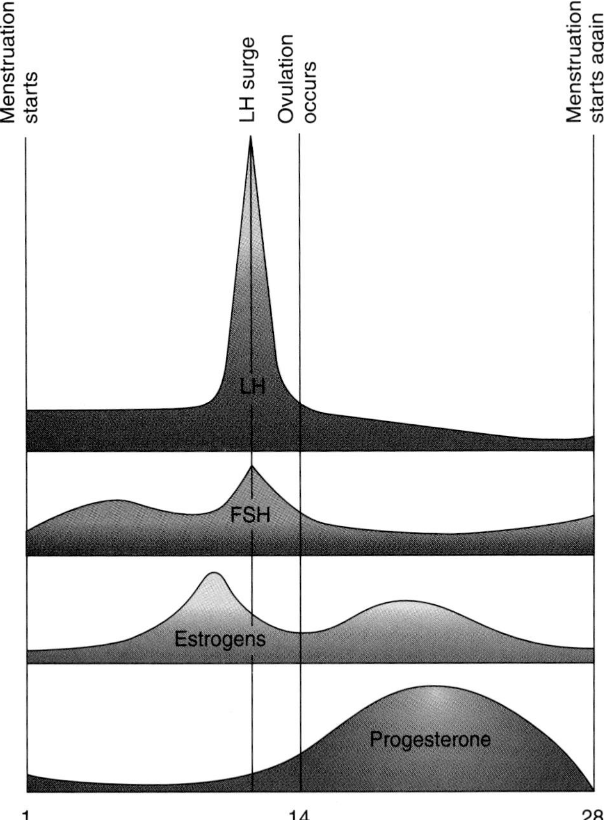

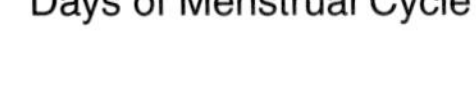

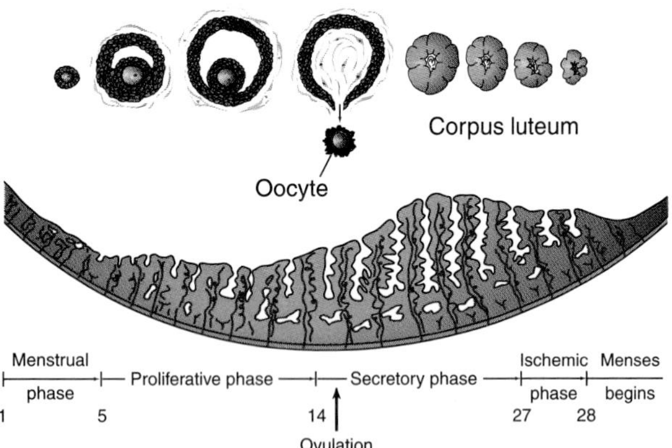

■ **Figure 2–12.** A diagram illustrating the blood levels of various hormones during the menstrual cycle. FSH stimulates the ovarian follicles to develop and produce estrogens. The level of estrogens rises to a peak just before the LH surge induces ovulation. Ovulation normally occurs 24 to 36 hours after the LH surge. If fertilization does not occur, the blood levels of circulating estrogens and progesterone fall. This hormone withdrawal causes the endometrium to regress and menstruation to start again.

Mittelschmerz and Ovulation

A variable amount of abdominal pain called mittelschmerz (Ger. *mittel*, mid + *schmerz*, pain), accompanies ovulation in some women. In these cases, ovulation results in slight bleeding into the peritoneal cavity, which results in sudden constant inferolateral pain in the abdomen. Mittelschmerz may be used as a symptom of ovulation, but there are better symptoms, such as the *basal body temperature*, which usually shows a slight drop followed by a sustained rise after ovulation.

Anovulation and Hormones

Some women do not ovulate because of an inadequate release of gonadotropins; as a result, they are unable to become pregnant in the usual way. In some of these women, *ovulation can be induced* by the administration of gonadotropins or an ovulatory agent such as *clomiphene citrate*. This drug stimulates the release of pituitary gonadotropins (FSH and LH), resulting in maturation of several ovarian follicles and multiple ovulations. The incidence of multiple pregnancy increases up to tenfold when ovulation is induced. Apparently, the fine control of FSH output is not present and multiple ovulations occur, leading to multiple pregnancies and often abortions because there is no chance that seven or more embryos can survive.

CORPUS LUTEUM

Shortly after ovulation, the walls of the ovarian follicle and theca folliculi collapse and are thrown into folds (Fig. 2-11*D*). Under LH influence they develop into a glandular structure known as the corpus luteum, which secretes *progesterone* but some estrogen also. These hormones, particularly progesterone, cause the endometrial glands to secrete and prepare the endometrium for implantation of the blastocyst.

If the oocyte is fertilized, the corpus luteum enlarges to form a *corpus luteum of pregnancy* and increases its hormone production. When pregnancy occurs, degeneration of the corpus luteum is prevented by *human chorionic gonadotropin* (hCG), a hormone secreted by the syncytiotrophoblast of the chorion (see Fig. 2-23*B*), which is rich in LH. The corpus luteum of pregnancy remains functionally active throughout the first 20 weeks of pregnancy. By this time the placenta has assumed the production of the estrogen and progesterone that is necessary for the maintenance of pregnancy (see Chapter 7).

If the oocyte is not fertilized, the corpus luteum begins to involute and degenerate about 10 to 12 days after ovulation. It is then called a *corpus luteum of menstruation*. The corpus luteum is subsequently transformed into white scar tissue in the ovary called a *corpus albicans* (atretic corpus luteum). Except during pregnancy, ovarian cycles normally persist throughout the reproductive life of women and terminate at **menopause**—permanent cessation of menstruation.

Menstrual Cycle

The menstrual cycle is the period during which the oocyte matures, is ovulated, and enters the uterine tube. The hormones produced by the ovarian follicles and corpus luteum (estrogen and progesterone) produce cyclic changes in the endometrium (Fig. 2-12). These monthly changes in the internal layer of the uterus constitute the **endometrial cycle**, commonly referred to as the menstrual cycle or period because **menstruation** (flow of blood from uterus) is an obvious event.

The normal endometrium is a mirror of the ovarian cycle because it responds in a consistent manner to the fluctuating concentrations of ovarian hormones. The average menstrual cycle is 28 days, with day 1 of the cycle designated as the day on which menstrual flow begins. Menstrual cycles can vary in length by several days in normal women. In 90% of women, the length of the cycles ranges between 23 and 35 days. Almost all these variations result from alterations in the duration of the proliferative phase of the cycle.

Anovulatory Menstrual Cycles

The typical reproductive cycle illustrated in Figure 2-12 is not always realized because the ovary may not produce a mature follicle and ovulation does not occur. In *anovulatory cycles* the endometrial changes are minimal; the proliferative endometrium develops as usual but no ovulation occurs and no corpus luteum forms. Consequently, the endometrium does not progress to the secretory phase; it remains in the proliferative phase until menstruation begins. Anovulatory cycles may result from *ovarian hypofunction* but they are commonly produced by self-administered sex hormones. The estrogen, with or without progesterone, in *birth control pills* acts on the hypothalamus and pituitary gland, resulting in inhibition of secretion of GnRH and FSH and LH, the secretion of which is essential for ovulation to occur. *Suppression of ovulation is the basis for the success of birth control pills.* In most cases, when no other method of contraception is used, the interval between cessation of *oral contraception* and the occurrence of pregnancy is 12 months; however, conception may occur after 1 month in some cases.

PHASES OF MENSTRUAL CYCLE

Changes in the estrogen and progesterone levels cause cyclic changes in the structure of the female reproductive tract, notably the endometrium. Although the menstrual cycle is divided into three main phases for descriptive purposes (Fig. 2-12), *the menstrual cycle is a continuous process*; each phase gradually passes into the next one.

Menstrual Phase. The first day of menstruation is the beginning of the menstrual cycle. The functional layer of the uterine wall (Fig. 2-6*C*) is sloughed off and discarded with the menstrual flow (L. *menses*, months), which usually lasts 4 to 5 days. The menstrual flow or **menses** discharged through the vagina consists of varying amounts of blood combined with small pieces of endometrial tissue. After menstruation the eroded endometrium is thin.

Proliferative Phase. The proliferative (estrogenic) phase, lasting about 9 days, coincides with growth of ovarian follicles and is controlled by estrogen secreted by these follicles. There is a two- to threefold increase in the thickness of the endometrium and in its water content during this *phase of repair and proliferation*. Early during this phase the surface epithelium reforms and covers the endometrium. The glands increase in number and length and the spiral arteries elongate.

Secretory Phase. The secretory (progestational) phase, lasting about 13 days, coincides with the formation, functioning, and growth of the corpus luteum. The progesterone produced by the corpus luteum stimulates the glandular epithelium to secrete a glycogen-rich material. The glands become wide, tortuous, and saccular, and the endometrium thickens because of the influence of progesterone and estrogen from the corpus luteum and partly as the result of increased fluid in the connective tissue. As the spiral arteries grow into the superficial compact layer, they become increasingly coiled (Fig. 2-6*C*). The venous network becomes complex and shows large *lacunae* (venous spaces). *Direct arteriovenous anastomoses* are prominent features of this stage.

If fertilization occurs:

- Cleavage of the zygote and blastogenesis (formation of the blastocyst) occur.
- The blastocyst begins to implant in the endometrium on about the sixth day of the secretory phase (day 20 of a 28-day cycle).
- hCG, a hormone produced by the syncytiotrophoblast of the chorion (see Fig. 2-23), keeps the corpus luteum secreting estrogens and progesterone.
- The secretory phase continues and menstruation does not occur.

If fertilization does not occur:

- The corpus luteum degenerates.
- Estrogen and progesterone levels fall and the secretory endometrium enters an *ischemic phase* during the last day of the secretory phase.
- Menstruation occurs.

Ischemia (reduced blood supply) occurs as the spiral arteries constrict, giving the endometrium a pale appearance. This constriction results from the decreasing secretion of hormones, primarily progesterone, by the degenerating corpus luteum. In addition to vascular changes, the hormone withdrawal results in the stoppage of glandular secretion, a loss of interstitial fluid, and a marked shrinking of the endometrium. Toward the end of the ischemic phase, the spiral arteries become constricted for longer periods. This results in *venous stasis* and patchy ischemic necrosis (death) in the superficial tissues. Eventually, rupture of damaged vessel walls follows and blood seeps into the surrounding connective tissue. Small pools of blood

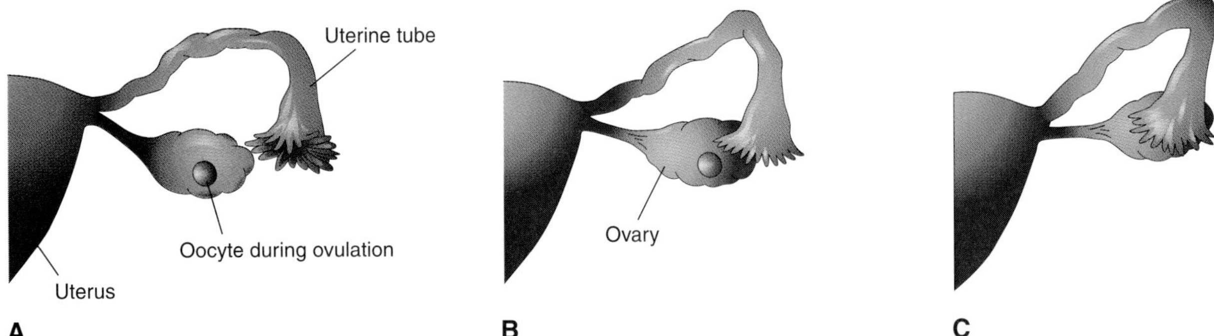

■ **Figure 2-13.** Drawings (*A-C*) illustrating the movement of the uterine tube that occurs during ovulation. Note that the fimbriated infundibulum of the tube becomes closely applied to the ovary. Its fingerlike fimbriae move back and forth over the ovary and "sweep" the secondary oocyte into the infundibulum as soon as it is expelled from the ovarian follicle and ovary during ovulation.

form and break through the endometrial surface, resulting in bleeding into the uterine lumen and from the vagina.

As small pieces of the endometrium detach and pass into the uterine cavity, the torn ends of the arteries bleed into the uterine cavity, resulting in a loss of 20 to 80 ml of blood. Eventually, over 3 to 5 days, the entire compact layer and most of the spongy layer of the endometrium are discarded in the *menses*. Remnants of the spongy and basal layers remain to undergo regeneration during the subsequent proliferative phase of the endometrium. It is obvious from the previous descriptions that the cyclic hormonal activity of the ovary is intimately linked with cyclic histological changes in the endometrium.

If pregnancy occurs, the menstrual cycles cease and the endometrium passes into a *pregnancy phase*. With the termination of pregnancy, the ovarian and menstrual cycles resume after a variable period (usually 6 to 10 weeks if the woman is not breast-feeding her baby). If pregnancy does not occur, the reproductive cycles normally continue until the end of a woman's reproductive life — *menopause*, the permanent cessation of the menses — usually between the ages of 48 and 55. The endocrine, somatic (body), and psychic changes occurring at the termination of the reproductive period are called the *climacteric*.

TRANSPORTATION OF GAMETES

Transportation of the gametes refers to the way the oocyte and sperms meet each other in the ampulla of the uterine tube, the usual site of fertilization.

Oocyte Transport

The secondary oocyte is expelled at ovulation from the ovarian follicle in the ovary with the escaping follicular fluid (Fig. 2-11). During ovulation the fimbriated end of the uterine tube becomes closely applied to the ovary. The fingerlike processes of the tube, the *fimbriae*, move back and forth over the ovary (Fig. 2-13). The sweeping action of the fimbriae and fluid currents produced by the cilia of the mucosal cells of the fimbriae "sweep" the secondary oocyte into the funnel-shaped infundibulum of the uterine tube. The oocyte then passes into the ampulla of the tube mainly as the result of gentle waves of *peristalsis* — movements of the wall of the tube characterized by alternate contraction and relaxation — that pass toward the uterus. The nature of oocyte transport through the rest of the uterine tube is extremely complex and involves many factors that are poorly understood (Egarter, 1990; Beer, 1991).

Sperm Transport

From their storage site in the epididymis, mainly in its tail, the sperms are rapidly transported to the urethra by peristaltic contractions of the thick muscular coat of the ductus deferens (Fig. 2-14). As the sperms pass by the accessory sex glands — *seminal vesicles, pros-*

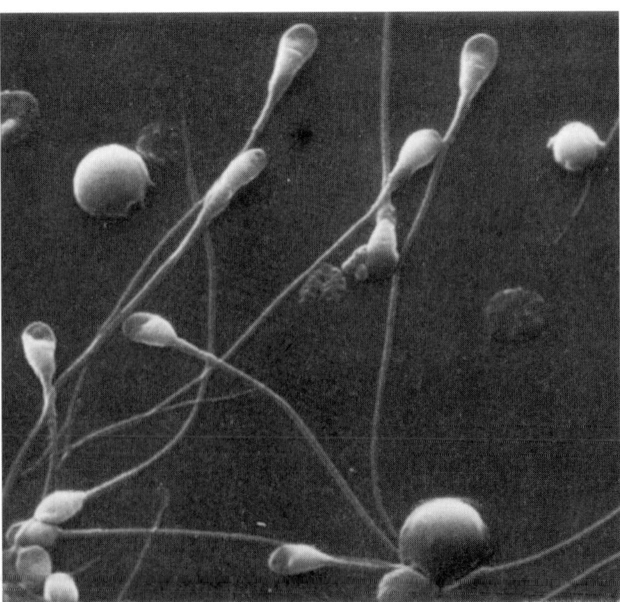

■ **Figure 2-14.** Scanning electron micrograph of human sperms. (From Page EW, Villee CA, Villee DB: *Human Reproduction. Essentials of Reproductive and Perinatal Medicine,* 3rd ed. Philadelphia, WB Saunders, 1981. Courtesy of J.E. Flechon and E.S.E. Hafez.)

tate, and *bulbourethral glands* — secretions from them are added to sperm-containing fluid in the ductus deferens and urethra (Fig. 2-15). From 200 to 600 million sperms are deposited around the external os of the cervix and in the fornix of the vagina during sexual intercourse. The sperms pass slowly by movements of their tails through the cervical canal. The enzyme *vesiculase*, produced by the seminal vesicles, coagulates some of the *semen* (seminal fluid containing sperms) and forms a vaginal plug that may prevent the backflow of semen into the vagina. At the time of ovulation, the cervical mucus increases in amount and becomes less viscid, making it more favorable for sperm transport.

The reflex ejaculation of sperms may be divided into two phases (Moore and Agur, 1995):

- *Emission* — semen is delivered to the prostatic part of the urethra through the ejaculatory ducts after peristalsis of the ductus deferentes (plural of ductus deferens) and seminal vesicles; emission is a sympathetic response.
- *Ejaculation* — semen is expelled from the urethra through the external urethral orifice; this results from closure of the vesical sphincter at the neck of the bladder, contraction of urethral muscle, and contraction of the bulbospongiosus muscles.

Passage of sperms through the uterus and uterine tubes results mainly from muscular contractions of the walls of these organs. *Prostaglandins* in the semen are thought to stimulate uterine motility at the time of intercourse and assist in the movement of sperms through the uterus and tubes to the site of fertilization in the ampulla of the tube. *Fructose* in the semen, secreted by the seminal vesicles, is an energy source for the sperms (Barratt and Cooke, 1991).

The **ejaculate** (sperms suspended in secretions from accessory sex glands) averages 3.5 ml, with a range of 2 to 6 ml. The sperms move 2 to 3 mm per minute but the speed varies with the pH of the environment. They are nonmotile during storage in the epididymis, but become motile in the ejaculate. They move slowly in the acid environment of the vagina, but move more rapidly in the alkaline environment of the uterus. It is not known how long it takes sperms to reach the fertilization site, but the time of transport is probably short. Settlage et al. (1973) found a few motile sperms in the ampulla of the uterine tube 5 minutes after their deposition near the external uterine os. Some sperms, however, took up to 45 minutes to complete the journey. Only about 200 sperms reach the fertilization site. Most sperms degenerate and are resorbed by the female genital tract.

MATURATION OF SPERMS

Freshly ejaculated sperms are unable to fertilize oocytes. They must undergo a *period of conditioning* —

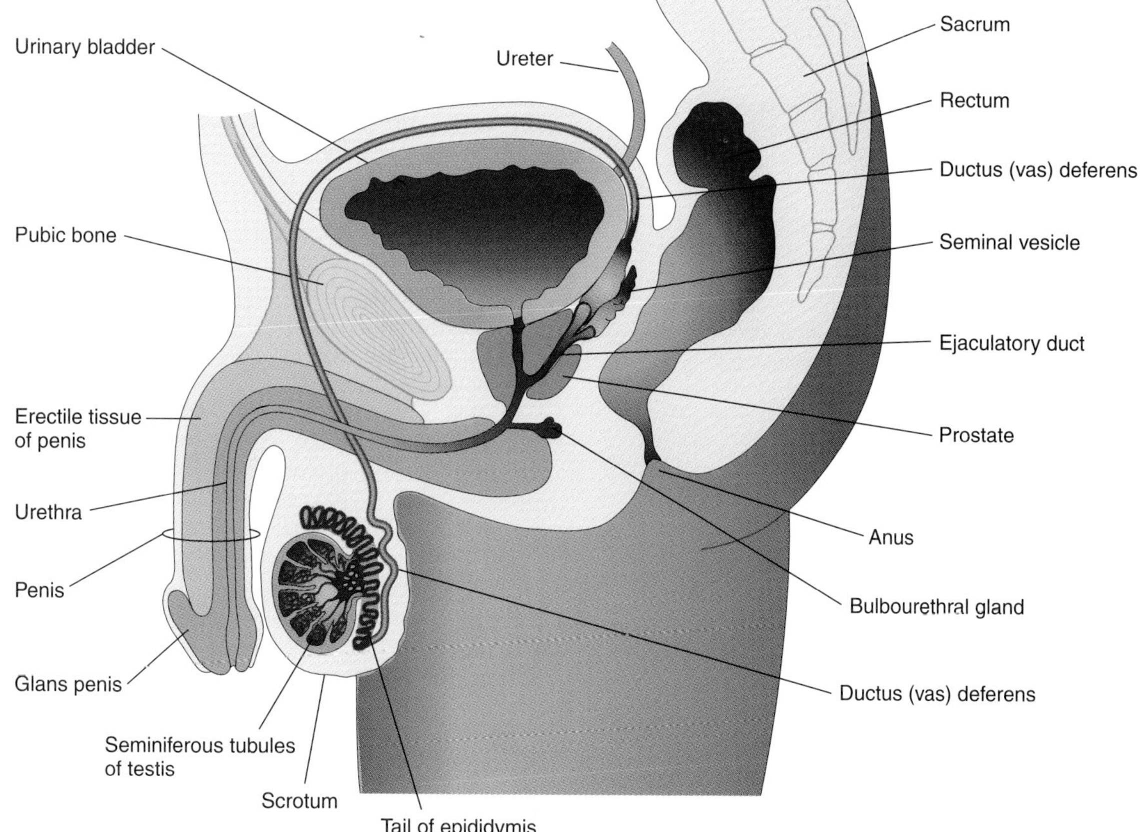

■ **Figure 2-15.** Sagittal section of the male pelvis primarily to show the male reproductive system.

capacitation—lasting about 7 hours. During this period a glycoprotein coat and seminal proteins are removed from the surface of the sperm's acrosome. The membrane cholesterol/phospholipid ratios, as well as the membrane potential, become altered. Capacitated sperms show no morphological changes but they are more active. Sperms are usually capacitated in the uterus or uterine tubes by substances secreted by these parts of the female genital tract. During *in vitro fertilization*—a process whereby several oocytes are placed in a medium to which sperms are added for fertilization (see Fig. 2-18)—capacitation is induced by incubating the sperms in a defined medium for several hours. Completion of capacitation permits the acrosome reaction to occur (Acosta, 1994).

Angiotensin converting enzyme (ACE) present in the acrosome of the sperm is probably involved in inducing the **acrosome reaction** and the fertilization process. The acrosome reaction of sperms must be completed before the sperm can fuse with the oocyte (Allen and Green, 1997). When capacitated sperms come into contact with the corona radiata surrounding a secondary oocyte (Fig. 2-16), they undergo changes that result in the development of perforations in the acrosome. Multiple point fusions of the plasma membrane of the sperm and the external acrosomal membrane occur. Breakdown of the membranes at these sites produces apertures. The changes induced by the acrosome reaction are associated with the release of enzymes, including *hyaluronidase and acrosin*, from the acrosome that facilitate fertilization.

Sperm Counts

During evaluation of male fertility, an analysis of semen is made. Sperms account for less than 10% of the semen. The remainder of the ejaculate consists of the secretions of the accessory sex glands: seminal vesicles (60%), prostate (30%), and bulbourethral glands (10%). There are usually more than 100 million sperms per ml of semen in the ejaculate of normal males. Although there is much variation in individual cases, men whose semen contains 20 million sperms per ml, or 50 million in the total specimen, are probably fertile (Comhaire et al., 1992). A man with less than 10 million sperms per ml of semen is likely to be sterile, especially when the specimen contains immotile and abnormal sperms. Thus, in assessing fertility potential, the total number and motility of sperms in the ejaculate are taken into consideration. For potential fertility, at least 40% of sperms should be motile after 2 hours and some should be motile after 24 hours. It is believed that male infertility is the cause of one-third to one-half of unintentional childless marriages. Male infertility may result from endocrine disorders, abnormal spermatogenesis, or obstruction of a genital duct such as in the ductus deferens (Fig. 2-15).

Deferentectomy (Vasectomy)

The most effective method of contraception in the male is *deferentectomy* (excision of a segment from each ductus deferens). This surgical procedure—*vasectomy*—is reversible in at least 50% of cases. Following deferentectomy there are no sperms in the ejaculate but the amount of seminal fluid is the same.

VIABILITY OF GAMETES

Studies on early stages of development indicate that **human oocytes** are usually fertilized within 12 hours after extrusion from the ovaries at ovulation. In vitro observations have shown that the oocyte cannot be fertilized after 24 hours and that it degenerates shortly thereafter.

Most **human sperms** probably do not survive for more than 48 hours in the female genital tract. Some sperms are stored in folds of the mucosa of the cervix and are gradually released into the cervical canal and pass through the uterus into the uterine tubes. The short-term storage of sperms in the cervix provides a gradual release of sperms and thereby increases the chances of fertilization. After being frozen to low temperatures, semen may be kept for many years. Children have been born to women who have been artificially inseminated with semen that had been stored for several years.

FERTILIZATION

The usual site of fertilization is the ampulla of the uterine tube, its longest and widest part (Fig. 2-6*B*). If the oocyte is not fertilized here, it slowly passes along the tube to the uterus, where it degenerates and is resorbed. Although fertilization may occur in other parts of the tube, it does not occur in the uterus.

Human development begins when a oocyte is fertilized. Fertilization is a complex sequence of "coordinated molecular events" (see Acosta, 1994 for details) that begins with contact between a sperm and a oocyte (Fig. 2-16) and ends with the intermingling of maternal and paternal chromosomes at metaphase of the first mitotic division of the zygote, a unicellular embryo (Fig. 2-17). Defects at any stage in the sequence of these events might cause the zygote to die (Asch et al., 1995). *Carbohydrate binding molecules* on the surface of the gametes are possibly involved in the process of fertilization through gamete recognition and union of the cells (Boldt et al., 1989). The fertilization process takes about 24 hours.

Phases of Fertilization

Fertilization is a complex sequence of coordinated events (Figs. 2-16 and 2-17):

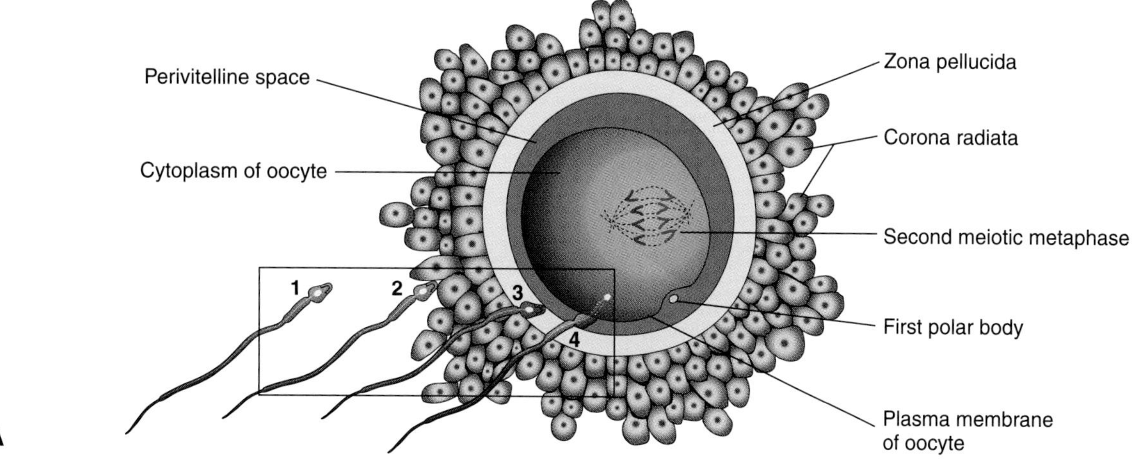

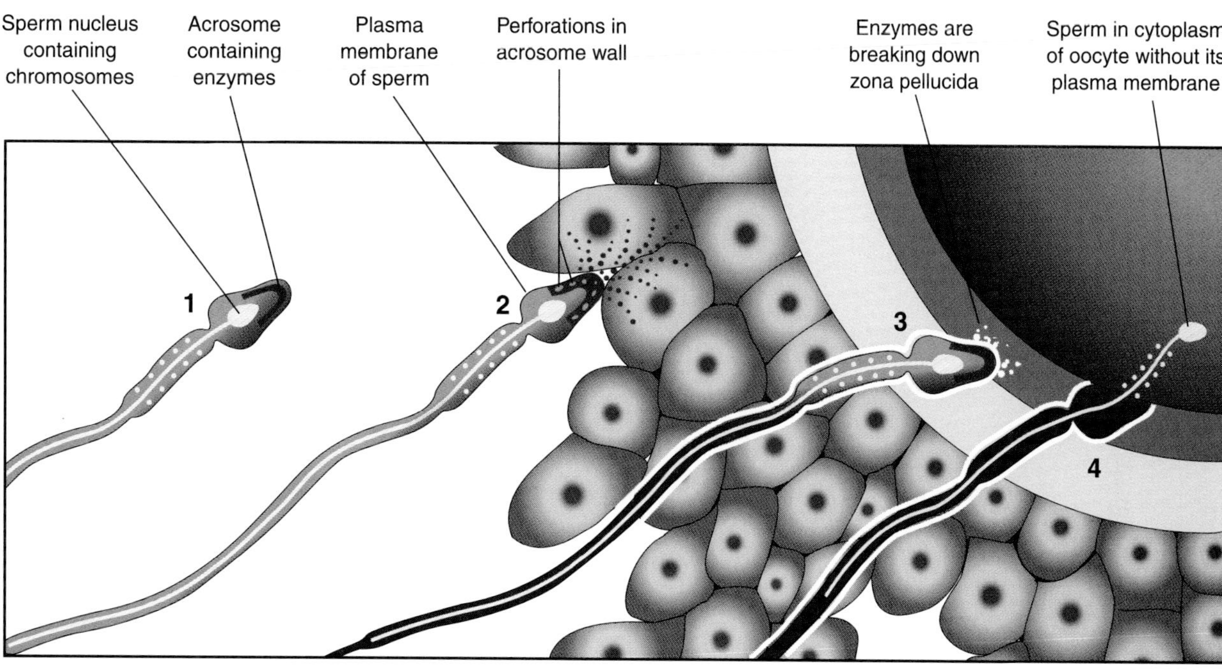

■ **Figure 2–16.** Diagrams illustrating the acrosome reaction and a sperm penetrating an oocyte. The detail of the area outlined in *A* is given in *B*. 1, Sperm during capacitation, a period of conditioning that occurs in the female reproductive tract. 2, Sperm undergoing the acrosome reaction, during which perforations form in the acrosome. 3, Sperm digesting a path through the zona pellucida by the action of enzymes released from the acrosome. 4, Sperm after entering the cytoplasm of the oocyte. Note that the plasma membranes of the sperm and oocyte have fused and that the head and tail of the sperm enter the oocyte, leaving the sperm's plasma membrane attached to the oocyte's plasma membrane.

- **Passage of sperm through corona radiata surrounding the zona pellucida of an oocyte**. Dispersal of the follicular cells of the corona radiata, which surrounds the oocyte and zona pellucida, appears to result mainly from the action of the enzyme *hyaluronidase* released from the acrosome of the sperm, but the evidence for this is not unequivocal (Carlson, 1994). *Tubal mucosal enzymes* also appear to assist hyaluronidase. Movements of the tail of the sperm are also important in its penetration of the corona radiata.
- **Penetration of zona pellucida surrounding the oocyte**. Penetration of the zona pellucida by a sperm is the important phase in the initiation of fertilization. The formation of a pathway through the zona pellucida also results from the action of

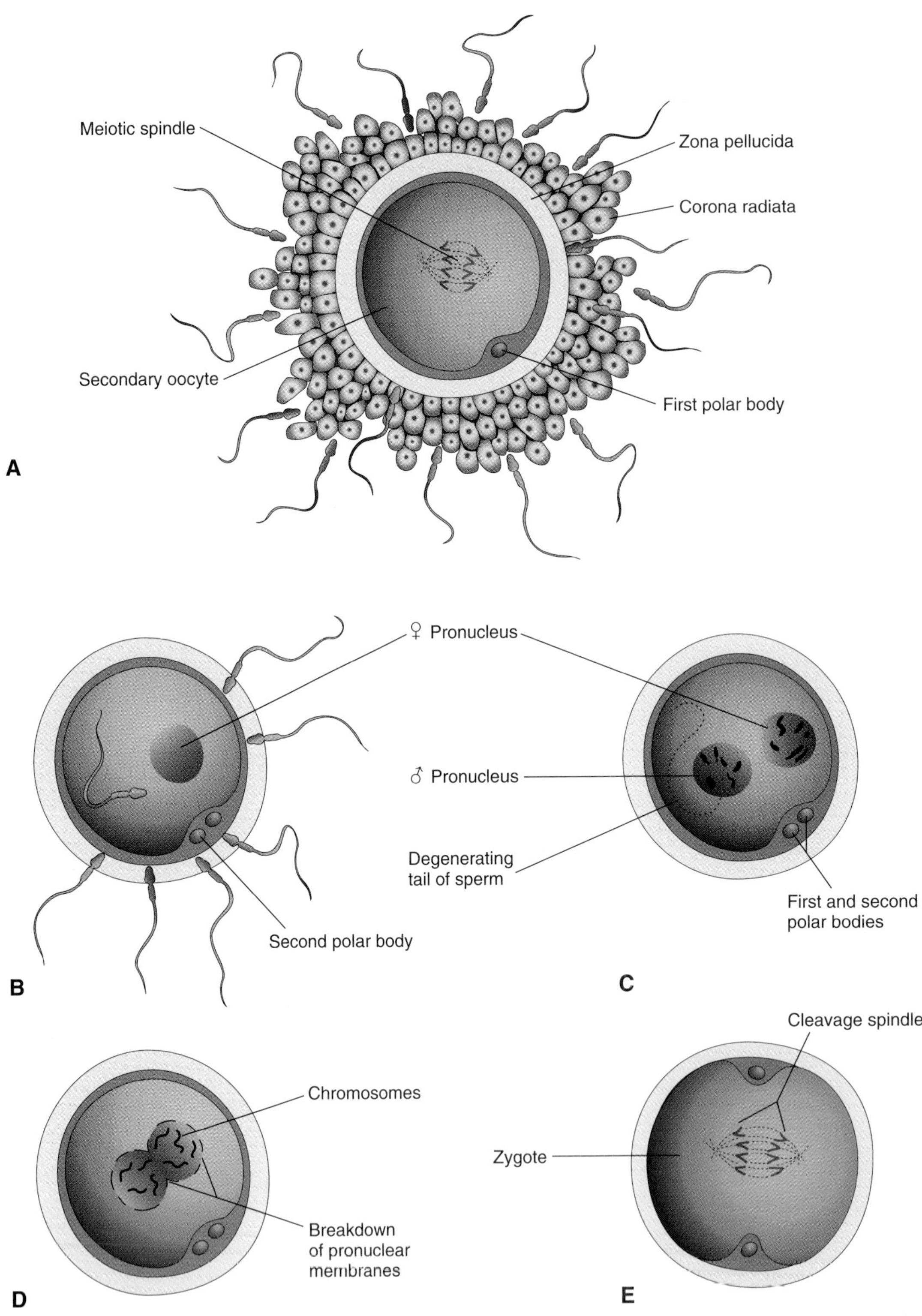

■ **Figure 2–17.** Diagrams illustrating fertilization, the procession of events beginning when the sperm contacts the secondary oocyte's plasma membrane and ending with the intermingling of maternal and paternal chromosomes at metaphase of the first mitotic division of the zygote. *A*, Secondary oocyte surrounded by several sperms. (Only four of the 23 chromosome pairs are shown.) *B*, The corona radiata has disappeared, a sperm has entered the oocyte, and the second meiotic division has occurred, forming a mature oocyte. The nucleus of the ovum is now the female pronucleus. *C*, The sperm head has enlarged to form the male pronucleus. *D*, The pronuclei are fusing. *E*, The zygote has formed; it contains 46 chromosomes, the diploid number.

enzymes released from the acrosome. The enzymes — *esterases, acrosin, and neuraminidase* — appear to cause lysis of the zona, thereby forming a path for the sperm to follow to the oocyte. The most important of these enzymes is *acrosin*, a proteolytic enzyme (Carlson, 1994). Once the sperm penetrates the zona pellucida, a **zona reaction** — a change in the properties of the zona pellucida — occurs in this amorphous layer that makes it impermeable to other sperms. The composition of this extracellular glycoprotein coat changes after fertilization (Moos et al., 1995). The zona reaction is believed to result from the action of lysosomal enzymes released by cortical granules near the plasma membrane of the oocyte. The contents of these granules, which are released into the perivitelline space (Fig. 2-16*A*), also cause changes in the plasma membrane of the oocyte that make it impermeable to sperms (Chen and Sathananthan, 1986; Wassarman, 1987; Bercegeay et al., 1995).

- **Fusion of plasma membranes of the oocyte and sperm**. The plasma or cell membranes of the oocyte and sperm fuse and break down at the area of fusion. The head and tail of the sperm enter the cytoplasm of the oocyte, but the sperm's plasma membrane remains behind (Fig. 2-16*B*).
- **Completion of second meiotic division of oocyte and formation of female pronucleus**. After entry of the sperm, the oocyte, which has been arrested in metaphase of the second meiotic division, completes this division and forms a mature oocyte and a second polar body (Fig. 2-17*B*). Following decondensation of the maternal chromosomes, the nucleus of the mature oocyte becomes the female pronucleus.
- **Formation of male pronucleus**. Within the cytoplasm of the oocyte, the nucleus of the sperm enlarges to form the male pronucleus and the tail of the sperm degenerates (Fig. 2-17*C*). Morphologically the male and female pronuclei are indistinguishable. During growth of the pronuclei, they replicate their DNA-1 n (haploid), 2 c (two chromatids).
- **Membranes of pronuclei break down, the chromosomes condense and become arranged for a mitotic cell division** — the first cleavage division (see Fig. 2-20*A*). The fertilized oocyte or **zygote** is a unicellular embryo (Fig. 2-17*E*). The combination of 23 chromosomes in each pronucleus results in a zygote with 46 chromosomes.

An immunosuppressant protein, the **early pregnancy factor** (EPF), is secreted by the trophoblastic cells and appears in the maternal serum within 24 to 48 hours after fertilization. EPF forms the basis of a pregnancy test during the first 10 days of development (Nahhas and Barnea, 1990).

Dispermy and Triploidy

Although several sperms begin to penetrate the zona pellucida, usually only one sperm enters the oocyte and fertilizes it. Two sperms may participate in fertilization during an abnormal process known as *dispermy*, resulting in a zygote with an extra set of chromosomes. Triploid conceptions account for about 20% of chromosomally abnormal abortions (Crane, 1994). The resulting **triploid embryos** (69 chromosomes) may appear normal, but they nearly always abort. Aborted triploid fetuses have severe *intrauterine growth retardation*, disproportionately small trunks, and many other anomalies in the central nervous system, for example. A few triploid infants have been born, but they all died shortly after birth (Carr, 1971). Livebirths are uncommon, occurring in fewer than 1 in 2500 pregnancies.

Results of Fertilization

Fertilization

- stimulates the secondary oocyte to complete the second meiotic division
- restores the normal diploid number of chromosomes (46) in zygote
- results in variation of the human species through mingling of maternal and paternal chromosomes
- determines chromosomal sex of embryo; an X-bearing sperm produces a female embryo and a Y-bearing sperm produces a male embryo
- causes metabolic activation of the oocyte and initiates cleavage (cell division of zygote)

The zygote is genetically unique because half of its chromosomes come from the mother and half from the father. The zygote contains a new combination of chromosomes that is different from that in the cells of either of the parents. *This mechanism forms the basis of biparental inheritance and variation of the human species.* Meiosis allows independent assortment of maternal and paternal chromosomes among the germ cells (Fig. 2-2). *Crossing over of chromosomes*, by relocating segments of the maternal and paternal chromosomes, "shuffles" the genes, thereby producing a recombination of genetic material.

The embryo's chromosomal sex is determined at fertilization by the kind of sperm (X or Y) that fertilizes the ovum; hence, it is the father rather than the mother whose gamete determines the sex of the embryo. Fertilization by an X-bearing sperm produces a 46, XX zygote, which normally develops into a female, whereas fertilization by a Y-sperm produces a 46, XY zygote, which normally develops into a male.

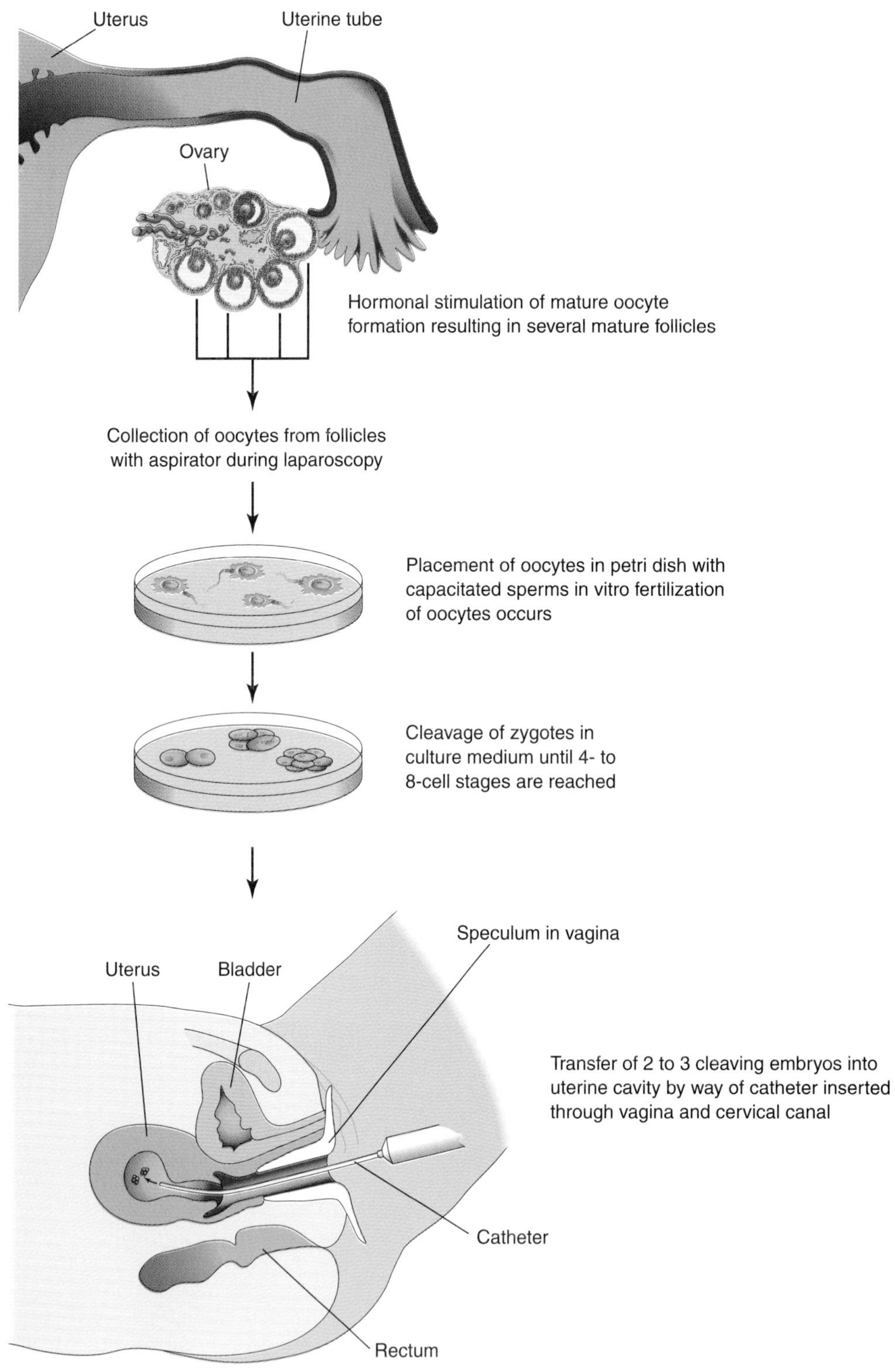

■ **Figure 2–18.** In vitro fertilization and embryo transfer procedures.

Parthenogenesis

Cleavage of an unfertilized oocyte may occur through a process known as *parthenogenesis* (Beatty, 1957); this may occur naturally or be artificially induced. Parthenogenesis is a normal event in some species; for example, some eggs laid by a queen bee are not fertilized but develop parthenogenetically. In a few other species (e.g., rabbits), an unfertilized ovum can be induced experimentally to undergo parthenogenetic development. *No verified case of parthenogenesis has occurred in humans*, but an embryo could develop by fusion of a secondary oocyte with the second polar body. These embryos, however, would not likely survive because they would probably contain lethal genes that would result in their death and early abortion.

Preselection of Embryo's Sex

Because the sex of the embryo is determined by whether the sperm contributes an X or a Y chromosome to the zygote, and because X and Y sperms are formed in equal numbers, the expectation is that the sex ratio at fertilization (*primary sex ratio*) would be 1.00 (100 boys per 100 girls). It is well known, however, that there are more male babies than female babies born in all countries. In North America, for example, the sex ratio at birth (*secondary sex ratio*) is about 1.05 (105 boys per 100 girls).

Various in vitro techniques have been developed in an attempt to separate X and Y sperms using:

- the differential swimming abilities of the two types of sperm
- different speeds of migration of sperms in an electric field
- microscopic differences in the appearance of X and Y sperms

The use of a selected sperm sample in artificial insemination may produce the desired sex. Others claim that the timing and management of sexual intercourse can enable a couple to choose the sex of their child. For example, a study of 3668 births found that the proportion of male births was higher when sexual intercourse occurred two or more days after ovulation than when it occurred at or near ovulation (Harlap, 1979); however, no method of controlling the human embryo's sex has been shown to change the sex ratio consistently.

In Vitro Fertilization and Embryo Transfer

In vitro fertilization (IVF) of oocytes and transfer of the dividing zygotes (cleaving embryos) into the uterus has provided an opportunity for many women who are sterile (e.g., owing to tubal occlusion) to bear children. The first of these IVF babies was born in 1978. Since then thousands of pregnancies have occurred using this technique and its modifications, especially *gamete intrafallopian transfer* (Steptoe and Edwards, 1978; Edwards and Brody, 1995). The steps involved during in vitro fertilization and embryo transfer are as follows (Figs. 2-18 to 2-20):

- Ovarian follicles are stimulated to grow and mature by the administration of gonadotropins.
- Several mature oocytes are aspirated from mature ovarian follicles during *laparoscopy*—viewing of ovaries with a laparoscope. Oocytes can also be removed by an ultrasound-guided large-gauge needle inserted through the vaginal wall into the ovarian follicles (Ritchie, 1994).
- The oocytes are placed in a Petri dish containing a special culture medium and capacitated sperms.
- Fertilization of the oocytes and cleavage of the zygotes are monitored microscopically.
- Dividing zygotes (cleaved embryos) during the four- to eight-cell stage are transferred by introducing a catheter through the vagina and cervical canal into the uterus; the probability of a successful pregnancy is enhanced by inserting up to three embryos.
- The patient remains in the supine position (face upward) for several hours.

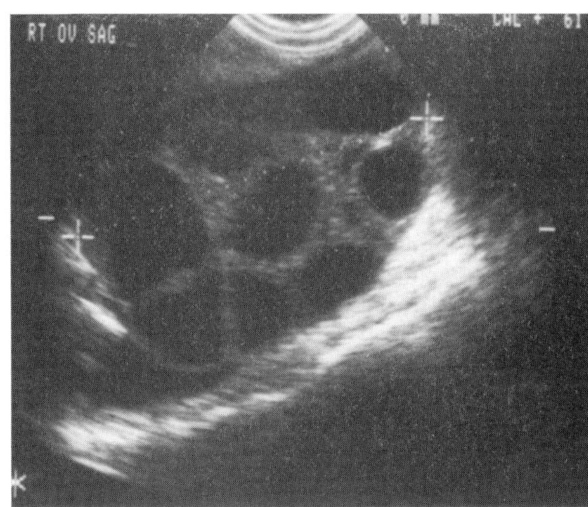

■ **Figure 2-19.** Induced follicular development. Following administration of hCG, sonograms through the ovary on day 14 of the menstrual cycle show the presence of several mature ovarian follicles. (From Ritchie WGM: Ultrasound evaluation of normal and induced ovulation. *In* Callen PW (ed): *Ultrasonography in Obstetrics and Gynecology,* 3rd ed. Philadelphia, WB Saunders, 1994.)

Obviously, the chances of multiple pregnancies are higher than when pregnancy results from normal ovulation and passage of the morula into the uterus via the uterine tube. The incidence of spontaneous abortion of transferred embryos is also higher than normal. This may result from the high incidence of chromosomal and other cellular abnormalities present in conceptuses fertilized in vitro (Winston, 1996).

Cryopreservation of Embryos

Embryos and blastocysts resulting from in vitro fertilization can be preserved for long periods by freezing them with a cryoprotectant (e.g., glycerol). Successful transfer of four- to eight-cell embryos and blastocysts to the uterus after thawing is now a common practice (Fugger et al., 1991).

Intracytoplasmic Sperm Injection

A sperm can be injected directly into the cytoplasm of a mature oocyte. This technique has been successfully used for the treatment of couples where IVF failed or in cases where there are too few sperms available for *in vitro insemination* (Palermo et al., 1995; Khalifeh et al., 1997).

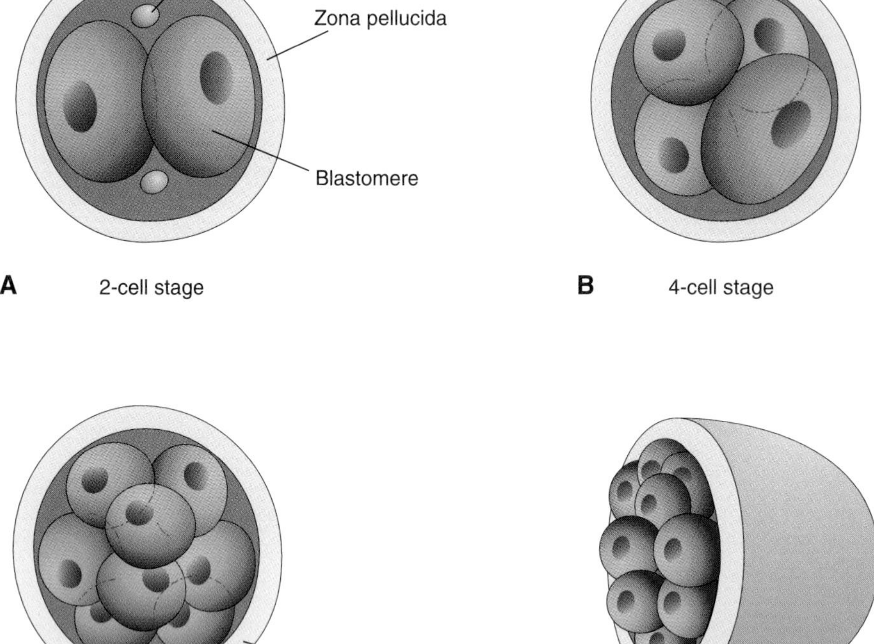

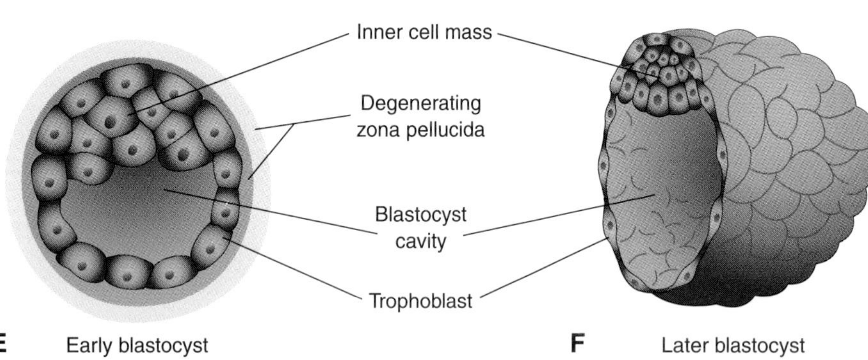

■ **Figure 2–20.** Drawings illustrating cleavage of the zygote and formation of the blastocyst. *A* to *D* show various stages of cleavage. The period of the morula begins at the 12- to 16-cell stage and ends when the blastocyst forms. *E* and *F* are sections of blastocysts. The zona pellucida has disappeared by the late blastocyst stage (5 days). The polar bodies shown in *A* are small, nonfunctional cells that soon degenerate. Cleavage of the zygote and formation of the morula occur as the dividing zygote passes along the uterine tube. Blastocyst formation normally occurs in the uterus. Although cleavage increases the number of blastomeres, note that each of the daughter cells is smaller than the parent cells. As a result there is no increase in the size of the developing embryo until the zona pellucida degenerates. The blastocyst then enlarges considerably. The inner cell mass or embryoblast gives rise to the tissues and organs of the embryo.

Assisted In Vivo Fertilization

A technique enabling fertilization to occur in the uterine (fallopian) tube is called *gamete intrafallopian* transfer (GIFT). It involves superovulation (similar to that used for IVF), oocyte retrieval, sperm collection, and laparoscopic placement of several oocytes and sperms into the uterine tubes. Using this technique, fertilization occurs in the ampulla, its usual location. For a description of GIFT and other assisted in vivo techniques, see Dooley et al. (1988) and Edwards (1994).

Surrogate Mothers

Some women can produce mature oocytes but are unable to become pregnant, e.g., a woman who has had her uterus excised (*hysterectomy*). In these cases IVF may be performed and the embryos transferred to another woman's uterus. The surrogate mother bears the fetus and delivers it to the natural mother at birth. For a discussion of ethical and legal issues related to surrogacy, see Robertson (1995).

CLEAVAGE OF ZYGOTE

Cleavage consists of repeated mitotic divisions of the zygote, resulting in a rapid increase in the number of cells. These cells — **blastomeres** — become smaller with each cleavage division (Figs. 2-20 and 2-21). First the zygote divides into two blastomeres, which then divide into four blastomeres, eight blastomeres, and so on. Cleavage normally occurs as the zygote passes along the uterine tube toward the uterus (see Fig. 2-24). During cleavage, the zygote is within the rather thick, jellylike zona pellucida (pellucid zone) that is translucent under the light microscope. Division of the zygote into blastomeres begins about 30 hours after fertilization. Subsequent divisions follow one another, forming progressively smaller blastomeres (Fig. 2-20).

After the nine-cell stage, the blastomeres change their shape and tightly align themselves against each other to form a compact ball of cells. This phenomenon — known as **compaction** — is probably mediated by cell surface adhesion glycoproteins (Gilbert, 1997). Compaction permits greater cell-to-cell interaction and is a prerequisite for segregation of the internal cells that form the inner cell mass (embryoblast) of the blastocyst (Fig. 2-20*E* and *F*). When there are 12 to 15 blastomeres, the developing human is called a **morula** (L. *morus*, mulberry). Internal cells of the morula (*inner cell mass*) are surrounded by a layer of cells that form the *outer cell layer*. The spherical morula forms about 3 days after fertilization and enters the uterus. It was given its name because of its resemblance to the fruit of the mulberry tree.

Nondisjunction of Chromosomes

If nondisjunction (failure of a chromosome pair to separate) occurs during an early cleavage division of a zygote, an embryo with two or more cell lines with different chromosome complements is produced. Such individuals in whom numerical mosaicism is present are termed *mosaics*; for example, a zygote with an additional chromosome 21 might lose the extra chromosome during an early division of the zygote into blastomeres. Consequently, some cells of the embryo would have a normal chromosome complement and others would have an additional chromosome 21. In general, individuals who are mosaic for a given trisomy, such as *mosaic Down syndrome*, are less severely affected than those with the usual nonmosaic condition (Thompson et al., 1991).

FORMATION OF BLASTOCYST (BLASTOGENESIS)

Shortly after the morula enters the uterus (about 4 days after fertilization), a fluid-filled space called the **blastocyst cavity** (blastocele) appears inside the morula (Fig. 2-20*E*). The fluid passes from the uterine cavity through the zona pellucida to form these spaces. As fluid increases in the blastocyst cavity, it separates the blastomeres into two parts:

- a thin, outer cell layer called the **trophoblast** (Gr. *trophe*, nutrition), which gives rise to the embryonic part of the placenta
- a group of centrally located blastomeres known as the **inner cell mass**, which gives rise to the embryo; because it is the primordium of the embryo, the inner cell mass is often called the *embryoblast*

At this stage of development, the conceptus is called a **blastocyst** (Fig. 2-22). The inner cell mass or embryoblast now projects into the blastocyst cavity and the trophoblast forms the wall of the blastocyst. After the blastocyst has floated in the uterine secretions for about 2 days, the zona pellucida gradually degenerates and disappears (Figs. 2-20*F* and 2-22*A*). *Shedding of the zona pellucida* and *"hatching of the blastocyst"* have been observed in vitro (Veeck, 1991).

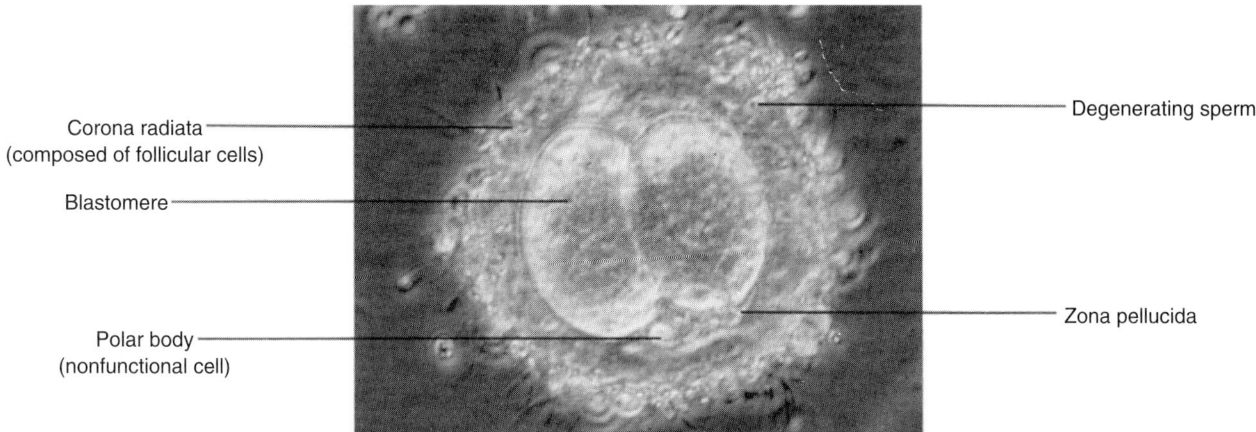

■ **Figure 2-21.** A two-cell stage of a cleaved zygote developing in vitro. Observe that it is surrounded by many sperms. (Courtesy of Dr. M.T. Zenzes, In Vitro Fertilization Program, Toronto Hospital, Toronto, Ontario, Canada.)

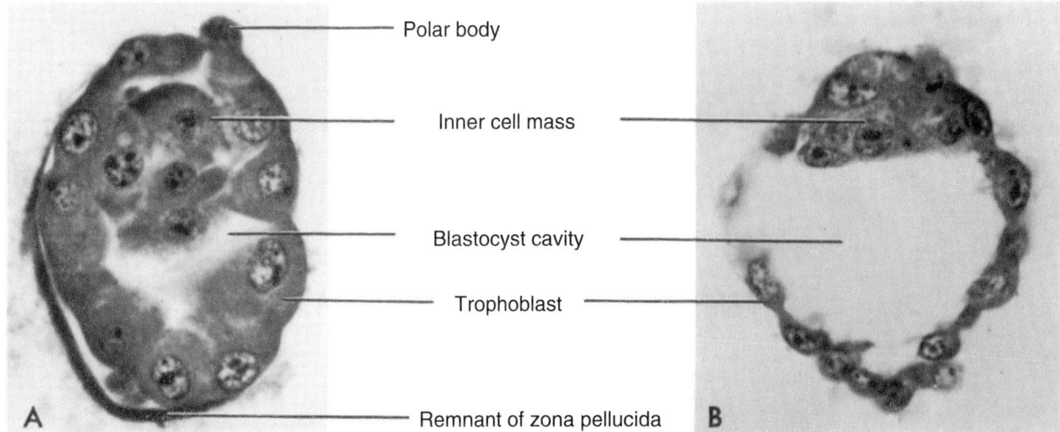

■ **Figure 2–22.** Photomicrographs of sections of human blastocysts recovered from the uterine cavity (×600). *A*, Four days; the blastocyst cavity is just beginning to form and the zona pellucida is deficient over part of the blastocyst. *B*, Four and a half days; the blastocyst cavity has enlarged and the inner cell mass and trophoblast are clearly defined. The zona pellucida has disappeared. (From Hertig AT, Rock, J, Adams EC: *Am J Anat 98*:435, 1956. Courtesy of Carnegie Institution of Washington.)

Shedding of the zona pellucida permits the blastocyst to increase rapidly in size. While floating freely in the uterus, the embryo derives nourishment from secretions of the uterine glands.

About 6 days after fertilization (day 20 of a 28-day menstrual cycle), the blastocyst attaches to the endometrial epithelium, usually adjacent to the inner cell mass, the *embryonic pole* (Fig. 2-23*A*). As soon as it attaches to the endometrial epithelium, the trophoblast starts to proliferate rapidly and gradually differentiates into two layers (Fig. 2-23*B*):

- an inner layer of *cytotrophoblast* (cellular trophoblast)
- an outer mass of *syncytiotrophoblast* (syncytial trophoblast) consisting of a multinucleated protoplasmic mass in which no cell boundaries can be observed

Both intrinsic and extracellular matrix factors modulate, in carefully timed sequences, the differentiation of the trophoblast (Aplin, 1991).

At about 6 days, the fingerlike processes of syncytiotrophoblast (syntrophoblast) extend through the endometrial epithelium and invade the connective tissue (stroma). By the end of the first week, the blastocyst is superficially implanted in the compact layer of the endometrium and is deriving its nourishment from the eroded maternal tissues (Fig. 2-23*B*). The highly invasive syncytiotrophoblast expands quickly adjacent to the inner cell mass, the area known as the *embryonic pole*. The syncytiotrophoblast produces enzymes that erode the maternal tissues, enabling the blastocyst to burrow into the endometrium.

At about 7 days, a layer of cells, the **hypoblast**, appears on the surface of the inner cell mass facing the blastocyst cavity (Fig. 2-23*B*). Comparative embryological data suggest that the hypoblast arises by delamination from the inner cell mass (Carlson, 1994).

Preimplantation Diagnosis of Genetic Disorders

Using currently available techniques of micromanipulation and DNA application, a dividing zygote known to be at risk for a specific genetic disorder may be diagnosed before implantation (Geber et al., 1995). Sex can be determined from one blastomere taken from a six- to eight-cell dividing zygote and analyzed by DNA amplification of sequences from the Y chromosome. This procedure has been used to detect female embryos during IVF in cases in which a male embryo would be at risk for a serious X-linked disorder (Handyside et al., 1990). For more information regarding the possibility of preimplantation genetic analysis for heritable diseases, see Kaufman et al., 1992.

Abnormal Embryos and Spontaneous Abortions

Many zygotes, morulae, and blastocysts abort spontaneously. Early implantation of the blastocyst is a critical period of development that may fail to occur owing to inadequate production of progesterone and estrogen by the corpus luteum. Clinicians occasionally see a patient who states that her last menstrual period was delayed by several days and that her last menstrual flow was unusually profuse. Very likely such patients have had an early spontaneous abortion; thus the overall *early spontaneous abortion rate* is thought to be about 45% (Rubin and Farber, 1988).

Early spontaneous abortions occur for a variety of reasons, one being the presence of chromosomal abnormalities in the zygote. Carr and Gedeon (1977) esti-

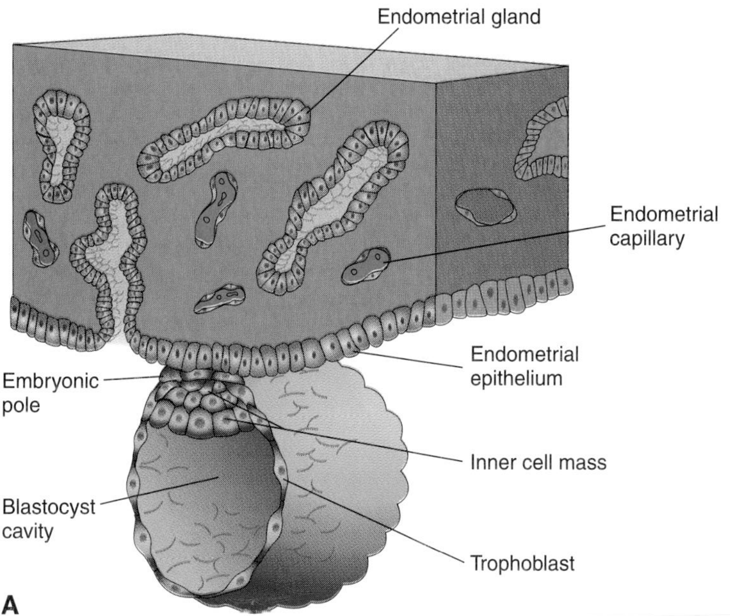

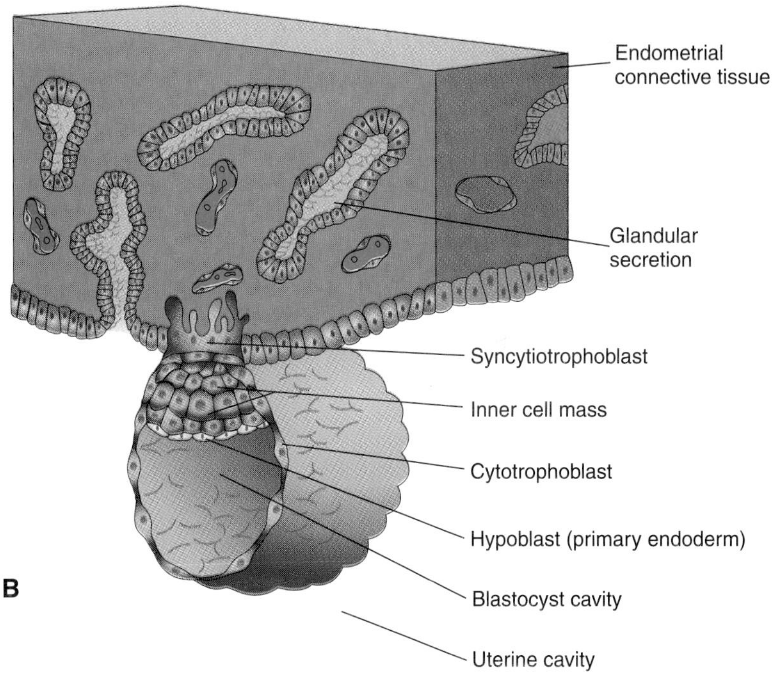

■ **Figure 2–23.** Drawings of sections illustrating the attachment of the blastocyst to the endometrial epithelium and the early stages of its implantation. *A*, Six days; the trophoblast is attached to the endometrial epithelium at the embryonic pole of the blastocyst. *B*, Seven days; the syncytiotrophoblast has penetrated the epithelium and has started to invade the endometrial stroma (framework of connective tissue). Some students have difficulty interpreting illustrations such as these because in histological studies it is conventional to draw the endometrial epithelium upward, whereas in embryological studies the embryo is usually shown with its dorsal surface upward. Because the embryo implants on its future dorsal surface, it would appear upside-down if the histological convention were followed. In this book, the histological convention is followed when the endometrium is the dominant consideration (e.g., Fig. 2–6*C*), and the embryological convention is used when the embryo is the center of interest, as in the adjacent illustrations.

mated that about half of all known spontaneous abortions occur because of chromosomal abnormalities. Hertig et al. (1959), while examining blastocysts recovered from early pregnancies, found several clearly defective dividing zygotes (cleavage stage embryos) and blastocysts. Some were so abnormal that survival would not have been likely. The early loss of embryos, once called *pregnancy wastage*, appears to represent a disposal of abnormal conceptuses that could not have developed normally, i.e., there is a natural screening of embryos. Without this screening, about 12% instead of 2 to 3% of infants would likely be congenitally malformed (Warkany, 1981).

SUMMARY OF FIRST WEEK OF DEVELOPMENT

Human development begins at fertilization but several important events happen before this process takes place (e.g., gametogenesis). Oocytes are produced by the ovary (*oogenesis*) and expelled from it during *ovulation*. The fimbriae of the uterine tube sweep the oocyte into the ampulla where it may be fertilized.

Sperms are produced in the seminiferous tubules of the testes (*spermatogenesis*) and are stored in the epididymis. Ejaculation of semen during sexual intercourse results in the deposit of millions of sperms in

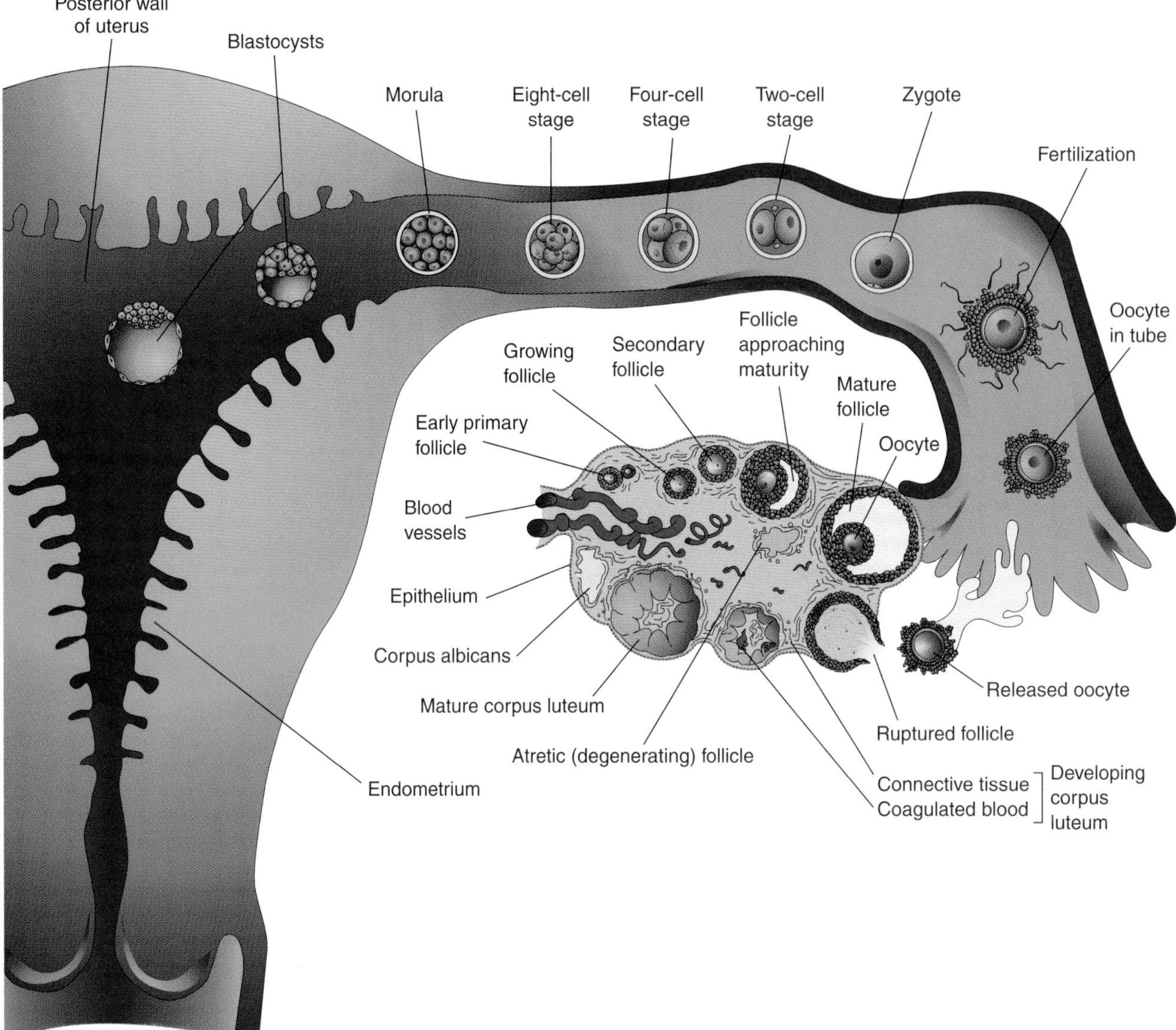

■ **Figure 2–24.** Diagrammatic summary of the ovarian cycle, fertilization, and human development during the first week. Stage 1 of development begins with fertilization in the uterine tube and ends when the zygote forms. Stage 2 (days 2 to 3) comprises the early stages of cleavage (from 2 to about 16 cells, the morula). Stage 3 (days 4 to 5) consists of the free unattached blastocyst. Stage 4 (days 5 to 6) is represented by the blastocyst attaching to the posterior wall of the uterus, the usual site of implantation. The blastocysts have been sectioned to show their structure.

the vagina around the external uterine os. Several hundred sperms pass through the uterus and enter the uterine tubes. Many of them surround the secondary oocyte if it is present. When an oocyte is contacted by a sperm, it completes the second meiotic division. As a result, a mature oocyte and a second polar body are formed. The nucleus of the mature oocyte constitutes the *female pronucleus*.

After the sperm enters the oocyte, the head of the sperm separates from the tail and enlarges to become the *male pronucleus*. Fertilization is complete when the pronuclei unite and the maternal and paternal chromosomes intermingle during metaphase of the first mitotic division of the *zygote*, the cell that is the primordium of a human being. As it passes along the uterine tube toward the uterus, the zygote undergoes *cleavage* (a series of mitotic cell divisions) into a number of smaller cells called *blastomeres*. About three days after fertilization, a ball of 12 or more blastomeres, called a *morula*, enters the uterus.

A cavity soon forms in the morula, converting it into a *blastocyst* consisting of:

- the *inner cell mass, or embryoblast*, which gives rise to the embryo and some extraembryonic tissues
- a *blastocyst cavity*, a fluid-filled space
- the *trophoblast*, a thin outer layer of cells

The trophoblast encloses the inner cell mass and blastocyst cavity and later forms extraembryonic structures and the embryonic part of the placenta. Four to five days after fertilization, the zona pellucida is shed and the trophoblast adjacent to the inner cell mass attaches to the endometrial epithelium. The trophoblast adjacent to the embryonic pole differentiates into two layers, an outer *syncytiotrophoblast* and an inner *cytotrophoblast*. The syncytiotrophoblast invades the endometrial epithelium and underlying connective tissue. Concurrently, a cuboidal layer of *hypoblast* forms on the deep surface of the inner cell mass. By the end of the first week, the blastocyst is superficially implanted in the endometrium.

Clinically Oriented Problems

1. What is the main cause of numerical aberrations of chromosomes? Define this process. What is the usual result of this abnormal chromosomal mechanism?
2. During in vitro cleavage of a zygote, all blastomeres of a morula were found to have an extra set of chromosomes. Explain how this could happen. Can such a morula develop into a viable fetus?
3. In infertile couples, the inability to conceive is attributable to some factor in the woman or the man. What is a major cause of (a) female infertility and (b) male infertility?
4. Some people have a mixture of cells with 46 and 47 chromosomes (e.g., some Down syndrome patients are *mosaics*). How do mosaics form? Would children with mosaicism and the Down syndrome have the same stigmata as other infants with this syndrome? At what stage of development does mosaicism develop? Can this chromosomal abnormality be diagnosed before birth?
5. A young woman who feared that she might be pregnant asked you about the so-called "morning after pills" (*postcoital birth control pills*). What would you tell her? Would termination of such an early pregnancy be considered an abortion?
6. What is the most common abnormality in early spontaneously aborted embryos?

Discussion of these problems appears at the back of the book.

REFERENCES AND SUGGESTED READING

Acosta AA: Process of fertilization in the human and its abnormalities: diagnostic and therapeutic possibilities. *Obstet Gynecol Surv 49*:567, 1994.

Adashi EY: Endocrinology of the ovary. *Hum Reprod 9(Supp 2)*:36, 1994.

Allen CA, Green DPL: The mammalian acrosome reaction: gateway to sperm fusion with the oocyte. *Bioessays 19*:241, 1997.

Angell R: Mechanism of chromosome nondisjunction in human oocytes. *Prog Clin Biol Res 393*:13, 1995.

Aplin JD: Implantation, trophoblast differentiation and hemochorial placentation: mechanistic evidence *in vivo* and *in vitro*. *J Cell Sci 99*:681, 1991.

Asch R, Simerly C, Ord T, Ord VA, Schatten G: The stages at which human fertilization arrests: microtubule and chromosome configurations in inseminated oocytes which failed to complete fertilization and development in humans. *Hum Reprod 10*:1897, 1995.

Austin CR: Membrane fusion events in fertilization. *J Reprod Fertil 44*:155, 1975.

Balasch J, Miro F, Burzaco I, et al: The role of luteinizing hormone in human follicle development and oocyte fertility: evidence from in vitro fertilization in a woman with long-standing hypogonadotrophic hypogonadism and using recombinant human follicle stimulating hormone. *Hum Reprod 10*:1678, 1995.

Barratt CLR, Cooke ID: Sperm transport in the human female reproductive tract—a dynamic interaction. *Int J Androl 14*:394, 1991.

Beatty RA: *Parthenogenesis and Polyploidy in Mammalian Development*. Cambridge, Cambridge University Press, 1957.

Beer E: Egg transport through the oviduct. *Am J Obstet Gynecol 165*:483, 1991.

Beier HM: Die molekulare Biologie der Befruchtungskaskade und der beginnenden Embryonalentwicklung. *Ann Anat 174*:491, 1992.

Bercegeay S, Jean M, Lucas H, Barriere P: Composition of human zona pellucida as revealed by SDS-PAGE after silver staining. *Mol Reprod Dev 41*:355, 1995.

Boldt J, Howe AM, Pererson JB, et al: Carbohydrate involvement in sperm-egg fusion in mice. *Biol Reprod 40*:887, 1989.

Carlson BM: *Human Embryology and Developmental Biology*. St Louis, Mosby, 1994.

Carr BR, Blackwell RE: *Textbook of Reproductive Medicine*. Norwalk, Appleton & Lange, 1993.

Carr DH: Chromosome studies on selected spontaneous abortions: polyploidy in man. *J Med Genet 8*:164, 1971.

Carr DH, Gedeon M: Population cytogenetics of human abortuses. In Hook EB, Porter IH (eds): *Population Cytogenetics: Studies in Humans*. New York, Academic Press, 1977.

Chandley AC: Meiosis in man. *Trends Genet 4*:79–83, 1988.

Chapman MG, Grudzinskas JG, Chard T (eds): *Implantation. Biological and Clinical Aspects*. Berlin, Springer Verlag, 1988.

Chen CM, Sathananthan AH: Early penetration of human sperm through the vestments of human egg *in vitro*. *Arch Androl 16*: 183, 1986.

Clermont Y, Trott M: Kinetics of spermatogenesis in mammals: seminiferous epithelium cycle and spermatogonial renewal. *Physiol Rev 52*:198, 1972.

Clouthier DE, Avarbock MR, Maika SD, et al: Rat spermatogenesis in mouse testis. *Nature 381*:418, 1996.

Comhaire FH, Huysse S, Hinting A, et al: Objective semen analysis: has the target been reached? *Human Reprod 7*:237, 1992.

Crane JP: Ultrasound evaluation of fetal chromosome disorders. *In* Callen PW: *Ultrasonography in Obstetrics and Gynecology*, 3rd ed. Philadelphia, WB Saunders, 1994.

Cumming DC, Cumming CE, Kieren DK: Menstrual mythology and sources of information about menstruation. *Am J Obstet Gynecol 164*:472, 1991.

Denis H: A parallel between development and evolution: germ cell recruitment by the gonads. *Bioessays 16*:933, 1994.

Dooley M, Lim-Howe D, Savros M, Studd JWW: Early experience with gamete intrafallopian transfer (GIFT) and direct intraperitoneal insemination (DIPT). *J Royal Soc Med 81*:637, 1988.

Dym M: Basement membrane regulation of sertoli cells. *Endocr Rev 15*:102, 1994.

Edwards RG (ed): New concepts in fertility control. *Hum Reprod 9(Suppl 2)*:1, 1994.

Edwards RG, Brody SA: *Principles and Practice of Assisted Human Reproduction*. Philadelphia, WB Saunders, 1995.

Egarter C: The complex nature of egg transport through the oviduct. *Am J Obstet Gynecol 163*:687, 1990.

Elstein M: Cervix and cervical barrier. *In* Ludwig H, Tauber PF (eds): *Human Fertilization*. Stuttgart, Georg Thieme, 1978.

Fugger EP, Bustillo M, Dorfmann AD, Schulman JD: Human preimplantation embryo cryopreservation: selected aspects. *Hum Reprod 6*:131, 1991.

Geber S, Winston RM, Handyside AH: Proliferation of blastomeres from biopsied cleavage stage human embryos in vitro: an alternative to blastocyst biopsy for preimplantation diagnosis. *Hum Reprod 10*:1492, 1995.

Gilbert SF: *Developmental Biology*, 5th ed. Sunderland, Sinauer Associates, 1997.

Handyside AH, Kontogianni EH, Hardy K, Winston RML: Pregnancies from biopsied human preimplantation embryos sexed by Y-specific DNA amplification. *Nature 344*:768, 1990.

Harlap S: Gender of infants conceived on different days of the menstrual cycle. *New Engl J Med 300:*1445, 1979.

Hertig AT, Adams EC, Mulligan WJ: On the preimplantation stages of the human ovum: A description of four normal and four abnormal specimens ranging from the second to the fifth day of development. *Contrib Embryol Carnegie Inst 35:*199, 1954.

Hertig AT, Rock J: Two human ova of the previllous stage, having a developmental age of about seven and nine days respectively. *Contrib Embryol Carnegie Inst 31:*65, 1945.

Hertig AT, Rock J, Adams EC: A description of 34 human ova within the first seventeen days of development. *Am J Anat 98:*435, 1956.

Hertig AT, Rock J, Adams EC, Menkin MC: Thirty-four fertilized human ova, good, bad, and indifferent, recovered from 210 women of known fertility. *Pediatrics 23:*202, 1959.

Hsueh AJW, Billig H, Tsafriri A: Ovarian follicle atresia: a hormonally controlled apoptotic process. *Endocr Rev 15:*707, 1994.

Kalthoff K: *Analysis of Biological Development*. New York, McGraw-Hill, 1995.

Kaufmann RA, Morsy M, Takeuchi K, Hodgen GD: Preimplantation genetic analysis. *J Reprod Med 37:*428, 1992.

Khalifeh FA, Sarraf M, Dabit ST: Full-term delivery following intracytoplasmic sperm injection with spermatozoa extracted from frozen-thawed testicular tissue. *Hum Reprod 12:*87, 1997.

Kierszenbaum AL: Mammalian spermatogenesis *in vivo* and *in vitro*: a partnership of spermatogenic and somatic cell lineages. *Endocr Rev 15:*116, 1994.

Leeson CR, Leeson TS, Paparo A: *Text/Atlas of Histology*. Philadelphia, WB Saunders, 1988.

Ludwig H, Tauber PF: *Human Fertilization*. Stuttgart, Georg Thieme Publishers, 1978.

Moore KL: *Clinically Oriented Anatomy*, 3rd ed. Baltimore, Williams & Wilkins, 1992.

Moore KL, Agur AMR: *Essential Clinical Anatomy*. Baltimore, Williams & Wilkins, 1995.

Moos J, Faundes D, Kopf GS, Schultz RM: Composition of the human zona pellucida and modifications following fertilization. *Hum Reprod 10:*2467, 1995.

Nahhas F, Barnea E: Human embryonic origin early pregnancy factor before and after implantation. *Am J Reprod Immunol 22:*105, 1990.

Nakayama T, Goto Y, Kanzaki H, et al: Developmental potential of frozen-thawed human blastocysts. *J Assist Reprod Genet 12:*239, 1995.

Oehninger S, Hodgen GD: Hypothalamic-pituitary-ovarian uterine axis. *In* Copeland LJ: *Textbook of Gynecology*. Philadelphia, WB Saunders, 1993.

O'Rahilly R: *Developmental Stages in Human Embryos. Part A. Embryos of the First Three Weeks (Stages 1 to 9)*. Washington, DC, Carnegie Institution of Washington, 1973.

Ombelet W, Vereecken A (eds): Modern Andrology. *Hum Reprod 10(Suppl 1):*1-178, 1995.

Oura C, Toshimori K: Ultrastructural studies on the fertilization of mammalian gametes. *Int Rev Cytol 122:*105, 1990.

Page EW, Villee CA, Villee DB: *Human Reproduction: Essentials of Reproductive and Perinatal Medicine*, 3rd ed. Philadelphia, WB Saunders, 1981.

Palermo GD, Cohen J, Alikani M, et al: Development and implementation of intracytoplasmic sperm injection (ICSI). *Reprod Fertil Dev 7:*211, 1995.

Poyser NL: The control of prostaglandin production by the endometrium in relation to luteolysis and menstruation. *Prostaglandins Leukot Essent Fatty Acids 53:*147, 1995.

Richards JS: Hormonal control of gene expression in the ovary. *Endocrin Rev 15:*574, 1994.

Ritchie WGM: Ultrasound Evaluation of Normal and Induced Ovulation. *In* Callen PW (ed): *Ultrasonography in Obstetrics and Embryology*, 3rd ed. Philadelphia, WB Saunders, 1994.

Robertson JA: Ethical and legal issues in human embryos donation. *Fertil Steril 64:*885, 1995.

Rock J, Hertig AT: The human conceptus during the first two weeks of gestation. *Am J Obstet Gynecol 55:*6, 1948.

Rosenbusch BE: Cytogenetics of human spermatozoa: what about the reproductive relevance of structural chromosomal aberrations? *J Assist Reprod Genet 12:*375, 1995.

Rubin E, Farber JL: *Pathology*. Philadelphia, JB Lippincott, 1988.

Sathananthan AH, Trounson A, Freeman L: The effects of cooling human oocytes. *Hum Reprod 3:*968, 1988.

Scott Jr, RT, Hodgen GD: The ovarian follicle: life cycle of a pelvic clock. *Clin Obstet Gynecol 33:*551, 1990.

Settlage DSF, Motoshima M, Tredway DR: Sperm transport from the external cervical os to the fallopian tubes in women. *Fertil Steril 24:*655, 1973.

Sidhu KS, Guraya SS: Current concepts in gamete receptors for fertilization in mammals. *Rev Cytol 127:*253, 1991.

Simon C, Pellicer A: Regulators of Human Implantation. *Hum Reprod 10(Suppl 2):*1, 1995.

Steinkampf MP, Kretzer PA, McElroy E, Conway-Myers BA: A simplified approach to in vitro fertilization. *J Reprod Med 37:*199, 1992.

Steptoe PC, Edwards RG: Birth after implantation of a human embryo. *Lancet ii:*36, 1978.

Stoll C, Roth MP, Bigel P: A re-examination of paternal age effect on the occurrence of new mutants for achondroplasia. *Prog Clin Biol Res 104:*419, 1982.

Talbot P: Sperm penetration through oocyte investments in mammals. *Am J Anat 174:*331, 1985.

Thompson MW, McInnes RR, Willard HF: *Thompson & Thompson Genetics in Medicine*, 5th ed. Philadelphia, WB Saunders, 1991.

Veeck LL: *Atlas of human oocyte and early conceptus*, vol 2. Baltimore, Williams & Wilkins, 1991.

Warkany J: Prevention of congenital malformations. *Teratology 23:* 175, 1981.

Wassarman PM: The biology and chemistry of fertilization. *Science 235:*553, 1987.

Wilmut I, Schnieke AE, McWhir J, et al: Viable offspring derived from fetal and adult mammalian cells. *Nature 385:*810, 1997.

Winston NJ: Developmental failure in preimplantation human conceptuses. *Int Rev Cytol 164:*139, 1996.

Wood C, Trounson A (eds): *Clinical In Vitro Fertilization,* 2nd ed. New York, Springer Verlag, 1989.

Zaneveld LJD: Capacitation of spermatozoa. *In* Ludwig H, Tauber PF (eds): *Human Fertilization*. Stuttgart, Georg Thieme Publishers, 1978.

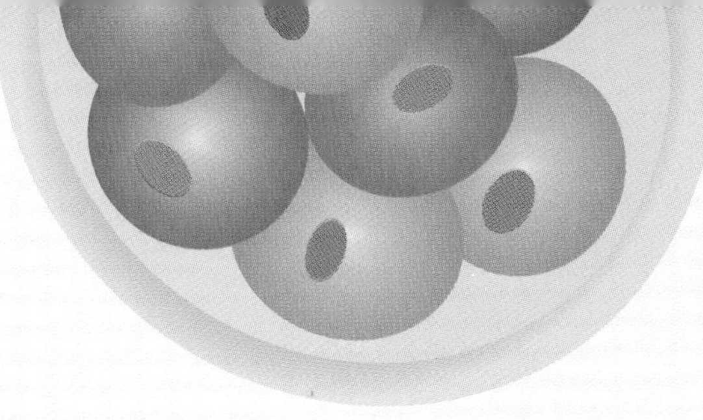

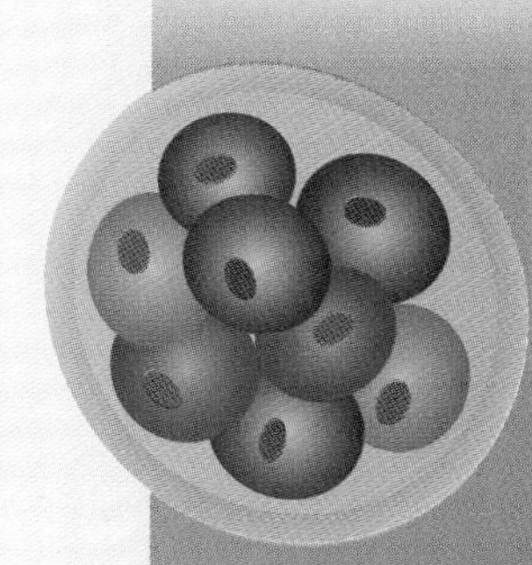

Formation of Bilaminar Embryonic Disc and Chorionic Sac: The Second Week

3

■ Implantation of the blastocyst is completed during the second week of embryonic development. As this crucial process occurs, morphological changes occur in the inner cell mass or embryoblast that produce a bilaminar embryonic disc composed of two layers, epiblast and hypoblast (Fig. 3-1). The **embryonic disc** gives rise to the germ layers that form all the tissues and organs of the embryo. Extraembryonic structures forming during the second week are the amniotic cavity, amnion, yolk sac, connecting stalk, and chorionic sac.

COMPLETION OF IMPLANTATION AND CONTINUATION OF EMBRYONIC DEVELOPMENT

Implantation of the blastocyst commences at the end of the first week and is completed by the end of the second week. The actively erosive **syncytiotrophoblast** invades the endometrial stroma (connective tissue framework), which supports the uterine capillaries and glands. As this occurs, the blastocyst slowly embeds itself in the endometrium. The blastocyst implants in the endometrial layer at its embryonic pole (site of inner cell mass). Syncytiotrophoblast cells from this region displace endometrial cells in the central part of the implantation site. *Proteolytic enzymes* produced by the syncytiotrophoblast promote *proteolysis* — dissolution of proteins — which facilitates the invasion of the maternal endometrium (Lindenberg et al., 1989). The stromal (connective tissue) cells around the implantation site become loaded with glycogen and lipids and assume a polyhedral appearance. Some of these new cells — **decidual cells** — degenerate adjacent to the penetrating syncytiotrophoblast. The syncytiotrophoblast engulfs these degenerating cells, providing a rich source of embryonic nutrition.

As the blastocyst implants, more trophoblast contacts the endometrium and differentiates into two layers (Fig. 3-1):

- the *cytotrophoblast*, a mononucleated layer of cells that is mitotically active and forms new trophoblast cells that migrate into the increasing mass of syncytiotrophoblast where they fuse and lose their cell membranes
- the *syncytiotrophoblast*, a rapidly expanding, multinucleated mass in which no cell boundaries are discernible

The syncytiotrophoblast begins to produce a hormone — *human chorionic gonadotrophin* (hCG) — which enters the maternal blood in the lacunae (L., hollow cavities) in the syncytiotrophoblast (Fig. 3-1*C*). hCG maintains the activity of the corpus luteum in the ovary during pregnancy and forms the basis for *pregnancy tests*. Highly sensitive radioimmune assays are available for detecting hCG and pregnancy. The antibodies used in these tests are specific for the beta subunit of the hormone (Filly, 1994a). Enough hCG is produced by the syncytiotrophoblast at the end of the second week to give a positive pregnancy test, even though the woman is probably unaware she is pregnant.

Formation of Amniotic Cavity, Embryonic Disc, and Yolk Sac

As implantation of the blastocyst progresses, a small cavity appears in the inner cell mass, which is the primordium of the **amniotic cavity** (Fig. 3-1*A*). Soon amniogenic (amnion-forming) cells — *amnioblasts* — separate from the epiblast and form a thin membrane, the **amnion**, which encloses the amniotic cavity (Fig. 3-1*B* and *C*). Concurrently, morphological changes occur in the inner cell mass (embryoblast) that result in the formation of a flattened, almost circular bilaminar plate of cells, the **embryonic disc**, consisting of two layers (Fig. 3-2*A*):

- **epiblast**, the thicker layer, consisting of high columnar cells related to the amniotic cavity
- **hypoblast**, or primary endoderm, consisting of small cuboidal cells adjacent to the exocoelomic cavity

The epiblast forms the floor of the amniotic cavity and is continuous peripherally with the amnion. The hypoblast forms the roof of the **exocoelomic cavity** and is continuous with the thin exocoelomic membrane (Fig. 3-1*B*). The exocoelomic membrane and cavity soon become modified to form the **primary yolk sac**. The embryonic disc now lies between the amniotic cavity and primary yolk sac (Fig. 3-1*C*). Cells from the yolk sac endoderm give rise to a layer of loosely arranged connective tissue, the **extraembryonic mesoderm** (Fig. 3-2*A*), which surrounds the amnion and yolk sac (Enders and King, 1988; Bianchi et al., 1993). Extraembryonic mesoderm is later formed by cells that arise from the primitive streak (see Chapter 4). The yolk sac and amniotic cavities make morphogenetic movements of the cells of the embryonic disc possible.

As the amnion, embryonic disc, and primary yolk sac form, isolated cavities — **lacunae** — appear in the syncytiotrophoblast (Figs. 3-1*C* and 3-2). The lacunae soon become filled with a mixture of maternal blood from ruptured endometrial capillaries and secretions from eroded uterine glands. The maternal blood in the lacunae also receives hCG produced by the syncytiotrophoblast, which maintains the **corpus luteum**, an endocrine glandular structure that secretes estrogen and progesterone to maintain the pregnancy. The fluid in the lacunar spaces, sometimes called *embryotroph* (*Gr. trophe*, nourishment), passes to the embryonic disc by diffusion.

The communication of the eroded endometrial capillaries with the lacunae represents *the beginning of uteroplacental circulation*. When maternal blood flows into the lacunae, oxygen and nutritive substances become available to the embryo. Because both arterial and venous branches of maternal blood vessels communicate with the lacunae, circulation of the blood is established. *Oxygenated blood* passes into

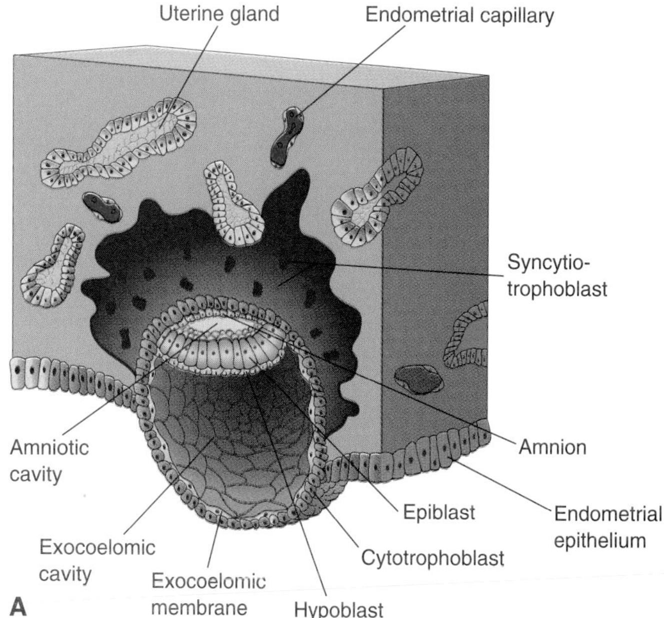

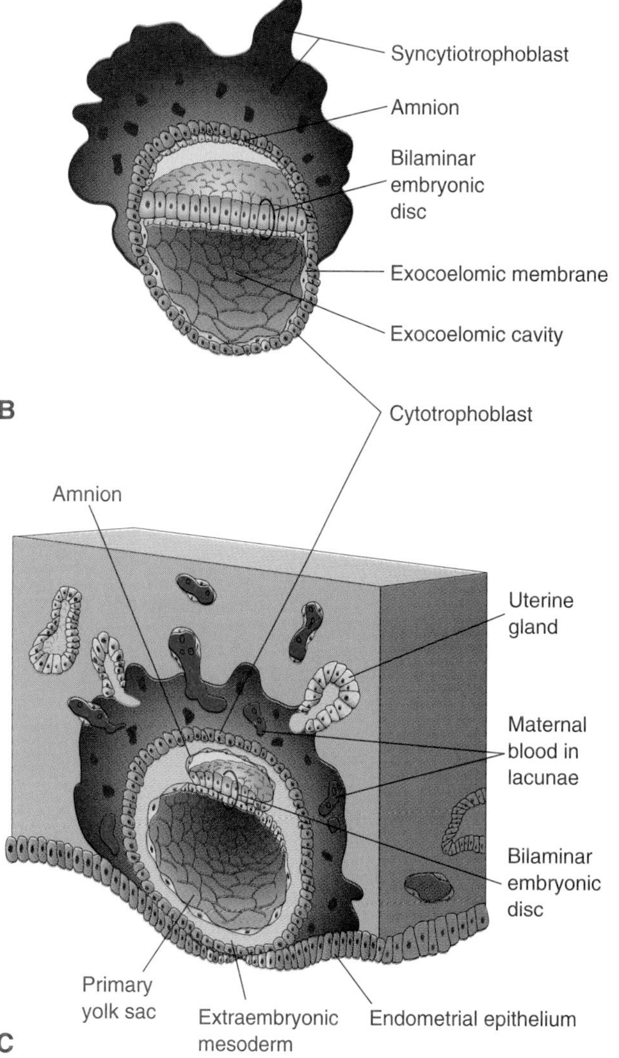

■ **Figure 3–1.** Drawings illustrating implantation of a blastocyst into the endometrium. The actual size of the conceptus is about 0.1 mm—about the size of the period at the end of this sentence. *A,* Drawing of a section through a blastocyst partially implanted in the endometrium (about 8 days). Note the slitlike amniotic cavity. *B,* An enlarged three-dimensional sketch of a slightly older blastocyst after removal from the endometrium. Note the extensive syncytiotrophoblast at the embryonic pole and the much larger amniotic cavity. *C,* Drawing of a section through a blastocyst of about 9 days implanted in the endometrium. Note the lacunae appearing in the syncytiotrophoblast. The type of implantation illustrated here, in which the blastocyst becomes completely embedded in the endometrium, is an *interstitial implantation.*

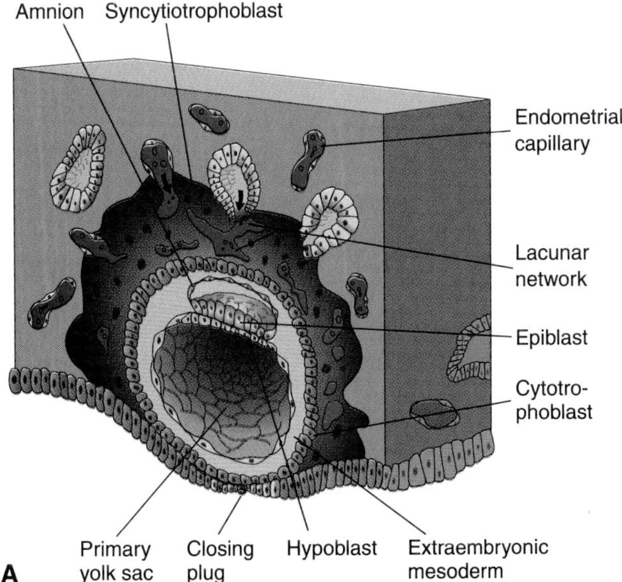

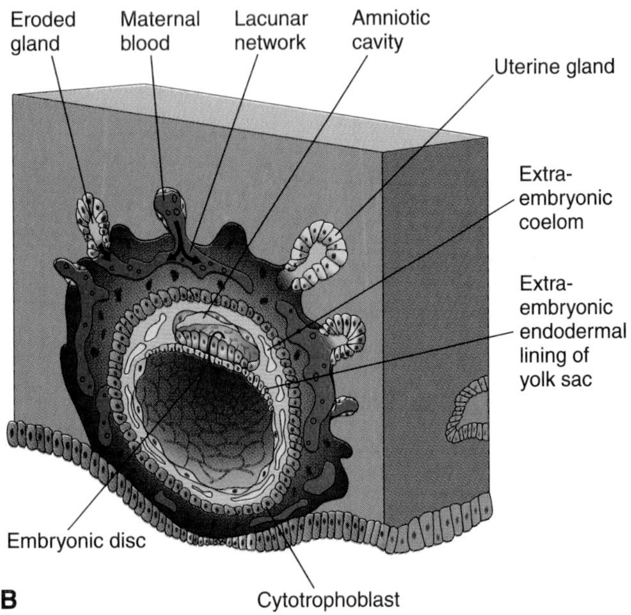

■ **Figure 3–2.** Drawings of sections through two implanted blastocysts. *A*, 10 days; *B*, 12 days. This stage of development is characterized by communication of the blood-filled lacunae. In *B* note cavities have appeared in the extraembryonic mesoderm, forming the beginning of the extraembryonic coelom.

the lacunae from the *spiral arteries* in the endometrium, and *deoxygenated blood* is removed from them through the endometrial veins (see Chapter 2).

The 10-day human conceptus (embryo and associated membranes) is completely embedded in the endometrium (Fig. 3-2*A*). For about 2 days, there is a defect in the endometrial epithelium that is filled by a **closing plug**, a fibrinous coagulum of blood. By day 12, an almost completely regenerated uterine epithelium covers the closing plug (Fig. 3-2*B*). As the conceptus implants, the endometrial connective tissue cells undergo a transformation known as the **decidual reaction**. After the cells swell because of the accumulation of glycogen and lipid in their cytoplasm, they are known as **decidual cells**. The primary function of the decidual reaction is to provide an immunologically privileged site for the conceptus (Carlson, 1994).

In a 12-day embryo, adjacent syncytiotrophoblastic lacunae have fused to form **lacunar networks** (Fig. 3-2*B*), giving the syncytiotrophoblast a spongelike appearance. The lacunar networks, particularly obvious around the embryonic pole, are the *primordia of the intervillous space of the placenta* (see Chapter 7). The endometrial capillaries around the implanted embryo become congested and dilated to form *sinusoids* — thin-walled terminal vessels that are larger than ordinary capillaries. The syncytiotrophoblast then erodes the sinusoids and maternal blood flows into the lacunar networks. Maternal blood flows in and out of the networks, establishing the *primitive uteroplacental circulation*. The degenerated endometrial stromal cells and glands, together with the maternal blood, provide a rich source of material for embryonic nutrition. Examination of Figures 3-1 and 3-2 shows that growth of the bilaminar embryonic disc (embryo) is slow compared with growth of the trophoblast. The implanted 12-day blastocyst produces a minute elevation on the endometrial surface that protrudes into the uterine lumen (Figs. 3-3 and 3-4).

As changes occur in the trophoblast and endometrium, the extraembryonic mesoderm increases and isolated spaces appear within it (Figs. 3-2 and 3-4). These spaces rapidly fuse to form a large isolated cavity, the **extraembryonic coelom** (Fig. 3-5*A*). This fluid-filled cavity surrounds the amnion and yolk sac, except where they are attached to the chorion by the connecting stalk. As the extraembryonic coelom forms, the primary yolk sac decreases in size and a smaller **secondary (definitive) yolk sac** forms (Fig. 3-5*B*). This smaller yolk sac is formed by extraem-

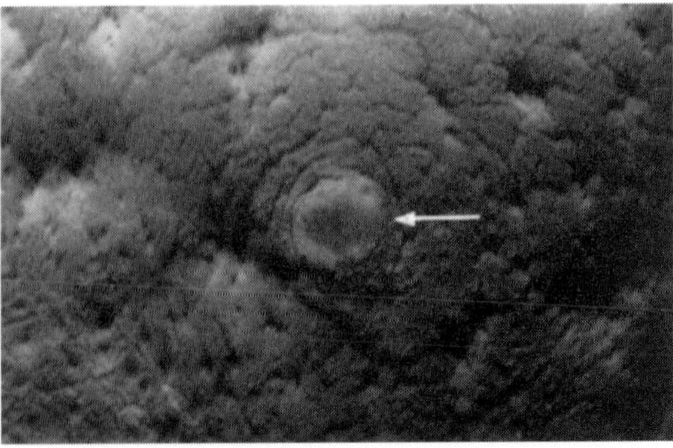

■ **Figure 3–3.** Photograph of the endometrial surface of the uterus, showing the implantation site of the 12-day embryo shown in Figure 3–4. The implanted conceptus produces a small elevation *(arrow)* (×8). (From Hertig AT, Rock J: *Contrib Embryol Carnegie Inst 29:*127, 1941. Courtesy of the Carnegie Institution of Washington.)

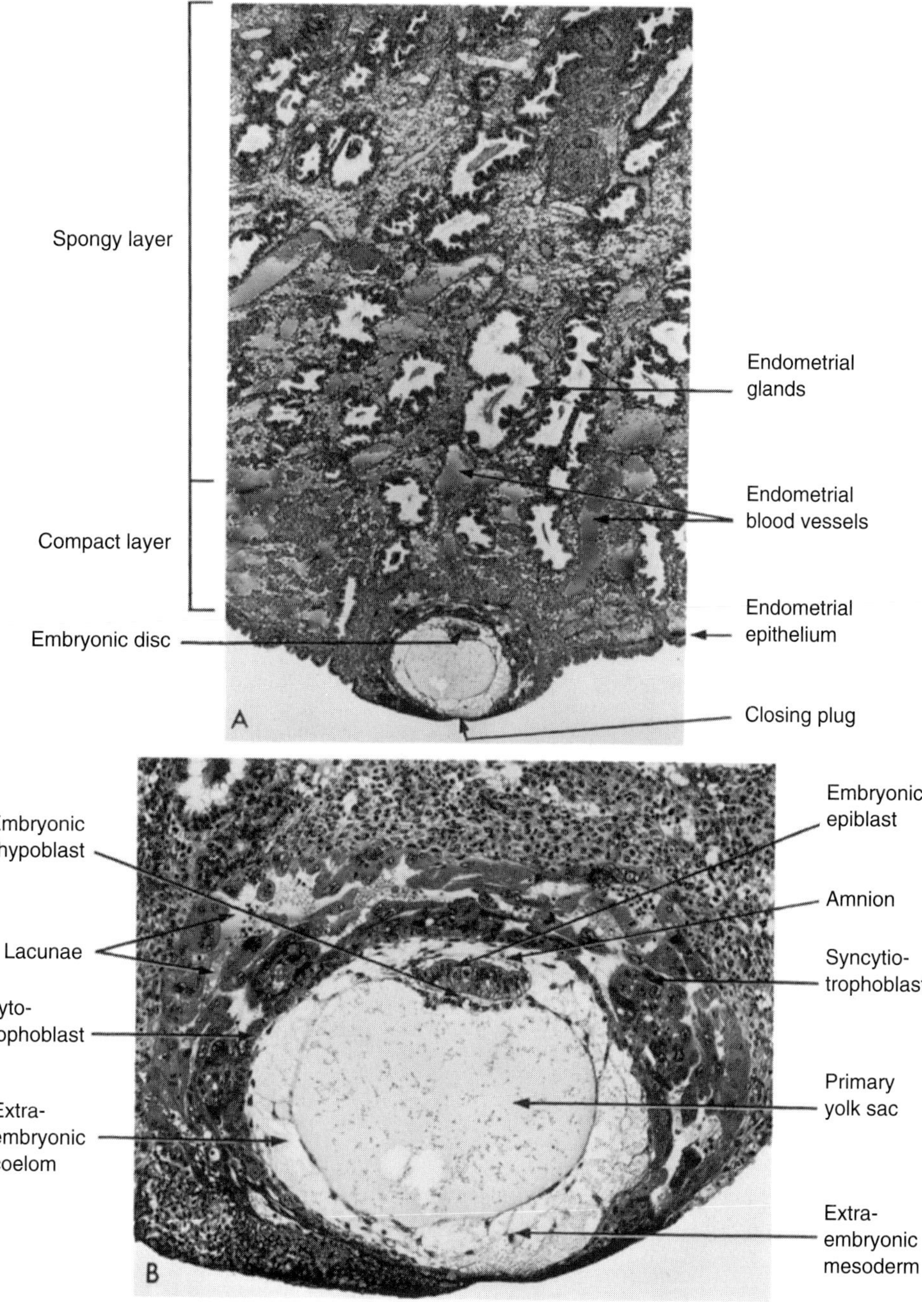

■ **Figure 3-4.** *A,* Section through the implantation site of the 12-day embryo shown in Figure 3–3. The embryo is embedded superficially in the endometrium (×30). *B,* Higher magnification of the conceptus and surrounding endometrium (×100). Lacunae containing maternal blood are visible in the syncytiotrophoblast. (From Hertig AT, Rock J: *Contrib Embryol Carnegie Inst 29:*127, 1941.)

bryonic endodermal cells that migrate inside the primary yolk sac from the hypoblast of the embryonic disc (Fig. 3-6). During formation of the secondary yolk sac, a large part of the primary yolk sac is pinched off (Fig. 3-5*B*). The yolk sac contains fluid but no yolk. It may have a role in the selective transfer of nutritive materials to the embryonic disc. The trophoblast absorbs nutritive fluid from the lacunar networks in the syncytiotrophoblast, which is transferred to the embryo.

DEVELOPMENT OF THE CHORIONIC SAC

The end of the second week is characterized by the appearance of **primary chorionic villi** (Figs. 3-5 and 3-7). Proliferation of cytotrophoblast cells produces cellular extensions that grow into the syncytiotrophoblast. The growth of the cytotrophoblastic extensions is thought to be induced by the underlying **extraembryonic somatic mesoderm**. The cellular

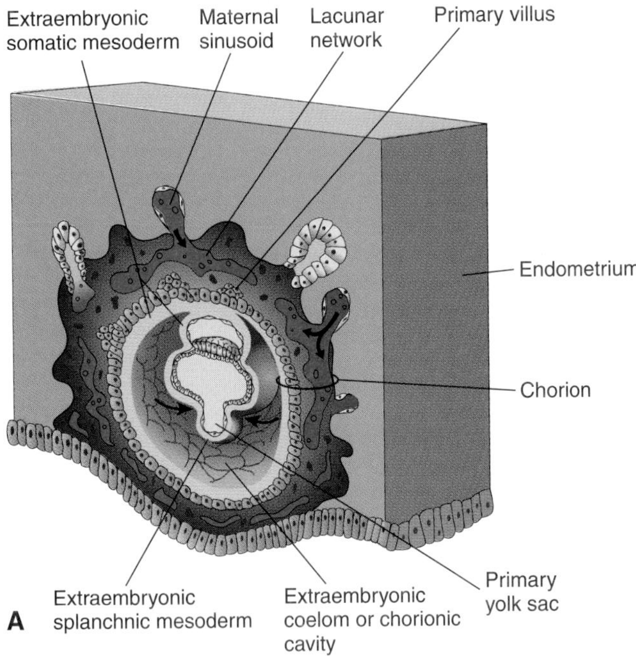

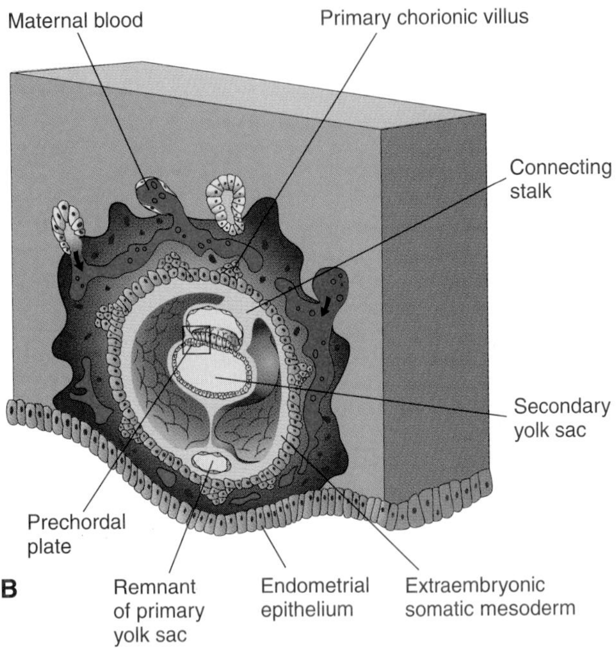

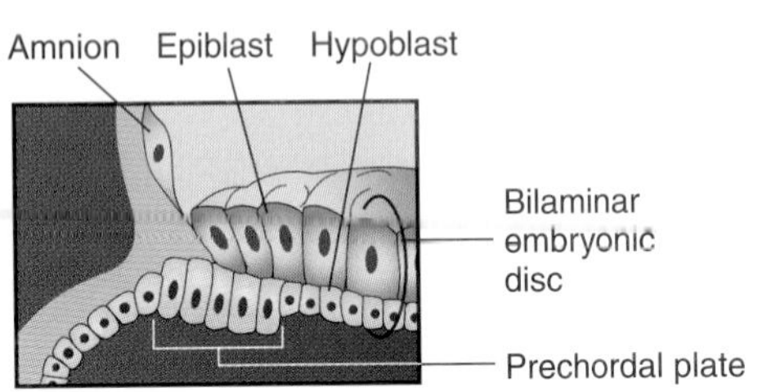

■ **Figure 3–5.** Drawings of sections through implanted human embryos, based mainly on Hertig et al., 1956. Observe: (1) the defect in the surface epithelium of the endometrium has disappeared; (2) a small secondary yolk sac has formed; (3) a large cavity, the extraembryonic coelom, now surrounds the yolk sac and amnion, except where the amnion is attached to the chorion by the connecting stalk; and (4) the extraembryonic coelom splits the extraembryonic mesoderm into two layers: extraembryonic somatic mesoderm lining the trophoblast and covering the amnion, and the extraembryonic splanchnic mesoderm around the yolk sac. *A,* 13 days, illustrating the decrease in relative size of the primary yolk sac and the early appearance of primary chorionic villi. *B,* 14 days, showing the newly formed secondary yolk sac and the location of the prechordal plate in its roof. *C,* Detail of the prechordal plate area outlined in *B.*

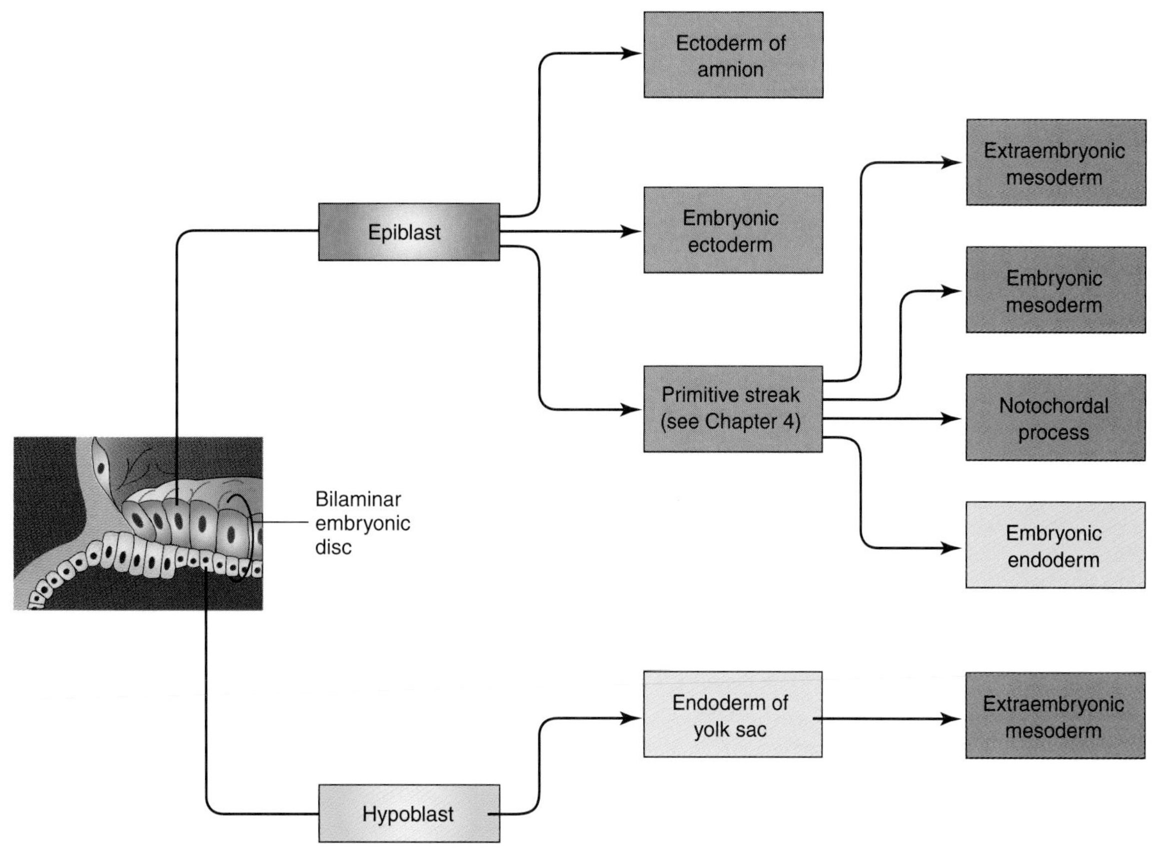

Figure 3–6. Origin of tissues in the embryo. The colors in the boxes are used in drawings of sections of conceptuses.

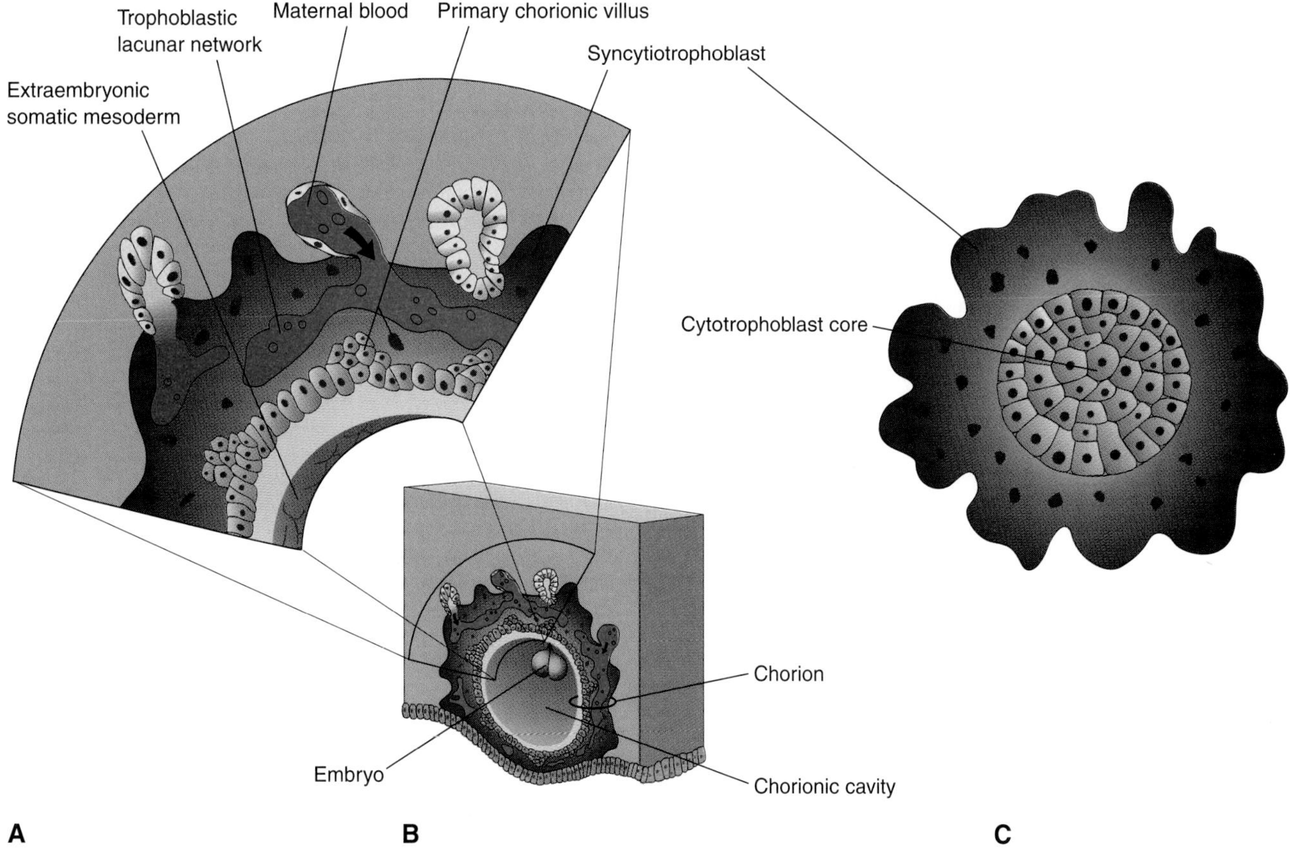

Figure 3–7. *A,* Detail of the section (outlined in *B*) of the wall of the chorionic sac. *B,* Sketch of a 14-day conceptus illustrating the chorionic sac and the shaggy appearance created by the primary villi (×6). *C,* Drawing of a transverse section through a primary chorionic villus (×400).

projections form primary chorionic villi, the first stage in the development of the chorionic villi of the placenta.

The Placenta as an Allograft

Because the chorionic sac forms part of the placenta, the conceptus, which inherits both paternal and maternal genes, can be regarded as an allograft in the uterus with respect to the mother. What protects the placenta from rejection by the mother's immune system? This question has puzzled embryologists and immunologists for a long time and remains an active area of research. Syncytiotrophoblast cells of the floating chorionic villi, although exposed to maternal immune cells within the blood sinusoids, lack major histocompatibility (MHC) antigens and thus do not evoke rejection responses (Faulk and Temple, 1976; Lala et al., 1984; Vince and Johnson, 1996). However, extravillous cytotrophoblast cells, which break out of the anchoring villi and invade uterine decidual tissue, express class 1 MHC antigens (Sunderland et al., 1981). These cells remain exposed to two types of maternal immune cells within the decidua—T lymphocytes and natural killer (NK) lymphocytes—and therefore are potential targets of immune attack (Lala, 1990). Protection of these cells is believed to be mediated by at least two mechanisms:

- First, the unique, nonpolymorphic nature of the class 1 MHC antigens (HLA-G) expressed by the extravillous trophoblast (Ellis et al., 1986; Kovats et al., 1990) makes these antigens poorly recognizable by T lymphocytes, and yet recognizable by NK cells, turning off their killer function (Carosella et al., 1996; Vince and Johnson, 1996; King et al., 1997).
- Second, decidual cells produce locally active immunosuppressor molecules such as prostaglandins E_2, which prevent activation of T cells and NK cells within the decidua (Parhar et al., 1988; Lala et al., 1988; Parhar et al., 1989; Lala, 1990). Indeed, the immunoregulatory function of decidual cells is consistent with their life history. It has been shown that uterine endometrial stromal cells, which differentiate into decidual cells during pregnancy, are derived from progenitor (stem) cells that migrate from the hemopoietic organs such as the fetal liver and bone marrow (Lysiak and Lala, 1992).

The extraembryonic coelom splits the extraembryonic mesoderm into two layers (Fig. 3-5*A* and *B*):

- *extraembryonic somatic mesoderm*, lining the trophoblast and covering the amnion
- *extraembryonic splanchnic mesoderm*, surrounding the yolk sac

The extraembryonic somatic mesoderm and the two layers of trophoblast constitute the **chorion** (Fig. 3-7*B*). *The chorion forms the wall of the chorionic*

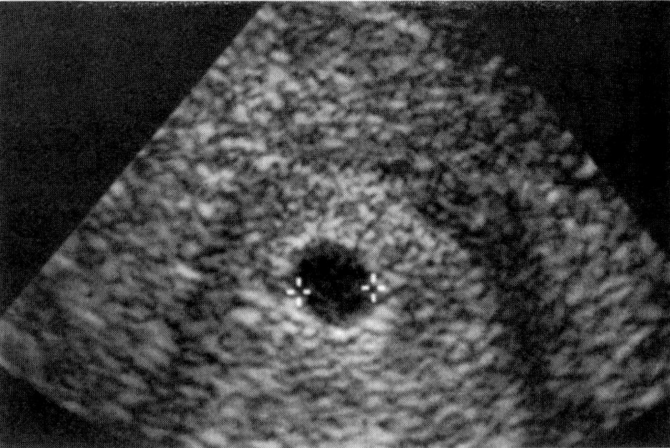

■ **Figure 3–8.** Transverse endovaginal sonogram of an early chorionic (gestational) sac. The mean sac diameter is the distance between the cursors (*). (From Callen PW [ed]: *Ultrasonography in Obstetrics and Gynecology,* 3rd ed. Philadelphia, WB Saunders, 1994.)

sac (gestational sac), within which the embryo and its amniotic and yolk sacs are suspended by the connecting stalk. The extraembryonic coelom is now called the **chorionic cavity**. The amniotic sac (with the embryonic epiblast forming its "floor") and the yolk sac (with the embryonic hypoblast forming its "roof") are analogous to two balloons pressed together (site of embryonic disc) and suspended by a cord (connecting stalk) from the inside of a larger balloon (chorionic sac).

Transvaginal ultrasound is used for measuring chorionic (gestational) sac diameter (Fig. 3-8). This measurement is valuable for evaluating very early embryonic development and pregnancy outcome (Dickey et al., 1994; Filly, 1994b). The 14-day embryo still has the form of a flat bilaminar embryonic disc, but the hypoblastic cells in a localized area are now columnar and form a thickened circular area, the **prechordal (prochordal) plate** (Fig. 3-5*B* and *C*). This plate indicates the future site of the mouth and *an important organizer of the head region*.

IMPLANTATION SITES OF THE BLASTOCYST

Implantation of the blastocyst usually occurs in the endometrium of the uterus, usually superiorly in the body of the uterus, slightly more often on the posterior than on the anterior wall. Implantation of a blastocyst can be detected by ultrasonography and highly sensitive radioimmune assays of hCG as early as the end of the second week.

Placenta Previa

Implantation of a blastocyst in the inferior segment of the uterus near the internal os (opening) results in *placenta previa*, a placenta that partially or completely covers the os (see Fig. 3-10). Placenta previa may cause bleeding because of premature separation of the placenta during pregnancy or at delivery of the fetus (see Chapter 7).

Extrauterine Implantation Sites

Blastocysts may implant outside the uterus. These implantations result in **ectopic pregnancies** (Filly, 1994a); 95 to 97% of ectopic implantations occur in the uterine tube. *Most ectopic pregnancies are in the ampulla and isthmus of the uterine tube* (Figs. 3-9 to 3-11). The incidence of tubal pregnancy varies from 1 in 80 to 1 in 250 pregnancies, depending on the socioeconomic level of the population (Page et al., 1981). The highest rates of ectopic pregnancy are in women 35 years of age or older and in women who are nonwhite (Rubin, 1983); however "all women of childbearing age are at risk of harboring an ectopic gestation" (Filly, 1994a).

A woman with a tubal pregnancy has signs and symptoms of pregnancy (e.g., misses her menstrual period). She may also experience abdominal pain and tenderness because of distention of the uterine tube, abnormal bleeding, and irritation of the pelvic peritoneum. The pain may be confused with *appendicitis* if the pregnancy is in the right uterine tube. Ectopic pregnancies produce hCG at a slower rate than normally implanted pregnancies (Cartwright and DiPietro, 1984); consequently assays may give false-negative tests if performed too early. *Endovaginal (intravaginal) sonography* is very helpful in the early detection of ectopic pregnancies (Ash et al., 1991; Fleischer et al., 1991; Filly, 1994a).

There are several causes of tubal pregnancy, but they are often related to factors that delay or prevent transport of the cleaving zygote to the uterus; for example, by mucosal adhesions or from blockage caused by scarring resulting from infection in the abdominopelvic cavity such as *pelvic inflammatory disease*. Ectopic tubal pregnancies usually result in rupture of the uterine tube and hemorrhage into the peritoneal cavity during the first 8 weeks, followed by death of the embryo. Tubal rupture and hemorrhage constitute a threat to the mother's life and consequently are of major clinical importance. The affected tube and conceptus are usually surgically removed (Fig. 3-11).

When blastocysts implant in the isthmus of the uterine tube (Fig. 3-10*D*), the tube tends to rupture early because this narrow part of the tube is relatively unexpandable. Abortion of an embryo from this site often results in extensive bleeding, probably because of the rich anastomoses between ovarian and uterine vessels in this area. When blastocysts implant in the intramural (uterine) part of the tube (Fig. 3-10*E*), they may develop into fetuses before expulsion occurs. When an *intramural tubal pregnancy ruptures*, it usually bleeds profusely.

Blastocysts that implant in the ampulla or in fimbriae of the uterine tube are often expelled into the peritoneal cavity where they commonly implant in the rectouterine pouch, a pouch of peritoneum between the rectum and the uterus (Fig. 3-12). In exceptional cases, an **abdominal pregnancy** may continue to full term and the fetus may be delivered alive through an abdominal incision. Usually, however, an abdominal

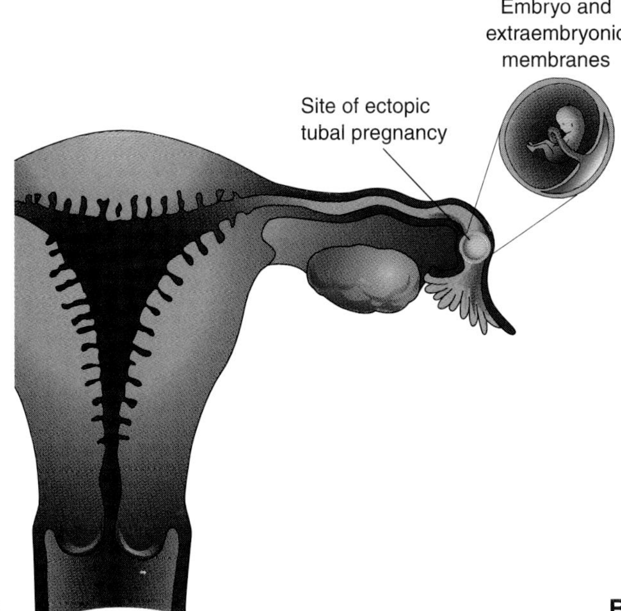

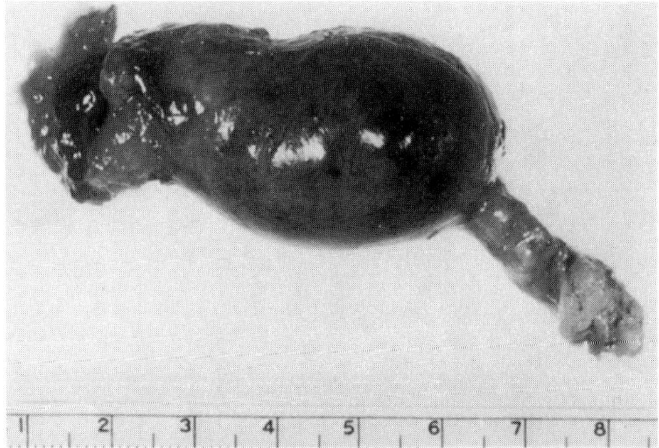

■ **Figure 3-9.** *A,* Coronal section of the uterus and left uterine tube, illustrating an ectopic tubal pregnancy. *B,* Photograph of an unruptured ectopic tubal pregnancy in the ampulla of the uterine tube. (From Page EW, Villee CA, Villee DB: *Human Reproduction. Essentials of Reproductive and Perinatal Medicine,* 3rd ed. Philadelphia, WB Saunders, 1981.)

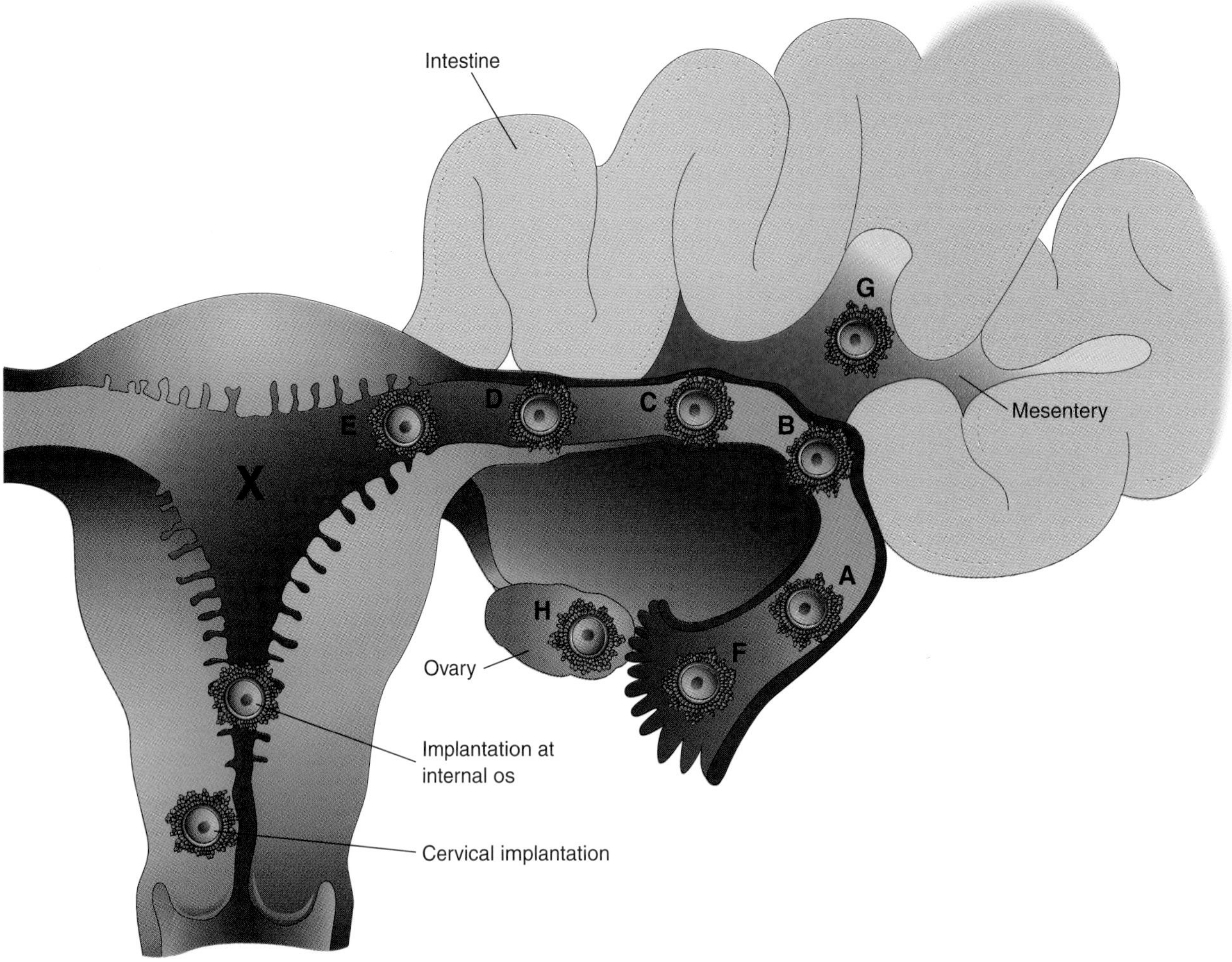

■ **Figure 3–10.** Drawing of the uterus and tubes illustrating various implantation sites of the blastocyst. The usual site in the posterior wall of the uterus is indicated by an **X.** The approximate order of frequency of ectopic implantations is indicated alphabetically (**A,** most common, **H,** least common). **A** to **F,** Tubal pregnancies. **G,** Abdominal pregnancy. **H,** Ovarian pregnancy. Tubal pregnancies are the most common type of ectopic pregnancy.

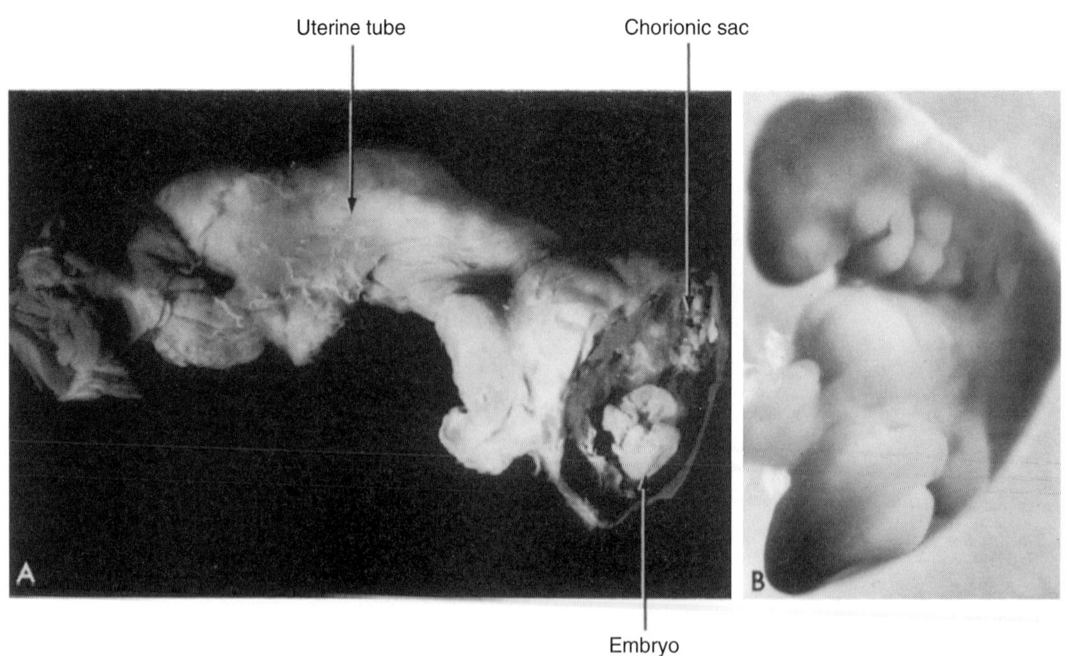

■ **Figure 3–11** Photographs of a tubal pregnancy. *A,* The uterine tube has been surgically removed and sectioned to show the conceptus implanted in the mucous membrane (×3). *B,* Enlarged photograph of the normal-appearing 4-week embryo (×13). (Photographed by Professor Jean Hay [retired], Department of Anatomy, University of Manitoba, Winnipeg, Canada.)

pregnancy creates a serious condition because the placenta attaches to abdominal organs and causes considerable intraperitoneal bleeding. Indeed, the leading cause of maternal death is from hemorrhage, and abdominal pregnancy increases the risk of maternal death by a factor of 90 when compared with intrauterine pregnancy, and seven times more than that for tubal pregnancy (Yu et al., 1995). In very unusual cases, an abdominal conceptus dies and is not detected; the fetus becomes calcified, forming a "stone fetus" or lithopedion (Gr. *lithos*, stone, + *paidion*, child).

Simultaneous intrauterine and extrauterine pregnancies are unusual, occurring about 1 in 7000 (Filly, 1994a; Rousso et al., 1997). The ectopic pregnancy is masked initially by the presence of the uterine pregnancy. Usually the ectopic pregnancy can be terminated by surgical removal of the involved uterine tube, for example, without interfering with the intrauterine pregnancy. *Cervical implantations* are unusual (Fig. 3-10); some of these pregnancies are not recognized because the conceptus is aborted during early gestation. In other cases, the placenta becomes firmly attached to fibrous and muscular parts of the cervix, often resulting in bleeding and subsequent surgical intervention, such as *hysterectomy* (excision of uterus).

Spontaneous abortion of an early embryo and its membranes implanted in the uterine tube may result in implantation of the conceptus in the ovary or in other organs or on mesenteries (Figs. 3-10 and 3-12), but ovarian and abdominal pregnancies are very uncommon. Bleeding from these ectopic implantation sites usually results in *intra-abdominal hemorrhage* and severe abdominal pain. Most of these cases are discovered during ultrasound studies and abdominal exploration of a presumed tubal pregnancy.

Spontaneous Abortion of Early Embryos

Abortion is commonly defined as the termination of pregnancy before 20 weeks' gestation, before the period of viability of the embryo or fetus. Most abortions of embryos during the first 3 weeks occur spontaneously. *Sporadic and recurrent spontaneous abortions* are two of the most common gynecological problems (Coulam et al., 1990; Hill, 1995). The frequency of early abortions is difficult to establish because they often occur before women are aware they are pregnant. An abortion occurring just after the first missed period is very likely to be mistaken for a delayed menstruation. Detection of a conceptus in the menses (menstrual blood) is very difficult become of its small size (see Fig. 3-13*E*).

Study of most early spontaneous abortions resulting from medical problems reveals abnormal conceptuses. Hertig et al. (1959) studied 34 early embryos recovered from women of known fertility, and found 10 of them so abnormal that they probably would have aborted spontaneously by the end of the second week of development. Hertig (1967) estimated that of the 70 to 75% of blastocysts that implant, only 58% survive to the end of the second week. He further estimated that 16% of this latter group would be abnormal and would abort in a week or so. The incidence of chromosomal abnormalities in early spontaneous abortions in one study was about 61% (Boué et al., 1975).

Summarizing the data of several studies, Carr and Gedeon (1977) estimated that 50% of all known spontaneous abortions result from chromosomal abnormali-

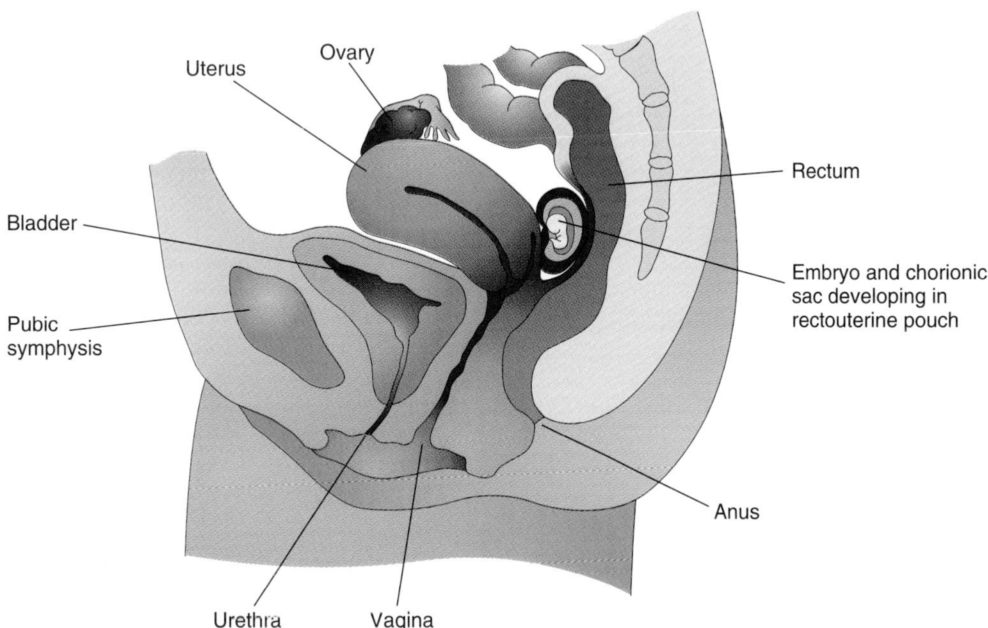

■ **Figure 3-12** Drawing of a median section of a female pelvis illustrating an abdominal pregnancy. Although a blastocyst expelled from the uterine tube may attach to any organ or to the mesentery of the intestines, it commonly attaches to the peritoneum in the rectouterine pouch.

ties. The higher incidence of early abortions in older women probably results from the increasing frequency of *nondisjunction of chromosomes* during oogenesis (see Chapter 2). It has been estimated that from one-third to one-half of all zygotes never become blastocysts and implant. Failure of blastocysts to implant may result from a poorly developed endometrium; however, in many cases there are probably lethal chromosomal abnormalities in the zygote that cause the abortion. Shepard et al. (1988) found a higher incidence of spontaneous abortion of fetuses with *neural tube defects*, cleft lip, and cleft palate, as well as other anomalies, than in newborns and induced abortuses.

Inhibition of Implantation

The administration of relatively large doses of estrogens ("morning-after pills") for several days, beginning shortly after unprotected sexual intercourse, usually does not prevent fertilization but often prevents implantation of the blastocyst. *Diethylstilbestrol*, given daily in high dosage for 5 to 6 days, may also accelerate passage of the dividing zygote along the uterine tube (Kalant et al., 1990). Normally, the endometrium progresses to the secretory phase of the menstrual cycle as the zygote forms, undergoes cleavage, and enters the uterus. The large amount of estrogen disturbs the normal balance between estrogen and progesterone that is necessary for preparation of the endometrium for implantation of the blastocyst. Postconception administration of hormones to prevent implantation of the blastocyst is sometimes used in cases of sexual assault or leakage of a condom, but this treatment is contraindicated for routine contraceptive use. The "abortion pill" *RU486* also destroys the conceptus by interrupting implantation because of interference with the hormonal environment of the implanting embryo.

An *intrauterine device* (IUD) inserted into the uterus through the vagina and cervix usually interferes with implantation by causing a local inflammatory reaction. Some IUDs contain progesterone that is slowly released and interferes with the development of the endometrium so that implantation does not usually occur.

SUMMARY OF IMPLANTATION OF THE BLASTOCYST

Implantation of the blastocyst begins at the end of the first week and is completed by the end of the second week. The molecular events relating to human implantation are just beginning to emerge. Cytokines, steroid hormones, and various growth factors are involved in implantation (Edwards, 1995; Loke et al., 1995). Implantation may be summarized as follows:

- The zona pellucida surrounding the oocyte degenerates (day 5). Its disappearance results from enlargement of the blastocyst and degeneration caused by enzymatic lysis. The lytic enzymes are released from the acrosomes of the sperms that surround and partially penetrate the zona pellucida.
- The blastocyst adheres to the endometrial epithelium (day 6).
- The trophoblast begins to differentiate into two layers — syncytiotrophoblast and cytotrophoblast (day 7).
- The syncytiotrophoblast erodes endometrial tissues (capillaries, glands, and connective tissue) and the blastocyst starts to embed in the endometrium (day 8).
- Blood-filled lacunae appear in the syncytiotrophoblast (day 9).
- The blastocyst sinks beneath the endometrial epithelium, and the defect in the endometrial epithelium is filled by a closing plug (day 10).
- Lacunar networks form by fusion of adjacent lacunae (days 10 and 11).
- The syncytiotrophoblast erodes endometrial blood vessels, allowing maternal blood to seep in and out of lacunar networks, thereby establishing a *primitive uteroplacental circulation* (days 11 and 12).
- The defect in the endometrial epithelium gradually disappears as the endometrial epithelium is repaired (days 12 and 13).
- Primary chorionic villi develop (days 13 and 14).

SUMMARY OF THE SECOND WEEK OF DEVELOPMENT

Rapid proliferation and differentiation of the trophoblast are important features of the second week (Figs. 3-13 and 3-14). These processes occur as the blastocyst completes its implantation in the endometrium. The various endometrial changes resulting from the adaptation of these tissues to implantation are known as the **decidual reaction**. Concurrently the *primary yolk sac* forms and extraembryonic mesoderm arises from the endoderm of the yolk sac. The extraembryonic coelom forms from spaces that develop in the *extraembryonic mesoderm*. The extraembryonic coelom later becomes the **chorionic cavity**. The primary yolk sac becomes smaller and gradually disappears as the secondary or definitive yolk sac develops. As these changes occur —

- The **amniotic cavity** appears as a space between the cytotrophoblast and the **inner cells mass** or embryoblast.
- The inner cell mass differentiates into a **bilaminar embryonic disc** consisting of *epiblast*, related to the amniotic cavity, and *hypoblast*, adjacent to the blastocyst cavity.
- The **prechordal plate** develops as a localized

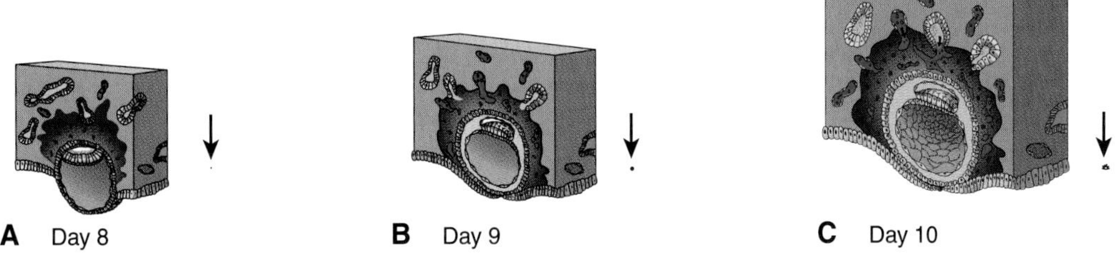

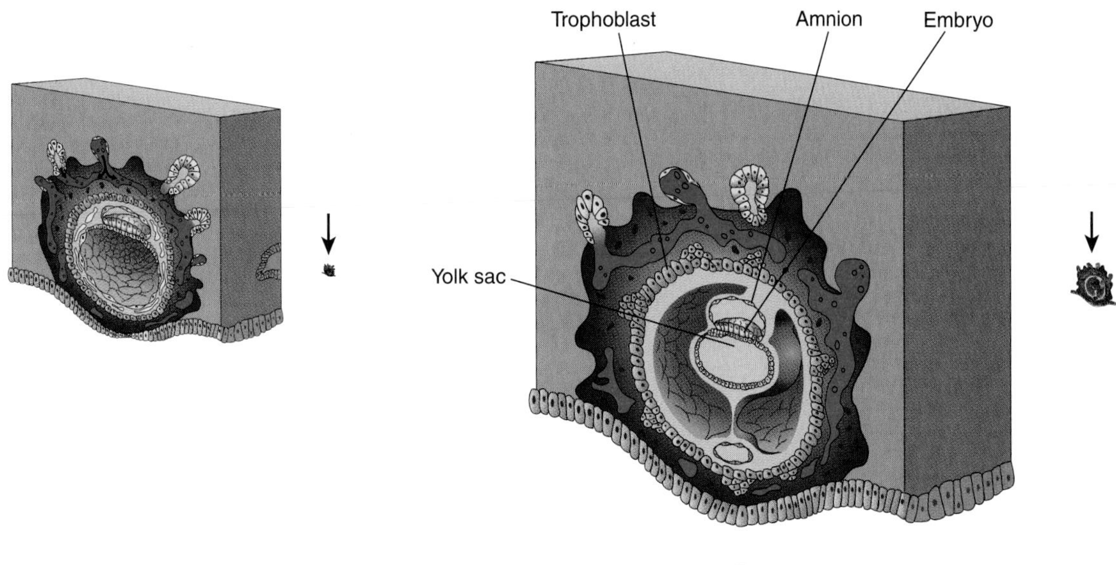

■ **Figure 3–13** Drawings of sections of human blastocysts during the second week, illustrating the rapid expansion of the trophoblast and the relatively minute size of the conceptuses (×25); the sketches indicated by arrows show the actual size of the blastocysts.

thickening of the hypoblast (primary endoderm), which indicates the future cranial region of the embryo and the future site of the mouth; the prechordal plate is also an important organizer of the head region.

Clinically Oriented Problems

Case 3–1

A 22-year-old woman who complained of a severe "chest cold" was sent for a radiograph of her thorax.

- Is it advisable to examine a healthy female's chest radiologically during the last week of her menstrual cycle?
- Are birth defects likely to develop in her conceptus if she happens to be pregnant?

Case 3–2

A woman who was sexually assaulted during her fertile period was given large doses of estrogen twice daily for five days to interrupt a possible pregnancy.

- If fertilization had occurred, what do you think would be the mechanism of action of this hormone?
- What do lay people call this type of medical treatment? Is this what the media refer to as the "abortion pill"? If not, explain the method of action of the hormonal treatment.
- How early can a pregnancy be detected?

Case 3–3

A 23-year-old woman consulted her physician about severe right lower abdominal pain. She said that she had missed two menstrual periods. A diagnosis of ectopic pregnancy was made.

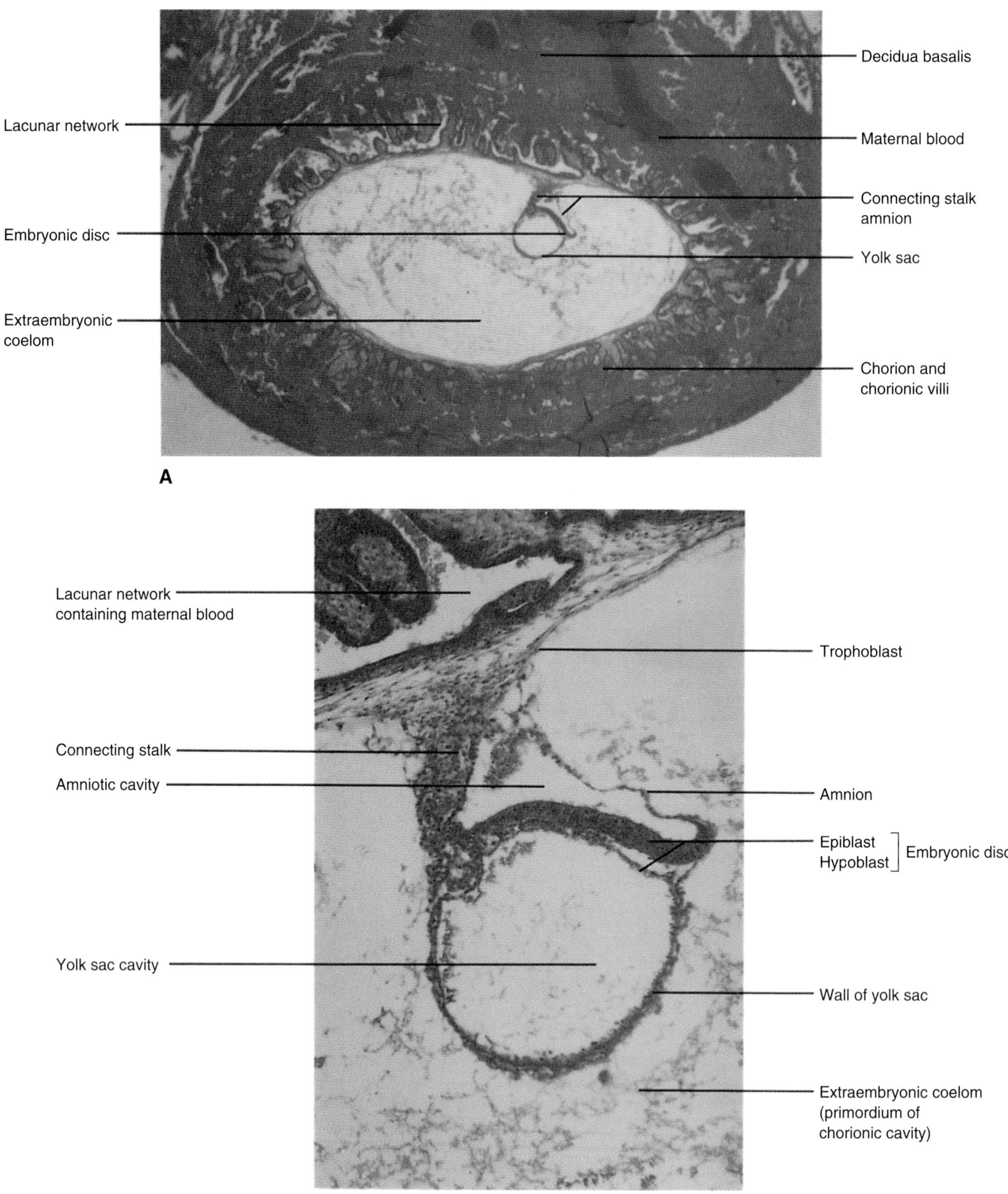

■ **Figure 3–14** Photomicrographs of longitudinal sections of an implanted embryo at Carnegie stage 6, about 14 days. Note the large size of the extraembryonic coelom. *A*, Low-power view (×18). *B*, High-power view (×95). The embryo is represented by the bilaminar embryonic disc composed of epiblast and hypoblast. (From Nishimura H [ed]: *Atlas of Human Prenatal Histology.* Tokyo, Igaku-Shoin, 1983.)

- What techniques might be used to enable this diagnosis to be made with certainty?
- What is the most likely site of the extrauterine gestation?
- How do you think the physician would likely treat the condition?

Case 3–4

A 30-year-old woman had an appendectomy toward the end of her menstrual cycle; 8 1/2 months later she had a child with a congenital anomaly of the brain.

- Could the surgery have produced this child's congenital anomaly?
- What is the basis for your views?

Case 3–5

A 42-year-old woman finally became pregnant after many years of trying to conceive. She was concerned about the development of her baby.

- What would the physician likely tell her?
- Can women over 40 have normal babies?
- What tests and diagnostic techniques would likely be performed?

Discussion of these problems appears at the back of the book.

REFERENCES AND SUGGESTED READING

Ash KM, Lyons ES, Levi CS, Lindsay DJ: Endovaginal sonographic diagnosis of ectopic twin gestation. *J Ultrasound Med 10:*497, 1991.

Bianchi DW, Wilkins-Haug LE, Enders AC, Hay ED: Origin of extraembryonic mesoderm in experimental animals: relevance to chorionic mosaicism in humans. *Am J Med Genet 46:*542, 1993.

Billington WD: Trophoblast. *In* Philipp EE, Barnes J, Newton M (eds): *Scientific Foundations of Obstetrics and Gynecology*. London, William Heinemann, 1970.

Boronow RC, McElin TW, West RH, Buckingham JC: Ovarian pregnancy. *Am J Obstet Gynecol 91:*1095, 1965.

Boué J, Boué A, Lazar P: Retrospective and prospective epidemiological studies of 1500 karyotyped spontaneous abortions. *Teratology 12:*11, 1975.

Carlson BM: *Human Embryology and Developmental Biology*. St Louis, Mosby, 1994.

Carosella ED, Dausset J, Kirszenbaum M: HLA-G revisted. *Immunology Today 17:*404, 1996.

Carr DH: Chromosome studies in selected spontaneous abortions. III. Early pregnancy loss. *Obstet Gynecol 37:*750, 1971.

Carr DH, Gedeon M: Population cytogenetics of human abortuses. *In* Hook EB, Porter IH (eds): *Population Cytogenetics: Studies in Humans*. New York, Academic Press, 1977.

Cartwright PS, DiPietro DL: Ectopic pregnancy: Changes in serum human chorionic gonadotropin concentration. *Obstet Gynecol 63:* 76, 1984.

Chapman MG, Grudzinskas JG, Chard T (eds): *Implantation: Biological and Clinical Aspects*. Berlin, Springer Verlag, 1988.

Coulam CB, Faulk WP, McIntyre JA: Spontaneous and recurrent abortions. *In* Quilligan EJ, Zuspan FP (eds): *Current Therapy in Obstetrics and Gynecology*, vol 3. Philadelphia, WB Saunders, 1990.

Coulam CG: Epidemiology of recurrent spontaneous abortion. *Am J Reprod Immunol 26:*23, 1991.

Cowchock S: Autoantibodies and fetal wastage. *Am J Reprod Immunol 26:*38, 1991.

Dickey RP, Gasser R, Olar TT, et al: Relationship of initial chorionic sac diameter to abortion and abortus karyotype based on new growth curves for the 16th to 49 post-ovulation day. *Hum Reprod 9:*559, 1994.

Dickey RP, Gasser RF, Olar TT, et al: The relationship of initial embryo crown-rump length to pregnancy outcome and abortus karyotype based on new growth curves for the 2–31 mm embryo. *Hum Reprod 9:*366, 1994.

Edwards RG: Physiological and molecular aspects of human implantation. *Hum Reprod 10(Suppl 2):*1, 1995.

Ellis SA, Sargent IL, Redman CWG, McMichael AJ: Evidence for a novel HLA antigen found on human extravillous trophoblast and a choriocarcinoma cell line. *Immunology 59:*595, 1986.

Enders AC, King, BF: Formation and differentiation of extraembryonic mesoderm in the rhesus monkey. *Am J Anat 181:*327, 1988.

Faulk WP, Temple A: Distribution of beta-2 microglobulin and HLA in chorionic villi of human placentae. *Nature 262:*799, 1976.

Filly RA: Ectopic pregnancy. *In* Callen PW (ed): *Ultrasonography in Obstetrics and Gynecology*, 3rd ed. Philadelphia, WB Saunders, 1994a.

Filly RA: Ultrasound evaluation during the first trimester. *In* Callen PW (ed): *Ultrasonography in Obstetrics and Gynecology*, 3rd ed. Philadelphia, WB Saunders, 1994b.

Fleischer AC, Cartwright PS, Pennell RG, Sacks GA: Sonograph of ectopic pregnancy with transabdominal and transvaginal scanning. *In* Fleischer AC, Romero R, Manning FA, et al (eds): *The Principles and Practice of Ultrasonography in Obstetrics and Gynecology*, 4th ed. Norwalk, Appleton & Kange, 1991.

Garcia-Martinez V, Darnell DK, Lopez-Sanchez C, et al: State of commitment of prospective neural plate and prospective mesoderm in late gastrula/early neural stages of avian embryos. *Dev Biol 181:* 102, 1997.

Gilbert SF: *Developmental Biology*, 5th ed. Sunderland, Sinauer Associates, 1997.

Hertig AT: The overall problem in man. *In* Benirschke K (ed): *Comparative Aspects of Reproductive Failure*. New York, Springer Verlag, 1967.

Hertig AT: *Human Trophoblast*. Springfield, IL, Charles C Thomas, 1968.

Hertig AT, Rock J: Two human ova of the previllous stage, having a developmental age of about eleven and twelve days respectively. *Contrib Embryol Carnegie Inst 29:*127, 1941.

Hertig AT, Rock J: Two human ova of the pre-villous stage, having a developmental age of about seven and nine days respectively. *Contrib Embryol Carnegie Inst 31:*65, 1945.

Hertig AT, Rock J: Two human ova of the pre-villous stage, having a developmental age of about eight and nine days, respectively. *Contrib Embryol Carnegie Inst 33:*169, 1949.

Hertig AT, Rock, J, Adams EC: A description of 34 human ova within the first seventeen days of development. *Am J Anat 98:*435, 1956.

Hertig AT, Rock J, Adams EC, Menkin MC: Thirty-four fertilized human ova, good, bad and indifferent, recovered from 210 women of known fertility. *Pediatrics 23:*202, 1959.

Hill JA: T-helper 1-type immunity to trophoblast: evidence for a new immunological mechanism for recurrent abortion in women. *Human Reprod 10(Suppl 2):*114, 1995.

Kalant H, Roschlau WHE, Hickie RA: *Essentials of Medical Pharmacology*. Toronto, BC Decker, 1990.

King A, Loke YW, Chaouat G: NK cells and reproduction. *Immunology Today 18:*64, 1997.

Kovats S, Main EK, Librach C, et al: A class 1 antigen, HLA-G, expressed in human trophoblasts. *Science 18:*220, 1990.

Lala PK: Similarities between immunoregulation in pregnancy and malignancy: the role of prostaglandin E_2 [Editorial]. *Am J Reprod Immunol 20:*147–152, 1990.

Lala PK, Kearns M, Colavincenzo V: Cells of the fetomaternal interface: their role in the maintenance of viviparous pregnancy. *Am J Anat 170:*501, 1984.

Lala PK, Kennedy TG, Parhar RS: Suppression of lymphocyte alloreactivity by early gestational human decidua. II. Characterization of suppressor mechanisms. *Cell Immunol 116:*411, 1988.

Li TC, Tristram A, Hill AS, Cooke ID: A review of 254 ectopic pregnancies in a teaching hospital in the Trent region, 1977–1990. *Hum Reprod 6:*1002, 1991.

Lindenberg G, Hyttel P, Sjogren A, Greve T: A comparative study of attachment of human, bovine and mouse blastocysts to uterine epithelia monolayer. *Hum Reprod 4:*446, 1989.

Lindsay DJ, Lovett IS, Lyons EA, et al: Endovaginal sonography: yolk sac diameter and shape as a predictor of pregnancy outcome in the first trimester. *Radiology 183:*115, 1992.

Loke YW, King A: *Human Implantation: Cell Biology and Immunology*. Cambridge, Cambridge University Press, 1995.

Loke YW, King A, Burrows TD: Decidua in human implantation. *Hum Reprod 10(Suppl 2):*14, 1995.

Luckett WP: The origin of extraembryonic mesoderm in the early human and rhesus monkey embryos. *Anat Rec 169:*369, 1971.

Luckett WP: Amniogenesis in the early human and rhesus monkey embryos. *Anat Rec 175:*375, 1973.

Luckett WP: Origin and differentiation of the yolk sac and extraembryonic mesoderm in presomite human and rhesus monkey embryos. *Am J Anat 152:*59, 1978.

Lysiak JJ, Lala PK: *In situ* localization and characterization of bone marrow-derived cells in the decidua of normal murine pregnancy. *Biol Reprod 47:*603, 1992.

Moore KL: *Clinically Oriented Anatomy*, 3rd ed. Baltimore, Williams & Wilkins, 1992.

Nogales FF (ed): *The Human Yolk Sac and Yolk Sac Tumors*. New York, Springer Verlag, 1993.

O'Rahilly R, Müller F: *Human Embryology & Teratology*, 2nd ed. New York, Wiley-Liss, 1996.

Page EW, Villee CA, Villee DB: *Human Reproduction. Essentials of Reproductive and Perinatal Medicine*, 3rd ed. Philadelphia, WB Saunders, 1981.

Parhar RS, Kennedy TG, Lala PK: Suppression of lymphocyte alloreactivity by early gestational human decidua. 1. Characterization of suppressor cells and suppressor molecules. *Cell Immunol 116:*392, 1988.

Parhar RS, Yagel S, Lala PK: PGE_2-mediated immunosuppression by first trimester human decidual cells blocks activation of maternal leukocytes in the decidua with potential anti-trophoblast activity. *Cell Immunol 120:*61, 1989.

Polan ML, Simón C, Frances A, et al: Role of embryonic factors in human implantation. *Hum Reprod 10(Suppl 2):*22, 1995.

Psychoyos A, Nika G, Gravanis A: The role of prostaglandins in blastocyst implantation. *Hum Reprod 10(Suppl 2):*30, 1995.

Rousso D, Klearchou N, Rousso I, et al: Combined intrauterine and abdominal pregnancy. *J Obstet Gynecol 17:*62, 1997.

Rubin GL: Ectopic pregnancy in the United States: 1970 through 1978. *JAMA 249:*1725, 1983.

Shepard TH, Fantel AG, Mirkes PE: Collection and scientific use of human embryonic and fetal material. *In* Kalter H (ed): *Issues and Reviews in Teratology,* vol 4, 1988.

Simón C, Pellicer A, Polan ML: Interleukin-1 system crosstalk between embryo and endometrium implantation. *Hum Reprod 10(Suppl 2):*43, 1995.

Streeter GL: Developmental horizons in human embryos. Description of age group XI, 13 to 20 somites, and age group XII, 21 to 29 somites. *Contrib Embryol Carnegie Inst 30:*211, 1942.

Sunderland CA, Redman CWG, Stirrat GM: HLA-A,B,C, antigens are expressed on nonvillous trophoblasts of the early human placenta. *J Immunol 127:*2614-2615, 1981.

Thom DH, Nelson LM, Vaughan TL: Spontaneous abortion and subsequent adverse birth outcomes. *Am J Obstet Gynecol 166:*111, 1992.

Vince GS, Johnson PM: Reproductive immunology, conception, contraception and consequences. *The Immunologist 4:*172-178, 1996.

Yu S, Pennisi JA, Moukhtar M, Friedman EA: Placental abruption in association with advanced abdominal pregnancy. *J Reprod Med 40:*731, 1995.

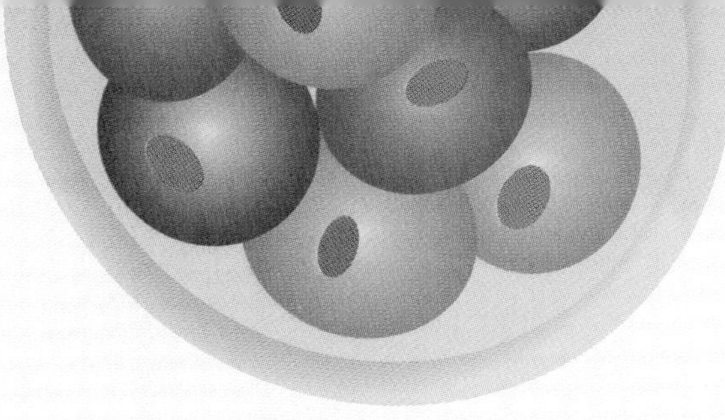

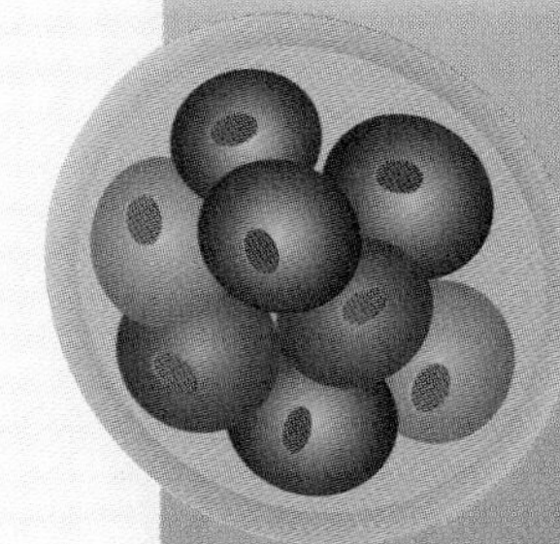

Formation of Germ Layers and Early Tissue and Organ Differentiation: The Third Week

4

■ Rapid development of the embryo from the embryonic disc during the early part of the third week is characterized by:

- appearance of the primitive streak
- development of the notochord
- differentiation of three germ layers from which all embryonic tissues and organs develop

The third week of embryonic development occurs during the week following the first missed menstrual period, that is, 5 weeks after the onset of the last normal menstrual period (LNMP).

Cessation of menstruation is often the first indication that a woman may be pregnant, but missing a menstrual period is not always a certain sign of pregnancy; for example, delay of menstruation may result from emotional shock or illness.

Pregnancy Tests

Relatively simple and rapid tests are now available for detecting pregnancy. Most tests depend on the presence of an *early pregnancy factor* (EPF) in the maternal serum and *human chorionic gonadotropin* (hCG), a hormone produced by the syncytiotrophoblast and excreted in the mother's urine. EPF can be detected 24 to 48 hours after fertilization and the production of hCG is sufficient to give a positive indication of pregnancy early in the second week of development. About 3 weeks after conception, approximately 5 weeks after the LNMP (Fig. 4-1), a normal pregnancy can be detected with ultrasonography (Filly, 1994).

A frequent symptom of pregnancy is nausea and vomiting, which may occur by the end of the third week; however, the time of onset of these symptoms is variable. Vaginal bleeding at the expected time of menstruation does not rule out pregnancy because there may be a slight loss of blood from the implantation site of the blastocyst. *Implantation bleeding* results from leakage of blood into the uterine cavity from disrupted endometrial blood vessels in the lacunae around the implanted blastocyst. When such bleeding is interpreted as menstruation, an error occurs initially in determining the *expected date of confinement (EDC)* and delivery date of the baby.

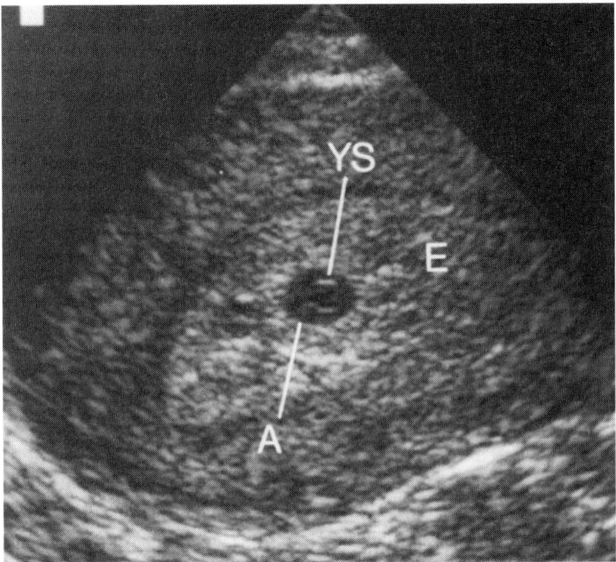

■ **Figure 4-1.** Endovaginal sonogram of a conceptus about 3 weeks after conception, showing the amnion (**A**) and yolk sac (**YS**). The endometrium (**E**) surrounding the conceptus is also visible. (From Filly RA: Ultrasound evaluation during the first trimester. *In* Callen PW [ed]: *Ultrasonography in Obstetrics and Gynecology,* 3rd ed. Philadelphia, WB Saunders, 1994.)

GASTRULATION: FORMATION OF GERM LAYERS

Gastrulation is the process by which the bilaminar embryonic disc is converted into a trilaminar embryonic disc. *Gastrulation* is the *beginning of morphogenesis* (development of body form) and is the significant event occurring during the third week. Gastrulation begins with formation of the **primitive streak** on the surface of the epiblast of the embryonic disc (Fig. 4-2*B*). Each of the three germ layers (ectoderm, mesoderm, and endoderm) gives rise to specific tissues and organs.

- *Ectoderm* gives rise to the epidermis, the central and peripheral nervous systems, the retina of the eye, and various other structures (see Chapter 5).
- *Endoderm* is the source of the epithelial linings of the respiratory passages and gastrointestinal (GI) tract, including the glands opening into the GI tract and the glandular cells of associated organs such as the liver and pancreas.
- Mesoderm gives rise to smooth muscular coats, connective tissues, and vessels associated with the tissues and organs; mesoderm also forms most of the cardiovascular system and is the source of blood cells and bone marrow, the skeleton, striated muscles, and the reproductive and excretory organs.

Formation of the primitive streak, germ layers, and notochord are the important processes occurring during gastrulation. During this period, the embryo is sometimes referred to as a *gastrula*.

Primitive Streak

The first sign of gastrulation is the appearance of the primitive streak at the caudal end of the embryo (Fig. 4-2*B*). At the beginning of the third week, an opacity formed by a thickened linear band of epiblast, known as the primitive streak, appears caudally in the median plane of the dorsal aspect of the embryonic disc (Figs. 4-2*C* and 4-3). The primitive streak results from the proliferation and migration of cells of the epiblast to the median plane of the embryonic disc. As the primitive streak elongates by addition of cells to its caudal end, its cranial end proliferates to form a **primitive node** (Figs. 4-2*B* and 4-3). Concurrently, a narrow **primitive groove** develops in the primitive streak

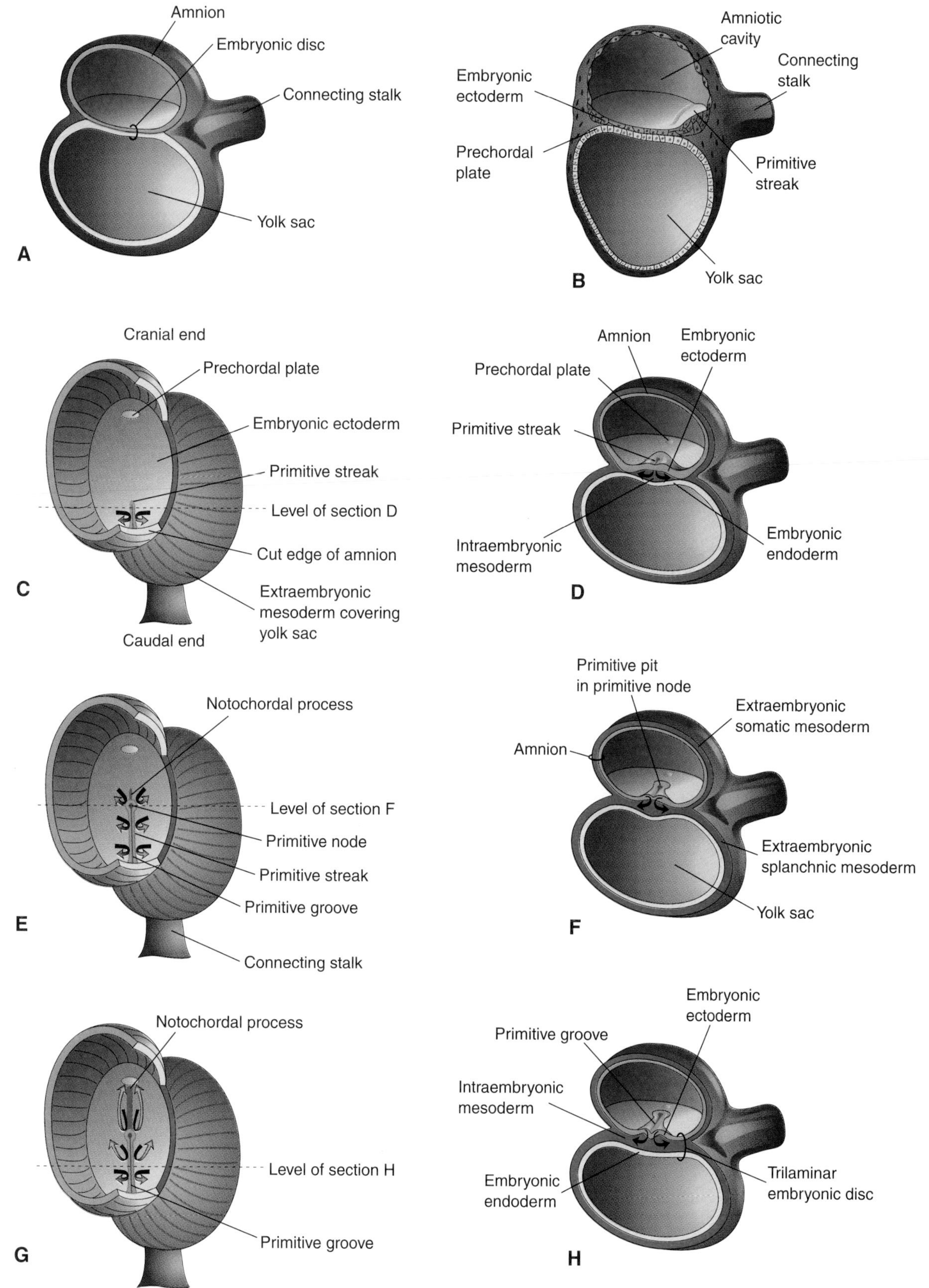

■ **Figure 4–2.** Drawings illustrating formation of the trilaminar embryonic disc (days 15 to 16). The arrows in the drawings indicate invagination and migration of mesenchymal cells from the primitive streak between the ectoderm and endoderm. *A, C, E,* and *G,* Dorsal views of the embryonic disc early in the third week, exposed by removal of the amnion. *B, D, F,* and *H,* Transverse sections through the embryonic disc. The levels of the sections are indicated in *C, E,* and *G.* The prechordal plate, indicating the head region, is indicated by a light blue oval because it is a thickening of endoderm that cannot be seen from the dorsal surface.

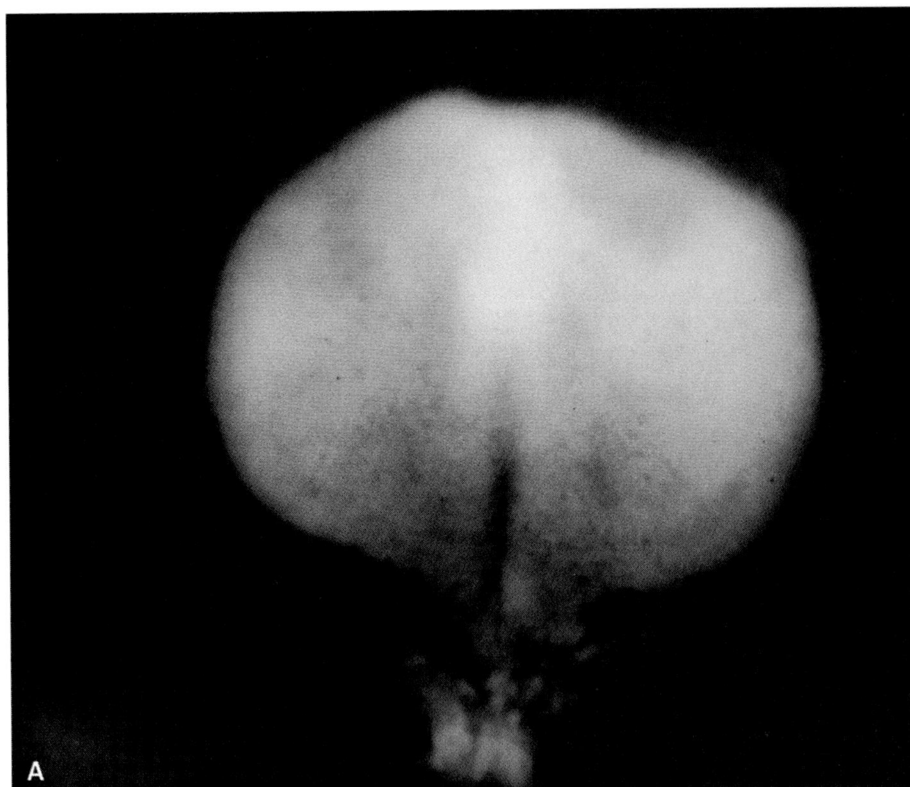

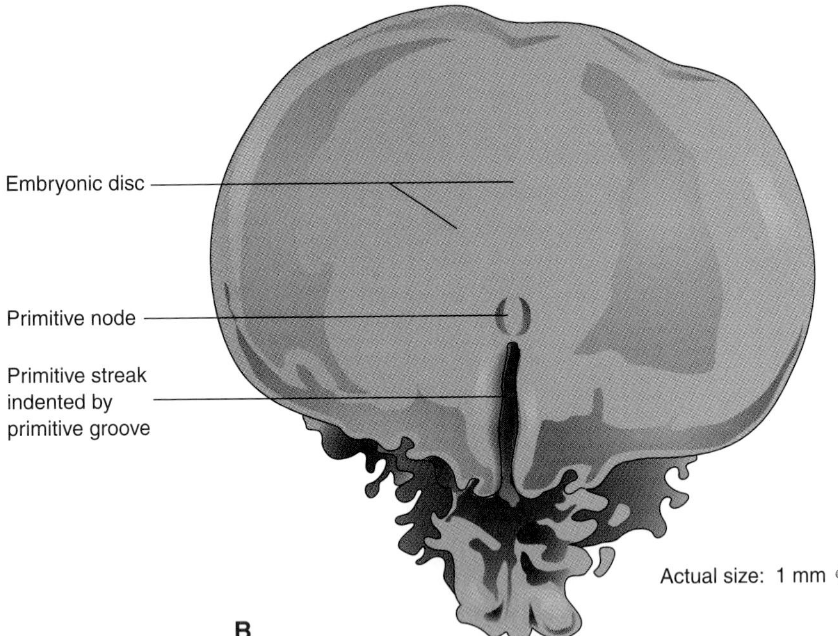

■ **Figure 4–3.** *A,* Photograph of a dorsal view of an embryo about 16 days old. *B,* Drawing indicating structures shown in *A.* (*A* From Moore KL, Persaud TVN, Shiota K: *Color Atlas of Clinical Embryology.* Philadelphia, WB Saunders, 1994.)

that is continuous with a small depression in the primitive node, the **primitive pit**. As soon as the primitive streak appears, it is possible to identify the embryo's craniocaudal axis, its cranial and caudal ends, its dorsal and ventral surfaces, and its right and left sides. The primitive groove and pit result from the invagination (an inward movement) of epiblastic cells, which is indicated by arrows in Figure 4–2*E*.

Shortly after the primitive streak appears, cells leave its deep surface and form a loose network of embryonic connective tissue called **mesenchyme** or mesoblast (Fig. 4–4*B*). Mesenchyme forms the supporting tissues of the embryo, such as most of the connective tissues of the body and the stromal components or framework of glands. Some mesenchyme forms a layer known as the **intraembryonic mesoderm** (Fig.

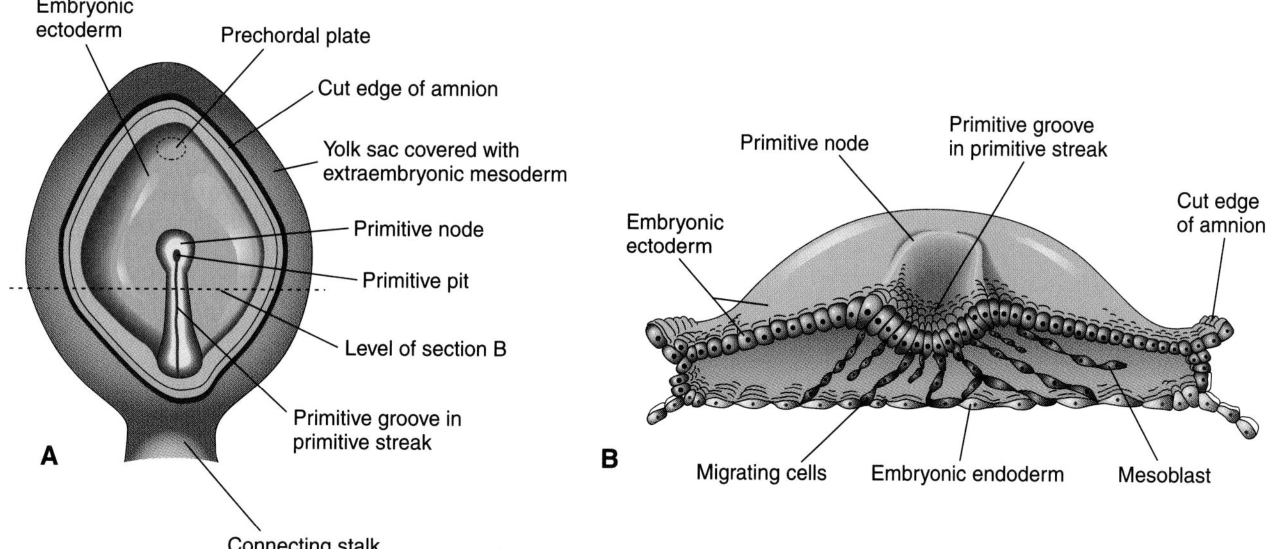

■ **Figure 4–4.** *A,* Drawing of a dorsal view of a 16-day embryo. The amnion has been removed to expose the embryonic disc. *B,* Drawing of the cranial half of the embryonic disc. The disc has been cut transversely to show the migration of mesenchymal cells from the primitive streak to form mesoblast or mesenchyme that soon organizes to form the intraembryonic mesoderm. This illustration also shows that most of the embryonic endoderm also arises from the epiblast. Most of the hypoblastic cells are displaced to extraembryonic regions such as the wall of the yolk sac.

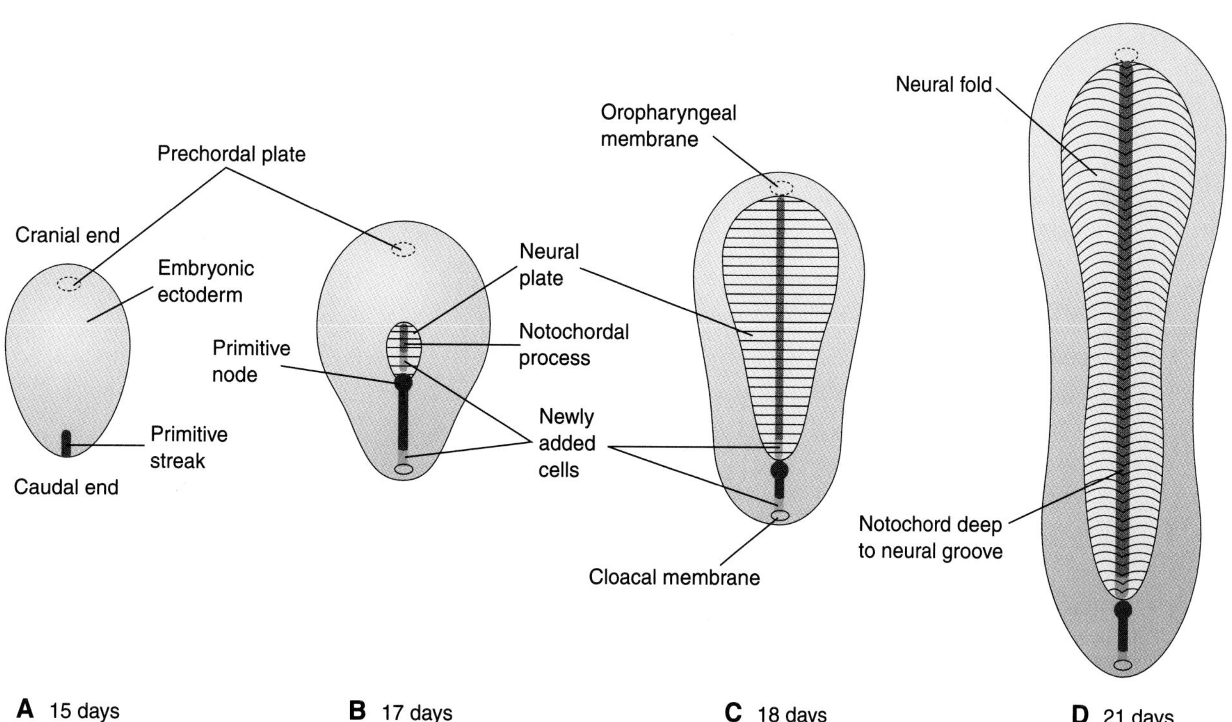

■ **Figure 4–5.** Diagrammatic sketches of dorsal views of the embryonic disc showing how it lengthens and changes shape during the third week. The primitive streak lengthens by addition of cells at its caudal end, and the notochordal process lengthens by migration of cells from the primitive node. The notochordal process and adjacent mesoderm induce the overlying embryonic ectoderm to form the neural plate, the primordium of the central nervous system. Observe that as the notochordal process elongates, the primitive streak shortens. At the end of the third week the notochordal process is transformed into the notochord. Note that the embryonic disc is originally egg-shaped but soon becomes pear-shaped and then slipperlike as the notochord develops.

4-2*D*). Some cells of the epiblast of the primitive streak also displace the hypoblast, forming the **intraembryonic** or **embryonic endoderm** in the roof of the yolk sac. Cells remaining in the epiblast form the **intraembryonic** or **embryonic ectoderm**. Under the influence of various *embryonic growth factors* (Slack, 1987; Tabin, 1991), the mesenchymal cells migrate widely from the primitive streak. These cells have the potential to proliferate and differentiate into diverse types of cells, such as fibroblasts, chondroblasts, and osteoblasts (see Chapter 5). In summary, cells of the epiblast, through the process of gastrulation, give rise to all three germ layers in the embryo, the primordia of all its tissues and organs.

FATE OF PRIMITIVE STREAK

The primitive streak actively forms mesoderm until the early part of the fourth week; thereafter production of mesoderm slows down. The primitive streak diminishes in relative size and becomes an insignificant structure in the sacrococcygeal region of the embryo (Fig. 4-5*D*). Normally the primitive streak undergoes degenerative changes and disappears by the end of the fourth week.

Sacrococcygeal Teratoma

Remnants of the primitive streak may persist and give rise to a large tumor known as a *sacrococcygeal teratoma* (Fig. 4-6). Because they are derived from pluripotent primitive streak cells, these tumors contain various types of tissues containing elements of the three germ layers in incomplete stages of differentiation. Sacrococcygeal teratomas are the most common tumor in newborns and have an incidence of about 1 in 35,000 (Holzgreve et al., 1991; Marina, 1996). The incidence of malignancy in sacrococcygeal teratomas increases from 10% at birth to 50 to 70% at 2 months of age (Marina, 1996). These tumors are usually surgically excised promptly and the prognosis is good.

NOTOCHORDAL PROCESS AND NOTOCHORD

Some mesenchymal cells migrate cranially from the primitive node and pit, forming a median cellular cord, the **notochordal process** (Fig. 4-7*C*). This process soon acquires a lumen, the **notochordal canal**. The notochordal process grows cranially between the ectoderm and endoderm until it reaches the **prechordal plate** (prochordal plate), a small circular area of columnar endodermal cells. The hollow, rodlike notochordal process can extend no farther because the prechordal plate is firmly attached to the overlying ectoderm. These fused germ layers form the **oropharyngeal membrane,** located at the future site of the oral cavity (mouth).

Some mesenchymal cells from the primitive streak and notochordal process migrate laterally and cranially between the ectoderm and mesoderm until they reach the margins of the embryonic disc. There, these cells are continuous with the extraembryonic mesoderm covering the amnion and yolk sac (Fig. 4-2*C*). This extraembryonic mesoderm is derived from the endoderm of the yolk sac (Enders and King, 1988; Bianchi et al., 1993; also see Chapter 3). Some cells from the primitive streak migrate cranially on each side of the notochordal process and around the prechordal plate. Here they meet cranially to form the cardiogenic mesoderm in the **cardiogenic area** where the primordium of the heart begins to develop at the end of the third week.

Caudal to the primitive streak there is a circular area known as the **cloacal membrane**, which indicates the future site of the anus (Fig. 4-7*E*). The embryonic disc remains bilaminar here and at the **oropharyngeal membrane** because the embryonic ectoderm and endoderm are fused at these sites, thereby preventing migration of mesenchymal cells between them

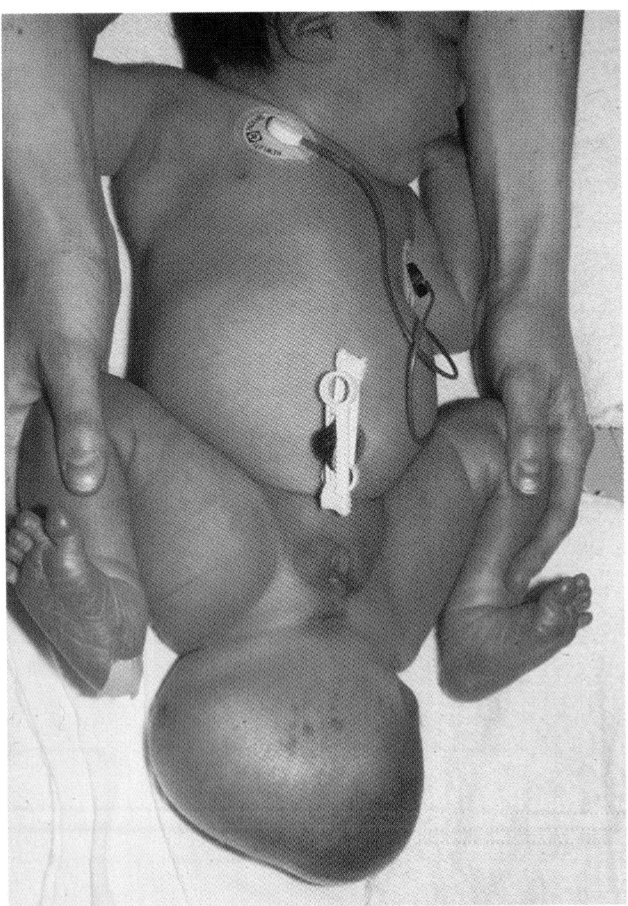

■ **Figure 4-6.** Female infant with a large sacrococcygeal teratoma that developed from remnants of the primitive streak. The tumor, a neoplasm made up of several different types of tissue, was surgically removed. About 75% of infants with these tumors are female; the reason for this preponderance is unknown. (Courtesy of A.E. Chudley, MD, Section of Genetics and Metabolism, Department of Pediatrics and Child Health, Children's Hospital and University of Manitoba, Winnipeg, Manitoba, Canada.)

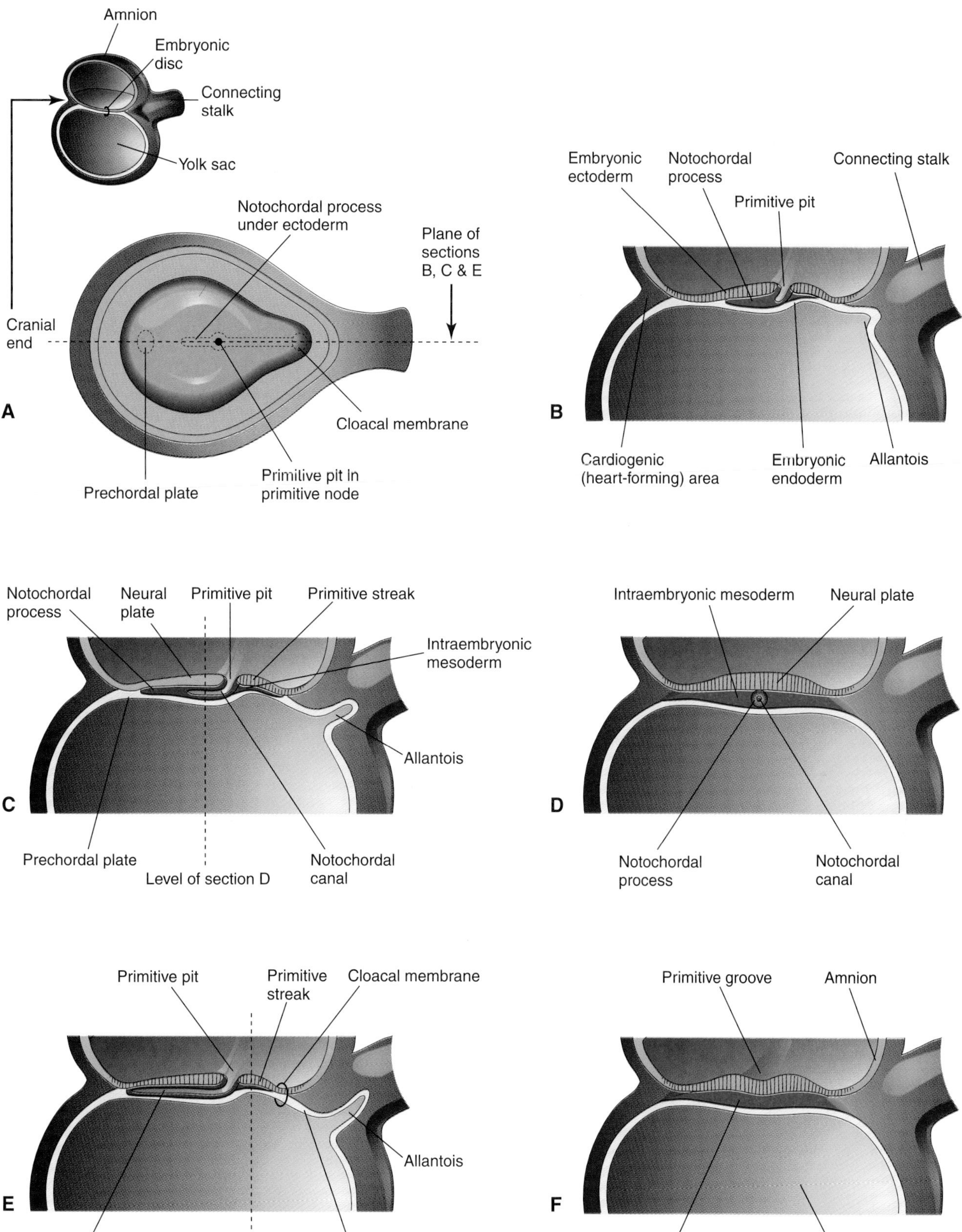

■ **Figure 4–7.** Drawings illustrating development of the notochordal process. The small sketch at the upper left is for orientation. *A,* Dorsal view of the embryonic disc (about 16 days), exposed by removal of the amnion. The notochordal process is shown as if it were visible through the embryonic ectoderm. *B, C,* and *E,* Median sections at the plane shown in *A,* illustrating successive stages in the development of the notochordal process and canal. The stages shown in *C* and *E* occur at about 18 days. *D* and *F,* Transverse sections through the embryonic disc at the levels shown in *C* and *E.*

(Fig. 4-8*C*). By the middle of the third week, intraembryonic mesoderm separates the ectoderm and endoderm everywhere except:

- at the oropharyngeal membrane cranially
- in the median plane cranial to the primitive node, where the notochordal process is located
- at the cloacal membrane caudally

The **notochord** is a cellular rod that develops by transformation of the notochordal process. The notochord

- defines the primordial axis of the embryo and gives it some rigidity
- serves as the basis for development of the axial skeleton (bones of head and vertebral column)
- indicates the future site of the vertebral bodies

The notochord develops as follows:

- The notochordal process elongates by invagination of cells from the primitive pit.
- The primitive pit extends into the notochordal process, forming a *notochordal canal* (Fig. 4-7*C*).
- The notochordal process is now a cellular tube that extends cranially from the primitive node to the prechordal plate.
- The floor of the notochordal process fuses with the underlying intraembryonic endoderm of the yolk sac.
- The fused layers gradually undergo degeneration, resulting in the formation of openings in the floor of the notochordal process, which brings the notochordal canal into communication with the yolk sac (Fig. 4-8*B*).
- The openings rapidly become confluent and the floor of the notochordal canal disappears (Fig. 4-8*C*); the remains of the notochordal process form a flattened, grooved *notochordal plate* (Fig. 4-8*D*).
- Beginning at the cranial end of the embryo, the notochordal cells proliferate and the notochordal plate infolds to form the rod-shaped notochord (Fig. 4-8*F* and *G*).
- The proximal part of the notochordal canal persists temporarily as the *neurenteric canal* (Fig. 4-8*C* and *E*), which forms a transitory communication between the amniotic and yolk sac cavities. When development of the notochord is complete, the neurenteric canal normally obliterates.
- The notochord becomes detached from the endoderm of the yolk sac, which again becomes a continuous layer (Fig. 4-8*G*).

Three-dimensional reconstruction studies on serial sections of human embryos revealed that the cranial end of the notochord is complex with a forked termination; the caudal end also appeared to be branching, with separated fragments of chordal tissue (Salisbury et al., 1993). The notochord is an intricate structure around which the vertebral column forms (see Chapter 15). It extends from the oropharyngeal membrane to the primitive node. The notochord degenerates and disappears as the bodies of the vertebrae form, but it persists as the *nucleus pulposus* of each intervertebral disc (Moore and Agur, 1995).

The notochord functions as the primary inductor in the early embryo; "it is a prime mover in a series of signal-calling episodes that ultimately transform unspecialized embryonic cells into definitive adult tissues and organs" (Carlson, 1994). The developing notochord induces the overlying embryonic ectoderm to thicken and form the **neural plate** (Fig. 4-8*C*), the primordium of the central nervous system (CNS).

The Allantois

The allantois (Gr. *allas*, sausage) appears on about day 16 as a small, sausage-shaped diverticulum (outpouching) from the caudal wall of the yolk sac that extends into the connecting stalk (Fig. 4-7*B*, *C*, and *E*). The allantois is a large sacklike structure in embryos of reptiles, birds, and some mammals, which has a respiratory function and/or acts as a reservoir for urine during embryonic life. The allantois remains very small in human embryos because the placenta and amniotic sac take over its functions. The allantois is involved with early blood formation in the human embryo and is associated with development of the urinary bladder (see Chapter 13). As the bladder enlarges, the allantois becomes the urachus, which is represented in adults by the *median umbilical ligament*. The blood vessels of the allantois become the umbilical arteries and veins (see Fig. 4-12).

Persistence of Neurenteric Canal

Uncommonly the neurenteric canal persists, giving rise to a very rare congenital anomaly in which the central canal of the spinal cord is connected with the lumen of the intestine.

Remnants of Notochordal Tissue

Both benign and malignant tumors arising from notochordal tissue have been reported (Salisbury et al., 1993). About one-third of *chordomas* that arise from vestigial remnants of the notochord occur at the base of the skull and extend to the nasopharynx (Rubin and Farber, 1988). Chordomas grow slowly and infiltrate bone.

Allantoic Cysts

Allantoic cysts, remnants of the extraembryonic portion of the allantois, are usually found between the fetal umbilical vessels and can be detected by ultraso-

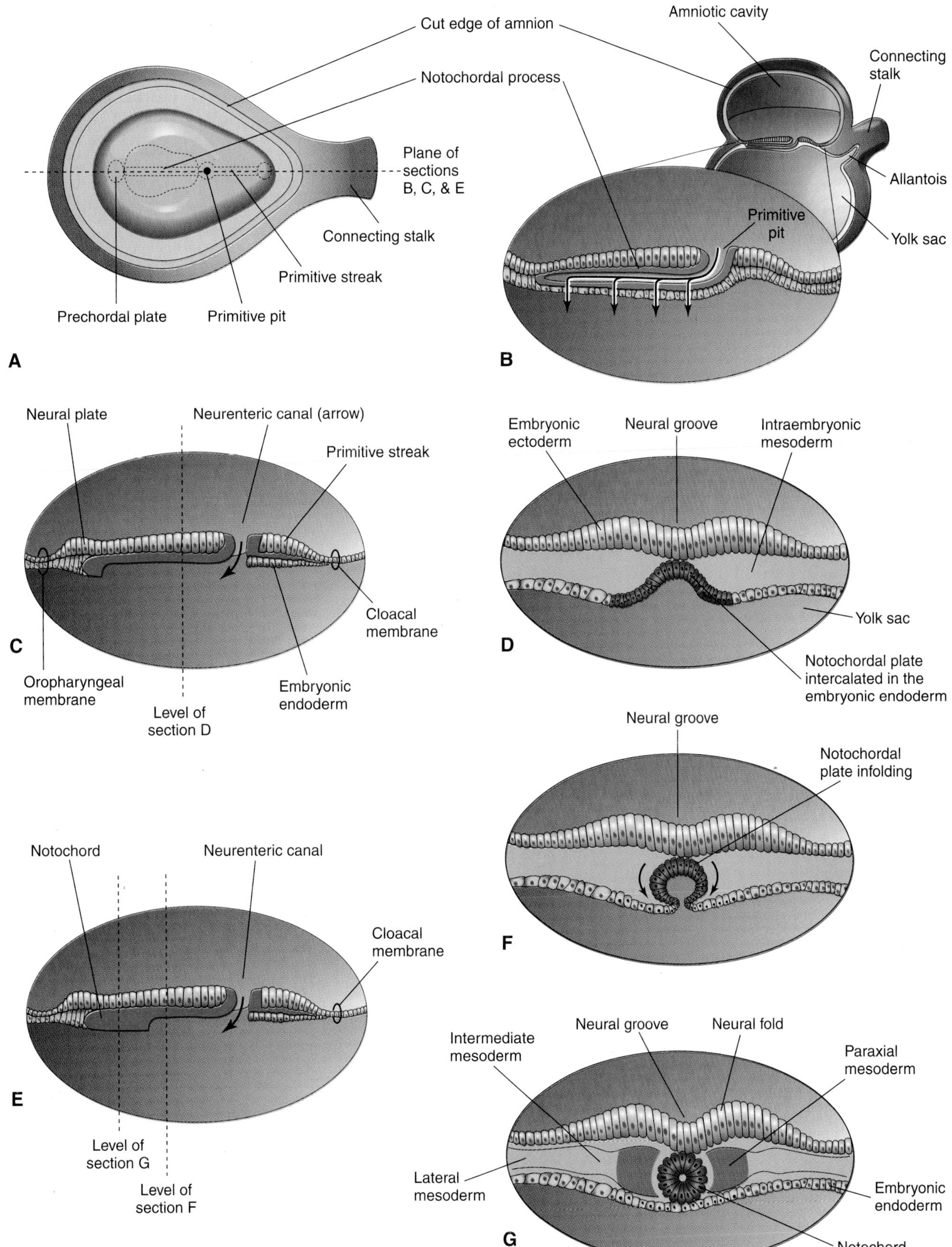

■ **Figure 4–8.** Drawings illustrating further development of the notochord by transformation of the notochordal process. *A,* Dorsal view of the embryonic disc (about 18 days), exposed by removing the amnion. *B,* Three-dimensional median section of the embryo. *C* and *E,* Similar sections of slightly older embryos. *D, F,* and *G,* Transverse sections of the trilaminar embryonic disc at the levels shown in *C* and *E.*

nography. They are most commonly detected in the proximal part of the umbilical cord, near its attachment to the ventral abdominal wall.

NEURULATION: FORMATION OF NEURAL TUBE

The processes involved in the formation of the neural plate and neural folds and closure of these folds to form the neural tube constitute neurulation. These processes are completed by the end of the fourth week, when closure of the caudal (posterior) **neuropore** occurs (see Chapter 5). During neurulation, the embryo is sometimes referred to as a *neurula*.

Neural Plate and Neural Tube

As the notochord develops, the embryonic ectoderm over it thickens to form an elongated, slipperlike plate of thickened epithelial cells, the **neural plate**. *Neural plate formation is induced by the developing notochord*. The ectoderm of the neural plate (neuroectoderm) gives rise to the **CNS**—the brain and spinal cord. Neuroectoderm also gives rise to various other structures, the retina, for example. At first the elongated neural plate corresponds precisely in length to the underlying notochord. It appears cranial to the primitive node and dorsal to the notochord and mesoderm adjacent to it (Fig. 4-5*B*). As the notochord elongates, the neural plate broadens and eventually extends cranially as far as the oropharyngeal membrane (Figs. 4-5*C* and 4-8*C*). Eventually the neural plate extends beyond the notochord. About the 18th day, the neural plate invaginates along its central axis to form a longitudinal median **neural groove**, which has neural folds on each side (Fig. 4-8*G*). The **neural folds** become particularly prominent at the cranial end of the embryo and are *the first signs of brain development*. By the end of the third week, the neural folds have begun to move together and fuse, converting the neural plate into a **neural tube**, the primordium of the CNS (Figs. 4-9 and 4-10).

Neural tube formation is a complex, multifactorial process involving extrinsic forces (Smith and Schoenwolf, 1991). The neural tube soon separates from the surface ectoderm and the free edges of the ectoderm fuse so that this layer becomes continuous over the neural tube and the back of the embryo (Fig. 4-10*E* and *F*). Subsequently, the surface ectoderm differentiates into the epidermis. Neurulation is completed during the fourth week (see Chapter 5).

Neural Crest Formation

As the neural folds fuse to form the neural tube, some neuroectodermal cells lying along the crest of each neural fold lose their epithelial affinities and attachments to neighboring cells (Fig. 4-10). As the neural tube separates from the surface ectoderm, **neural crest cells** migrate dorsolaterally on each side of the neural tube. They soon form a flattened irregular mass, the **neural crest**, between the neural tube and the overlying surface ectoderm (Fig. 4-10*E*). The neural crest soon separates into right and left parts that migrate to the dorsolateral aspects of the neural tube; here they give rise to the sensory ganglia of the spinal and cranial nerves. Many neural crest cells migrate in various directions and disperse within the mesenchyme. Although these cells are difficult to identify, special tracer techniques have revealed that neural crest cells disseminate widely.

Neural crest cells give rise to the spinal ganglia (dorsal root ganglia) and the ganglia of the autonomic nervous system. The ganglia of cranial nerves V, VII, IX, and X are also partly derived from neural crest cells. In addition to forming ganglion cells, neural crest cells form the neurolemmal sheaths of peripheral nerves (composed of Schwann cells) and the meningeal coverings of the brain and spinal cord (at least the pia mater and arachnoid mater). They also contribute to the formation of pigment cells, cells of the suprarenal (adrenal) medulla, and several skeletal and muscular components in the head (see Chapter 10).

Congenital Anomalies Resulting From Abnormal Neurulation

Because the neural plate, the primordium of the CNS, appears during the third week and gives rise to the neural folds and the beginning of the neural tube, disturbance of neurulation may result in severe abnormalities of the brain and spinal cord (see Chapter 18). **Neural tube defects** (NTDs) are among the most common congenital anomalies (Filly, 1991). The incidence of NTDs has been estimated to be as high as 16 per 10,000 births in the eastern United States (Greenberg et al., 1983). *Meroanencephaly or anencephaly*—partial absence of the brain—is the most severe defect and is also the most common anomaly affecting the CNS (see Chapter 18). Although the term anencephaly (Gr. *an*, without + *enkephalos*, brain) is commonly used, it is a misnomer because the brain is not completely absent. Available evidence suggests that the primary disturbance (e.g., a teratogenic drug; see Chapter 8) affects the neuroectoderm, resulting in failure of the neural folds to fuse and form the neural tube in the brain region.

DEVELOPMENT OF SOMITES

As the notochord and neural tube form, the intraembryonic mesoderm on each side of them proliferates to form a thick, longitudinal column of **paraxial mesoderm** (Figs. 4-8*G* and 4-9*B*). Each column is continuous laterally with the **intermediate mesoderm**, which gradually thins into a layer of lateral mesoderm. The **lateral mesoderm** is continuous with the extraembryonic mesoderm covering the yolk sac and amnion.

Toward the end of the third week, the paraxial mesoderm differentiates and begins to divide into paired cuboidal bodies, the **somites** (Gr. *soma*, body). These blocks of mesoderm are located on each side of

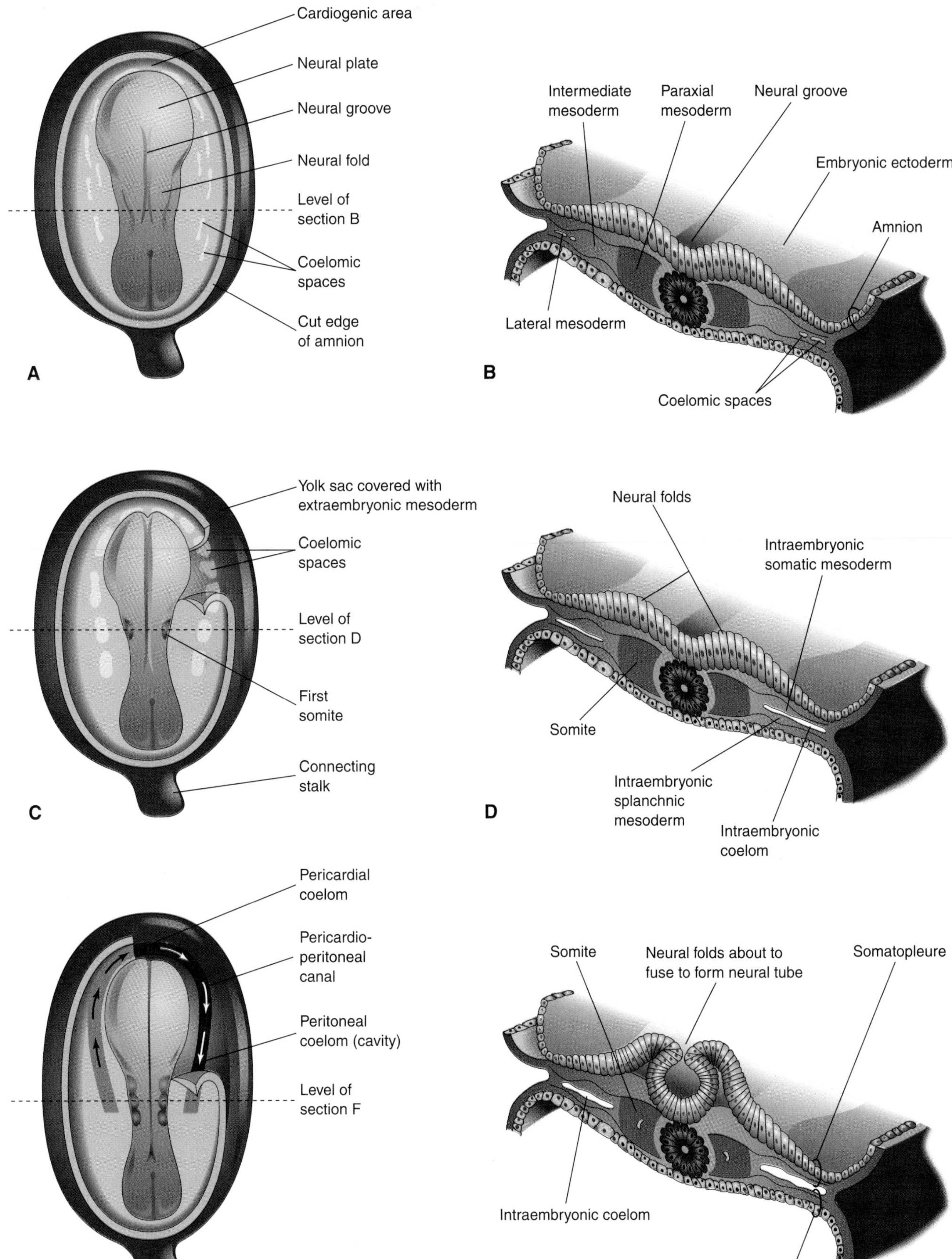

■ **Figure 4–9.** Drawings of embryos of 19 to 21 days, illustrating development of the somites and intraembryonic coelom. *A, C,* and *E,* Dorsal views of the embryo, exposed by removal of the amnion. *B, D,* and *F,* Transverse sections through the embryonic disc at the levels shown. *A,* Presomite embryo of about 18 days. *C,* An embryo of about 20 days, showing the first pair of somites. Part of the somatopleure on the right has been removed to show the isolated coelomic spaces in the lateral mesoderm. *E,* A three-somite embryo (about 21 days), showing the horseshoe-shaped intraembryonic coelom, exposed on the right by removal of part of the somatopleure.

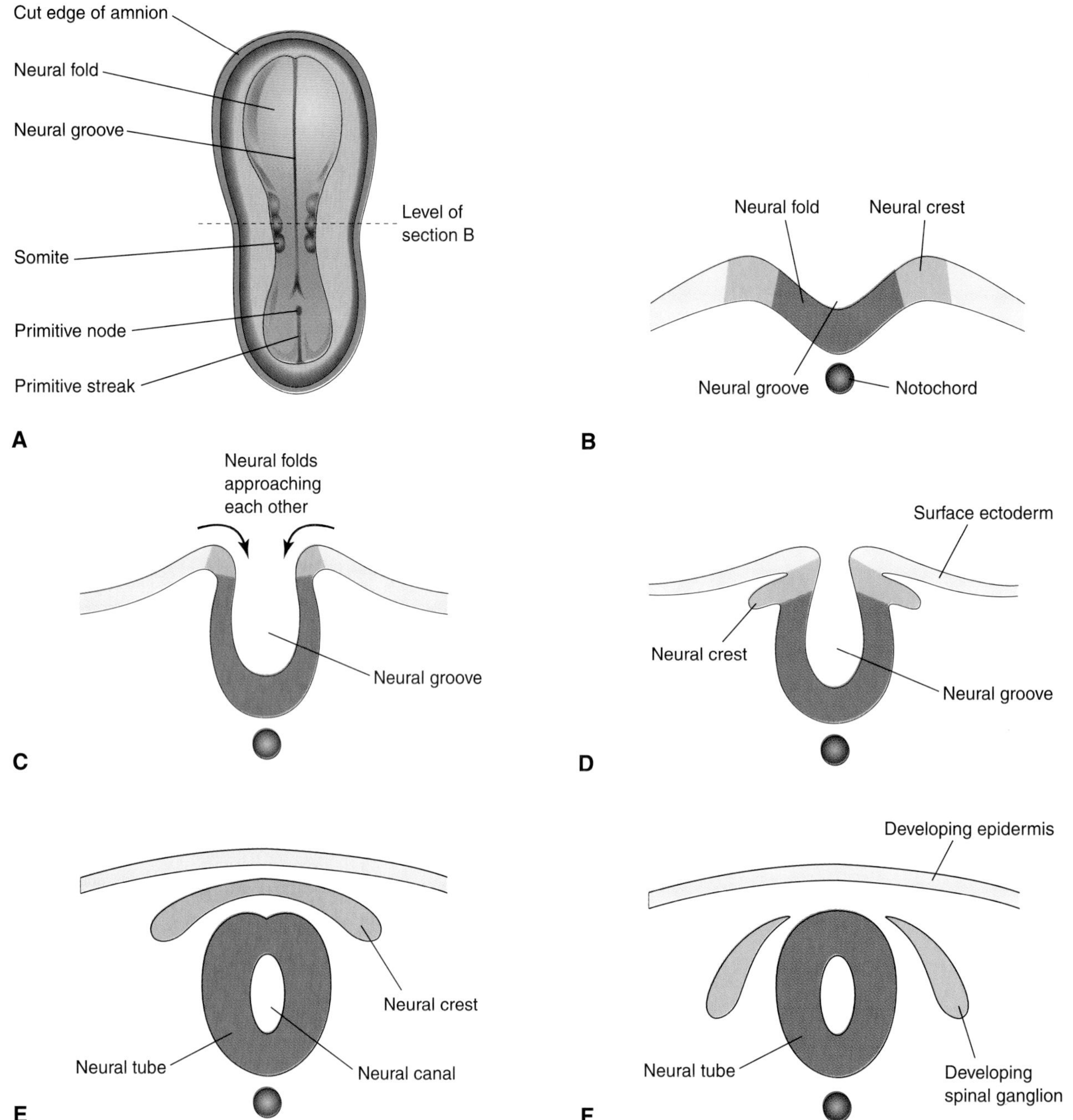

■ **Figure 4–10.** Diagrammatic transverse sections through progressively older embryos, illustrating formation of the neural groove, neural tube, and neural crest.

the developing neural tube (Fig. 4-9*C* to *F*). About 38 pairs of somites form during the *somite period of development* (days 20 to 30). By the end of the fifth week, 42 to 44 pairs of somites are present. The somites form distinct surface elevations on the embryo and are somewhat triangular in transverse section (Fig. 4-9*C* to *F*). An unimportant slitlike cavity, the myocoele, appears within each somite but soon disappears. Because the somites are so prominent during the fourth and fifth weeks, they are used as one of several criteria for determining an embryo's age (see Chapter 5, Table 5-1).

The somites first appear in the future occipital region of the embryo. They soon develop craniocaudally and give rise to most of the *axial skeleton* (bones of the cranium, vertebral column, ribs, and sternum) and associated musculature, as well as to the adjacent dermis of the skin (see Chapters 15, 16, and 20). The first pair of somites appears at the end of the third week (Fig. 4-9*C*) a short distance caudal to the cranial end of the notochord. Subsequent pairs form in a craniocaudal sequence.

DEVELOPMENT OF INTRAEMBRYONIC COELOM

The primordium of the intraembryonic coelom (embryonic body cavity) appears as small, isolated *coe-*

lomic spaces or vesicles in the lateral mesoderm and cardiogenic (heart-forming) mesoderm (Fig. 4-9*A*). These spaces soon coalesce to form a single horseshoe-shaped cavity, the **intraembryonic coelom** (Fig. 4-9*E*), which divides the lateral mesoderm into two layers (Fig. 4-9*D*):

- a somatic or *parietal layer* continuous with the extraembryonic mesoderm covering the amnion
- a splanchnic or *visceral layer* continuous with the extraembryonic mesoderm covering the yolk sac

The somatic mesoderm and overlying embryonic ectoderm form the embryonic body wall or **somatopleure** (Fig. 4-9*F*), whereas the splanchnic mesoderm and underlying embryonic endoderm form the embryonic gut wall or **splanchnopleure**. During the second month, the intraembryonic coelom is divided into three body cavities:

- *pericardial cavity*
- *pleural cavities*
- *peritoneal cavity*

For a description of these divisions of the intraembryonic coelom, see Chapter 9.

EARLY DEVELOPMENT OF CARDIOVASCULAR SYSTEM

At the beginning of the third week, **angiogenesis** (Gr. *angeion*, vessel, + *genesis*, production), or blood vessel formation, begins in the extraembryonic mesoderm of the yolk sac, connecting stalk, and chorion (Fig.

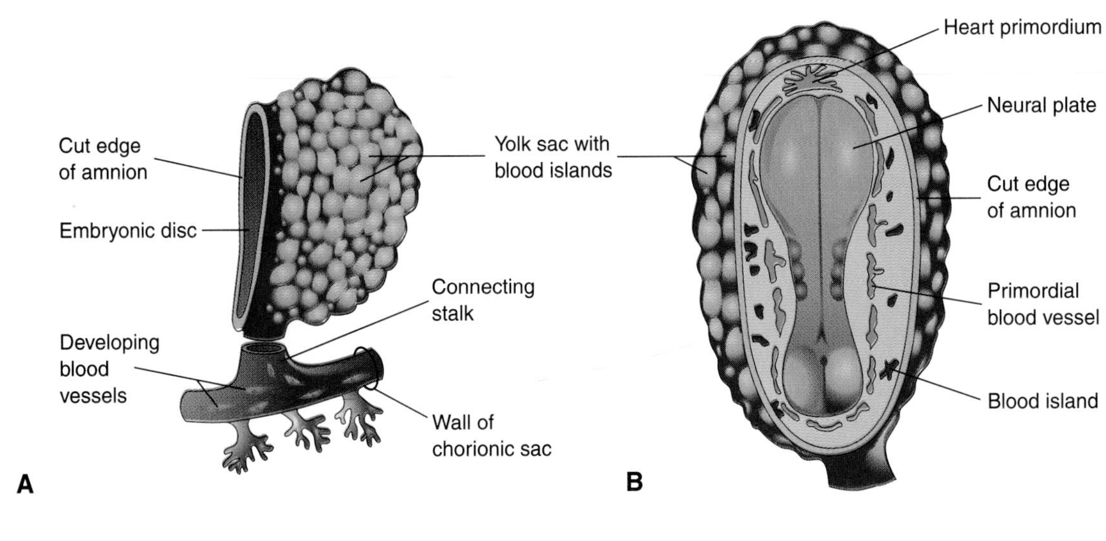

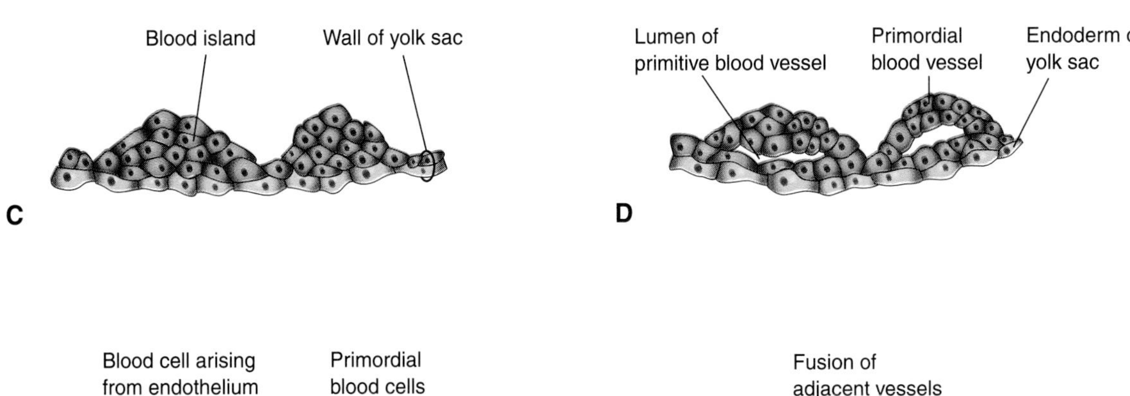

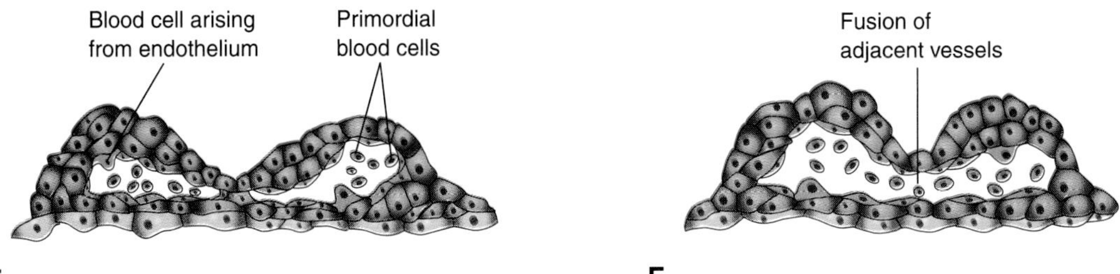

■ **Figure 4–11.** Successive stages in the development of blood and blood vessels. *A,* Lateral view of the yolk sac and part of the chorionic sac (about 18 days). *B,* Dorsal view of the embryo exposed by removing the amnion. *C* to *F,* Sections of blood islands showing progressive stages in the development of blood and blood vessels.

4-11). Embryonic blood vessels begin to develop about 2 days later. The early formation of the cardiovascular system is correlated with the absence of a significant amount of yolk in the ovum and yolk sac, and the consequent urgent need for blood vessels to bring oxygen and nourishment to the embryo from the maternal circulation through the placenta. At the end of the second week, embryonic nutrition is obtained from the maternal blood by diffusion through the extraembryonic coelom and yolk sac. During the third week a primordial uteroplacental circulation develops (Fig. 4-12).

Angiogenesis and Hematogenesis

Blood vessel formation (angiogenesis) in the embryo and extraembryonic membranes during the third week may be summarized as follows (Fig. 4-11):

- Mesenchymal cells, **angioblasts** — vessel-forming cell — aggregate to form isolated angiogenic cell clusters — the **blood islands**.
- Small cavities appear within the blood islands by confluence of intercellular clefts.
- Angioblasts flatten to form endothelial cells that arrange themselves around the cavities in the blood island to form the endothelium.
- These endothelial-lined cavities soon fuse to form networks of endothelial channels.
- Vessels extend into adjacent areas by endothelial budding and fusion with other vessels.

Blood cells develop from the endothelial cells (*hemocytoblasts*) as the vessels develop in the walls of the yolk sac and allantois at the end of the third week (Fig. 4-11*E* and *F*). Blood formation does not begin in the embryo until the fifth week. It occurs first in various parts of the embryonic mesenchyme, chiefly the

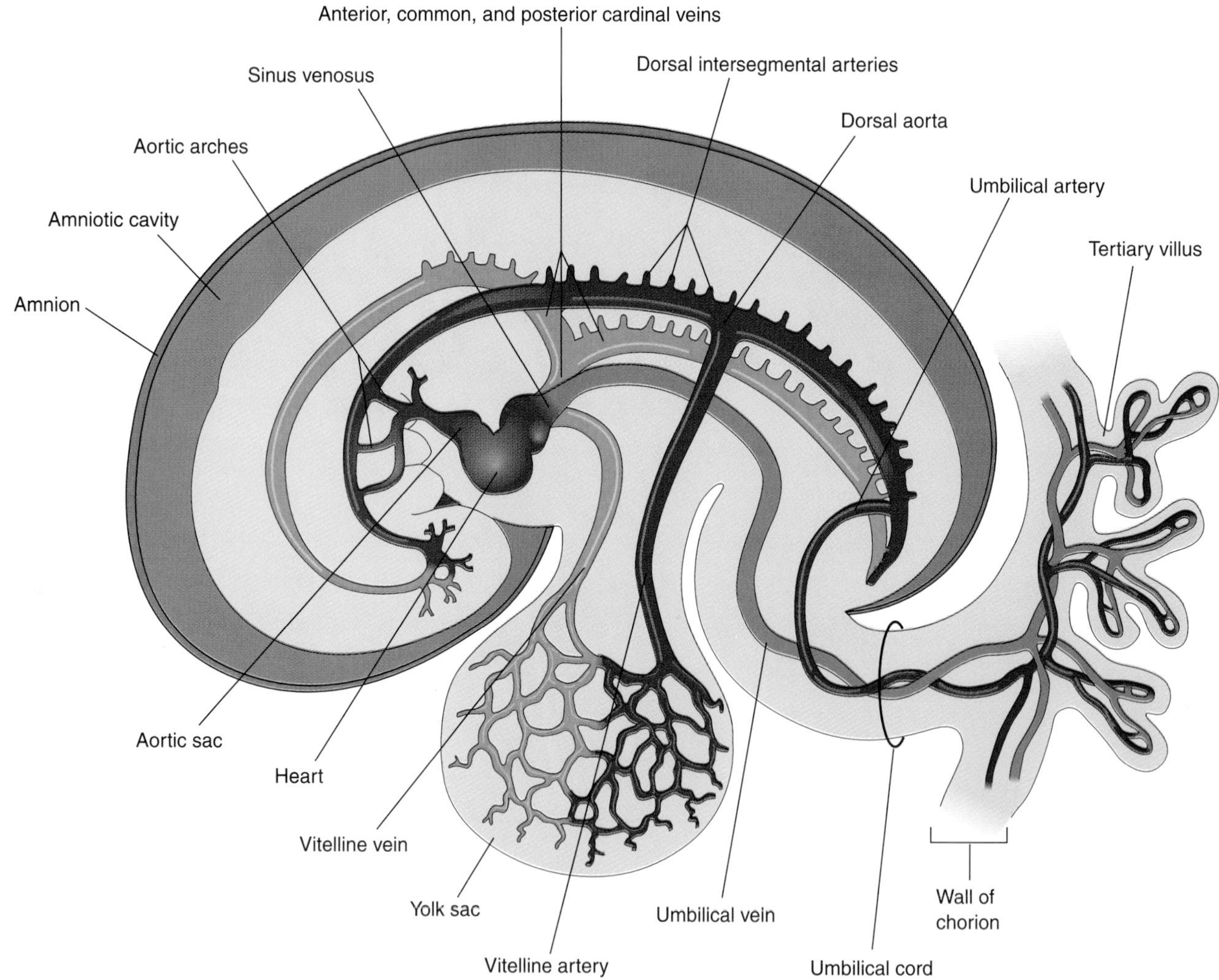

■ **Figure 4-12.** Diagram of the primordial cardiovascular system in an embryo of about 21 days, viewed from the left side. Observe the transitory stage of paired symmetrical vessels. Each heart tube continues dorsally into a dorsal aorta that passes caudally. Branches of the aortae are: (1) umbilical arteries, establishing connections with vessels in the chorion; (2) vitelline arteries to the yolk sac; and (3) dorsal intersegmental arteries to the body of the embryo. The umbilical vein returns well-oxygenated blood from the chorion. Vessels on the yolk sac form a vascular plexus that is connected to the heart tubes by vitelline veins. The cardinal veins return blood from the body of the embryo. The umbilical vein carries oxygenated blood and nutrients from the chorion. The arteries carry poorly oxygenated blood and waste products to the chorionic villi for transfer to the mother's blood.

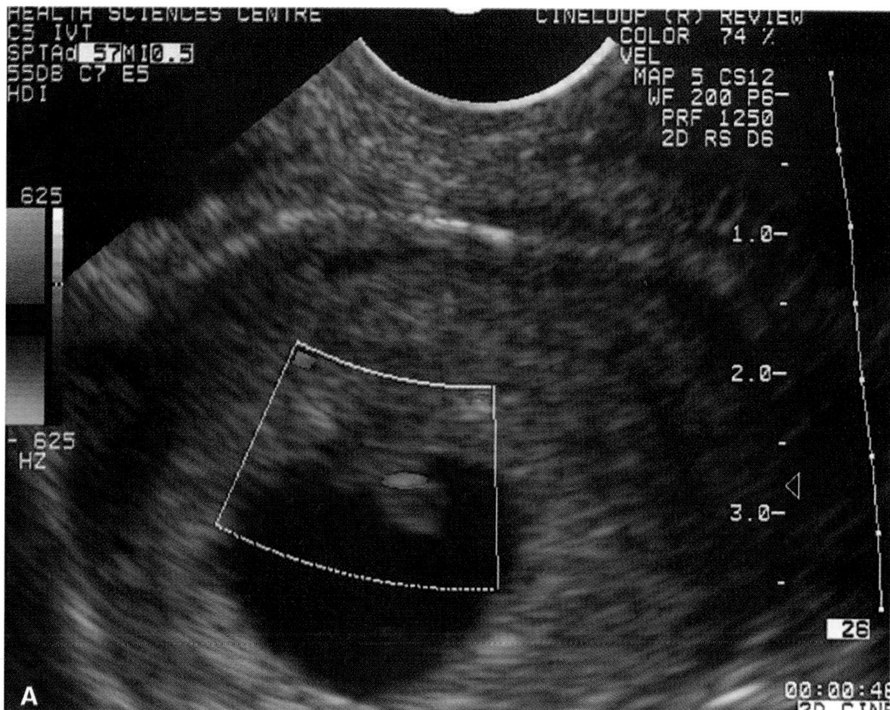

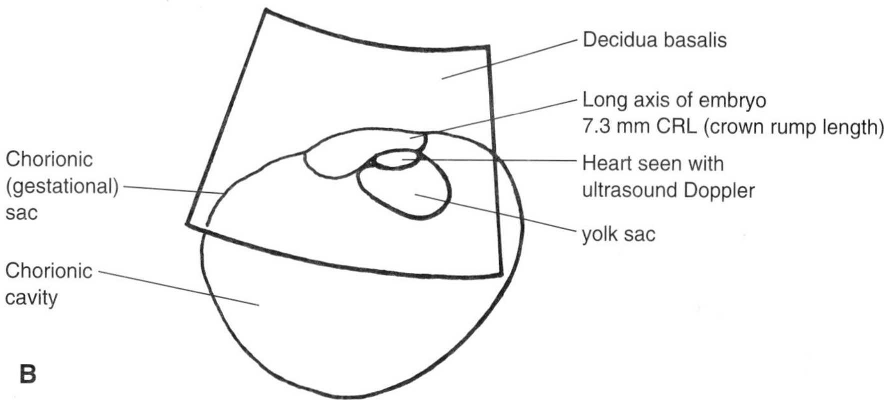

■ **Figure 4-13.** *A,* Sonogram of a 5-week embryo (7.2 mm) and its attached yolk sac within its chorionic (gestational) sac. The red pulsating heart of the embryo was visualized using Doppler ultrasound. *B,* Sketch of the sonogram for orientation and identification of structures. (Courtesy of E.A. Lyons, MD, Professor of Radiology and Obstetrics and Gynecology, Health Sciences Centre, University of Manitoba, Winnipeg, Manitoba, Canada.)

liver, and later in the spleen, bone marrow, and lymph nodes. Fetal and adult erythrocytes are probably derived from different hematopoietic precursors (Nakano et al., 1996). The mesenchymal cells surrounding the primordial endothelial blood vessels differentiate into the muscular and connective tissue elements of the vessels (for details, see Schwartz et al., 1990 and Navaratnam, 1991).

Primordial Cardiovascular System

The heart and great vessels form from mesenchymal cells in the cardiogenic area (Fig. 4-11*B*). Paired, longitudinal endothelial-lined channels — the **endocardial heart tubes** — develop during the third week and fuse to form a primitive **heart tube**. The tubular heart joins with blood vessels in the embryo, connecting stalk, chorion, and yolk sac to form a primordial cardiovascular system (Fig. 4-12). By the end of the third week, the blood is circulating and the heart begins to beat on the twenty-first or twenty-second day (about 5 weeks after LNMP). The cardiovascular system is thus the first organ system to reach a functional state. The embryonic heartbeat can be detected ultrasonographically using Doppler technology during the fifth week, about 7 weeks after LNMP (Fig. 4-13).

FURTHER DEVELOPMENT OF CHORIONIC VILLI

Shortly after the **primary chorionic villi** appear at the end of the second week, they begin to branch. Early in the third week, mesenchyme grows into the primary villi, forming a core of loose mesenchymal (connective) tissue. The villi at this stage — **secondary chorionic villi** — cover the entire surface of the chorionic sac (Fig. 4-14*A* and *B*). Some mesenchymal cells in the villi soon differentiate into capillaries and

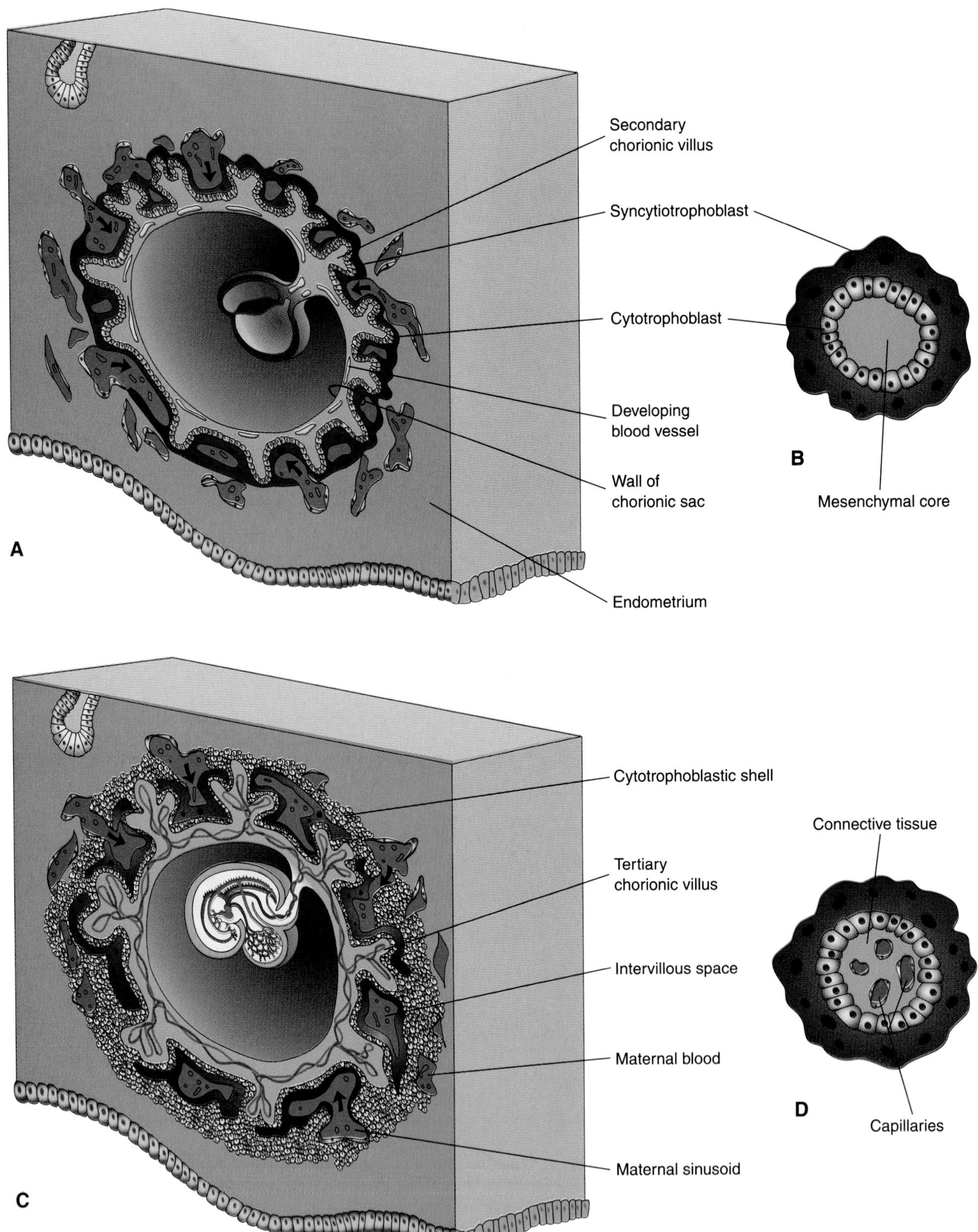

■ **Figure 4–14.** Diagrams illustrating development of secondary chorionic villi into tertiary chorionic villi. Early formation of the placenta is also shown. *A,* Sagittal section of an embryo (about 16 days). *B,* Section of a secondary chorionic villus. *C,* Section of an implanted embryo (about 21 days). *D,* Section of a tertiary chorionic villus. The fetal blood in the capillaries is separated from the maternal blood surrounding the villus by the placental membrane, composed of the endothelium of the capillary, embryonic connective tissue, cytotrophoblast, and syncytiotrophoblast.

blood cells (Fig. 4-14*C* and *D*). They are **tertiary chorionic villi** when blood vessels are visible in the villi. The capillaries in the chorionic villi fuse to form **arteriocapillary networks**, which soon become connected with the embryonic heart through vessels that differentiate in the mesenchyme of the chorion and connecting stalk (Fig. 4-12). By the end of the third week, embryonic blood begins to flow slowly through the capillaries in the chorionic villi. Oxygen and nutrients in the maternal blood in the intervillous space diffuse through the walls of the villi and enter the embryo's blood (Fig. 4-14*C* and *D*). Carbon dioxide and waste products diffuse from blood in the fetal capillaries through the wall of the villi into the maternal blood.

Concurrently, cytotrophoblast cells of the chorionic villi proliferate and extend through the syncytiotrophoblast to form a **cytotrophoblastic shell** (Fig. 4-14*C*), which gradually surrounds the chorionic sac and attaches it to the endometrium. Villi that attach to the maternal tissues through the cytotrophoblastic shell are **stem villi** (anchoring villi). The villi that grow from the sides of the stem villi are **branch villi** (terminal villi). It is through the walls of the branch villi that the main exchange of material between the blood of the mother and the embryo takes place. The branch villi are bathed in continually changing maternal blood in the intervillous space.

Abnormal Growth of Trophoblast

Sometimes the embryo dies and the chorionic villi do not complete their development, that is, they do not become vascularized to form tertiary villi. These degenerating villi soon form cystic swellings—**hydatidiform moles**—which resemble a bunch of grapes (Copeland, 1993). The mole exhibits variable degrees of trophoblastic proliferation and produces excessive amounts of hCG. Complete hydatidiform moles are of paternal origin. Three to five per cent of moles develop into malignant trophoblastic lesions—**choriocarcinomas**. Some moles develop after spontaneous abortions and others occur after normal deliveries. Choriocarcinomas invariably metastasize (spread) by way of the bloodstream to various sites, such as the lungs, vagina, liver, bone, intestine, and brain (Berkowitz and Goldstein, 1996).

The main mechanisms for development of complete hydatidiform moles are:

- fertilization of an empty oocyte by a sperm, followed by duplication (monospermic mole)
- fertilization of an empty oocyte by two sperms (dispermic mole).

A complete (monospermic) hydatidiform mole results from fertilization of an oocyte in which the female pronucleus is absent or inactive—an empty oocyte. A *partial (dispermic) hydatidiform mole* usually results from fertilization of an oocyte by two sperms (dispermy). More than 90% of complete hydatidiform moles are monospermic (Wake et al., 1984). For both types, the genetic origin of the nuclear DNA is paternal.

SUMMARY OF THE THIRD WEEK OF DEVELOPMENT

Major changes occur in the embryo as the bilaminar embryonic disc is converted into a trilaminar embryonic disc during **gastrulation.** These changes begin with the appearance of the primitive streak.

Primitive Streak

The primitive streak appears at the beginning of the third week as a localized thickening of the epiblast at the caudal end of the embryonic disc. The primitive streak results from migration of epiblastic cells to the median plane of the embryonic disc. Invagination of epiblastic cells from the primitive streak gives rise to mesenchymal cells that migrate ventrally, laterally, and cranially between the epiblast and hypoblast. As soon as the primitive streak begins to produce mesenchymal cells, the epiblast layer is known as the embryonic ectoderm. Some cells of the epiblast displace the hypoblast and form the embryonic endoderm. Mesenchymal cells produced by the primitive streak soon organize into a third germ layer, the *intraembryonic mesoderm*. Cells of the intraembryonic mesoderm migrate to the edges of the embryonic disc, where they join the *extraembryonic mesoderm* covering the amnion and yolk sac. By the end of the third week, mesoderm exists between the ectoderm and endoderm everywhere except at the oropharyngeal membrane, in the median plane occupied by the notochord, and at the cloacal membrane.

Notochord Formation

Early in the third week, mesenchymal cells arising from the primitive node of the primitive streak form the **notochordal process**, which extends cranially from the primitive node as a rod of cells between the embryonic ectoderm and endoderm. The primitive pit extends into the notochordal process and forms a *notochordal canal*. When fully developed, the notochordal process extends from the primitive node to the prechordal plate. Openings develop in the floor of the notochordal canal and soon coalesce, leaving a *notochordal plate*. The notochordal plate infolds to form the **notochord**, the primordial axis of the embryo around which the axial skeleton forms.

Neural Tube Formation

The *neural plate* appears as a thickening of the embryonic ectoderm, cranial to the primitive node. The neural plate is induced to form by the developing notochord. A longitudinal *neural groove* develops in the neural plate, which is flanked by *neural folds*. Fusion of the folds forms the neural tube, the primordium of the central nervous system. The process of neural plate formation and its infolding to form the neural tube is called *neurulation*.

Neural Crest Formation

As the neural folds fuse to form the neural tube, neuroectodermal cells migrate dorsolaterally to form a neural crest between the surface ectoderm and the neural tube. The neural crest soon divides into two cell masses that give rise to the sensory ganglia of the cranial and spinal nerves. Other neural crest cells migrate from the neural tube and give rise to various other structures, the retina for example (see Chapter 5).

Somite Formation

The mesoderm on each side of the notochord thickens to form longitudinal columns of paraxial mesoderm. Division of these paraxial columns into pairs of somites begins cranially by the end of the third week. The somites are compact aggregates of mesenchymal cells from which cells migrate to give rise to the vertebrae, ribs, and axial musculature. During the third week the number of somites present is an indicator of the age of the embryo.

Formation of Intraembryonic Coelom

The coelom (body cavity) within the embryo arises as isolated spaces or vesicles in the lateral mesoderm and cardiogenic mesoderm. The coelomic vesicles subsequently coalesce to form a single, horseshoe-shaped cavity that eventually gives rise to the body cavities, the peritoneal cavity, for example.

Formation of Blood Vessels and Blood

Blood vessels first appear in the wall of the yolk sac, allantois, and in the chorion. They develop within the embryo shortly thereafter. Spaces appear within aggregations of mesenchyme, known as *blood islands*. The spaces soon become lined with endothelium derived from the mesenchymal cells. These primordial vessels unite with other vessels to form a *primordial cardiovascular system*. Toward the end of the third week, the heart is represented by paired endothelial heart tubes that are joined to blood vessels in the embryo and in the extraembryonic membranes (yolk sac, umbilical cord, and chorionic sac). By the end of the third week, the endothelial heart tubes have fused to form a tubular heart that is joined to vessels in the embryo, yolk sac, chorion, and connecting stalk to form a *primordial cardiovascular system*. The primordial blood cells — hemocytoblasts — are derived mainly from the endothelial cells of blood vessels in the walls of the yolk sac and allantois. Fetal and adult erythrocytes probably develop from different hematopoietic precursors.

Completion of Chorionic Villi Formation

Primary chorionic villi become secondary chorionic villi as they acquire mesenchymal cores. Before the end of the third week capillaries develop in the *secondary chorionic villi,* transforming them into tertiary chorionic villi. Cytotrophoblastic extensions from these stem villi join to form a **cytotrophoblastic shell** that anchors the chorionic sac to the endometrium. The rapid development of chorionic villi during the third week greatly increases the surface area of the chorion for the exchange of oxygen and nutrients and other substances between the maternal and embryonic circulations.

Clinically Oriented Problems

Case 4–1

A 30-year-old woman became pregnant 2 months after discontinuing use of birth control pills. About three weeks later she had an early spontaneous abortion.

- How do the hormones in these pills affect the ovarian and menstrual cycles?
- What might have caused the abortion?
- What would the physician likely have told this patient?

Case 4–2

A 25-year-old woman with a history of regular menstrual cycles was 5 days overdue on menses. Owing to her mental distress related to the abnormal bleeding and the undesirability of a possible pregnancy, the doctor decided to do a menstrual extraction or uterine evacuation. The tissue removed was examined for evidence of a pregnancy.

- Would a highly sensitive radioimmune assay have detected pregnancy at this early stage?
- What findings would indicate an early pregnancy?
- How old would the products of conception be?

Case 4–3

A woman who had just missed her menstrual period was concerned that a glass of wine she had consumed the week before may have harmed her embryo.

- What major organ systems undergo early development during the third week?
- What severe congenital anomaly might result from teratological factors (see Chapter 8) acting during this period of development?

Case 4–4

A female infant was born with a large tumor situated between her rectum and sacrum. A diagnosis of *sacrococcygeal teratoma* was made and the mass was surgically removed.

- What is the probable embryological origin of this tumor?
- Explain why these tumors often contain various types of tissue derived from all three germ layers.

- Does an infant's sex make him or her more susceptible to the development of one of these tumors?

Case 4–5

A woman with a history of early spontaneous abortions had an ultrasound examination to determine if her embryo was still implanted.

- Is ultrasonography any value in assessing pregnancy during the third week?
- What structures might be recognizable?
- If a pregnancy test is negative, is it safe to assume that the woman is not pregnant?
- Could an extrauterine gestation be present?

Discussion of these problems appears at the back of the book.

REFERENCES AND SUGGESTED READING

Adra A, Cordero D, Mejldes A, et al: Caudal regression syndrome: etiopathogenesis, prenatal diagnosis, and prenatal management. *Obstet Gynecol Surv 49:*508, 1994.

Amaya E, Musci TJ, Kirschner AW: Expression of a dominant negative mutant of the FGF receptor disrupts mesoderm formation in Xenopus embryos. *Cell 66:*257, 1991.

Anderson CK, Deiter RW, Motz MJ, Goldstein JA: Complete hydatidiform mole with a coexistent healthy, viable fetus near term. *J Reprod Med 41:*55, 1996.

Avery ME, Taeusch, HW (eds): *Schaffer's Diseases of the Newborn,* 5th ed. Philadelphia, WB Saunders, 1984.

Beddington RSP: The origin of the foetal tissues during gastrulation in the rodent. *In* Johnson MH (ed): *Development in Mammals.* New York, Elsevier, 1983.

Bellairs R, Sanders EJ, Lash JW (eds): *Formation and Differentiation of Early Embryonic Mesoderm.* New York, Plenum, 1992.

Berkowitz RS, Goldstein DP: Chorionic tumors. *N Engl J Med 335:* 1740, 1996.

Bessis M: The blood cells and their formation. In Brachet J, Mirsky AE (eds): *The Cell,* vol 5. New York, Academic Press, 1961.

Bianchi DW, Wilkins-Haug LE, Enders AC, Hay ED: Origin of extraembryonic mesoderm in experimental animals: relevance to chorionic mosaicism in humans. *Am J Med Genet 46:*542, 1993.

Boué J, Boué A, Lazar P: Retrospective and prospective epidemiological studies of 1500 karyotyped spontaneous abortions. *Teratology 12:*11, 1975.

Callen PW: *Ultrasonography in Obstetrics and Gynecology,* 3rd ed. Philadelphia, WB Saunders, 1994, p 615.

Callen PW: Ultrasound evaluation of gestational trophoblastic disease. *In* Callen PW (ed): Ultrasonography in Obstetrics and Gynecology, 3rd ed. Philadelphia, WB Saunders, 1994.

Candia AF, Hu J, Crosby J, et al: Mox-1 and Mox-2 define a novel homeobox gene subfamily and are differentially exposed during early mesodermal patterning in mouse embryos. *Development 116:*1123, 1992.

Carlson BM: *Human Embryology and Developmental Biology.* St Louis, Mosby, 1994.

Carr DH: Chromosomes and abortion. *Adv Hum Genet 2:*201, 1971.

Cooke J: The early embryo and the formation of body pattern. *American Scientist 76:*35, 1988.

Copeland LJ (ed): *Textbook of Gynecology.* Philadelphia, WB Saunders, 1993.

Enders AC, King BF: Formation and differentiation of extraembryonic tissue in the rhesus monkey. *Am J Anat 181:*327, 1988.

Filly RA: The fetus with a CNS malformation: Ultrasound evaluation. *In* Harrison MR, Golbus MS, Filly RA (eds): *The Unborn Patient. Prenatal Diagnosis and Treatment,* 2nd ed. Philadelphia, WB Saunders, 1991.

Filly RA: Ectopic pregnancy. *In* Callen PW (ed): *Ultrasonography in Obstetrics and Gynecology,* 3rd ed. Philadelphia, WB Saunders, 1994.

Garcia-Martinez V, Darnell DK, Lopez-Sanchez C, et al: State of commitment of prospective neural plate and prospective mesoderm in late gastrula/early neural stages of avian embryos. *Dev Biol 181:* 102, 1997.

Gilbert SF: *Developmental Biology,* 5th ed. Sunderland, Sinauer Associates, 1997.

Gordon R, Björklund NK, Nieuwkoop PD: Appendix: dialogue on embryonic induction and differentiation waves. *Int Rev Cytol 150:* 373, 1994.

Gravenson AC: Neural crest contributions to the development of the vertebrate head. *Am Zool 33:*424, 1993.

Greenberg F, James LM, Oakley GP: Estimates of birth prevalence rates of spina bifida in the United States from computer generated maps. *Am J Obstet Gynecol 145:*570, 1983.

Guthrie S: Horizontal and vertical pathways in neural induction. *Trends Neurosc 14:*123, 1991.

Hall BK, Hörstadius S: *The Neural Crest.* Oxford, Oxford University Press, 1988.

Hamilton WJ, Boyd JD: Development of the human placenta. *In* Philipp EE, Barnes J, Newton M (eds): *Scientific Foundations of Obstetrics and Gynecology.* London, William Heinemann, 1970.

Hertig AT: Angiogenesis in the early human chorion and in the primary placenta of the macaque monkey. *Contrib Embryol Carnegie Inst 25:*37, 1935.

Holzgreve W, Flake AW, Langer JC: The fetus with sacrococcygeal teratoma. *In* Harrison MR, Golbus MS, Filly RA (eds): *The Unborn Patient. Prenatal Diagnosis and Treatment,* 2nd ed. Philadelphia, WB Saunders, 1991.

Horowitz T: *The Human Notochord. A Study of Its Development and Regression, Variations and Pathogenic Derivative, Chordoma.* Indianapolis, Limited Private Printing, 1977.

Jacobson AG, Sater AK: Features of embryonic induction. *Development 104:*341, 1988.

Jacobson M: *Developmental Neurobiology,* 2nd ed. New York, Plenum Press, 1989.

Keller R, Danilchick M: Regional expression, pattern and timing of convergence and extension during gastrulation of Xenopus laevis. *Development 103:*193, 1988.

Kratochwil K: Embryonic induction. *In* Yamada KM (ed): *Cell Interactions and Development.* New York, John Wiley & Sons, 1982.

Kurtz AB, Needleman L: Ultrasound assessment of fetal age. *In* Callen PW (ed): *Ultrasonography in Obstetrics and Gynecology,* 2nd ed. Philadelphia, WB Saunders, 1988.

Lecuit T, Brook WJ, Ng M, et al: Two distinct mechanisms for long-range patterning by Decapentaplegic in Drosophilia wing. *Nature 381:*387, 1996.

Luton D, Sibony O, Oury JF, et al: The C-24ets 1 protooncogene is expressed in human trophoblast during the first trimester of pregnancy. *Early Hum Dev 47:*147, 1997.

Luckett WP: Origin and differentiation of the yolk sac and extraembryonic mesoderm in presomite human and rhesus monkey embryos. *Am J Anat 152:*59, 1978.

Marina N: Gonadal and germ cell neoplasms. *In* Behrman RE, Kliegman RM, Arvin AM (eds): *Nelson Textbook of Pediatrics,* 15th ed. Philadelphia, WB Saunders, 1996.

Marx J: How embryos tell heads from tails. *Science 254:*1586, 1991.

Moore KL, Agur AMR: *Essential Clinical Anatomy.* Baltimore, Williams & Wilkins, 1995.

Nakano T, Kodama H, Hojo T: In vitro development of primitive and definitive erythrocytes from different precursors. *Science 272:*772, 1996.

Navaratnam V: Organization and reorganization of blood vessels in embryonic development. *Eye 5(Pt 2):*147, 1991.

Nieuwkoop PD, Albers B: The role of competence in the craniocaudal segregation of the central nervous system. *Develop Growth & Differ 32:*23, 1990.

Noden DM: Spatial integration among cells forming the cranial peripheral neurons. *J Neurobiol 24:*248, 1993.

O'Connor JF, Birken S, Lustbader JW, et al: Recent advances in the chemistry and immunochemistry of human chorionic gonadotropin: impact on clinical measurements. *Endocr Rev 15:*650, 1994.

O'Rahilly R: The manifestation of the axes of the human embryo. *Z Anat Entwicklungsgesch 132:*50, 1970.

O'Rahilly R, Müller F: *Developmental Stages in Human Embryos.* Washington, Carnegie Institute of Washington, 1987.

Placzek M, Tessier-Lavigne M, Yamada T, et al: Mesodermal control of neural cell identity: floor plate induction by the notochord. *Science 250:*985, 1990.

Rohrer H: The role of growth factors in the control of neurogenesis. *Eur J Neurosci 2:*1005, 1990.

Rubin R, Farber JL: *Pathology*. Philadelphia, JB Lippincott, 1988.

Salisbury JR, Deverell MH, Cookson MJ, Whimster WF: Three-dimensional reconstruction of human embryonic notochords: clue to pathogenesis of chordoma. *J Pathol 17:*59, 1993.

Sasai U, DeRobertis EM: Ectodermal patterning in vertebrate embryos. *Dev Biol 182:*5, 1997.

Sausedo RA, Schoenwolf GC: Quantitative analyses of cell behaviors underlying notochord formation and extension in mouse embryos. *Anat Rec 239:*103, 1994.

Schoenwolf GC, Smith JL: Mechanisms of neurulation: traditional viewpoint and recent advances. *Development 109:*243, 1990.

Schwartz SM, Heimark RL, Majesky MW: Developmental mechanisms underlying pathology of arteries. *Physiol Rev 70:*117, 1990.

Slack JMW: We have a morphogen! *Nature 327:*553, 1987.

Smith J: How to tell a cell where it is. *Nature 381:*367, 1996.

Smith JL, Schoenwolf GC: Further evidence of extrinsic forces in bending of the neural plate. *J Comp Neurol 307:*225, 1991.

Springer M: Die Canalis neurentericus beim Menschen. *Z Kinderchir 11:*183, 1972.

Tabin CJ: Retinoids, homeoboxes, and growth factors: toward molecular models for limb development. *Cell 66:*199, 1991.

Wake N, Seki T, Fujita H, et al: Malignant potential of homozygous and heterozygous complete moles. *Cancer Res 44:*1226, 1984.

Weston JA: Regulation of neural crest cell migration and differentiation. *In* Yamada KM (ed): *Cell Interactions and Development*. New York, John Wiley & Sons, 1982.

Wilson KM: A normal human ovum of 16 days development, the Rochester ovum. *Contrib Embryol Carnegie Inst 31:*103, 1945.

Wolpert L: *The Triumph of the Embryo*. Oxford, Oxford University Press, 1991.

Yuan S, Darnell DK, Schoenwolf GC: Identification of inducing, responding, and suppressing regions in an experimental model of notochord formation in avian embryos. *Dev Biol 172:*567, 1995.

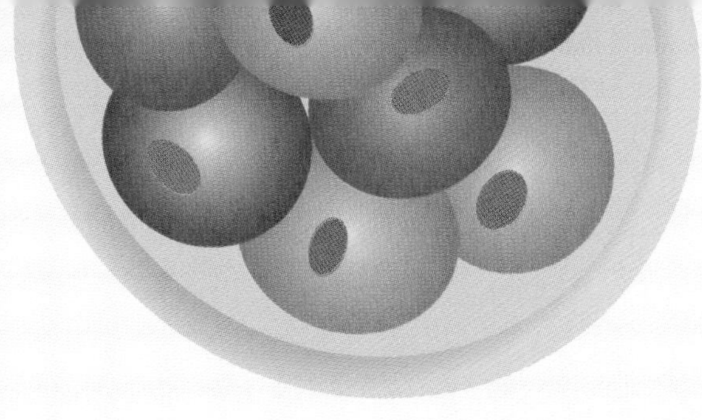

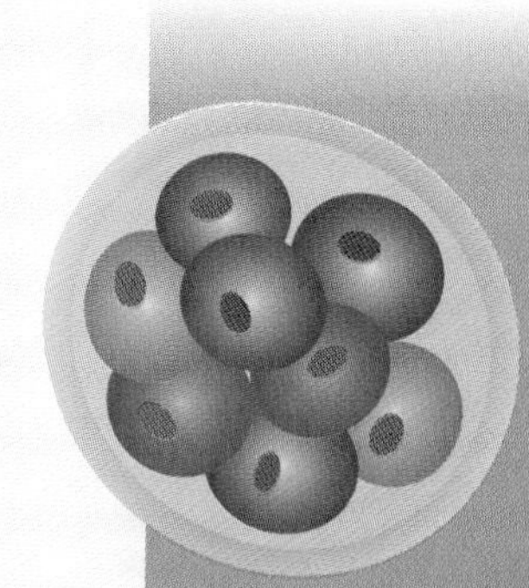

Organogenetic Period: The Fourth to Eighth Weeks

5

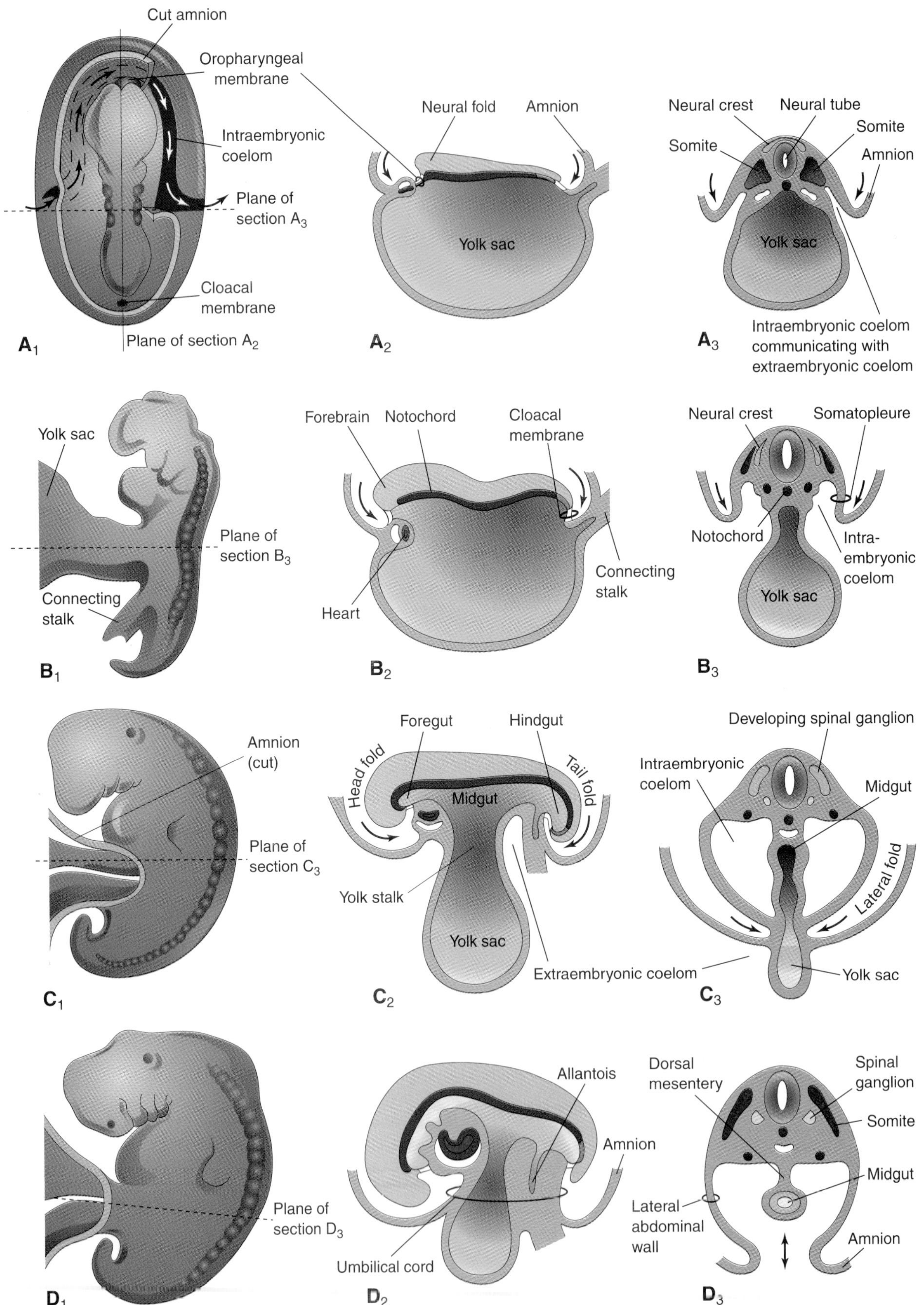

■ **Figure 5–1.** Drawings illustrating folding of embryos during the fourth week. A_1, Dorsal view of an embryo at the beginning of the fourth week. Three pairs of somites are visible. The continuity of the intraembryonic coelom and extraembryonic coelom is illustrated on the right side by removal of a part of the embryonic ectoderm and mesoderm. B_1, C_1, and D_1, Lateral views of embryos at 22, 26 and 28 days, respectively. A_2 to D_2, Sagittal sections at the plane shown in A_1. A_3 to D_3, Transverse sections at the levels indicated in A_1 to D_1.

■ The fourth to eight weeks of development constitute most of the embryonic period; however, critical developmental events also occur during the first three weeks, such as *cleavage of the zygote, blastogenesis,* and early development of the nervous and cardiovascular systems. All major external and internal structures are established during fourth to eighth weeks. By the end of this **organogenetic period**, all the main organ systems have begun to develop; however, the function of most of them is minimal, except for the cardiovascular system. As the tissues and organs form, the shape of the embryo changes so that by the eighth week it has a distinctly human appearance.

PHASES OF EMBRYONIC DEVELOPMENT

Human development may be divided into three phases, which to some extent are interrelated:

- The first phase of development is **growth** (increase in size), which involves cell division and the elaboration of cell products.
- The second phase of development is **morphogenesis** (development of form), which includes mass cell movements. Morphogenesis is an elaborate process during which many complex interactions occur in an orderly sequence (Cooke, 1988; Wolpert, 1991). The movement of cells allows them to interact with each other during the formation of tissues and organs.
- The third phase of development is **differentiation** (maturation of physiological processes). Completion of differentiation results in the formation of tissues and organs that are capable of performing specialized functions.

Because the tissues and organ systems are developing rapidly during the fourth to eighth weeks, exposure of embryos to teratogens during this period may cause major congenital anomalies. **Teratogens** are agents such as drugs and viruses that produce or raise the incidence of congenital anomalies (see Chapter 8). Teratogens act during the stage of active differentiation of a tissue or organ.

FOLDING OF THE EMBRYO

A significant event in the establishment of body form is folding of the flat trilaminar embryonic disc into a somewhat cylindrical embryo (Fig. 5-1). Folding occurs in both the median and horizontal planes and results from rapid growth of the embryo, particularly of its brain and spinal cord (central nervous system). The growth rate at the sides of the embryonic disc fails to keep pace with the rate of growth in the long axis as the embryo increases rapidly in length. As a result, folding of the embryo occurs. Folding at the cranial and caudal ends and sides of the embryo occurs simultaneously. Concurrently, there is relative constriction at the junction of the embryo and yolk sac.

Folding of the Embryo in the Median Plane

Folding of the ends of the embryo ventrally produces head and tail folds that result in the cranial and caudal

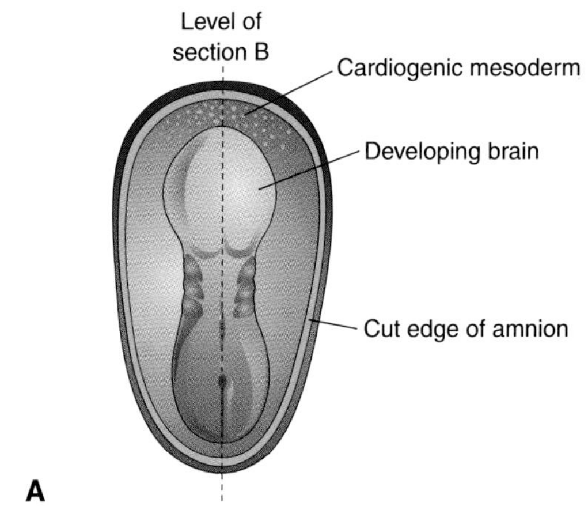

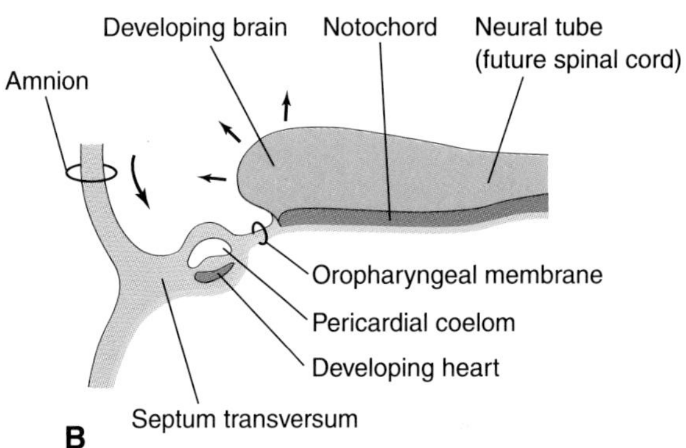

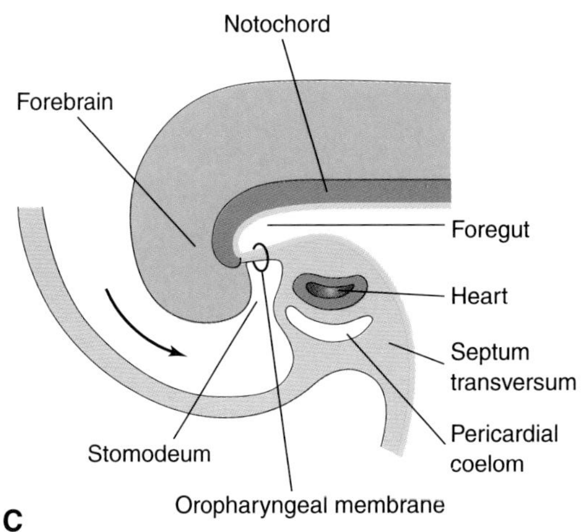

■ **Figure 5-2.** Folding of the cranial end of the embryo. *A,* Dorsal view of an embryo at 21 days. *B,* Sagittal section of the cranial part of the embryo at the plane shown in *A.* Observe the ventral movement of the heart. *C,* Sagittal section of an embryo at 26 days. Note that the septum transversum, heart, pericardial coelom, and oropharyngeal membrane have moved onto the ventral surface of the embryo. Observe also that part of the yolk sac is incorporated into the embryo as the foregut.

regions move ventrally as the embryo elongates cranially and caudially (Fig. 5-1A_2 to D_2).

THE HEAD FOLD

By the beginning of the fourth week, the neural folds in the cranial region have thickened to form the primordium of the brain. Initially, the developing brain projects dorsally into the amniotic cavity. Later the developing forebrain grows cranially beyond the oropharyngeal membrane and overhangs the developing heart. Concomitantly, the **septum transversum** (transverse mesodermal septum), primordial heart, pericardial coelom, and oropharyngeal membrane move onto the ventral surface of the embryo (Fig. 5-2). During longitudinal folding, part of the endoderm of the yolk sac is incorporated into the embryo as the **foregut** (primordium of pharynx, esophagus, etc.; see Chapter 12). The foregut lies between the brain and heart and the *oropharyngeal membrane* separates the foregut from the *stomodeum* (Fig. 5-2*C*). After folding, the septum transversum lies caudal to the heart where it subsequently develops into the *central tendon of the diaphragm* (see Chapter 9). The head fold also affects the arrangement of the embryonic coelom (primordium of body cavities). Before folding, the coelom consists of a flattened, horseshoe-shaped cavity (Fig. 5-1A_1). After folding, the pericardial coelom lies ventral to the heart and cranial to the septum transversum (Fig. 5-2*C*). At this stage the intraembryonic coelom communicates widely on each side with the extraembryonic coelom (Figs. 5-1A_3 and 5-3).

THE TAIL FOLD

Folding of the caudal end of the embryo results primarily from growth of the distal part of the neural tube—the primordium of the spinal cord (Fig. 5-4). As the embryo grows, the tail region projects over the *cloacal membrane* (future site of the anus). During folding, part of the endodermal germ layer is incorporated into the embryo as the **hindgut** (primordium of the descending colon). The terminal part of the hindgut soon dilates slightly to form the **cloaca** (primordium of the urinary bladder and rectum; see Chapters 12 and 13). Before folding, the primitive streak lies cranial to the cloacal membrane (Fig. 5-4*B*); after folding, it lies caudal to it (Fig. 5-4*C*). The connecting stalk (primordium of the umbilical cord) is now attached to the ventral surface of the embryo, and the *allantois*—a diverticulum of the yolk sac—is partially incorporated into the embryo.

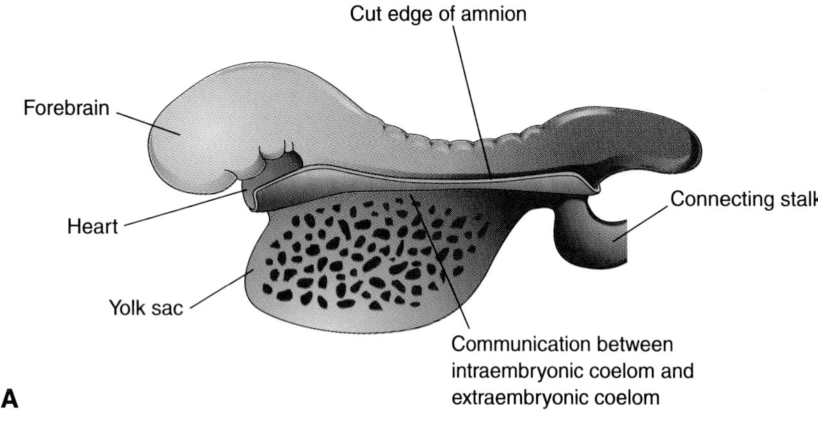

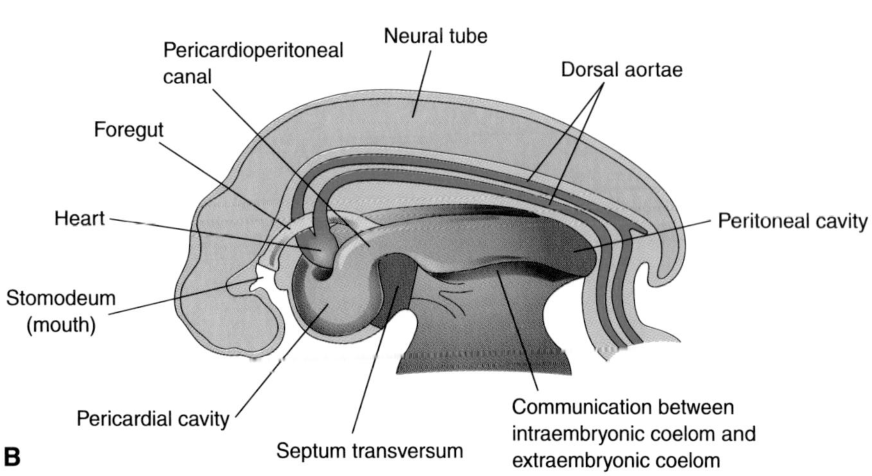

■ **Figure 5-3.** Drawings illustrating the effect of the head fold on the intraembryonic coelom. *A,* Lateral view of an embryo (24 to 25 days) during folding, showing the large forebrain, ventral position of the heart, and communication between the intraembryonic and extraembryonic parts of the coelom. *B,* Schematic drawing of an embryo (26 to 27 days) after folding, showing the pericardial cavity ventrally, the pericardioperitoneal canals running dorsally on each side of the foregut, and the peritoneal cavity (coelom) in communication with the extraembryonic coelom.

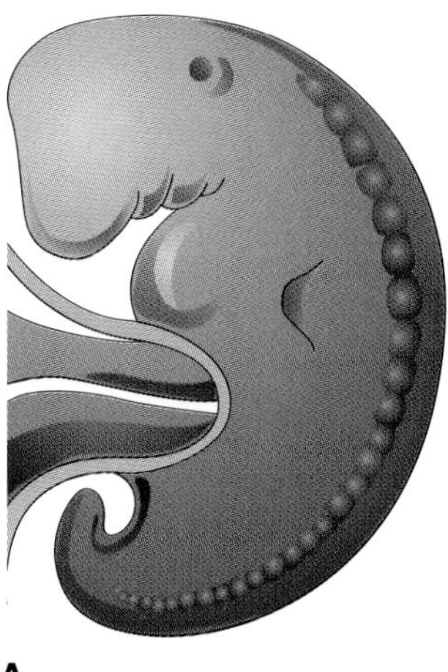

A

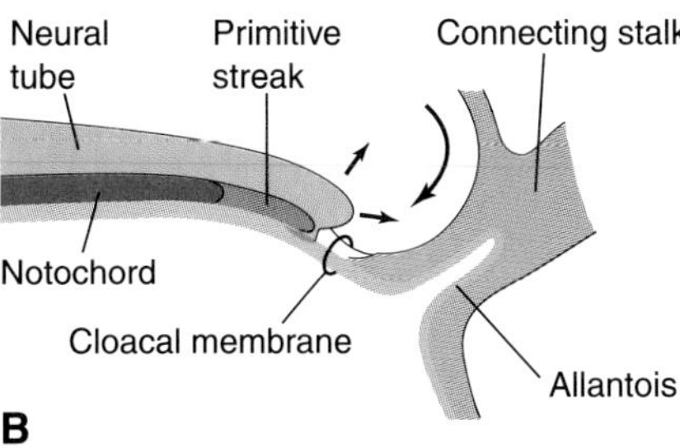

B

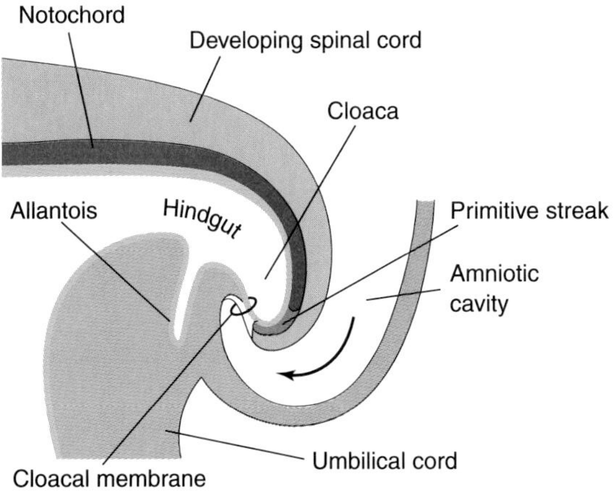

C

Figure 5-4. Folding of the caudal end of the embryo. *A,* Lateral view of a 4-week-old embryo. *B,* Sagittal section of the caudal part of the embryo at the beginning of the fourth week. *C,* Similar section at the end of the fourth week. Note that part of the yolk sac is incorporated into the embryo as the hindgut and that the terminal part of the hindgut has dilated to form the cloaca. Observe also the change in position of the primitive streak, allantois, cloacal membrane, and connecting stalk.

Folding of the Embryo in the Horizontal Plane

Folding of the sides of the embryo produces right and left **lateral folds** (Fig. 5-1A_3 to D_3). Lateral folding is produced by the rapidly growing spinal cord and somites. The primordia of the ventrolateral wall fold toward the median plane, rolling the edges of the embryonic disc ventrally and forming a roughly cylindrical embryo. As the abdominal walls form, part of the endoderm germ layer is incorporated into the embryo as the *midgut* (primordium of the small intestine, etc; see Chapter 12). Initially, there is a wide connection between the midgut and yolk sac (Fig. 5-1A_2), but after lateral folding the connection is reduced to a *yolk stalk* (Fig. 5-1C_2). The region of attachment of the amnion to the ventral surface of the embryo is also reduced to a relatively narrow umbilical region (Figs. 5-1D_2 and D_3). As the **umbilical cord** forms from the connecting stalk, ventral fusion of the lateral folds reduces the region of communication between the intraembryonic and extraembryonic coelomic cavities to a narrow communication (Fig. 5-1C_2). As the amniotic cavity expands and obliterates most of the extraembryonic coelom, the amnion forms the epithelial covering of the umbilical cord (Fig. 5-1D_2). Body folding abnormalities are uncommon. Early diagnosis by antenatal ultrasonography is essential for the management of these cases (Hiett et al., 1992).

GERM LAYER DERIVATIVES

The three germ layers (ectoderm, mesoderm, and endoderm), formed during gastrulation (see Chapter 4) give rise to the primordia of all the tissues and organs. The specificity of the germ layers, however, is not rigidly fixed. The cells of each germ layer divide, migrate, aggregate, and differentiate in rather precise patterns as they form the various organ systems (*organogenesis*). The main germ layer derivatives are as follows (Fig. 5-5):

- **Ectoderm** gives rise to the central nervous system (CNS), peripheral nervous system, sensory epithelia of the eye, ear, and nose, epidermis and its appendages (hair and nails), mammary glands, pituitary gland, subcutaneous glands, and enamel of teeth.

  Neural crest cells, derived from neuroectoderm, give rise to the cells of the spinal, cranial (CNs V, VII, IX, and X), and autonomic ganglia; ensheathing cells of the peripheral nervous system; pigment cells of the dermis; muscle, connective tissues, bone of pharyngeal (branchial) arch origin (see Chapter 10); suprarenal (adrenal) medulla, and meninges (coverings) of the brain and spinal cord.
- **Mesoderm** gives rise to connective tissue, cartilage, bone, striated and smooth muscles, heart, blood and lymphatic vessels, kidneys, ovaries and testes, genital ducts, serous membranes lining the body cavities (pericardial, pleural, and peritoneal), spleen, and cortex of the suprarenal (adrenal) glands.
- **Endoderm** gives rise to the epithelial lining of the gastrointestinal and respiratory tracts, parenchyma of the tonsils, thyroid and parathyroid glands, thy-

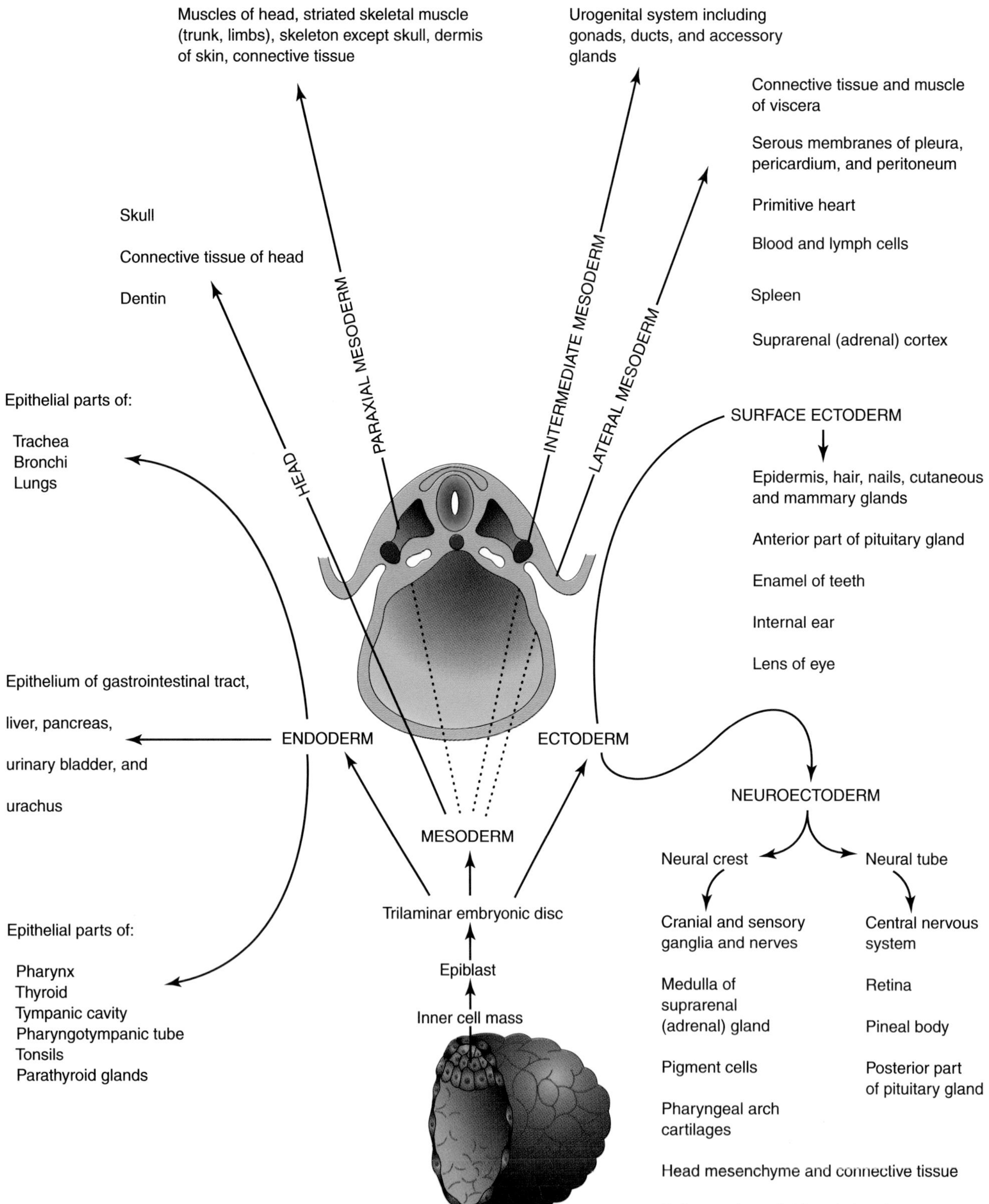

■ **Figure 5–5.** Schematic drawing illustrating the derivatives of the three germ layers: ectoderm, endoderm, and mesoderm. Cells from these layers make contributions to the formation of different tissues and organs; e.g., the endoderm forms the epithelial lining of the gastrointestinal tract and the mesoderm gives rise to connective tissues and muscles.

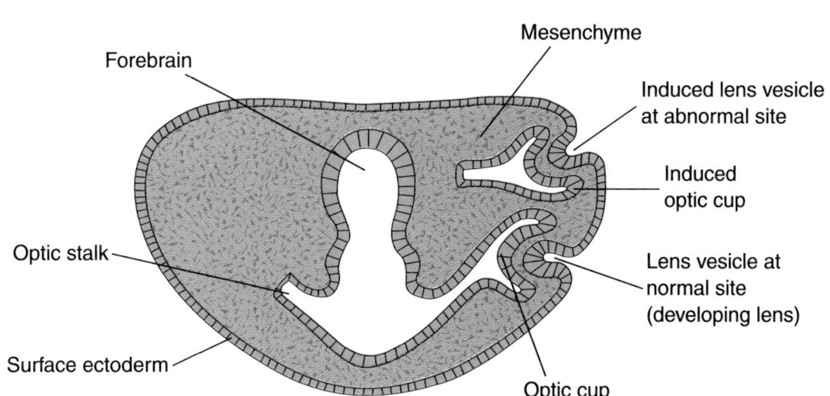

■ **Figure 5–6.** Schematic transverse section through the head of an embryo in the region of the developing eyes to illustrate inductive tissue interaction. At the normal site (lower right), observe that the optic vesicle, the precursor of the optic cup, has acted on the surface ectoderm of the head to induce formation of a lens vesicle, the primordium of the lens of the eye. On the opposite side, the optic stalk was cut and the optic vesicle removed. As a result, no lens placode (first indication of the lens) developed. At the abnormal site (upper right), the optic vesicle removed from the right side was inserted deep to the skin. Here, it acted on the surface ectoderm to induce the formation of a lens vesicle that has induced the formation of an optic cup (primordium of the eyeball).

mus, liver, and pancreas, epithelial lining of the urinary bladder and most of the urethra, and the epithelial lining of the tympanic cavity, tympanic antrum, and pharyngotympanic or auditory tube.

CONTROL OF EMBRYONIC DEVELOPMENT*

Development results from genetic plans in the chromosomes. Knowledge of the genes or hereditary units that control human development is increasing. Most information about developmental processes has come from studies in other organisms, especially *Drosophila* and mice, because of ethical problems associated with the use of human embryos for laboratory studies. For a discussion of the molecular genetics of mammalian development, see Thompson et al. (1991). Most developmental processes depend upon a precisely coordinated interaction of genetic and environmental factors. Several control mechanisms guide differentiation and ensure synchronized development, such as tissue interactions, regulated migration of cells and cell colonies, controlled proliferation, and programmed cell death (England, 1990; Wolpert, 1991). Each system of the body has its own developmental pattern, but most processes of morphogenesis are similar and are relatively simple. Underlying all these changes are basic regulating mechanisms (Cooke, 1988).

Embryonic development is essentially a process of growth and increasing complexity of structure and function. Growth is achieved by mitosis (process of somatic reproduction of cells) together with the production of extracellular matrices; whereas complexity is achieved through morphogenesis and differentiation. The cells that make up the tissues of very early embryos are pluripotential, which under different circumstances are able to follow more than one pathway of development. This broad developmental potential becomes progressively restricted as tissues acquire the specialized features necessary for increasing their sophistication of structure and function. Such restriction presumes that choices must be made in order to achieve tissue diversification. At present, most evidence indicates that these choices are determined, not as a consequence of cell lineage, but rather in response to cues from the immediate surroundings, including the adjacent tissues. As a result, the architectural precision and coordination that are often required for the normal function of an organ appear to be achieved by the interaction of its constituent parts during development.

The interaction of tissues during development is a recurring theme in embryology (Guthrie, 1991). The interactions that lead to a change in the course of development of at least one of the interactants are termed **inductions**. Numerous examples of such inductive interactions can be found in the literature; for example, during development of the eye, the optic vesicle is believed to induce the development of the lens from the surface ectoderm of the head. When the optic vesicle is absent, the eye fails to develop. Moreover, if the optic vesicle is removed and placed in association with surface ectoderm that is not usually involved in eye development, lens formation can be induced (Fig. 5-6). Clearly then, development of a lens is dependent on the ectoderm acquiring an association with a second tissue. In the presence of the neuroectoderm of the optic vesicle, the surface ectoderm of the head adopts a pathway of development that it would not otherwise have taken. In a similar fashion, many of the morphogenetic tissue movements that play such important roles in shaping the embryo also provide for the changing tissue associations that are fundamental to inductive tissue interactions.

The fact that one tissue can influence the developmental pathway adopted by another tissue presumes that a signal passes between the two interactants. The precise nature of the signal is not known; however, the mechanism of signal transfer appears to vary with

* The authors are grateful to Dr. Michael Wiley, Associate Professor of Anatomy and Cell Biology, Faculty of Medicine, University of Toronto, for his assistance in preparing this section.

the specific tissues involved. In some cases, the signal appears to take the form of a diffusible molecule, such as sonic hedgehog (Placzek and Furley, 1996; Tanabe et al., 1995), that passes from the inductor to the reacting tissue (Fig. 5-7*A*). In others, the message appears to be mediated through a nondiffusible extracellular matrix that is secreted by the inductor and with which the reacting tissue comes into contact (Fig. 5-7*B*). In still other cases, the signal appears to require that physical contacts occur between the inducing and responding tissues (Fig. 5-7*C*). Regardless of the mechanism of intercellular transfer involved, the signal is translated into an intracellular message that influences the genetic activity of the responding cells.

Laboratory studies have established that the signal can be relatively nonspecific in some interactions. Under experimental conditions, the role of the natural inductor in a variety of interactions has been shown to be mimicked by a number of heterologous tissue sources and, in some instances, even by a variety of cell-free preparations. These studies suggest that the specificity of a given induction is a property of the reacting tissue rather than that of the inductor. Inductions should not be thought of as isolated phenomena. Often they occur in a sequential fashion that results in the orderly development of a complex structure; for example, following induction of the lens by the optic vesicle, the lens induces the development of the cornea from the surface ectoderm and adjacent mesenchyme. This ensures the formation of component parts that are appropriate in size and relationship for the function of the organ. In other systems, there is evidence that the interactions between tissues are reciprocal. During development of the kidney, for instance, the ureteric bud induces the formation of tubules in the metanephric mesoderm (see Chapter 13). This mesoderm, in turn, induces branching of the ureteric bud that results in the development of the collecting tubules and calices of the kidney.

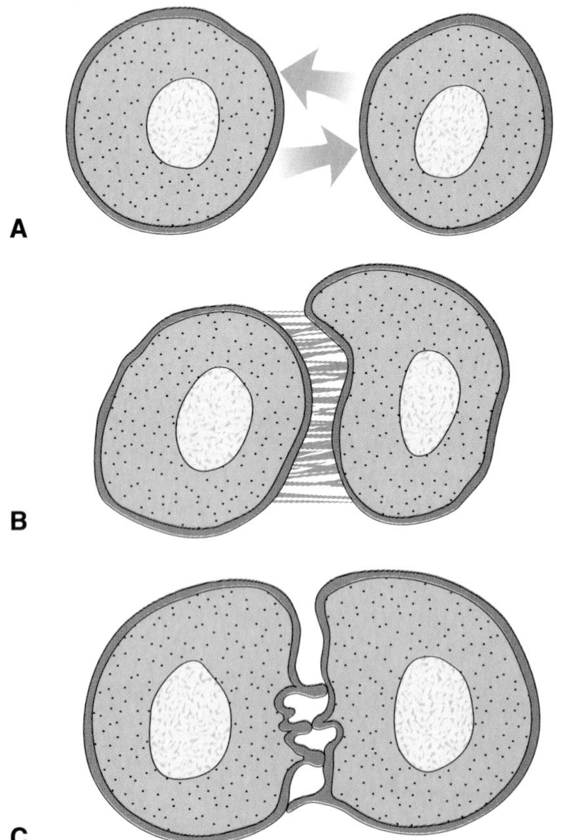

■ **Figure 5-7.** A series of sketches illustrating three possible methods of transmission of signal substances in inductive cell interactions. *A,* Diffusion of signal substances. The signal appears to take the form of a diffusible molecule that passes from the inductor to the reacting tissue. *B,* Matrix-mediated interaction. The signal is mediated through a nondiffusible extracellular matrix, secreted by the inductor, with which the reacting tissue comes in contact. *C,* Cell contact-mediated interaction. The signal requires physical contact between the inducing and responding tissues. (Modified from Grobstein C: *Adv Cancer Res 4:*187, 1956, and Saxen L: *In* Tarin D [ed]: *Tissue Interactions in Carcinogenesis.* London, Academic Press, 1972.)

The ability of the reacting system to respond to an inducing stimulus is not unlimited. Most inducible tissues appear to pass through a transient, but more or less sharply delimited physiological state in which they are competent to respond to an inductive signal from the neighboring tissue. Because this state of receptiveness is limited in time, a delay in the development of one or more components in an interacting system may lead to failure of an inductive interaction. Regardless of the signal mechanism employed, inductive systems seem to have the common feature of close proximity between the interacting tissues. Experimental evidence has demonstrated that interactions may fail if the interactants are too widely separated. Consequently, inductive processes appear to be limited in space as well as by time. Because tissue induction plays such a fundamental role in ensuring the orderly formation of precise structure, failed interactions can be expected to have drastic developmental consequences (e.g., congenital anomalies such as absence of the lens of the eye).

HIGHLIGHTS OF THE FOURTH TO EIGHTH WEEKS

The following descriptions summarize the main developmental events and changes in external form of the embryo during the fourth to eighth weeks. The details of organ formation are given with descriptions of the various systems in Chapters 11 to 20. Criteria for estimating developmental stages in human embryos are listed in Table 5-1.

Fourth Week

Major changes in body form occur during the fourth week. At the beginning, the embryo (2.0 to 3.5 mm long) is almost straight and has 4 to 12 somites that

Table 5-1 ■ **Criteria for Estimating Developmental Stages in Human Embryos**

Age (Days)	Figure Reference	Carnegie Stage	No. of Somites	Length (mm)*	Main External Characteristics†
20-21	5-1A_1	9	1-3	1.5-3.0	*Flat embryonic disc. Deep neural groove and prominent neural folds. One to three pairs of somites present.* Head fold evident.
22-23	5-8*A* 5-8*B* 5-9	10	4-12	2.0-3.5	*Embryo straight or slightly curved.* Neural tube forming or formed opposite somites, but widely open at rostral and caudal neuropores. First and second pairs of branchial arches visible.
24-25	5-8*C* 5-10	11	13-20	2.5-4.5	*Embryo curved owing to head and tail folds.* Rostral neuropore closing. Otic placodes present. Optic vesicles formed.
26-27	5-8*D* 5-11	12	21-29	3.0-5.0	*Upper limb buds appear.* Rostral neuropore closed. Caudal neuropore closing. Three pairs of branchial arches visible. Heart prominence distinct. Otic pits present.
28-30	5-8*E* 5-12	13	30-35	4.0-6.0	*Embryo has C-shaped curve.* Caudal neuropore closed. Upper limb buds are flipper-like. Four pairs of branchial arches visible. Lower limb buds appear. *Otic vesicles* present. Lens placodes distinct. Attenuated *tail* present.
31-32	5-16	14	‡	5.0-7.0	*Upper limbs are paddle-shaped.* Lens pits and nasal pits visible. Optic cups present.
33-36		15		7.0-9.0	*Hand plates formed; digital rays present.* Lens vesicles present. Nasal pits prominent. *Lower limbs are paddle-shaped.* Cervical sinuses visible.
37-40		16		8.0-11.0	*Foot plates formed.* Pigment visible in retina. Auricular hillocks developing.
41-43	5-17	17		11.0-14.0	*Digital rays clearly visible in hand plates.* Auricular hillocks outline future auricle of external ear. Trunk beginning to straighten. Cerebral vesicles prominent.
44-46		18		13.0-17.0	*Digital rays clearly visible in foot plates.* Elbow region visible. Eyelids forming. Notches between the digital rays in the hands. Nipples visible.
47-48	5-18	19		16.0-18.0	*Limbs extend ventrally.* Trunk elongating and straightening. Midgut herniation prominent.
49-51		20		18.0-22.0	*Upper limbs longer and bent at elbows. Fingers distinct but webbed.* Notches between the digital rays in the feet. Scalp vascular plexus appears.
52-53	5-19	21		22.0-24.0	*Hands and feet approach each other. Fingers are free and longer. Toes distinct but webbed.* Stubby tail present.
54-55		22		23.0-28.0	*Toes free and longer.* Eyelids and auricles or external ears more developed.
56	5-20	23		27.0-31.0	*Head more rounded and shows human characteristics.* External genitalia still have sexless appearance. Distinct bulge still present in umbilical cord, caused by herniation of intestines. *Tail has disappeared.*

* The embryonic lengths indicate the usual range. In stages 9 and 10, the measurement is greatest length (*GL*); in subsequent stages crown-rump (*CR*) measurements are given (Fig. 5-23).

† Based on Nishimura et al. (1974), O'Rahilly and Müller (1987), and Shiota (1991).

‡ At this and subsequent stages, the number of somites is difficult to determine and so is not a useful criterion.

produce conspicuous surface elevations (Fig. 5-8*A*). The neural tube is formed opposite the somites, but it is widely open at the rostral (anterior) and caudal (posterior) neuropores (Figs. 5-8*B* and 5-9). By 24 days the pharyngeal (branchial) arches are visible. The first or mandibular arch and the second or hyoid arch are distinct (Figs. 5-8*C* and 5-10). The major part of the first arch gives rise to the mandible (lower jaw), and a rostral extension of the arch, the maxillary prominence, contributes to the maxilla (upper jaw). The embryo is now slightly curved because of the head and tail folds. The heart produces a large ventral prominence and pumps blood.

Three pairs of **pharyngeal arches** are visible by 26 days (Figs. 5-8*D* and 5-11), and the rostral neuropore is closed. The **forebrain** produces a prominent elevation of the head, and folding of the embryo has given the embryo a characteristic C-shaped curvature. A long, *curved tail* is present. **Upper limb buds** become recognizable by day 26 or 27 as small swellings on the ventrolateral body walls (Figs. 5-8*D* and *E*). The **otic pits**, the primordia of the internal ears, are also visible. Ectodermal thickenings indicating the future lenses of the eyes called **lens placodes** are visible on the sides of the head. The fourth pair of pharyngeal arches and the **lower limb buds** are visible by the end of the fourth week (Fig. 5-8*E*). Toward the end of the fourth week, an *attenuated tail* is a characteristic feature (Figs. 5-11 and 5-12). Rudiments of many of the organ systems, especially the

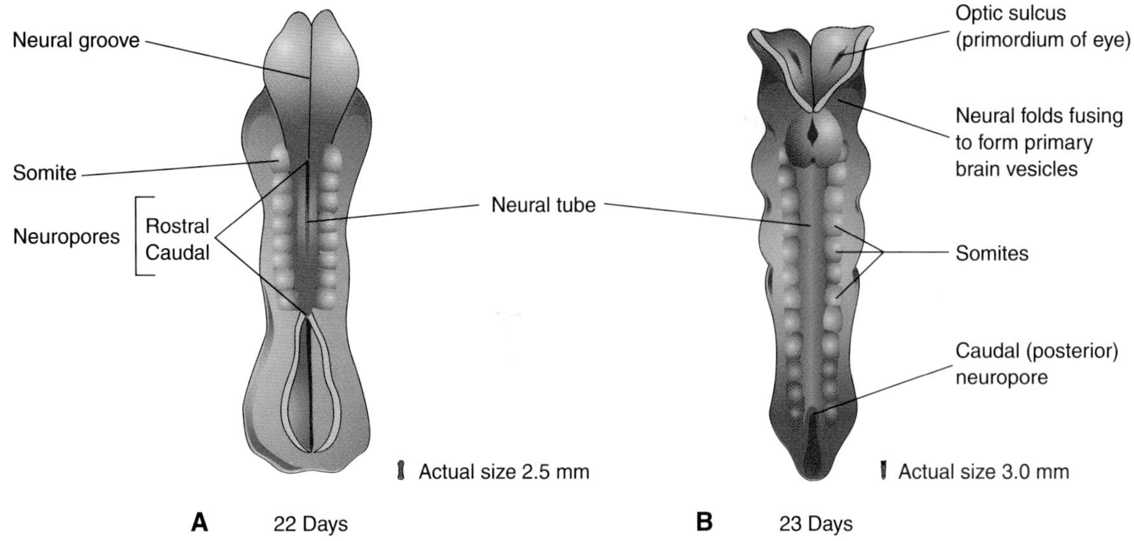

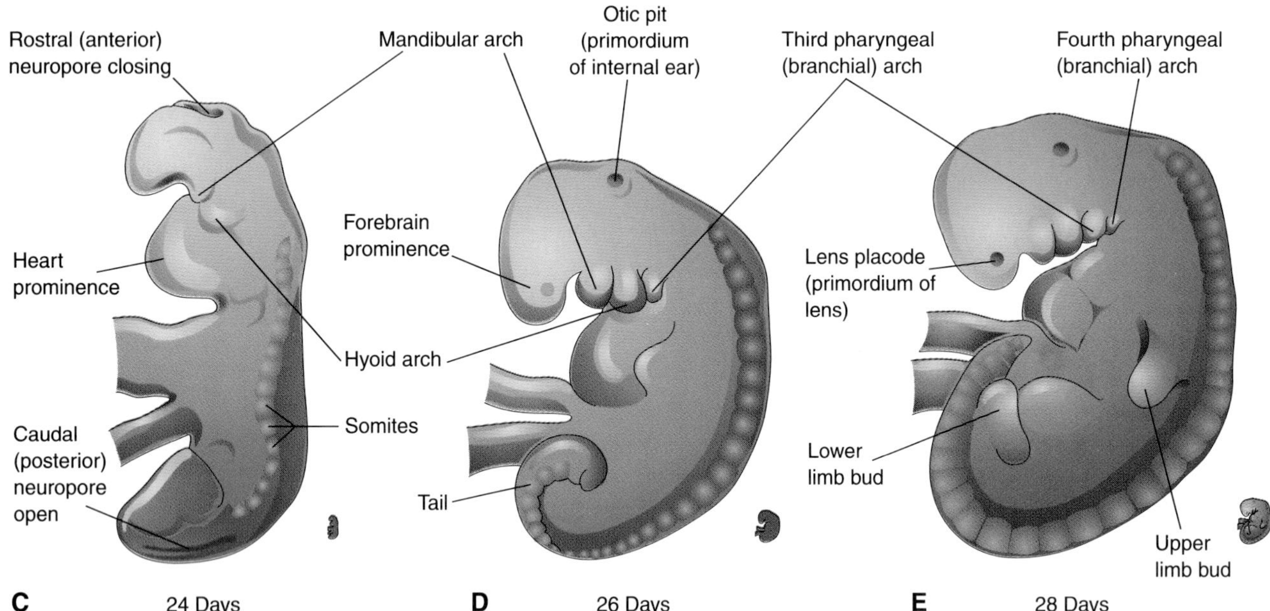

■ **Figure 5–8.** *A* and *B,* Drawings of dorsal views of embryos early in the fourth week showing 8 and 12 somites, respectively. *C, D,* and *E,* Lateral views of older embryos showing 16, 27, and 33 somites, respectively. The rostral neuropore is normally closed by 25 to 26 days and the caudal neuropore is usually closed by the end of the fourth week.

cardiovascular system, are established (Figs. 5-13 and 5-14). By the end of the fourth week the caudal neuropore is usually closed.

Fifth Week

Changes in body form are minor during the fifth week compared with those that occurred during the fourth week, but growth of the head exceeds that of other regions (Figs. 5-15 and 5-16). Enlargement of the head is caused mainly by the rapid development of the brain and facial prominences. The face soon contacts the heart prominence. The rapidly growing second (hyoid) pharyngeal arch overgrows the third and fourth arches, forming a lateral ectodermal depression on each side—the **cervical sinus**. The upper limb buds are paddle-shaped and the lower limb buds are flipperlike. The *mesonephric ridges* indicate the site of the mesonephric kidneys, which are interim kidneys in humans.

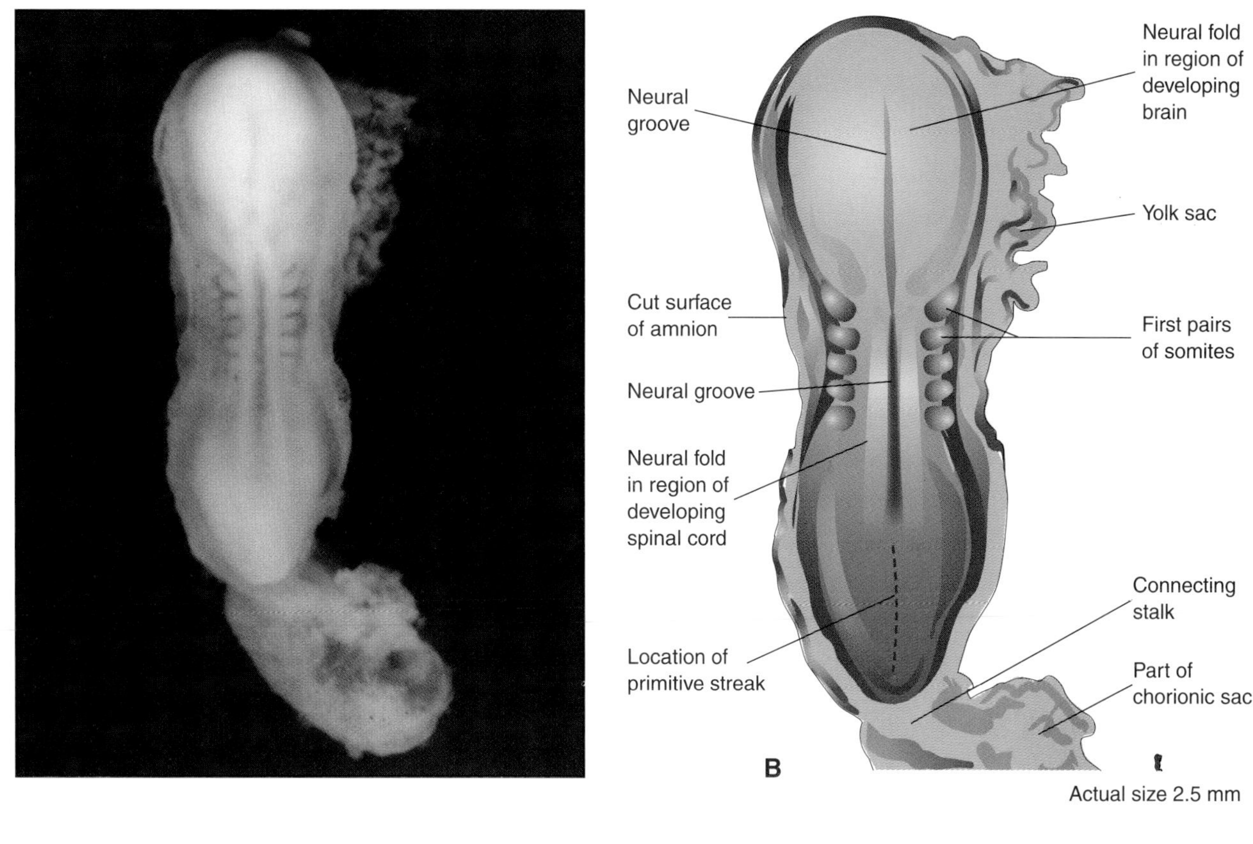

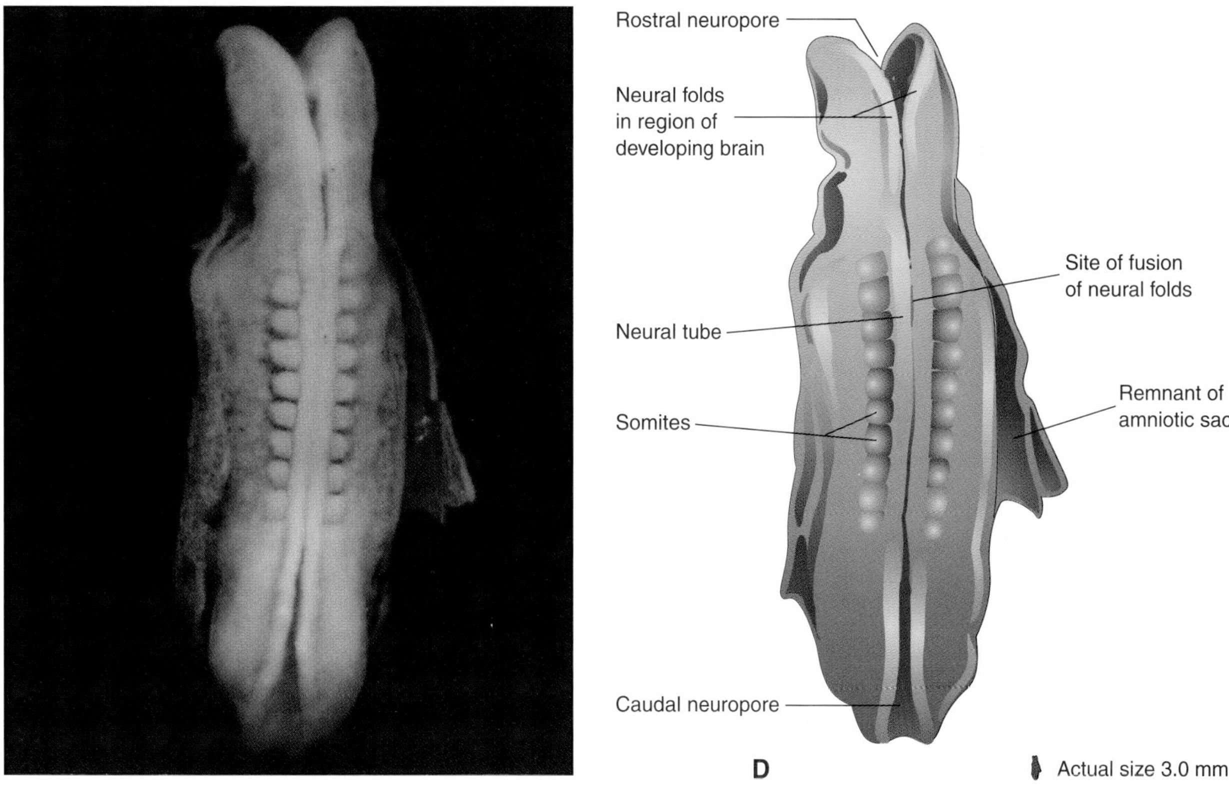

■ **Figure 5–9.** *A,* Dorsal view of a five-somite embryo at Carnegie stage 10, about 22 days. Observe the neural folds and deep neural groove. The neural folds in the cranial region have thickened to form the primordium of the brain. *B,* Drawing indicating the structures shown in *A.* Most of the amniotic and chorionic sacs have been cut away to expose the embryo. *C,* Dorsal view of an 8-somite embryo at Carnegie stage 10, about 22 days. The neural tube is in open communication with the amniotic cavity at the cranial and caudal ends through the rostral and caudal neuropores, respectively. *D,* Diagram indicating the structures shown in *C.* The neural folds have fused opposite the somites to form the neural tube (primordium of the spinal cord in this region). (*A* and *C* from Moore KL, Persaud TVN, Shiota K: *Color Atlas of Clinical Embryology.* Philadelphia, WB Saunders, 1994.)

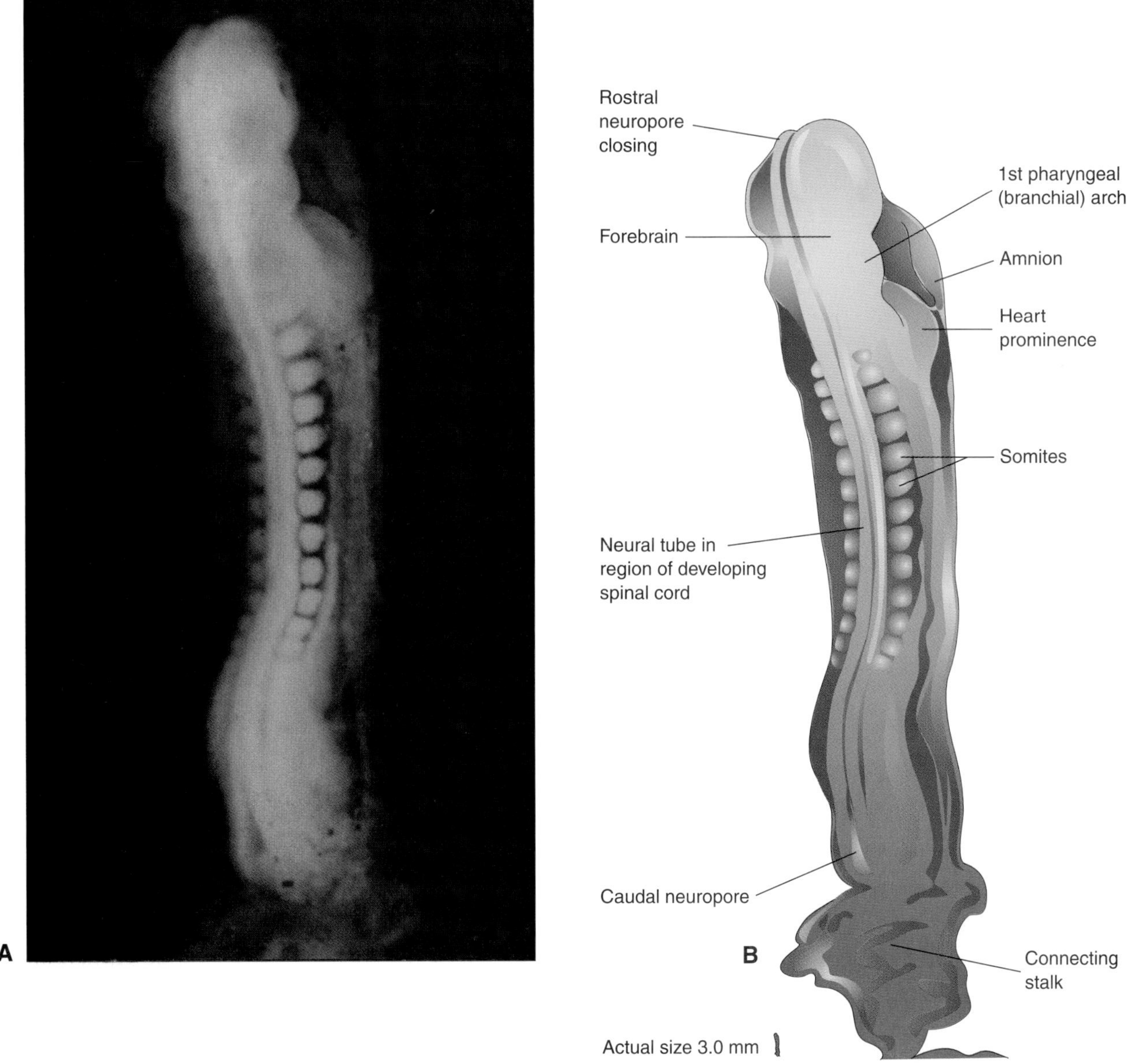

■ **Figure 5-10.** *A,* Dorsal view of a 13-somite embryo at Carnegie stage 11, about 24 days. The rostral neuropore is closing but the caudal neuropore is wide open. (From Moore KL, Persaud TVN, Shiota K: *Color Atlas of Clinical Embryology.* Philadelphia, WB Saunders, 1994.) *B,* Drawing indicating the structures shown in *A.* The embryo is curved because of folding at the cranial and caudal ends.

Sixth Week

The upper limbs begin to show regional differentiation as the elbows and large **hand plates** develop (Fig. 5-17). The primordia of the digits (fingers), called **digital rays**, begin to develop in the hand plates, which indicate the formation of digits. It has been reported that embryos in the sixth week show spontaneous movements, such as twitching of the trunk and limbs. Development of the lower limbs occurs somewhat later than that of the upper limbs. Several small swellings called **auricular hillocks** develop around the pharyngeal (branchial) groove or cleft between the first two pharyngeal arches. This groove becomes the **external acoustic meatus** (external auditory canal) and the auricular hillocks around it fuse to form the auricle, the shell-shaped part of the external ear. Largely because retinal pigment has formed, the eye is now obvious. The head is now much larger relative to the trunk and is bent over the *large heart prominence*. This head position results from bending in the cervical (neck) region. The trunk and neck have begun to straighten. It has been reported that embryos during the sixth week show reflex responses to touch.

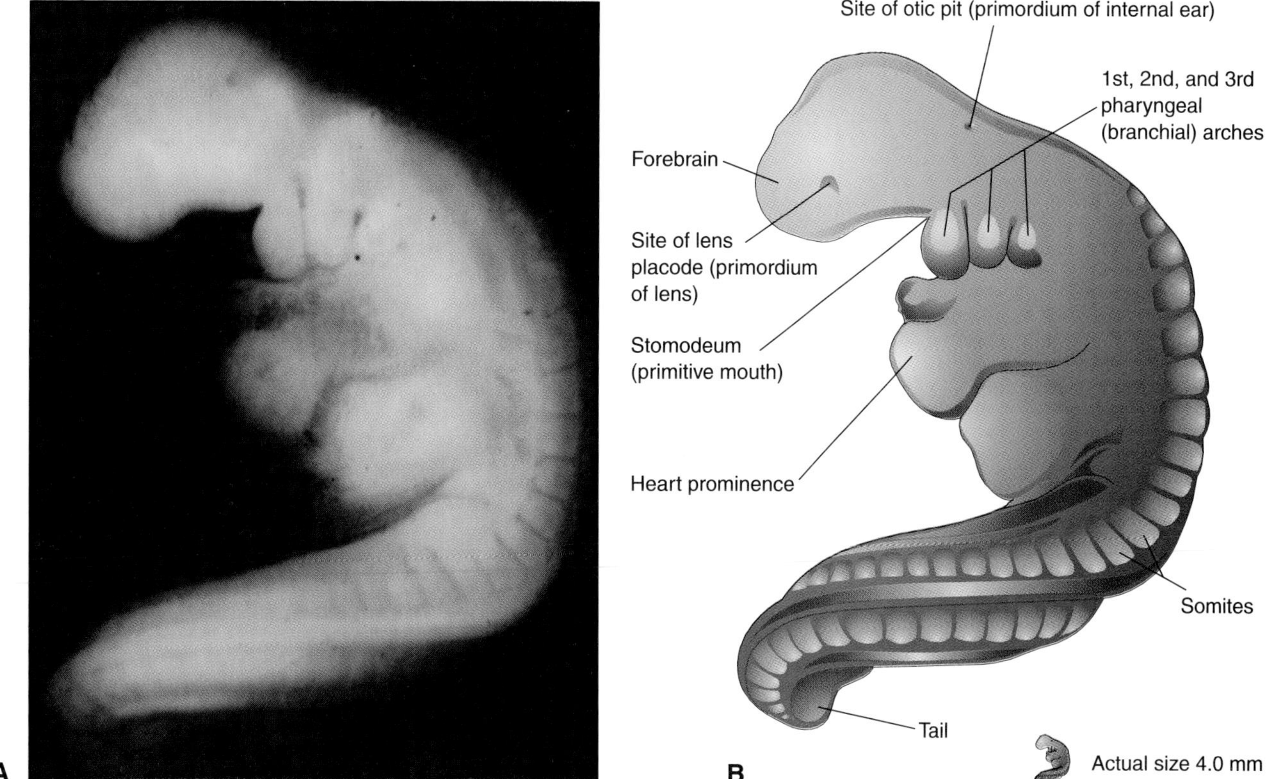

■ **Figure 5–11.** *A,* Lateral view of a 27-somite embryo at Carnegie stage 12, about 26 days. The embryo is very curved, especially its long tail. Observe the lens placode (primordium of the lens of the eye) and the otic pit indicating early development of the internal ear. (From Nishimura H, Semba R, Tanimura T, Tanaka O: *Prenatal Development of the Human with Special Reference to Craniofacial Structures: An Atlas.* Washington DC, National Institutes of Health, 1977.) *B,* Drawing indicating the structures shown in *A,* The rostral neuropore is closed and three pairs of pharyngeal arches are present.

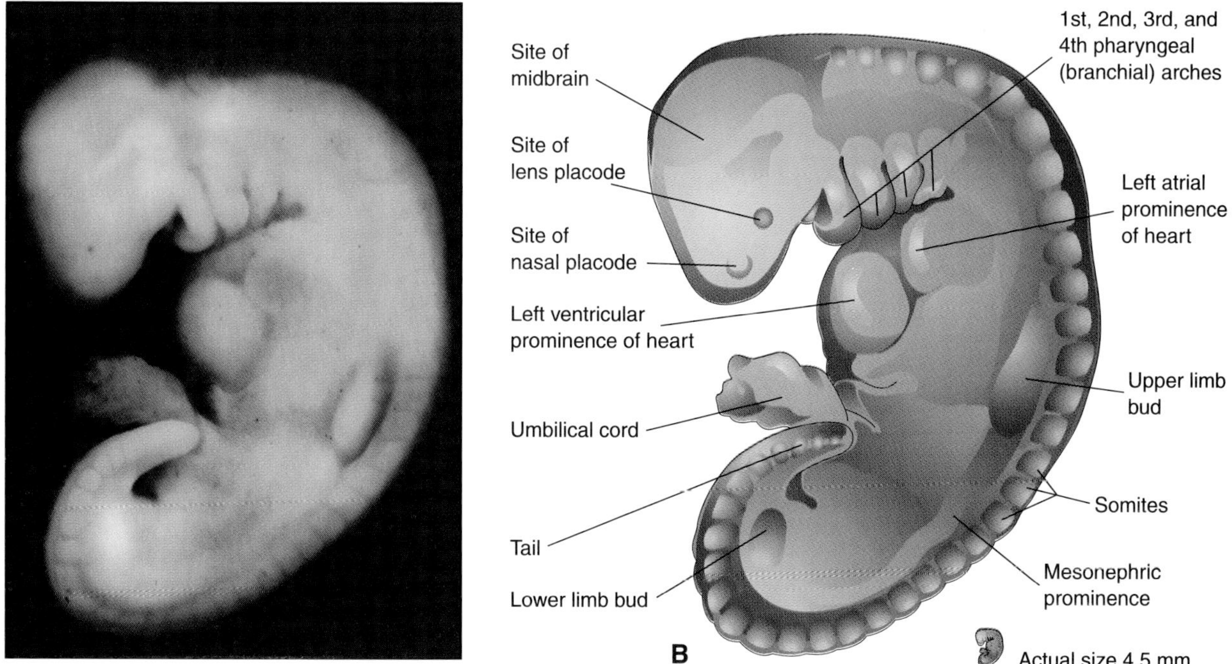

■ **Figure 5–12.** *A,* Lateral view of an embryo at Carnegie stage 13, about 28 days. The heart is large and its division into a primordial atrium and ventricle is visible. The rostral and caudal neuropores are closed. (From Nishimura H, Semba R, Tanimura T, Tanaka O: *Prenatal Development of the Human with Special Reference to Craniofacial Structures: An Atlas.* Washington DC, National Institutes of Health, 1977.) *B,* Drawing indicating the structures shown in *A.* The embryo has a characteristic C-shaped curvature, four pharyngeal arches, and upper and lower limb buds.

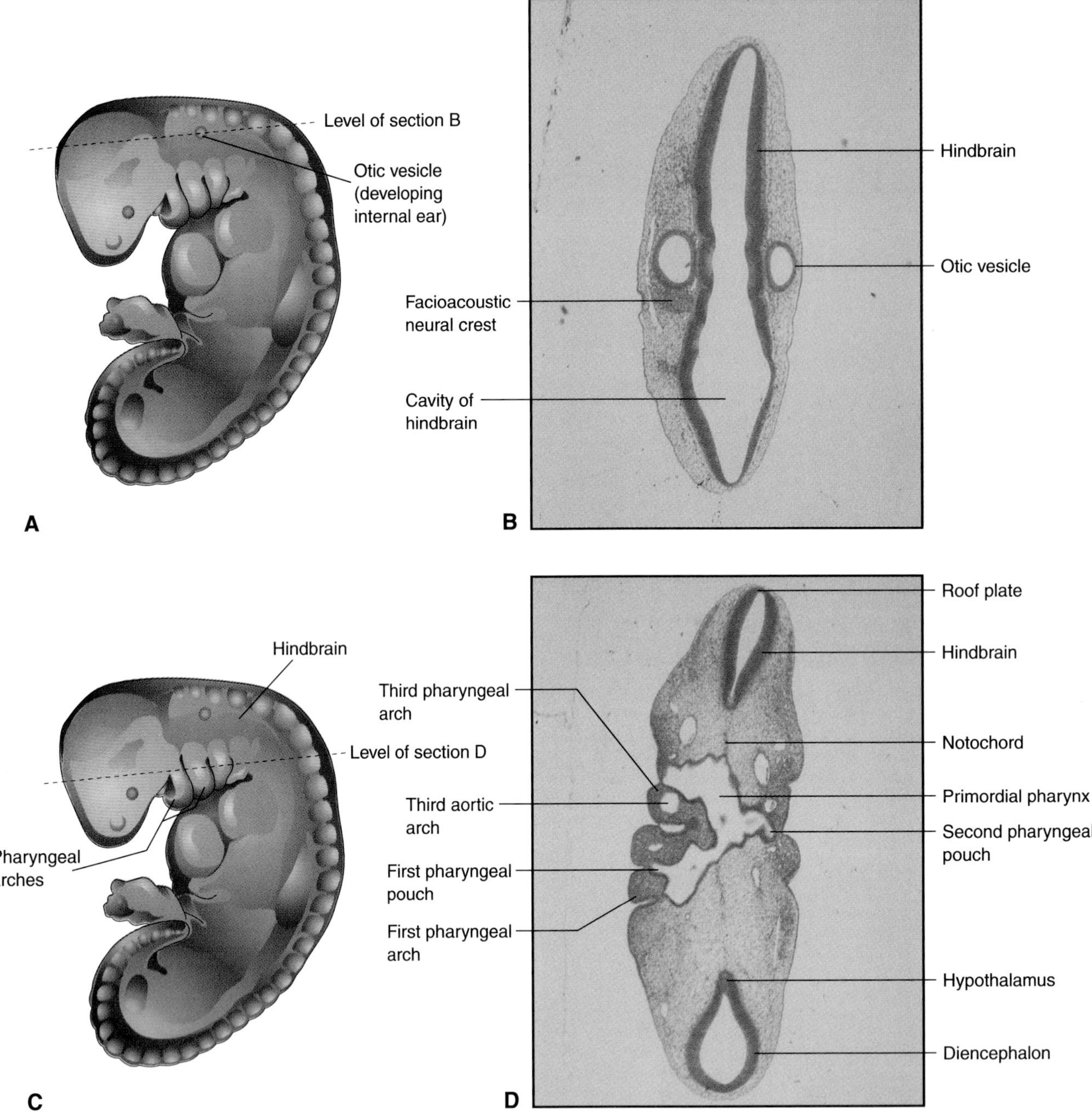

■ **Figure 5–13.** *A,* Drawing of an embryo at Carnegie stage 13, about 28 days *B,* Photomicrograph of a section of the embryo at the level shown in *A.* Observe the hindbrain and otic vesicle (primordium of the internal ear). *C,* Drawing of the same embryo showing the level of the section in *D.* Observe the primordial pharynx and pharyngeal arches. (*B* and *D* from Moore KL, Persaud TVN, Shiota K: *Color Atlas of Clinical Embryology.* Philadelphia, WB Saunders, 1994.)

Seventh Week

The limbs undergo considerable change during the seventh week. Notches appear between the digital rays in the hand plates, clearly indicating the future digits (Fig. 5-18). Communication between the primitive gut and yolk sac is now reduced to a relatively slender duct, the *yolk stalk.* The intestines enter the extraembryonic coelom in the proximal part of the umbilical cord. This **umbilical herniation** is a normal event in the embryo. The herniation occurs because the abdominal cavity is too small at this age to accommodate the rapidly growing intestine. By the end of the seventh week, ossification of the bones of the upper limbs has begun.

Eighth Week

At the beginning of this final week of the embryonic period, the digits of the hand are separated but noticeably webbed (Fig. 5-19). Notches are now clearly visible between the digital rays of the fan-shaped feet. The tail is still present but stubby. The **scalp vascular plexus** has appeared and forms a characteristic band around the head. By the end of the eighth week, all regions of the limbs are apparent, the digits have lengthened and are completely separated (Fig. 5-20). Purposeful limb movements first occur during this week. Ossification begins in the lower limbs during the eighth week and is first recognizable in the femur. All evidence of the tail has disappeared by the end of

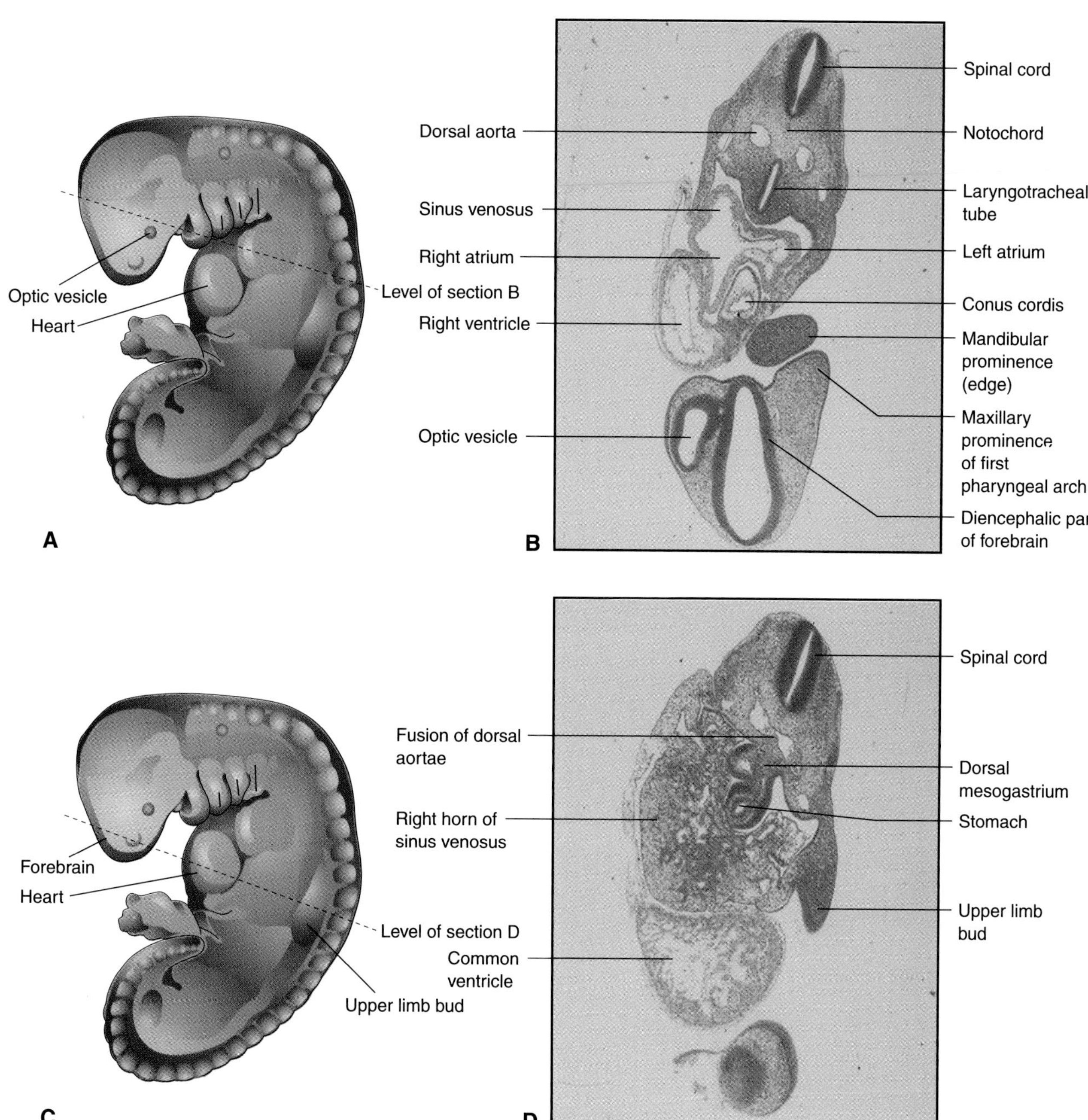

■ **Figure 5-14.** *A,* Drawing of an embryo at Carnegie stage 13, about 28 days. *B,* Photomicrograph of a section of the embryo at the level shown in *A.* Observe the parts of the primordial heart. *C,* Drawing of the same embryo showing the level of section in *D.* Observe the heart and primordium of the stomach. (*B* and *D* from Moore KL, Persaud TVN, Shiota K: *Color Atlas of Clinical Embryology.* Philadelphia, WB Saunders, 1994.)

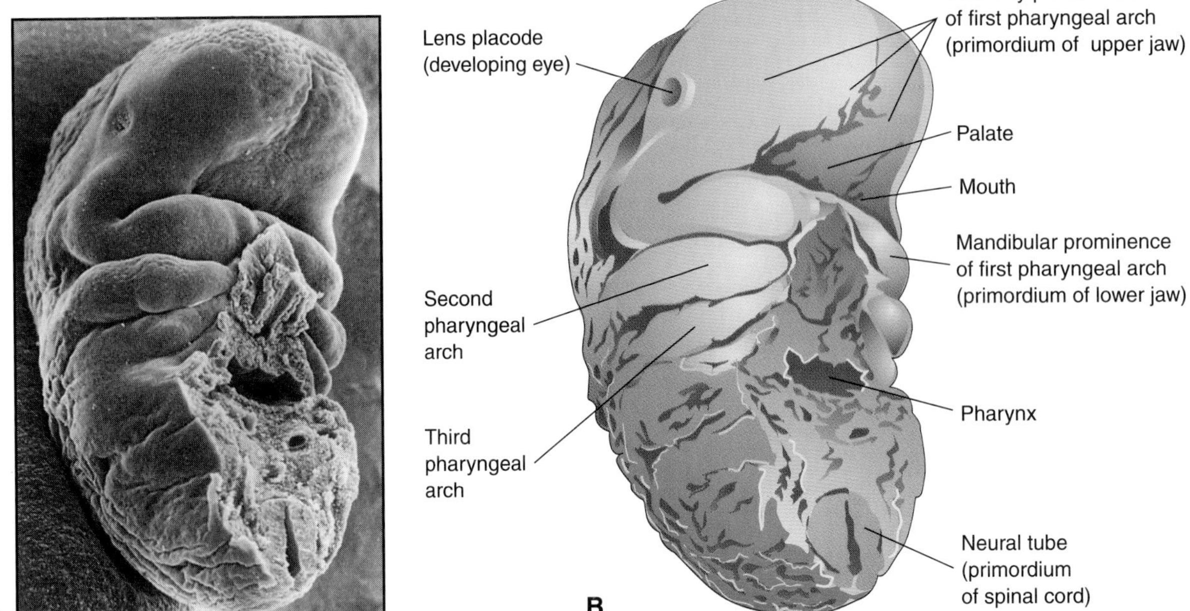

■ **Figure 5–15.** *A,* Scanning electron micrograph (SEM) of the craniofacial region of a human embryo of about 32 days (Carnegie stage 14, 6.8 mm). Three pairs of pharyngeal arches are present. The maxillary and mandibular prominences of the first arch are clearly delineated. Observe the mouth located between the maxillary prominences and the fused mandibular prominences. (Courtesy of Professor K. Hinrichsen, Ruhr-Universität, Bochum, Germany.) *B,* Drawing of the SEM indicating the structures shown in *A.*

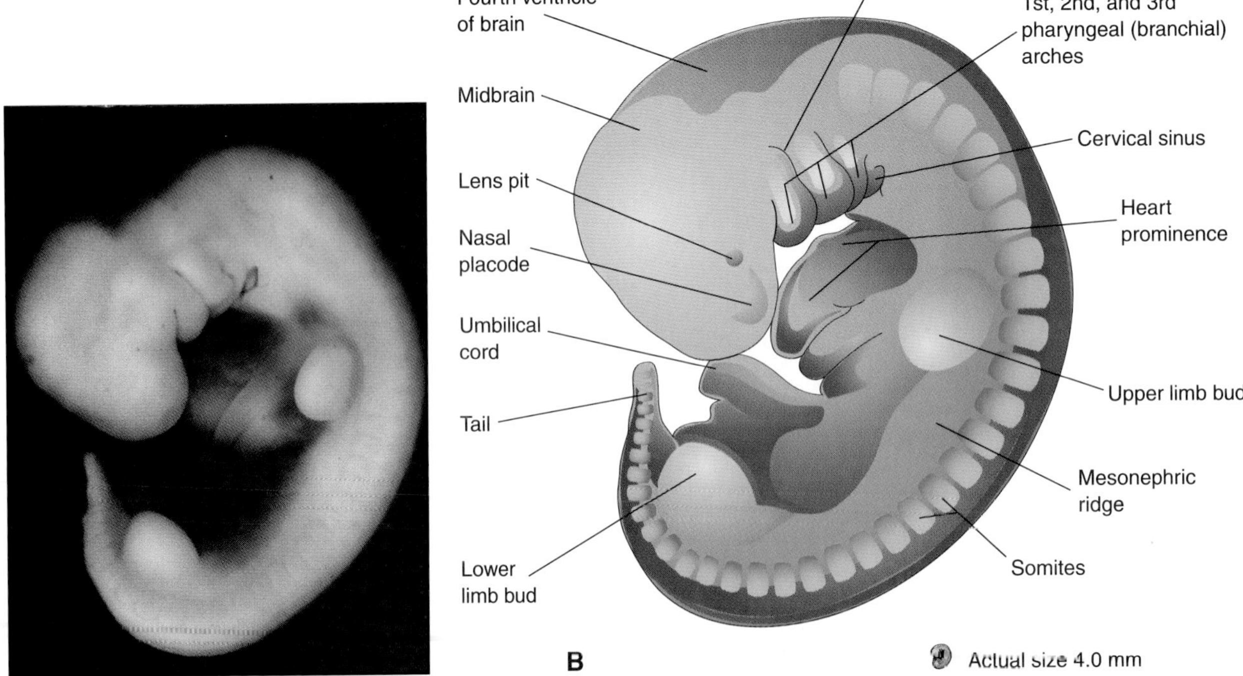

■ **Figure 5–16.** *A,* Lateral view of an embryo at Carnegie stage 14, about 32 days. The second pharyngeal arch has overgrown the third arch, forming a depression known as the cervical sinus. The mesonephric ridge indicates the site of the mesonephric kidney, an interim kidney (see Chapter 13). (From Nishimura H, Semba R, Tanimura T, Tanaka O: *Prenatal Development of the Human with Special Reference to Craniofacial Structures: An Atlas.* Washington DC, National Institutes of Health, 1977.) *B,* Drawing indicating the structures shown in *A.* The upper limb buds are paddle-shaped and the lower limb buds are flipperlike.

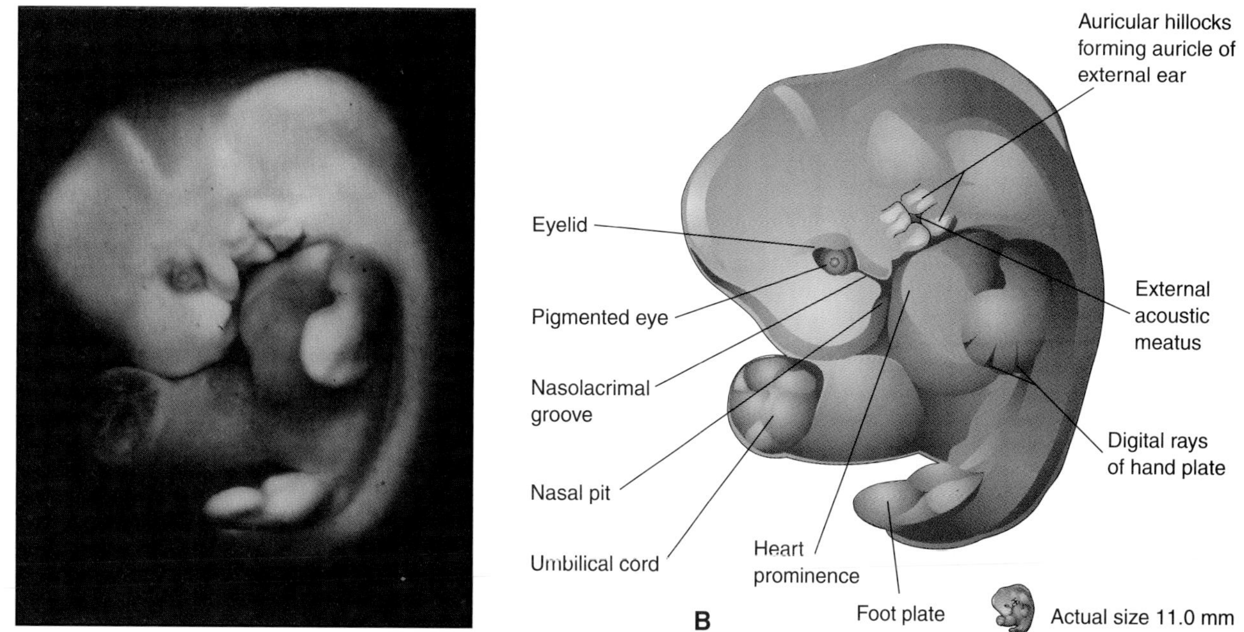

■ **Figure 5–17.** *A,* Lateral view of an embryo at Carnegie stage 17, about 42 days. Digital rays are visible in the large hand plate, indicating the future site of the digits. (From Moore KL, Persaud TVN, Shiota K: *Color Atlas of Clinical Embryology.* Philadelphia, WB Saunders, 1994.) *B,* Drawing indicating the structures shown in *A.* The eye, auricular hillocks, and external acoustic meatus (auditory canal) are now obvious.

the eighth week. The *scalp vascular plexus* now forms a band near the vertex (crown) of the head. The hands and feet approach each other ventrally.

At the end of the eighth week, the embryo has distinct human characteristics (Fig. 5-21); however, the head is still disproportionately large, constituting almost half of the embryo. The neck region is established and the eyelids are more obvious. The eyelids

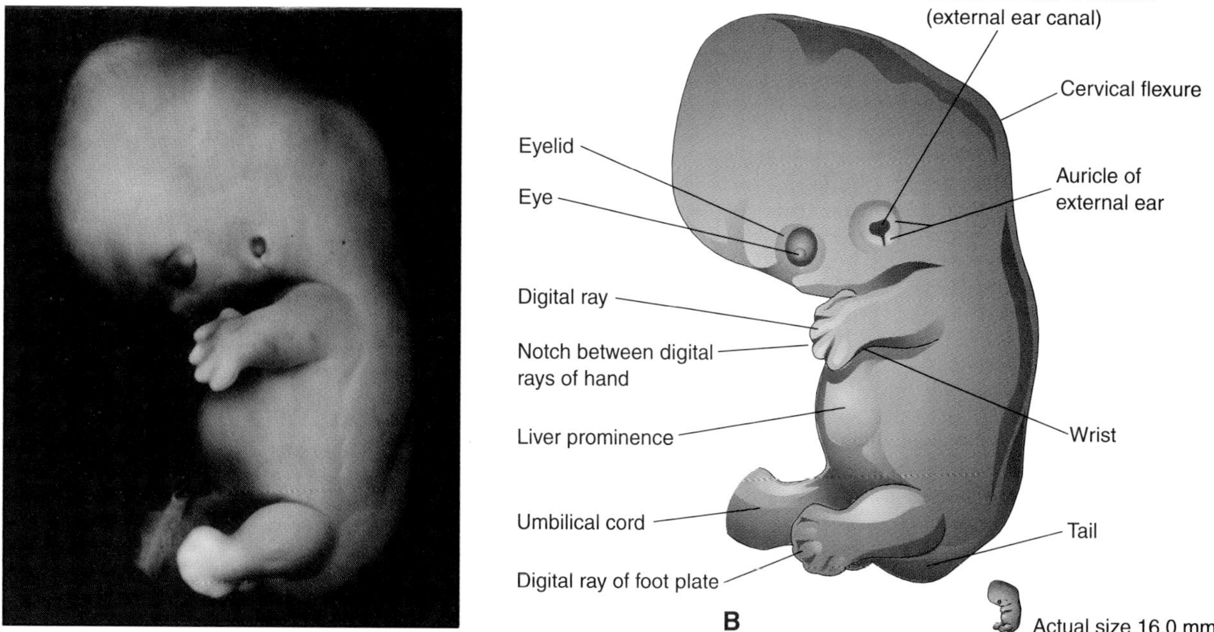

■ **Figure 5–18.** *A,* Lateral view of an embryo at Carnegie stage 19, about 48 days. The auricle and external acoustic meatus are now clearly visible. Note the relatively low position of the ear at this stage. Digital rays are now visible in the large foot plate. The prominence of the abdomen is caused mainly by the large size of the liver. (From Moore KL, Persaud TVN, Shiota K: *Color Atlas of Clinical Embryology.* Philadelphia, WB Saunders, 1994.) *B,* Drawing indicating the structures shown in *A.* Observe the large hand and the notches between the digital rays, which clearly indicate the developing digits.

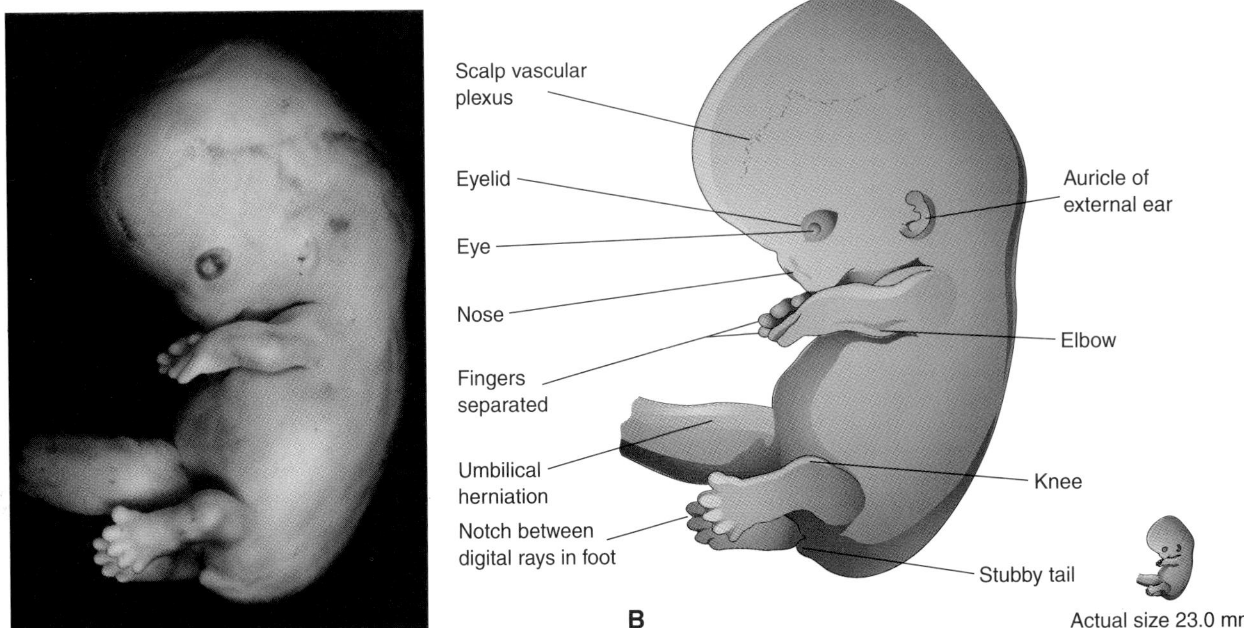

■ **Figure 5–19.** *A,* Lateral view of an embryo at Carnegie stage 21, about 52 days. Note that the feet are fan-shaped and that the tail is very short. The scalp vascular plexus now forms a characteristic band across the head. The nose is stubby and the eye is heavily pigmented. (From Nishimura H, Semba R, Tanimura T, Tanaka O: *Prenatal Development of the Human with Special Reference to Craniofacial Structures: An Atlas.* Washington DC, National Institutes of Health, 1977.) *B,* Drawing indicating the structures shown in *A.* The fingers are separated and the toes are beginning to separate.

are closing and by the end of the eighth week they begin to unite by epithelial fusion. The intestines are still in the proximal portion of the umbilical cord. The auricles of the external ears begin to assume their final shape but they are still low-set on the head. Although sex differences exist in the appearance of the external genitalia, they are not distinctive enough to permit accurate sexual identification (see Chapter 13).

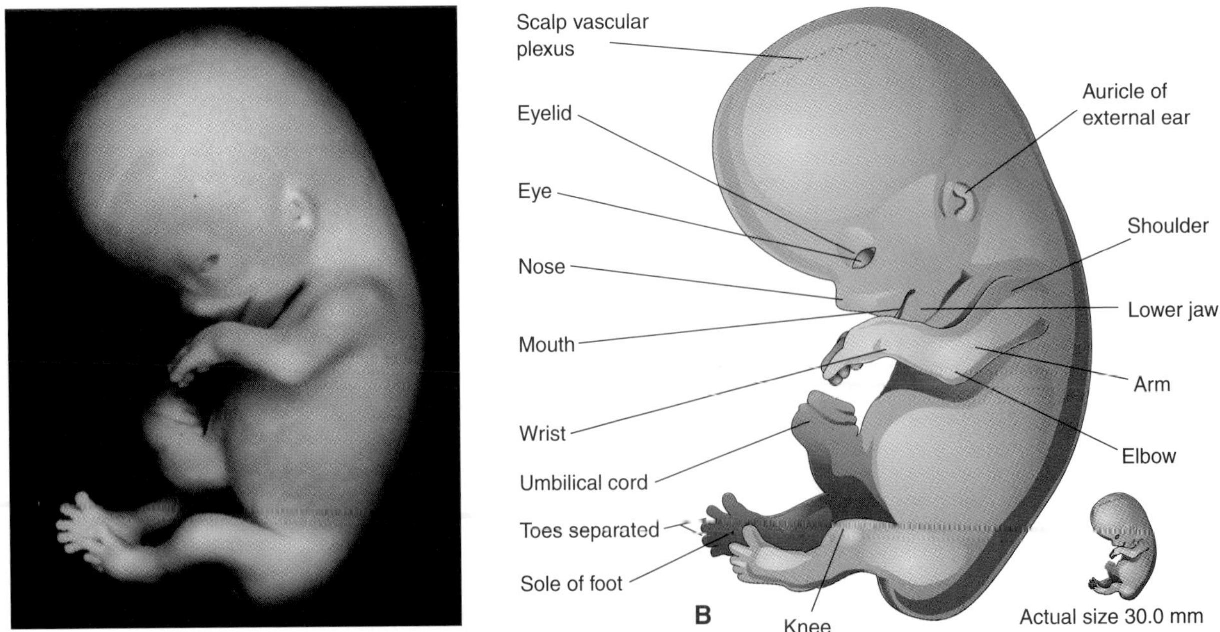

■ **Figure 5–20.** *A,* Lateral view of an embryo at Carnegie stage 23, about 56 days. The embryo has a distinct human appearance. (From Nishimura H, Semba R, Tanimura T, Tanaka O: *Prenatal Development of the Human with Special Reference to Craniofacial Structures: An Atlas.* Washington DC, National Institutes of Health, 1977.) *B,* Drawing indicating the structures shown in *A.*

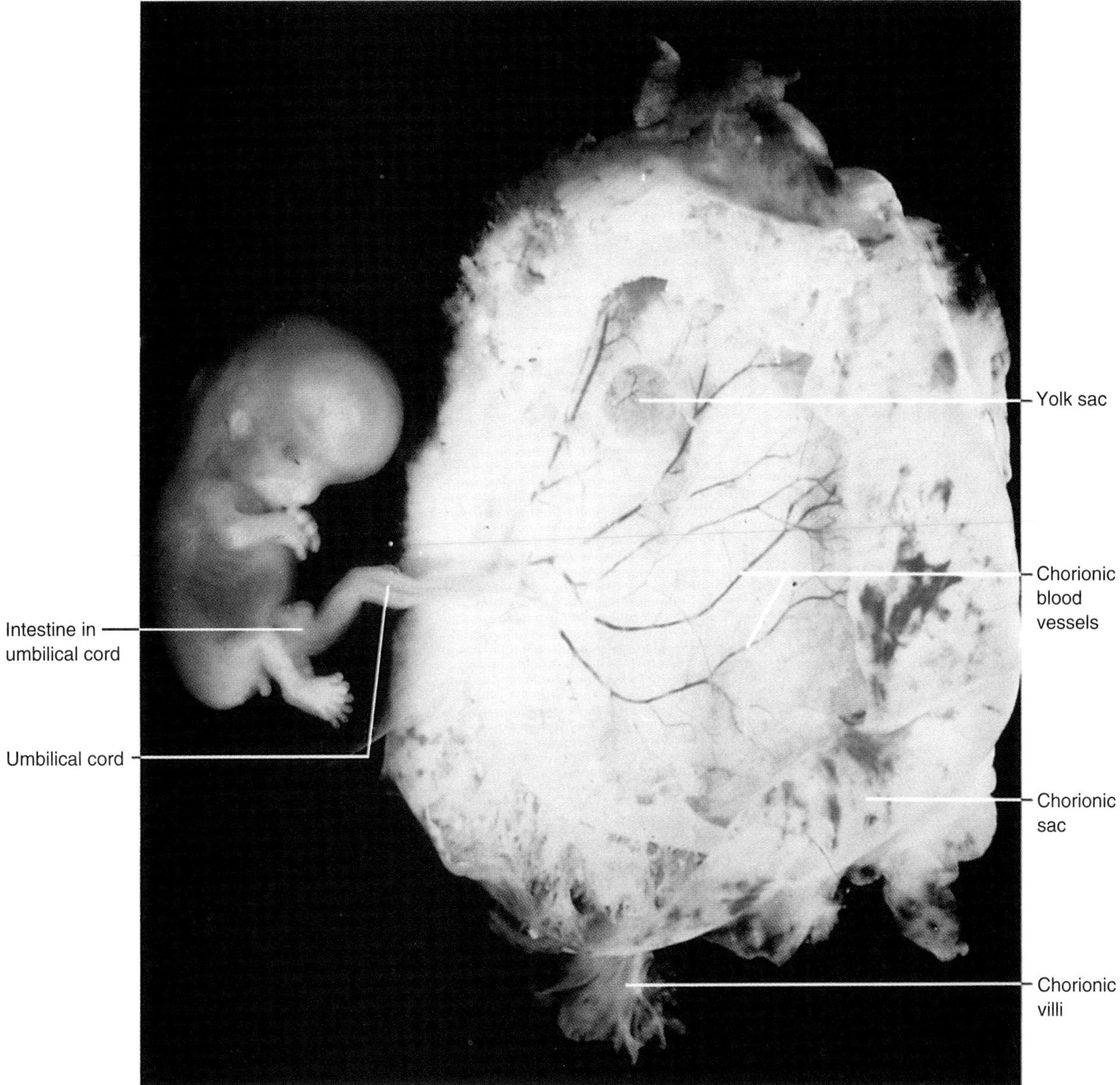

■ **Figure 5–21.** Lateral view of an embryo and its chorionic sac at Carnegie stage 23, about 56 days. Observe the human appearance of the embryo. (From Nishimura H, Semba R, Tanimura T, Tanaka O: *Prenatal Development of the Human with Special Reference to Craniofacial Structures: An Atlas.* Washington DC, National Institutes of Health, 1977.)

Estimation of Gestational Age

By convention, obstetricians date pregnancy in menstrual weeks, beginning from the first day of the last normal menstrual period (LNMP) (Hadlock, 1994). This is the *menstrual age* or gestational age. Embryonic or *fetal age* begins at fertilization or conception, about two weeks after LNMP. *Conceptional age* is used when the actual date of conception is known in patients who have undergone IV fertilization or artificial insemination (see Chapter 2). Determination of the starting date of a pregnancy may be difficult in some instances, partly because it depends on the mother's memory of an event that occurred several weeks before she realized she was pregnant. In summary, two reference points are commonly used for estimating age:

- onset of LNMP
- probable time of fertilization (conception)

Knowledge of embryonic age is important to obstetricians because it affects clinical management (Hadlock, 1994), especially when invasive procedures such as chorionic villus sampling and amniocentesis are necessary (see Chapter 6).

In some women, estimation of gestational age from the menstrual history alone may be unreliable. The probability of error in establishing LNMP is highest in women who become pregnant after cessation of oral contraception because the interval between discontinuance of hormones and the onset of ovulation is highly variable. In addition, slight uterine bleeding

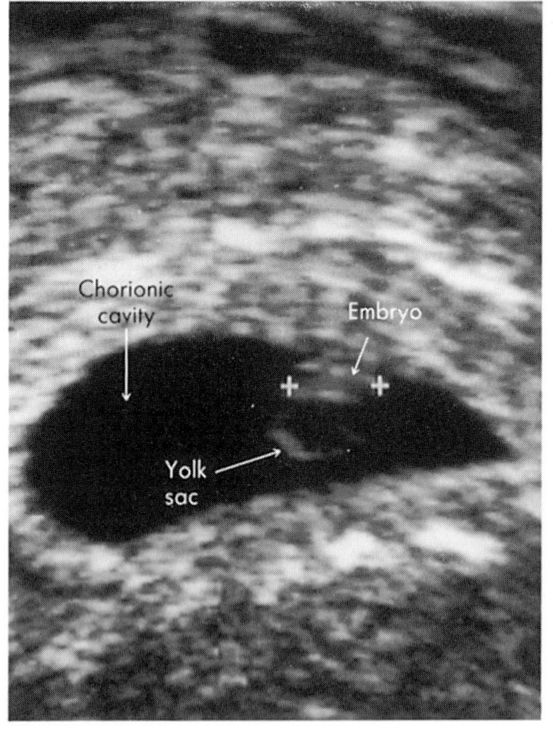

A

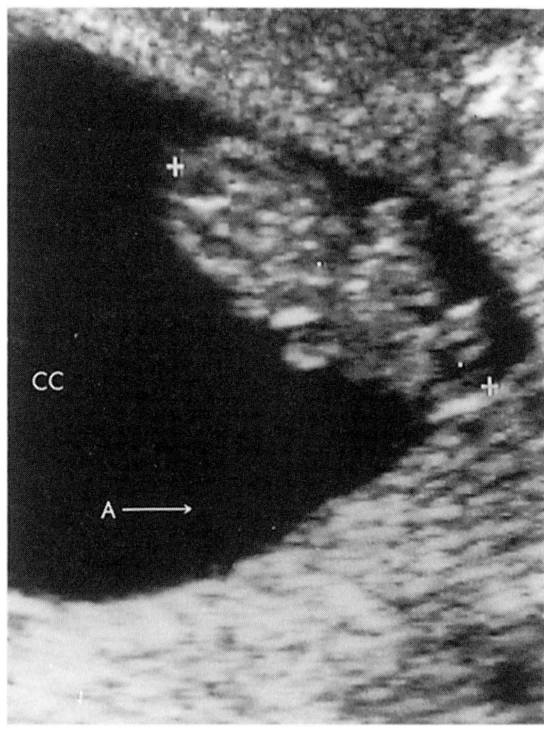

B

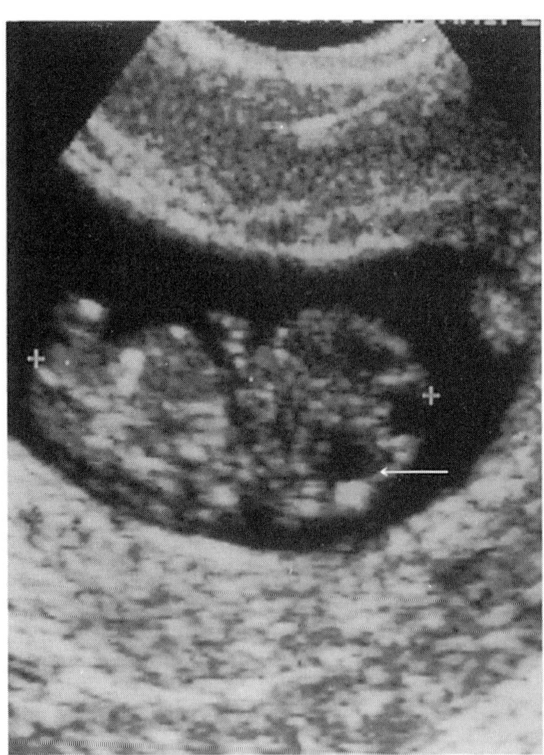

C

■ **Figure 5–22.** Ultrasound images of embryos. *A,* Crown-rump length (CRL) 4.8 mm. The 4.5-week-old embryo is indicated by the measurement cursors (+). Ventral to the embryo is the yolk sac. The chorionic cavity appears black. *B,* Coronal scan of 5-week-old embryo (CRL 2.09 cm). The upper limbs are clearly shown. The embryo is surrounded by a thin amnion (**A**). The fluid in the chorionic cavity (**CC**) is more particulate than the amniotic fluid. *C,* Sagittal scan of a 7-week-old embryo (CRL of 2.14 cm.) demonstrating the eye, limbs, and the developing fourth ventricle *(arrow)* of the brain. (Courtesy of E.A. Lyons, MD, Professor of Radiology and Obstetrics & Gynecology, Health Sciences Centre, University of Manitoba, Winnipeg, Manitoba, Canada.)

("spotting"), which sometimes occurs after implantation of the blastocyst, may be incorrectly regarded by a woman as light menstruation. Other contributing factors may include *oligomenorrhea* (scanty menstruation), pregnancy in the postpartum period (i.e., several weeks after childbirth), and use of intrauterine devices (IUDs). Despite possible sources of error, LNMP is commonly used by clinicians to estimate the age of embryos and it is a reliable criterion in most cases.

Ultrasound assessment of the size of the chorionic (gestational) cavity and its embryonic contents (Fig. 5-22) enables clinicians to obtain an accurate estimate of the date of conception (Filly, 1994; Lyons and Levi, 1991). The zygote does not form until about 2 weeks after LNMP; consequently, 14 ± 2 days must be deducted from the so-called menstrual (gestational) age to obtain the actual or fertilization age of an embryo.

The day fertilization occurs is the most accurate reference point for estimating age; this is commonly calculated from the estimated time of ovulation because the ovum is usually fertilized within 12 hours after ovulation. Because it may be important to know the actual age of an embryo (for determining its sensitivity to teratogenic agents—see Chapter 8), all statements about age should indicate the reference point used, that is, days after LNMP or after the estimated time of fertilization.

ESTIMATION OF EMBRYONIC AGE

Estimates of the age of recovered embryos after a spontaneous abortion, for example, are determined from their external characteristics and measurements of their length (Fig. 5-23, Table 5-1). Size alone may be an unreliable criterion because some embryos undergo a progressively slower rate of growth prior to death. The appearance of the developing limbs is a very helpful criterion for estimating embryonic age.

Methods of Measuring Embryos

Because embryos of the third and early fourth weeks are straight (Fig. 5-23*A*), measurements of them indicate the greatest length (GL). The sitting height or crown-rump length (CRL) is most frequently used for older embryos (Fig. 5-23*B*). Because no anatomical marker clearly indicates the crown or rump, one assumes that the longest CRL is the most accurate (Filly, 1994). In embryos with greatly flexed necks, the CRL is actually a head-rump measurement. Standing height, or crown-heel length (CHL), is sometimes measured for 8-week-old embryos. The CHL of formalin-fixed embryos may be difficult to determine because their limbs are not easy to straighten; these embryos should be measured as shown in Figure 5-23*D*. Because the length of an embryo is only one criterion for establishing age (Table 5-1), one should not refer to a 5-mm stage embryo. The *Carnegie Embryonic Staging System* is used internationally (Table 5-1); its usage enables comparisons to be made between the findings of one person and those of another.

Ultrasound Examination of Embryos

Most women seeking obstetrical care have at least one ultrasound examination during their pregnancy for one or more of the following reasons (Callen, 1994):

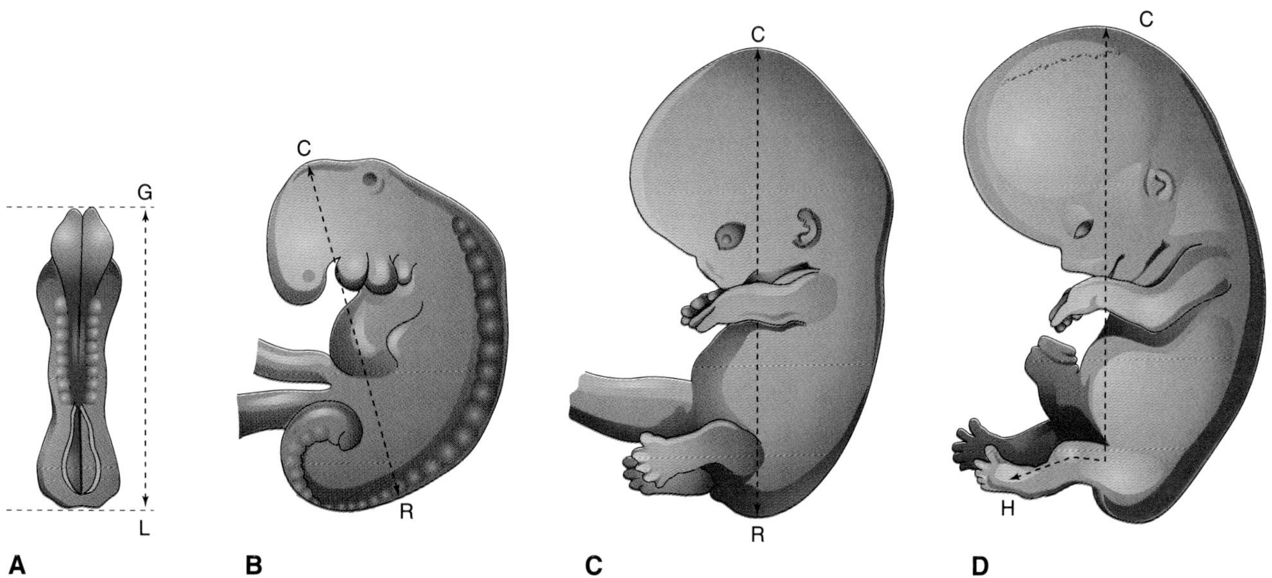

■ **Figure 5-23.** Sketches showing the methods used to measure the length of embryos. *A,* Greatest length. *B* and *C,* Crown-rump length. *D,* Crown-heel length.

- estimation of gestational and conceptional age for confirmation of clinical dating, which is usually calculated from the first day of the LNMP
- evaluation of embryonic growth when intrauterine growth retardation is suspected
- guidance during chorionic villus sampling (see Chapter 6)
- examination of a clinically detected pelvic mass
- suspected ectopic pregnancy (see Chapter 3)
- possible uterine abnormality
- detection of congenital anomalies

Current data indicate that there are no confirmed biological effects of ultrasound on embryos or fetuses from the use of diagnostic ultrasound evaluation (Reece et al., 1990).

The size of an embryo in a pregnant woman can be estimated using ultrasound measurements. *Transvaginal or endovaginal sonography* permits an earlier and more accurate measurement of CRL in early pregnancy. The embryonic CRL was determined as early as 25 days after follicle aspiration in pregnancies resulting from in vitro fertilization (Schats et al., 1991). Early in the fifth week (7 weeks after LNMP), the embryo is 4 to 7 mm long (Figs. 5-16 and 5-22*A*). During the sixth and seventh weeks, discrete embryonic structures can be visualized (e.g., parts of the limbs), and crown-rump measurements are predictive of embryonic age with an accuracy of 1 to 4 days. Furthermore, after the sixth week (8 weeks after LNMP), dimensions of the head and trunk can be obtained and used for assessment of embryonic age (Manning, 1989; Schats et al., 1991; Callen, 1994; Filly, 1994). There is, however, considerable variability in early embryonic growth (size) and development. Differences are greatest before the end of the first 4 weeks of development, but less so by the end of the embryonic period (Dickey and Gasser, 1993).

SUMMARY OF THE FOURTH TO EIGHTH WEEKS

During these 5 weeks, representing the major part of the embryonic period, *all major organs and systems of the body form* from the three germ layers (Fig. 5-5). At the beginning of the fourth week, folding in the median and horizontal planes converts the flat trilaminar embryonic disc into a C-shaped, cylindrical embryo. The formation of head, tail, and lateral folds is a continuous sequence of events that results in a constriction between the embryo and the yolk sac. During folding, the endodermal-lined yolk sac is incorporated into the embryo and gives rise to the primordial gut (foregut, midgut, and hindgut). As the head region folds ventrally, part of the endodermal layer is incorporated into the developing embryonic head as the *foregut*. Folding of the head region also results in the oropharyngeal membrane and heart being carried ventrally, and the developing brain becoming the most cranial part of the embryo.

As the tail region folds ventrally, part of the endodermal germ layer is incorporated into the caudal end of the embryo as the *hindgut*. The terminal part of the hindgut expands to form the *cloaca*. Folding of the tail region also results in the cloacal membrane, allantois, and connecting stalk being carried to the ventral surface of the embryo. Folding of the embryo in the horizontal plane incorporates part of the endodermal germ layer into the embryo as the *midgut*. The yolk sac remains attached to the midgut by a narrow *yolk stalk*. During folding in the horizontal plane, the primordia of the lateral and ventral body walls are formed. As the amnion expands, it envelops the connecting stalk, yolk stalk, and allantois, thereby forming an epithelial covering for the *umbilical cord*. The three germ layers differentiate into various tissues and organs, so that by the end of the embryonic period the beginnings of all the main organ systems have been established.

The external appearance of the embryo is greatly affected by the formation of the brain, heart, liver, somites, limbs, ears, nose, and eyes. As these structures develop, the appearance of the embryo changes so that it has unquestionably human characteristics at the end of the eighth week. Because the beginnings of most essential external and internal structures are formed during the fourth to eighth weeks, this is the most critical period of development. Developmental disturbances during this period may give rise to major congenital anomalies of the embryo (see Chapter 8).

Reasonable estimates of the age of embryos can be determined from

- the day of onset of the LNMP
- the estimated time of fertilization or conception
- ultrasound measurements of the chorionic sac and embryo
- examination of the external characteristics of the embryo.

Clinically Oriented Problems

Case 5–1

A 28-year-old woman, who has been a heavy cigarette smoker since her teens, was informed that she was in the second month of pregnancy.

- What would the doctor likely tell the patient about her smoking habit and the use of other drugs (e.g., alcohol)?

Case 5–2

Physicians usually explain the critical period of development to their patients.

- Why is the embryonic period such a critical stage of development?

Case 5–3

A patient was concerned about what she had read in the newspaper about recent effects of drugs in laboratory animals.

- Can one predict the possible harmful effects of drugs on the human embryo from studies performed in experimental animals?
- Discuss germ layer formation and organogenesis.

Case 5–4

A 30-year-old woman was unsure when her LNMP was. She stated that her periods were irregular.

- Why may information about the starting date of a pregnancy provided by a patient be unreliable?
- What clinical techniques are now available for evaluating embryonic (gestational) age?

Case 5–5

A woman who had just become pregnant told her doctor that she had accidentally taken a sleeping pill given to her by a friend. She wondered if it could harm her baby.

- Would a drug known to cause severe limb defects be likely to cause these abnormalities if it was administered during the eighth week?
- Discuss the mechanism of the action of these teratogens (see Chapter 8).

Discussion of these problems appears at the back of the book.

REFERENCES AND SUGGESTED READING

Bard J: *Morphogenesis. The Cellular and Molecular Processes of Developmental Anatomy*. Cambridge, Cambridge University Press, 1992.

Barnea ER, Hustin J, Jauniaux E (eds): *The First Twelve Weeks of Gestation*. Berlin, Springer Verlag, 1992.

Biggers JD: Arbitrary Partitions of Prenatal life. *Hum Reprod 5*:1, 1990.

Callen PW (ed): *Ultrasonography in Obstetrics and Gynecology*, 3rd ed. Philadelphia, WB Saunders, 1994.

Chapman MG, Grudzinskas JG, Chard T (eds): *The Embryo. Normal and Abnormal Development and Growth*. New York, Springer Verlag, 1990.

Cooke J: The early embryo and the formation of body pattern. *American Scientist 76*:35, 1988.

De Haan R, Ursprung H: *Organogenesis*. New York, Holt, Rinehart and Winston, 1965.

Dickey RP, Gasser RF: Computer analysis of the human embryo growth curve: differences between published ultrasound findings on living embryos in utero and data on fixed specimens. *Anat Rec 237*:400, 1993.

Dickey RP, Gasser RF: Ultrasound evidence for variability in the size and development of normal human embryos before the tenth post-insemination week after assisted reproductive technologies. *Hum Reprod 8*:331, 1993.

Eichele G: Retinoids and vertebrate limb pattern formation. *Trends Genet 5*:246, 1990.

England MA: Cellular processes and tissue interactions in developmental pathology. *In* Harrison MR, Golbus MS, Filly RA (eds): *The Unborn Patient. Prenatal Diagnosis and Treatment*, 2nd ed. Philadelphia, WB Saunders, 1990.

Filly RA: Ultrasound evaluation during the first trimester. *In* Callen PW (ed): *Ultrasonography in Obstetrics and Gynecology*, 3rd ed. Philadelphia, WB Saunders, 1994.

Guthrie S: Horizontal and vertical pathways in neural induction. *Trends Neurosci 14*:123, 1991.

Hadlock FP: Ultrasound determination of menstrual age. *In* Callen PW (ed): *Ultrasonography in Obstetrics and Gynecology*, 3rd ed. Philadelphia, WB Saunders, 1994.

Hiett AK, Devoe LD, Falls DG, Martin SA: Ultrasound diagnosis of a twin gestation with concordant body stalk anomaly. *J Reprod Med 37*:944, 1992.

Hinrichsen KV (ed): *Humanembryologie*. Berlin, Springer Verlag, 1990.

Iffy L, Shepard TH, Jakobovits A, et al: The rate of growth in young human embryos of Streeter's horizons XIII and XXIII. *Acta Anat 66*:178, 1967.

Kalousek DK, Fitch N, Paradice BA: *Pathology of the Human Embryo and Previable Fetus: An Atlas*. New York, Springer Verlag, 1990.

Kerner P: The rate of growth in young human embryos of Streeter's horizons XIII and XXIII. *Acta Anat 66*:178, 1967.

Khong TY: Pathology of intrauterine growth retardation. *Am J Reprod Immunol 21*:132, 1989.

Kurtz AB, Needleman L: Ultrasound assessment of fetal age. *In* Callen PW (ed) *Ultrasonography in Obstetrics and Gynecology*, 3rd ed. Philadelphia, WB Saunders, 1994.

Lyons EA, Levi CS: Ultrasound of the normal first trimester of pregnancy. Syllabus. Special Course. Ultrasound, Radiological Society of North America, Inc., 1991.

Manning FA: General principles and applications of ultrasound. *In* Creasy RK, Resnik R (eds): *Maternal-Fetal Medicine*, 2nd ed. Philadelphia, WB Saunders, 1989.

Muragaki Y, Mundlos S, Upton J, Olsen BR: Altered growth and branching patterns in synpolydactyly caused by mutations in HOXD13. *Science 272*:548, 1996.

Nieuwkoop PD, Johnen AG, Albers B: *The Epigenetic Nature of Early Chordate Development. Inductive Interaction and Competence*. London, Cambridge University Press, 1985.

Nishimura H, Takano K, Tanimura T, Yasuda M: Normal and abnormal development of human embryos. *Teratology 1*:281, 1968.

Nishimura H, Tanimura T, Semba R, Uwabe C: Normal development of early human embryos: Observation of 90 specimens at Carnegie stages 7 to 13. *Teratology 10*:1, 1974.

Oppenheimer JM: The non-specificity of the germ layers. *Q Rev Biol 15*:1-27, 1940.

O'Rahilly R, Müller F: *Developmental Stages in Human Embryos*. Washington, Carnegie Institute of Washington, 1987.

Persaud TVN: *Environmental Causes of Human Birth Defects*. Springfield, Charles C Thomas, 1990.

Placzek M, Furley A: Neural development: patterning cascades in the neural tube. *Curr Biol 6*:526, 1996.

Reece EA, Assimakopoulos E, Zheng X-Z, et al: The safety of obstetric ultrasonography: concern for the fetus. *Obstet Gynecol 6*:139, 1990.

Rossomando EF, Alexander S (eds): *Morphogenesis. An Analysis of the Development of Biological Form*. New York, Dekker, 1992.

Ruberte E, Dolle P, Krust A, et al: Specific spatial and temporal distribution of retinoic acid receptor gamma transcripts during mouse embryogenesis. *Development 108*:213, 1990.

Sasai Y, DeRobertis EM: Ectodermal patterning in vertebrate embryos. *Dev Biol 182*:5, 1997.

Saxen L: Interactive mechanisms in morphogenesis. *In* Tarin D (ed): *Tissue Interactions in Carcinogenesis*. London, Academic Press, 1972.

Schats R, Van Os HC, Jansen CAM, Wladimiroff JW: The crown-rump length in early human pregnancy: a reappraisal. *Br J Obstet Gynaecol 98*:460, 1991.

Senterre J (ed): Intrauterine Growth Retardation: Nestle Nutrition Workshop Series, vol 18. New York, Raven Press, 1989.

Shepard TH: Normal and abnormal growth patterns. *In* Gardner LI (ed): *Endocrine and Genetic Diseases of Childhood and Adolescence*, 2nd ed. Philadelphia, WB Saunders, 1975.

Shiota K: Development and intrauterine fate of normal and abnormal human conceptuses. *Congen Anom 31*:67, 1991.

Streeter GL: Developmental horizons in human embryos: description of age group XI, 13 to 20 somites, and age group XII, 21 to 29 somites. *Contrib Embryol Carnegie Inst 30*:211, 1942.

Streeter GL: Developmental horizons in human embryos: description of age group XIII, embryos of 4 or 5 millimeters long, and age group XIV, period of identification of the lens vesicle. *Contrib Embryol Carnegie Inst 31*:27, 1945.

Streeter GL: Developmental horizons in human embryos: description of age groups XV, XVI, XVII, and XVIII. *Contrib Embryol Carnegie Inst 32:*133, 1948.

Streeter GL, Heuser CH, Corner GW: Developmental horizons in human embryos: Description of age groups XIX, XX, XXI, XXII and XXIII. *Contrib Embryol Carnegie Inst 34:*165, 1951.

Tanabe Y, Roelink H, Jessell T: Induction of motor neurons by sonic hedgehog is independent of foreplate differentiation. *Curr Biol 5:* 651, 1995.

Thompson MW, McInnes RR, Willard HF: *Thompson & Thompson Genetics in Medicine*, 5th ed. Philadelphia, WB Saunders, 1991.

Torry DS, Cooper GM: Proto-oncogenes in development and cancer. *Am J Reprod Immunol 25:*129, 1991.

Wolpert L: *The Triumph of the Embryo*. Oxford, Oxford University Press, 1991.

Yamada KM (ed): *Cell Interactions and Development.* New York, John Wiley & Sons, 1983.

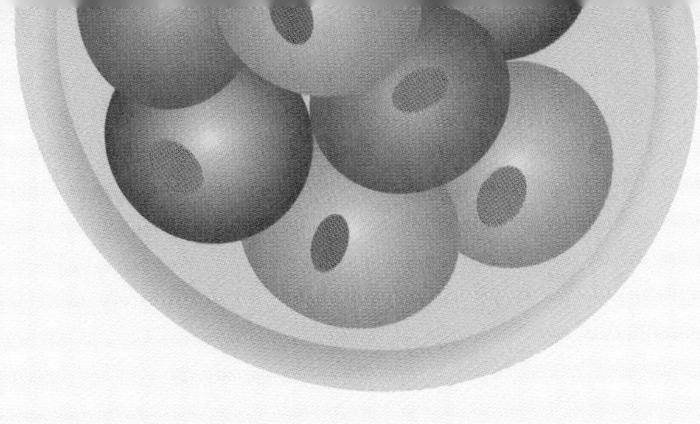

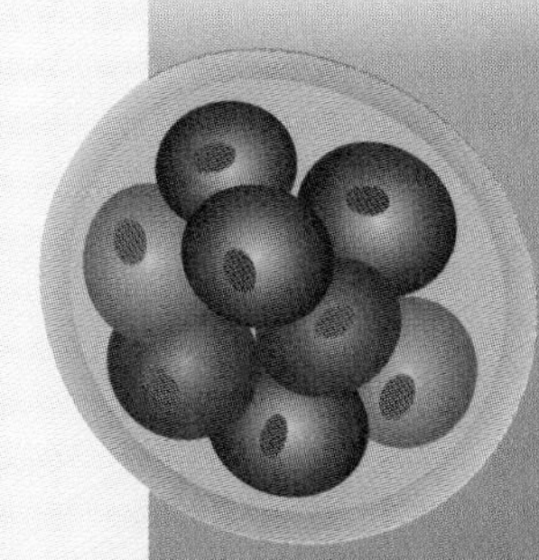

The Fetal Period:
Ninth Week to Birth

6

■ The transformation of an embryo to a fetus is gradual, but the name change is meaningful because it signifies that the embryo has developed into a recognizable human being, and that all major systems have formed. Development during the fetal period is primarily concerned with rapid body growth and differentiation of tissues, organs, and systems. A notable change occurring during the fetal period is the relative slowdown in the growth of the head compared with the rest of the body (England, 1983; Barnea et al., 1992; Hadlock, 1994a). The rate of body growth during the fetal period is very rapid (Fig. 6-1, Table 6-1), and

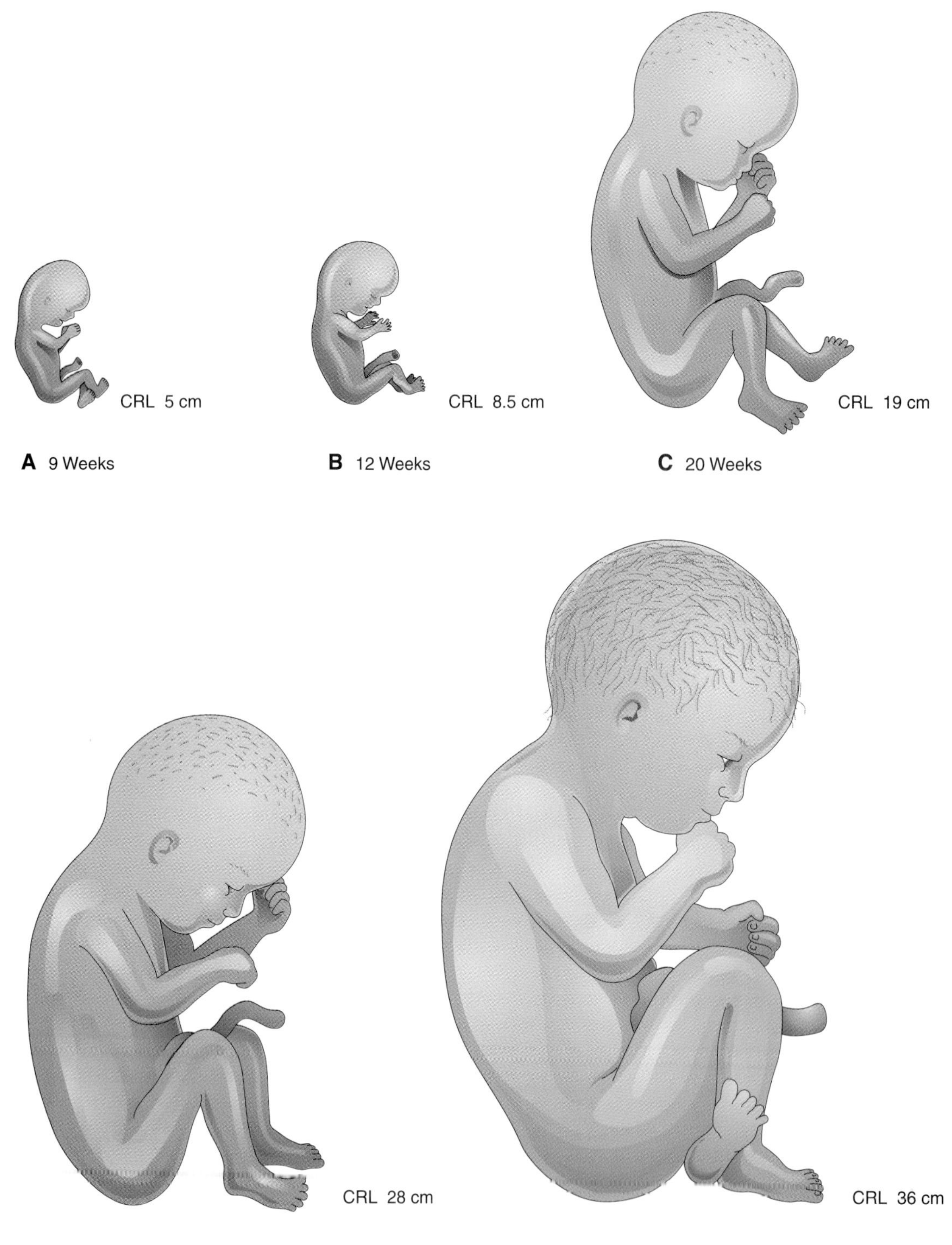

■ **Figure 6–1.** Drawings of fetuses at various stages of development. Head hair begins to appear at about 20 weeks and eyebrows and eyelashes are usually recognizable at about 24 weeks. The eyes are open at about 26 weeks. (CRL, crown-rump length.)

Table 6–1 ■ Criteria for Estimating Fertilization Age During the Fetal Period

Age (weeks)	CR Length (mm)*	Foot Length (mm)*	Fetal Weight (gm)†	Main External Characteristics
Previable Fetuses				
9	50	7	8	*Eye closing or closed.* Head large and more rounded. External genitalia still not distinguishable as male or female. Intestines in proximal part of umbilical cord. Ears are low-set.
10	61	9	14	*Intestines in the abdomen.* Early fingernail development.
12	87	14	45	*Sex distinguishable externally.* Well-defined neck.
14	120	20	110	*Head erect.* Eyes face anteriorly. Ears are closed to their definitive position. Lower limbs well-developed. Early toenail development.
16	140	27	200	*External ears stand out* from head.
18	160	33	320	*Vernix caseosa covers skin.* Quickening (signs of life) felt by mother.
20	190	39	460	*Head and body hair (lanugo) visible.*
Viable Fetuses‡				
22	210	45	630	*Skin wrinkled,* translucent, and pink to red.
24	230	50	820	*Fingernails present.* Lean body.
26	250	55	1000	*Eyes partially open.* Eyelashes present.
28	270	59	1300	*Eyes wide open.* Good head of hair often present. Skin slightly wrinkled.
30	280	63	1700	*Toenails present.* Body filling out. Testes descending.
32	300	68	2100	*Fingernails reach finger tips.* Skin pink and smooth.
36	340	79	2900	*Body usually plump.* Lanugo hairs almost absent. Toenails reach toe tips. Flexed limbs; firm grasp.
38	360	83	3400	*Prominent chest;* breasts protrude. Testes in scrotum or palpable in inguinal canals. Fingernails extend beyond finger tips.

CR, crown-rump

* These measurements are averages and so may not apply to specific cases; dimensional variations increase with age.

† These weights refer to fetuses that have been fixed for about 2 weeks in 10% formalin. Fresh specimens usually weigh about 5% less.

‡ There is no sharp limit of development, age, or weight at which a fetus automatically becomes viable or beyond which survival is assured, but experience has shown that it is rare for a baby to survive whose weight is less than 500 gm or whose fertilization age is less than 22 weeks. Even fetuses born between 26 and 28 weeks have difficulty surviving, mainly because the respiratory system and the central nervous system are not completely differentiated. The term *abortion* refers to all pregnancies that terminate before the period of viability.

fetal weight gain is phenomenal during the terminal weeks. Periods of normal continuous growth alternate with prolonged intervals of absent growth (Bernstein et al., 1995).

Viability of Fetuses

Viability is defined as the ability of fetuses to survive in the extrauterine environment (i.e., after a premature birth). Fetuses weighing less than 500 gm at birth usually do not survive; however, Muraskas et al. (1992) have reported an infant who weighed 280 gm at birth with intact (unimpaired) survival. The infant was delivered by cesarean section at 26.9 weeks gestation (about 24.9 weeks after fertilization). At 2 years of age the child was developmentally normal (Muraskas et al., 1992). Many full-term, *low-birth weight babies* result from intrauterine growth retardation (IUGR). Consequently, if given expert postnatal care, some fetuses weighing less than 500 gm may survive; they are referred to as *extremely low birth weight* (ELBW) or *immature infants.* Most fetuses weighing between 1500 and 2500 gm survive but have difficulties; they are *premature infants.* Prematurity is one of the most common causes of morbidity and perinatal death (Behrman et al., 1996).

ESTIMATION OF FETAL AGE

If doubt arises about the age of a fetus in patients with an uncertain medical history, ultrasound measurements of the crown-rump length (CRL) can be taken to determine its size and probable age, and to provide a reliable prediction of the *expected date of confinement* (EDC) for delivery of the fetus (Hadlock, 1994b). Fetal head measurements and femur length are also used to evaluate the age of the fetus. *Gestational age* is commonly used clinically and it may be confusing because the term seems to imply the actual age of the fetus from fertilization or conception (Callen, 1994b). In fact this term is most often meant to be synonymous with menstrual age — the length of time calculated from the first day of the last normal menstrual period (LNMP). *It is important that the person ordering the ultrasound examination and the ultrasonographer use the same terminology* (Callen, 1994b).

The intrauterine period may be divided into days, weeks, or months (Table 6–2), but confusion arises if it is not stated whether the age is calculated from the onset of the LNMP, or the estimated day of fertilization or conception. Most uncertainty about age arises when months are used, particularly when it is not stated whether calendar months (28 to 31 days) or lunar months (28 days) are meant. Unless otherwise stated, fetal age in this book is calculated from the

Table 6-2 ▪ Comparison of Gestational Time Units

Reference Point	Days	Weeks	Calendar Months	Lunar Months
Fertilization*	266	38	8¾	9½
LNMP	280	40	9¼	10

* The date of birth is calculated as 266 days after the estimated day of fertilization, or 280 days after the onset of the last normal menstrual period (*LNMP*). From fertilization to the end of the embryonic period (8 weeks), age is best expressed in days; thereafter age is often given in weeks.

estimated time of fertilization, and months refer to calendar months. It is best to express fetal age in weeks and to state whether the beginning or end of a week is meant, because statements such as "in the tenth week" are nonspecific.

Trimesters of Pregnancy

Clinically the gestational period is divided into three *trimesters*, each lasting 3 months. At the end of the first trimester, all major systems are developed (see Fig. 7-1*B*). Recently, it has been proposed that embryonic and developmental landmarks be used in defining progressive stages of fetal development (Sawin and Morgan, 1996). In the second trimester the fetus grows sufficiently in size so that good anatomical detail can be visualized during ultrasonography. During this period most major fetal anomalies can be detected using high-resolution real-time ultrasound (Hadlock, 1994b). By the end of the second trimester, the fetus may survive if born prematurely. The fetus reaches a major developmental landmark at 35 weeks of gestation. It weighs about 2500 gm, which is used to define the level of fetal maturity. At this stage the fetus usually survives if born prematurely.

External Characteristics of Fetuses

Various measurements and external characteristics are useful for estimating fetal age (Table 6-1). CRL is the method of choice for estimating fetal age until the end of the first trimester because there is very little variability in fetal size during this period. In the second and third trimesters, several structures can be identified and measured ultrasonographically (Hadlock, 1994b), but the basic measurements are:

- biparietal diameter (BPD) — diameter of the head between the two parietal eminences
- head circumference
- abdominal circumference
- femur length
- foot length

Foot length correlates well with CRL and is particularly useful for estimating the age of incomplete or macerated fetuses (see Fig. 6-12). *Fetal weight* is often a useful criterion for estimating age, but there may be a discrepancy between the age and the weight of a fetus, particularly when the mother had metabolic disturbances during pregnancy such as diabetes mellitus. In these cases, fetal weight often exceeds values considered normal for CRL.

Freshly expelled fetuses have a shiny translucent appearance, whereas those that have been dead for several days prior to spontaneous abortion have a tanned appearance and lack normal resilience. Fetal dimensions obtained from ultrasound measurements of fetuses closely approximate CRL measurements obtained from aborted fetuses. Cheek-to-cheek (Abramowicz et al., 1991) and transverse cerebellar measurements (Lee et al., 1991) have also been used for assessment of fetal growth and gestational age, respectively. Determination of the size of a fetus, especially of its head, is of great value to the obstetrician for the management of patients; e.g., women with small pelves and/or fetuses with IUGR and/or congenital anomalies.

HIGHLIGHTS OF THE FETAL PERIOD

There is no formal staging system for the fetal period; however, it is helpful to consider the changes that occur in periods of 4 to 5 weeks.

Nine to Twelve Weeks

At the beginning of the ninth week, the head constitutes half the CRL of the fetus (Figs. 6-1*A* to 6-3). Subsequently, growth in body length accelerates rapidly and by the end of 12 weeks the CRL has more than doubled (Table 6-1). Although growth of the head slows down considerably by the twelfth week, it is still disproportionately large compared with the rest of the body. At 9 weeks the face is broad, the eyes are widely separated, the ears are low-set, and the eyelids are fused. By the end of 12 weeks, *primary ossification centers* appear in the skeleton, especially in the

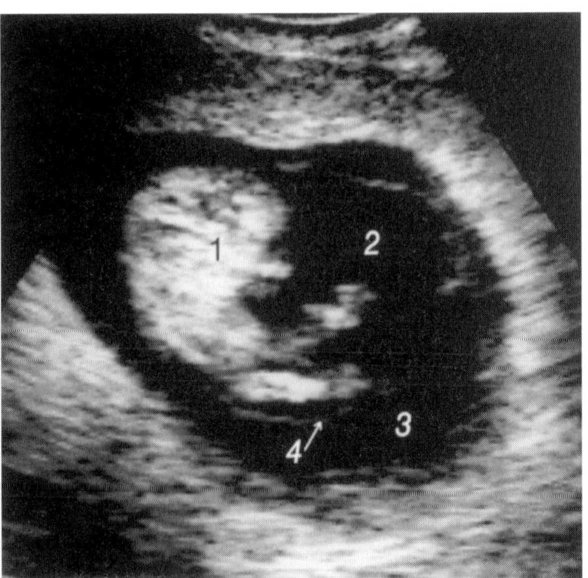

■ **Figure 6-2.** Transvaginal ultrasound scan of a fetus **(1)** early in the ninth week showing its relationship to the amniotic cavity **(2)**, the extrafetal or chorionic cavity **(3)**, and amnion **(4)**. (From Wathen NC, Cass PL, Kitan MJ, Chard T: *Prenatal Diagnosis 11*:145, 1991.)

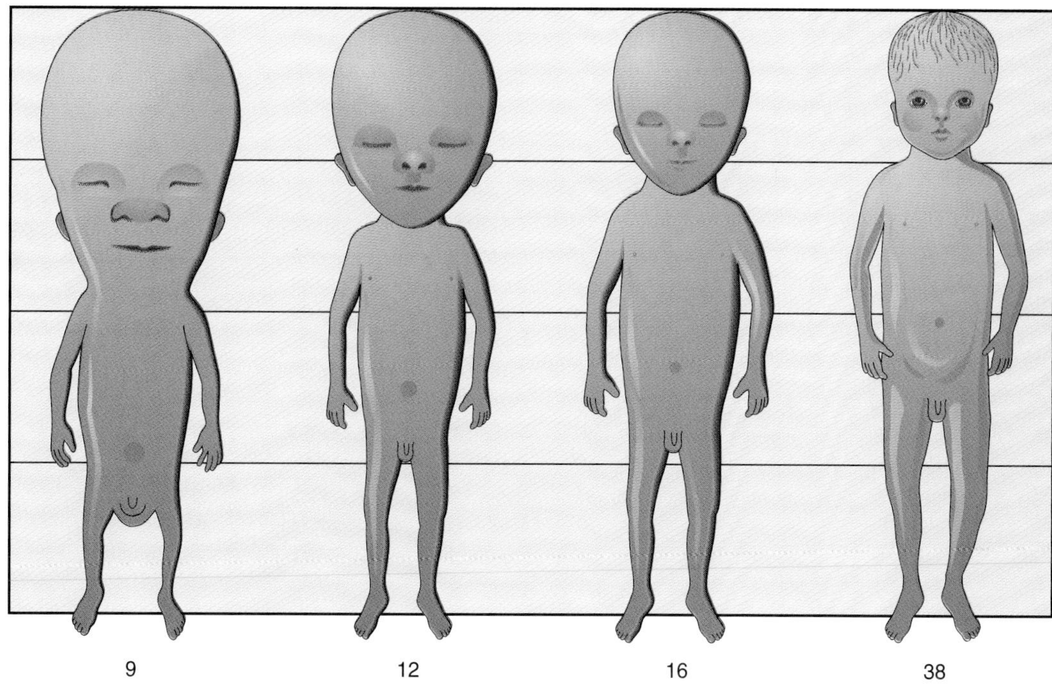

■ **Figure 6–3.** Diagram illustrating the changing proportions of the body during the fetal period. At 9 weeks the head is about half the crown-rump length of the fetus. By 36 weeks, the circumferences of the head and the abdomen are approximately equal. After this, the circumference of the abdomen may be greater. All stages are drawn to the same total height.

skull and long bones. The eyelids are fused throughout this period (Fig. 6-4*A* and *B*).

Early in the ninth week, the legs are short and the thighs are relatively small. By the end of 12 weeks, the upper limbs have almost reached their final relative lengths, but the lower limbs are still not so well developed and are slightly shorter than their final relative lengths. The external genitalia of males and females

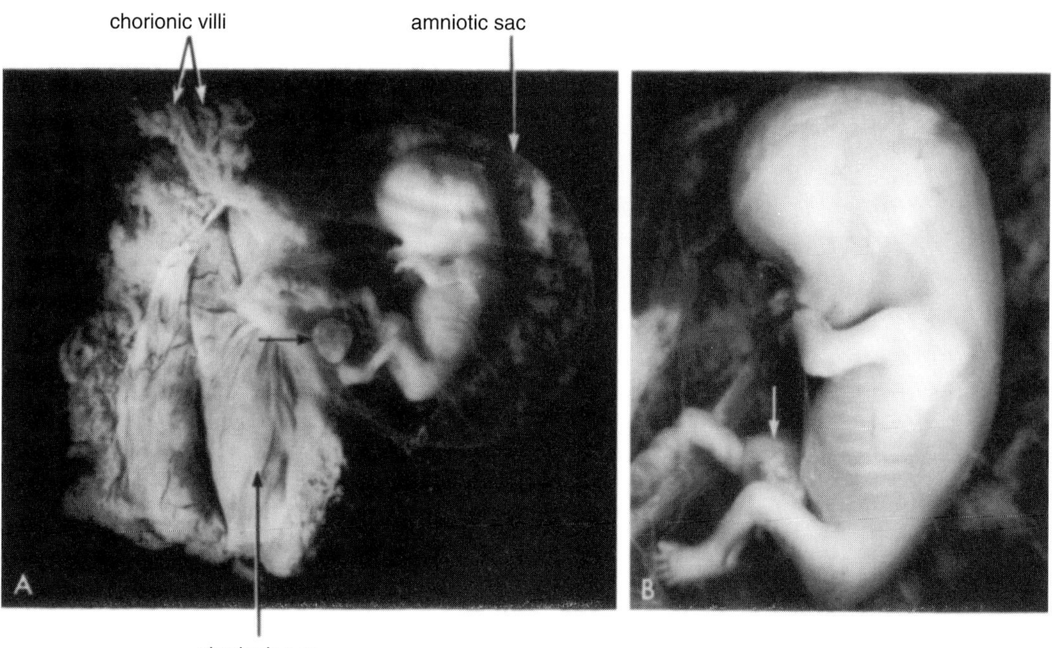

■ **Figure 6–4.** Photographs of a 9-week fetus in the amniotic sac exposed by removal from its chorionic sac. *A,* Actual size. The remnant of the yolk sac is indicated by an arrow. *B,* Enlarged photograph of the fetus (×2). Note the following features: large head, cartilaginous ribs, and intestines in the umbilical cord *(arrow).* (Courtesy of Professor Jean Hay [Retired], Department of Anatomy, University of Manitoba, Winnipeg, Manitoba, Canada.)

appear similar until the end of the ninth week. Their mature fetal form is not established until the twelfth week. Intestinal coils are clearly visible in the proximal end of the umbilical cord until the middle of the tenth week (Fig. 6-4*B*). By the eleventh week the intestines have returned to the abdomen (Fig. 6-5).

At the beginning of the fetal period, the liver is the major site of *erythropoiesis* (formation of red blood cells). By the end of the twelfth week, this activity has decreased in the liver and has begun in the spleen. *Urine formation* begins between the ninth and twelfth weeks and urine is discharged into the amniotic fluid. The fetus reabsorbs some of this fluid after swallowing it. Fetal waste products are transferred to the maternal circulation by passing across the placental membrane (see Chapter 7).

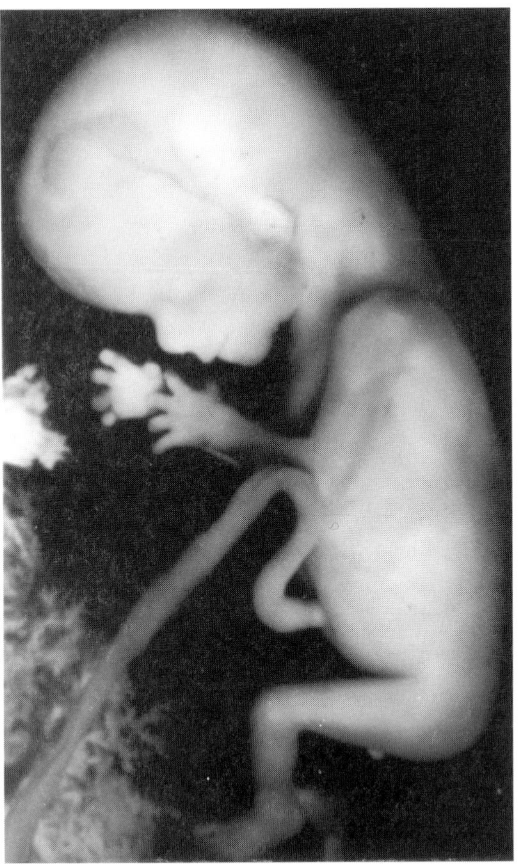

■ **Figure 6-5.** Photograph of an 11-week fetus exposed by removal from its chorionic and amniotic sacs (×1.5). Note the relatively large head and that the intestines are no longer in the umbilical cord. (Courtesy of Professor Jean Hay [Retired], Department of Anatomy, University of Manitoba, Winnipeg, Manitoba, Canada.)

Thirteen to Sixteen Weeks

Growth is very rapid during this period (Figs. 6-6 and 6-7; Table 6-1). By 16 weeks the head is relatively small compared with that of the 12-week fetus and the lower limbs have lengthened. Limb movements, which first occur at the end of the embryonic period (8 weeks), become coordinated by the fourteenth week but are too slight to be felt by the mother. These movements are visible during ultrasound examinations.

Ossification of the fetal skeleton is active during this period and the bones are clearly visible in ultrasound images of the mother's abdomen by the beginning of the sixteenth week. Birnholz (1981) revealed by ultrasonography that *slow eye movements occur at 14 weeks* (16 weeks after LNMP). Scalp hair patterning is also determined during this period. By 16 weeks

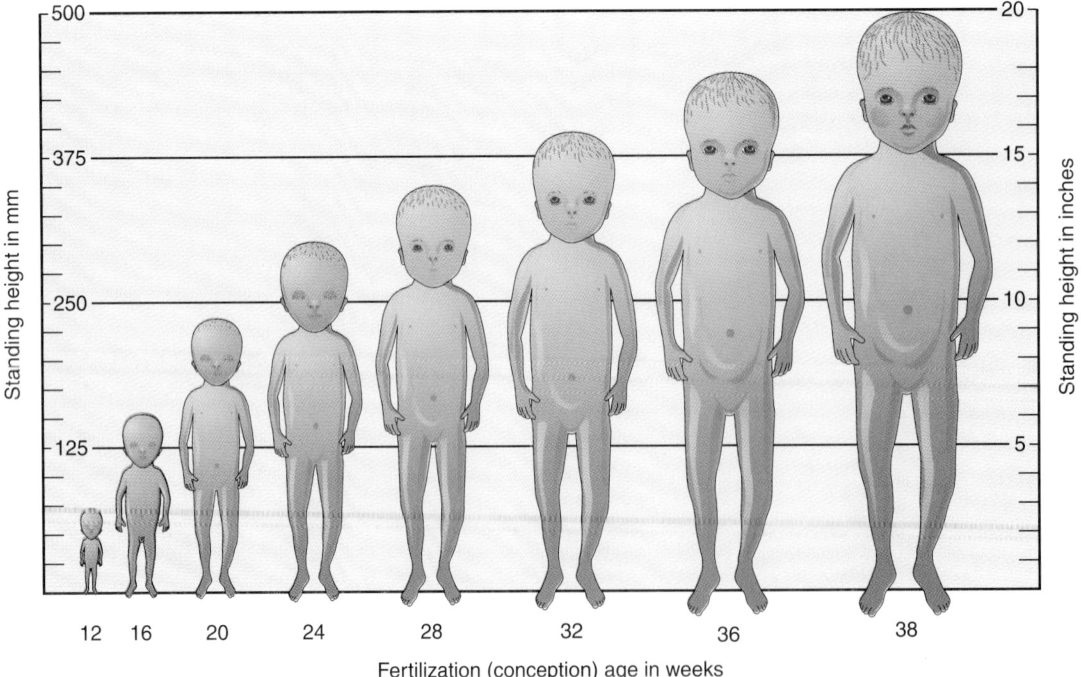

■ **Figure 6-6.** Diagram, drawn to scale, illustrating the changes in the size of the human fetus.

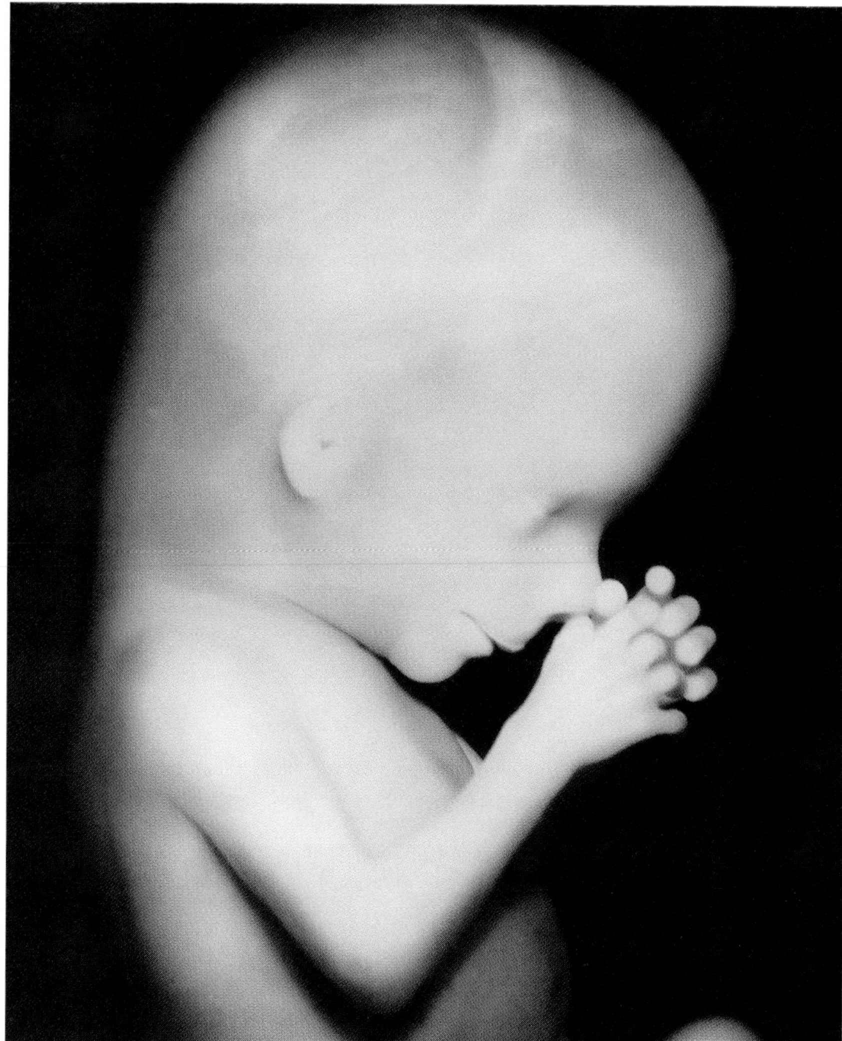

■ **Figure 6–7.** Enlarged photograph of the head and shoulders of a 13-week fetus. (Courtesy of Professor Jean Hay [Retired], Department of Anatomy, University of Manitoba, Winnipeg, Manitoba, Canada.)

the ovaries are differentiated and contain primordial follicles that have oogonia (see Chapter 13). The external genitalia can be recognized by 14 weeks, and by 16 weeks the appearance of the fetus is even more human because its eyes face anteriorly rather than anterolaterally. In addition, the external ears are close to their definitive position on the sides of the head.

Seventeen to Twenty Weeks

Growth slows down during this period but the fetus still increases its CRL by about 50 mm (Figs. 6-6 and 6-8; Table 6-1). The limbs reach their final relative proportions and fetal movements — **quickening** — are commonly felt by the mother. The mean time that intervenes between a mother's first detection of fetal movements and delivery is 147 days, with a standard deviation of ± 15 days (Page et al., 1981). The skin is now covered with a greasy cheeselike material — **vernix caseosa**. It consists of a mixture of a fatty secretion from the fetal sebaceous glands and dead epidermal cells. The vernix caseosa protects the delicate fetal skin from abrasions, chapping, and hardening that could result from exposure to the amniotic fluid. Eyebrows and head hair are also visible at 20 weeks. The bodies of 20-week fetuses are usually completely covered with fine downy hair — **lanugo** — which helps to hold the vernix caseosa on the skin.

Brown fat forms during this period and is the site of heat production, particularly in the newborn infant. This specialized adipose tissue produces heat by oxidizing fatty acids. Brown fat is chiefly found at the root of the neck, posterior to the sternum, and in the perirenal area (England, 1983). Brown fat has a high content of mitochondria, giving it a definite brown hue. By 18 weeks the uterus is formed and canalization of the vagina has begun. By this time many *primordial ovarian follicles* containing oogonia have formed. By 20 weeks the *testes* have begun to descend, but they are still located on the posterior abdominal wall, as are the *ovaries* in female fetuses.

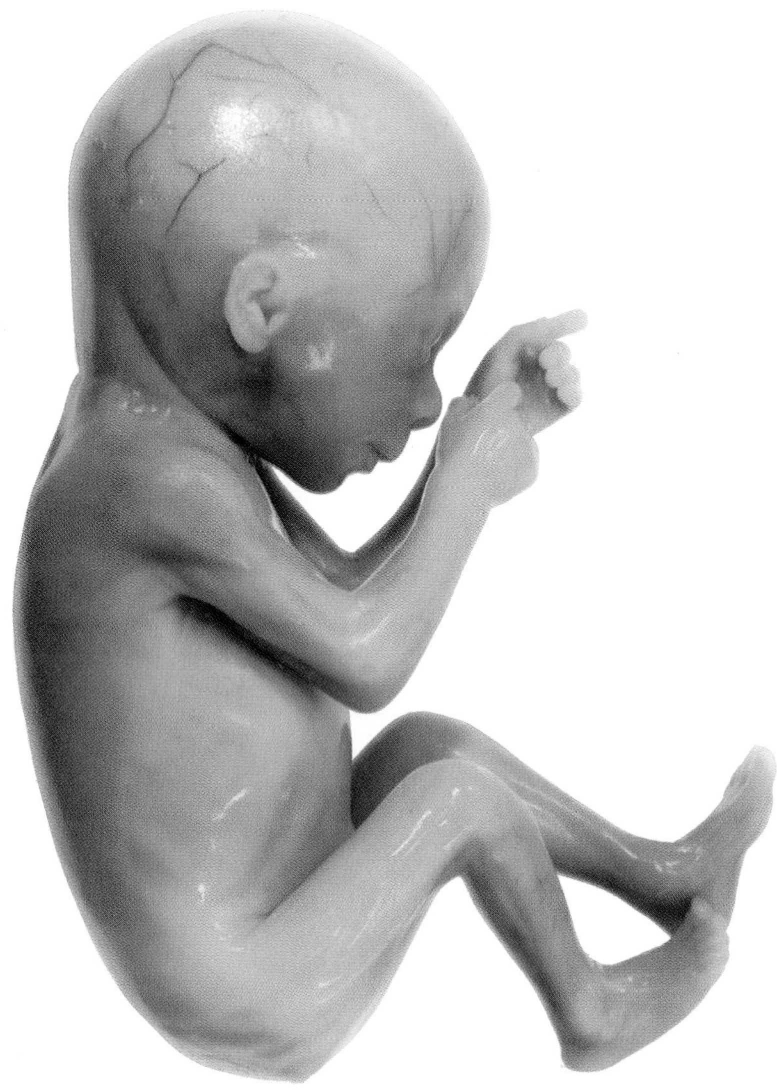

■ **Figure 6–8.** Photograph of a 17-week fetus. Actual size. Because there is no subcutaneous fat and the skin is thin, the blood vessels of the scalp are visible. Fetuses at this age are unable to survive if born prematurely, mainly because their respiratory systems are immature. (From Moore KL, Persaud TVN, Shiota K: *Color Atlas of Clinical Embryology.* Philadelphia, WB Saunders, 1994.)

Twenty-One to Twenty-Five Weeks

There is a substantial weight gain during this period. Although still somewhat lean, the fetus is better proportioned (Fig. 6-9). The skin is usually wrinkled and more translucent, particularly during the early part of this period. The skin is pink to red in fresh specimens because blood is visible in the capillaries. At 21 weeks rapid eye movements begin and *blink-startle responses* have been reported at 22 to 23 weeks following application of a vibroacoustic noise source to the mother's abdomen (Birnholz and Benaceraff, 1983). By 24 weeks the secretory epithelial cells (type II pneumocytes) in the interalveolar walls of the lung have begun to secrete *surfactant*, a surface-active lipid that maintains the patency of the developing alveoli of the lungs (see Chapter 11). *Fingernails* are also present by 24 weeks. Although a 22- to 25-week fetus born prematurely may survive if given intensive care, it may die during early infancy because its respiratory system is still immature.

Twenty-Six to Twenty-Nine Weeks

At this age a fetus often survives if born prematurely and given intensive care because its *lungs are now capable of breathing air*. The lungs and pulmonary vasculature have developed sufficiently to provide adequate gas exchange. In addition, the central nervous system has matured to the stage where it can direct rhythmic breathing movements and control body temperature. The greatest neonatal losses occur in infants of low (2500 gm or less) and very low (1500 gm or less) birth weight (Behrman et al., 1996).

The eyes are open at 26 weeks and lanugo and head hair are well developed (Fig. 6-10). Toenails become visible and considerable subcutaneous fat is now present under the skin, smoothing out many of the wrinkles. During this period the quantity of white fat increases to about 3.5% of body weight. *The fetal spleen is now an important site of hematopoiesis*— the process of formation and development of various types of blood cells and other formed elements. Erythropoiesis in the spleen ends by 28 weeks, by which time bone marrow has become the major site of this process (Boles, 1991).

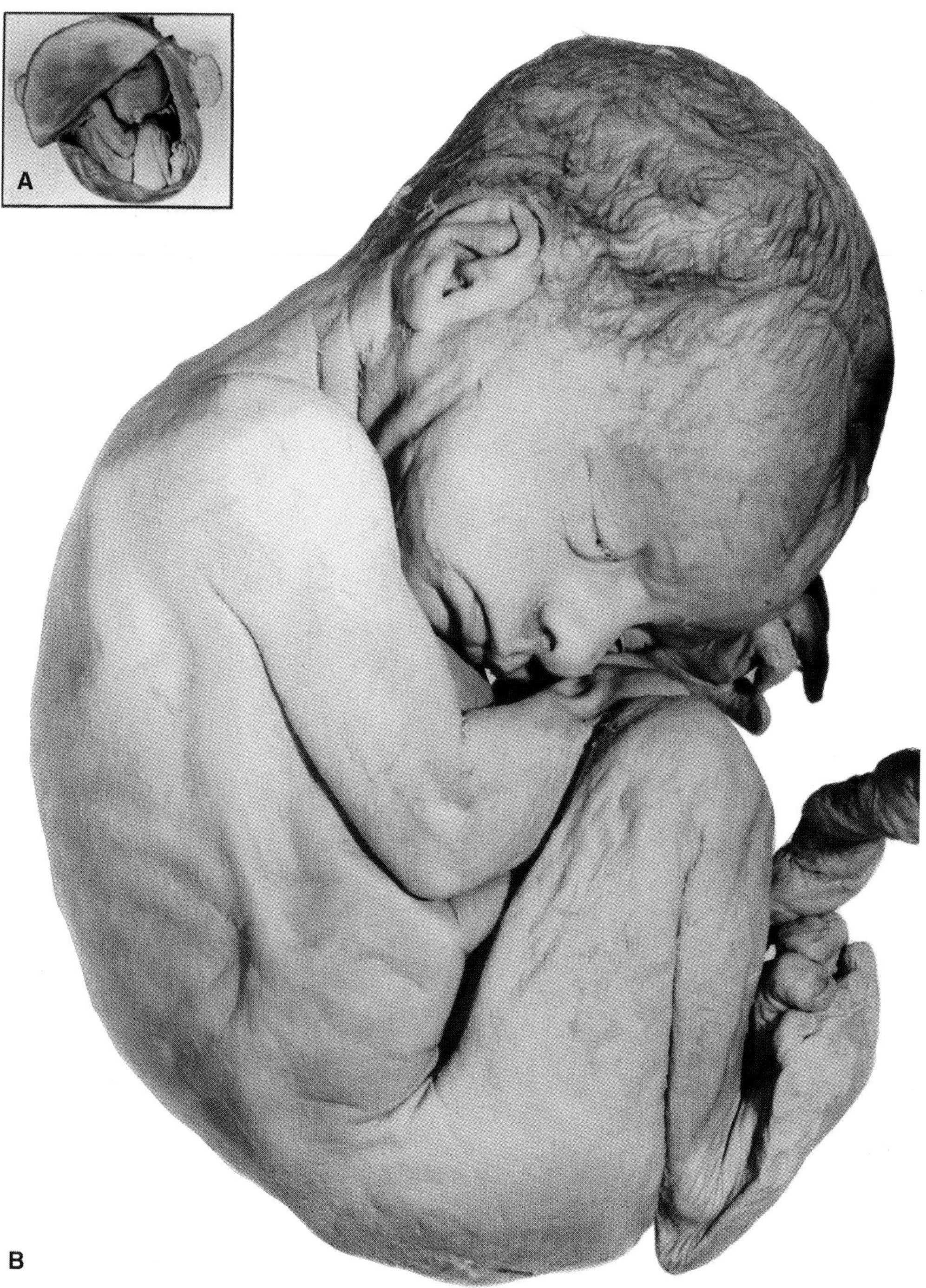

■ **Figure 6–9.** Photographs of a 25-week fetus. *A,* In the uterus. *B,* Actual size. Note the wrinkled skin and rather lean body caused by the scarcity of subcutaneous fat. Observe that the eyes are beginning to open. A fetus of this size might survive if born prematurely; hence it is considered a viable fetus. (*B* from Moore KL, Persaud TVN, Shiota K: *Color Atlas of Clinical Embryology.* Philadelphia, WB Saunders, 1994.)

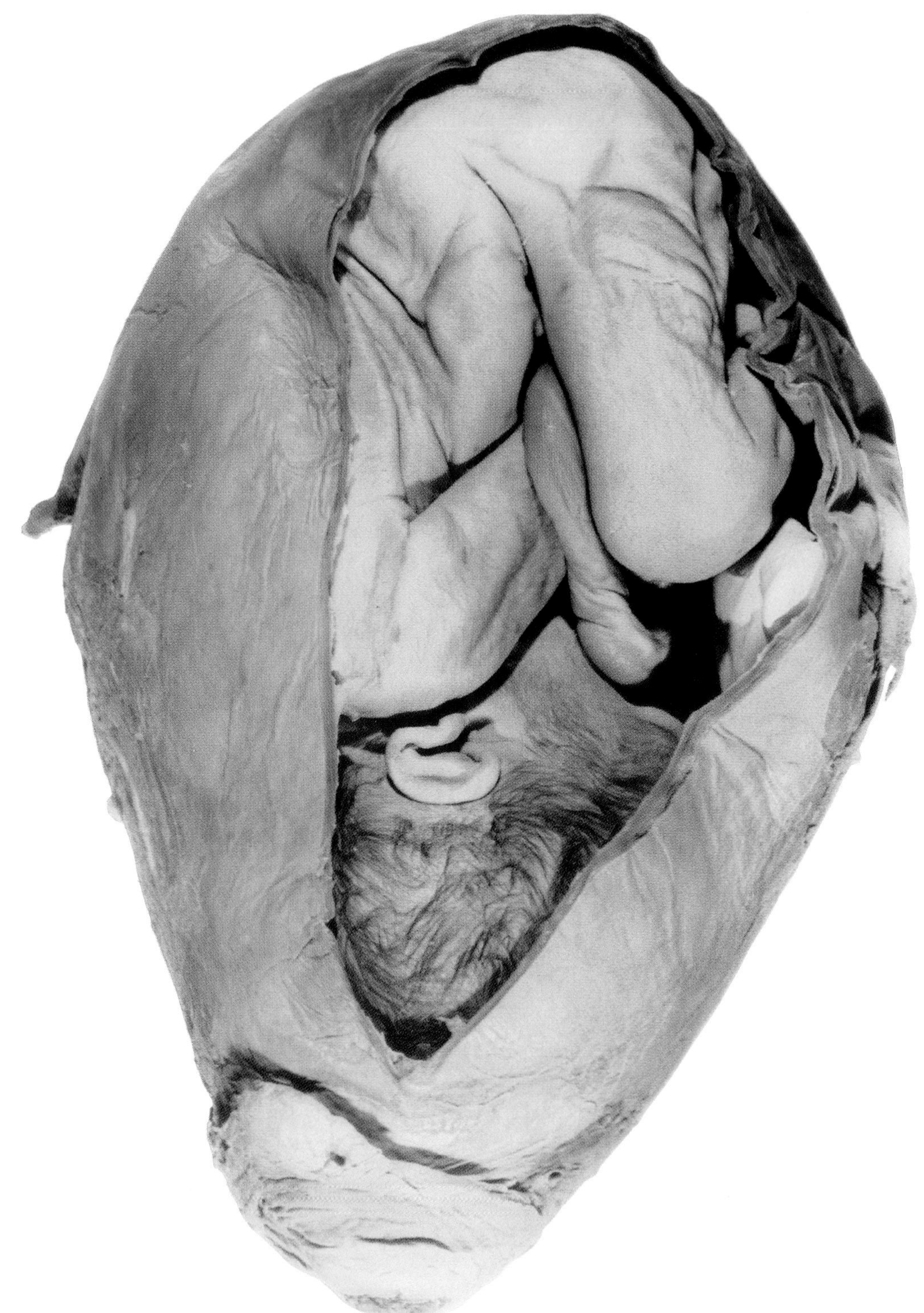

■ **Figure 6–10.** Photograph of a 29-week fetus in the uterus. Actual size. Note that the fetus is in a longitudinal lie and cephalic (head) presentation, which is normal at this period of gestation. Part of the wall of the uterus and parts of the chorion and amnion have been removed to show the fetus. This fetus and the mother died as the result of injuries sustained in an automobile accident. (From Moore KL, Persaud TVN, Shiota K: *Color Atlas of Clinical Embryology*. Philadelphia, WB Saunders, 1994.)

Thirty to Thirty-Four Weeks

The pupillary light reflex of the eyes can be elicited by 30 weeks. Usually by the end of this period, the skin is pink and smooth and the upper and lower limbs have a chubby appearance. At this age, the quantity of white fat is about 8% of body weight. Fetuses 32 weeks and older usually survive if born prematurely. If a normal-weight fetus is born during this period, it is "premature by date" as opposed to being "premature by weight."

Thirty-Five to Thirty-Eight Weeks

Fetuses at 35 weeks have a firm grasp and exhibit a spontaneous orientation to light. As term approaches (37-38 weeks), the nervous system is sufficiently mature to carry out some integrative functions (Drife, 1985). Most fetuses during this "finishing period" are plump (Fig. 6-11). By 36 weeks the circumferences of the head and abdomen are approximately equal. After this, the circumference of the abdomen may be greater than that of the head. The fetal foot measure-

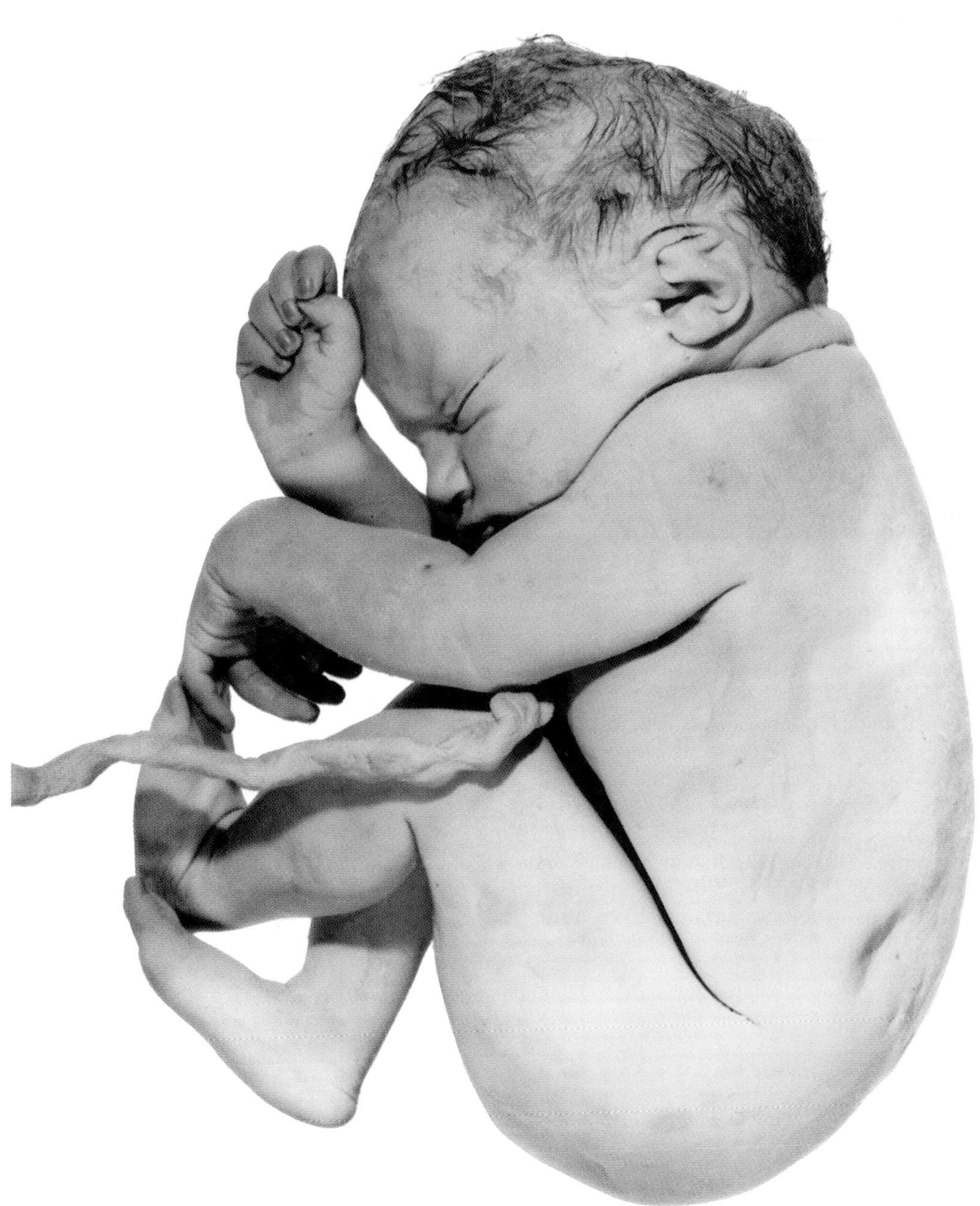

■ **Figure 6–11.** Photograph of a 36-week fetus. Half actual size. Fetuses at this size and age usually survive. Note the plump body resulting from the deposition of subcutaneous fat. This fetus's mother was killed in an automobile accident and the fetus died before it could be delivered by cesarean section. (From Moore KL, Persaud TVN, Shiota K: *Color Atlas of Clinical Embryology.* Philadelphia, WB Saunders, 1994.)

■ **Figure 6–12.** Ultrasound scan of the foot of a fetus at 37 weeks' gestation (Courtesy of Dr. C. R. Harman, Department of Obstetrics, Gynecology and Reproductive Sciences, Women's Hospital and University of Manitoba, Winnipeg, Manitoba, Canada.)

ment is usually slightly larger than femoral length at 37 weeks, and is an alternative parameter for confirmation of fetal age (Fig. 6-12). There is a slowing of growth as the time of birth approaches (Fig. 6-13).

By full term, normal fetuses usually reach a CRL of 360 mm and weigh about 3400 gm. The amount of white fat is about 16% of body weight. A fetus adds about 14 gm of fat a day during these last weeks of gestation. In general, male fetuses are longer and weigh more at birth than females. By full term (38 weeks after fertilization; 40 weeks after LNMP), the skin is normally bluish-pink. The chest is prominent and the breasts often protrude slightly in both sexes. The testes are usually in the scrotum in full-term male infants; premature male infants commonly have undescended testes. Although the head is smaller at full term in relation to the rest of the body than it was earlier in fetal life, it still is one of the largest regions of the fetus. This is an important consideration related to its passage through the birth canal (cervix and vagina; see Chapter 7).

Low Birth Weight

Not all low-weight babies are premature. About one-third of those with a birth weight of 2500 gm or less are actually small or undergrown for their gestational age. These "small for dates" infants may be underweight because of *placental insufficiency* (see Chapter 7). The placentas are often small and/or poorly attached. Placental insufficiency often results from degenerative changes in the placenta that progressively reduce the oxygen supply and nourishment to the fetus (Behrman et al., 1996).

It is important to distinguish between *full-term infants* who have a low birth weight because of IUGR and *preterm infants* who are underweight because of a shortened gestation (i.e., premature by date). IUGR may be caused by placental insufficiency, multiple gestations (e.g., triplets), infectious diseases, cardiovascular anomalies, inadequate maternal nutrition, and maternal and fetal hormones. Teratogens (drugs, chemicals, and viruses) and genetic factors are also known to cause IUGR (see Chapter 8). Infants with IUGR show a characteristic lack of subcutaneous fat and their skin is wrinkled, suggesting that white fat has actually been lost.

EXPECTED DATE OF DELIVERY

The expected date of delivery (EDD) of a fetus is 266 days or 38 weeks after fertilization; i.e., 280 days or 40 weeks after LNMP (see Table 6-2). About 12% of

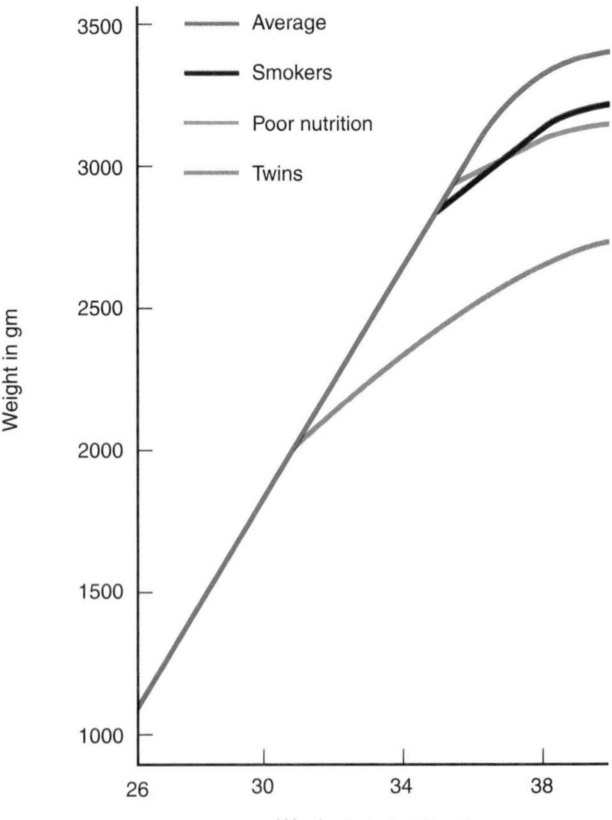

■ **Figure 6–13.** Graph showing the rate of fetal growth during the last trimester. Average refers to babies born in the United States. After 36 weeks the growth rate deviates from the straight line. The decline, particularly after full term (38 weeks), probably reflects inadequate fetal nutrition caused by placental changes. (Adapted from Gruenwald P: *Am J Obstet Gynecol 94:*1112, 1966.)

babies, however, are born 1 to 2 weeks after the expected time of birth.

Expected Date of Delivery (EDD)

The common delivery date rule (*Nägele's rule*) for determining the EDD or the expected date of confinement (EDC) is to count back 3 months from the first day of the LNMP, and add a year and 7 days. For example:

- first day of LNMP—January 4, 1998
- subtract 3 months = October 4, 1997
- add a year and 7 days = October 11, 1998—the EDD

In women with regular menstrual cycles, this method gives a reasonably accurate EDD. However, if the woman's cycles were irregular, miscalculations of 2 to 3 weeks may occur. In addition, *implantation bleeding* occurs in some pregnant women at the time of the first missed period (about 2 weeks after fertilization). Should the woman interpret this bleeding as a normal menstruation, the estimated time of birth could be miscalculated by 2 or more weeks. Ultrasound examinations of the fetus, in particular CRL measurements during the first trimester, are commonly used for a more reliable prediction of the EDD.

Postmaturity Syndrome

Prolongation of pregnancy for 3 or more weeks beyond the EDD occurs in 5 to 6% of women. Some infants in prolonged pregnancies develop the *postmaturity syndrome*. They have dry parchmentlike skin and are often overweight. These infants are characterized by absence of lanugo hair, decreased or absent vernix caseosa, long nails, and increased alertness. "When delivery is delayed three weeks or more beyond term, there is a significant increase in mortality" (Behrman et al., 1996). Because of this, labor is often induced (see Chapter 7).

FACTORS INFLUENCING FETAL GROWTH

The fetus requires substrates for growth and production of energy. Gases and nutrients pass freely to the fetus from the mother through the placental membrane (see Chapter 7). **Glucose** is a primary source of energy for fetal metabolism and growth; *amino acids* are also required. These substances pass from the mother's blood to the fetus through the placental membrane. **Insulin** required for the metabolism of glucose is secreted by the fetal pancreas; no significant quantities of maternal insulin reach the fetus because the placental membrane is relatively impermeable to this hormone. Insulin, human growth hormone, and some small polypeptides (such as somatomedin C) are believed to stimulate fetal growth. For a comprehensive account of human fetal growth, see Miller and Merritt (1979) and Hadlock (1994a).

Many factors may affect prenatal growth: maternal, fetal, and environmental. In general, factors operating throughout pregnancy, such as *cigarette smoking and consumption of alcohol*, tend to produce IUGR and small infants, whereas factors operating during the last trimester, such as maternal malnutrition, usually produce underweight infants with normal length and head size. IUGR is usually defined as infant weight within the lowest tenth percentile for gestational age (Hadlock, 1994a; Behrman et al., 1996; Ghidini, 1996). Severe malnutrition resulting from a poor-quality diet is known to cause reduced fetal growth (Fig. 6-13). Poor nutrition and faulty food habits are common during pregnancy and are not restricted to mothers belonging to poverty groups (Illsley and Mitchell, 1984; Creasy and Resnik, 1989).

Cigarette Smoking

Smoking is a well-established cause of IUGR (Nash and Persaud, 1988). The growth rate for fetuses of mothers who smoke cigarettes is less than normal during the last 6 to 8 weeks of pregnancy (Fig. 6-13). On average, the birth weight of infants whose mothers smoke heavily during pregnancy is 200 gm less than normal, and *perinatal morbidity* is increased when adequate medical care is unavailable (Behrman et al., 1996). The effect of maternal smoking is greater on fetuses whose mothers also receive inadequate nutrition. Presumably there is an additive effect of heavy smoking and poor-quality diet.

Multiple Pregnancy

Individuals of twin, triplet, and other multiple births usually weigh considerably less than infants resulting from a single pregnancy (Fig. 6-13). It is evident that the total requirements of two or more fetuses exceed the nutritional supply available from the placenta during the third trimester.

Social Drugs

Infants born to alcoholic mothers often exhibit IUGR as part of the *fetal alcohol syndrome* (see Chapter 8). Similarly, the use of *marijuana* and other illicit drugs (e.g., *cocaine*) can cause IUGR and other obstetrical complications (Persaud, 1988, 1990).

Impaired Uteroplacental and Fetoplacental Blood Flow

Maternal placental circulation may be reduced by conditions that decrease uterine blood flow (e.g., small chorionic or umbilical vessels, severe hypotension, and renal disease). Chronic reduction of uterine blood flow can cause *fetal starvation* resulting in IUGR (Harding and Charlton, 1991; Ghidini, 1996). Placental dysfunction or defects (e.g., infarction; see Chapter 7) can also cause IUGR. The net effect of these placental abnormalities is a reduction of the total area for exchange of nutrients between the fetal and maternal blood streams. It is very difficult to separate the effect of these placental changes from the effect of reduced maternal blood flow to the placenta. In some instances of chronic maternal disease, the maternal vascular changes in the uterus are primary and the placental defects are secondary (Harding and Charlton, 1991).

Genetic Factors and Growth Retardation

It is well established that genetic factors can cause IUGR. Repeated cases of this condition in one family indicate that recessive genes may be the cause of the abnormal growth. In recent years, structural and numerical chromosomal aberrations have also been shown to be associated with cases of retarded fetal growth (Thompson et al., 1991). IUGR is pronounced in infants with Down syndrome and is very characteristic of fetuses with trisomy 18 syndrome (see Chapter 8).

PROCEDURES FOR ASSESSING FETAL STATUS

By accepting the shelter of the uterus, the fetus also takes the risk of maternal disease or malnutrition and of biochemical, immunological and hormonal adjustment.

—GEORGE W. CORNER, AMERICAN EMBRYOLOGIST, 1888–1981

Perinatology is the branch of medicine that is concerned with the well-being of the fetus and newborn infant, generally covering the period from about 26 weeks after fertilization to 4 weeks after birth. The subspecialty of *perinatal medicine* combines aspects of obstetrics and pediatrics. A third-trimester fetus is commonly regarded as an *unborn patient* on whom diagnostic and therapeutic procedures may be performed (Harrison et al., 1991). Several techniques are now available for assessing the status of the fetus and providing prenatal treatment if required (Soothill, 1996). Fetal activity felt by the mother or palpated by the physician were the first clues to fetal well-being. Then the fetal heartbeat was detected, first by auscultation and later by electronic monitors. These techniques indicated when there was fetal stress and distress. Later gonadotrophic hormones were detected in maternal blood. Many new procedures for assessing the status of the fetus have been developed in the last two decades. It is now possible to treat many fetuses whose lives are in jeopardy (Harrison, 1991; Harman, 1995; Manning, 1995).

Diagnostic Amniocentesis

This is the most common invasive prenatal diagnostic procedure (Wilson, 1991; Elias and Simpson, 1993). For prenatal diagnosis, amniotic fluid is sampled by inserting a hollow needle through the mother's anterior abdominal and uterine walls into the amniotic cavity by piercing the chorion and amnion (Fig. 6-14*A*).

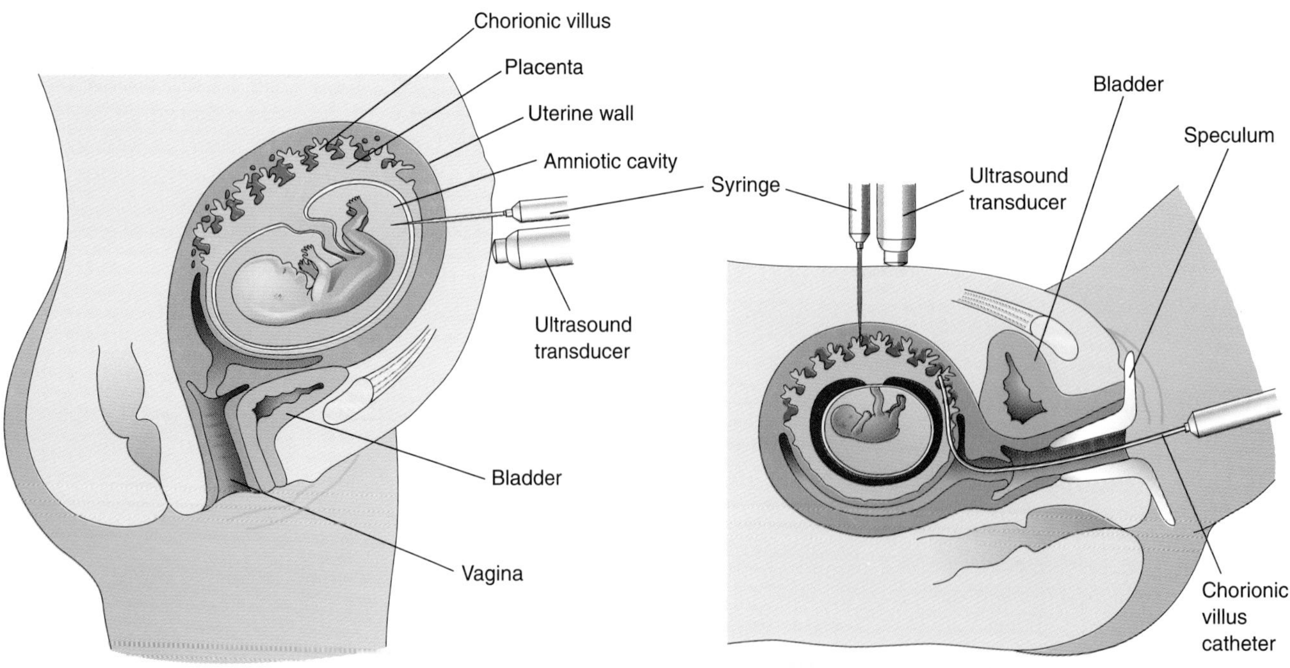

■ **Figure 6–14.** *A,* Drawing illustrating the technique of amniocentesis. A needle is inserted through the lower abdominal wall and uterine wall into the amniotic cavity. A syringe is attached and amniotic fluid is withdrawn for diagnostic purposes. *B,* Drawing illustrating chorionic villus sampling (CVS). This technique is usually performed at about the ninth week after the last menstrual period. Two sampling approaches are illustrated: through the maternal anterior abdominal wall with a spinal needle, and through the vagina and cervical canal using a malleable cannula.

A syringe is attached and amniotic fluid is withdrawn. Bevis (1952) introduced diagnostic amniocentesis with his report on the antenatal prediction of hemolytic disease in the newborn (HDN). Because there is relatively little amniotic fluid prior to the fourteenth week after LNMP, amniocentesis is difficult to perform prior to this time. The amniotic fluid volume is approximately 200 ml, and 20 to 30 ml can be safely withdrawn. The procedure is relatively devoid of risk, especially when the procedure is performed by an experienced physician who is guided by ultrasonography for outlining the position of the fetus and placenta.

Transabdominal Amniocentesis

Amniocentesis is a common technique for detecting genetic disorders (e.g., Down syndrome). Complications associated with amniocentesis are relatively uncommon. There is a small risk of inducing an abortion, estimated to be about 0.5% (Goldberg, 1994).

The common *indications for amniocentesis*:

- advanced maternal age (38 years or older)
- previous birth of a trisomic child (e.g., Down syndrome)
- chromosome abnormality in either parent (e.g., a chromosome translocation; see Chapter 8)
- women who are carriers of X-linked recessive disorders (e.g., *hemophilia*)
- history of neural tube defects (NTDs) in the family (e.g., spina bifida cystica; see Chapter 18)
- carriers of inborn errors of metabolism (Elias and Simpson, 1993)

Alpha-Fetoprotein (AFP) Assay

Alpha-fetoprotein (AFP) is a glycoprotein that is synthesized in the fetal liver, yolk sac, and gut (Filly et al., 1994). AFP is found in high concentration in fetal serum, peaking 14 weeks after the LNMP. Small amounts of AFP normally enter the amniotic fluid. Large amounts of AFP escape from the circulation into the amniotic fluid from fetuses with open NTDs, such as spina bifida with myeloschisis or meroanencephaly, or anencephaly (see Chapter 18). Open NTDs refer to lesions that are not covered with skin. AFP also enters the amniotic fluid from open ventral wall defects (VWDs) such as gastroschisis and omphalocele (see Chapter 12).

AFP and Fetal Anomalies

The concentration of AFP in the amniotic fluid surrounding fetuses with open NTDs and VWDs is remarkably high. Thus it is possible to detect the presence of these severe anomalies of the central nervous system and ventral wall by measuring the concentration of AFP in amniotic fluid (Haddow, 1991; Filly et al., 1994). *Amniotic fluid AFP* concentration is measured by immunoassay, and, when used with ultrasonographic scanning, about 99% of fetuses with these severe defects can be diagnosed prenatally. When a fetus has an open NTD, the concentration of AFP is also likely to be higher than normal in the maternal serum. *Maternal serum AFP* (MSAFP) concentration is low when the fetus has Down syndrome, trisomy 18, and other chromosome defects (Merkatz et al., 1984; Thompson et al., 1991).

Spectrophotometric Studies

Examination of amniotic fluid by this method may be used for assessing the degree of *erythroblastosis fetalis*—also called hemolytic disease of newborn (HDN). HDN results from destruction of fetal red blood cells by maternal antibodies (see Chapter 7).

Chorionic Villus Sampling (CVS)

Biopsies of chorionic villi (mostly trophoblast) may be obtained by inserting a needle, guided by ultrasonography, through the mother's abdominal and uterine walls into the uterine cavity (Fig. 6-14*B*). CVS is also performed transcervically using real-time ultrasound guidance (Hogge, 1991; Harman, 1995).

Diagnostic Value of CVS

Biopsies of chorionic villi are used for detecting chromosomal abnormalities, inborn errors of metabolism, and X-linked disorders. CVS can be performed as early as the ninth week of gestation (7 weeks after fertilization). The rate of fetal loss is about 1%, slightly more than the risk from amniocentesis (Thompson et al., 1991). Reports regarding an increased risk of limb defects after CVS are conflicting (Hsieh et al., 1995; Evans and Hamerton, 1996; Froster and Jackson, 1996). The major advantage of CVS over amniocentesis is that it allows the results of chromosomal analysis to be available several weeks earlier than when performed by amniocentesis.

Sex Chromatin Patterns

Fetal sex can be determined by noting the presence or absence of sex chromatin in the nuclei of cells recovered from amniotic fluid. These tests were developed after it was discovered that sex chromatin was visible in nuclei of normal female cells but not in normal male cells (Moore, 1966) (Fig. 6-15*A* and *B*). Females with three X chromosomes (46, XXX) have two masses of sex chromatin (Fig. 6-15*C*). By use of a special staining technique, the Y chromosome can also be identified in cells recovered from the amniotic fluid surrounding male fetuses (Fig. 6-15*D*). Knowledge of *fetal sex* can be useful in diagnosing the presence of severe sex-linked hereditary diseases, such as *hemo-*

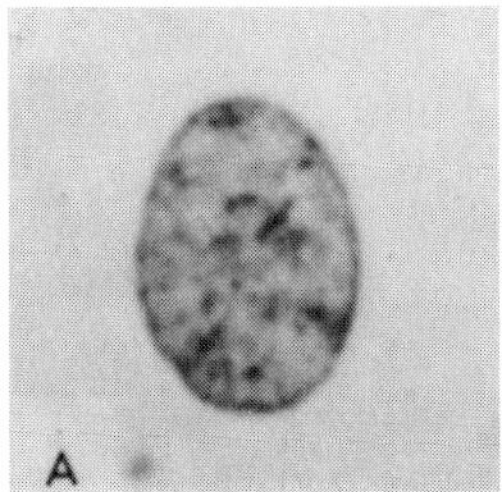

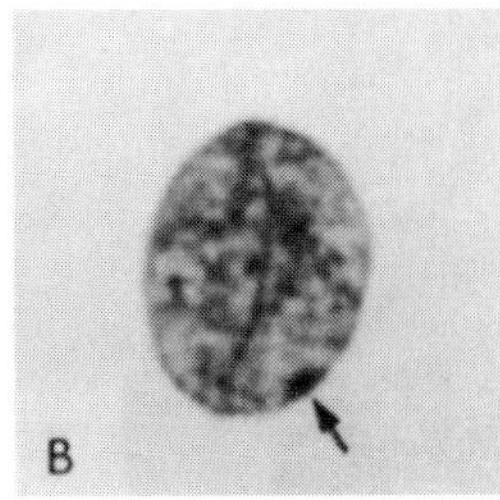

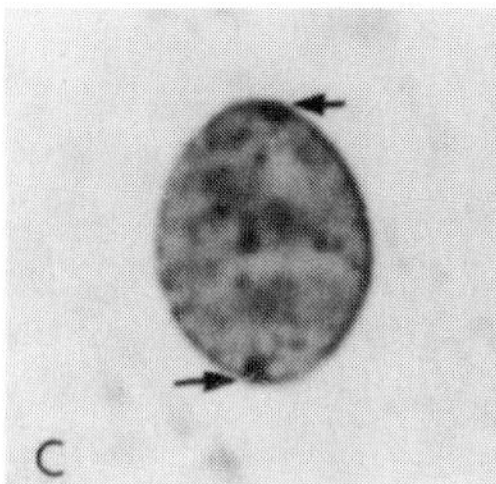

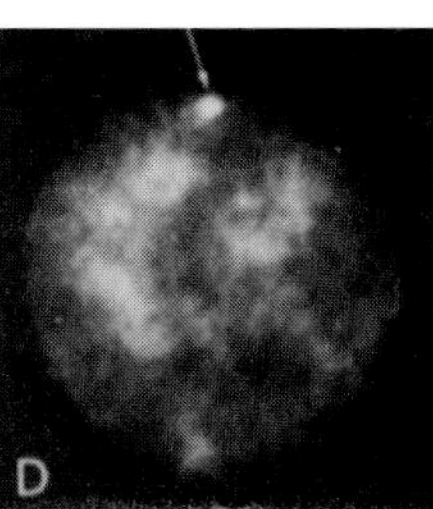

■ **Figure 6–15.** Oral epithelial nuclei stained with cresylecht violet (*A, B,* and *C*) and quinacrine mustard *(D)* (×2000). *A,* From normal male. No sex chromatin is visible (chromatin negative). *B,* From normal female. The arrow indicates a typical mass of sex chromatin (chromatin positive). *C,* From female with XXX trisomy. The arrows indicate two masses of sex chromatin. *D,* From normal male. The arrow indicates a mass of Y chromatin as an intensely fluorescent body. (*A* and *B* from Moore KL, Barr ML: *Lancet 2*:57, 1955).

philia and muscular dystrophy (Simpson and Elias, 1989, 1993; Thompson et al., 1991). Sex chromatin tests are not routine and should not be performed to satisfy the parents' curiosity about the sex of a fetus.

Cell Cultures

Fetal sex and chromosomal aberrations can also be determined by studying the sex chromosomes in cultured fetal cells obtained during amniocentesis. These cultures are commonly done when an autosomal abnormality such as occurs in the Down syndrome is suspected. *Inborn errors of metabolism* in fetuses can also be detected by studying cell cultures. Enzyme deficiencies can be determined by incubating cells recovered from amniotic fluid and then detecting the specific enzyme deficiency in the cells (Polin and Mennuti, 1987; Weaver, 1989).

Intrauterine Fetal Transfusion

Some fetuses with HDN can be saved by receiving intrauterine blood transfusions. The blood is injected through a needle inserted into the fetal peritoneal cavity (Bowman, 1989). Over a period of 5 to 6 days, most of the injected blood cells pass into the fetal circulation through the diaphragmatic lymphatics. With recent advances in percutaneous *umbilical cord puncture*, blood can be transfused directly into the fetal cardiovascular system.

In addition to red blood cell alloimmunization (or HDN), intrauterine fetal transfusion therapy with either red blood cells or platelets is now used for the management of other fetal cytopenias, including alloimmune thrombocytopenia and fetal parvovirus B19 infection (Skupski et al., 1996; Soothill, 1996). The need for fetal blood transfusions is reduced nowadays owing to the treatment of Rh-negative mothers of Rh-positive fetuses with anti-Rh immunoglobulin. Consequently *HDN is relatively uncommon now* because Rh immune globulin usually prevents development of this disease of the Rh system (Thompson et al., 1991).

Fetoscopy

Using fiberoptic lighting instruments, parts of the fetal body may be directly observed (Reece et al., 1993). It is possible to scan the entire fetus looking for congenital anomalies such as cleft lip and limb defects. The fetoscope is usually introduced through the anterior abdominal and uterine walls into the amniotic cavity, similar to the way the needle is inserted during amniocentesis. Fetoscopy is usually carried out between 17 and 20 weeks of gestation, but with new approaches such as *transabdominal thin-gauge embryofetoscopy* (TSEF), it is possible to detect certain anomalies in the embryo or fetus during the first trimester (Quintero et al., 1993). Because of the risk to the fetus compared with other prenatal diagnostic procedures, fetoscopy now has few indications for routine prenatal diagnosis or treatment of the fetus. For certain disorders, however, prenatal diagnosis depends on the availability of fetal tissues, such as skin, liver, and muscle samples (for more details, see Simpson and Elias, 1993).

Percutaneous Umbilical Cord Blood Sampling (PUBS)

Fetal blood samples may be obtained from the umbilical vessels for chromosome analysis by PUBS. Ultrasonographic scanning facilitates the procedure by outlining the location of the vessels. PUBS is often used about 20 weeks after LNMP for chromosome analysis when ultrasonographic or other examinations have shown characteristics of a severe fetal anomaly, such as trisomy 13 (see Chapter 8).

Ultrasonography

Ultrasonography is the primary imaging modality in the evaluation of the fetus because of its wide availability, low cost, and lack of known adverse effects (Feldstein and Popovitch, 1994). The chorionic (gestational) sac and its contents may be visualized by ultrasonography during the embryonic and fetal periods. Placental and fetal size, multiple births, abnormalities of placental shape, and abnormal presentations can also be determined (Townsend, 1994).

Ultrasound scans give accurate measurements of the biparietal diameter (BPD) of the fetal skull, from which close estimates of fetal age and length can be made (Hadlock, 1994b). Figures 6-12 and 6-16 illustrate how details of the fetus can be observed in ultrasound scans. Ultrasound examinations are also helpful

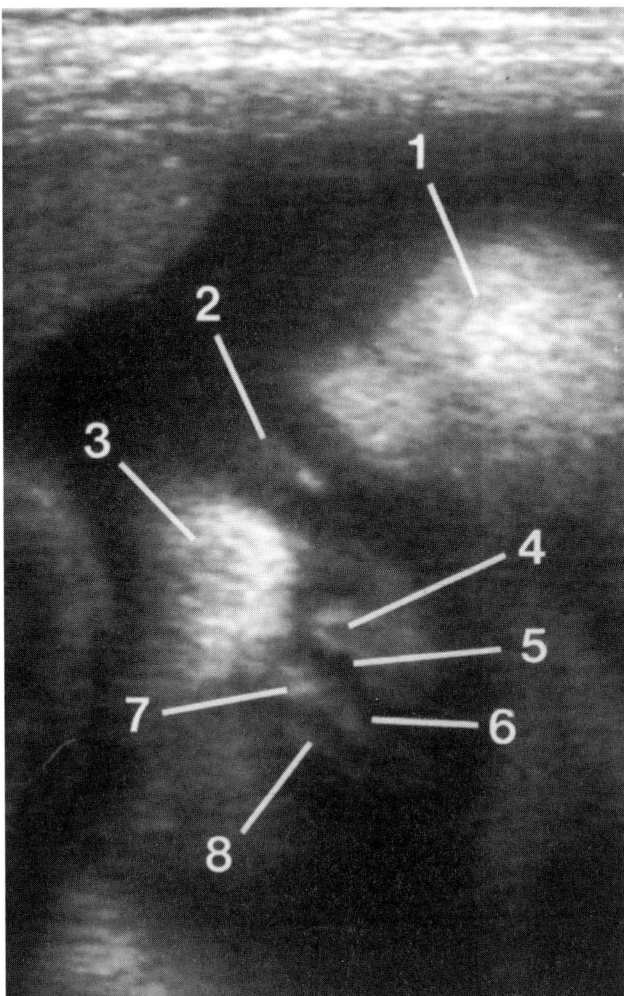

■ **Figure 6–16.** Sonogram of a third trimester fetus showing that the face can be viewed with considerable clarity: **1,** forehead (brow); **2,** eyelid; **3,** cheek; **4,** ala (side) of nose; **5,** nostril; **6,** philtrum (depression) in upper lip; **7,** right side of lip; **8,** lower lip. Amniotic fluid surrounding the face provides "contrast" for visualization. (From Filly RA: Sonographic anatomy of the normal fetus. *In* Harrison MR, Globus MS, Filly RA [eds]: *The Unborn Patient. Prenatal Diagnosis and Treatment,* 2nd ed. Philadelphia, WB Saunders, 1991.)

for diagnosing abnormal pregnancies at a very early stage (Filly, 1991b), e.g., the "blighted embryo." Rapid advances in ultrasonography have made this technique a major tool for prenatal diagnosis of fetal abnormalities, i.e., meroanencephaly (anencephaly), hydrocephaly, microcephaly, fetal ascites, and renal agenesis (Spirt et al., 1987; Callen, 1994a; Ploeckinger-Ulm et al., 1996). Because of the possibility of a harmful effect on the fetus, it is prudent to restrict prenatal ultrasound examinations to cases where there are clinical indications (Campbell et al., 1993; Newnham et al., 1993).

Computed Tomography (CT) and Magnetic Resonance Imaging (MRI)

When planning fetal treatment (e.g., surgery [Filly, 1991a and b]), one may use CT and MRI to provide more information about an abnormality that has been detected in ultrasonic images. The disadvantages of current MRI include high cost, fixed planes of section, and limited fetal resolution (Fig. 6-17). CT is helpful for differentiating between monoamniotic and diamniotic twins, i.e., in one or two amniotic sacs (see Chapter 7). This is important to know for management of the pregnancy because the perinatal mortality of monoamniotic twins is high — 30 to 50% risk of death (Finberg, 1994).

Amniography and Fetography

When performing these techniques, a radiopaque substance is injected into the amniotic cavity to outline the amniotic sac and the external features of the fetus. A water-soluble contrast medium is used in amniography, and an oil-soluble contrast medium is injected during fetography. The latter medium is apparently absorbed by the vernix caseosa. These procedures increase the risk of premature rupture of the membranes and preterm labor. Like fetoscopy, these procedures have been more or less replaced by noninvasive, high-resolution ultrasonic imaging techniques, which give an even more accurate delineation of fetal structures.

Fetal Monitoring

Continuous fetal heart rate monitoring in high-risk pregnancies is routine and provides information about the oxygenation of the fetus. Fetal distress, e.g., indicated by an abnormal heart rate or rhythm, suggests that the fetus is in jeopardy.

Fetal Distress

There are various causes of prenatal antepartum fetal distress such as maternal diseases that reduce oxygen transport to the fetus (e.g., cyanotic heart disease). The external mode of monitoring uses transducers placed on the mother's abdomen. For example, an ultrasound transducer picks up high-frequency sound waves that reflect the mechanical action of the fetal heart. For more information on fetal distress and continuous fetal heart monitoring, see Harman (1995) and Manning (1995).

SUMMARY OF FETAL PERIOD

The fetal period begins 9 weeks after fertilization (11 weeks after LNMP) and ends at birth. It is characterized by rapid body growth and differentiation of tissues and organ systems. An obvious change in the fetal period is the relative slowing of head growth compared with that of the rest of the body. By the beginning of the twentieth week, lanugo and head hair appear, and the skin is coated with vernix caseosa. The eyelids are closed during most of the fetal

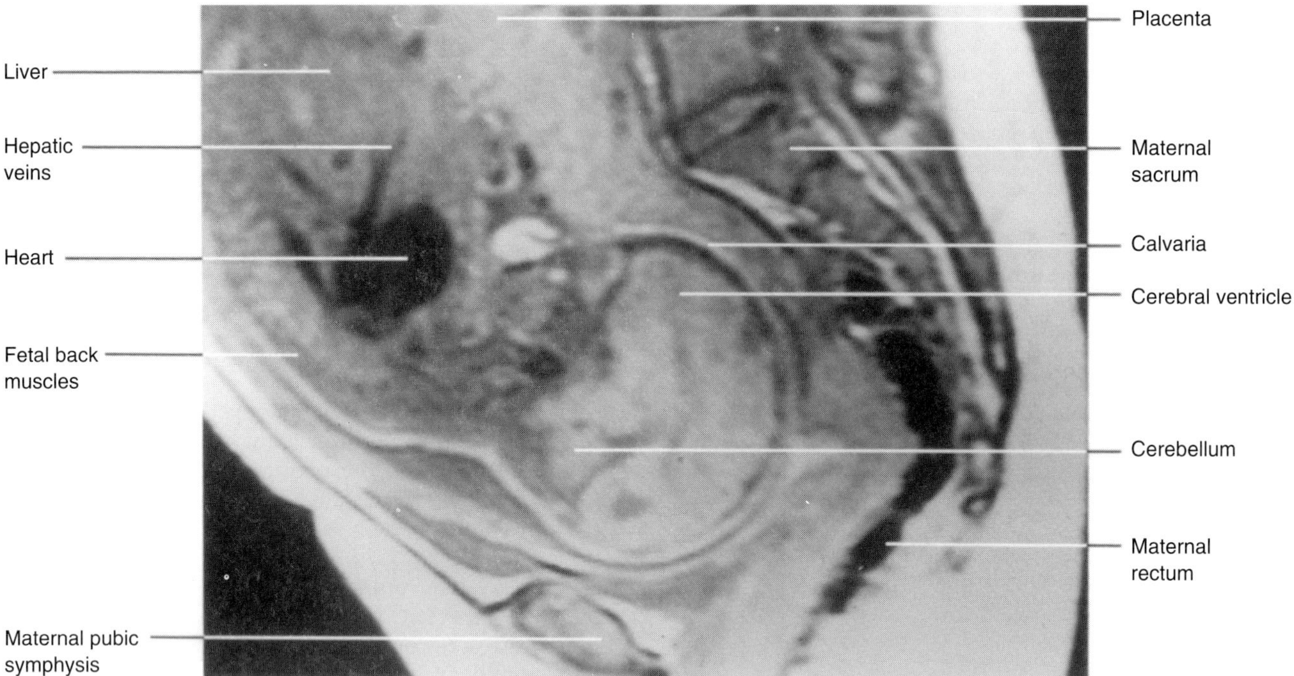

■ **Figure 6–17.** Sagittal magnetic resonance image (MRI) of the pelvis of a pregnant woman. The fetus is in the cephalic presentation. The brain, heart, liver, and hepatic veins are well shown, as is the placenta. (Courtesy of Dr. Shirley McCarthy, Director of MRI, Department of Diagnostic Radiology, Yale University School of Medicine, New Haven, Connecticut.)

period but begin to reopen at about 26 weeks. At this time the fetus is usually capable of extrauterine existence, mainly because of the maturity of its respiratory system.

Until about 30 weeks, the fetus appears reddish and wizened because of the thinness of its skin and the relative absence of subcutaneous fat. Fat usually develops rapidly during the last 6 to 8 weeks, giving the

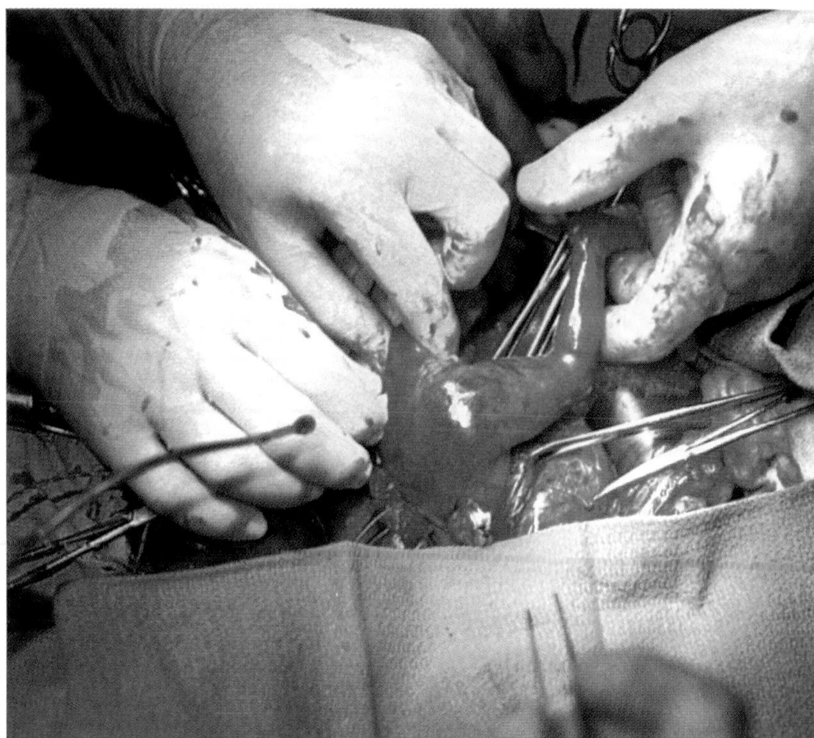

■ **Figure 6–18.** Fetus at 21 weeks undergoing bilateral ureterostomies, the establishment of external openings of the ureters into the bladder. (From Harrison MR, Globus MS, Filly RA [eds]: *The Unborn Patient. Prenatal Diagnosis and Treatment,* 2nd ed. Philadelphia, WB Saunders, 1991.)

fetus a smooth, plump appearance. This terminal ("finishing") period is devoted mainly to building up of tissues and preparing systems involved in the transition from intrauterine to extrauterine environments, primarily the respiratory and cardiovascular systems. Changes occurring during the fetal period are not so dramatic as those appearing in the embryonic period, but they are very important. The fetus is less vulnerable to the teratogenic effects of drugs, viruses, and radiation, but these agents may interfere with growth and normal functional development, especially of the brain and eyes (see Chapter 8).

Various techniques are available for assessing the status of the fetus and for diagnosing certain diseases and developmental anomalies before birth. The physician can now determine whether or not a fetus has a particular disease or a congenital anomaly by using various diagnostic techniques, e.g., amniocentesis and ultrasonography. Prenatal diagnosis can be made early enough to allow early termination of the pregnancy if elected, e.g., when serious anomalies incompatible with postnatal life are diagnosed. In selected cases, various treatments can be given to the fetus (Soothill, 1996), e.g., the administration of drugs to correct cardiac arrhythmia or thyroid disorders. Surgical correction of congenital anomalies in utero is also possible (Fig. 6-18), such as ureterostomies on fetuses that have ureters that do not open into the bladder (Harrison, 1991).

Clinically Oriented Problems

Case 6–1

A woman in the twentieth week of a high-risk pregnancy was scheduled for a repeat Cesarean section. Her physician wanted to establish an EDC.

- How would an EDC be established?
- When would labor likely be induced?
- How could this be accomplished?

Case 6–2

A 42-year-old pregnant woman was worried that she might be carrying a fetus with major congenital anomalies.

- How could the status of her fetus be obtained?
- What chromosomal abnormality would most likely be found?
- What other chromosomal aberrations might be detected?
- If this was of clinical interest, how could the sex of the fetus be determined in a family known to have hemophilia or muscular dystrophy?

Case 6–3

A 19-year-old woman in the second trimester of pregnancy asked a physician whether her fetus was vulnerable to "over-the-counter drugs" and street drugs. She also wondered about the effect of her heavy drinking and cigarette smoking on her fetus.

- What would the physician likely tell her?

Case 6–4

An ultrasound examination of a pregnant woman revealed IUGR.

- What factors may cause IUGR? Discuss them.
- Which factors can the mother eliminate?

Case 6–5

A woman in the first trimester of pregnancy who was to undergo amniocentesis expressed concerns about a miscarriage and the possibility of injury to her fetus.

- What are the risks of these complications?
- What procedures are used to minimize these risks?
- What other technique might be used for obtaining cells for chromosome study?
- What does the acronym "PUBS" mean?
- Describe how this technique is performed and how it is used to assess the status of a fetus.

Case 6–6

A pregnant woman is told that she is going to have an AFP test to determine if there are any fetal anomalies.

- What types of fetal anomalies can be detected by an AFP assay of maternal serum? Explain.
- What is the significance of high and low levels of AFP?

Discussion of these problems appears at the back of the book.

REFERENCES AND SUGGESTED READING

Abramowicz JS, Sherer DM, Bar-Tov E, Woods JR Jr: The cheek-to-cheek diameter in the ultrasonographic assessment of fetal growth. *Am J Obstet Gynecol 165:*846, 1991.

Anderson EM, Jones DRE, Liu DTY, Pipkin FB: Does angiotensin play a role in human fetal erythropoiesis. *Biol Neonate 71:*194, 1997.

Anonymous: Canadian Guidelines for Prenatal Diagnosis of Genetic Disorders: An Update. A Joint Document of the Canadian College of Medical Geneticists and the Society of Obstetricians and Gynaecologists of Canada. *SOGC 13:*13, 1991.

Barnea ER, Hustin J, Jauniaux E (eds): *The First Twelve Weeks of Gestation*. Berlin, Springer-Verlag, 1992.

Beck F: Structural development of the embryo and fetus. *In* Chamberlain G (ed): *Turnbull's Obstetrics*, 2nd ed. Edinburgh, Churchill Livingstone, 1995.

Behrman RE, Kleigman RM, Arvin AM (eds): *Nelson Textbook of Pediatrics*, 15th ed. Philadelphia, WB Saunders, 1996.

Benson CB, Doubilet PM: Sonographic prediction of gestational age '91—Accuracy of second-trimester and third-trimester fetal measurements. *AJR 157:*1275, 1991.

Bernstein IM, Blake K, Wall B, Badger GJ: Evidence that normal fetal growth can be noncontinuous. *J Maternal-Fetal Med 4:*197, 1995.

Bevis DCA: The antenatal prediction of hemolytic disease of the newborn. *Lancet 1:*395, 1952.

Biggers JD: Arbitrary partitions of prenatal life. *Hum Reprod 5:*1, 1990.

Birnholz JC: The development of human fetal eye movement patterns. *Science 213:*679, 1981.

Birnholz JC, Benaceraff BR: The development of human fetal hearing. *Science 222:*516, 1983.

Boehm CD, Kazazian HH Jr: Prenatal diagnosis by DNA analysis. *In* Harrison MR, Golbus MS, Filly RA (eds): *The Unborn Patient. Prenatal Diagnosis and Treatment*, 2nd ed. Philadelphia, WB Saunders, 1991.

Boles ET Jr: The spleen. *In* Schiller M (ed): *Pediatric Surgery of the Liver, Pancreas and Spleen*. Philadelphia, WB Saunders, 1991.

Boué A (ed): *Fetal Medicine: Prenatal Diagnosis and Management*. Translated by M Vekemans and L Cartier. Oxford, Oxford University Press, 1995.

Bowman JM: Hemolytic disease (Erythroblastosis fetalis). *In* Creasy RK, Resnik R (eds): *Maternal-Fetal Medicine. Principles and Practice*, 2nd ed. Philadelphia, WB Saunders, 1989.

Callen PW: The obstetric ultrasound examination. *In* Callen PW (ed): *Ultrasonography in Obstetrics and Gynecology*, 3rd ed. Philadelphia, WB Saunders, 1994a.

Callen PW (ed): *Ultrasonography in Obstetrics and Gynecology*, 3rd ed. Philadelphia, WB Saunders, 1994b.

Campbell JD, Eford W, Brant RF: Case-control study of prenatal ultrasonography exposure in children with delayed speech. *Can Med Assoc J 149:*1435, 1993.

Carlson DE, Platt LD: Ultrasound detection of genetic anomalies. *J Reprod Med 37:*419, 1992.

Cooke RWI: The low birth weight baby. *In* Lister J, Irving IM (eds): *Neonatal Surgery*, 3rd ed. London, Butterworths, 1990.

Creasy RK, Resnik R: Intrauterine growth retardation. *In* Creasy RK, Resnik R (eds): *Maternal-Fetal Medicine. Principles and Practice*, 2nd ed. Philadelphia, WB Saunders, 1989.

Drife JO: Can the fetus listen and learn. *Br J Obstet Gynaecol 92:* 777, 1985.

Elias S, Simpson JL: Amniocentesis. *In* Simpson JL, Elias S (eds): *Essentials of Prenatal Diagnosis*. New York, Churchill Livingstone, 1993.

Evans JA, Hamerton JL: Limb defects and chorionic villus sampling. *Lancet 347:*484, 1996.

England MA: *Color Atlas of Life Before Birth*. Chicago, Year Book Medical Publishers, 1983.

Feldstein VA, Popovitch MJ: The role of computed tomography and magnetic resonance imaging in obstetrics. *In* Callen PW (ed): *Ultrasonography in Obstetrics and Gynecology*, 3rd ed. Philadelphia, WB Saunders, 1994.

Filly RA: Alternative imaging techniques: computed tomography and magnetic resonance imaging. *In* Harrison MR, Golbus MS, Filly RA (eds): *The Unborn Patient. Prenatal Diagnosis and Treatment*. 2nd ed. Philadelphia, WB Saunders, 1991a.

Filly RA: Sonographic anatomy of the normal fetus. *In* Harrison MR, Golbus MS, Filly RA (eds): *The Unborn Patient. Prenatal Diagnosis and Treatment*, 2nd ed. Philadelphia, WB Saunders, 1991b.

Filly RA: Ultrasound evaluation during the first trimester. *In* Callen PW (ed): *Ultrasonography in Obstetrics and Gynecology*, 3rd ed. Philadelphia, WB Saunders, 1994.

Filly RA, Callen PW, Goldstein RB: Alpha-fetoprotein screening programs: What every obstetric sonologist should know. *In* Callen PW (ed): *Ultrasonography in Obstetrics and Gynecology*, 3rd ed. Philadelphia, WB Saunders, 1994.

Finberg HJ: Ultrasound evaluations in multiple gestation. *In* Callen PW (ed): *Ultrasonography in Obstetrics and Gynecology*, 3rd ed. Philadelphia, WB Saunders, 1994.

Froster VG, Jackson L: Limb defects and chorionic villus sampling: results from an international registry, 1992–94. *Lancet 347:*489, 1996.

Ghidini A: Idiopathic fetal growth restriction: a pathophysiologic approach. *Obstet Gynecol Surv 51:*376, 1996.

Goldberg JD: The role of genetic screening in the obstetric patient. *In* Callen PW (ed): *Ultrasonography in Obstetrics and Gynecology*, 3rd ed. Philadelphia, WB Saunders, 1994.

Haddow JE: Alpha-fetoprotein. *In* Harrison MR, Golbus MS, Filly RA (eds): *The Unborn Patient. Prenatal Diagnosis and Treatment*, 2nd ed. Philadelphia, WB Saunders, 1991.

Hadlock FP: Fetal growth. *In* Callen PW (ed): *Ultrasonography in Obstetrics and Gynecology*, 3rd ed. Philadelphia, WB Saunders, 1994a.

Hadlock FP: Ultrasound determination of menstrual age. *In* Callen PW (ed): *Ultrasonography in Obstetrics and Gynecology*, 3rd ed. Philadelphia, WB Saunders, 1994b.

Harding JE, Charlton V: Experimental nutritional supplementation for intrauterine growth retardation. *In* Harrison MR, Golbus MS, Filly RA (eds): *The Unborn Patient. Prenatal Diagnosis and Treatment*, 2nd ed. Philadelphia, WB Saunders, 1991.

Harman CR (ed): *Invasive Fetal Testing and Treatment*. Boston, Blackwell Scientific Publications, 1995.

Harrison MR: Selection for treatment: Which defects are correctable. *In* Harrison MR, Golbus MS, Filly RA (eds): *The Unborn Patient. Prenatal Diagnosis and Treatment*, 2nd ed. Philadelphia, WB Saunders, 1991.

Harrison MR, Globus MS, Filly RA (eds): *The Unborn Patient. Prenatal Diagnosis and Treatment*, 2nd ed. Philadelphia, WB Saunders, 1991.

Hay W Jr, Catz CS, Grave GD, Yaffe SY: Workshop summary: fetal growth: its regulation and disorders. *Pediatrics 99:*585, 1997.

Hinrichsen KV (ed): *Humanembryologie*. Berlin, Springer-Verlag, 1990.

Hobbins JC: Amniocentesis. *In* Harrison MR, Golbus MS, Filly RA (eds): *The Unborn Patient. Prenatal Diagnosis and Treatment*, 2nd ed. Philadelphia, WB Saunders, 1991.

Hogge WA: Chorionic villus sampling. *In* Harrison MR, Golbus MS, Filly RA (eds): *The Unborn Patient. Prenatal Diagnosis and Treatment*, 2nd ed. Philadelphia, WB Saunders, 1991.

Hsieh FJ, Shyu MK, Sheu BC, et al: Limb defects after chorionic villus sampling. *Obstet Gynecol 85:*84, 1995.

Hull D: Brown adipose tissue in the new born. *In* Philipp EE, Barnes J, Newton M (eds): *Scientific Foundations of Obstetrics and Gynecology*. London, William Heinemann, 1970.

Illingworth RS: *The Development of the Infant and Young Child*, 9th ed. New York, Churchill Livingstone, 1987.

Illsley R, Mitchell RG: The developing concept of low birth weight and the present state of knowledge. *In* Illsley R, Mitchell RGF (eds): *Low Birth Weight. A Medical, Psychological and Social Study*. New York, John Wiley & Sons, 1984.

Jeantry P, Romero R: *Obstetrical Ultrasound*. New York, McGraw-Hill, 1984.

Kalousek DK, Fitch N, Paradice BA: *Pathology of the Human Embryo and Previable Fetus. An Atlas*. New York, Springer-Verlag, 1990.

Kolata G: Finding biological clocks in fetuses. *Science 230:*929, 1985.

La Pine TR, Jackson JC, Bennett FC: Outcome of infants weighing less than 800 grams at birth: 15 years' experience. *Pediatrics 96:* 479, 1995.

Lee W, Barton S, Comstock CH, et al: Transverse cerebellar diameter: a useful predictor of gestational age for fetuses with asymmetric growth retardation. *Am J Obstet Gynecol 165:*1044, 1991.

Liley AW: The use of amniocentesis and fetal transfusion in erythroblastosis fetalis. *Pediatrics 35:*876, 1965.

Lucey JF: Conditions and diseases of the newborn. *In* Reid DE, Ryan KJ, Benirschke K (eds): *Principles and Management of Human Reproduction*. Philadelphia, WB Saunders, 1972.

Lyons EA, Levi CS: *Ultrasound of the normal first trimester of pregnancy*. Syllabus: Special Course Ultrasound. Radiological Society of North America, 1991.

MacIntyre M: Chromosomal problems of intrauterine diagnosis. *In* Bergsma D, Motulsky AG, Jackson C, Sitter J (eds): *Symposium on Intrauterine Diagnosis. Birth Defects 7:*10, 1971.

Manning F: Fetal assessment. *Manitoba Medicine 61:*63, 1991.

Manning FA: *Fetal Medicine. Principles and Practice*. Norwalk, Appleton & Lange, 1995.

Merkatz IR, Nitowsky HM, Macri JN: An association between low maternal serum alpha-fetoprotein and fetal chromosome abnormalities. *Am J Obstet Gynecol 148:*886, 1984.

Miller HC, Merritt TA: *Fetal Growth in Humans*. Chicago, Year Book Medical Publishers, 1979.

Moore KL (ed): *The Sex Chromatin*. Philadelphia, WB Saunders, 1966.

Muraskas JK, Myers TF, Lambert GH, Anderson CL: Intact survival of a 280-g infant: an extreme case of growth retardation with normal cognitive development at two years of age. *Acta Paediatr (Suppl) 382:*16, 1992.

Nash JE, Persaud TVN: Embryopathic risks of cigarette smoking. *Exp Pathol 33:*65, 1988.

Nathanielsz PW: *Life Before Birth. The Challenges of Fetal Development*. New York, WH Freeman and Company, 1996.

Nava S, Bocconi L, Zuliani G, et al: Aspects of fetal physiology from 18 to 37 weeks' gestation as assessed by blood sampling. *Obstet Gynecol 87*:975, 1996.

Newnham JP, Evans SF, Michael CA, et al: Effects of frequent ultrasound during pregnancy: a randomised controlled trial. *Lancet 342*:887, 1993.

O'Rahilly R, Müller F: *Developmental Stages in Human Embryos*. Publication 637. Washington, Carnegie Institution of Washington, 1987.

Page EW, Villee CA, Villee DB: *Human Reproduction: Essentials of Reproductive and Perinatal Medicine*, 3rd ed. Philadelphia, WB Saunders, 1981.

Persaud TVN: *Prenatal Pathology. Fetal Medicine*. Springfield, Charles C Thomas, 1979.

Persaud TVN: Fetal alcohol Syndrome. *CRC Critical Rev in Anatomy & Cell Biology 1*:277, 1988.

Persaud TVN: *Environmental Causes of Human Birth Defects*. Springfield, Charles C Thomas, 1990.

Platek DN, Divon MY, Anyaegbunam A, Merkatz IR: Intrapartum ultrasonographic estimates of fetal weight by the house staff. *Am J Obstet Gynecol 165*:842, 1991.

Ploeckinger-Ulm B, Ulm MR, Lee A, et al: Antenatal depiction of fetal digits with three-dimensional ultrasonography. *Am J Obstet Gynecol 175*:571, 1996.

Polin RA, Mennuti MTP: Genetic disease and chromosomal abnormalities. *In* Fanaroff AA, Martin RJ (eds): *Neonatal-Perinatal Medicine. Diseases of the Fetus and Infant*. St Louis, CV Mosby, 1987.

Quilligan EJ, Zuspan FP (eds): *Current Therapy in Obstetrics and Gynecology*, vol 3. Philadelphia, WB Saunders, 1990.

Quintero RA, Puder KS, Cotton DB: Embryoscopy and fetoscopy. *Obstet Gynecol Clin North Am 20*:563, 1993.

Reece EA, Whetham J, Rotmensch S, Wiznitzer A: Gaining access to the embryonic-fetal circulation via first-trimester endoscopy: a step into the future. *Obstet Gynecol 82*:876, 1993.

Resnick R: Post-term pregnancy. *In* Quilligan EJ, Zuspan FP (eds): *Current Therapy in Obstetrics and Gynecology*, vol 3. Philadelphia, WB Saunders, 1990.

Riis P, Fuchs F: Sex chromatin and antenatal sex diagnosis. *In* Moore KL (ed): *The Sex Chromatin*. Philadelphia, WB Saunders, 1966.

Roberts L: Fishing cuts the angst in amniocentesis. *Science 254*:378, 1991.

Robinson JS: Fetal growth and development. *In* Chamberlain G (ed): *Turnbull's Obstetrics*, 2nd ed. Edinburgh, Churchill Livingstone, 1995.

Rosen M: Anesthesia and monitoring for fetal intervention. *In* Harrison MR, Golbus MS, Filly RA (eds): *The Unborn Patient. Prenatal Diagnosis and Treatment*, 2nd ed. Philadelphia, WB Saunders, 1991.

Sawin SW, Morgan MA: Dating of pregnancy by trimesters: a review and reappraisal. *Obstet Gynecol Surv 51*:261, 1996.

Scammon RE, Calkins HA: *Development and Growth of the External Dimensions of the Human Body in the Fetal Period*. Minneapolis, University of Minnesota Press, 1929.

Schats R, Van Os HC, Jansen CAM, Wladimiroff JW: The crown-rump length in early human pregnancy: a reappraisal. *Br J Obstet Gynaecol 98*:460, 1991.

Sciscioine AC, Gorman R, Callan NA: Adjustment of birth weight standards for maternal and infant characteristics improves the prediction of outcome in the small-for-gestational age infant. *Am J Obstet Gynecol 175*:544, 1996.

Scott F, Beeby P, Abbott J, et al: New formula for estimating fetal weight below 1000 g: comparison with existing formulas. *J Ultrasound Med 15*:669, 1996.

Senterre J (ed): *Intrauterine Growth Retardation*: Nestle Nutrition Workshop Series, vol 18. New York, Raven Press, 1989.

Shepard TH: Normal and abnormal growth patterns. *In* Gardner LI (ed): *Endocrine and Genetic Diseases of Childhood and Adolescence*, 2nd ed. Philadelphia, WB Saunders, 1975.

Shiota K: Development and intrauterine fate of normal and abnormal human conceptuses. *Congen Anom 31*:67, 1991.

Simpson JL, Elias S: *Essentials of Prenatal Diagnosis*. New York, Churchill Livingstone, 1993.

Simpson JL, Elias S: Prenatal diagnosis of genetic disorders. *In* Creasy RK, Resnik R (eds): *Maternal-Fetal Medicine. Principles and Practice*, 2nd ed. Philadelphia, WB Saunders, 1989.

Sinclair D: *Human Growth After Birth*. Oxford, Oxford University Press, 1985.

Skupsi DW, Wolf CFW, Bussel JB: Fetal transfusion therapy. *Obstet Gynecol Surv 51*:181, 1996.

Smith DW, Gong BT: Scalp hair patterning as a clue to early fetal brain development. *J Pediatr 83*:379, 1973.

Soothill P: Fetal and perinatal medicine. *Br J Hosp Med 56*:141, 1996.

Spence WC, Maddalena A, Demers DB, et al: Molecular analysis of the RHD genotype in fetuses at risk for RHD hemolytic disease. *Obstet Gynecol 85*:296, 1995.

Spirt BA, Gordon LP, Oliphant M: *Prenatal Ultrasound. A Color Atlas with Anatomic and Pathologic Correlation*. New York, Churchill Livingstone, 1987.

Stevenson RE: *The Fetus and Newly Born Infant. Influences of the Prenatal Environment*. St Louis, CV Mosby, 1973.

Streeter GL: Weight, sitting height, head size, foot length and menstrual age of the human embryo. *Contrib Embryol Carnegie Inst 11*:143, 1920.

Suzumori K, Tanemura M, Adachi R: Molecular genetic techniques for prenatal diagnosis. *Congen Anom 34*:161, 1994.

Thompson MW, McInnes RR, Willard HF: *Thompson & Thompson Genetics in Medicine*, 5th ed. Philadelphia, WB Saunders, 1991.

Townsend RR: Ultrasound evaluation of the placenta and umbilical cord. *In* Callen PW (ed): *Ultrasonography in Obstetrics and Gynecology*, 3rd ed. Philadelphia, WB Saunders, 1994.

Tulchinsky D, Ryan KJ: *Maternal-Fetal Endocrinology*. Philadelphia, WB Saunders, 1980.

Usher RH, McLean FH: Normal fetal growth and the significance of fetal growth retardation. *In* Davis JA, Dobbing J (eds): *Scientific Foundation of Paediatrics*. Philadelphia, WB Saunders, 1974.

Wald NJ, Cuckle HS: APF screening in early pregnancy. *In* Spencer JAD (ed): *Fetal Monitoring*. Oxford, Oxford University Press, 1991.

Wald NJ, Cuckle HS, Densem JW, et al: Maternal serum screening for Down's syndrome in early pregnancy. *Br Med J 297*:883, 1988.

Wathen NC, Cass PL, Kitau MJ, Chard T: Human chorionic gonadotrophin and alpha-fetoprotein levels in matched samples of amniotic fluid, extraembryonic coelomic fluid, and maternal serum in the first trimester of pregnancy. *Prenatal Diagnosis 11*:145, 1991.

Weaver DD: Inborn errors of metabolism. *In* Weaver DD (ed): *Catalogue of Prenatally Diagnosed Conditions*. Baltimore, The John Hopkins University Press, 1989.

Wilson RD: How to perform genetic amniocentesis. *Journal SOGC 13*:61, 1991.

Yen SSC, Jaffe RB: *Reproductive Endocrinology. Physiology, Pathophysiology and Clinical Management*, 3rd ed. Philadelphia, WB Saunders, 1991.

Young SR, Shipley CF, Wade RV, et al: Single-center comparison of results of 1000 prenatal diagnoses with chorionic villus sampling and 1000 diagnoses with amniocentesis. *Am J Obstet Gynecol 165*:255, 1991.

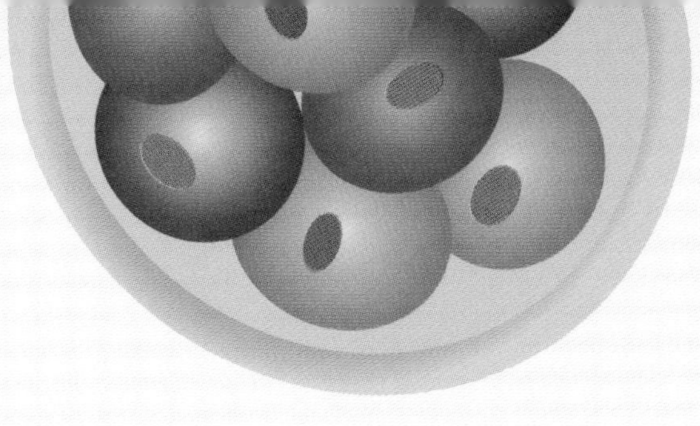

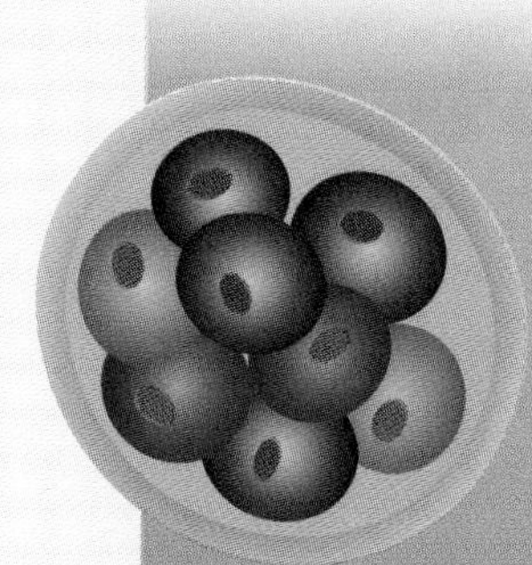

Placenta and Fetal Membranes

7

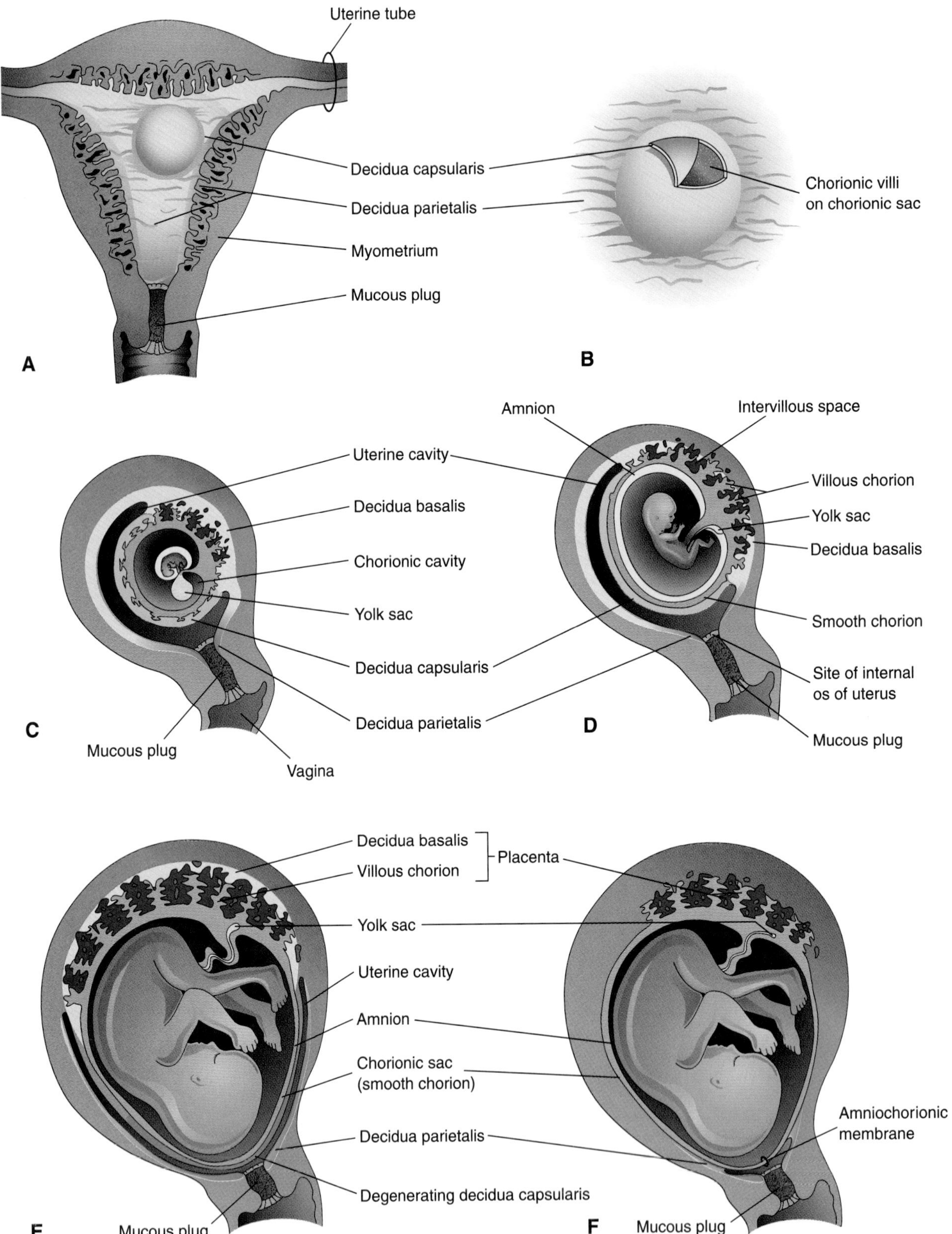

■ **Figure 7–1.** Drawings illustrating development of the placenta and fetal membranes. *A,* Coronal section of the uterus showing elevation of the decidua capsularis by the expanding chorionic sac of a 4-week embryo, implanted in the endometrium on the posterior wall. *B,* Enlarged drawing of the implantation site. The chorionic villi were exposed by cutting an opening in the decidua capsularis. *C* to *F,* Sagittal sections of the gravid uterus from the fifth to twenty-second week, showing the changing relations of the fetal membranes to the decidua. In *F,* the amnion and chorion are fused with each other and the decidua parietalis, thereby obliterating the uterine cavity. Note in *D* to *F* that the chorionic villi persist only where the chorion is associated with the decidua basalis.

■ The fetal part of the placenta and the fetal membranes separate the fetus from the endometrium of the uterus. There is an interchange of substances such as nutrients and oxygen between the maternal and fetal blood streams through the placenta. The vessels in the umbilical cord connect the placental circulation with the fetal circulation.

The chorion, amnion, yolk sac, and allantois constitute the fetal membranes. They develop from the zygote but do not participate in the formation of the embryo or fetus, except for parts of the yolk sac and allantois. Part of the yolk sac is incorporated into the embryo as the primordium of the gut. The allantois forms a fibrous cord that is known as the urachus in the fetus and the median umbilical ligament in the adult. It extends from the apex of the urinary bladder to the umbilicus.

THE PLACENTA

The placenta is the primary site of nutrient and gas exchange between the mother and fetus. The placenta is a **fetomaternal organ** that has two components:

- a **fetal portion** that develops from the chorionic sac
- a **maternal portion** that is derived from the endometrium

The placenta and umbilical cord function as a *transport system* for substances passing between the mother and fetus. Nutrients and oxygen pass from the maternal blood through the placenta to the fetal blood, and waste materials and carbon dioxide pass from the fetal blood through the placenta to the maternal blood. The placenta and fetal membranes perform the following functions and activities:

- protection
- nutrition
- respiration
- excretion
- hormone production

Shortly after birth of a baby, the placenta and fetal membranes are expelled from the uterus as the *afterbirth*.

The Decidua

The decidua (L. *deciduus*, a falling off) refers to the *gravid endometrium*—the functional layer of the endometrium in a pregnant woman. The term decidua is appropriate because this part of the endometrium separates ("falls away") from the remainder of the uterus after *parturition* (childbirth).

Three regions of the decidua are named according to their relation to the implantation site (Fig. 7-1):

- The **decidua basalis** is the part of the decidua deep to the conceptus that forms the maternal component of the placenta.
- The **decidua capsularis** is the superficial part of the decidua overlying the conceptus.
- The **decidua parietalis** (decidua vera) is all the remaining parts of the decidua.

In response to increasing progesterone levels in the maternal blood, the stromal (connective tissue) cells of the decidua enlarge to form pale-staining **decidual cells**. These cells enlarge as glycogen and lipid accumulate in their cytoplasm. The decidual cellular and vascular changes resulting from pregnancy are referred to as the **decidual reaction**. Many decidual cells degenerate near the chorionic sac in the region of the *syncytiotrophoblast* and, together with maternal blood and uterine secretions, provide a rich source of nutrition for the embryo. The full significance of decidual cells is not understood, but it has also been suggested that they protect the maternal tissue against uncontrolled invasion by the syncytiotrophoblast, and that they may be involved in hormone production. Decidual regions, clearly recognizable during *ultrasonography*, are important in diagnosing early pregnancy (Filly, 1994; Townsend, 1994).

Development of the Placenta

Previous descriptions of early placental development traced the rapid proliferation of the trophoblast and development of the chorionic sac and chorionic villi (see Chapters 3 and 4). By the end of the third week, the anatomical arrangements necessary for physiological exchanges between the mother and embryo are established. A complex vascular network is established in the placenta by the end of the fourth week which facilitates maternal-embryonic exchanges of gases, nutrients, and metabolic waste products. For more information about angiogenesis in the placenta, see Gordon et al. (1995).

Chorionic villi cover the entire chorionic sac until the beginning of the eighth week (Figs. 7-1*C*, 7-2, and 7-3). As this sac grows, the villi associated with the decidua capsularis are compressed, reducing the blood supply to them. These villi soon degenerate (Figs. 7-1*D* and 7-3*B*), producing a relatively avascular bare area, the **smooth chorion**, or chorion laeve (L. *levis*, smooth). As the villi disappear, those associated with the decidua basalis rapidly increase in number, branch profusely, and enlarge (Fig. 7-4). This bushy part of the chorionic sac is the **villous chorion** or chorion frondosum (L. *frondosus*, leafy).

Ultrasonography of Chorionic Sac

The size of the chorionic sac is useful in determining *gestational age* of embryos in patients with uncertain menstrual histories (Filly, 1994). The early chorionic sac is filled with *chorionic fluid* because the amniotic sac containing the embryo and the yolk sac are relatively small (Fig. 7-1*C*). Growth of the chorionic sac is extremely rapid between the fifth and tenth weeks. Modern ultrasound equipment, especially instruments equipped with intravaginal transducers, enables sonolo-

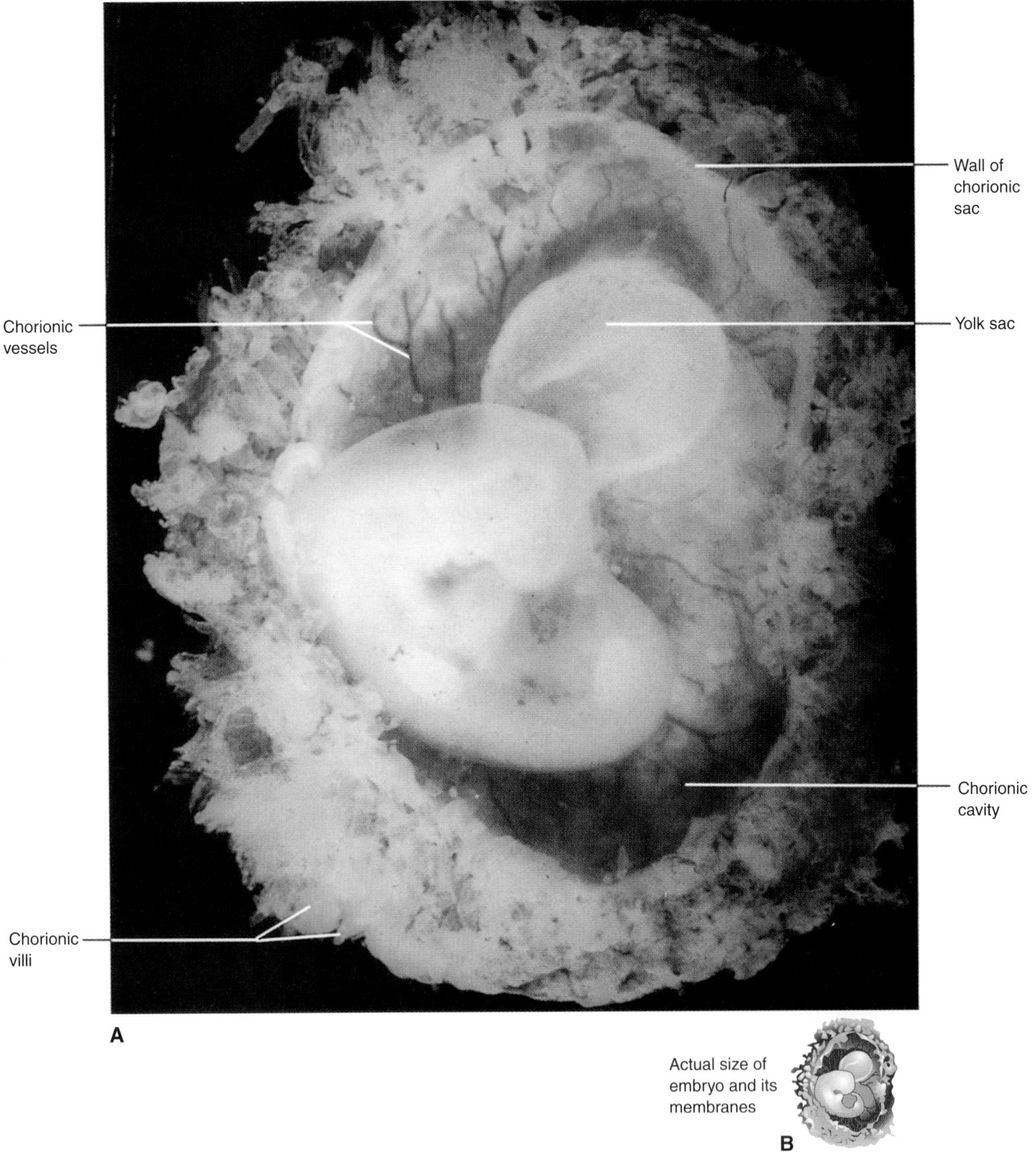

■ **Figure 7–2.** *A,* Lateral view of a spontaneously aborted embryo at Carnegie stage 14, about 32 days. The chorionic and amniotic sacs have been opened to show the embryo. Note the large size of the yolk sac at this stage. (From Moore KL, Persaud TVN, Shiota K: *Color Atlas of Clinical Embryology.* Philadelphia, WB Saunders, 1994.) *B,* The sketch shows the actual size of the embryo and its membranes.

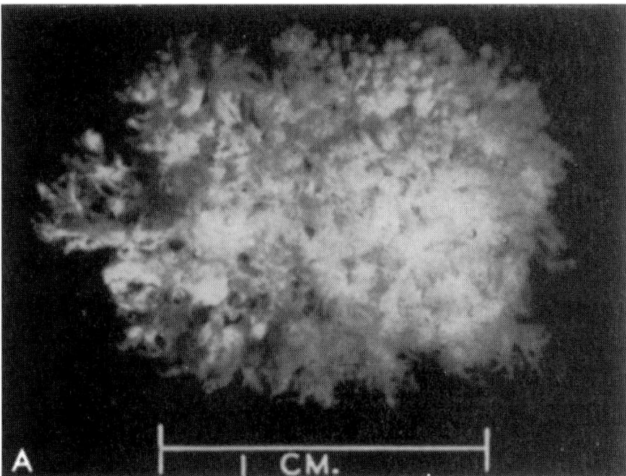

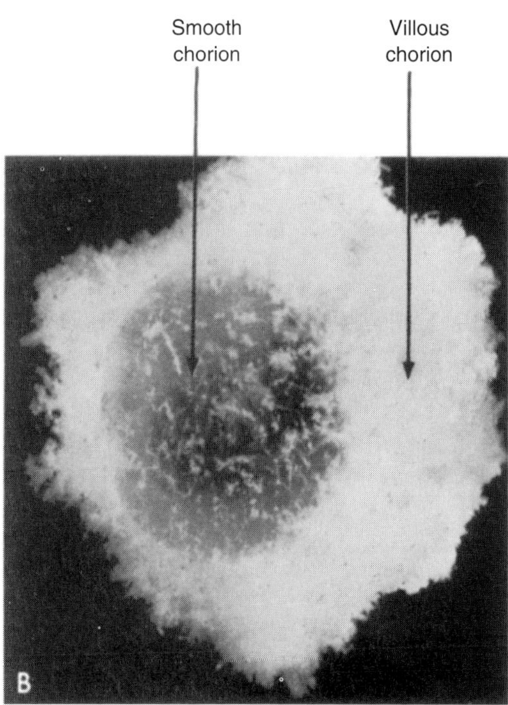

■ **Figure 7–3.** Photographs of spontaneously aborted human chorionic sacs. *A,* 21 days. The entire sac is covered with chorionic villi (×4). *B,* 8 weeks. Actual size. As the decidua capsularis becomes stretched and thin, the chorionic villi on the corresponding part of the chorionic sac gradually degenerate and disappear, leaving a smooth chorion. The remaining villous chorion forms the fetal part of the placenta. (From Potter EL, Craig JM: *Pathology of the Fetus and the Infant,* 3rd ed. Copyright 1975 by Year Book Medical Publishers, Chicago.)

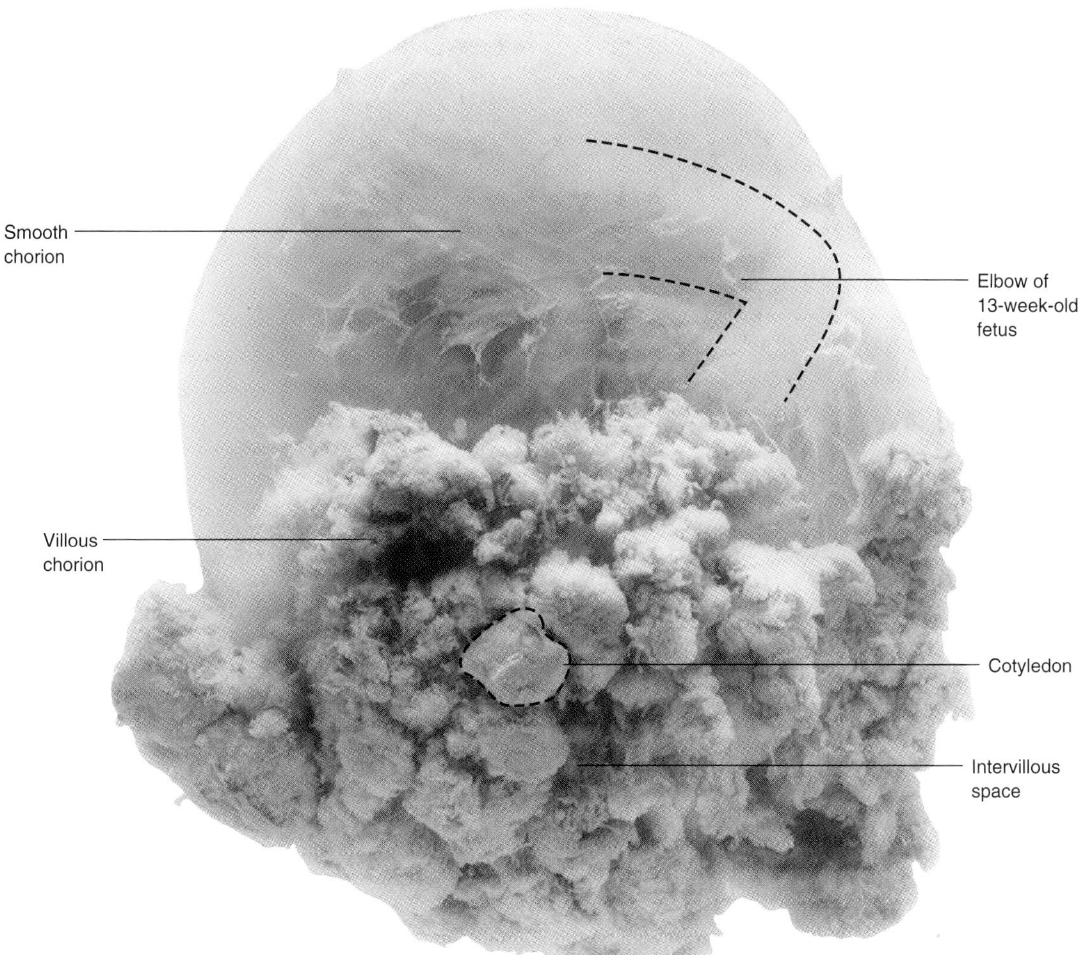

■ **Figure 7–4.** Photograph of a human chorionic sac containing a 13-week-old fetus. The smooth chorion formed when the chorionic villi degenerated and disappeared from this area of the chorionic sac. The villous chorion (chorion frondosum) is where chorionic villi persist and form the fetal part of the placenta. In situ the cotyledons were attached to the decidua basalis and the intervillous space was filled with maternal blood. (From Moore KL, Persaud TVN, Shiota K: *Color Atlas of Clinical Embryology.* Philadelphia, WB Saunders, 1994.)

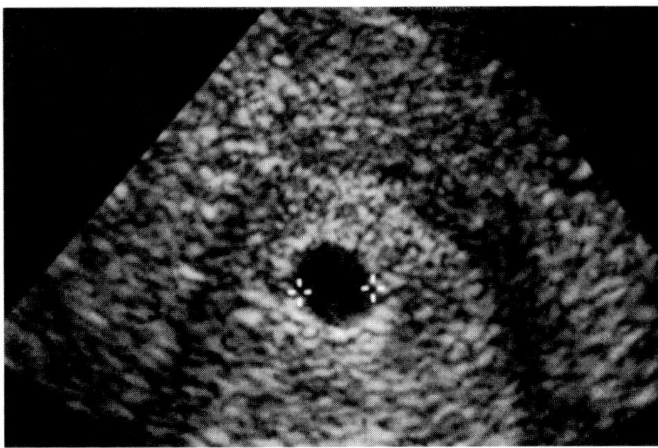

■ **Figure 7–5.** Transverse endovaginal sonograph of an early chorionic sac (before visualization of a yolk sac), showing how the mean sac diameter is measured. This image depicts the transverse diameter—between the white cursors—measured from the chorionic tissue-fluid interfaces. (From Filly RA: Ultrasound Evaluation During the First Trimester. *In* Callen PW [ed]: *Ultrasonography in Obstetrics and Gynecology,* 3rd ed. Philadelphia, WB Saunders, 1994.)

gists to detect the chorionic sac, or gestational sac, when it has a *median sac diameter* (MSD) of 2 to 3 mm (Fig. 7-5). Chorionic sacs with this diameter indicate that the gestational age is 4 weeks and 3 to 4 days (Filly, 1994); i.e., about 18 days after fertilization.

The uterus, chorionic sac, and placenta enlarge as the fetus grows. Growth in the size and thickness of the placenta continues rapidly until the fetus is about 18 weeks old (20 weeks' gestation). The fully developed placenta covers 15 to 30% of the decidua and weighs about one-sixth that of the fetus. The placenta has two parts (Figs. 7-1*E* and *F* and 7-6):

- **The fetal component of the placenta** is formed by the *villous chorion*. The stem villi that arise from it project into the intervillous space containing maternal blood.
- **The maternal component of the placenta** is formed by the *decidua basalis*, the part of the decidua related to the fetal component of the placenta. By the end of the fourth month, the decidua basalis is almost entirely replaced by the fetal component of the placenta.

THE FETOMATERNAL JUNCTION

The fetal part of the placenta (villous chorion) is attached to the maternal part of the placenta (decidua basalis) by the **cytotrophoblastic shell**—the external layer of trophoblastic cells on the maternal surface of the placenta (Fig. 7-7). **Stem chorionic villi** (anchoring villi) attach firmly to the decidua basalis through the cytotrophoblastic shell and anchor the *chorionic sac* to the decidua basalis. Endometrial arteries and veins pass freely through gaps in the cyto-

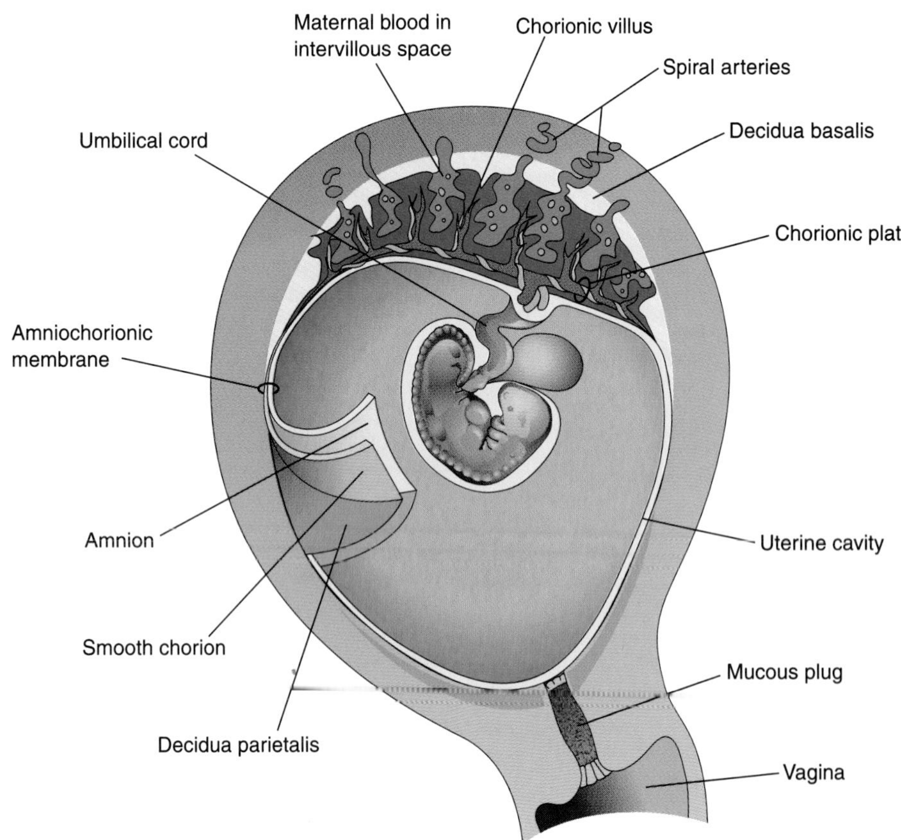

■ **Figure 7–6.** Drawing of a sagittal section of a gravid uterus at 4 weeks showing the relation of the fetal membranes to each other and to the decidua and embryo. The amnion and smooth chorion have been cut and reflected to show their relationship to each other and the decidua parietalis.

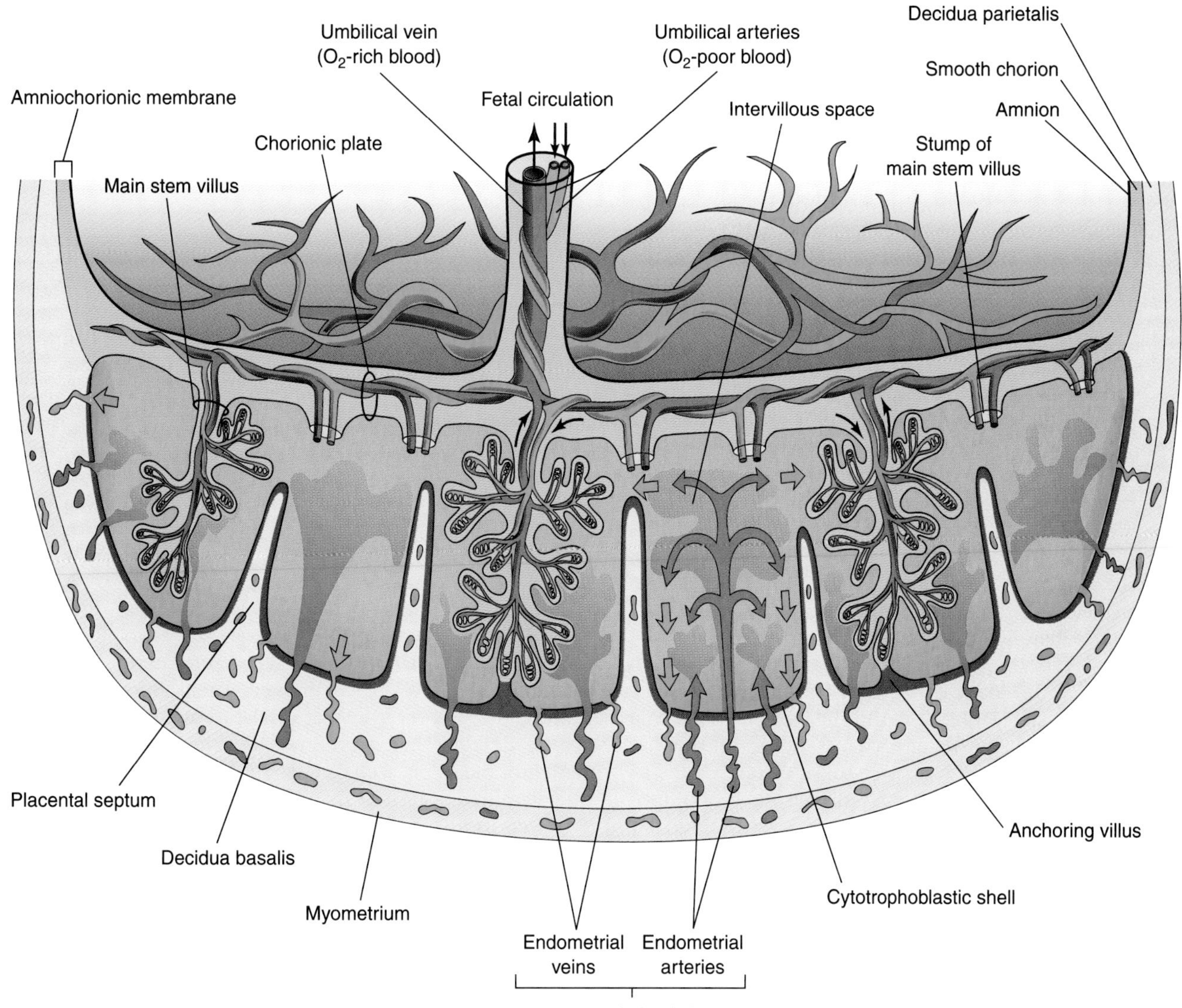

■ **Figure 7–7.** Schematic drawing of a transverse section through a full-term placenta, showing: (1) the relation of the villous chorion (fetal part of placenta) to the decidua basalis (maternal part of placenta), (2) the fetal placental circulation, and (3) the maternal placental circulation. Maternal blood flows into the intervillous spaces in funnel-shaped spurts from the spiral arteries, and exchanges occur with the fetal blood as the maternal blood flows around the branch villi. It is through the branch villi that the main exchange of material between the mother and embryo/fetus occurs. The inflowing arterial blood pushes venous blood out of the intervillous space into the endometrial veins, which are scattered over the entire surface of the decidua basalis. Note that the umbilical arteries carry poorly oxygenated fetal blood (shown in blue) to the placenta and that the umbilical vein carries oxygenated blood (shown in red) to the fetus. Note that the cotyledons are separated from each other by placental septa, projections of the decidua basalis. Each cotyledon consists of two or more main stem villi and their many branches. In this drawing, only one stem villus is shown in each cotyledon, but the stumps of those that have been removed are indicated.

trophoblastic shell and open into the intervillous space.

The **shape of the placenta** is determined by the shape of the persistent area of chorionic villi (Fig. 7-1*F*). Usually this is a circular area, giving the placenta a discoid shape. As the chorionic villi invade the decidua basalis during placental formation, decidual tissue is eroded to enlarge the intervillous space. This erosion process produces several wedge-shaped areas of decidua, placental septa, that project toward the **chorionic plate**—the part of the chorionic wall related to the placenta (Fig. 7-7). The **placental septa** divide the fetal part of the placenta into irregular convex areas called **cotyledons** (Fig. 7-4). Each cotyledon, visible on the maternal surface of the placenta, consists of two or more stem villi and their many branch villi. By the end of the fourth month, the decidua basalis is almost entirely replaced by the cotyledons.

The **decidua capsularis**, the layer of decidua overlying the implanted chorionic sac, forms a capsule over the external surface of the sac (Fig. 7-1*A* to *D*). As the conceptus enlarges, the decidua capsularis bulges into the uterine cavity and becomes greatly attenuated. Eventually the decidua capsularis contacts and fuses with the decidua parietalis, thereby slowly obliterating the uterine cavity (Fig. 7-1*E* and *F*). By 22-24 weeks, the reduced blood supply to the decidua capsularis causes it to degenerate and disappear. After disappearance of the decidua capsularis, the smooth part of the chorionic sac fuses with the decidua parietalis. This fusion can be separated and usually occurs when blood escapes from the intervillous space (Fig. 7-6). The collection of blood (*hematoma*) pushes the chorionic membrane away from the decidua parietalis, thereby reestablishing the potential space of the uterine cavity.

THE INTERVILLOUS SPACE

The intervillous space containing maternal blood is derived from the lacunae that developed in the syncytiotrophoblast during the second week of development (see Chapter 3). This large blood-filled space results from the coalescence and enlargement of the lacunar networks. The intervillous space of the placenta is divided into compartments by the *placental septa*; however, there is free communication between the compartments because the septa do not reach the *chorionic plate* (Fig. 7-7).

Maternal blood enters the intervillous space from the *spiral endometrial arteries* in the decidua basalis. See Foidart et al. (1992) for new insights on maternal blood circulation in the intervillous space of the human placenta. The spiral arteries pass through gaps in the cytotrophoblastic shell and discharge blood into the intervillous space. This large space is drained by endometrial veins that also penetrate the cytotrophoblastic shell. Endometrial veins are found over the entire surface of the decidua basalis. The numerous **branch villi**—arising from stem chorionic villi—are continuously showered with maternal blood that circulates through the intervillous space. The blood carries oxygen and nutritional materials that are necessary for fetal growth and development. The maternal blood also contains fetal waste products such as carbon dioxide, salts, and products of protein metabolism.

THE AMNIOCHORIONIC MEMBRANE

The amniotic sac enlarges faster than the chorionic sac. As a result, the amnion and smooth chorion soon fuse to form the amniochorionic membrane (Fig. 7-7). This composite membrane fuses with the decidua capsularis and, after disappearance of this capsular part of the decidua, adheres to the decidua parietalis (Fig. 7-1*F*). It is the amniochorionic membrane that ruptures during labor. Preterm rupture of this membrane is the most common event leading to premature labor. When the amniochorionic membrane ruptures, amniotic fluid escapes through the cervix and vagina to the exterior.

Placental Circulation

The many *branch chorionic villi* of the placenta provide a large surface area where materials may be exchanged across the very thin **placental membrane** ("barrier") interposed between the fetal and maternal circulations (Figs. 7-7 and 7-8). It is through the numerous *branch villi*, which arise from the *stem villi*, that the main exchange of material between the mother and fetus takes place. The circulations of the fetus and the mother are separated by the placental membrane consisting of extrafetal tissues (Fig. 7-8*B* and *C*).

FETAL PLACENTAL CIRCULATION

Poorly oxygenated blood leaves the fetus and passes through the **umbilical arteries** to the placenta. At the site of attachment of the cord to the placenta, these arteries divide into a number of radially disposed **chorionic arteries** that branch freely in the chorionic plate before entering the chorionic villi (Fig. 7-7). The blood vessels form an extensive **arterio-capillary-venous system** within the chorionic villi (Fig. 7-8*A*), which brings the fetal blood extremely close to the maternal blood. This system provides a very large area for the exchange of metabolic and gaseous products between the maternal and fetal blood streams.

There is normally no intermingling of fetal and maternal blood; however, very small amounts of fetal blood may enter the maternal circulation through minute defects that sometimes develop in the placental membrane. The well-oxygenated fetal blood in the fetal capillaries passes into thin-walled veins that follow the chorionic arteries to the site of attachment of the umbilical cord, where they converge to form the **umbilical vein**. This large vessel carries oxygen-rich blood to the fetus (Fig. 7-7).

MATERNAL PLACENTAL CIRCULATION

The blood in the intervillous space is temporarily outside the maternal circulatory system. It enters the intervillous space through 80 to 100 **spiral endometrial arteries** in the decidua basalis. These vessels discharge into the intervillous space through gaps in the cytotrophoblastic shell. The blood flow from the spiral arteries is pulsatile and is propelled in jetlike fountains by the maternal blood pressure (Fig. 7-7). The entering blood is at a considerably higher pressure than that in the intervillous space and spurts toward the **chorionic plate** forming the "roof" of the intervillous space. As the pressure dissipates, the blood flows slowly around the branch villi, allowing an exchange of metabolic and gaseous products with the fetal blood. The blood eventually returns through the endometrial veins to the maternal circulation.

The welfare of the embryo and fetus depends more on the adequate bathing of the branch villi with maternal blood than on any other factor. Reductions of uteroplacental circulation result in fetal hypoxia and IUGR (Werler et al., 1986). Severe reductions of uteroplacental circulation may result in fetal death. The intervillous space of the mature placenta contains about 150 ml of blood that is replenished three or four times per minute. The intermittent contractions of the

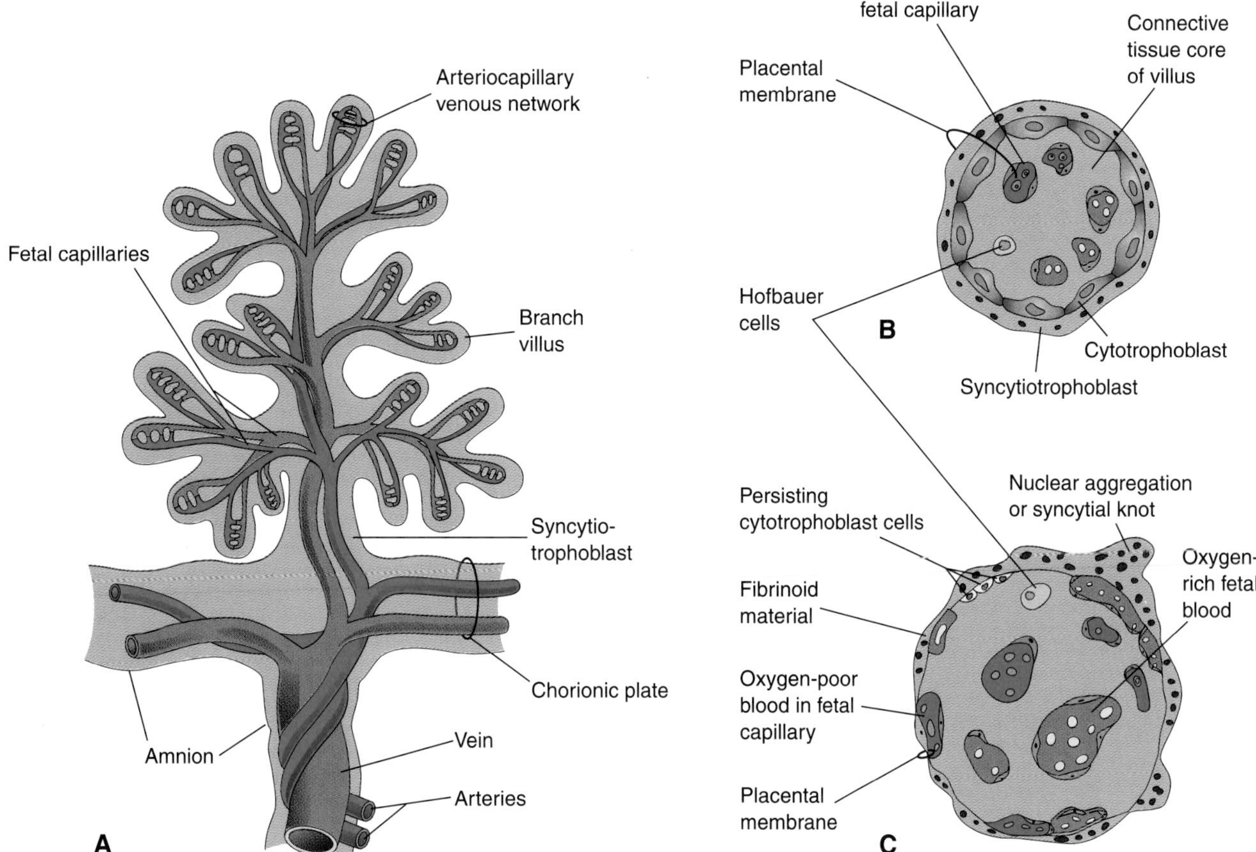

■ **Figure 7–8.** *A,* Drawing of a stem chorionic villus showing its arteriocapillary-venous system. The arteries carry poorly oxygenated fetal blood and waste products from the fetus, whereas the vein carries oxygenated blood and nutrients to the fetus. *B* and *C,* Drawings of sections through a branch villus at 10 weeks and full term, respectively. The placental membrane, composed of extrafetal tissues, separates the maternal blood in the intervillous space from the fetal blood in the capillaries in the villi. Note that the placental membrane becomes very thin at full term. Hofbauer cells are thought to be phagocytic cells.

uterus during pregnancy decrease uteroplacental blood flow slightly; however, they do not force significant amounts of blood out of the intervillous space. Consequently, oxygen transfer to the fetus is decreased during uterine contractions, but does not stop.

THE PLACENTAL MEMBRANE

The placental membrane is a composite membrane that *consists of the extrafetal tissues separating the maternal and fetal blood.* Until about 20 weeks, the placental membrane consists of four layers (Figs. 7-8 and 7-9):

- syncytiotrophoblast
- cytotrophoblast
- connective tissue of villus
- endothelium of fetal capillaries

After the twentieth week, histological changes occur in the branch villi that result in the cytotrophoblast in many of the villi becoming attenuated. Eventually cytotrophoblast cells disappear over large areas of the villi leaving only thin patches of syncytiotrophoblast. As a result, the placental membrane consists of three layers in most places (Fig. 7-8*C*). In some areas the placental membrane becomes markedly thinned and attenuated. At these sites the syncytiotrophoblast comes in direct contact with the endothelium of the fetal capillaries to form a *vasculosyncytial placental membrane.* The placental membrane was formerly called the *placental barrier,* an inappropriate term because there are only a few substances, endogenous or exogenous, that are unable to pass through the placental membrane in detectable amounts (Kraemer and Noerr, 1997). The placental membrane acts as a true barrier only when the molecule has a certain size, configuration, and charge such as heparin and bacteria. Some metabolites, toxins, and hormones, though present in the maternal circulation, do not pass through the placental membrane in sufficient concentrations to affect the embryo/fetus.

Most drugs and other substances in the maternal plasma pass through the placental membrane and enter the fetal plasma (Fig. 7-9). Electronmicrographs of the syncytiotrophoblast show that its free surface has many *microvilli*—over 1 billion/cm^2 at term (Benirschke and Kaufman, 1990)—that increase the surface area for exchange between the maternal

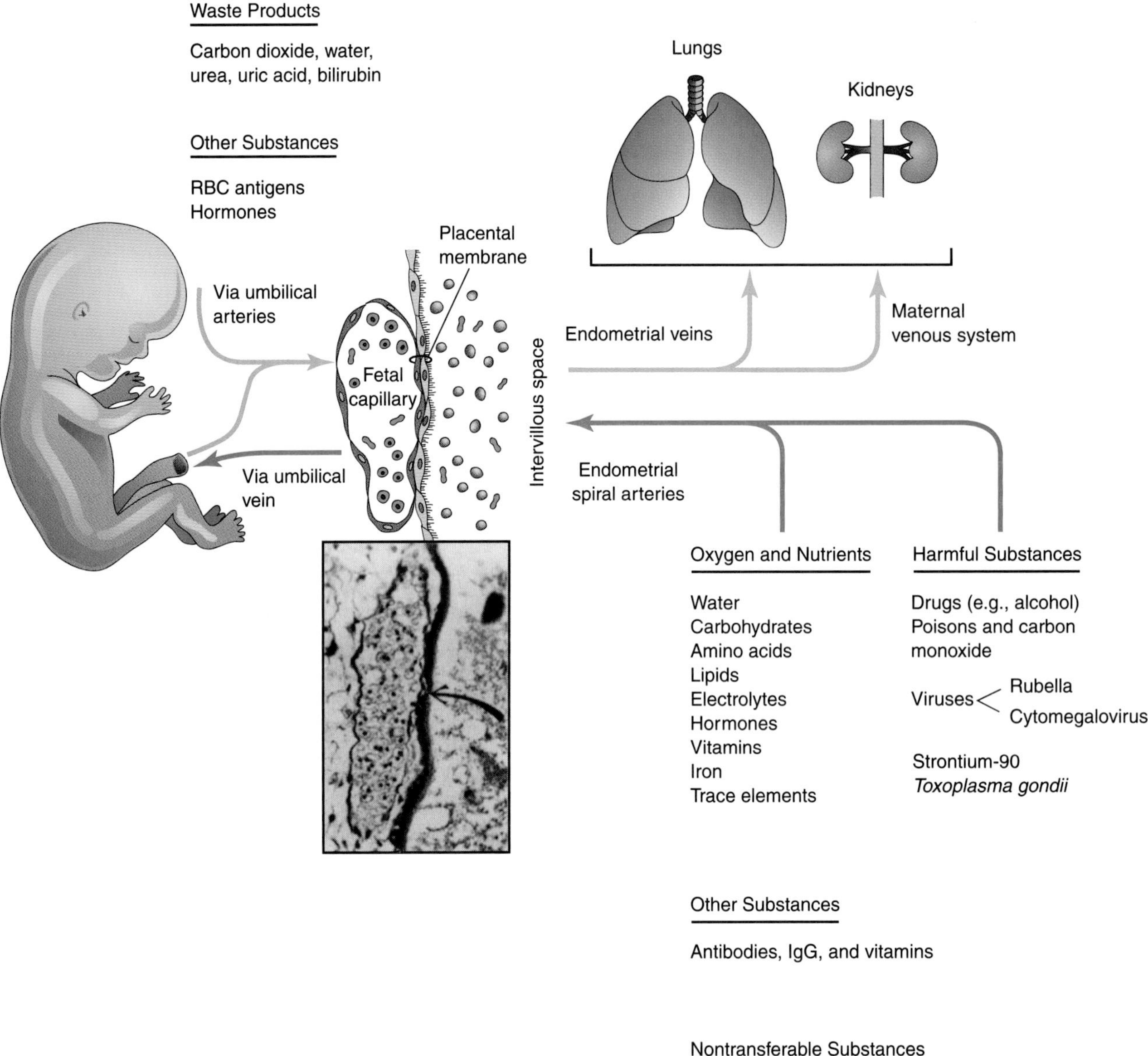

■ **Figure 7–9.** Diagrammatic illustration of transfer across the placental membrane (barrier). The extrafetal tissues, across which transport of substances between the mother and fetus occurs, collectively constitute the placental membrane. (Inset photomicrograph from Javert CT: *Spontaneous and Habitual Abortion.* 1957. Courtesy of the Blakiston Division, McGraw-Hill Book Co. Copyright 1957 by McGraw-Hill. Used by permission of McGraw-Hill Book Company.)

and fetal circulations. As pregnancy advances, the placental membrane becomes progressively thinner so that blood in many fetal capillaries is extremely close to the maternal blood in the intervillous space (Fig. 7-8*C*).

During the third trimester, numerous nuclei in the syncytiotrophoblast aggregate to form multinucleated protrusions or nuclear aggregations—**syncytial knots**. These aggregations continually break off and are carried from the intervillous space into the maternal circulation. Some knots lodge in capillaries of the maternal lung where they are rapidly destroyed by local enzyme action. Toward the end of pregnancy, **fibrinoid material** forms on the surfaces of villi. This material consists of fibrin and other unidentified substances that stain intensely with eosin. Fibrinoid material results mainly from aging and appears to reduce placental transfer.

Functions of the Placenta

The placenta has three main functions:

- metabolism (e.g., synthesis of glycogen)
- transport of gases and nutrients
- endocrine secretion (e.g., hCG)

These comprehensive activities are essential for maintaining pregnancy and promoting normal fetal development.

PLACENTAL METABOLISM

The placenta, particularly during early pregnancy, synthesizes glycogen, cholesterol, and fatty acids, which serve as sources of nutrients and energy for the embryo/fetus. Many of its metabolic activities are undoubtedly critical for its other two major placental activities (transport and endocrine secretion).

PLACENTAL TRANSFER

The transport of substances in both directions between the placenta and maternal blood is facilitated by the great surface area of the placental membrane. Almost all materials are transported across the placental membrane by one of the following *four main transport mechanisms*:

- simple diffusion
- facilitated diffusion
- active transport
- pinocytosis

Passive transport by simple diffusion is usually characteristic of substances moving from areas of higher to lower concentration until equilibrium is established. In *facilitated diffusion* there is transport through electrical charges. *Active transport* against a concentration gradient requires energy. Such systems may involve enzymes that temporarily combine with the substances concerned. *Pinocytosis* is a form of endocytosis in which the material being engulfed is a small sample of extracellular fluid. This method of transport is usually reserved for large molecules. Some proteins are transferred very slowly through the placenta by pinocytosis.

Other Placental Transport Mechanisms

There are three other methods that substances use to cross the placental membrane. In the first, fetal red blood cells pass into the maternal circulation, particularly during parturition, through microscopic breaks in the placental membrane. Labeled maternal red blood cells have also been found in the fetal circulation. Consequently, red blood cells may pass in either direction through very small defects or breaks in the placental membrane. In the second method of transport, cells cross the placental membrane under their own power; e.g., maternal leukocytes and *Treponema pallidum*—the organism that causes syphilis. In the third method of transport, some bacteria and protozoa such as *Toxoplasma gondii* (see Chapter 8) infect the placenta by creating lesions and then cross the placental membrane through the defects that are created.

Transfer of Gases. Oxygen, carbon dioxide, and carbon monoxide cross the placental membrane by simple diffusion. The exchange of oxygen and carbon dioxide is limited more by blood flow than by the efficiency of diffusion (Carlson, 1994). *Interruption of oxygen transport for several minutes endangers survival of the embryo or fetus.* The placental membrane approaches the efficiency of the lungs for gas exchange. The quantity of oxygen reaching the fetus is primarily flow-limited rather than diffusion-limited; hence, fetal hypoxia (decreased levels of oxygen) results primarily from factors that diminish either the uterine blood flow or fetal blood flow. Inhaled anesthetics can also cross the placental membrane and affect fetal breathing if used during parturition.

Nutritional Substances. Nutrients constitute the bulk of substances transferred from the mother to the fetus. **Water** is rapidly and freely exchanged by simple diffusion between the mother and fetus, and in increasing amounts as pregnancy advances. **Glucose** produced by the mother and placenta is quickly transferred to the embryo or fetus by diffusion. There is little or no transfer of maternal cholesterol, triglycerides, or phospholipids. Although there is transport of free fatty acids, the amount transferred appears to be relatively small. **Vitamins** cross the placental membrane and are essential for normal development. Water-soluble vitamins cross the placental membrane more quickly than fat-soluble ones.

Hormones. *Protein hormones* do not reach the embryo or fetus in significant amounts, except for a slow transfer of thyroxine and triiodothyronine. *Unconjugated steroid hormones* cross the placental membrane rather freely. Testosterone and certain synthetic progestins cross the placental membrane and may cause masculinization of female fetuses (see Chapter 8).

Electrolytes. These compounds are freely exchanged across the placental membrane in significant quantities, each at its own rate. When a mother receives *intravenous fluids*, they also pass to the fetus and affect its water and electrolyte status.

Maternal Antibodies. The fetus produces only small amounts of antibodies because of its immature immune system. Some passive immunity is conferred upon the fetus by the placental transfer of maternal antibodies. The alpha and beta globulins reach the fetus in very small quantities but many gamma globulins, such as the IgG (7S) class are readily transported to the fetus by pinocytosis. **Maternal antibodies confer fetal immunity** to diseases such as diphtheria, smallpox, and measles; however, no immunity is acquired to pertussis (whooping cough) or varicella (chickenpox). A maternal protein, *transferrin*, crosses the placental membrane and carries iron to the embryo or fetus. The placental surface contains special receptors for this protein (Carlson, 1994).

Hemolytic Disease of the Newborn

Small amounts of fetal blood may pass to the maternal blood through microscopic breaks in the placental membrane. If the fetus is Rh-positive and the mother Rh-negative, the fetal blood cells may stimulate the formation of anti-Rh antibody by the immune system of the mother. This passes to the fetal blood and causes hemolysis of fetal Rh-positive blood cells and anemia in the fetus. Some fetuses with **hemolytic disease of the newborn** (HDN), or *fetal erythroblastosis*, fail to make a satisfactory intrauterine adjustment and may die unless delivered early or given intrauterine, intraperitoneal, or intravenous transfusions of packed Rh-negative blood cells in order to maintain the fetus until after birth (see Chapter 6). HDN is relatively uncommon now because Rh immunoglobulin given to the mother usually prevents development of this disease in the fetus (Behrman et al., 1996).

Waste Products. Urea and uric acid pass through the placental membrane by simple diffusion and bilirubin is quickly cleared.

Drugs and Drug Metabolites. Most drugs and drug metabolites cross the placenta by simple diffusion (Kraemer and Noerr, 1997), the exception being those with a structural similarity to amino acids, such as methyldopa and antimetabolites. Some drugs cause major congenital anomalies (see Chapter 8). **Fetal drug addiction** may occur after maternal use of drugs such as heroin and 50 to 75% of newborns experience withdrawal symptoms (Behrman et al., 1996). Because psychic dependence on these drugs is not developed during the fetal period, no liability to subsequent narcotic addiction exists in the infant after withdrawal is complete. Except for muscle relaxants such as succinylcholine and curare, most agents used for the management of labor readily cross the placental membrane. Depending on the dose and its timing in relation to delivery, these drugs may cause respiratory depression of the newborn infant. All sedatives and analgesics affect the fetus to some degree. Drugs taken by the mother can affect the embryo/fetus directly or indirectly by interfering with maternal or placental metabolism. The amount of drug or metabolite reaching the placenta is controlled by the maternal blood level and blood flow through the placenta (Kraemer and Noerr, 1997).

Infectious Agents. Cytomegalovirus, rubella and Coxsackie viruses, and viruses associated with variola, varicella, measles, and poliomyelitis may pass through the placental membrane and cause *fetal infection*. In some cases, such as the **rubella virus**, severe congenital anomalies may be produced (see Chapter 8). Microorganisms such as *Treponema pallidum* that causes syphilis and *Toxoplasma gondii* that produces destructive changes in the brain and eyes also cross the placental membrane. These organisms enter the fetal blood, often causing congenital anomalies and/or death of the embryo or fetus.

PLACENTAL ENDOCRINE SYNTHESIS AND SECRETION

Using precursors derived from the fetus and/or the mother, the syncytiotrophoblast of the placenta synthesizes protein and steroid hormones. The **protein hormones** synthesized by the placenta are:

- human chorionic gonadotropin (hCG)
- human chorionic somatomammotropin (hCS), or human placental lactogen (hPL)
- human chorionic thyrotropin (hCT)
- human chorionic corticotropin (hCACTH)

The glycoprotein hCG, similar to luteinizing hormone (LH), is first secreted by the syncytiotrophoblast during the second week. *Human chorionic gonadotropin maintains the corpus luteum*, preventing the onset of menstrual periods. The concentration of hCG in the maternal blood and urine rises to a maximum by the eighth week and then declines. The placenta also plays a major role in the production of the **steroid hormones**—*progesterone* and *estrogens*. Progesterone can be obtained from the placenta at all stages of gestation, indicating that it is essential for the maintenance of pregnancy. The placenta forms progesterone from maternal cholesterol or pregnenolone. The ovaries of a pregnant woman can be removed after the first trimester without causing an abortion because the placenta takes over the production of progesterone from the corpus luteum of the ovary. Estrogens are also produced in large quantities by the syncytiotrophoblast. The placenta forms them from 19 carbon precursors, many of which are supplied by the fetus (Nathanielsz, 1996).

UTERINE GROWTH DURING PREGNANCY

The uterus of a nonpregnant woman lies in the pelvis minor or true pelvis (Fig. 7-10*A*). To accommodate the growing conceptus, the uterus increases in size. It also increases in weight and its walls become thinner (Fig. 7-10*B* and *C*). During the first trimester, the uterus moves out of the pelvic cavity and by 20 weeks reaches the level of the umbilicus. By 28 to 30 weeks, it reaches the epigastric region—the area between the xiphoid process of the sternum and the umbilicus. The increase in size of the uterus largely results from hypertrophy of preexisting smooth muscular fibers, and partly from the development of new fibers.

PARTURITION (CHILDBIRTH)

Parturition (L. *parturitio*, childbirth) is the process during which the fetus, placenta, and fetal membranes are expelled from the mother's reproductive tract (Fig.

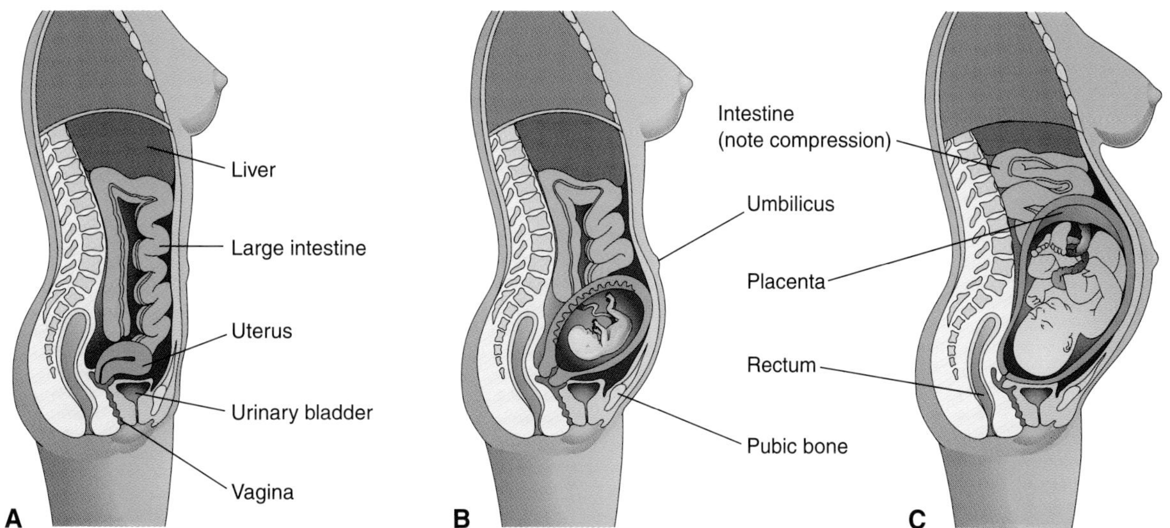

■ **Figure 7–10.** Drawings of median sections of a woman's body. *A,* Not pregnant. *B,* 20 weeks pregnant. *C,* 30 weeks pregnant. Note that as the conceptus enlarges, the uterus increases in size to accommodate the rapidly growing fetus. By 20 weeks the uterus and fetus reach the level of the umbilicus and by 30 weeks they reach the epigastric region. The mother's abdominal viscera are displaced and compressed and the skin and muscles of her anterior abdominal wall are greatly stretched.

7-11). **Labor** is the *sequence of involuntary uterine contractions that result in dilation of the cervix* and delivery of the fetus and placenta from the uterus. The factors that trigger labor are not completely understood, but several hormones are related to the initiation of contractions. The fetal hypothalamus secretes **corticotropin-releasing hormone** (CRH), which stimulates the anterior cerebral hypophysis or pituitary gland to produce **adrenocorticotropin** (ACTH). ACTH causes the secretion of corticol from the suprarenal (adrenal) cortex. **Corticol** is involved in the synthesis of estrogens. These steroids stimulate uterine contraction (Turnbull, 1995; Nathanielsz, 1996).

Peristaltic contractions of uterine smooth muscle are elicited by **oxytocin**, which is released by the posterior cerebral hypophysis. This hormone is administered clinically when it is necessary to induce labor. Oxytocin also stimulates release of **prostaglandins** from the decidua that stimulate myometrial contractility by sensitizing the myometrial cells to oxytocin. **Estrogens** also increase myometrial contractile activity and stimulate the release of oxytocin and prostaglandins. From studies carried out in sheep and nonhuman primates, it seems that the duration of pregnancy and the process of birth are under the direct control of the fetus. Indeed, it is the fetal hypothalamus that initiates the birth process (Nathanielsz, 1996).

The Stages of Labor

There are four stages of labor:

- **The first stage of labor** (dilation stage) begins when there is objective evidence of progressive dilation of the cervix (Fig. 7-11*A* and *B*). This is mediated by changes in the circulating hormones and other regulatory factors, such as prostaglandins. *The first stage begins when regular painful contractions of the uterus occur less than 10 minutes apart.* The first stage ends with complete dilation of the cervix and is by far the most time-consuming stage of labor. The average duration is about 12 hours for first pregnancies (nulliparous patients or *primigravidas*), and about 7 hours for women who have had a child previously (multiparous patients or *multigravidas*).
- **The second stage of labor** (expulsion stage) begins when the cervix is fully dilated and ends with delivery of the baby (Figs. 7-11*C* to *E* and 7-12). *During the second stage the fetus descends through the cervix and vagina.* As soon as the fetus is outside the mother, it is called a *newborn infant* or neonate. The average duration of the second stage is 50 minutes for primigravidas and 20 minutes for multigravidas.
- **The third stage of labor** (placental stage) begins as soon as the baby is born and ends when the placenta and membranes are expelled. Uterine contractions begin again shortly after parturition. The duration of the third stage is 15 minutes in about 90% of pregnancies. *Retraction of the uterus and manual compression of the abdomen reduce the area of placental attachment* (Fig. 7-11*G*). A ***hematoma*** — a localized mass of extravasated blood — soon forms deep to the placenta and separates it from the uterine wall. The placenta and fetal membranes separate from the uterine wall and are expelled through the vagina and pudendal cleft — the slit between the labia majora into which the vagina opens. The placenta separates through the spongy layer of the decidua basalis (see Chapter 2). After delivery of the baby the uterus continues to contract.

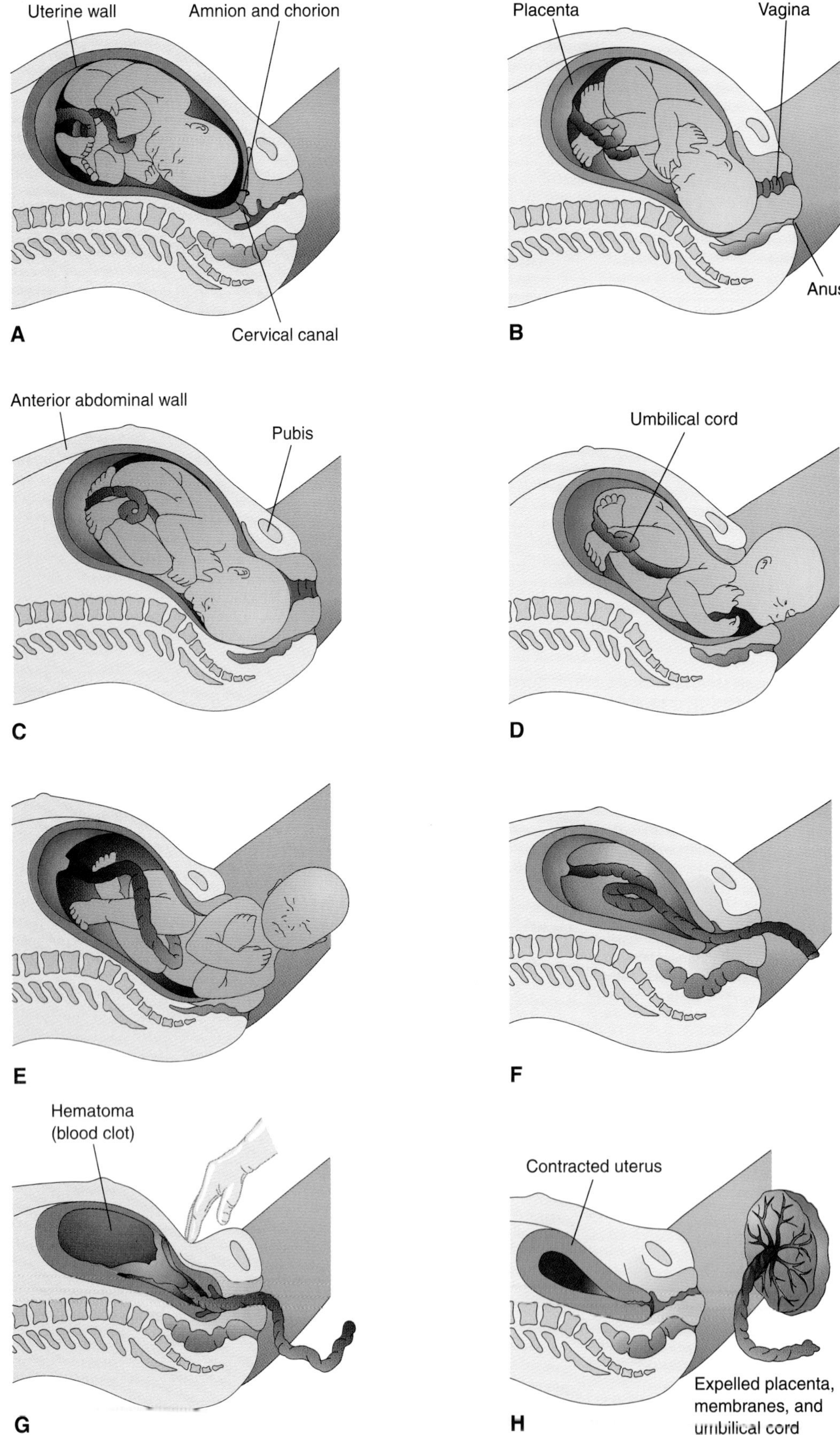

■ **Figure 7–11.** Drawings illustrating parturition. *A* and *B,* The cervix is dilating during the first stage of labor. *C* to *E,* The fetus is passing through the cervix and vagina during the second stage of labor. *F* and *G,* As the uterus contracts during the third stage of labor, the placenta folds and pulls away from the uterine wall. Separation of the placenta results in bleeding and the formation of a large hematoma (mass of blood). Pressure on the abdomen facilitates placental separation. *H,* The placenta is expelled and the uterus contracts during the fourth stage of labor.

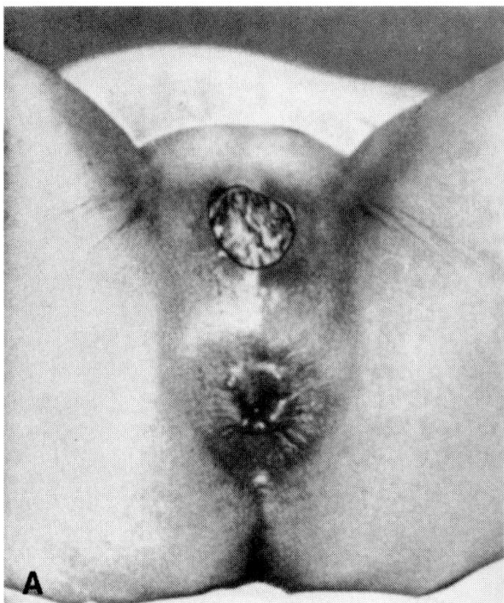

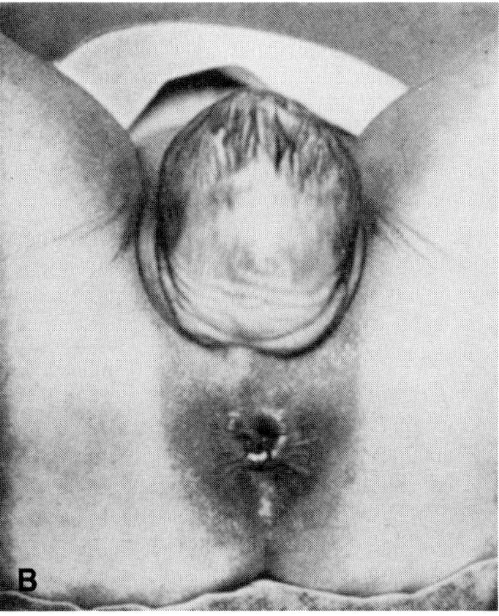

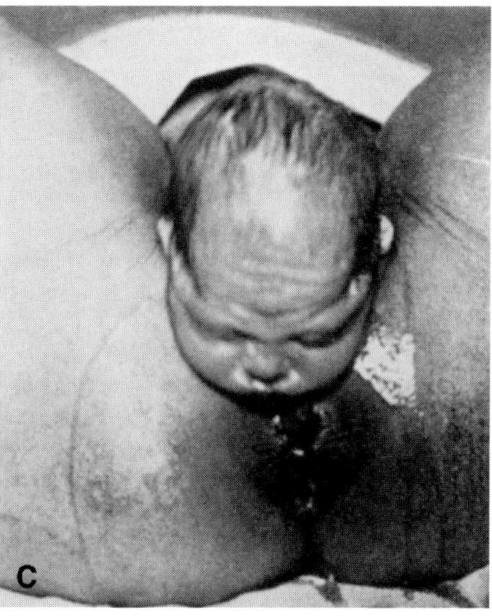

■ **Figure 7–12.** Photographs illustrating delivery of the baby's head during the second stage of labor. *A,* The crown of the head distends the mother's perineum. *B,* The perineum slips over the head and face. *C,* The head is delivered; subsequently the body of the fetus is expelled. Episiotomy—surgical incision of the perineum to facilitate birth—is often performed as the fetal head distends the perineum. (From Greenhill JB, Friedman EA: *Biological Principles and Modern Practice of Obstetrics.* Philadelphia, WB Saunders, 1974).

- **The fourth stage of labor** (recovery stage) begins as soon as the placenta and fetal membranes are expelled. This stage lasts about 2 hours. The myometrial contractions constrict the spiral arteries that formerly supplied blood to the intervillous space. These contractions prevent excessive uterine bleeding.

The Placenta and Fetal Membranes After Birth

The placenta and fetal membranes that are extruded from the uterus after birth are the **secundina** (L., following or afterbirth). The **placenta** (Gr. *plakuos*, a flat cake) commonly has a discoid shape, with a diameter of 15 to 20 cm and a thickness of 2 to 3 cm (Fig. 7-13). It weighs 500 to 600 gm, which is about one-sixth the weight of the average fetus. The margins of the placenta are continuous with the ruptured amniotic and chorionic sacs.

VARIATIONS IN PLACENTAL SHAPE

As the placenta develops, chorionic villi usually persist only where the villous chorion is in contact with the decidua basalis. This usually produces a discoid placenta (Fig. 7-13). When villi persist on the entire surface of the chorionic sac, a thin layer of placenta attaches to a large area of the uterus. This very rare type of placenta is a diffuse or membranous placenta—*placenta membranacea* (Townsend, 1994). When villi persist elsewhere, several variations in placental shape occur: *accessory placenta* (Fig. 7-14), bidiscoid placenta, and horseshoe placenta. Although there are many variations in the size and shape of the placenta, most of them are of little physiological or clinical significance.

Examination of the placenta prenatally by ultrasound or magnetic resonance imaging (Fig. 7-15), or postnatally by gross and microscopic study, may provide clinical information about the causes of:

- intrauterine growth retardation (IUGR)
- placental dysfunction
- fetal distress and death
- neonatal illness

Placental studies can also determine whether the placenta is complete. *Retention of a cotyledon* or an accessory placenta in the uterus may cause severe *uterine hemorrhage*.

Gestational Choriocarcinoma

Abnormal proliferation of the trophoblast results in *gestational trophoblastic disease*, a spectrum of lesions including highly malignant tumors (Freedman et al., 1996). The cells invade the decidua basalis, penetrate its blood vessels and lymphatics, and metastasize to the maternal lungs, bone marrow, liver, and other organs. *Gestational choriocarcinomas* are highly sensitive to chemotherapy and cures are usually achieved (see Berkowitz and Goldstein [1996] for more details).

MATERNAL SURFACE OF THE PLACENTA

The characteristic **cobblestone appearance** of the maternal surface is produced by slightly bulging villous areas—**cotyledons**—which are separated by grooves

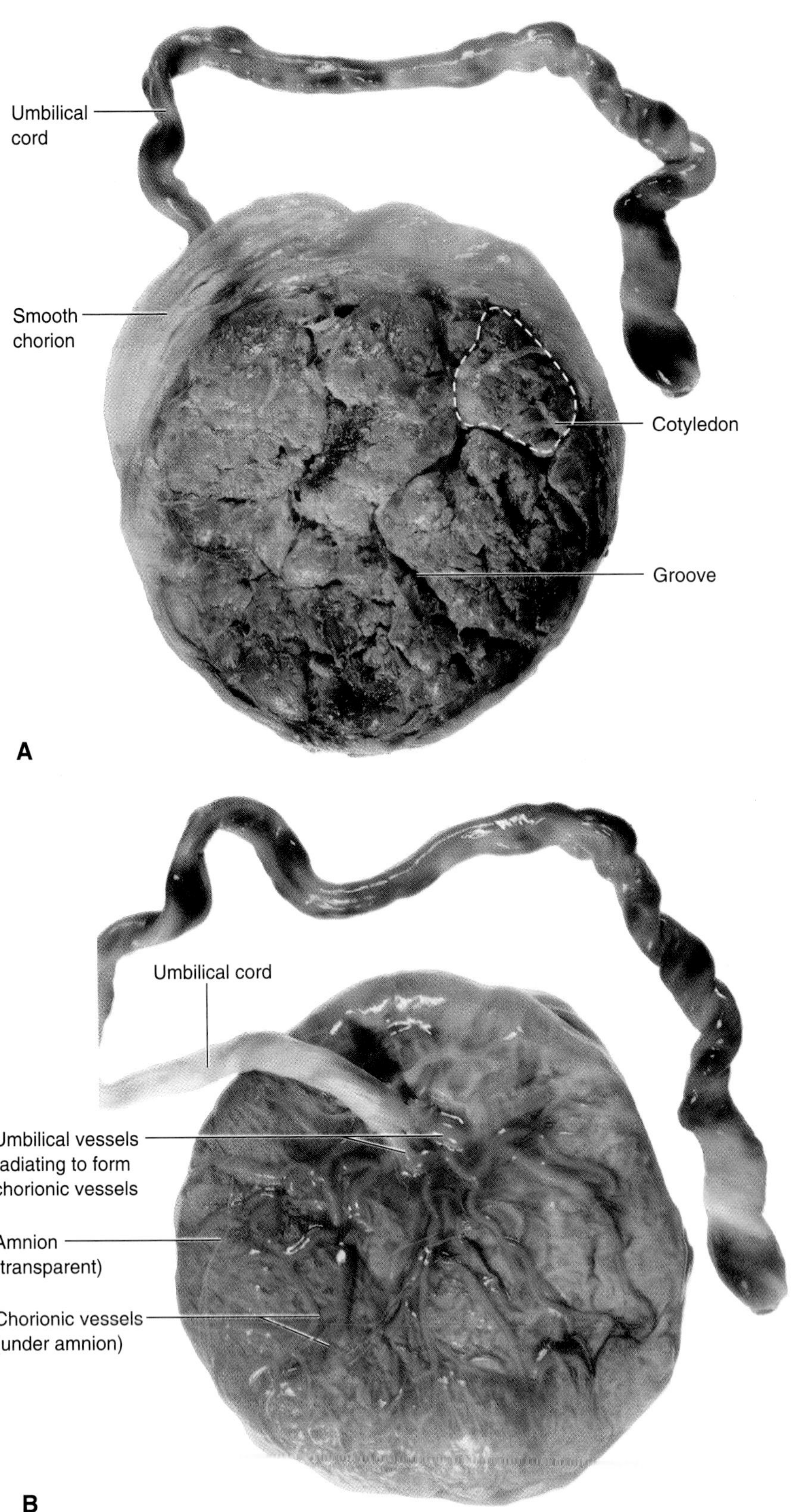

■ **Figure 7–13.** Photographs of placentas and fetal membranes after birth, about one-third actual size. *A,* Maternal surface, showing cotyledons and the grooves around them. Each convex cotyledon consists of a number of main stem villi with their many branch villi. The grooves were occupied by the placental septa when the maternal and fetal parts of the placenta were together (Fig. 7–7). *B,* Fetal surface, showing blood vessels running in the chorionic plate deep to the amnion and converging to form the umbilical vessels at the attachment of the umbilical cord.

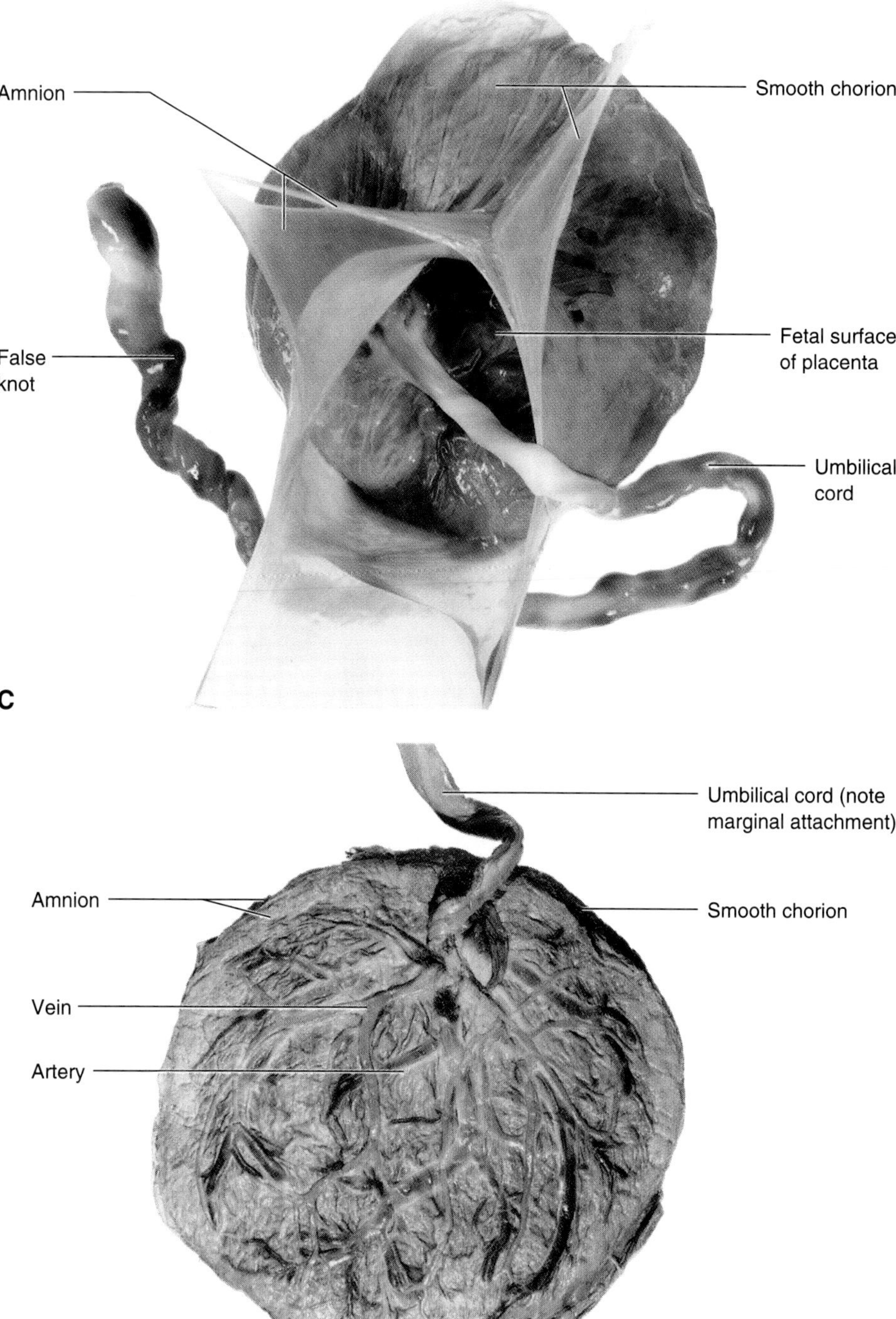

■ **Figure 7-13.** *Continued.* *C,* The amnion and smooth chorion are arranged to show that they are fused and continuous with the margins of the placenta. *D,* Placenta with a marginal attachment of the cord, often called a battledore placenta because of its resemblance to the bat used in the medieval game of battledore and shuttlecock. (From Moore KL, Persaud TVN, Shiota K: *Color Atlas of Clinical Embryology.* Philadelphia, WB Saunders, 1994.)

that were formerly occupied by *placental septa* (Figs. 7-7 and 7-13*A*) The surface of the cotyledons is covered by thin grayish shreds of decidua basalis that separated from the uterine wall when the placenta was extruded. These shreds of tissue are recognizable in sections of the placenta that are examined under a microscope. Most of the decidua is temporarily retained in the uterus and is shed with subsequent uterine bleeding.

FETAL SURFACE OF THE PLACENTA

The **umbilical cord** usually attaches to the fetal surface, and its epithelium is continuous with the amnion adhering to the fetal surface of the placenta (Figs. 7-7 and 7-13*B* and *C*). The fetal surface of a freshly delivered placenta is smooth and shiny because it is covered by the amnion. The chorionic vessels radiating to and from the umbilical cord are clearly visible through

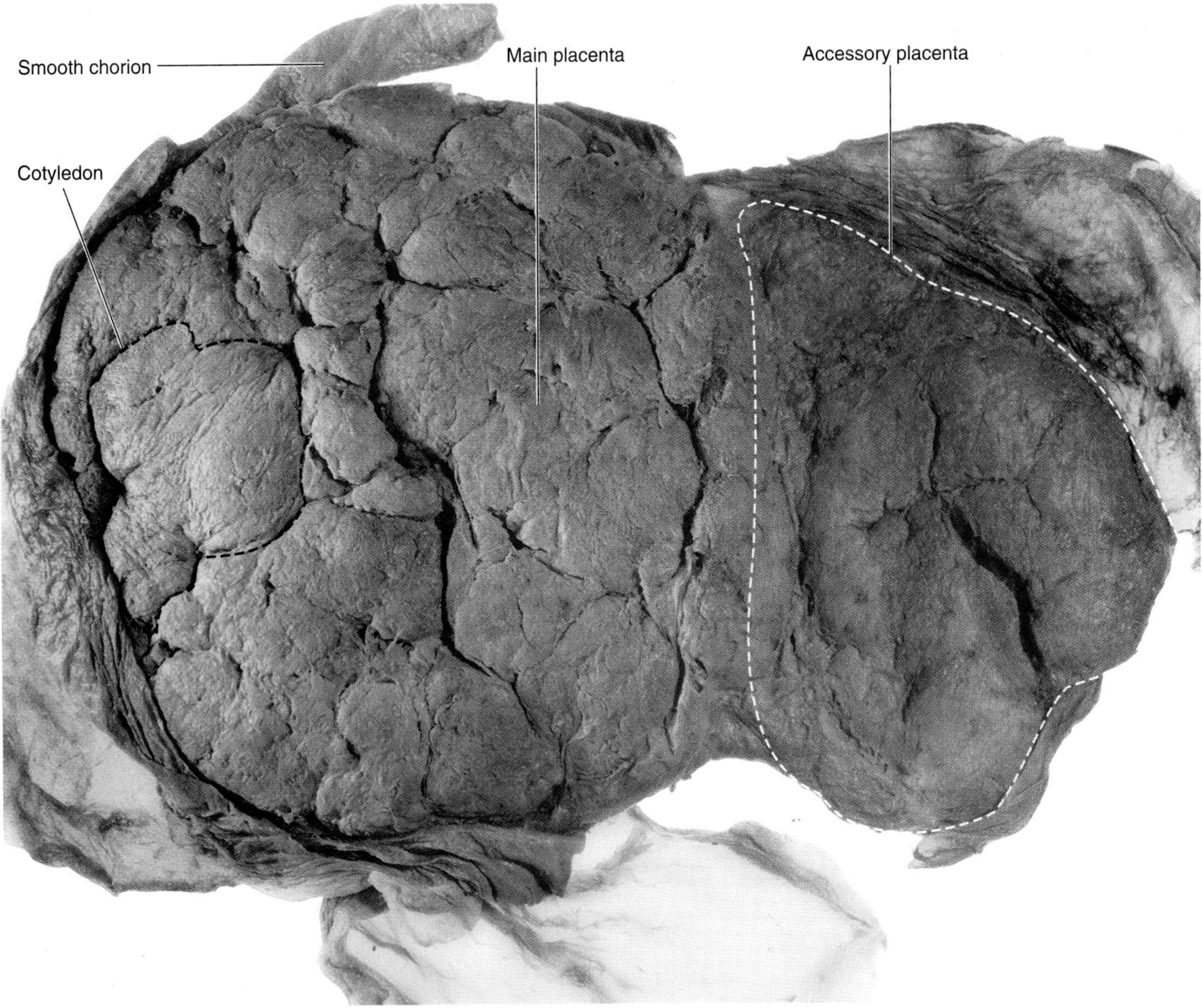

■ **Figure 7–14.** Photograph of the maternal surface of a full-term placenta and an accessory placenta; about one-half actual size. The accessory placenta developed from a patch of chorionic villi that persisted a short distance from the main placenta. (From Moore KL, Persaud TVN, Shiota K: *Color Atlas of Clinical Embryology.* Philadelphia, WB Saunders, 1994.)

the transparent amnion. The *umbilical vessels* branch on the fetal surface to form the *chorionic vessels,* which enter the chorionic villi.

Placental Abnormalities

Abnormal adherence of chorionic villi to part or all of the uterine wall, with partial or complete absence of the decidua basalis, especially the spongy layer, is called **placenta accreta** (Fig. 7-16). When chorionic villi penetrate the myometrium all the way to the perimetrium (peritoneal covering), the abnormality is called **placenta percreta**. The villi are normal and show no evidence of trophoblastic proliferation (Rubin and Farber, 1988). *Third trimester bleeding is the common presenting sign of these placental abnormalities.* Most patients with placenta accreta have normal pregnancies and labors. After birth the placenta fails to separate from the uterine wall, and attempts to remove it may cause hemorrhage that is difficult to control. When the blastocyst implants close to or overlying the internal os of the uterus, the abnormality is called **placenta previa.** Late pregnancy bleeding can result from this placental abnormality. The fetus has to be delivered by Cesarean section because the placenta blocks the entrance to the cervical canal.

Umbilical Cord

The attachment of the umbilical cord, connecting the embryo/fetus to the placenta, is usually near the center of the fetal surface of this fetomaternal organ (Fig. 7-13*B*), but it may attach at any point. For example, insertion of it at the placental margin produces a *battledore placenta* (Fig. 7-13*D*), and its attachment to the membranes is a *velamentous insertion of the cord*

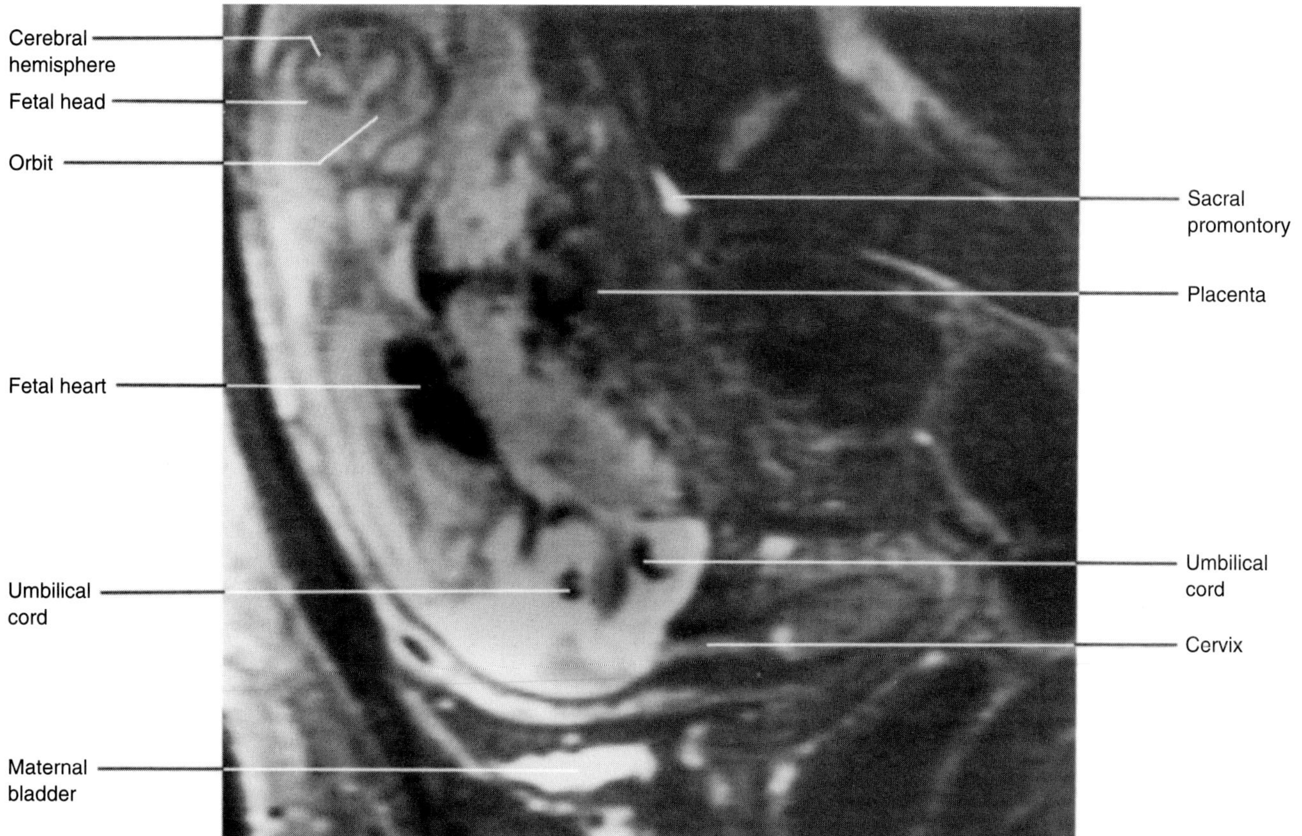

■ **Figure 7–15.** Sagittal magnetic resonance image (MRI) of the pelvis of a pregnant woman. The fetus, placenta, and umbilical cord are visible. (Courtesy of Dr. Shirley McCarthy, Director of MRI, Department of Diagnostic Radiology, Yale University School of Medicine, New Haven, Connecticut.)

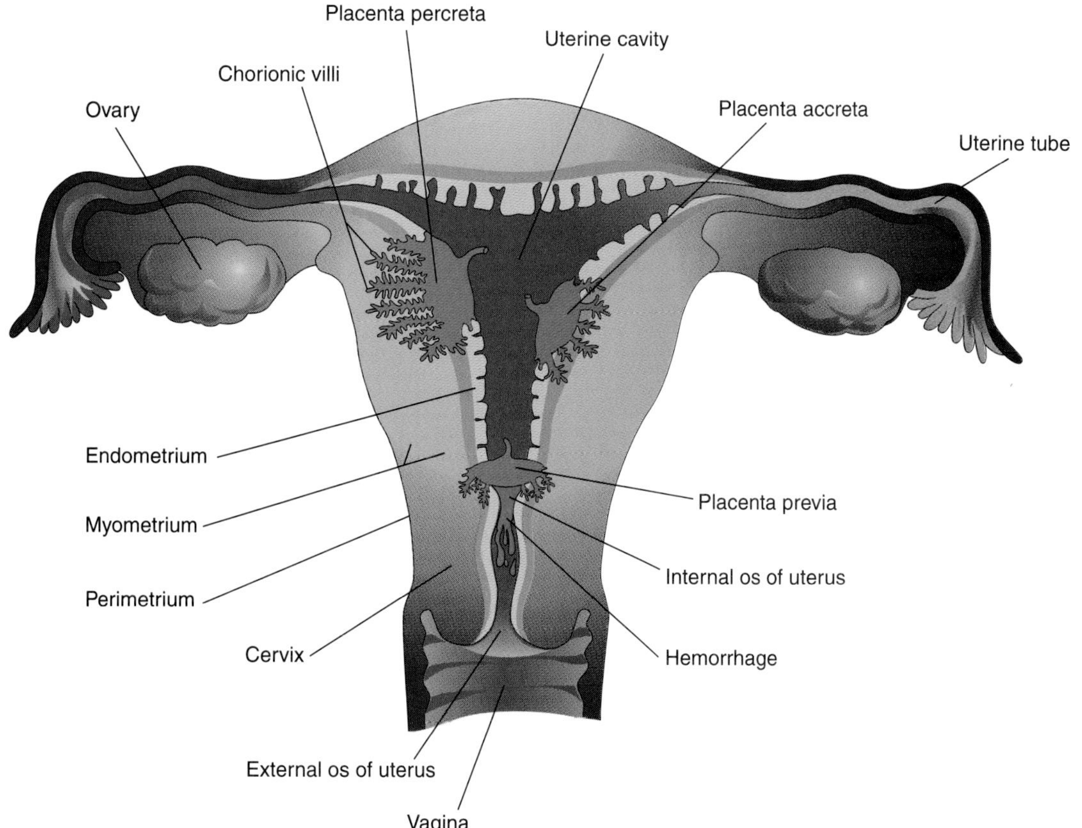

■ **Figure 7–16.** Placental abnormalities. In *placenta accreta* there is abnormal adherence of the placenta to the myometrium. In *placenta percreta* the placenta has penetrated the full thickness of the myometrium. In *placenta previa* the placenta overlies the internal os of the uterus and blocks the cervical canal.

(Fig. 7-17). **Color flow Doppler ultrasonography** may be used for the prenatal diagnosis of the position and structural abnormalities of the umbilical cord and its vessels (Raga et al., 1995; Heinonen et al., 1996). The umbilical cord is usually 1 to 2 cm in diameter and 30 to 90 cm in length (average 55 cm). The length of the umbilical cord is believed to be under the influence of genetic and other factors. Excessively long or short cords are uncommon. Long cords have a tendency to prolapse and/or to coil around the fetus (see Fig. 7-21). Prompt recognition of *prolapse of the cord* is important because the cord may be compressed between the presenting body part of the fetus and the mother's bony pelvis, causing *fetal hypoxia* or anoxia. If the deficiency of oxygen persists for more than 5 minutes, the baby's brain may be damaged, producing mental retardation. A very short cord may cause premature separation of the placenta from the wall of the uterus during delivery.

The umbilical cord usually has two arteries and one vein that are surrounded by mucoid connective tissue (*Wharton jelly*). Because the umbilical vessels are longer than the cord, twisting and bending of the vessels are common. They frequently form loops, producing *false knots* that are of no significance; however, in about 1% of pregnancies, **true knots** form in the cord, which may tighten and cause fetal death resulting from *fetal anoxia* (Fig. 7-18). In most cases the knots form during labor as a result of the fetus passing through a loop of the cord. Because these knots are usually loose, they have no clinical significance. Simple *looping of the cord around the fetus* occasionally occurs (Fig. 7-21*B*). In about one-fifth of deliveries, the cord is loosely looped around the neck without increased fetal risk. See Benirschke (1994) for more details regarding abnormalities of the umbilical cord that are obstetrically important.

Percutaneous Umbilical Cord Blood Sampling

Percutaneous umbilical cord blood sampling (PUBS) may be performed to assess fetal acid-base status for monitoring the fetus and newborn (Thorp et al., 1996). Refer to Chapter 6 for more information about PUBS.

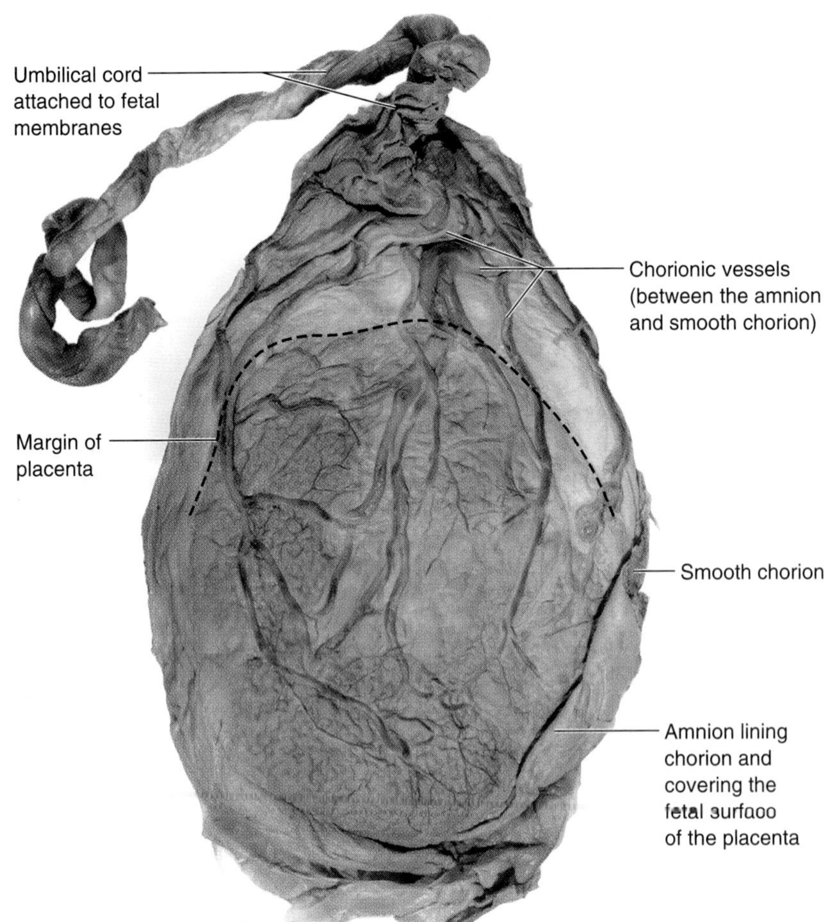

■ **Figure 7-17.** Photograph of a placenta with a velamentous insertion of the umbilical cord. The cord is attached to the membranes (amnion and chorion), not to the placenta. The umbilical vessels leave the cord and run between the amnion and chorion before spreading over the placenta. The vessels are easily torn in this location, especially when they cross over the inferior uterine segment; the latter condition is known as *vasa previa.* If the vessels rupture before birth, the fetus loses blood and could be near exsanguination when born. (From Moore KL, Persaud TVN, Shiota K: *Color Atlas of Clinical Embryology.* Philadelphia, WB Saunders, 1994.)

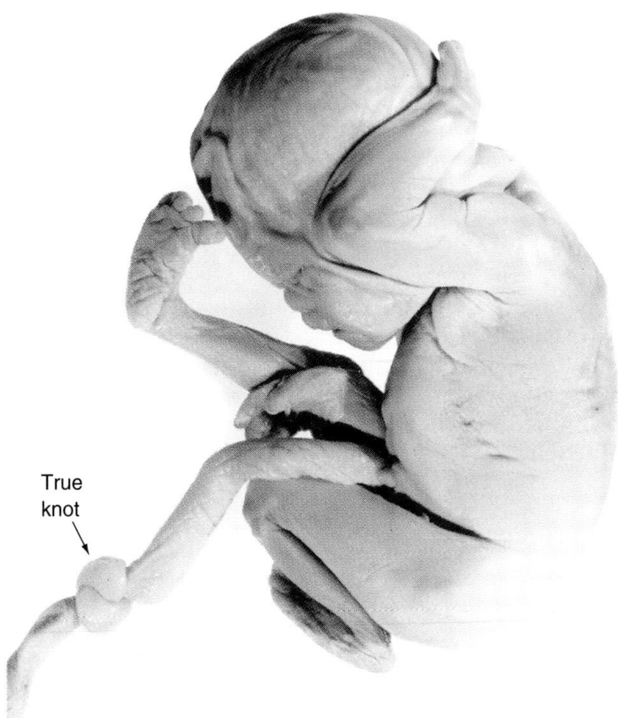

■ **Figure 7–18.** Photograph of a 20-week fetus with a true knot *(arrow)* in its umbilical cord. Half actual size. The diameter of the cord is greater in the part closest to the fetus, indicating that there was an obstruction of blood flow from the fetus in the umbilical arteries and compression of the umbilical vein. Undoubtedly, this knot caused severe anoxia (decreased oxygen in the fetal tissues and organs) and was a major cause of the fetus's death. (From Moore KL, Persaud TVN, Shiota K: *Color Atlas of Clinical Embryology.* Philadelphia, WB Saunders, 1994.)

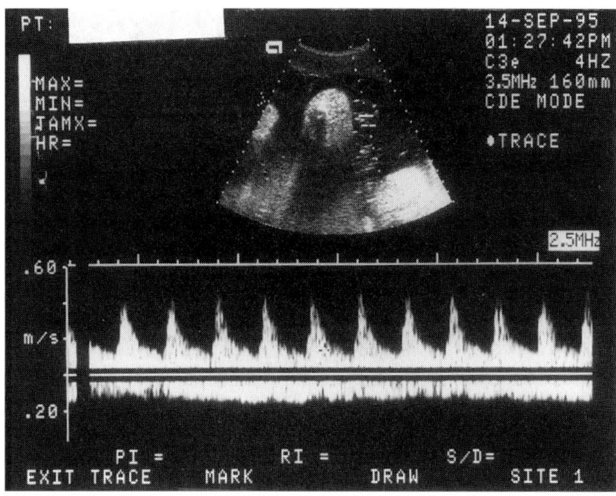

■ **Figure 7–19.** Doppler velocimetry of the umbilical cord. The arterial waveform (top) illustrates pulsatile forward flow, with high peaks and low velocities during diastole. This combination suggests high resistance in the placenta to placental blood flow. Because this index changes over gestation, it is important to know that the pregnancy was 18 weeks' gestation. For this period, the flow pattern is normal. The nonpulsatile flow in the opposite, negative direction represents venous return from the placenta. Both waveforms are normal for this gestational age. (Courtesy of Dr. CR Harman, Department of Obstetrics, Gynecology and Reproductive Sciences, Women's Hospital and University of Manitoba, Winnipeg, Manitoba, Canada.)

Umbilical Artery Doppler Velocimetry

As gestation and trophoblastic invasion of the decidua basalis progress, there is a progressive increase in the diastolic flow velocity in the umbilical arteries (Fleischer et al., 1994). Doppler velocimetry of the uteroplacental and fetoplacental circulation is used to investigate complications of pregnancy such as intrauterine growth retardation (IUGR) and fetal distress resulting from fetal hypoxemia and asphyxia (Fig. 7-19). For example, there is a statistically significant association between IUGR and abnormally increased resistance in an umbilical artery (Worrell et al., 1991).

Absence of an Umbilical Artery

In about one in 200 newborns, only *one umbilical artery* is present (Fig. 7-20), a condition that may be

■ **Figure 7–20.** Transverse section of an umbilical cord. Observe that the cord is covered by a single-layered epithelium derived from the enveloping amnion. It has a core of mucous connective tissue (Wharton jelly). Observe also that the cord has one umbilical artery and one vein. Usually there are two umbilical arteries. The vein, which carries oxygenated blood from the placenta, is unusual in that its wall, unlike that of most veins, consists principally of a tunica media. (Courtesy of Professor V Becker, Pathologisches Institut der Universität, Erlangen, Germany.)

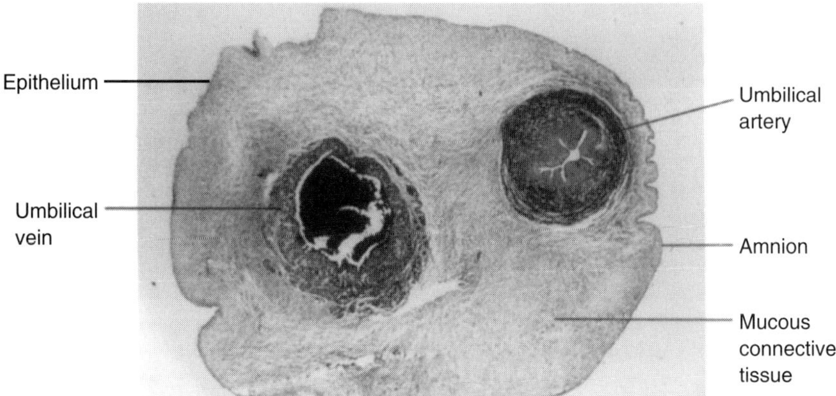

associated with chromosomal and fetal abnormalities, particularly of the cardiovascular system. *Absence of an umbilical artery is accompanied by a 15 to 20% incidence of cardiovascular anomalies in the fetus.* Absence of an artery results from either agenesis or degeneration of this vessel early in development. A single umbilical artery and the anatomical defects associated with it can be detected before birth by ultrasonography (Parilla et al., 1995).

AMNION AND AMNIOTIC FLUID

The **amnion** forms a fluid-filled, membranous *amniotic sac* that surrounds the embryo and fetus (Fig. 7-21). Because the amnion is attached to the margins of the embryonic disc, its junction with the embryo (future umbilicus) is located on the ventral surface after embryonic folding (Fig. 7-22*B*). As the amnion enlarges, it gradually obliterates the chorionic cavity and forms the epithelial covering of the umbilical cord (Fig. 7-22*C* and *D*).

Amniotic Fluid

Amniotic fluid plays a major role in fetal growth and development (Doubilet and Benson, 1994). Initially, some amniotic fluid may be secreted by amniotic cells; however, most fluid is derived from *maternal tissue (interstitial) fluid* by diffusion across the amniochorionic membrane from the decidua parietalis (Fig. 7-7). Later there is diffusion of fluid through the chorionic plate from blood in the intervillous space of the placenta. Before keratinization of the skin occurs, a major pathway for passage of water and solutes in tissue fluid from the fetus to the amniotic cavity is through the skin (Callen and Filly, 1990); thus, amniotic fluid is similar to fetal tissue fluid. Fluid is also secreted by the fetal respiratory tract and enters the amniotic cavity. Bissonnette (1986) estimated that the daily rate of contribution of fluid to the amniotic cavity from the respiratory tract was 300 to 400 ml. Beginning in the eleventh week, the fetus contributes to the amniotic fluid by expelling urine into the amniotic cavity. By late pregnancy about a half-liter of urine is added daily. The volume of amniotic fluid normally increases slowly, reaching about 30 ml at 10 weeks, 350 ml at 20 weeks, and 700 to 1000 ml by 37 weeks.

CIRCULATION OF AMNIOTIC FLUID

The water content of amniotic fluid changes every 3 hours. Large amounts of water pass through the amniochorionic membrane into the maternal tissue fluid and enter the uterine capillaries. An exchange of fluid with fetal blood also occurs through the umbilical cord and where the amnion adheres to the chorionic plate on the fetal surface of the placenta (Figs. 7-7 and 7-13*B*); thus, amniotic fluid is in balance with the fetal circulation. *Amniotic fluid is swallowed by the*

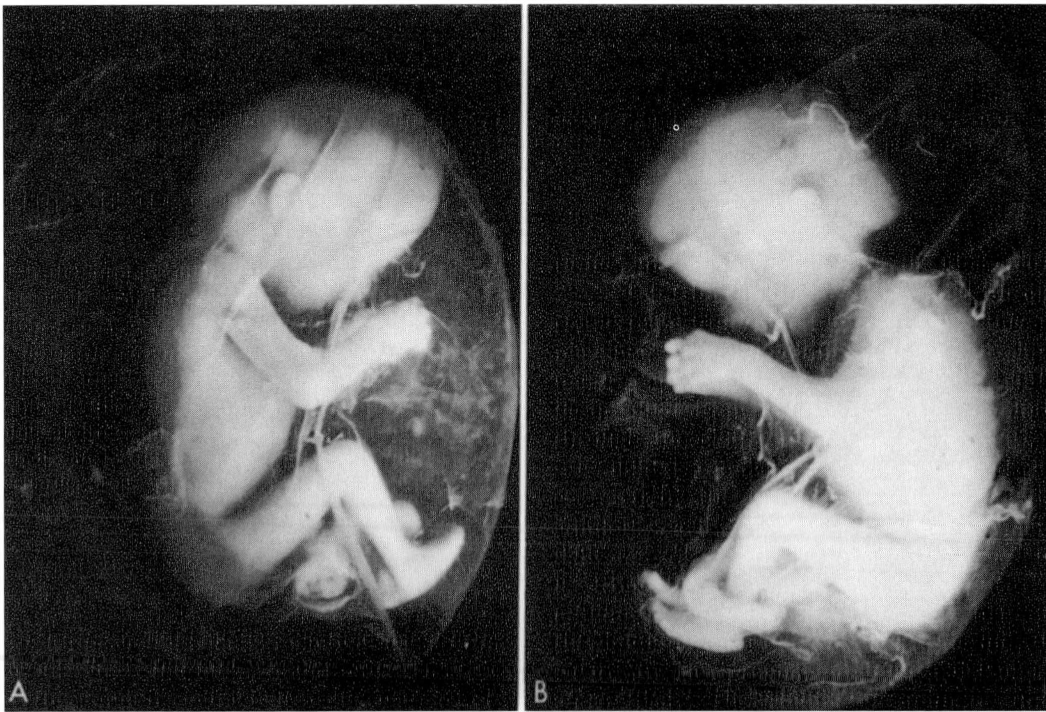

■ **Figure 7–21.** Photographs of a 12-week-old fetus within its amniotic sac. The fetus and its membranes aborted spontaneously. It was removed from its chorionic sac with its amniotic sac intact. Actual size. In *B,* note that the umbilical cord is looped around the left ankle of the fetus. Coiling of the cord around parts of the fetus affects their development when the coils are so tight that the circulation to the parts is affected.

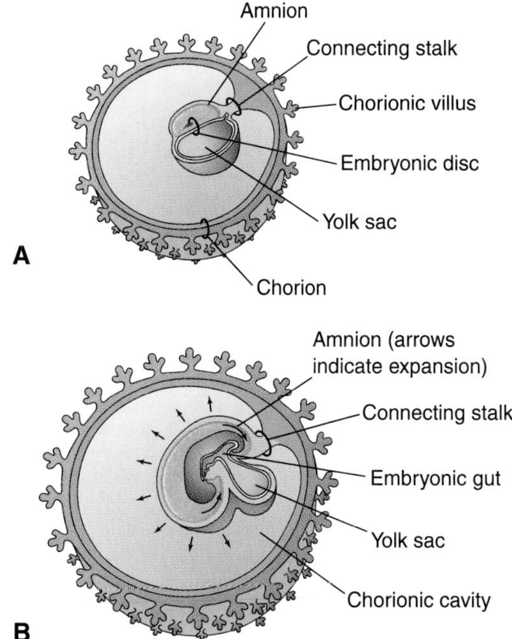

■ **Figure 7–22.** Drawings illustrating how the amnion enlarges, fills the chorionic sac, and envelops the umbilical cord. Observe that part of the yolk sac is incorporated into the embryo as the primitive gut. Formation of the fetal part of the placenta and degeneration of chorionic villi are also shown. *A,* 3 weeks. *B,* 4 weeks. *C,* 10 weeks. *D,* 20 weeks.

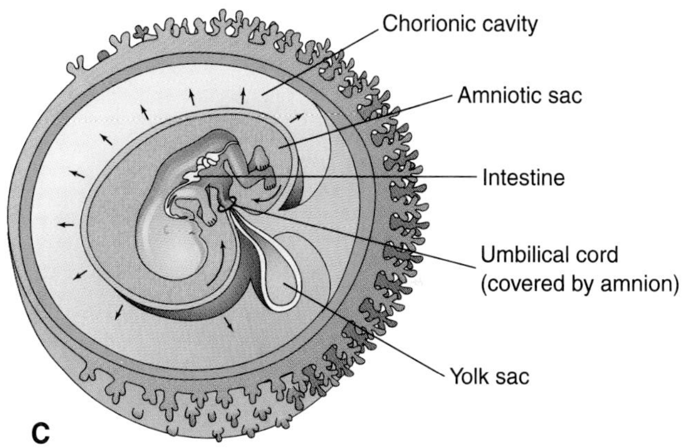

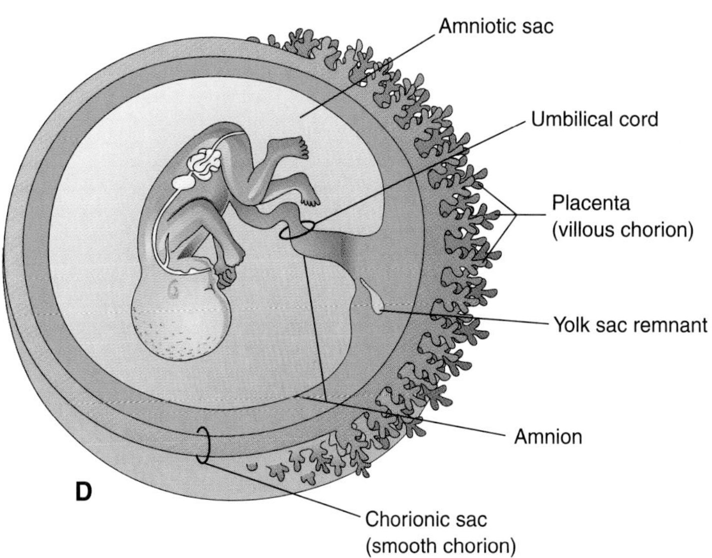

fetus and absorbed by the fetus's respiratory and digestive tracts. It has been estimated that during the final stages of pregnancy, the fetus swallows up to 400 ml of amniotic fluid per day. The fluid passes into the fetal blood stream and the waste products in it cross the placental membrane and enter the maternal blood in the intervillous space. Excess water in the fetal blood is excreted by the fetal kidneys and returned to the amniotic sac through the fetal urinary tract.

Disorders of Amniotic Fluid Volume

Low volumes of amniotic fluid for any particular gestational age — **oligohydramnios** — (e.g., 400 mL in the third trimester) result in most cases from placental insufficiency with diminished placental blood flow. Preterm rupture of the amniochorionic membrane occurs in approximately 10% of pregnancies and is the most common cause of oligohydramnios (Callen and Filly, 1990). When there is **renal agenesis** (failure of kidney formation), the absence of fetal urine contribution to the amniotic fluid is the main cause of oligohydramnios. A similar decrease in fluid occurs when there is **obstructive uropathy** (urinary tract obstruction). Complications of oligohydramnios include fetal abnormalities (pulmonary hypoplasia, facial defects, and limb defects), which are caused by fetal compression by the uterine wall. Compression of the umbilical cord is also a potential complication of severe oligohydramnios (Doubilet and Benson, 1994).

High volumes of amniotic fluid — **polyhydramnios (hydramnios)** — in excess of 2000 ml, result when the fetus does not swallow the usual amount of amniotic fluid. Most cases of polyhydramnios (60%) are idiopathic (unknown cause), 20% are caused by maternal factors, and 20% are fetal in origin (Fig. 7-23). Polyhydramnios may be associated with severe anomalies of the central nervous system, such as meroanencephaly or anencephaly. When there are other anomalies, **esophageal atresia** (blockage) for example, the fetus is unable to swallow amniotic fluid (see Chapters 11 and 12), which accumulates because it is unable to pass to the fetal stomach and intestines for absorption. *Ultrasonography* has become the technique of choice for diagnosing polyhydramnios (Callen and Filly, 1990; Doubilet and Benson, 1994).

EXCHANGE OF AMNIOTIC FLUID

Large volumes of amniotic fluid move in both directions between the fetal and maternal circulations, mainly through the placental membrane. Fetal swallowing of amniotic fluid is also a normal occurrence. Most fluid passes into the gastrointestinal tract but some passes into the lungs. In either case, the fluid is absorbed and enters the fetal circulation. It then passes into the maternal circulation through the placental membrane. For more details on amniotic fluid dynamics, see Mann et al. (1996).

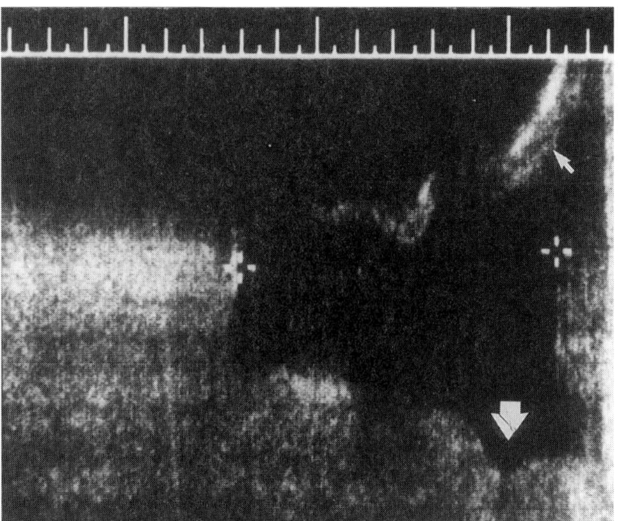

■ **Figure 7-23.** Sonogram performed at 22 weeks' gestation. Severe Rh isoimmunization produces multiple effects. Observe the polyhydramnios (hydramnios), with amniotic fluid pockets measuring 10 cm or more (between white cursors). The placenta (right and bottom) is grossly buckled with edema *(large arrow)*. The fetus has anasarca (generalized infiltration of edema fluid in subcutaneous tissues), with scalp edema (shown at small arrow). (Courtesy of CR Harman, MD, Department of Obstetrics, Gynecology and Reproductive Sciences, Women's Hospital and University of Manitoba, Winnipeg, Manitoba, Canada.)

COMPOSITION OF AMNIOTIC FLUID

About 99% of the fluid in the amniotic cavity is water. Amniotic fluid is a solution in which undissolved material is suspended; e.g., desquamated fetal epithelial cells and approximately equal portions of organic and inorganic salts. Half the organic constituents are protein; the other half consist of carbohydrates, fats, enzymes, hormones, and pigments. As pregnancy advances, the composition of the amniotic fluid changes as fetal excreta (*meconium* [fetal feces] and urine) are added. Because fetal urine enters the amniotic fluid, studies of fetal enzyme systems, amino acids, hormones, and other substances can be conducted on fluid removed by **amniocentesis** (see Chapter 6). Studies of cells in the amniotic fluid permit diagnosis of the sex of the fetus and detection of fetuses with chromosomal abnormalities such as in trisomy 21, the Down syndrome. Moreover, molecular diagnostic studies can be carried out on the DNA extracted from fetal cells if there is a family history or clinical indication of certain diseases. *High levels of alpha-fetoprotein* (AFP) in the amniotic fluid usually indicate the presence of a severe neural tube defect (e.g., meroanencephaly). *Low levels of AFP* may indicate chromosomal aberrations such as trisomy 21 (see Chapter 8).

SIGNIFICANCE OF AMNIOTIC FLUID

The embryo, suspended in amniotic fluid by the umbilical cord, floats freely. Amniotic fluid has critical functions in the normal development of the fetus; see Doubilet and Benson (1994) for more details regarding the physiology of amniotic fluid production, consumption, and disorders associated with amniotic fluid volume.

The buoyant amniotic fluid:

- permits symmetrical external growth of the embryo and fetus
- acts as a barrier to infection
- permits normal fetal lung development
- prevents adherence of the amnion to the embryo and fetus
- cushions the embryo and fetus against injuries by distributing impacts the mother receives
- helps control the embryo's body temperature by maintaining a relatively constant temperature
- enables the fetus to move freely, thereby aiding muscular development in the limbs, for example
- is involved in maintaining homeostasis of fluid and electrolytes

Premature Rupture of Fetal Membranes

Rupture of the amniochorionic membrane is the most common event leading to premature labor and delivery and the most common complication resulting in oligohydramnios. The absence of amniotic fluid also removes the major protection the fetus has against infection. Rupture of the amnion may cause various fetal anomalies that constitute the *amniotic band syndrome* (ABS), or the *amniotic band disruption complex* (ABDC). The incidence of the ABS is about 1 in every 1200 live births (Seed et al., 1982). Prenatal ultrasound diagnosis of ABS is now possible (Filly and Golbus, 1990). The malformations caused by ABS vary from digital constriction to major scalp, craniofacial, and visceral defects (Callen and Filly, 1990). The cause of these anomalies is probably related to constriction by encircling amniotic bands (Fig. 7-24). Other het-

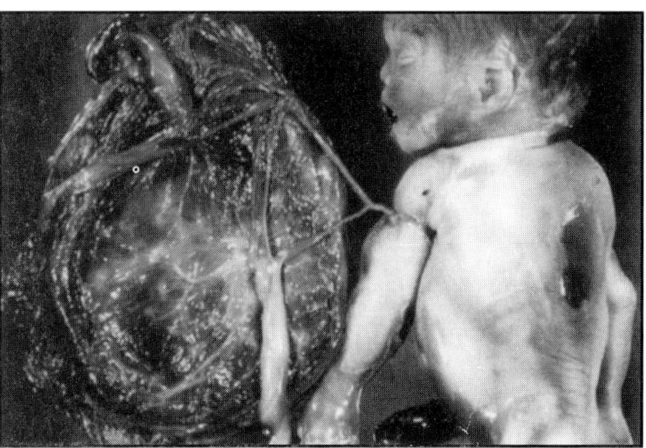

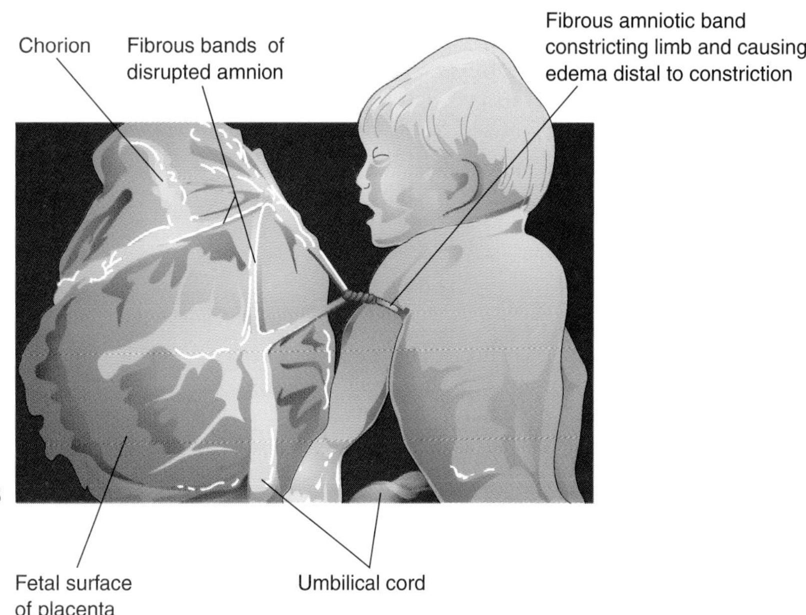

■ **Figure 7-24.** *A,* Photograph of a fetus with the amniotic band syndrome (ABS), showing amniotic bands constricting the left arm. (Courtesy of Professor V Becker, Pathologisches Institut der Universität, Erlangen, Germany.) *B,* Drawing indicating the structures shown in *A.*

erogeneous factors may be involved (Bamforth, 1992). The pathogenesis of these anomalies remains unknown.

YOLK SAC

Early development of the yolk sac was described in Chapters 3 and 5. At 32 days the yolk sac is large (Fig. 7-2). By 10 weeks the yolk sac has shrunk to a pear-shaped remnant about 5 mm in diameter (Fig. 7-22*C*) and is connected to the midgut by a narrow *yolk stalk*. By 20 weeks the yolk sac is very small (Fig. 7-22*D*); thereafter it is usually not visible. The yolk sac can be observed sonographically early in the fifth week (see Chapter 5). The presence of the amnion and yolk sac enables early recognition and measurement of the embryo. The yolk sac is recognizable in ultrasound examinations until the end of the first trimester (Filly, 1994).

Significance of the Yolk Sac

Although the yolk sac is nonfunctional as far as yolk storage is concerned, its presence is essential for several reasons:

- It has a role in the *transfer of nutrients* to the embryo during the second and third weeks when the uteroplacental circulation is being established.
- *Blood development* first occurs in the well-vascularized extraembryonic mesoderm covering the wall of the yolk sac beginning in the third week (see Chapter 4) and continues to form there until hemopoietic activity begins in the liver during the sixth week.
- During the fourth week the endoderm of the yolk sac is incorporated into the embryo as the *primitive gut* (see Fig. 5-1). Its endoderm, derived from epiblast, gives rise to the epithelium of the trachea, bronchi, lungs, and digestive tract.
- *Primordial germ cells* appear in the endodermal lining of the wall of the yolk sac in the third week and subsequently migrate to the developing sex glands (see Chapter 13). They differentiate into the germ cells (spermatogonia in males and oogonia in females).

FATE OF THE YOLK SAC

At 10 weeks the small yolk sac lies in the chorionic cavity between the amnion and chorionic sac (Fig. 7-22*C*). It atrophies as pregnancy advances, eventually becoming very small (Fig. 7-22*D*). In very unusual cases, the yolk sac persists throughout pregnancy and appears under the amnion as a small structure on the fetal surface of the placenta near the attachment of the umbilical cord. Persistence of the yolk sac is of no significance. The *yolk stalk* usually detaches from the midgut loop by the end of the sixth week. In about 2% of adults, the proximal intra-abdominal part of the yolk stalk persists as an ***ileal diverticulum*** or a ***Meckel diverticulum*** (see Chapter 12).

ALLANTOIS

Early development of the allantois was described in Chapter 4. During the third week it appears as a sausagelike diverticulum from the caudal wall of the yolk sac that extends into the connecting stalk (Fig. 7-25*A*). During the second month the extraembryonic part of the allantois degenerates (Fig. 7-25*B*). Although the allantois is not functional in human embryos, it is important for four reasons:

- Blood formation occurs in its wall during the third to fifth weeks.
- Its blood vessels persist as the umbilical vein and arteries.
- Fluid from the amniotic cavity diffuses into the umbilical vein and enters the fetal circulation for transfer to the maternal blood through the placental membrane.
- The intraembryonic portion of the allantois runs from the umbilicus to the urinary bladder, with which it is continuous. As the bladder enlarges, the allantois involutes to form a thick tube, the *urachus*. After birth the urachus becomes a fibrous cord, the *median umbilical ligament*, that extends from the apex of the urinary bladder to the umbilicus. For a discussion of urachal anomalies and their clinical significance, see Chapter 13.

Allantoic Cysts

A cystic mass in the umbilical cord may represent the remains of the extraembryonic part of the allantois (Fig. 7-26). These cysts resolve but *they may be associated with omphalocele*—congenital herniation of viscera into the proximal part of the umbilical cord (Townsend, 1994; see Chapter 12).

MULTIPLE PREGNANCIES

Multiple gestations have higher risks of fetal morbidity and mortality than single gestations (Finberg, 1994). The risks are progressively greater as the number of fetuses increases. Multiple births are more common now due to the stimulation of ovulation that occurs when exogenous gonadotropins are administered to women with ovulatory failure, and to those being treated for infertility by in vitro fertilization and embryo transfer. In North America, **twins** normally occur about once in every 85 pregnancies; **triplets** about once in 90^2 pregnancies, **quadruplets** about once in 90^3, and **quintuplets** about once in 90^4. These estimates increase when ovulations have been primed with hormones, a technique that is in general use for women who are sterile because of tubal occlusion.

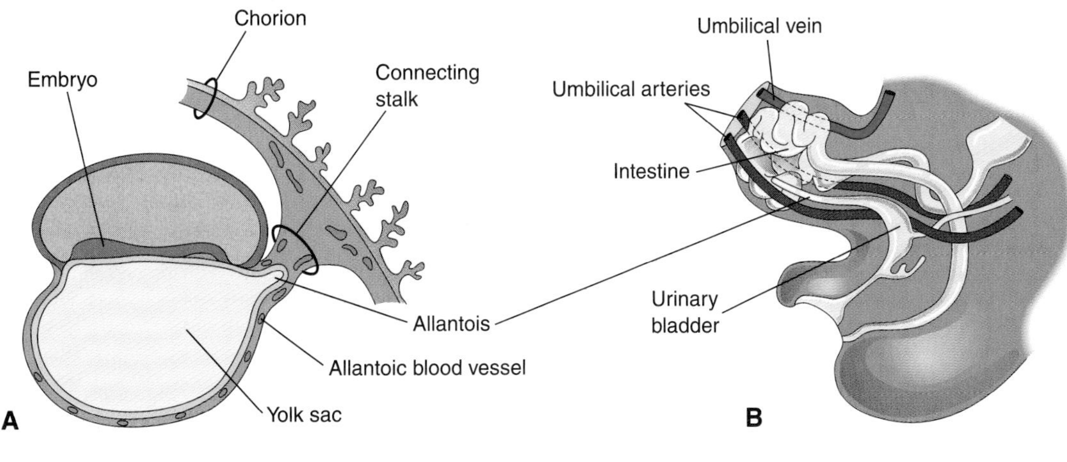

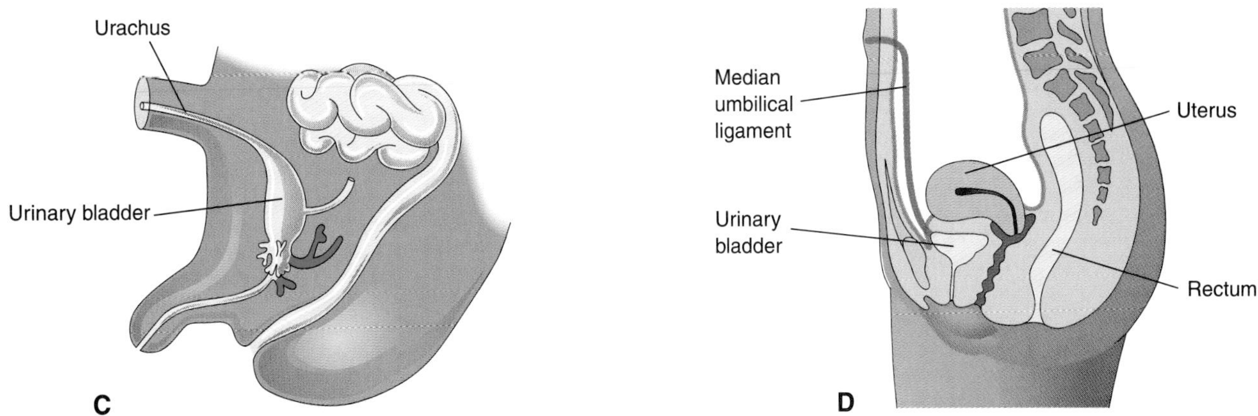

■ **Figure 7–25.** Drawings illustrating the development and usual fate of the allantois. *A,* 3-week-old embryo. *B,* 9-week-old fetus. *C,* 3-month-old male fetus. *D,* Adult female. The nonfunctional allantois forms the urachus in the fetus and the median umbilical ligament in the adult.

Twins and Fetal Membranes

Twins that originate from two zygotes are **dizygotic (DZ) twins** or fraternal twins (Fig. 7-27), whereas twins that originate from one zygote are **monozygotic (MZ) twins** or identical twins (Fig. 7-28). The fetal membranes and placentas vary according to the origin of the twins (Table 7-1), and, in the case of MZ twins, the type of placenta and membranes formed depends on when the twinning process occurs. *About two-thirds of twins are DZ.* The frequency of DZ twinning shows marked racial differences, but *the incidence of MZ twinning is about the same in all populations* (Thompson et al., 1991). In addition, the rate of MZ twinning shows little variation with the mother's age, whereas *the rate of DZ twinning increases with maternal age.*

The study of twins is important in human genetics because it is useful for comparing the effects of genes and environment on development. If an abnormal condition does not show a simple genetic pattern, com-

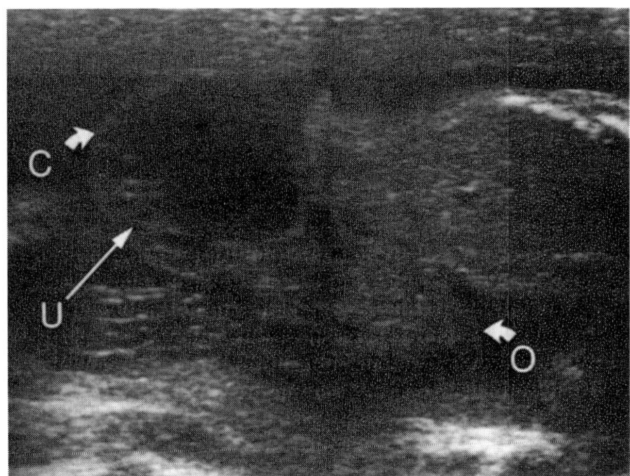

■ **Figure 7–26.** Sonogram of the umbilical cord **(U)** of a fetus exhibiting an allantoic cyst **(C)**, which is associated with an omphalocele **(O)**. (From Townsend RR: Ultrasound evaluation of the placenta and umbilical cord. *In* Callen PW [ed]: *Ultrasonography in Obstetrics and Gynecology,* 3rd ed. Philadelphia, WB Saunders, 1994.)

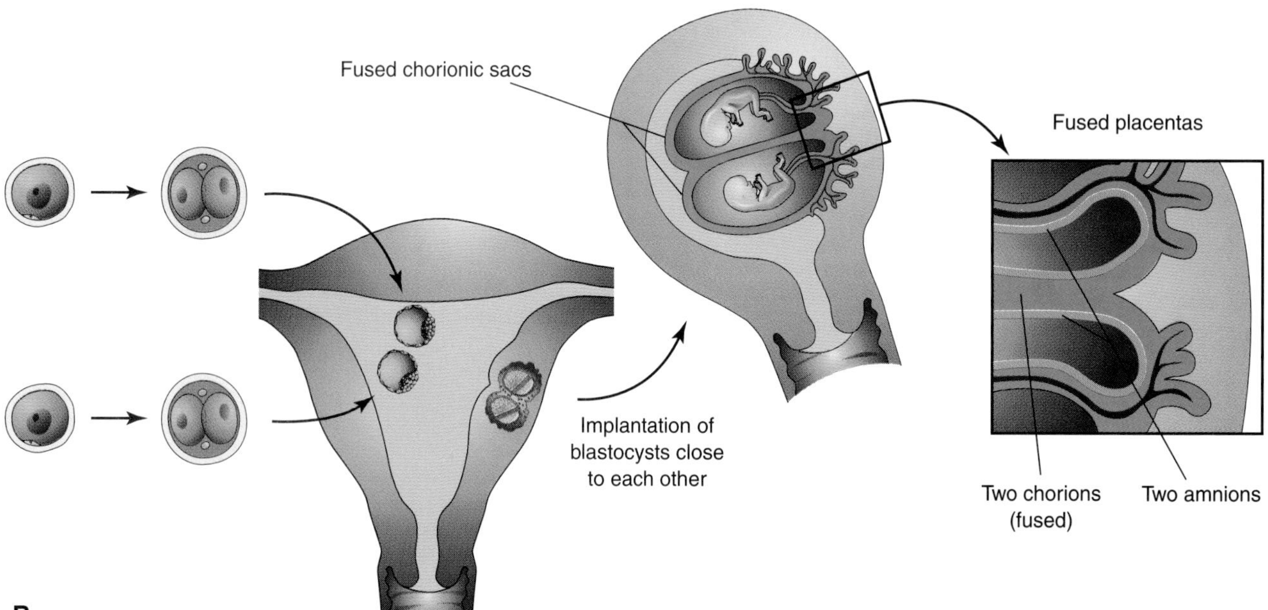

■ **Figure 7–27.** Diagrams illustrating how dizygotic (DZ) twins develop from two zygotes. The relations of the fetal membranes and placentas are shown for instances in which *A*, the blastocysts implant separately, and *B*, the blastocysts implant close together. In both cases there are two amnions and two chorions. The placentas are usually fused when they implant close together.

parison of its incidence in MZ and DZ twins may reveal that heredity is involved. The tendency for DZ but not MZ twins to repeat in families is evidence of hereditary influence (Thompson et al., 1991). Studies in a Mormon population showed that the genotype of the mother affects the frequency of DZ twins, but the genotype of the father has no effect (Page et al., 1981). It has also been observed that if the firstborn are twins, a repetition of twinning or some other form of multiple birth is about five times more likely to occur at the next pregnancy than in the general population.

Anastomosis of Placental Blood Vessels

Anastomoses between blood vessels of fused placentas of DZ twins may occur and result in **erythrocyte mosaicism**. The members of these DZ twins have red blood cells of two different types because red cells were exchanged between the circulations of the twins. Anastomosis of placental blood vessels commonly oc-

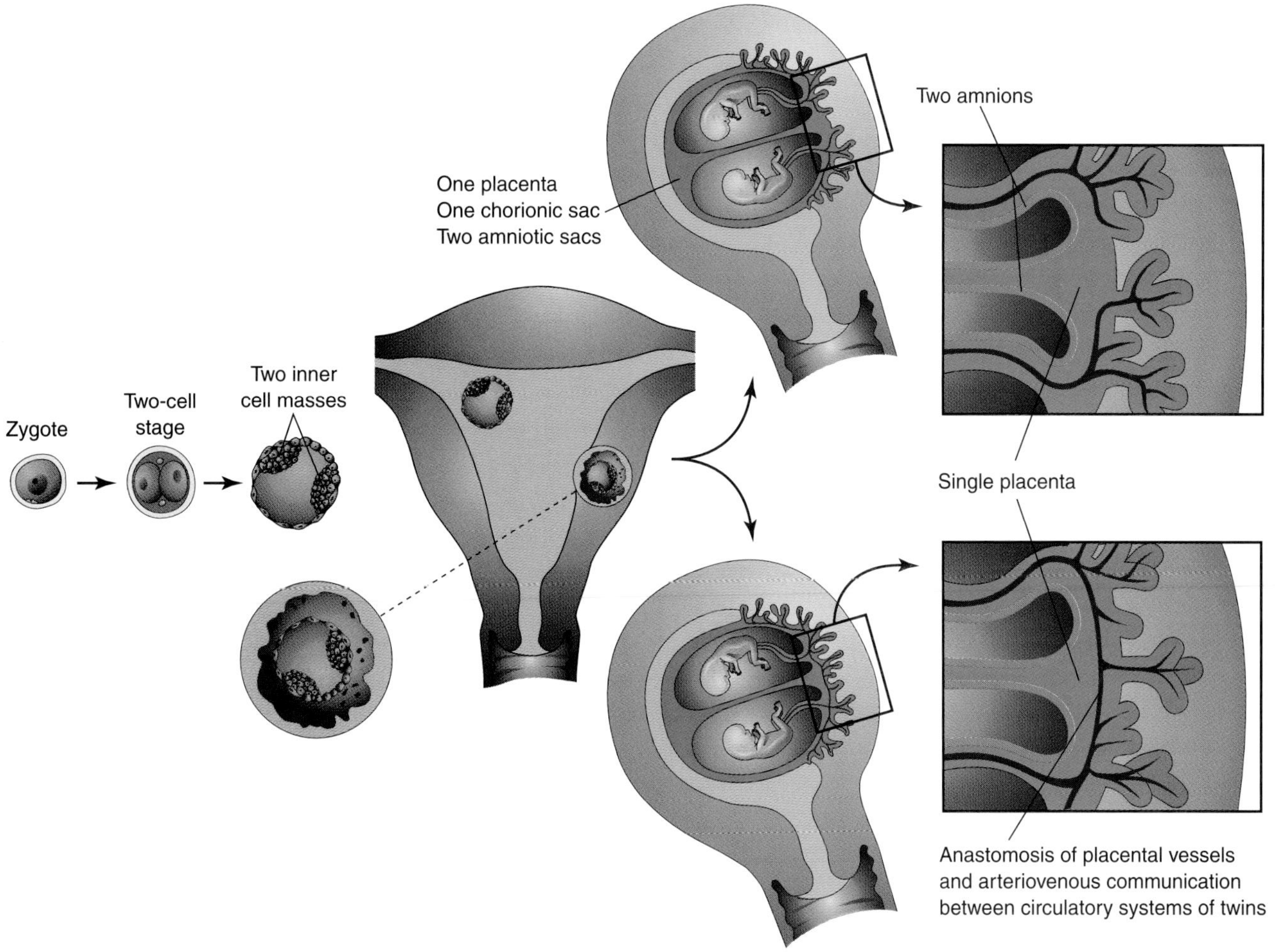

■ **Figure 7–28.** Diagrams illustrating how about 65% of monozygotic (MZ) twins develop from one zygote by division of the inner cell mass of the blastocyst. These twins always have separate amnions, a single chorionic sac, and a common placenta. If there is anastomosis of the placental vessels, one twin may receive most of the nutrition from the placenta.

curs in cattle and causes *freemartinism* (Moore, 1966). Freemartins are intersexual female calves born as twins with male calves. They are intersexual because of male hormones that reach them through anastomosed placental vessels. When placental vascular anastomoses occur in human DZ twins, in cases in which one fetus is a male and the other is female, masculinization of the female fetus does not occur, but

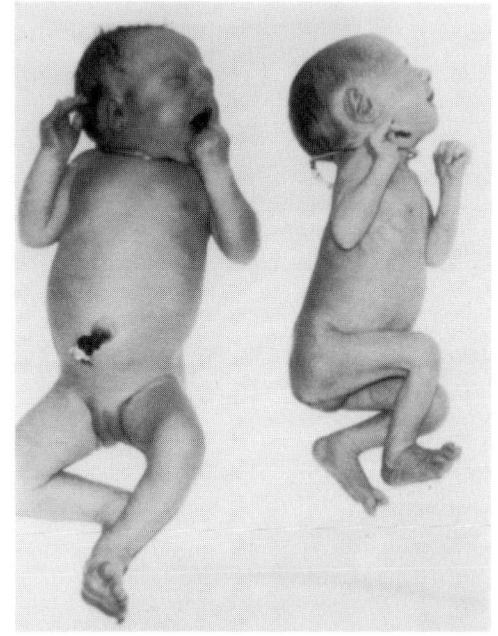

■ **Figure 7–29.** Monozygotic (MZ), monochorionic, diamniotic twins showing a wide discrepancy in size resulting from an uncompensated arteriovenous anastomosis of placental vessels. Blood was shunted from the smaller twin to the larger one, producing the fetal transfusion syndrome.

Table 7–1 ■ Frequency of Types of Placentas and Fetal Membranes in Monozygotic (MZ) and Dizygotic (DZ) Twins

	Single Chorion		Two Chorions	
Zygosity	*Single Amnion*	*Two Amnions*	*Fused Placentas**	*Two Placentas*
MZ	Very rare	65%	25%	10%
DZ	—	—	40%†	60%

Modified slightly from Thompson MW, McInnes RR, Willard HF: *Thompson & Thompson Genetics in Medicine,* 5th ed. Philadelphia, WB Saunders, 1991.
* Results from secondary fusion.
† DZ twins, the most common type, have their own amniotic and chorionic sacs, but the placentas may be fused (see Fig. 7-27*B*).

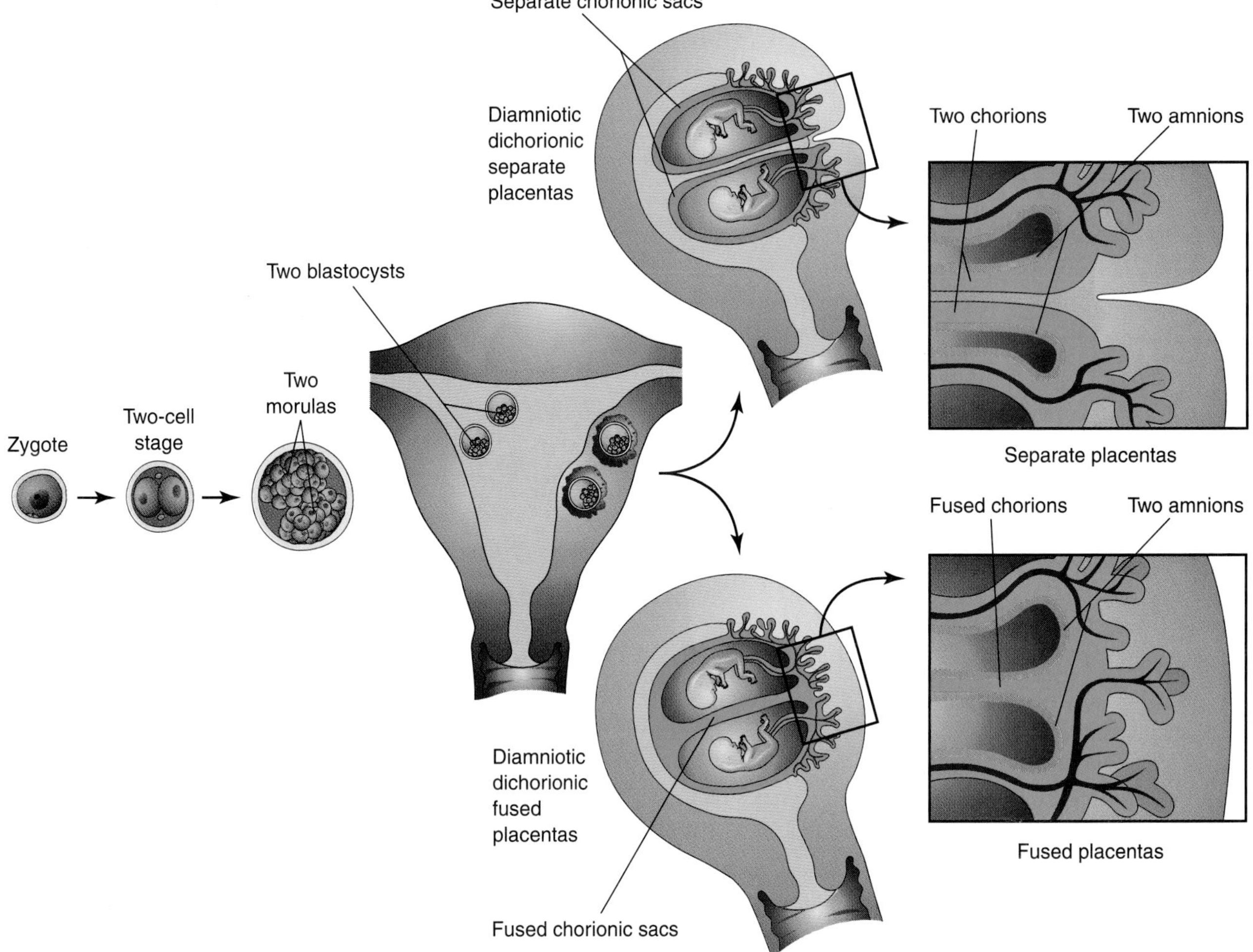

■ **Figure 7-30.** Diagrams illustrating how about 35% of monozygotic (MZ) twins develop from one zygote. Separation of the blastomeres may occur anywhere from the two-cell (blastomere) stage to the morula stage, producing two identical blastocysts. Each embryo subsequently develops its own amniotic and chorionic sacs. The placentas may be separate or fused. In 25% of cases there is a single placenta resulting from secondary fusion and in 10% of cases there are two placentas. In the latter cases, examination of the placenta would suggest that they were dizygotic (DZ) twins. This explains why some MZ twins are wrongly stated to be DZ twins at birth.

the anastomotic condition may give rise to *blood group chimeras*—persons with populations of blood cells of two genotypes that are from different zygotes (Thompson et al., 1991).

Twin-Transfusion Syndrome

This syndrome occurs in 15 to 30% of monochorionic-diamniotic MZ twins. There is a shunt of arterial blood from one twin through arteriovenous anastomoses into the venous circulation of the other twin (Behrman et al., 1996). The donor twin is small, pale, and anemic (Fig. 7-29), whereas the recipient twin is large and *polycythemic*—an increase above the normal in the number of red blood cells. The placenta shows similar abnormalities; the part of the placenta supplying the anemic twin is pale, whereas the part supplying the polycythemic twin is dark red. In lethal cases, death results from anemia in the donor twin and congestive heart failure in the recipient twin.

DIZYGOTIC (DZ) TWINS

Because they result from fertilization of two oocytes by two different sperms, DZ twins develop from two zygotes and may be of the same sex or different sexes (Fig. 7-27). For the same reason, they are no more alike genetically than brothers or sisters born at different times. The only thing they have in common is that they were in their mother's uterus at the same time (i.e., "they were womb-mates"). *DZ twins always have two amnions and two chorions*, but the chorions and placentas may be fused. **DZ twinning shows a hereditary tendency**. The recurrence risk in families is about triple the general population risk. The incidence of DZ twinning shows considerable variation, being about 1 in 500 in Asians, 1 in 125 in Caucasians, and as high as 1 in 20 in some African populations (Thompson et al., 1991).

MONOZYGOTIC (MZ) TWINS

Because they result from the fertilization of one oocyte and develop from one zygote (Fig. 7-28), *MZ twins are of the same sex, genetically identical, and very similar in physical appearance*. Physical differences between MZ twins are environmentally induced; e.g., because of anastomosis of placental vessels. MZ twinning usually begins in the blastocyst stage, around the end of the first week, and results from division of the inner cell mass or embryoblast into two embryonic primordia. Subsequently, two embryos, each in its own amniotic sac, develop within the same chorionic sac and share a **common placenta**—a monochorionic-diamniotic twin placenta. Uncommonly, early separation of embryonic blastomeres (e.g., during the two- to eight-cell stages) results in MZ twins with two amnions, two chorions, and two placentas that may or may not be fused (Fig. 7-30). In such cases it is impossible to determine from the membranes alone whether the twins are MZ or DZ. To determine the relationship of twins of the same sex with similar blood groups, one must wait until other characteristics such as eye color and fingerprints develop.

Establishing the Zygosity of Twins

Establishment of the zygosity of twins is important, particularly since tissue and organ transplantation was introduced (e.g., *bone marrow transplants*). The determination of twin zygosity is now done by *molecular diagnosis* because any two people who are not MZ twins are virtually certain to show differences in some of the large number of DNA markers that can be studied (Thompson et al., 1991).

About 35% of MZ twins result from early separation of the embryonic blastomeres; i.e., during the first 3 days of development (Fig. 7-30). The other 65% of MZ twins originate at the end of the first week of development; i.e., right after the blastocyst has formed (Fig. 7-28). Late division of early embryonic cells, such as division of the embryonic disc during the second week, results in MZ twins that are in one amniotic sac and one chorionic sac (Fig. 7-31*A*). A *monochorionic-monoamniotic twin placenta* is associated

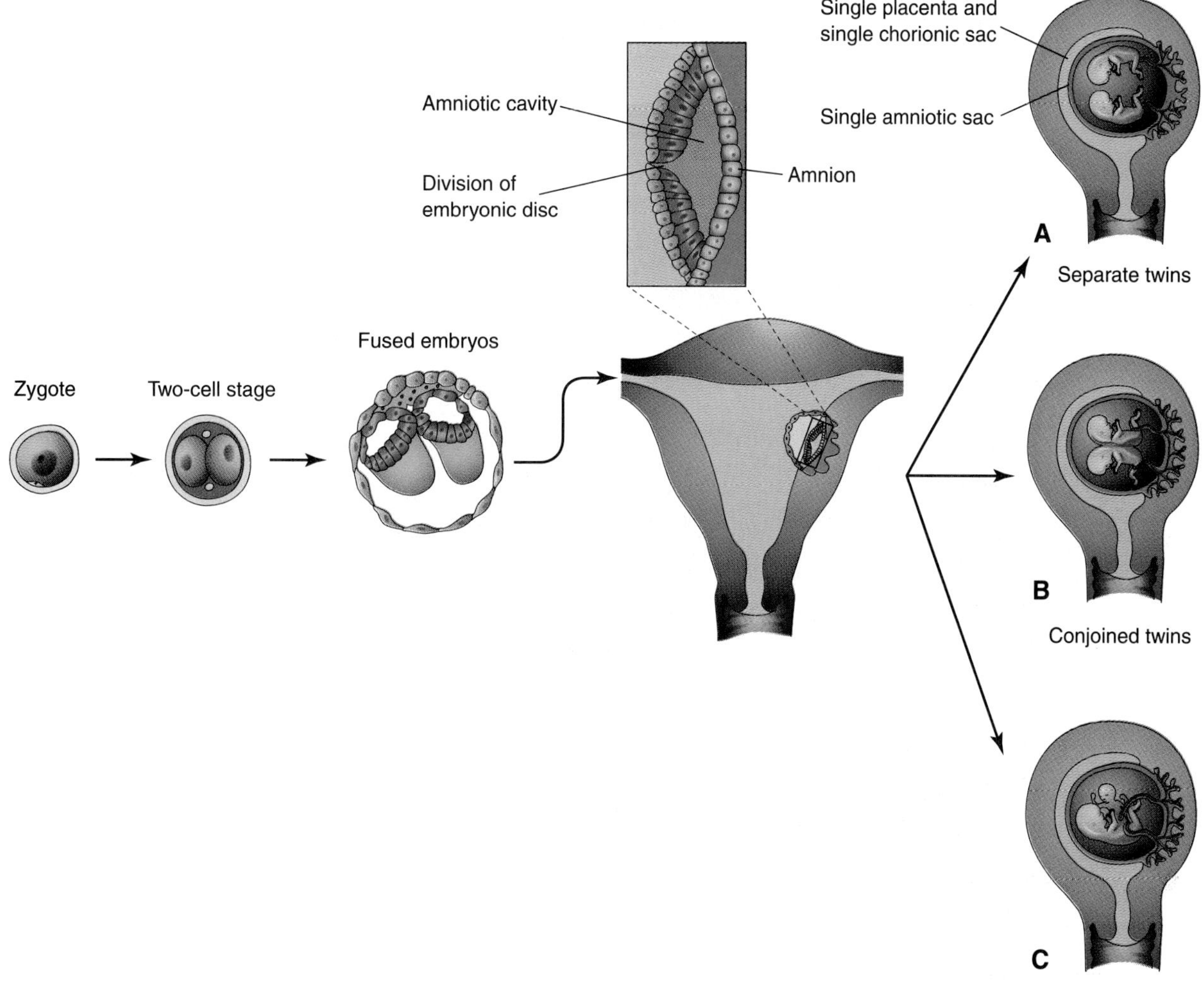

■ **Figure 7-31.** Diagrams illustrating how some monozygotic (MZ) twins develop. This method of development is very uncommon. Division of the embryonic disc results in two embryos within one amniotic sac. *A,* Complete division of the embryonic disc gives rise to twins. Such twins rarely survive because their umbilical cords are often so entangled that interruption of the blood supply to the fetuses occurs. *B* and *C,* Incomplete division of the disc results in various types of conjoined twins.

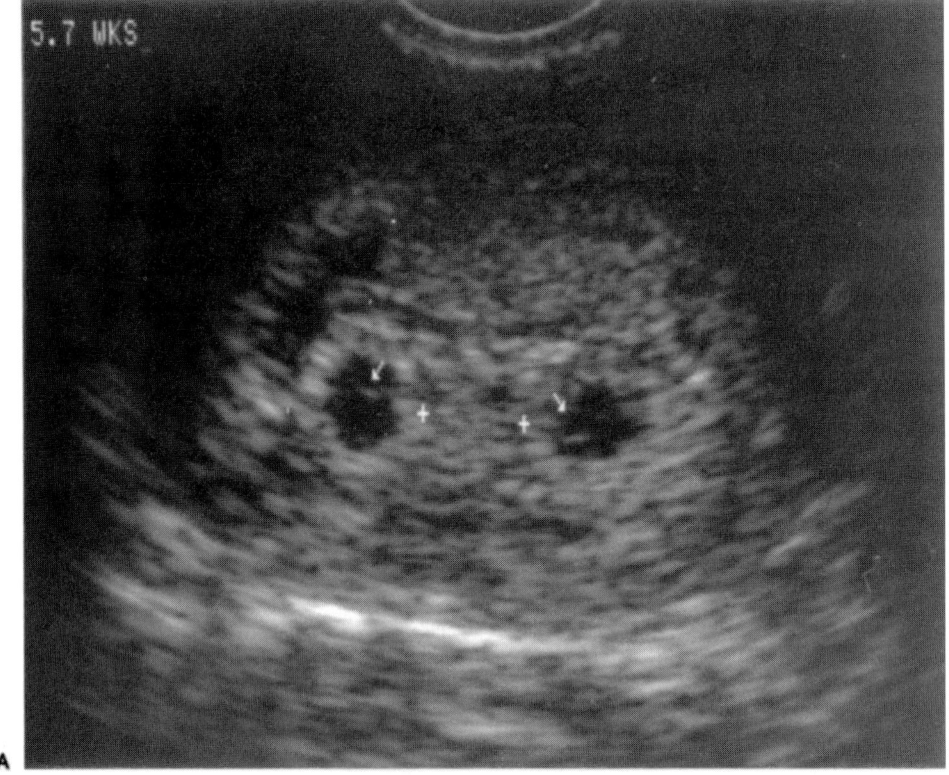

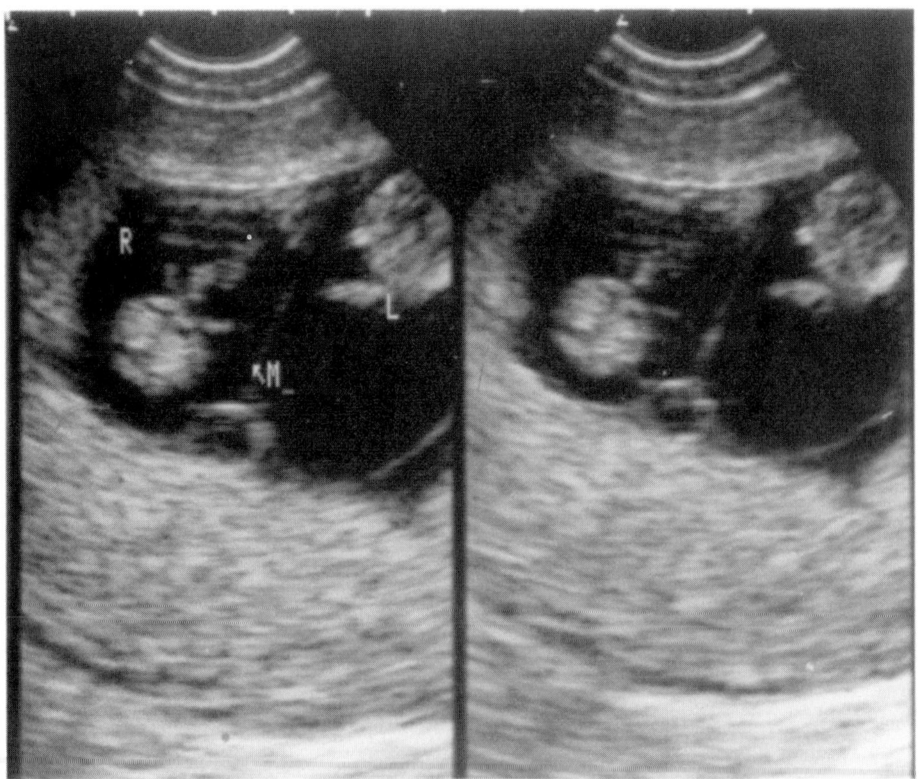

■ **Figure 7-32.** Ultrasound scans of pregnant women. *A,* Diamniotic/dichorionic twin gestation at 5.7 weeks—3.7 weeks after fertilization. The *arrows* indicate the yolk sacs of the dizygotic (DZ) twins in their chorionic sacs. *B,* Diamniotic/monochorionic twin gestation at 11 weeks—9 weeks after fertilization. The fused amnions **(M)** separate the MZ fetuses (**R** and **L**). (Courtesy of Dr. Lyndon M Hill, Department of Obstetrics and Gynecology, Division of Maternal-Fetal Medicine, University of Pittsburgh, Pittsburgh, PA.)

with a fetal mortality rate approaching 50%. These MZ twins are rarely delivered alive because the umbilical cords are frequently so entangled that circulation of blood through their vessels ceases and one or both fetuses die. *Sonography plays an important role in the diagnosis and management of twin pregnancies* (Fig. 7-32). Ultrasound evaluation is necessary to identify various conditions that may complicate MZ twinning such as intrauterine growth retardation, fetal distress, and premature labor (Finberg, 1994).

MZ twins may be discordant for a variety of birth defects and genetic disorders, despite their origin from the same zygote. In addition to environmental differences and chance variation, the following reasons given by Thompson et al. (1991) are recognized:

- mechanisms of embryological development, such as *vascular abnormalities*, that can lead to discordance for anomalies
- postzygotic changes such as *somatic mutation* leading to discordance for cancer, or somatic rearrangement of immunoglobulin or T-cell receptor genes
- *chromosome aberrations* originating in one blastocyst after the twinning event
- uneven *X chromosome inactivation* between female MZ twins, with the result that one twin preferentially expresses the paternal X, the other the maternal X.

Early Death of a Twin

Because ultrasonographic studies are a common part of prenatal care, it is known that early death and resorption of one member of a twin pair is fairly common (Filly, 1994; Liu et al., 1992). Awareness of this possibility must be considered when discrepancies occur between prenatal cytogenetic findings and the karyotype of an infant. Errors in prenatal diagnosis may arise if extraembryonic tissues (e.g., part of a chorionic villus) from the resorbed twin are examined.

Conjoined MZ Twins

If the embryonic disc does not divide completely, or adjacent embryonic discs fuse, various types of conjoined MZ twins may form (Figs. 7-31*B* and *C*, 7-33, and 7-34). These attached (Gr. *pagos,* fixed) twins are named according to the regions that are attached; e.g., *thoracopagus* indicates that there is anterior union of the thoracic regions. It has been estimated that the incidence of conjoined (Siamese) twins is 1 in 50,000 to 100,000 births (Finberg, 1994). In some cases, the

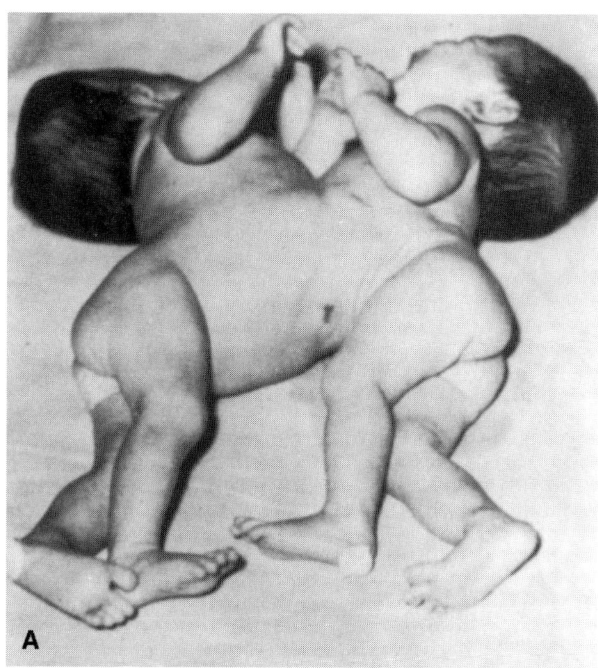

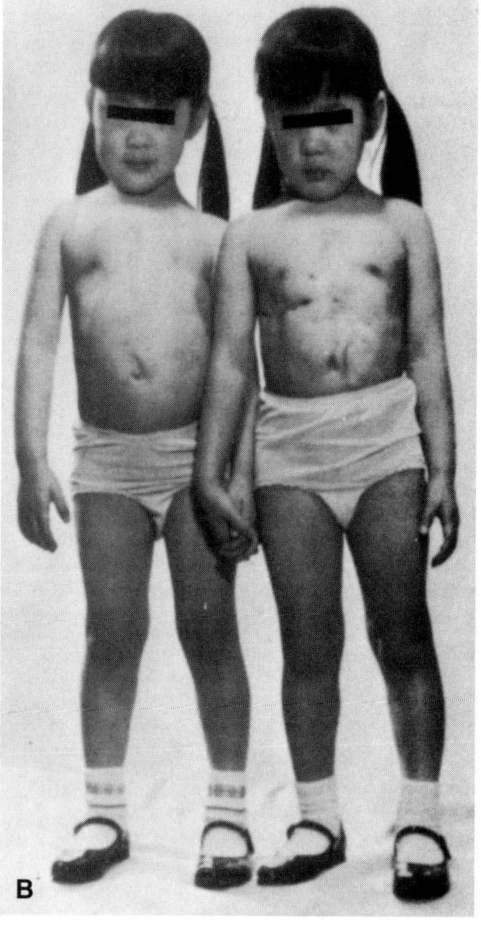

■ **Figure 7-33.** *A,* Photograph of newborn MZ conjoined twins showing union in the thoracic regions (thoracopagus). *B,* The twins about 4 years after separation. (From deVries PA: Case history—the San Francisco twins. *In* Bergsma D [ed]: *Conjoined Twins.* New York, Alan R Liss for the National Foundation–March of Dimes, DBOAS III [1], 141–142, 1967, with permission of the copyright holder.)

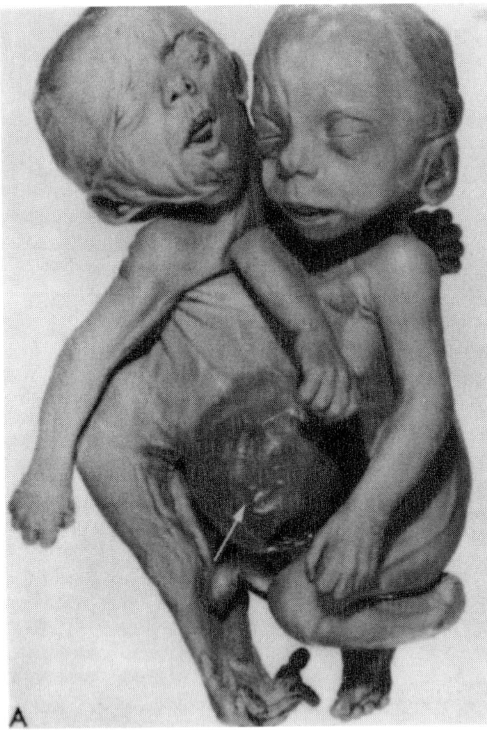

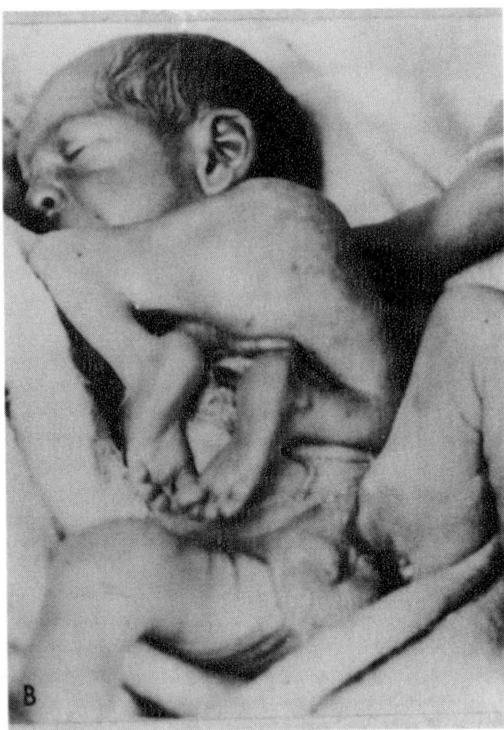

■ **Figure 7-34.** *A*, Photograph of conjoined MZ twins showing extensive anterior fusion and an omphalocele *(arrow)*. This hernia contained intestines from both fetuses. These fetuses died before they could be delivered. The lower limbs of the left fetus are fused, a condition known as sirenomelia. *B*, Parasitic fetus with well-developed lower limbs and pelvis attached to the thorax of an otherwise normal male infant.

twins are connected to each other by skin only or by cutaneous and other tissues, e.g., fused livers (Fig. 7-34*A*). Some conjoined twins can be successfully separated by surgical procedures (Fig. 7-33*B*); however, the anatomical relations in most conjoined twins do not permit surgical separation with sustained viability. For a discussion of the theoretical basis of conjoined twins, see Spencer (1992).

Other Types of Multiple Birth

Triplets may be derived from:

- one zygote and be identical
- two zygotes and consist of identical twins and a singleton
- three zygotes and be of the same sex or of different sexes (Fig. 7-35)

In the last case, the infants are no more similar than infants from three separate pregnancies. Similar combinations occur in quadruplets (Fig. 7-36), quintuplets, sextuplets, and septuplets.

Superfecundation

Superfecundation is the fertilization of two or more oocytes around the same time by sperms from different men. This phenomenon commonly occurs in some mammals (e.g., cats and dogs). DZ human twins with different fathers have been confirmed by genetic markers (Terasaki et al., 1978).

SUMMARY OF PLACENTA AND FETAL MEMBRANES

In addition to the embryo and fetus, the fetal membranes and the major part of the placenta originate from the zygote. The placenta consists of two parts:

- a larger fetal part derived from the villous chorion
- a smaller maternal part developed from the decidua basalis

The two parts are held together by stem chorionic villi that attach to the cytotrophoblastic shell surrounding the chorionic sac, which attaches the sac to the decidua basalis.

The principal *activities of the placenta* are:

- metabolism such as synthesis of glycogen, cholesterol, and fatty acids
- respiratory gas exchange (oxygen, carbon dioxide, and carbon monoxide)
- transfer of nutrients such as vitamins, hormones, and antibodies
- elimination of waste products
- endocrine secretion (e.g., hCG) for maintenance of pregnancy

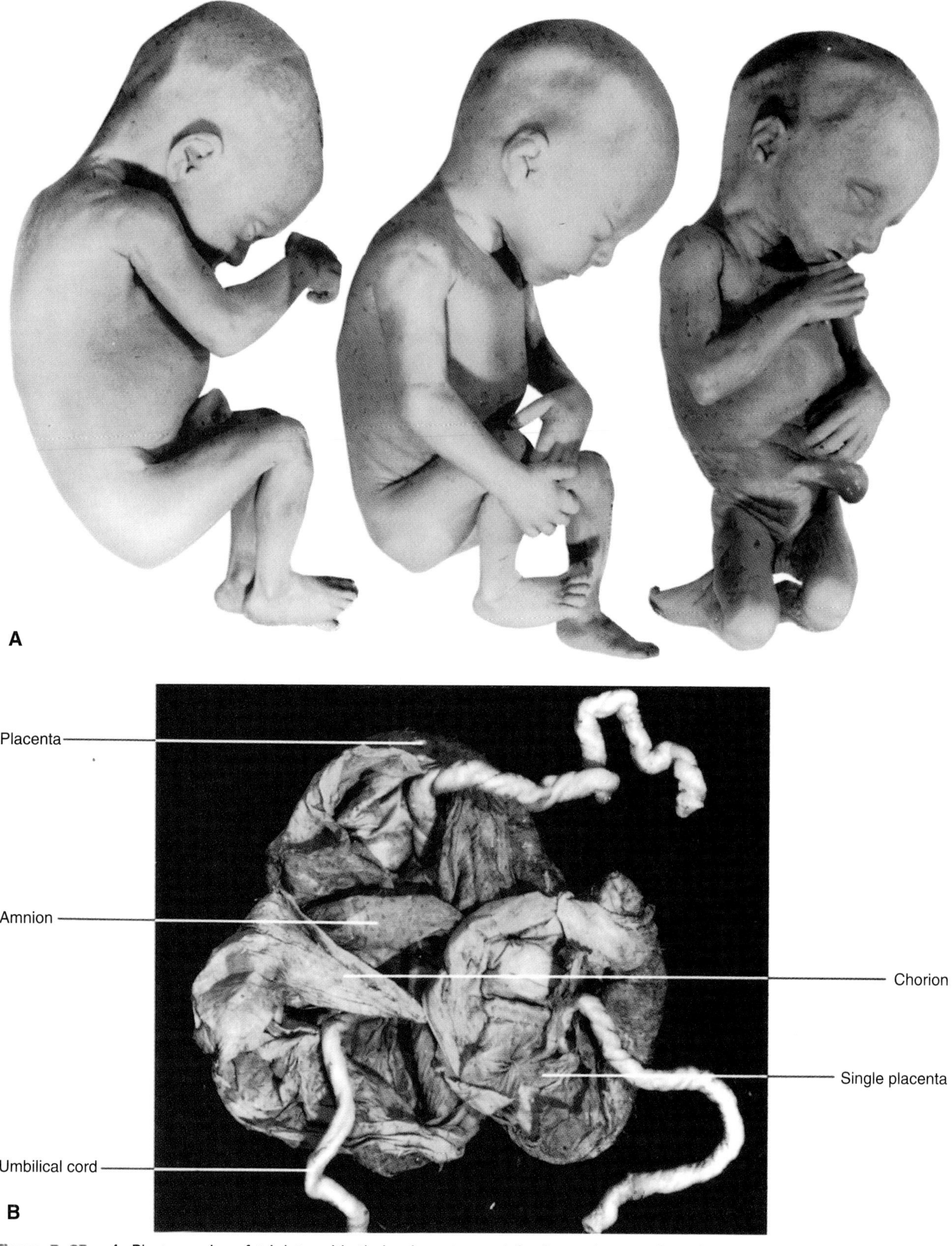

■ **Figure 7–35.** *A*, Photographs of triplets with their placentas and fetal membranes. Examination of the placentas and membranes revealed that the two fetuses on the left were identical and the one on the right was a singleton. *B*, The diamniotic/monochorionic placenta is on the left and the single placenta is on the right. Thus, these three fetuses developed from two zygotes. (From Moore KL, Persaud TVN, Shiota K: *Color Atlas of Clinical Embryology,* Philadelphia, WB Saunders, 1994.)

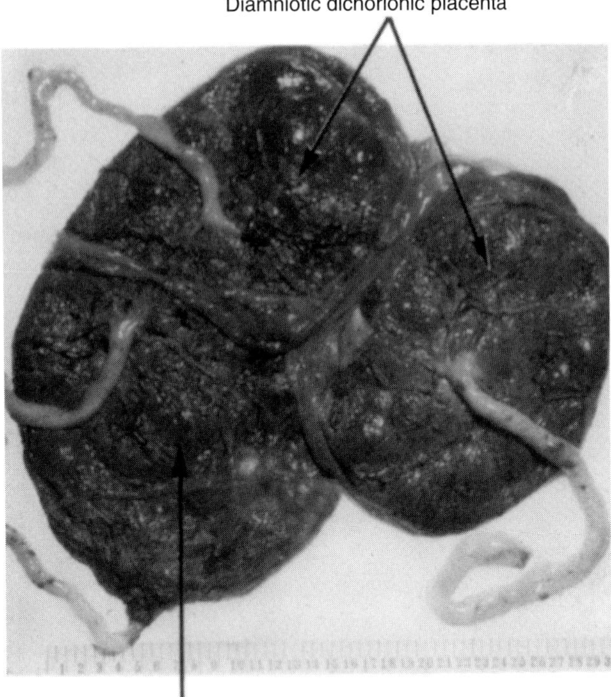

■ **Figure 7–36.** Photograph of the placentas from quadruplets. The upper two placentas (and the dizygotic fetuses associated with them) were derived from two zygotes, whereas the lower fused placenta was attached to monozygotic twins. (Reprinted with permission from The American College of Obstetrics and Gynecologists [*Obstetrics and Gynecology* 18:309, 1961].)

All these activities are essential for maintaining pregnancy and promoting normal fetal development.

The fetal circulation is separated from the maternal circulation by a thin layer of extrafetal tissues—the **placental membrane**. It is a permeable membrane that allows water, oxygen, nutritive substances, hormones, and noxious agents to pass from the mother to the embryo or fetus. Excretory products pass through the placental membrane from the fetus to the mother.

The fetal membranes and placenta(s) in *multiple pregnancies* vary considerably, depending on the derivation of the embryos and the time when division of embryonic cells occurs. The common type of twins is *dizygotic twins (DZ)*, with two amnions, two chorions, and two placentas that may or may not be fused. *Monozygotic twins (MZ)*, the less common type, represent about a third of all twins; they are derived from one zygote. MZ twins commonly have one chorion, two amnions, and one placenta. Twins with one amnion, one chorion, and one placenta are always monozygotic, and their umbilical cords are often entangled. Other types of multiple birth (triplets, etc.) may be derived from one or more zygotes.

The *yolk sac* and *allantois* are vestigial structures; however, their presence is essential to normal embryonic development. Both are early sites of blood formation and both are partly incorporated into the embryo. Primordial germ cells also originate in the wall of the yolk sac.

The *amnion* forms a sac for amniotic fluid and provides a covering for the umbilical cord. The amniotic fluid has three main functions:

- to provide a protective buffer for the embryo or fetus
- to allow room for fetal movements
- to assist in the regulation of fetal body temperature

Clinically Oriented Problems

Case 7–1

A physician is concerned about the effects of a drug on the embryo of one of his patients.

- How is the estimated date of confinement (EDC) or estimated delivery date (EDD) of a baby determined?
- How could the EDD be confirmed in a high-risk obstetrical patient?

Case 7–2

A physician told a pregnant woman that she had *polyhydramnios*.

- If you were asked to explain the meaning of this clinical condition, what would be your answer?
- What conditions are often associated with polyhydramnios?
- Explain why polyhydramnios occurs.

Case 7–3

A physician was asked, "Does twinning run in families?"

- Is maternal age a factor?
- If uncertainty exists about the origin of twins, how would you determine whether they were MZ or DZ?

Case 7–4

A pathologist asked you to examine a section of an umbilical cord. You observed that there was only one umbilical artery.

- How often does this anomaly occur?
- What kind of fetal abnormalities might be associated with this condition?

Case 7–5

An ultrasonographic examination revealed a twin pregnancy with a single placenta. Chorionic villus sampling and chromosome analysis revealed that the twins were likely female. At birth the twins were of different sexes.

- How could this error have occurred?

Case 7–6

An ultrasound examination of a pregnant woman during the second trimester revealed multiple amniotic bands associated with the fetus.

- What produces these bands?
- What congenital defects may result from them?
- What is the syndrome called?

Discussion of these problems appears at the back of the book.

REFERENCES AND SUGGESTED READING

Aplin JD: Implantation, trophoblast differentiation and haemochorial placentation: mechanistic evidence *in vivo* and *in vitro*. *J Cell Sci 99:*681, 1991.

Bamforth JS: Amniotic band sequence: Streeter's hypothesis re-examined. *Am J Med Genet 44:*280, 1992.

Bassett JM: Current perspectives on placental development and its integration with fetal growth. *Proc Nutr Soc 50:*311, 1991.

Beck F, Moffat DB, Davies DP: *Human Embryology,* 2nd ed. Oxford, Blackwell Scientific Publications, 1985.

Beck T: Placental morphometry using a computer assisted measuring programme. Reference values for normal pregnancies at term. *Arch Gynecol Obstet 249:*135, 1991.

Beebe LA, Cowan LD, Alshuler G: The epidemiology of placental features: associations with gestational age and neonatal outcome: *Obstet Gynecol 87:*771, 1996.

Behrman RE, Kliegman RM, Arvin AM (eds): *Nelson Textbook of Pediatrics,* 15th ed. Philadelphia, WB Saunders, 1996.

Benirschke K: Implantation, placental development, uteroplacental blood flow. *In* Reid DE, Ryan KJ, Benirschke K (eds): *Principles and Management of Human Reproduction*. Philadelphia, WB Saunders, 1992.

Benirschke K: Obstetrically important lesions of the umbilical cord. *J Reprod Med 39:*262, 1994.

Benirschke K, Kaufman P: *The Pathology of the Human Placenta*. Berlin, Springer Verlag, 1990.

Bergsma D (ed): *Conjoined Twins. Birth Defects III(1):*1-147, 1967.

Berkowitz RS, Goldstein DP: Chorionic tumors. *N Engl J Med 335:* 1740, 1996.

Billington WB: Trophoblast. *In* Philipp EE, Barnes J, Newton M (eds): *Scientific Foundations of Obstetrics and Gynecology*. London, William Heinemann, 1970.

Bissonnette J: Placental and fetal physiology. *In* Gabbe SG, Neibyl JR, Simpson JL (eds): *Obstetrics, Normal and Problem Pregnancies*. New York, Churchill Livingstone, 1986, p 109.

Bohn H, Winckler W, Grundmann U: Immunochemically detected placental proteins and their biological functions. *Arch Gynecol Obstet 249:*107, 1991.

Boura ALA, Walters WAW: Autocoids and the control of vascular tone in the human umbilical-placental circulation. *Placenta 12:* 453, 1991.

Bulmer MG: *The Biology of Twinning in Man*. Oxford, Clarendon Press, 1970.

Callen PW, Filly RA: Amniotic fluid evaluation. *In* Harrison MR, Golbus MS, Filly RA (eds): *The Unborn Patient. Prenatal Diagnosis and Treatment*, 2nd ed. Philadelphia, WB Saunders, 1990.

Carlson BM: *Human Embryology and Developmental Biology*. St Louis, Mosby, 1994.

Carr BR: Fertilization, implantation, and endocrinology of pregnancy. *In* Griffin JE, Ojeda SR (eds): *Textbook of Endocrine Physiology*. New York and Oxford, Oxford University Press, 1988.

Chamberlain G, Wilkinson A (eds): *Placental Transfer*. Baltimore, University Park Press, 1979.

Cotran RS, Kumar V, Robbins SL: *Robbins Pathologic Basis of Disease,* 4th ed. Philadelphia, WB Saunders, 1989.

Cunningham FG, MacDonald PC, Grant NF (eds): *Williams Obstetrics,* 19th ed. Norwalk, Appleton & Lange, 1993.

Demir R, Kaufmann P, Castellucci M, et al: Fetal vasculogenesis and angiogenesis in human placenta villi. *Acta Anat 136:*190, 1989.

DeSilva N: Zygosity and umbilical cord length. *J Reprod Med 37:*850, 1992.

deVries PA: Case history—the San Francisco twins. *In* Bergsma D (ed): *Conjoined Twins. Birth Defects III(1):*141, 1967.

Doubilet PM, Benson CB: Ultrasound evaluation of amniotic fluid. *In* Callen PW: *Ultrasonography in Obstetrics and Gynecology,* 3rd ed. Philadelphia, WB Saunders, 1994.

Dungy LJ, Siddigi TA, Khan S: Transforming growth factor-expression during placental development. *Am J Obstet Gynecol 165:*853, 1991.

Enders AC: Structural responses of the primate endometrium to implantation. *Placenta 12:*309, 1991.

Filly RA: Ultrasound evaluation during the first trimester. *In* Callen PW (ed): *Ultrasonography in Obstetrics and Gynecology*, 3rd ed. Philadelphia, WB Saunders, 1994.

Filly RA, Golbus MS: The fetus with amniotic band syndrome. *In* Harrison MR, Golbus MS, Filly RA (eds): *The Unborn Patient. Prenatal Diagnosis and Treatment*, 2nd ed. Philadelphia, WB Saunders, 1990.

Finberg HJ: Ultrasound evaluation in multiple pregnancy. *In* Callen PW (ed): *Ultrasonography in Obstetrics and Gynecology*, 3rd ed. Philadelphia, WB Saunders, 1994.

Fleischer AC, Goldstein RB, Bruner JP, Worrell JA: Doppler sonography in obstetrics and gynecology. *In* Callen PW (ed): *Ultrasonography in Obstetrics and Gynecology,* 3rd ed. Philadelphia, WB Saunders, 1994.

Foidart J-M, Hustin J, Dubois M, Schaaps J-P: The human placenta becomes haemochorial at the 13th week of pregnancy. *Int J Dev Biol 36:*451, 1992.

Fox H: *Pathology of the Placenta*. Philadelphia, WB Saunders, 1978.

Fox H: Trophoblastic pathology. *Placenta 12:*479, 1991.

Fox H: The placenta, membranes and umbilical cord. *In* Chamberlain G (ed): *Turnbull's Obstetrics,* 2nd ed. Edinburgh, Churchill Livingstone, 1995.

Freedman RS, Tortolero-Luna G, Pandey DK, et al: Gestational trophoblastic disease. *Obstet Gynecol Clin North Am 23:*545, 1996.

Gadd RL: The liquor amnii. *In* Philipp EE, Barnes J, Newton M (eds): *Scientific Foundations of Obstetrics and Gynecology*. London, William Heinemann, Ltd, 1970.

Glasser SR, Bullock DW (eds): *Cellular and Molecular Aspects of Implantation*. New York, Plenum Press, 1981.

Gordon JF, Shifren JL, Foulk RA, et al: Angiogenesis in the human female reproductive tract. *Obstet Gynecol Surv 50:*688, 1995.

Green JR: Placenta previa and abruptio placentae. *In* Creasy RK, Resnik R (eds): *Maternal-Fetal Medicine. Principles and Practice,* 2nd ed. Philadelphia, WB Saunders, 1989.

Heinonen S, Ryynänen M, Kirkinen P, Saarikoski S: Perinatal diagnostic evaluation of velamentous umbilical cord insertion: clinical, doppler, and ultrasonic findings. *Obstet Gynecol 87:*112, 1996.

Hay WW: In vivo measurements of placental transport and metabolism. *Proc Nutr Soc* 50:355, 1991.

Haugen G, Stray-Pedersen S, Bjoro K: Prostanoid production in umbilical arteries from preterm and term deliveries perfused in vitro. *Early Hum Develop 24:*153, 1990.

Jaffe R, Jauniaux E, Hustin J: Maternal circulation in the first-trimester human placenta—myth or reality? *Am J Obstet Gynecol 176:* 695, 1997.

Jauniaux E, Jurkovic D, Henriet Y, et al: Development of the secondary human yolk sac—correlation of sonographic and anatomical features. *Hum Reprod 6:*309, 1991.

Javert CT: *Spontaneous and Habitual Abortion*. New York, The Blakiston Division, McGraw-Hill, 1957.

Johnson MH, Everitt B: *Essential Reproduction*. Oxford, Blackwell Scientific Publications, 1984.

Jollie WP: Development, morphology and function of the yolk-sac placenta of laboratory rodents. *Teratology 41:*361, 1990.

Jones JM, Sbarra AJ, Cetrulo CL: Twin transfusion syndrome. *J Reprod Med 4:*11, 1996.

Kelly RV: Pregnancy maintenance and parturition: the role of prostaglandin in manipulating the immune and inflammatory response. *Endocr Rev 15:*684, 1994.

Kennedy LA, Persaud TVN: Pathogenesis of developmental defects induced in the rat by amniotic sac puncture. *Acta Anat 97:*23, 1977.

Klopper A, Chard T (eds): *Placental Proteins*. Berlin, Springer Verlag, 1978.

Kraemer K, Noerr B: Placental transfer of drugs. *J Obstet Gynecol Neonatal Nurs (Neonatal Network) 16:*65, 1997.

Lichnovsky V, Lojda Z, Bocek M, Vlkova M: Histochemistry of some enzymes in human embryonic and fetal placentae. *Acta Univ Palacki Olomuc Fac Med 126:*11, 1990.

Liu S, Benirschke K, Scioscia AL, Mannino FL: Intrauterine death in multiple gestation. *Acta Genet Med Gemellol Roma 41:*5, 1992.

Love CDB: Pregnancies complicated by placenta praevia: what is appropriate management. *Br J Obstet Gynaecol 103:*864, 1996.

Luton D, Sibony O, Oury JF, et al: The C-*ets* 1 protooncogene is expressed in human trophoblast during the first trimester of pregnancy. *Early Hum Dev 47:*147, 1997.

Mäkilä U-M, Jouppila P, Kirkinen P, et al: Placental membrane and prostacyclin in the regulation of placental blood flow. *Obstet Gynecol 68:*537, 1986.

Mann SE, Nijland MJM, Ross MG: Mathematic modeling of human amniotic fluid dynamics. *Am J Obstet Gynecol 175:*937, 1986.

Moore KL: The sex chromatin of freemartins and other animal intersexes. *In* Moore KL (ed): *The Sex Chromatin*. Philadelphia, WB Saunders, 1966.

Moore KL: *Clinically Oriented Anatomy,* 3rd ed. Baltimore, Williams & Wilkins, 1992.

Mossman HW: Classics revisited: comparative morphogenesis of fetal membranes and accessory uterine structures. *Placenta 12:*1, 1991.

Naeye RL: *Disorders of the Placenta, Fetus, and Neonate*. St Louis, Mosby-Year Book, 1992.

Nash JE, Persaud TVN: Embryopathic risks of cigarette smoking. *Exp Pathol 33:*65, 1988.

Nathanielsz PW: *Life Before Birth. The Challenges of Fetal Development.* New York, WH Freeman and Company, 1996.

Oxorn H: *Human Labor and Birth,* 5th ed. Norwalkco, Appleton-Century-Crofts, 1989.

Page EW, Villee CA, Villee DB: *Human Reproduction. Essentials of Reproductive and Perinatal Medicine,* 3rd ed. Philadelphia, WB Saunders, 1981.

Parilla V, Tamura RK, MacGregor SN, et al: The clinical significance of a single umbilical artery as an isolated finding on prenatal ultrasound. *Obstet Gynecol 85:*570, 1995.

Peipert JF, Donnenfeld AE: Oligohydramnios: a review. *Obstet Gynecol 46:*325, 1991.

Persaud TVN, Tiess D: *Plazentare Übertragung von Aethylbarbital Naturwissenschaften 53:*385, 1966.

Petraglia F, Angioni S, Coukos G, et al: Neuroendocrine mechanisms regulating placental hormone production. *Contr Gynecol Obstet 18:*147, 1991.

Raga R, Ballester MJ, Osborne NG, Barilla-Musoles F: Role of color flow doppler ultrasonography in diagnosing velamentous insertion of the umbilical cord and vas previa. *J Reprod Med 40:*804, 1995.

Rubin E, Farber JL: *Pathology*. Philadelphia, JB Lippincott, 1988.

Rosso P: Placental growth, development, and function in relation to maternal nutrition. *Fed Proc 39:*250, 1980.

Schmidt W: *The Amniotic Fluid Compartment: The Fetal Habitat.* Berlin, Springer, 1992.

Schnaufer L: Conjoined twins. *In* Raffensperger JG (ed): *Swenson's Pediatric Surgery,* 5th ed. Norwalkco, Appleton & Lange, 1990.

Schneider H: Placental transport function. *Reprod Fert Develop 3:* 345, 1991.

Schumacher GH, Gill H, Persaud TVN, Gill H: Historical documents concerning craniopagi and conjoined twins. *Gregenbaurs Morphol Jahrb 134:*541, 1988.

Scott JR, DiSaia PJ, Hammond CB, Spellacy WN (eds): *Danforth's Obstetrics and Gynecology,* 6th ed. Philadelphia, JB Lippincott, 1990.

Seed JW, Cefalo RC, Herbert WNP: Amniotic band syndrome. *Am J Obstet Gynecol 144:*243, 1982.

Seeds AE Jr: Amniotic fluid and fetal water metabolism. *In* Barnes AC (ed): *Intra-Uterine Development.* Philadelphia, Lea & Febiger, 1968.

Spencer R: Conjoined twins: theoretical embryologic basis. *Teratology 45:*591, 1992.

Terasaki PI, Gjertson D, Bernoco D, et al: Twins with two different fathers identified by HLA. *N Engl J Med 299:*590, 1978.

Thompson MW, McInnes RR, Willard HF: *Thompson & Thompson Genetics in Medicine,* 5th ed. Philadelphia, WB Saunders, 1991.

Thorp JA, Dildy GA, Yeomans ER, et al: Umbilical cord blood gas analysis at delivery. *Am J Obstet Gynecol 175:*517, 1996.

Townsend RR: Ultrasound evaluation of the placenta and umbilical cord. *In* Callen PW (ed): *Ultrasonography in Obstetrics and Gynecology,* 3rd ed. Philadelphia, WB Saunders, 1994.

Turksoy RN, Toy BL, Rogers J, Papageorge W: Birth of septuplets following human gonadotropin administration in Chiari-Frommel syndrome. *Obstet Gynecol 30:*692, 1967.

Turnbull A: The endocrine control of labour. *In* Chamberlain G (ed): *Turnbull's Obstetrics,* 2nd ed. Edinburgh, Churchill Livingstone, 1995.

Waisman HA, Kerr G: *Fetal Growth and Development.* New York, McGraw-Hill, 1970.

Wald NJ, Cuckle HS: AFP screening in early pregnancy. *In* Spencer JAD (ed): *Fetal Monitoring*. Oxford, Oxford University Press, 1991.

Watson WJ, Chescheir NC, Katz VL, Seeds JW: The role of ultrasound in evaluation of patients with elevated maternal serum alpha-fetoprotein: a review. *Obstet Gynecol 78:*123, 1991.

Werler MM, Pober BR, Holmes LB: Smoking and pregnancy. *In* Sever JL, Brent RL (eds): *Teratogen Update. Environmentally Induced Birth Defect Risks.* New York, Alan R Liss, 1986.

Worrell JA, Fleischer AC, Drolshagen LF, et al: Duplex Doppler sonography of the umbilical arteries: Predictive value in IUGR and correlation with birth weight. *Ultrasound Med Biol 17:*207, 1991.

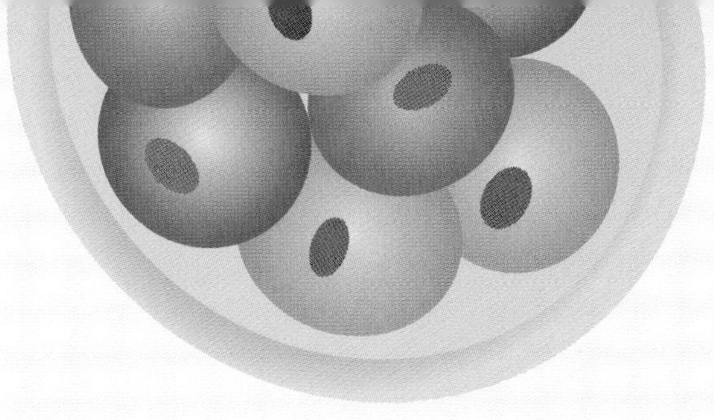

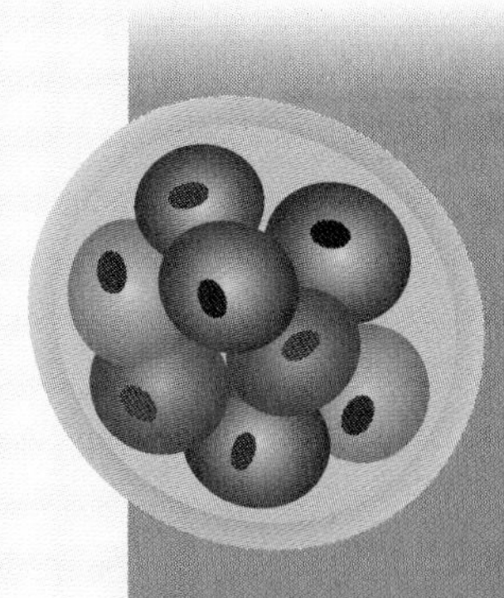

Human Birth Defects

8

We ought not to set them aside with idle thoughts or idle words about "curiosities" or "chances." Not one of them is without meaning; not one that might not become the beginning of excellent knowledge, if only we could answer the question — why is it rare, or being rare, why did it in this instance happen?

—JAMES PAGET, *LANCET* 2:1017, 1882

■ Congenital anomalies, birth defects, and congenital malformations are terms currently used to describe developmental disorders present at birth (L. *congenitus*, born with). Birth defects are the leading cause of infant mortality and may be structural, functional, metabolic, behavioral, or hereditary (Persaud et al., 1985).

The most widely used reference guide for classifying birth defects is the *International Classification of Diseases* (Medicodes' Hospital and Payer, 1995); however, no single classification or nomenclature has universal appeal. Each is limited, having been designed for a particular purpose. Attempts to classify human birth defects, especially those resulting from errors of morphogenesis, reveal the frustration and obvious difficulties in the formulation of concrete proposals that could be used in medical practice (Persaud et al., 1985). A practical classification system for developmental defects, which takes into consideration the time of onset of the injury, possible etiology, and pathogenesis, is now widely accepted among clinicians (Jones, 1996; Spranger et al., 1982).

Glossary of Terms

A **congenital anomaly** is a structural abnormality of any type; however, *not all variations of development are anomalies*. Anatomical variations are common; e.g., bones vary among themselves, not only in their basic shape but in lesser details of surface structure (Moore, 1992). *There are four clinically significant types of congenital anomaly*: malformation, disruption, deformation, and dysplasia.

- **Malformation:** A morphological defect of an organ, part of an organ, or larger region of the body that *results from an intrinsically abnormal developmental process*. Intrinsic implies that the developmental potential of the primordium is abnormal from the beginning, such as chromosome abnormality of a gamete at fertilization. Most malformations are considered to be a *defect of a morphogenetic or developmental field* "which responds as a coordinated unit to embryonic interaction and results in complex or multiple malformations."
- **Disruption:** A morphological defect of an organ, part of an organ, or a larger region of the body that *results from the extrinsic breakdown of, or an interference with, an originally normal developmental process*. Thus, morphological alterations following exposure to **teratogens**—agents such as drugs and viruses—should be considered as disruptions. *A disruption cannot be inherited*, but "inherited factors can predispose to and influence the development of a disruption."
- **Deformation:** An abnormal form, shape, or position of a part of the body that *results from mechanical forces*. Intrauterine compression that results from oligohydramnios—insufficient amount of amniotic fluid—produces an equinovarus foot or *clubfoot* (see Chapter 17), an example of a deformation produced by extrinsic forces. Some central nervous system defects, such as *meningomyelocele*—a severe type of spina bifida—produce intrinsic functional disturbances that also cause fetal deformation.
- **Dysplasia:** An abnormal organization of cells into tissue(s) and its morphological result(s). Dysplasia is the process and the consequence of *dyshistogenesis* (abnormal tissue formation). All abnormalities relating to histogenesis are therefore classified as dysplasias, e.g., *congenital ectodermal dysplasia* (see Chapter 20). Dysplasia is causally nonspecific and often affects several organs because of the nature of the underlying cellular disturbances.

Other descriptive terms are used to describe infants with multiple anomalies and terms have evolved to express causation and pathogenesis.

- A **polytopic field defect** is a pattern of anomalies derived from the disturbance of a single developmental field.
- A **sequence** is a pattern of multiple anomalies derived from a single known or presumed structural defect or mechanical factor.
- A **syndrome** is a pattern of multiple anomalies thought to be pathogenetically related and not known to represent a single sequence or a polytopic field defect.
- An **association** is a nonrandom occurrence in two or more individuals of multiple anomalies not known to be a polytopic field defect, sequence, or syndrome.

Whereas a *sequence* is a pathogenetic and not causal concept, a *syndrome* often implies a single cause, such as trisomy 21 (Down syndrome). In both cases, however, the pattern of anomalies is known or considered to be pathogenetically related. In the case of a sequence, the primary initiating factor and cascade of secondary developmental complications are known. For example, the **Potter sequence**, attributed to oligohydramnios, results from either renal agenesis or leakage of amniotic fluid. An *association*, in contrast, refers to statistically, not pathogenetically or causally, related defects. One or more sequences, syndromes, or field defects may very well constitute an *association* (Jones, 1996; Spranger et al., 1982).

- **Dysmorphology** is an area of clinical genetics that is concerned with the diagnosis and interpretation of patterns of structural defects. "The diagnosis of a malformation syndrome is made on the basis of the overall pattern of anomalies in a patient; however, problems in interpretation may arise because the characteristic abnormalities of any syndrome vary to some extent from patient to patient" (Thompson et al., 1991).

TERATOLOGY—STUDY OF ABNORMAL DEVELOPMENT

Teratology is the branch of science that studies the causes, mechanisms, and patterns of abnormal development. A fundamental concept in teratology is that certain stages of embryonic development are more vulnerable to disruption than others. Until the 1940s it was generally believed that human embryos were protected from environmental agents such as drugs and viruses by their extraembryonic/fetal membranes (amnion and chorion) and their mothers' abdominal and uterine walls. Gregg (1941) presented the first well-

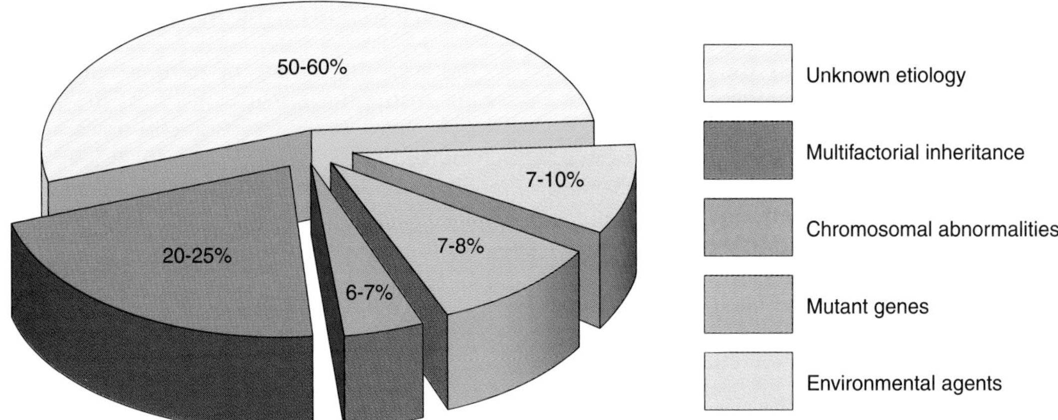

■ **Figure 8–1.** Graphic illustration of the causes of human congenital anomalies. Note that the causes of most anomalies are unknown and that 20 to 25% of them are caused by a combination of genetic and environmental factors (multifactorial inheritance).

documented evidence that an environmental agent (rubella virus) could produce severe developmental disruptions such as cataracts if it was present during the critical period of human development of the eyes, heart, and ears. It was, however, the observations of Lenz (1961) and McBride (1961) that focused attention on the role of drugs in the etiology of human birth defects. They described severe limb anomalies and other developmental disruptions that were caused by **thalidomide** during early pregnancy (see Newman, 1986a; Brent and Holmes, 1988; Kliegman, 1996). It is estimated that 7 to 10% of human birth defects result from the disruptive actions of drugs, viruses, and other environmental factors (Persaud et al., 1985; Persaud, 1990; Thompson et al., 1991). According to data from the *U.S. Centers for Disease Control* in 1989, the leading cause of death for white infants is birth defects.

More than 20% of infant deaths in North America are attributed to birth defects. Major structural anomalies, e.g., spina bifida cystica—a severe type of vertebral defect in which the neural tube fails to fuse—are observed in about 3% of newborn infants. Additional anomalies can be detected after birth; thus, the incidence reaches about 6% in 2-year-olds and 8% in 5-year-olds (Connor and Ferguson-Smith, 1987; Nelson and Holmes, 1989). For the contributions of epidemiology to the study of birth defects (registries, surveillance systems, prevention), see Khoury (1995).

The causes of congenital anomalies are divided into:

- *genetic factors* such as chromosome abnormalities
- *environmental factors* such as drugs and viruses

However, many common congenital anomalies are caused by genetic and environmental factors acting together—**multifactorial inheritance**.

For 50 to 60% of congenital anomalies, the causes are unknown (Fig. 8-1). Congenital anomalies may be single or multiple and of major or minor clinical significance. Single *minor anomalies* are present in about 14% of newborns (Jones, 1997). Anomalies of the external ear, for example, are of no serious medical significance, but they indicate to the clinician the possible presence of associated major anomalies; for example, the presence of a single umbilical artery alerts the clinician to the possible presence of cardiovascular and renal anomalies. Ninety per cent of infants with three or more minor anomalies also have one or more major defects (Connor and Ferguson-Smith, 1987; Jones, 1997). Of the 3% born with clinically significant congenital anomalies, 0.7% have multiple major anomalies. Most of these infants die during infancy. Major developmental defects are much more common in early embryos (10 to 15%), but most of them abort spontaneously during the first 6 weeks. Chromosome abnormalities are present in 50 to 60% of spontaneously aborted conceptuses (Shiota et al., 1987; Shepard et al., 1989; Kaufman, 1991).

ANOMALIES CAUSED BY GENETIC FACTORS*

Numerically, genetic factors are the most important causes of congenital anomalies. It has been estimated that they cause about a third of all birth defects (Fig. 8-1) and nearly 85% of anomalies with known causes. Any mechanism as complex as mitosis or meiosis may occasionally malfunction. *Chromosomal aberrations are common and are present in 6 to 7% of zygotes* (Fig. 8-1). Many of these early embryos never undergo normal cleavage to become blastocysts. *In vitro studies* of cleaving zygotes less than 5 days old have revealed a high incidence of abnormalities. More than 60% of day two cleaving zygotes were found to be abnormal (Winston et al., 1991). Many defective zygotes, blastocysts, and 3-week old embryos abort spontaneously, and the overall frequency of chromosome abnormalities in these embryos is at least 50% (Thompson et al., 1991).

*The authors are grateful to A. E. Chudley, M.D., F.R.C.P.C., F.C.C.M.G., Professor of Pediatrics and Child Health; Head, Section of Genetics and Metabolism, Children's Hospital, Health Sciences Centre, University of Manitoba, Winnipeg, Manitoba, Canada, for assistance with the preparation of this section.

Two kinds of change occur in chromosome complements: numerical and structural. The changes may affect the sex chromosomes and/or the autosomes—chromosomes other than sex chromosomes. In some instances, both kinds of chromosome are affected. Persons with chromosome abnormalities usually have characteristic phenotypes such as the physical characteristics of infants with Down syndrome (Hall, 1996; Jones, 1997). They often look more like other persons with the same chromosome abnormality than their own siblings (brothers or sisters). This characteristic appearance results from genetic imbalance. Genetic factors initiate anomalies by biochemical or other means at the subcellular, cellular, or tissue level. The abnormal mechanisms initiated by the genetic factor may be identical or similar to the causal mechanisms initiated by a teratogen, a drug for example.

Numerical Chromosome Abnormalities

Numerical aberrations of chromosomes usually result from **nondisjunction**, an error in cell division in which there is failure of a chromosome pair or two chromatids of a chromosome to disjoin during mitosis or meiosis. As a result, the chromosome pair or chromatids pass to one daughter cell and the other daughter cell receives neither (Fig. 8-2). Nondisjunction may occur during maternal or paternal gametogenesis (see Chapter 2). The chromosomes in somatic (body) cells are normally paired; the homologous chromosomes making up a pair are *homologs*. Normal human females have 22 pairs of autosomes plus two X chromosomes; whereas, normal males have 22 pairs of autosomes plus one X and one Y chromosome.

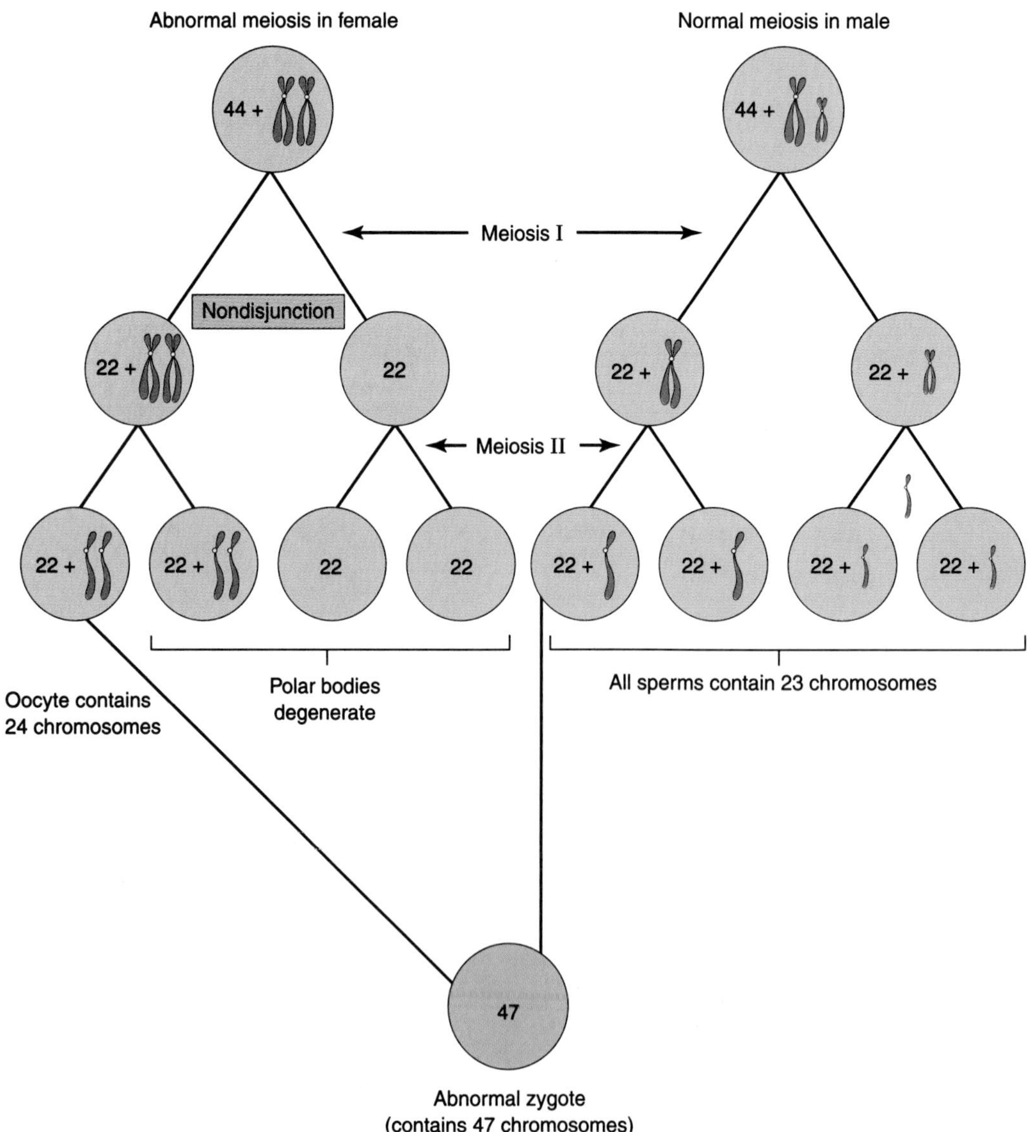

■ **Figure 8-2.** Diagram showing nondisjunction of chromosomes during the first meiotic division of a primary oocyte resulting in an abnormal oocyte with 24 chromosomes. Subsequent fertilization by a normal sperm produces a zygote with 47 chromosomes—aneuploidy—deviation from the human diploid number of 46.

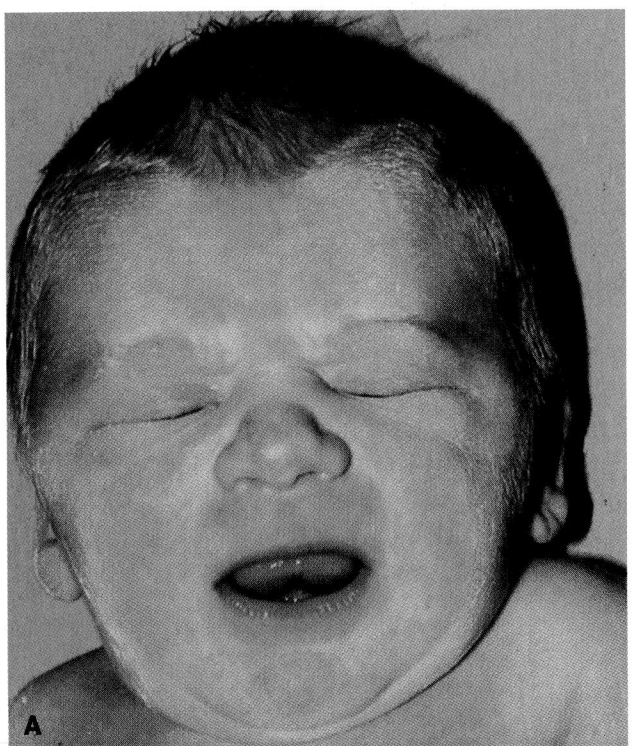

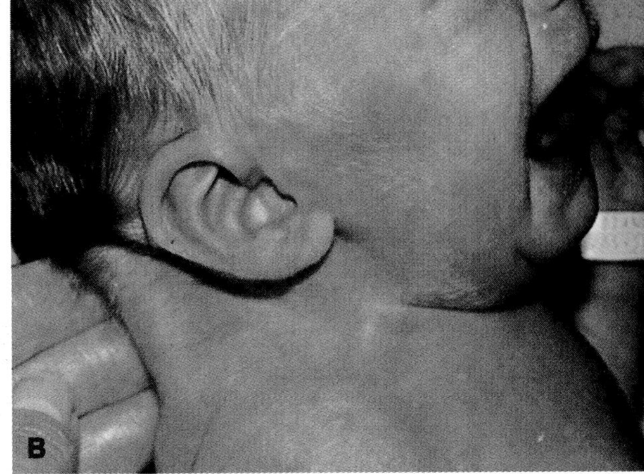

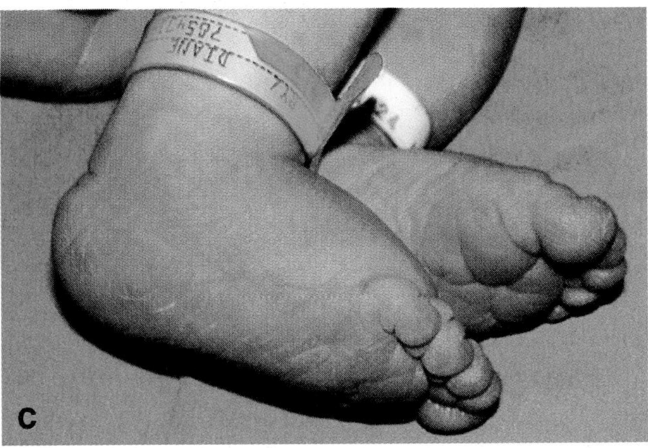

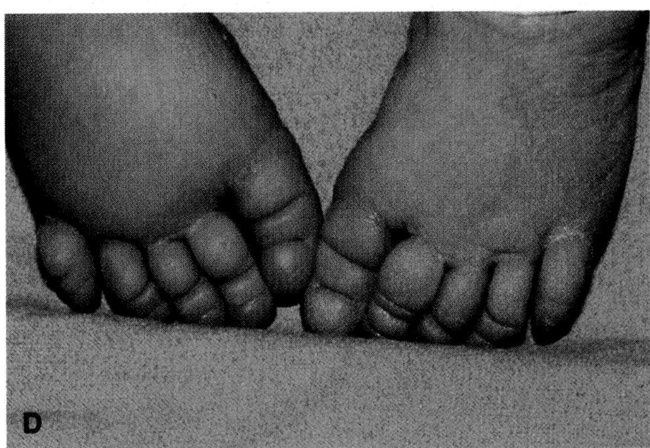

■ **Figure 8–3.** *A,* Face of a female infant with Turner syndrome (45, X). *B,* Lateral view of the infant's head and neck, showing a short neck, prominent ears, and redundant skin at the back of the neck. These infants have defective gonadal development (gonadal dysgenesis). *C,* Photographs of the infant's feet showing the characteristic lymphedema (puffiness and swelling), a useful diagnostic sign. *D,* Lymphedema of the toes, a condition that usually leads to nail hypoplasia. (Courtesy of Dr. AE Chudley, Professor of Pediatrics and Child Health, Children's Hospital, Winnipeg, Manitoba, Canada.)

Inactivation of Genes

During embryogenesis one of the two X chromosomes in female somatic cells is randomly inactivated and appears as a mass of **sex chromatin** (see Chapter 6). Inactivation of genes on one X chromosome in somatic cells of female embryos occurs during implantation (Thompson et al., 1991). *X-inactivation is important clinically* because it means that each cell from a carrier of an X-linked disease has the mutant gene causing the disease, either on the active X chromosome or on the inactivated X chromosome that is represented by sex chromatin. Uneven X-inactivation in monozygotic (MZ) twins is one reason given for discordance for a variety of congenital anomalies. The genetic basis for discordance is that one twin preferentially expresses the paternal X, the other the maternal X.

Aneuploidy and Polyploidy

Changes in chromosome number represent either aneuploidy or polyploidy. **Aneuploidy** is any deviation from the human diploid number of 46 chromosomes.

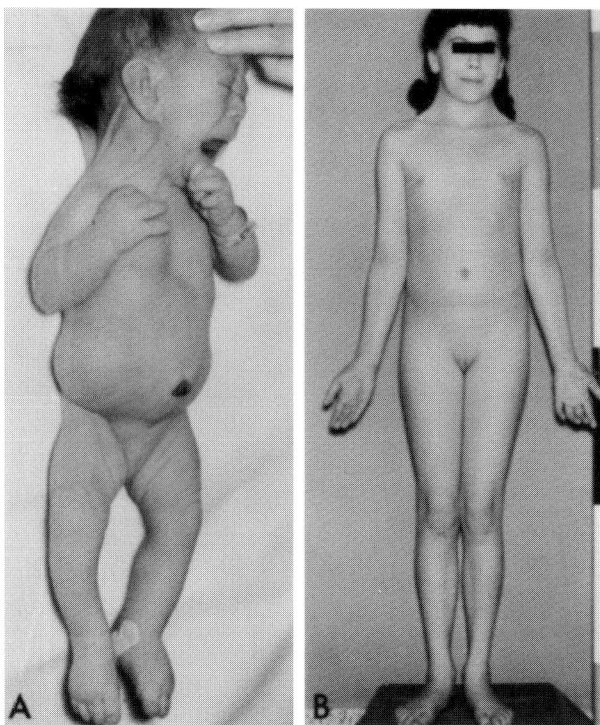

■ **Figure 8-4.** Female individuals with Turner syndrome. *A,* Newborn infant. Note the webbed neck and lymphedema of the hands and feet. *B,* 13-year-old girl showing the classic features of the syndrome in older females: short stature, webbed neck, absence of sexual maturation, and broad, shieldlike chest with widely spaced nipples. (From Moore KL: *The Sex Chromosome.* Philadelphia, WB Saunders, 1966.)

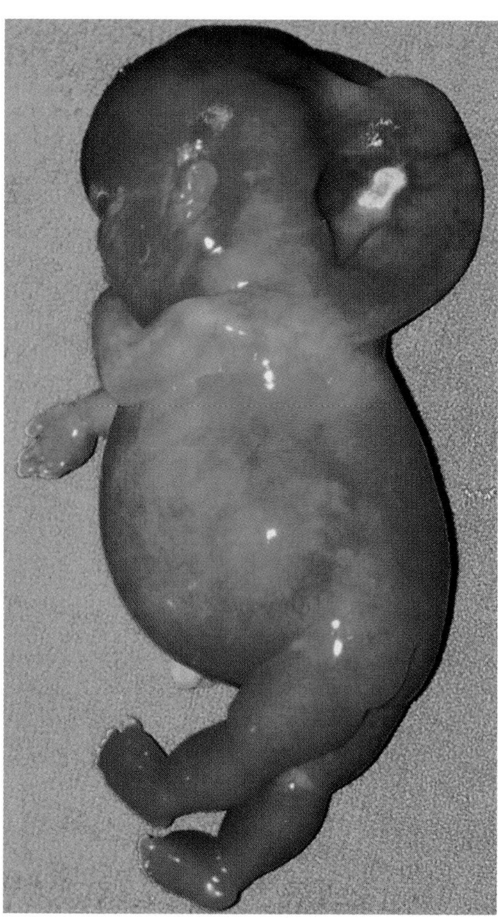

■ **Figure 8-5.** Female fetus (16 weeks) with Turner syndrome; 99% of fetuses with 45, X karyotype are spontaneously aborted. Note the excessive accumulation of watery fluid (hydrops) and the large cystic hygroma (lymphangioma) in the posterior cervical region. The hygroma causes the loose neck skin and webbing seen postnatally (Fig. 8-4). (Courtesy of Dr. AE Chudley, Professor of Pediatrics and Child Health, Children's Hospital, Winnipeg, Manitoba, Canada.)

An *aneuploid* is an individual that has a chromosome number that is not an exact multiple of the haploid number of 23 (e.g., 45 or 47). A polyploid is an individual that has a chromosome number that is a multiple of the haploid number of 23 other than the diploid number (e.g., 69; see Fig. 8-10). The principal cause of aneuploidy is nondisjunction during cell division (Fig. 8-2), resulting in an unequal distribution of one pair of homologous chromosomes to the daughter cells. One cell has two chromosomes and the other has neither chromosome of the pair. As a result, the embryo's cells may be *hypodiploid* (45, X, as in *Turner syndrome* [Fig. 8-3]), or *hyperdiploid* (usually 47, as in trisomy 21 or *Down syndrome* [Fig. 8-4]). Embryos with **monosomy**—missing a chromosome—usually die. About 99% of embryos lacking a sex chromosome (45, X) abort spontaneously (Connor and Ferguson-Smith, 1987).

Table 8-1 ■ **Trisomy of the Autosomes**

Chromosomal Aberration/ Syndrome	Incidence	Usual Clinical Manifestations	Figures
Trisomy 21 or Down syndrome*	1:800	Mental deficiency; brachycephaly, flat nasal bridge; upward slant to palpebral fissures; protruding tongue; simian crease, clinodactyly of 5th digit; congenital heart defects.	8-6
Trisomy 18 syndrome†	1:8000	Mental deficiency; growth retardation; prominent occiput; short sternum; ventricular septal defect; micrognathia; low-set malformed ears; flexed digits, hypoplastic nails; rocker-bottom feet.	8-7
Trisomy 13 syndrome†	1:25,000	Mental deficiency; severe central nervous system malformations; sloping forehead; malformed ears, scalp defects; microphthalmia; bilateral cleft lip and/or palate; polydactyly; posterior prominence of the heels.	8-8

* The importance of this disorder in the overall problem of mental retardation is indicated by the fact that persons with Down syndrome represent 10 to 15% of institutionalized mental defectives (Breg, 1975). *The incidence of trisomy 21 at fertilization is greater than at birth;* however, 75% of embryos are spontaneously aborted and at least 20% are stillborn.

† Infants with this syndrome rarely survive beyond 6 months.

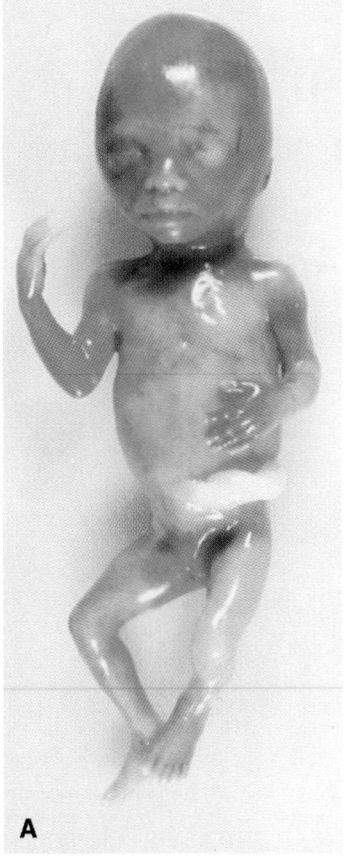

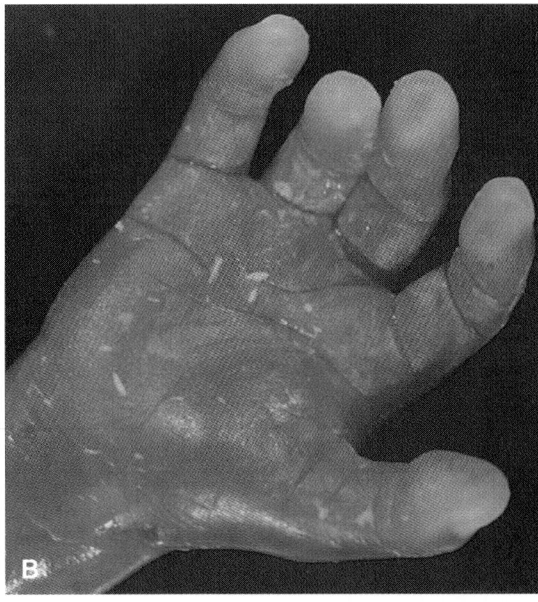

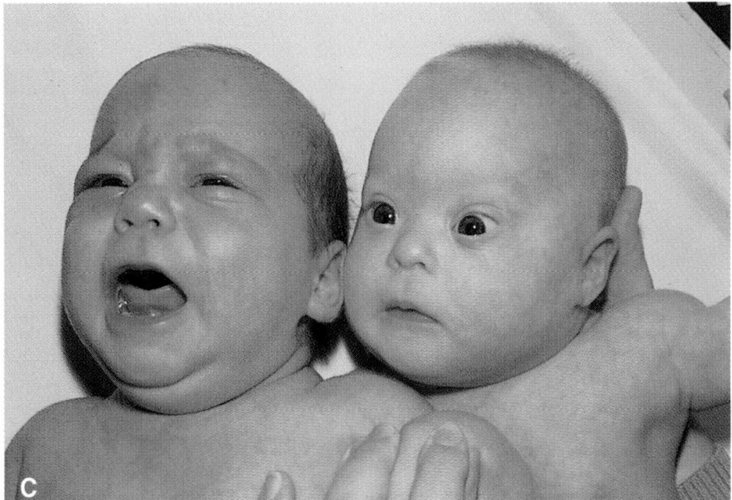

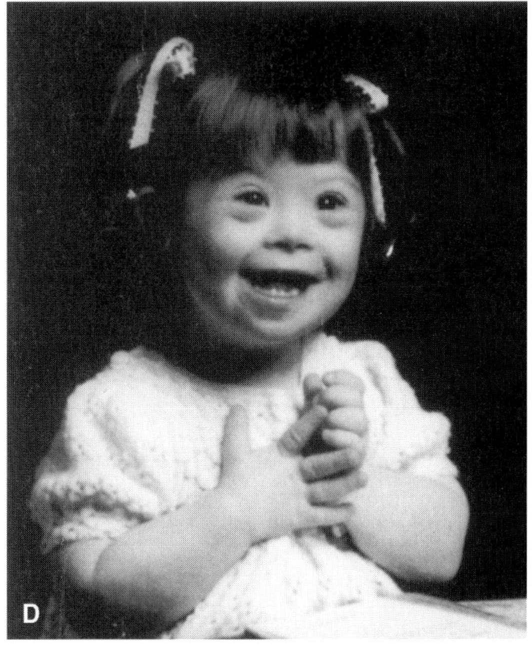

■ **Figure 8–6.** *A,* Anterior view of a female fetus (16.5 weeks) with Down syndrome. *B,* Hand of the fetus. Note the single, transverse palmar, flexion ("simian") crease and the clinodactyly (incurving) of the fifth digit. *C,* Anterior view of the faces of dizygotic male twins that are discordant for Down syndrome (trisomy 21). The one on the right is smaller and hypotonic compared with the unaffected twin. The twin on the right developed from a zygote that contained an extra 21 chromosome. Note the characteristic facial features of Down syndrome in this infant: upslanting, palpebral fissures, epicanthal folds, and flat nasal bridge. *D,* 2½-year-old girl with Down syndrome. (*A,* Courtesy of Dr. DK Kalousek, Professor, Department of Pathology, University of British Columbia, Vancouver, BC, Canada. *B,* Courtesy of Dr. AE Chudley, Professor of Pediatrics and Child Health, Children's Hospital, Winnipeg, Manitoba, Canada.)

TURNER SYNDROME

About 1% of monosomy X female embryos survive. The incidence of 45, X or Turner syndrome in newborn females is approximately one in 8000 livebirths (Hall, 1996). Half the affected individuals have 45, X; the other half have a variety of abnormalities of a sex chromosome. *The phenotype of Turner syndrome is female* and is illustrated in Figures 8-3 and 8-4. Secondary sexual characteristics do not develop in 90% of affected girls and hormonal replacement is required (Hall, 1996). **Phenotype** refers to the morphological characteristics of an individual as determined by the genotype and the environment in which it is expressed (Thompson et al., 1991). The *monosomy X chromosome abnormality* is the most common cytogenetic abnormality observed in liveborn humans and fetuses that abort spontaneously (Fig. 8-5), and it accounts for about 18% of all abortions caused by chromosome abnormalities. The error in gametogenesis (nondisjunction) that causes monosomy X, when it can be traced, is in the paternal gamete in about 75% of cases; i.e., it is the paternal X chromosome that is usually missing. The most frequent chromosome constitution in Turner syndrome is 45, X; however, nearly 50% of these people have other karyotypes (Hook and Warburton, 1983). For the clinical significance of these chromosome constitutions, e.g., a mosaic karyotype of 45, X / 46, XX, see Thompson et al. (1991).

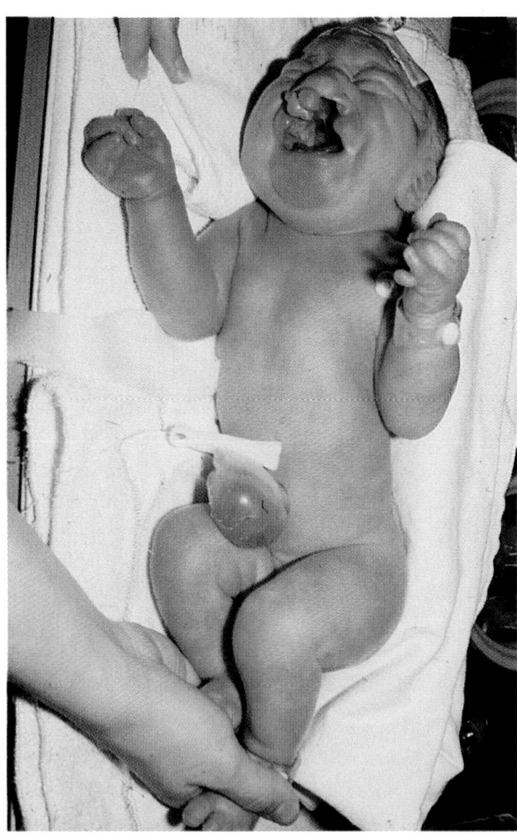

■ **Figure 8–8.** Female neonate with trisomy 13. Note particularly the bilateral cleft lip, low-set malformed ear, and polydactyly (extra digits). A small omphalocele (herniation of viscera into the umbilical cord) is also present. (Courtesy of Dr. AE Chudley, Professor of Pediatrics and Child Health, Children's Hospital, Winnipeg, Manitoba, Canada.)

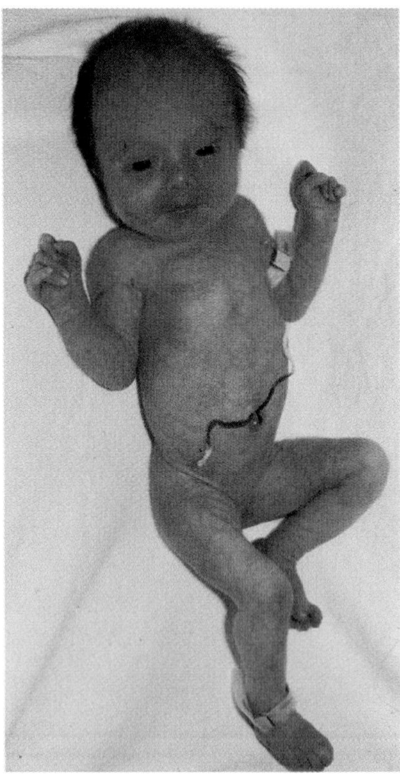

■ **Figure 8–7.** Female neonate with trisomy 18. Note the growth retardation, clenched fists with characteristic positioning of the fingers (second and fifth digits overlapping the third and fourth), short sternum, and narrow pelvis. (Courtesy of Dr. AE Chudley, Professor of Pediatrics and Child Health, Children's Hospital, Winnipeg, Manitoba, Canada.)

TRISOMY OF THE AUTOSOMES

If three chromosomes are present instead of the usual pair, the abnormality is trisomy. Trisomies are the most common abnormalities of chromosome number (Hall, 1996). The usual cause of this numerical error is **meiotic nondisjunction of chromosomes** (Fig. 8-2), resulting in a gamete with 24 instead of 23 chromosomes and subsequently in a zygote with 47 chromosomes. Trisomy of the autosomes is associated with three main syndromes (Table 8-1):

- trisomy 21 or Down syndrome (Fig. 8-6)
- trisomy 18 or Edwards syndrome (Fig. 8-7)
- trisomy 13 or Patau syndrome (Fig. 8-8)

Infants with trisomy 13 and trisomy 18 are severely malformed and mentally retarded and usually die early in infancy. More than half of trisomic conceptions spontaneously abort early.

Trisomy of the autosomes occurs with increasing frequency as maternal age increases; for example, trisomy 21 syndrome occurs once in about 1400 births

Table 8–2 ■ Incidence of Down Syndrome in Newborn Infants

Maternal Age (Years)	Incidence
20-24	1:1400
25-29	1:1100
30-34	1:700
35	1:350
37	1:225
39	1:140
41	1:85
43	1:50
45+	1:25

in mothers aged 20 to 24 years, but once in about 25 births in mothers 45 years and over (Table 8-2). Molecular studies have confirmed that errors in meiosis occur with increasing maternal age. Because of the current trend of increasing maternal age, it has been estimated that by the end of this decade, children born to women older than 34 years will account for 39% of infants with trisomy 21 (Goodwin and Huether, 1987). *Mosaicism*—two or more cell types containing different numbers of chromosomes (normal and abnormal)—leads to a less severe phenotype and the IQ may be nearly normal. For more information on trisomies, see Hall (1996).

TRISOMY OF THE SEX CHROMOSOMES

Trisomy of the sex chromosomes is a common condition (Table 8-3); however, because there are no characteristic physical findings in infants or children, this disorder is not usually detected before puberty (Fig. 8-9). **Sex chromatin studies** were useful in the past in detecting some types of trisomy of the sex chromosomes because two masses of sex chromatin are present in nuclei of XXX females (Moore, 1966), and nuclei of XXY males contain a mass of sex chromatin (see Chapter 6). Today, diagnosis is best achieved by chromosome analysis.

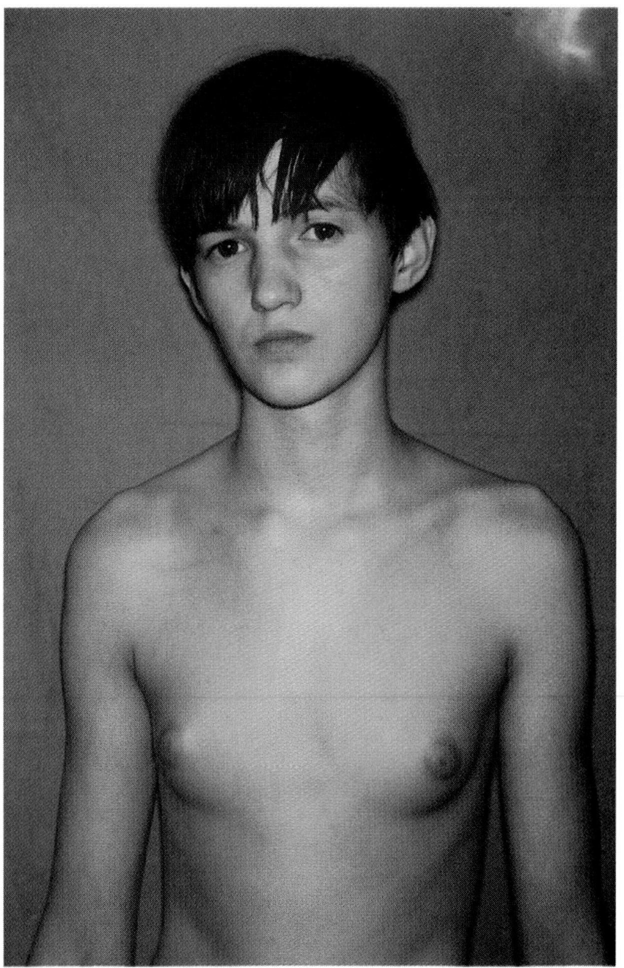

■ **Figure 8–9.** Young male with Klinefelter syndrome (XXY trisomy). Note the presence of breasts; about 40% of males with this syndrome have gynecomastia (excessive development of male mammary glands) and small testes.

Tetrasomy and Pentasomy

Tetrasomy and pentasomy of the sex chromosomes also occur. Persons with these abnormalities have four or five sex chromosomes; the following chromosome complexes have been reported *in females*: 48, XXXX and 49, XXXXX; and *males*: 48, XXXY, 48, XXYY, 49, XXXYY, and 49, XXXXY. The extra sex chromosomes do not accentuate sexual characteristics; however, usually the greater the number of sex chromosomes present, the greater the severity of mental retardation and physical impairment (Neu and Gardner, 1975; Thompson et al., 1991).

Table 8–3 ■ Trisomy of the Sex Chromosomes

Chromosome Complement*	Sex	Incidence†	Usual Characteristics
47, XXX	Female	1:960	Normal in appearance; usually fertile; 15-25% are mildly mentally retarded.
47, XXY	Male	1:1080	Klinefelter syndrome: small testes, hyalinization of seminiferous tubules; aspermatogenesis; often tall with disproportionately long lower limbs. Intelligence is less than in normal siblings. About 40% of these males have gynecomastia (Fig. 8-9).
47, XYY	Male	1:1080	Normal in appearance; usually tall; often exhibit aggressive behavior.

* The numbers designate the total number of chromosomes including the sex chromosomes shown after the comma.

† Data from Hook EB, Hamerton JL: The frequency of chromosome abnormalities detected in consecutive newborn studies—Differences between studies—Results by sex and by severity of phenotypic involvement. *In* Hook EB, Porter IH (eds): *Population Cytogenetics: Studies in Humans.* New York, Academic Press, 1977.

Mosaicism

A person who has at least two cell lines with *two or more different genotypes* (genetic constitutions) is a **mosaic**. Either the autosomes or sex chromosomes may be involved. Usually the anomalies are less serious than in persons with monosomy or trisomy; e.g., the features of Turner syndrome are not as evident in 45, X / 46, XX mosaic females as in the usual 45, X females (Thompson et al., 1991). Mosaicism usually results from nondisjunction during early cleavage of the zygote (see Chapter 2). Mosaicism resulting from loss of a chromosome by *anaphase lagging* also occurs; the chromosomes separate normally but one of them is delayed in its migration and is eventually lost.

Triploidy

The most common type of polyploidy is **triploidy** (69 chromosomes). Triploid fetuses have severe intrauterine growth retardation with a disproportionately small trunk (Fig. 8-10). Several other anomalies are common. Triploidy could result from the second polar body failing to separate from the oocyte during the second meiotic division (see Chapter 2); but more likely, triploidy results when an oocyte is fertilized by two sperms (dispermy) almost simultaneously (Crane, 1994). Triploidy occurs in about 2% of embryos but most of them abort spontaneously. Triploid fetuses account for about 20% of chromosomally abnormal miscarriages. Although *triploid fetuses* have been born alive, this is exceptional (Crane, 1994). These infants all died within a few days because of multiple anomalies and low birth weight (Connor and Ferguson-Smith, 1987).

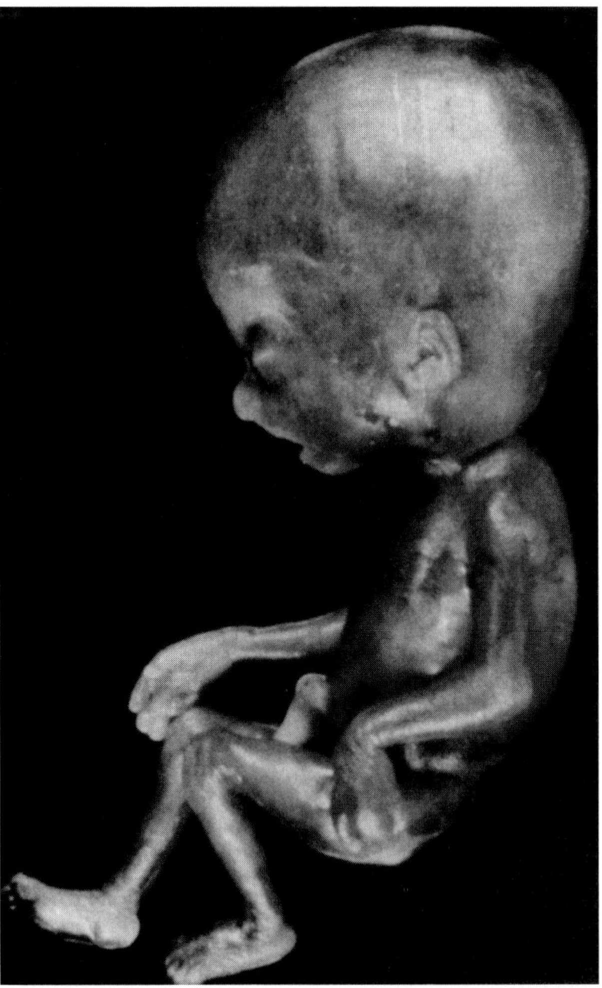

■ **Figure 8-10.** Mid-trimester triploid fetus illustrating severe head-to-body disproportion. Triploidy is characterized by a complete extra set of chromosomes. Triploid fetuses account for nearly 20% of chromosomally abnormal miscarriages. (From Crane JP: Ultrasound evaluation of fetal chromosome disorders. *In* Callen PW [ed]: *Ultrasonography in Obstetrics and Gynecology,* 3rd ed. Philadelphia, WB Saunders, 1994.)

Tetraploidy

Doubling the diploid chromosome number to 92 (*tetraploidy*) probably occurs during the first cleavage division. Division of this abnormal zygote would subsequently result in an embryo with cells containing 92 chromosomes. *Tetraploid embryos* abort very early and often all that is recovered is an empty chorionic sac, which is often referred to as a "blighted embryo" (Carr, 1971; Kaufman, 1991).

Structural Chromosome Abnormalities

Most abnormalities of chromosome structure result from chromosome breakage followed by reconstitution in an abnormal combination (Fig. 8-11). **Chromosome breaks** may be induced by various environmental factors, e.g., radiation, drugs, chemicals, and viruses (Connor and Ferguson-Smith, 1987; Hall, 1996). The resulting type of structural chromosome abnormality depends upon what happens to the broken pieces. The only two aberrations of chromosome structure that are likely to be transmitted from parent to child are structural rearrangements, such as inversion and translocation (Thompson et al., 1991).

TRANSLOCATION

This is the transfer of a piece of one chromosome to a nonhomologous chromosome. If two nonhomologous chromosomes exchange pieces, it is a *reciprocal translocation* (Fig. 8-11*A* and *G*). Translocation does not necessarily cause abnormal development. Persons with a translocation between a number 21 and a number 14 chromosome, for example (Fig. 8-11*G*), are phenotypically normal. Such persons are called *balanced translocation carriers*. They have a tendency, independent of age, to produce germ cells with an abnormal translocation chromosome. Three to four per cent of persons with Down syndrome have translocation trisomies; i.e., the extra 21 chromosome is attached to another chromosome.

DELETION

When a chromosome breaks, a portion of the chromosome may be lost (Fig. 8-11*B*). A partial terminal deletion from the short arm of chromosome 5 causes the **cri du chat syndrome** (Fig. 8-12). Affected infants have a weak catlike cry, microcephaly (abnormally small head), severe mental retardation, and congenital heart disease. A **ring chromosome** is a type of deletion chromosome from which both ends have been lost, and the broken ends have rejoined to form a ring-shaped chromosome (Fig. 8-11*C*). Ring chromosomes are very rare but they have been found for all chromosomes. These abnormal chromosomes have been described in persons with Turner syndrome, trisomy 18, and other abnormalities (Hall, 1996).

Microdeletions and Microduplications

High-resolution banding techniques have allowed detection of very small interstitial and terminal deletions in a number of disorders. Normal resolution chromosome banding reveals 350 bands per haploid set,

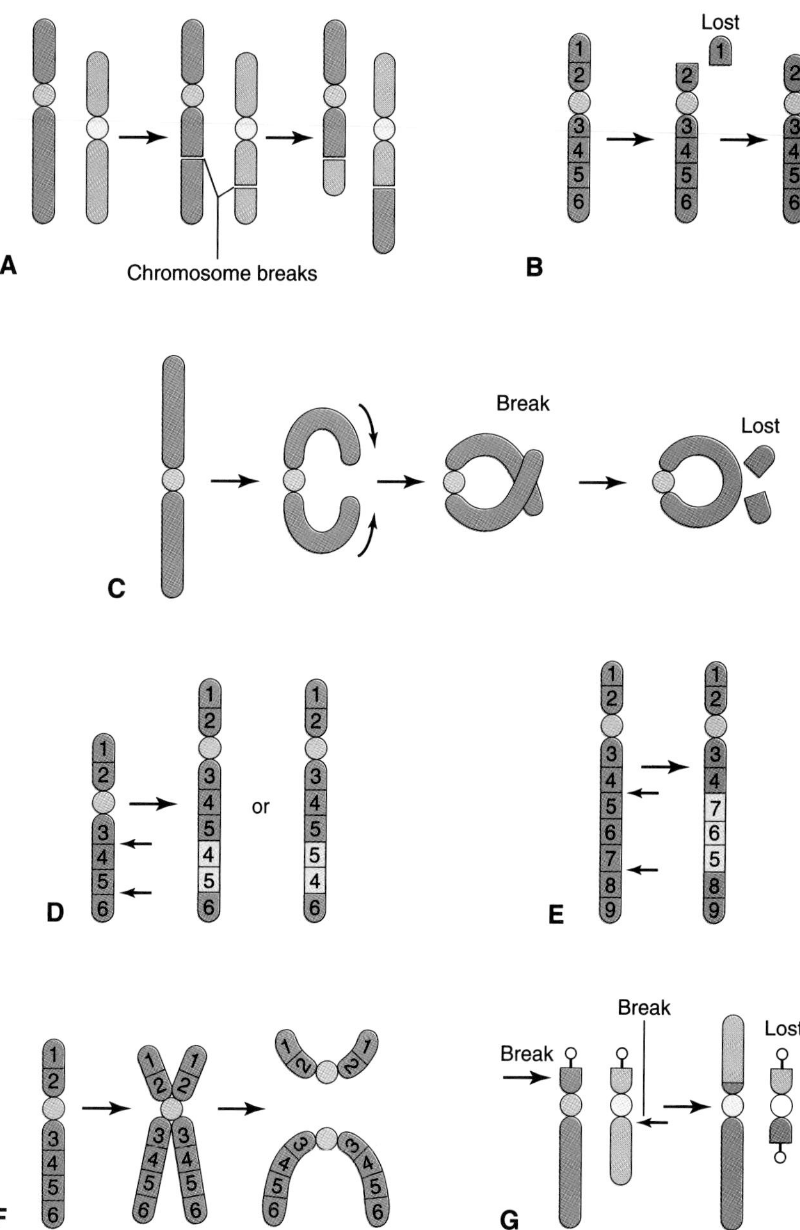

■ **Figure 8-11.** Diagrams illustrating various structural abnormalities of chromosomes. *A,* Reciprocal translocation. *B,* Terminal deletion. *C,* Ring chromosome. *D,* Duplication. *E,* Paracentric inversion. *F,* Isochromosome. *G,* Robertsonian translocation.

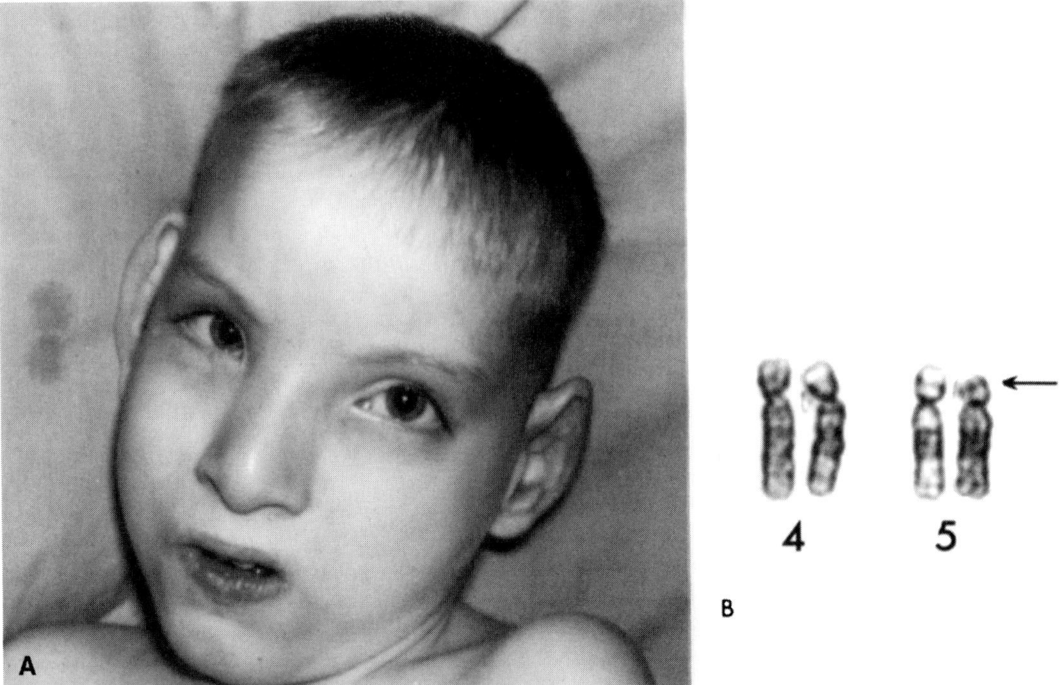

■ **Figure 8–12.** *A,* Male child with cri du chat syndrome. (From Gardner EJ: *Principles of Genetics,* 5th ed. New York, John Wiley & Sons, Inc., 1975.) *B,* Partial karyotype of this child showing a terminal deletion of the short arm (end) of chromosome number 5. The arrow indicates the site of the deletion. (Courtesy of Dr. M Ray, Department of Human Genetics, University of Manitoba, Winnipeg, Canada.)

whereas *high-resolution chromosome banding* reveals up to 1300 bands per haploid set. Because the deletions span several contiguous genes, these disorders, as well as those with microduplications, are referred to as **contiguous gene syndromes** (Table 8–4). Two examples are:

- *Prader-Willi syndrome* (PWS), a sporadically occurring disorder associated with short stature, mild mental retardation, obesity, hyperphagia (overeating), and hypogonadism (inadequate gonadal function).
- *Angelman syndrome* (AS), characterized by severe mental retardation, microcephaly, brachycephaly (shortness of head), seizures, and ataxic (jerky) movements of the limbs and trunk.

Both PWS and AS are often associated with a visible deletion of band q12 on chromosome 15. The clinical phenotype is determined by the parental origin of the deleted chromosome 15. If the deletion arises in the mother, AS occurs; if passed on by the father, the child exhibits the PW phenotype. This suggests the phenomenon of **genetic imprinting** whereby differential expression of genetic material is dependent on the sex of the transmitting parent (Knoll et al., 1989; Kirkilionis et al., 1991).

Table 8–4 ■ Examples of Contiguous Gene Syndromes (Microdeletion or Microduplication Syndromes)

Syndrome	Clinical Features	Chromosome Findings	Parental Origin
Prader-Willi	Hypotonia, hypogonadism, obesity with hyperphagia, distinct face, short stature, small hands and feet, mild developmental delay.	del 15 q12 (most cases)	Paternal
Angelman	Microcephaly, macrosomia, ataxia, excessive laughter, seizures, severe mental retardation.	del 15 q12 (most cases)	Maternal
Miller-Dieker	Type I lissencephaly, dysmorphic face, seizures, severe developmental delay, cardiac anomalies.	del 17 p13.3 (most cases)	Either parent
DiGeorge	Thymic hypoplasia, parathyroid hypoplasia, conotruncal cardiac defects, facial dysmorphism.	del 22 q11 (some cases)	Either parent
Velocardiofacial (Shprintzen)	Palatal defects, hypoplastic alae nasi, long nose, conotruncal cardiac defects, speech delay, learning disorder, schizophreniclike disorder.	del 22 q11 (most cases)	Either parent
Smith-Magenis	Brachycephaly, broad nasal bridge, prominent jaw, short broad hands, speech delay, mental retardation.	del 17 p11.2	Either parent
Williams	Short stature, hypercalcemia, cardiac anomalies, especially supravalvular aortic stenosis, characteristic elfinlike face, mental retardation.	del 17 q11.23 (most cases)	Either parent
Beckwith-Wiedemann (some cases)	Macrosomia, macroglossia, omphalocele, hypoglycemia, hemihypertrophy, transverse ear lobes.	dup 11 p15 (some cases)	Paternal

Molecular Cytogenetics

Several new methods for merging classical cytogenetics with DNA technology have facilitated a more precise definition of chromosome abnormalities, location, or origins, including unbalanced translocations, accessory or marker chromosomes, as well as *gene mapping*. One new approach to chromosome identification is based on *fluorescent in situ hybridization* (FISH), whereby chromosome-specific DNA probes can adhere to complementary regions located on specific chromosomes (Pinkel et al., 1986). This allows improved identification of chromosome location and number in metaphase spreads or even in interphase cells (Manuelidis, 1985). FISH techniques using interphase cells may soon obviate the need to culture cells for specific chromosome analysis, such as in the case of prenatal diagnosis of fetal trisomies.

Duplications

These abnormalities may be represented as a duplicated part of a chromosome, within a chromosome (Fig. 8-11*D*), attached to a chromosome, or as a separate fragment. *Duplications are more common than deletions and they are less harmful* because there is no loss of genetic material. Duplication may involve part of a gene, whole genes, or a series of genes (Thompson et al., 1991).

Inversion

This is a chromosomal aberration in which a segment of a chromosome is reversed. *Paracentric inversion* is confined to a single arm of the chromosome (Fig. 8-11*E*), whereas *pericentric inversion* involves both arms and includes the centromere. Carriers of pericentric inversions are at risk of having offspring with abnormalities because of unequal crossing over and malsegregation at meiosis (Thompson et al., 1991).

Isochromosomes

The abnormality resulting in these chromosomes occurs when the centromere divides transversely instead of longitudinally (Fig. 8-11*E*). An isochromosome is a chromosome in which one arm is missing and the other duplicated. It appears to be the *most common structural abnormality of the X chromosome.* Persons with this chromosomal abnormality are often short in stature and have other stigmata of Turner syndrome. These characteristics are related to the loss of an arm of an X chromosome (Thompson et al., 1991).

Anomalies Caused by Mutant Genes

Seven to 8% of congenital anomalies are caused by gene defects (Fig. 8-1). A mutation usually involves a loss or change in the function of a gene and is any permanent, heritable change in the sequence of genomic DNA (Thompson et al., 1991). Because a random change is unlikely to lead to an improvement in development, *most mutations are deleterious and some are lethal.* The mutation rate can be increased by a number of environmental agents, e.g., large doses of radiation and some chemicals, especially carcinogenic (cancer-inducing) ones. Anomalies resulting from gene mutations are inherited according to mendelian laws; consequently, predictions can be made about the probability of their occurrence in the affected person's children and other relatives.

An example of a dominantly inherited congenital anomaly—**achondroplasia** (Fig. 8-13)—is due to a G to A transition mutation at nucleotide 1138 of the cDNA in the *Fibroblast Growth Factor Receptor 3 (FGFR3) gene* on chromosome 4p. Other congenital anomalies are attributed to *autosomal recessive inheritance,* e.g., congenital adrenal hyperplasia (see Fig. 8-18) and microcephaly. Autosomal recessive

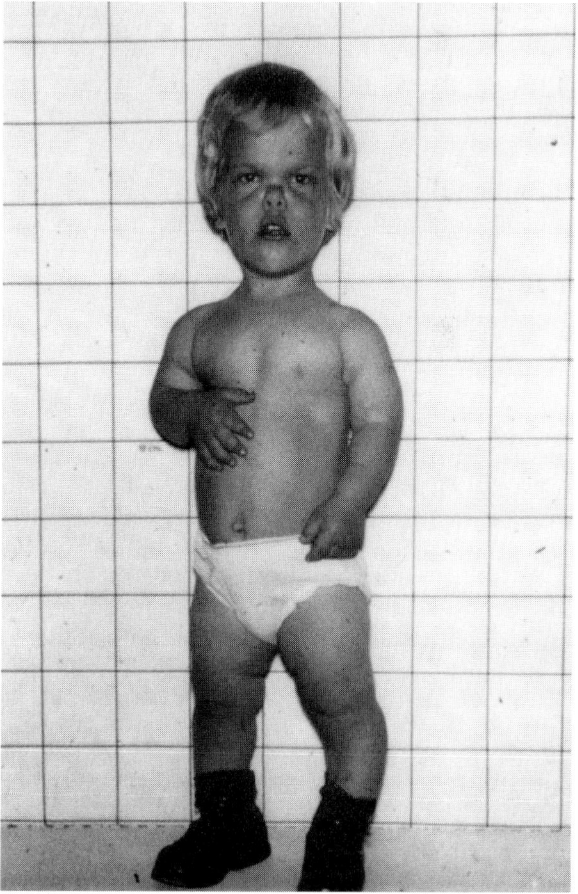

■ **Figure 8-13.** A boy with achondroplasia showing short stature, short limbs and fingers, normal length of the trunk, bowed legs, a relatively large head, prominent forehead, and depressed nasal bridge. (Courtesy of Dr. AE Chudley, Professor of Pediatrics and Child Health, Children's Hospital, Winnipeg, Manitoba, Canada.)

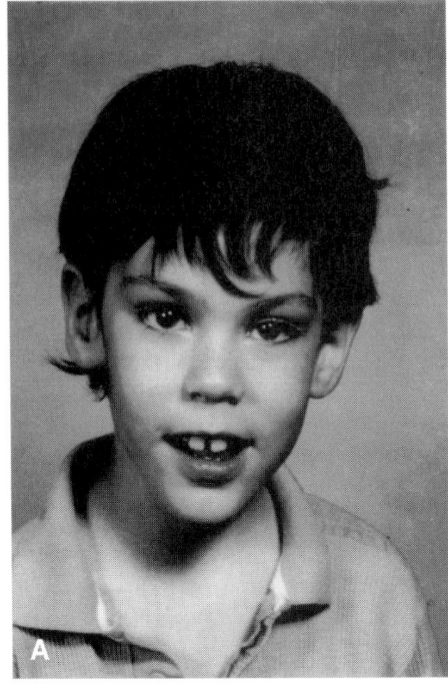

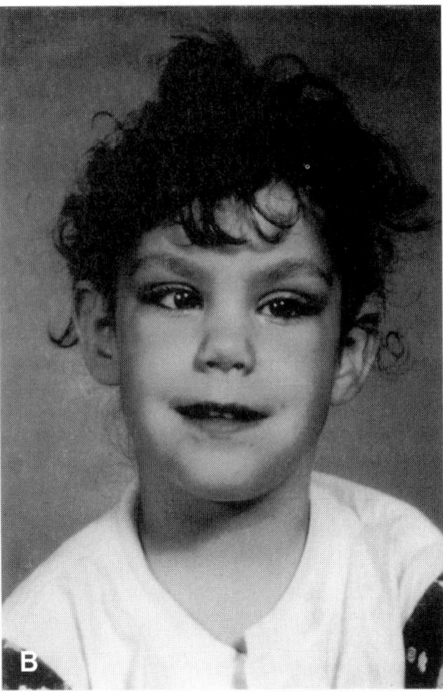

■ **Figure 8–14.** Fragile X syndrome. *A,* An 8-year-old, mentally retarded boy exhibiting a relatively normal appearance with a long face and prominent ears. *B,* His 6-year-old sister also has this syndrome. She has a mild learning disability and similar features of long face and prominent ears. Note the strabismus (crossed right eye). Although an X-linked disorder, sometimes female carriers have expression of the disease. (Courtesy of Dr. AE Chudley, Professor of Pediatrics and Child Health, Children's Hospital, Winnipeg, Manitoba, Canada.)

genes manifest themselves only when homozygous; as a consequence, many carriers of these genes (heterozygous persons) remain undetected.

The **fragile X syndrome** is the most common inherited cause of moderate mental retardation (Fig. 8-14), and is *second only to Down syndrome among all causes of moderate mental retardation in males* (Chudley and Hagerman, 1987; Hall, 1996). The fragile X syndrome has a frequency of 1 in 1500 male births and may account for much of the excess of males in the mentally retarded population (Thompson et al., 1991). The diagnosis can be confirmed by chromosome analysis demonstrating the fragile X chromosome at x927.3, or by DNA studies showing an expression of CGG nucleotides in a specific region of the FMRI gene. Several genetic disorders have been confirmed to be due to expansion of trinucleotides in specific genes. Other examples include myotonic dystrophy, Huntington chorea, spinobulbar atrophy (Kennedy disease), Friedreich ataxia, and others. X-linked recessive genes are usually manifest in affected (hemizygous) males and occasionally in carrier (heterozygous) females, e.g., fragile X syndrome (Chudley and Hagerman, 1987; Heitz et al., 1991).

The **human genome** contains an estimated 50,000 to 100,000 structural genes per haploid set, or three billion base pairs. Many disease-causing genes are being identified because of international collaborations and the Human Genome Project. It is expected that most genetic diseases will be mapped and all genes sequenced by the early part of the twenty-first century. It is plausible that the majority of infants with congenital anomalies of unknown etiology will be determined to result from gene mutations. Molecular analysis has already confirmed this for many disorders.

Genomic imprinting is an epigenetic process whereby the female and male germline confer a sex-specific mark on a chromosome subregion, so that only the paternal or maternal allele of a gene is active in the offspring. In other words, the sex of the transmitting parent will influence expression or nonexpression of certain genes in the offspring (Table 8-4). This is the reason for Prader-Willi syndrome (PWS) and Angelman syndrome (AS), in which case the phenotype is determined by whether the microdeletion is transmitted by the father (PWS) or by the mother (AS). In a substantial number of cases of PWS and AS, as well as several other genetic disorders, the condition

Table 8-5 ■ Examples of Disorders in Humans Associated With Homeobox Mutations

Name	Clinical Features	Gene
Waardenburg Syndrome Type I	White forelock, lateral displacement of inner canthus of the eyes, cochlear deafness, heterochromia, tendency to facial clefting, autosomal dominant inheritance.	HuP2 gene in humans, homolog of Pax3 gene of mouse
Synpolydactyly (Type II syndactyly)	Webbing and duplication of fingers, supernumerary metacarpal, autosomal dominant inheritance.	HOX D 13 mutation
Holoprosencephaly (one form)	Incomplete separation of lateral cerebral ventricles, anophthalmia or cyclopia, midline facial hypoplasia or clefts, single maxillary central incisors, hypotelorism, autosomal dominant inheritance with widely variable expression.	HPE 3 (Sonic Hedgehog) mutation gene which is homologous to the *Drosophila* segment polarity gene hedgehog
Schizencephaly (Type II)	Full-thickness cleft within the cerebral ventricles often leading to seizures, spasticity and mental retardation.	Germline mutation in the EMX2 homeobox gene, homologous to the mouse EMX2

arises from a phenomenon referred to as *uniparental disomy*. In the situation with PWS and AS, both chromosomes 15s originate from only one parent. PWS occurs when both chromosomes 15s are derived from the mother, and AS occurs when both are paternally derived. The mechanism for this is believed to begin with a trisomic conceptus, followed by a loss of the extra chromosome in an early postzygotic cell division. This results in a "rescued" cell, in which both chromosomes have been derived from one parent.

Homeobox genes are a group of genes found in all vertebrates. They have highly conserved sequences and order. They are involved in early embryonic development and specify identity and spatial arrangements of body segments. Protein products of these genes bind to DNA and form transcriptional factors which regulate gene expression. Disorders associated with homeobox mutations are described in Table 8-5.

ANOMALIES CAUSED BY ENVIRONMENTAL FACTORS

Although the human embryo is well protected in the uterus, certain environmental agents—**teratogens**—may cause developmental disruptions following maternal exposure to them (Table 8-6). A teratogen is any

Table 8-6 ■ **Teratogens Known to Cause Human Birth Defects**

Agents	Most Common Congenital Anomalies
Drugs	
Alcohol	*Fetal alcohol syndrome (FAS):* intrauterine growth retardation *(IUGR);* mental retardation, microcephaly; ocular anomalies; joint abnormalities; short palpebral fissures.
Androgens and high doses of progestogens	Varying degrees of masculinization of female fetuses: ambiguous external genitalia resulting in labial fusion and clitoral hypertrophy.
Aminopterin	IUGR; skeletal defects, malformations of the central nervous system (CNS), notably meroanencephaly (most of the brain is absent).
Busulfan	Stunted growth; skeletal abnormalities; corneal opacities; cleft palate; hypoplasia of various organs.
Cocaine	IUGR; microcephaly; cerebral infarction; urogenital anomalies; neurobehavioral disturbances.
Diethystilbesterol	Abnormalities of the uterus and vagina; cervical erosion and ridges.
Isotretinoin (13-cis-retinoic acid)	Craniofacial abnormalities; neural tube defects *(NTDs)*, such as spina bifida cystica; cardiovascular defects.
Lithium carbonate	Various anomalies usually involving the heart and great vessels.
Methotrexate	Multiple anomalies, especially skeletal, involving the face, skull, limbs, and vertebral column.
Phenytoin (Dilantin)	*Fetal hydantoin syndrome (FHS):* IUGR; microcephaly; mental retardation; ridged metopic suture; inner epicanthal folds; eyelid ptosis; broad depressed nasal bridge; phalangeal hypoplasia.
Tetracycline	Stained teeth; hypoplasia of enamel.
Thalidomide	Abnormal development of limbs, e.g., meromelia (partial absence) and amelia (complete absence); facial anomalies; systemic anomalies, e.g., cardiac and kidney defects.
Trimethadione	Developmental delay; V-shaped eyebrows; low-set ears; cleft lip and/or palate.
Valproic acid	Craniofacial anomalies; NTDs; often hydrocephalus; heart and skeletal defects.
Warfarin	Nasal hypoplasia; stippled epiphyses; hypoplastic phalanges; eye anomalies; mental retardation.
Chemicals	
Methylmercury	Cerebral atrophy; spasticity; seizures; mental retardation.
Polychlorinated biphenyls (PCBs)	IUGR; skin discolorization.
Infections	
Cytomegalovirus	Microcephaly; chorioretinitis; sensorineural loss; delayed psychomotor/mental development; hepatosplenomegaly; hydrocephaly; cerebral palsy; brain (periventricular) calcification.
Herpes simplex virus	Skin vesicles and scarring; chorioretinitis; hepatomegaly; thrombocytopenia; petechiae; hemolytic anemia; hydranencephaly.
Human immunodeficiency virus (HIV)	Growth failure; microcephaly; prominent boxlike forehead; flattened nasal bridge; hypertelorism; triangular philtrum and patulous lips.
Human parvovirus B19	Eye defects; degenerative changes in fetal tissues.
Rubella virus	IUGR; postnatal growth retardation; cardiac and great vessel abnormalities; microcephaly; sensorineural deafness; cataract; microphthalmos; glaucoma; pigmented retinopathy; mental retardation; newborn bleeding, hepatosplenomegaly; osteopathy.
Toxoplasma gondii	Microcephaly; mental retardation; microphthalmia; hydrocephaly; chorioretinitis; cerebral calcifications; hearing loss; neurological disturbances.
Treponema pallidum	Hydrocephalus; congenital deafness; mental retardation; abnormal teeth and bones.
Venezuelan equine encephalitis virus	Microcephaly; microphthalmia; cerebral agenesis; CNS necrosis; hydrocephalus.
Varicella virus	Cutaneous scars (dermatome distribution); neurological anomalies (limb paresis, hydrocephaly, seizures, etc.); cataracts; microphthalmia; Horner syndrome; optic atrophy; nystagmus; chorioretinitis; microcephaly; mental retardation; skeletal anomalies (hypoplasia of limbs, fingers, and toes, etc.); urogenital anomalies.
High Levels of Ionizing Radiation	Microcephaly; mental retardation; skeletal anomalies; growth retardation; cataracts.

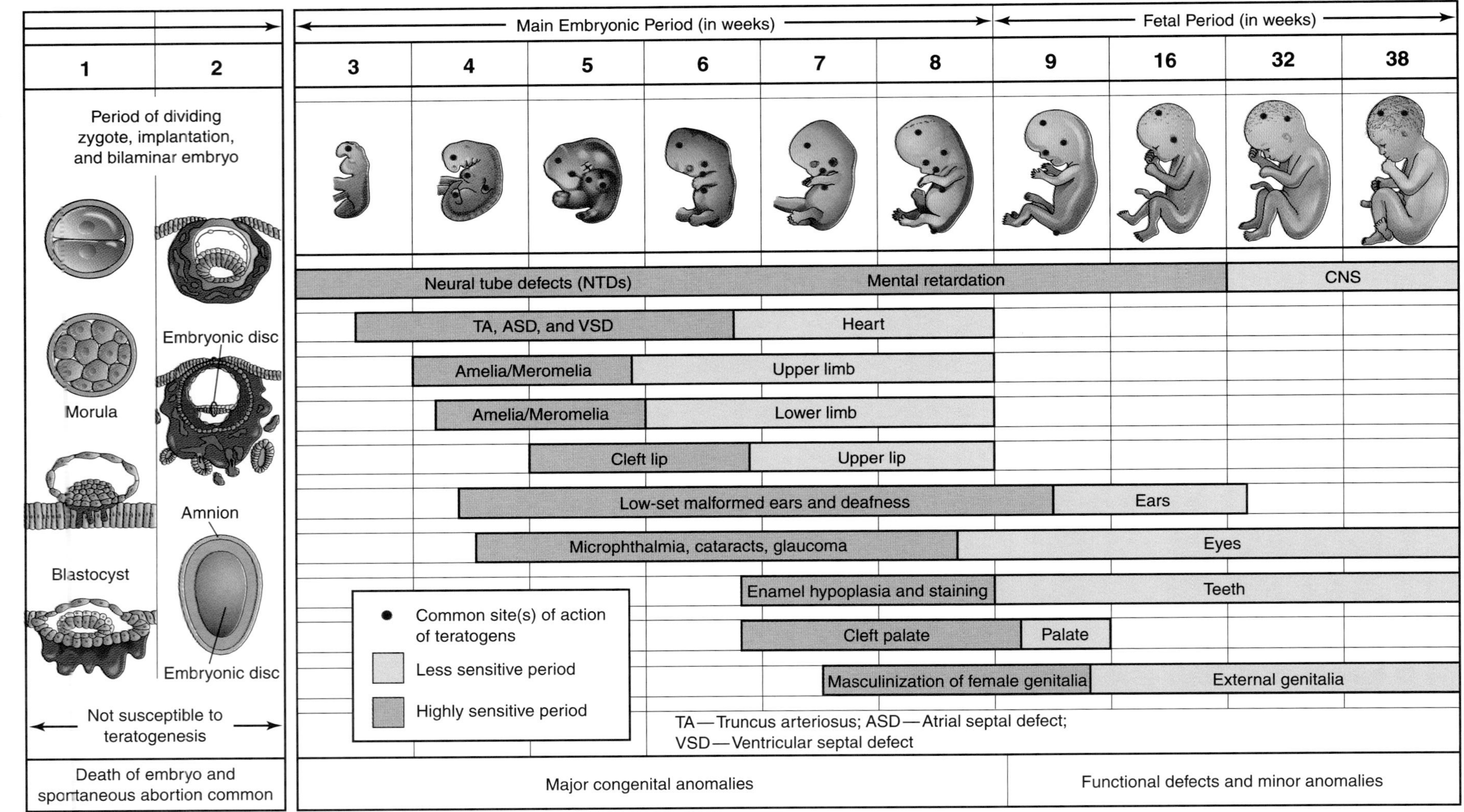

Figure 8–15. Schematic illustration of critical periods in human prenatal development. During the first 2 weeks of development, the embryo is usually not susceptible to teratogens; a teratogen either damages all or most of the cells, resulting in death of the embryo, or damages only a few cells, allowing the conceptus to recover and the embryo to develop without birth defects. *Mauve denotes highly sensitive periods* when major defects may be produced (e.g., amelia, absence of limbs). *Green* indicates stages that are less sensitive to teratogens when minor defects may be induced (e.g., hypoplastic thumbs).

agent that can produce a congenital anomaly or raise the incidence of an anomaly in the population (Persaud, 1990; Kliegman, 1996). Environmental factors, such as infection and drugs, may simulate genetic conditions, e.g., when two or more children of normal parents are affected. The *important principle* is that "not everything that is familial is genetic." The organs and parts of an embryo are most sensitive to teratogenic agents during periods of rapid differentiation (Fig. 8-15).

Environmental factors cause 7 to 10% of congenital anomalies (Fig. 8-1). Because biochemical differentiation precedes morphological differentiation, the period during which structures are sensitive to interference by teratogens often precedes the stage of their visible development by a few days. Teratogens do not appear to be effective in causing anomalies until cellular differentiation has begun; however, their early actions may cause the death of the embryo, e.g., during the first 2 weeks of development. The exact *mechanisms* by which drugs, chemicals, and other environmental factors disrupt embryonic development and induce abnormalities still remain obscure. Even thalidomide's mechanisms of action on the embryo are a "mystery," and more than 20 hypotheses have been postulated to explain how it disrupts development of the embryo (Stephens, 1988; Castella et al., 1996).

Many studies have shown that certain hereditary and environmental influences may adversely affect embryonic development by altering such fundamental processes as the intracellular compartment, surface of the cell, extracellular matrix, and fetal environment. There is no fundamental hypothesis to explain the underlying mechanisms (Persaud et al., 1985). It has been suggested that the initial cellular response may take more than one form (genetic, molecular, biochemical, biophysical), resulting in different sequences of cellular changes (cell death, faulty cellular interaction-induction, reduced biosynthesis of substrates, impaired morphogenetic movements, and mechanical disruption). Eventually these different types of pathological lesion could possibly lead to the final defect (intrauterine death, developmental anomalies, fetal growth retardation, or functional disturbances) through a common pathway (Beckman and Brent, 1984).

Rapid progress in molecular biology is providing more information on the genetic control of differentiation, as well as the cascade of events involved in the expression of homeobox genes and pattern formation. It is reasonable to speculate that disruption of gene activity at any critical stage could lead to a developmental defect. This view is supported by recent experimental studies which showed that exposure of mouse and amphibian embryos to the teratogen *retinoic acid* altered the domain of gene expression and disrupted normal morphogenesis. Researchers are now directing increasing attention to the molecular mechanisms of abnormal development in an attempt to understand the pathogenesis of congenital anomalies better (DeLuca, 1991).

Basic Principles in Teratogenesis

When considering the possible teratogenicity of an agent such as a drug or chemical, *three important principles* must be considered:

- critical periods of development
- dosage of the drug or chemical
- genotype (genetic constitution) of the embryo

CRITICAL PERIODS OF HUMAN DEVELOPMENT

The stage of development of an embryo when an agent, such as a drug or virus, is present determines its susceptibility to a teratogen (Fig. 8-15). The most critical period in development is when cell division, cell differentiation, and morphogenesis are at their peak. Table 8-7 indicates the relative frequencies of anomalies for certain organs. *The most critical period for brain development is from 3 to 16 weeks*, but its development may be disrupted after this because the brain is differentiating and growing rapidly at birth and continues to do so throughout the first 2 years after birth. Teratogens (e.g., alcohol) may produce mental retardation during the embryonic and fetal periods. *Tooth development continues long after birth* (see Chapter 20); hence, development of permanent teeth may be disrupted by *tetracyclines* from 18 weeks (prenatal) to 16 years. *The skeletal system has a prolonged critical period of development* extending into childhood; hence, the growth of skeletal tissues provides a good gauge of general growth.

Environmental disturbances during the first 2 weeks after fertilization may interfere with cleavage of the zygote and implantation of the blastocyst and/or cause early death and spontaneous abortion of the embryo; however, they are not known to cause congenital anomalies in human embryos (Fig. 8-15). Teratogens acting during the first 2 weeks either kill the embryo or their disruptive effects are compensated for by powerful regulatory properties of the early embryo (Carlson, 1994). Most development during the first 2 weeks is concerned with the formation of extraembryonic structures such as the amnion, yolk sac, and chorionic sac (see Chapter 3); however, the early embryo also develops.

Development of the embryo is most easily disrupted when the tissues and organs are forming

Table 8-7 ■ Incidence of Major Anomalies in Human Organs at Birth*

Organ	Incidence
Brain	10:1000
Heart	8:1000
Kidneys	4:1000
Limbs	2:1000
All other	6:1000
Total	30:1000

* Data from Connor JM, Ferguson-Smith MA: *Essential Medical Genetics,* 2nd ed. Oxford, Blackwell Scientific Publications, 1987.

(Figs. 8-15 and 8-16). During this **organogenetic period**, teratogenic agents may induce major congenital anomalies. Physiological defects, minor morphological anomalies of the external ear for example, and functional disturbances such as mental retardation are likely to result from disruption of development during the fetal period. Some microorganisms, ***Toxoplasma gondii*** for example, are known to cause serious congenital anomalies, particularly of the brain and eyes, when they infect the fetus (see Figs. 8-24 and 8-25; Table 8-6). If present during the embryonic period, microorganisms often kill the embryo.

Each part, tissue, and organ of an embryo has a critical period during which its development may be disrupted (Fig. 8-15). The type of congenital anomalies produced depends on which parts, tissues, and organs are most susceptible at the time the teratogen is active. The following examples illustrate that teratogens may affect different organ systems that are developing at the same time:

- *High levels of radiation* produce anomalies of the central nervous system and eyes.
- *The rubella virus* causes eye defects (glaucoma and cataracts), deafness, and cardiac anomalies.
- *Thalidomide* induces limb defects and several other anomalies. Early in the critical period of limb development, it causes severe limb defects such as *meromelia*—absence of part of the upper and/or lower limbs (see Fig. 8-22). Later in the sensitive period, thalidomide causes mild to moderate limb defects, e.g., hypoplasia of radius and ulna. There is no clinical evidence that thalidomide was capable of damaging the embryo when it was administered after the critical period of development (Newman, 1986a).

Embryological timetables, shown in Figure 8-15, are helpful when considering the cause of human birth defects; however, it is wrong to assume that anomalies always result from a single event occurring during the critical period, or that one can determine from these tables the day on which the anomaly was produced. All one can state is that the teratogen would have had to disrupt development before the end of the critical period of the tissue, part, or organ concerned. *The critical period for limb development, for example, is 24 to 36 days after fertilization.*

DOSAGE OF THE DRUG OR CHEMICAL

Animal research has shown that there is a dose-response relationship for teratogens; however, *the dose used in animals to produce anomalies is often at levels much higher than human exposures. Consequently, animal studies are not readily applicable to human pregnancies.* For a drug to be considered a human teratogen, a dose-response relationship has to be observed; i.e., the greater the exposure during pregnancy, the more severe the phenotypic effect.

GENOTYPE OF THE EMBRYO

There are numerous examples in experimental animals and several suspected cases in humans that show that there are genetic differences in response to a teratogen. *Phenytoin*, for example, is a well-known human teratogen (Table 8-6). Five to 10% of embryos exposed to this anticonvulsant medication develop the *fetal hydantoin syndrome* (see Fig. 8-19). About one-third of exposed embryos, however, have only some congenital anomalies, and more than half of the embryos are unaffected. It appears, therefore, that the genotype of the embryo determines whether a teratogenic agent will disrupt its development.

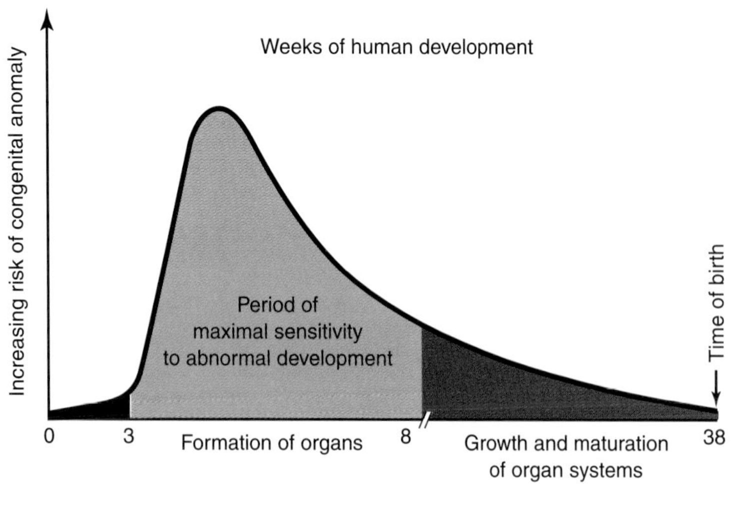

■ **Figure 8-16.** Schematic illustration showing the increasing risk of congenital anomalies developing during organogenesis.

Known Human Teratogens

Awareness that certain agents can disrupt human prenatal development offers the opportunity to prevent some congenital anomalies; for example, if women are aware of the harmful effects of drugs such as alcohol, environmental chemicals (e.g., polychlorinated biphenyls [PCBs]), and viruses, most of them will not expose their embryos to these teratogenic agents. The general objective of teratogenicity testing of drugs, chemicals, food additives, and pesticides is to identify agents that may be teratogenic during human development and to alert physicians and pregnant women of their possible danger to the embryo/fetus.

Proof of Teratogenicity

To prove that an agent is a teratogen, one must show either that the frequency of anomalies is increased above the spontaneous rate in pregnancies in which the mother is exposed to the agent (*the prospective approach*), or that malformed infants have a history of maternal exposure to the agent more often than normal children (*the retrospective approach*). Both types of data are difficult to obtain in an unbiased form (Shepard, 1994). *Case reports are not convincing* unless both the agent and type of anomaly are so uncommon that their association in several cases can be judged not coincidental (e.g., thalidomide).

Drug Testing in Animals

Although testing of drugs in pregnant animals is important, the results are of limited value for predicting drug effects on human embryos. *Animal experiments can suggest only that similar effects may occur in humans.* If a drug or chemical produces teratogenic effects in two or more species, the probability of potential human hazard must be considered to be high; however, the dosage of the drug has to be considered.

DRUGS AS TERATOGENS

Drugs vary considerably in their teratogenicity. Some teratogens such as thalidomide cause severe disruption of development if administered during the organogenetic period of certain parts of the embryo (e.g., thalidomide and limb development). Other teratogens cause mental and growth retardation and other anomalies if used excessively throughout development (e.g., alcohol). *The use of prescription and nonprescription drugs during pregnancy is surprisingly high.* From 40 to 90% of pregnant women consume at least one drug during pregnancy. Several studies have indicated that some pregnant women take an average of four drugs, excluding nutritional supplements, and about half of these women take them during the first trimester. Drug consumption also tends to be higher during the critical period of development among heavy smokers and drinkers (Persaud, 1990). Despite this, *less than 2% of congenital anomalies are caused by drugs and chemicals* (Brent, 1986a). Only a few drugs have been positively implicated as human teratogenic agents (Table 8-6).

While only 7 to 10% of anomalies are caused by recognizable teratogens (Fig. 8-1; Table 8-6), new agents continue to be identified (Behrman et al., 1996). It is best for women to avoid using all medication during the first trimester, unless there is a strong medical reason for its use, and then only if it is recognized as reasonably safe for the human embryo. The reason for this caution is that, even though well-controlled studies of certain drugs (e.g., *marijuana*) have failed to demonstrate a teratogenic risk to human embryos, it does harm the embryo; i.e., it causes a decrease in birth weight.

Cigarette Smoking. *Maternal smoking is a well-established cause of intrauterine growth retardation (IUGR).* Despite warnings that cigarette smoking is harmful to the fetus, more than 25% of women continue to smoke during their pregnancies. In heavy cigarette smokers (20 or more per day), premature delivery is twice as frequent as in mothers who do not smoke, and their infants weigh less than normal (see Fig. 6-12). *Low birth weight (below 2000 gm) is the chief predictor of infant death.* In a case-control study, there was a modest increase in the incidence of infants with conotruncal heart defects and limb deficiencies associated with both maternal and paternal smoking (Wasserman et al., 1996). Moreover there is some evidence that maternal smoking may cause urinary tract anomalies (Li et al., 1996), behavioral problems, and decreased physical growth (Milberger et al., 1996).

Nicotine constricts uterine blood vessels, causing a decrease in uterine blood flow, lowering the supply of oxygen and nutrients available to the embryo/fetus from the maternal blood in the intervillous space of the placenta. The resulting deficiency in the embryo impairs cell growth and may have an adverse effect on mental development. High levels of *carboxyhemoglobin*, resulting from cigarette smoking, appear in the maternal and fetal blood and may alter the capacity of the blood to transport oxygen. As a result, chronic *fetal hypoxia* (decrease below normal oxygen levels) may occur and affect fetal growth and development (Nash and Persaud, 1988a).

Caffeine. Caffeine is the most popular drug in North America because it is present in several widely consumed beverages (e.g., coffee, tea, and cola drinks), chocolate products, and some drugs. *Caffeine is not known to be a human teratogen* (Nash and Persaud, 1988b; Barr and Streissguth, 1991); however, there is no assurance that heavy maternal consumption of it is safe for the embryo.

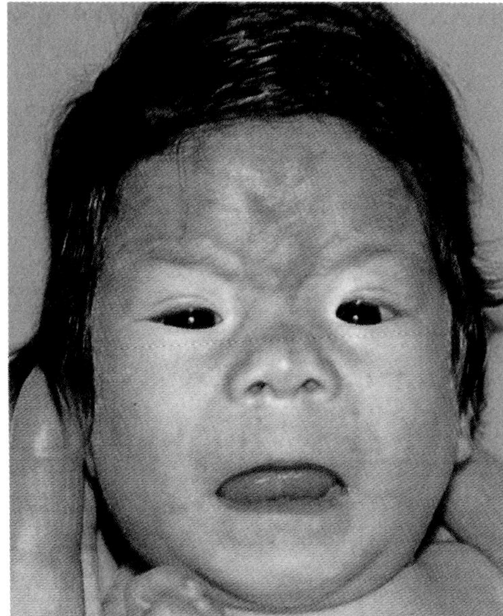

■ **Figure 8–17.** Infant with the fetal alcohol syndrome. Note the thin upper lip, short palpebral fissures, flat nasal bridge, short nose, and elongated and poorly formed philtrum (vertical groove in medial part of upper lip). Maternal alcohol abuse is thought to be the most common environmental cause of mental retardation. (Courtesy of Dr. AE Chudley, Professor of Pediatrics and Child Health, Children's Hospital, Winnipeg, Manitoba, Canada.)

Alcohol. Alcoholism is a drug abuse problem that affects 1 to 2% of women of childbearing age. Both moderate and high levels of alcohol intake during early pregnancy may result in alterations in growth and morphogenesis of the fetus (Behrman et al., 1996); the greater the intake, the more severe the signs. Infants born to chronic alcoholic mothers exhibit a specific pattern of defects (Persaud, 1988, 1990; Aase, 1994), including prenatal and postnatal growth deficiency, mental retardation, and other anomalies (Fig. 8-17; Table 8-6). Microcephaly, short palpebral fissures, epicanthal folds, maxillary hypoplasia, short nose, thin upper lip, abnormal palmar creases, joint anomalies, and congenital heart disease are also present in most infants. This pattern of anomalies—**the fetal alcohol syndrome (FAS)**—is detected in 1 to 2 infants/1000 livebirths (Behrman et al., 1996). The incidence of FAS is related to the population studied. Clinical experience is often necessary in order to make an accurate diagnosis of FAS because the physical anomalies in affected children are nonspecific. Nonetheless, the overall pattern of clinical features present is unique, but may vary from subtle to severe (Aase, 1994).

Maternal alcohol abuse is now thought to be the most common cause of mental retardation. Even moderate maternal alcohol consumption (e.g., 1 to 2 ounces per day) may produce **fetal alcohol effects (FAE)**, children with behavioral and learning difficulties, for example, especially if the drinking is associated with malnutrition. *Binge drinking* (heavy consumption of alcohol for 1 to 3 days during pregnancy) is very likely to produce FAE. The susceptible period of brain development spans the major part of gestation; therefore, the safest advice is total abstinence from alcohol during pregnancy (Hankin, 1994).

Androgens and Progestogens. The terms "progestogens" and "progestins" are used for substances, natural or synthetic, that induce some or all the biological changes produced by progesterone, a hormone secreted by the corpus luteum that promotes and maintains a gravid endometrium (see Chapter 7). Some of these substances have androgenic or masculinizing properties that may affect the female fetus, producing masculinization of the external genitalia (Fig. 8-18). The incidence of anomalies varies with the hormone and the dosage. Preparations that should be avoided are the progestins *ethisterone* and *norethisterone.* From a practical standpoint, the teratogenic risk of these hormones is low (Jones, 1997; Persaud, 1990). Progestin exposure during the critical period of development is also associated with an increased prevalence of cardiovascular abnormalities, and exposure of male fetuses during this period may double the incidence of *hypospadias* in the newborn (see Chapter 13). Obviously, the administration of *testosterone* will also produce masculinizing effects in female fetuses.

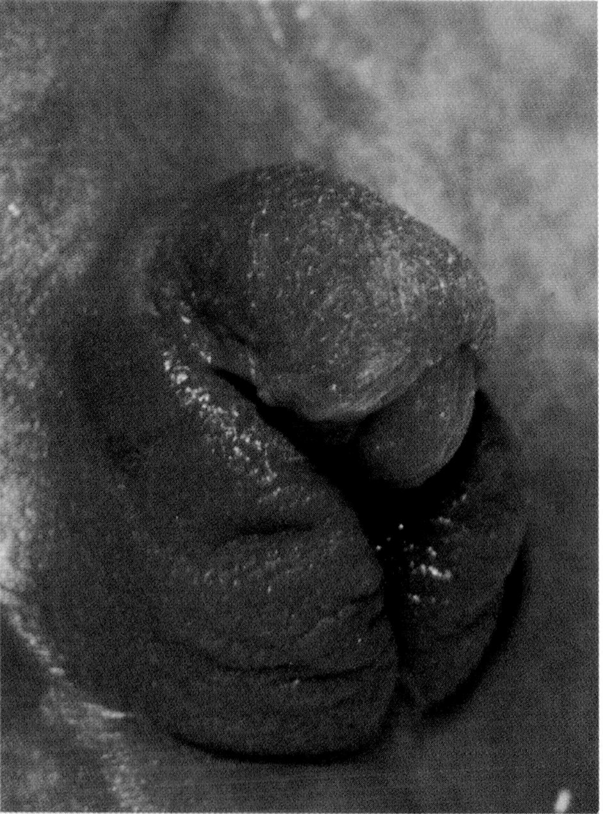

■ **Figure 8–18.** Masculinized external genitalia of a 46,XX female infant. Observe the enlarged clitoris and fused labia majora. Just below the clitoris, there is a single orifice of a urogenital sinus. The virilization was caused by excessive androgens produced by the suprarenal (adrenal) glands during the fetal period (congenital adrenal hyperplasia). (Courtesy of Dr. Heather Dean, M.D., Department of Pediatrics and Child Health, University of Manitoba, Winnipeg, Canada.)

Many women use contraceptive hormones —"birth control pills" (Forrest and Fordyce, 1988). *Oral contraceptives* containing progestogens and estrogens, taken during the early stages of an unrecognized pregnancy, are suspected of being teratogenic agents, but the results of several recent epidemiological studies are conflicting (Persaud, 1990). The infants of 13 of 19 mothers who had taken *progestogen-estrogen birth control pills* during the critical period of development exhibited the VACTERL syndrome (Nora and Nora, 1975). The acronym VACTERL stands for **v**ertebral, **a**nal, **c**ardiac, **t**rachea, **e**sophageal, **r**enal, and **l**imb anomalies. As a precaution, use of oral contraceptives should be stopped as soon as pregnancy is detected because of these possible teratogenic effects.

Diethylstilbestrol (DES) (stilbestrol) is a human teratogen. Both gross and microscopic congenital abnormalities of the uterus and vagina have been detected in women who were exposed to diethylstilbestrol *in utero* (Ulfelder, 1986). Three types of lesion were observed: vaginal adenosis, cervical erosions, and transverse vaginal ridges. A number of young women aged 16 to 22 years have developed *adenocarcinoma of the vagina* after a common history of exposure to the synthetic estrogen *in utero* (Herbst et al., 1974; Hart et al., 1976). However, the probability of cancers developing at this early age in females exposed to DES *in utero* now appears to be low. The risk of cancer from DES exposure in utero is estimated to be less than 1 in 1000 (Ulfelder, 1986); for more information see Mittendorf (1995). Males who were exposed to DES *in utero*, following maternal treatment before the eleventh week of gestation, had a higher incidence of genital tract anomalies, including epididymal cysts and hypoplastic testes. However, fertility in the men exposed to DES *in utero* seems to be unaffected (Wilcox et al., 1995).

Antibiotics. Tetracyclines cross the placental membrane and are deposited in the embryo's bones and teeth at sites of active calcification. As little as 1 gm per day of **tetracycline** during the third trimester of pregnancy can produce yellow staining of the primary and/or deciduous teeth (Cohlan, 1986). Tetracycline therapy during the fourth to tenth months of pregnancy may also cause tooth defects (e.g., enamel hypoplasia), yellow to brown discoloration of the teeth, and diminished growth of long bones. Calcification of the secondary (permanent) teeth begins at birth and, except for the third molars, is complete by 7 to 8 years of age; hence, long-term tetracycline therapy during childhood can affect the permanent teeth.

Deafness has been reported in infants of mothers who have been treated with high doses of streptomycin and dihydrostreptomycin as *antituberculosis agents*. More than 30 cases of hearing deficit and eighth cranial nerve damage have been reported in infants exposed to **streptomycin derivatives** in utero (Ganguin and Rempt, 1970; Warkany, 1986). *Penicillin* has been used extensively during pregnancy and appears to be harmless to the human embryo and fetus. *Acetohydroxamic acid* can be used for the treatment of chronic cervicitis resulting from a chronic infection with *Ureaplasma urealyticum*. Although no case of human teratogenicity involving hydroxamic acid has been reported, it is recommended that this antibiotic not be used during pregnancy because it is potentially a human teratogen (Holmes, 1996).

Anticoagulants. All anticoagulants except heparin cross the placental membrane and may cause hemorrhage in the embryo or fetus. Warfarin and other coumarin derivatives are antagonists of vitamin K. Warfarin is used for the treatment of thromboembolitic disease and for patients with artificial heart valves. **Warfarin is definitely a teratogen**. There are reports of infants with hypoplasia of the nasal cartilage, stippled epiphyses, and various central nervous system defects whose mothers took this anticoagulant during the critical period of their embryo's development (Holzgreve et al., 1976). The period of greatest sensitivity is between 6 and 12 weeks after fertilization—8 to 14 weeks after last normal menstrual period (LNMP) (Behrman et al., 1996). Second- and third-trimester exposure may result in mental retardation, optic atrophy, and microcephaly. **Heparin is not a teratogen**. Furthermore, it does not cross the placental membrane and so is the drug of choice for pregnant women requiring anticoagulant therapy (Turrentine et al., 1995).

Anticonvulsants. Approximately 1 of 200 pregnant women is epileptic and requires treatment with an anticonvulsant. Of the anticonvulsant drugs available, there is strong evidence that **trimethadione** (Tridione) is a teratogen (Goldman et al., 1986). The main features of the *fetal trimethadione syndrome* are prenatal and postnatal growth retardation, developmental delay, V-shaped eyebrows, low-set ears, cleft lip and/or palate, and cardiac, genitourinary, and limb defects. Use of this drug is contraindicated during pregnancy (Paulson and Paulson, 1990). **Phenytoin (Dilantin, Novophenytoin) is definitely a teratogen** (Fig. 8-19). The *fetal hydantoin syndrome* occurs in 5 to 10% of children born to mothers treated with phenytoins or hydantoin anticonvulsants. The usual pattern of anomalies consists of intrauterine growth retardation (IUGR), microcephaly, mental retardation, ridged metopic (frontal) suture, inner epicanthal folds, eyelid ptosis, broad depressed nasal bridge, nail and/or distal phalangeal hypoplasia, and hernias (Hanson, 1986; Chodirker et al., 1987; Behrman et al., 1996).

Valproic acid has been the drug of choice for the management of different types of epilepsy; however, its use by pregnant women has led to a *pattern of anomalies* consisting of craniofacial, heart, and limb defects. There is also an increased risk of neural tube defects (Paulson and Paulson, 1990; Kliegman, 1996). *Phenobarbital is considered to be a safe, antiepileptic drug for use during pregnancy* (Persaud, 1990). Magnesium sulfate and diazepam are also widely used for seizure prophylaxis; however, more controlled clinical trials are required to establish whether these combinations are free of teratogenic risks.

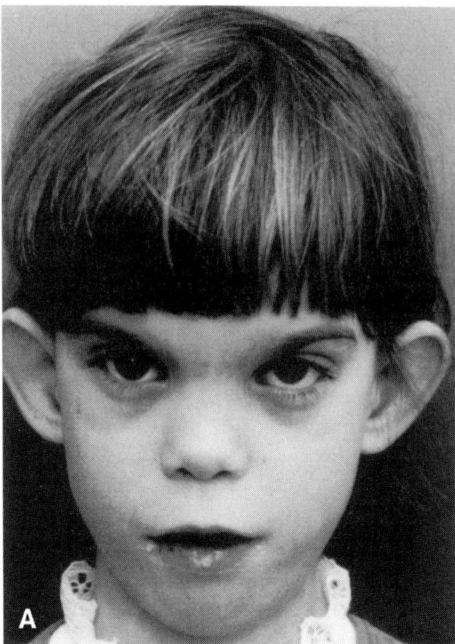

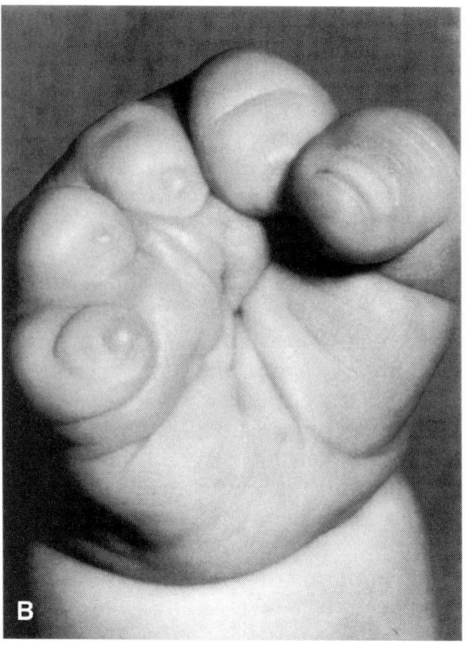

■ **Figure 8–19.** Fetal hydantoin syndrome. *A,* This young girl has a learning disability. Note the unusual ears, wide space between the eyes, epicanthal folds, short nose, and long philtrum. Her mother has epilepsy and took Dilantin throughout her pregnancy. (Courtesy of Dr. AE Chudley, Professor of Pediatrics and Child Health, Children's Hospital, Winnipeg, Manitoba, Canada.) *B,* Right hand of infant with severe digital hypoplasia (short fingers) born to a mother who took Dilantin throughout her pregnancy. (From Chodirker BN, Chudley AE, Reed MH, Persaud TVN: *Am J Med Genet 27*:373, copyright © 1987. Reprinted by permission of Wiley-Liss, a division of John Wiley and Sons, Inc.)

Antinauseants. There has been extensive debate in the lay press and in the courts as to whether *Bendectin* (Debendox, Lenotan, Diclectin) is a human teratogenic drug. *Teratologists consider Bendectin to be nonteratogenic in humans* because large-scale epidemiologic studies of infants have failed to show an increased risk of birth defects after its administration to pregnant woman (Fortin and Lalonde, 1995; Holmes, 1986).

Antineoplastic Agents. About 20 cytotoxic agents are currently available for clinical use. With the exception of the folic acid antagonist **aminopterin**, few well-documented reports of teratogenic effects are available for assessment. Because the data available on the possible teratogenicity of antineoplastic drugs are inadequate, it is recommended that they should be avoided, especially during the first trimester of pregnancy. **Tumor-inhibiting chemicals are highly teratogenic.** This is not surprising because these agents inhibit mitosis in rapidly dividing cells. The use of aminopterin during the embryonic period often results in intrauterine death of the embryos, but the 20 to 30% of those that survive are severely malformed. *Busulfan and 6-mercaptopurine* administered in alternating courses throughout pregnancy have produced multiple severe abnormalities, but neither drug alone appears to cause major anomalies (Table 8-6). For information on the long-term development of children exposed in utero to antineoplastic drugs, see Garber (1989).

Aminopterin is a potent teratogen that produces major congenital anomalies (Fig. 8-20), especially of the skeletal and central nervous systems (Thiersch, 1952; Kliegman, 1996). Aminopterin, an antimetabolite, is a *folic acid antagonist.* Multiple skeletal and other congenital anomalies were found in an infant born to a mother who attempted to terminate her pregnancy by taking *methotrexate* (Milunsky et al., 1968), a derivative of aminopterin that is also a folic acid antagonist.

Corticosteroids. Cortisone causes cleft palate and cardiac defects in susceptible strains of mice and rabbits. *Cortisone does not induce cleft palate or any other congenital anomaly in human embryos.* The teratogenic risk of corticosteroids is minimal, if at all (Fraser and Sajoo, 1995).

Angiotensin-Converting Enzyme (ACE) Inhibitors. Exposure of the fetus to ACE inhibitors as antihypertensive agents causes oligohydramnios, fetal death, long-lasting hypoplasia of the bones of the calvaria, IUGR, and renal dysfunction. During early pregnancy the risk to the embryo is apparently less, and there is no indication in such a case to terminate a wanted pregnancy. Because of the high incidence of serious perinatal complications, it is recommended that ACE inhibitors not be prescribed during pregnancy (Brent and Beckman, 1991; Hanssens et al., 1991; Barr, 1994).

Insulin and Hypoglycemic Drugs. Insulin is not teratogenic in human embryos except possibly in maternal insulin coma therapy. Hypoglycemic drugs (e.g., tolbutamide) have been implicated, but evidence for their teratogenicity is very weak; consequently, despite their marked teratogenicity in rodents, there is no convincing evidence that oral hypoglycemic agents (particularly sulfonylureas) are teratogenic in human embryos. The incidence of congenital anomalies (e.g., **sacral agenesis**) is increased two to three times in the offspring of diabetic mothers, and about 40% of all perinatal deaths among diabetic infants are the result of congenital anomalies. The teratogenic mechanism of diabetic embryopathy is not known (Reece and Eriksson, 1996). Women with insulin-dependent diabetes mellitus may significantly decrease their risk of having infants with birth defects by achieving good control of their disease *before conception* (Behrman et al., 1996).

Retinoic Acid (Vitamin A). Retinoic acid is a well-established teratogen in animals, and its teratogenicity in humans was recognized over a decade ago (Lammer et al., 1985; Kochhar, 1995). **Isotretinoin (13-cis-retinoic acid) is teratogenic at very low doses in humans**. This drug is used for treating severe cystic acne. The critical period for exposure appears to be from the third week to the fifth week (5 to 7 weeks after LNMP). The risk of spontaneous abortion and birth defects after exposure to retinoic acid is high. The most common major anomalies observed are: craniofacial dysmorphism (microtia, micrognathia), cleft palate and/or thymic aplasia defects, cardiovascular anomalies, and neural tube defects. Postnatal longitudinal follow-up of children exposed in utero to isotretinoin revealed significant neuropsychological impairment (Persaud, 1990). Vitamin A is a valuable and necessary nutrient during pregnancy, but long-term exposure to large doses is unwise. Pregnant women should avoid high levels of vitamin A because an increased risk of birth defects among the offspring of women who took more than 10,000 IU of vitamin A daily was reported recently (Rothman et al., 1995).

Salicylates. There is some evidence that large doses of *acetylsalicylic acid* (ASA) or *aspirin*, the most commonly ingested drug during pregnancy, are potentially harmful to the embryo or fetus (Corby, 1978). Epidemiological studies indicate that aspirin is not a teratogenic agent but large doses of ASA should be avoided, especially during the first trimester.

Thyroid Drugs. *Potassium iodide* in cough mixtures and large doses of *radioactive iodine* may cause congenital goiter (Shepard, 1992). Iodides readily cross the placental membrane and interfere with thyroxin production. They may also cause thyroid enlargement and **cretinism** (arrested physical and mental development and dystrophy of bones and soft parts). *Maternal iodine deficiency* may cause congenital cretinism. Pregnant women have been advised to avoid douches or creams containing povidone-iodine because it is absorbed by the vagina, enters the maternal blood, and may be teratogenic (Vorherr et al., 1980). *Propylthiouracil* interferes with thyroxin formation in the fetus and may cause goiter. The administration of *antithyroid substances* for the treatment of maternal thyroid disorders may cause congenital goiter (Fig. 8-21) if the mother is given the substances in excess of requirements to control the disease.

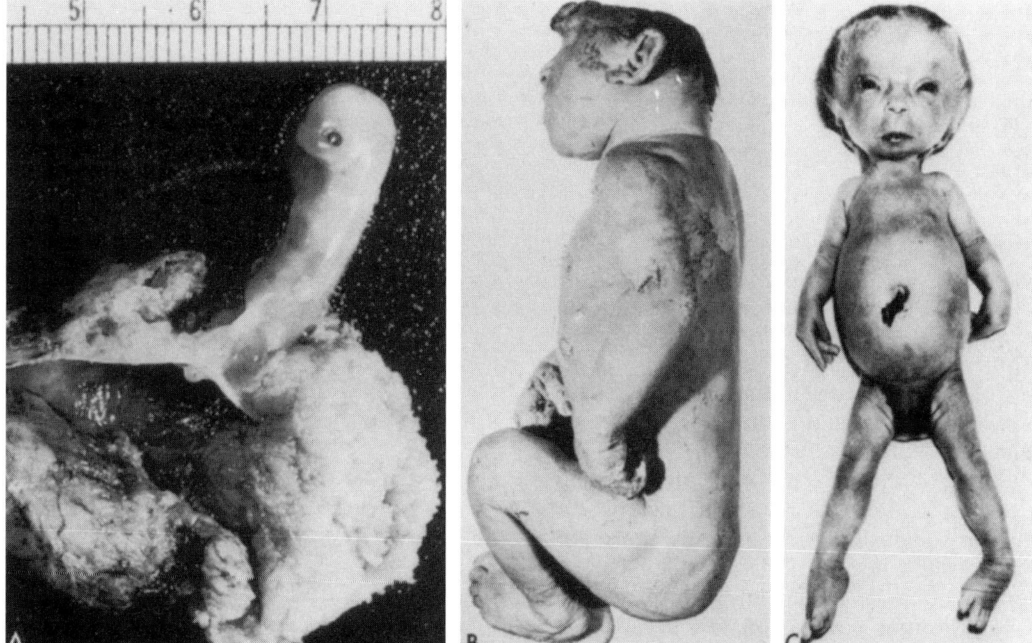

■ **Figure 8-20.** Aminopterin-induced congenital anomalies. *A,* Grossly malformed embryo and its membranes. (Courtesy of Dr. JB Thiersch, Seattle, Washington.) *B,* Newborn infant with meroanencephaly—partial absence of the brain. (From Thiersch JB: *In* Wolstenholme GEW, O'Connor CM [eds]: *Ciba Foundation Symposium on Congenital Malformation.* London, J & A Churchill, Ltd, 1960.) *C,* Newborn infant showing marked IUGR, a large head, a small mandible, deformed ears, clubhands, and clubfeet. (From Warkany J, Beaudry PH, Hornstein S: Attempted abortion with 4-aminoplerolyglutamic acid (Aminopterin): Malformations of the child. *Am J Dis Child 97:*274, 1960.)

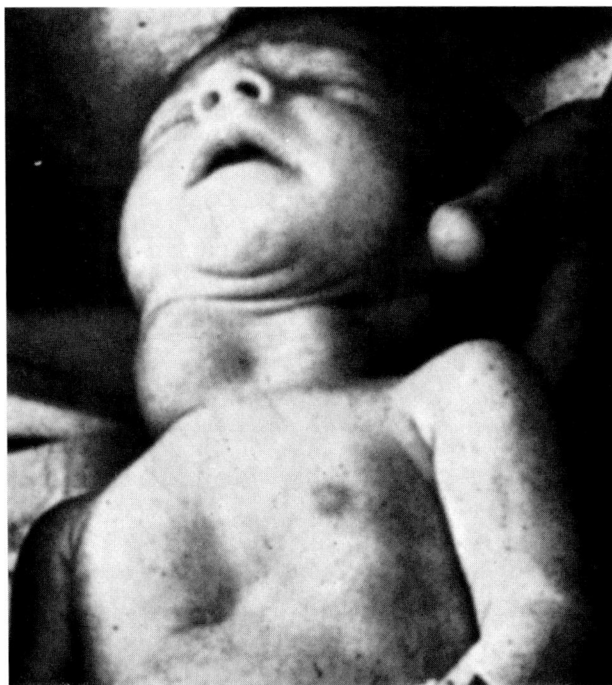

■ **Figure 8–21.** Newborn infant with congenital enlargement of the thyroid gland (goiter). The condition resulted from the administration of antithyroid drugs to the mother in excess of the amount needed to control the disease. (From Reid DF, Ryan KJ, Benirschke K: *Principles and Management of Human Reproduction.* Philadelphia, WB Saunders, 1972. Courtesy of Dr. Keith Russell.)

Tranquilizers. *Thalidomide is a potent teratogen.* This hypnotic agent was once widely used in West Germany and Australia as a tranquilizer and sedative, but is now used because of its immunosuppressive properties (Behrman et al., 1996). The **thalidomide epidemic** started in 1959. It has been estimated that nearly 12,000 infants were born with defects caused by this drug (Randall, 1990). Because thalidomide was not approved by the Food and Drug Administration (FDA) in the United States, relatively few anomalies occurred. The characteristic feature of the **thalidomide syndrome** is *meromelia*, phocomelia or "seal limbs" for example (Fig. 8-22), but the anomalies ranged from *amelia* (absence of limbs) through intermediate stages of development (rudimentary limbs) to *micromelia* (abnormal small and/or short limbs).

Thalidomide also caused anomalies of other organs, e.g., absence of the external and internal ears, hemangioma on the forehead, heart defects, and anomalies of the urinary and alimentary systems (Persaud, 1990). It is well established clinically that the period when thalidomide caused congenital anomalies was from 24 to 36 days after fertilization (38 to 50 days after LNMP). This sensitive period coincides with the critical periods for the development of the affected parts and organs (Fig. 8-16). *Thalidomide is absolutely contraindicated in women of childbearing age* (Behrman et al., 1996).

Lithium is the drug of choice for the long-term maintenance of patients with manic-depressive psychosis; however, it has caused congenital anomalies, mainly of the heart and great vessels, in infants born to mothers given the drug early in pregnancy. Although **lithium carbonate is a known human teratogen** (Warkany, 1988), the FDA has stated that the agent may be used during pregnancy if "in the opinion of the physician the potential benefits outweigh the possible hazards." **Benzodiazepine derivatives** are psychoactive drugs frequently used by pregnant women. These include *diazepam* and *ozazepam,* which readily cross the placental membrane. The use of these drugs during the first trimester of pregnancy is associated with transient withdrawal symptoms and **craniofacial anomalies** in the newborn. Patients are warned not to take these drugs during pregnancy because of their possible teratogenic effects (Laegreid et al., 1989).

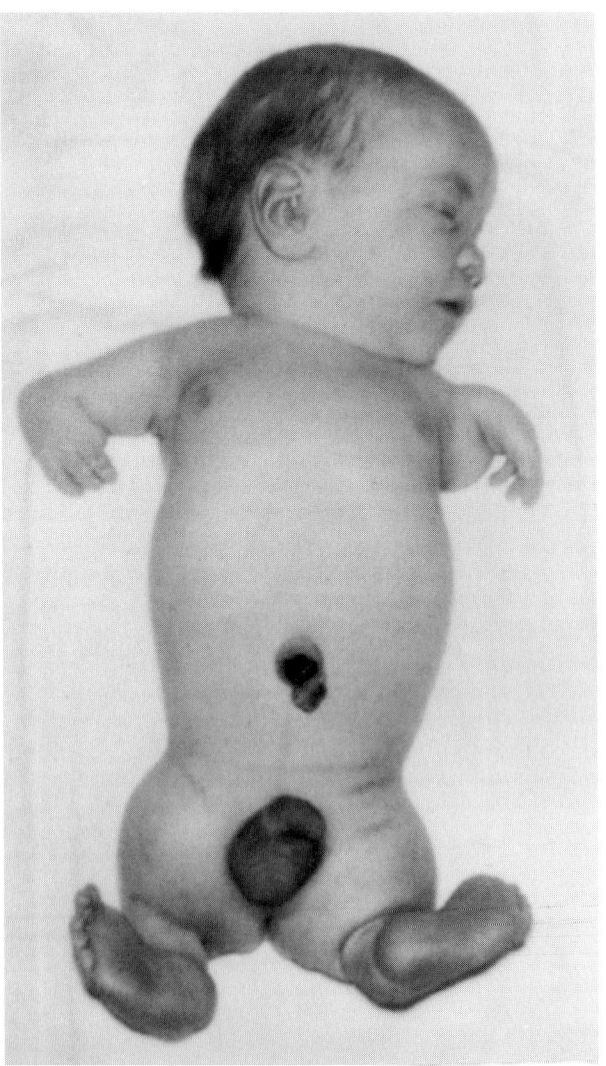

■ **Figure 8–22.** Newborn male infant showing typically malformed limbs (meromelia—limb reduction) caused by thalidomide ingested by his mother during the critical period of limb development. (From Moore KL: *Manit Med Rev 43:*306, 1963.)

Illicit Drugs. Several currently popular street drugs are used for their hallucinogenic properties. Long (1972) reviewed the literature on 161 infants born to mothers who ingested *lysergic acid diethylamide* **(LSD)** before conception and/or during pregnancy. Five infants had limb defects similar to those caused by thalidomide. Jacobson and Berlin (1972) also found limb defects and noted a 9.6% incidence of nervous system defects. There is no strong evidence to indicate that LSD is teratogenic; however, in view of the reported cases, it should be avoided during pregnancy (Persaud, 1990). There is no evidence that **marijuana** is a human teratogen (Nahas, 1986); however, there is an indication that marijuana use during the first 2 months of pregnancy affects fetal length and birth weight. In addition, sleep and EEG patterns in newborns exposed prenatally to marijuana were altered. For these reasons, women should not use marijuana during pregnancy (Day et al., 1991).

Golden and colleagues (1980) reported a case of an infant with several birth defects and behavioral disturbances whose mother used *phencyclidine (PCP, angel dust)* throughout her pregnancy. This suggests, but does not prove, a causal association. **Cocaine** is one of the most commonly abused illicit drugs in North America, and its increasing use by women of childbearing age is of major concern. There are many reports dealing with the prenatal effects of cocaine. These include spontaneous abortion, prematurity, IUGR, microcephaly, cerebral infarction, urogenital anomalies, and neurobehavioral disturbances. The use of cocaine during pregnancy should be avoided because of its teratogenic effects (Behrman et al., 1996; Little et al., 1996).

Methadone, used for the treatment of heroin addiction, is considered to be a "behavioral teratogen," as is heroin (Persaud, 1990). Infants born to narcotic-dependent women maintained on methadone therapy were found to have central nervous system dysfunction and smaller birth weights and head circumferences than nonexposed infants. There is also concern about the long-term, postnatal developmental effects of methadone. The problem, however, is difficult to resolve because other drugs are often used in combination with methadone, and heavy use of alcohol and cigarettes is prevalent among narcotic-dependent women (Kaltenbach and Finnegan, 1989).

ENVIRONMENTAL CHEMICALS AS TERATOGENS

In recent years there has been increasing concern about the possible teratogenicity of environmental chemicals, including industrial and agricultural chemicals (Nurminen et al., 1995), pollutants, and food additives. Most of these chemicals have not been positively implicated as teratogens in humans (Persaud, 1990).

Organic Mercury. Infants of mothers whose main diet during pregnancy consists of fish containing abnormally high levels of organic mercury acquire fetal **Minamata disease** and exhibit neurological and behavioral disturbances resembling cerebral palsy (Matsumoto et al., 1965). Severe *brain damage*, mental retardation, and blindness have been detected in infants of mothers who received *methylmercury* in their food (Amin-Zaki et al., 1974). Similar observations have been made in infants whose mothers ate pork that became contaminated when the pigs ate corn grown from seeds sprayed with a mercury-containing fungicide (Snyder, 1971). **Methylmercury is a teratogen** that causes cerebral atrophy, spasticity, seizures, and *mental retardation* (Melkonian and Baker, 1988; Burbacher et al., 1990; Behrman et al., 1996).

Lead. Abundantly present in the workplace and environment, lead passes through the placental membrane and accumulates in fetal tissues. Prenatal exposure to lead is associated with increased abortions, fetal anomalies, IUGR, and functional deficits. Several reports have indicated that children born to mothers who were exposed to subclinical levels of lead revealed neurobehavioral and psychomotor disturbances (Persaud, 1990; Bellinger, 1994).

Polychlorinated Biphenyls (PCBs). These teratogenic chemicals produce IUGR and skin discoloration. The main dietary source of PCBs in North America is probably sport fish caught in contaminated waters (Rogan, 1986). In Japan and Taiwan, the teratogenic chemical was detected in contaminated cooking oil.

INFECTIOUS AGENTS AS TERATOGENS

Throughout prenatal life the embryo and fetus are endangered by a variety of microorganisms. In most cases the assault is resisted; in some cases, an abortion or stillbirth occurs, and in others the infants are born with IUGR, congenital anomalies, or neonatal diseases (Table 8-6). Many of these congenital defects can be detected in utero by sonography (Drose et al., 1991). The microorganisms cross the placental membrane and enter the fetal blood stream. Inasmuch as there is a propensity for the central nervous system (CNS) to be affected, the fetal blood-brain barrier also apparently offers little resistance to microorganisms.

Rubella (German or Three-Day Measles). The virus that causes rubella, a communicable disease, is the prime example of an *infective teratogen* (Korones, 1986). In cases of primary maternal infection during the first trimester of pregnancy, the overall risk of embryonic/fetal infection is about 20% (Gibbs and Sweet, 1989). The **rubella virus** crosses the placental membrane and infects the embryo/fetus. The usual features of **congenital rubella syndrome (CRS)** are *cataract, cardiac defects*, and *deafness*; however, the following abnormalities are occasionally observed: mental deficiency, chorioretinitis, glaucoma (Fig. 8-23), microphthalmia, and tooth defects. The earlier in pregnancy the maternal rubella infection occurs, the greater the danger that the embryo will be malformed (Isada et al., 1990; Behrman et al., 1996).

Most infants have congenital anomalies if the disease

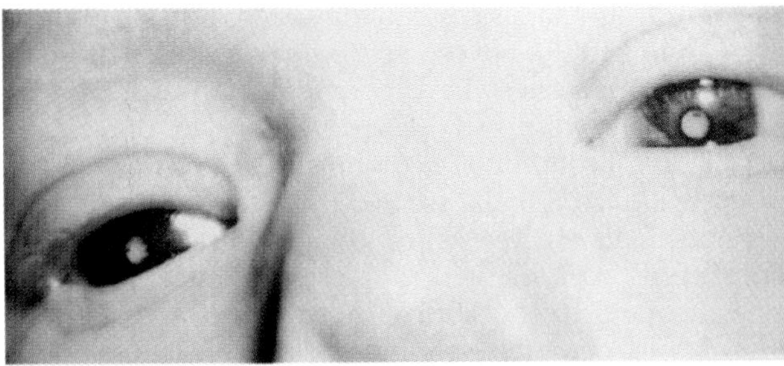

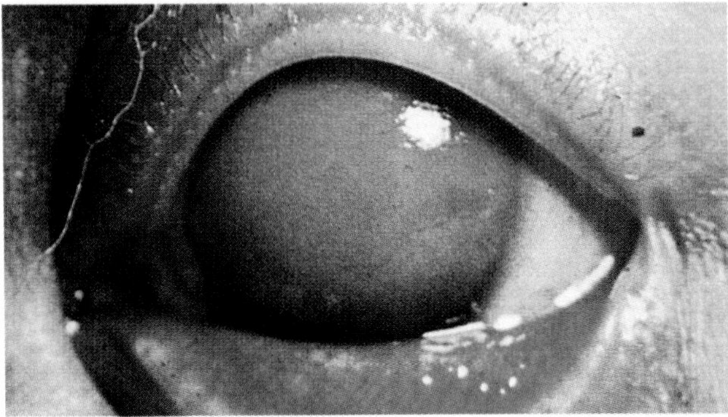

■ **Figure 8-23.** *A,* Typical bilateral congenital cataracts caused by the rubella virus. Cardiac defects and deafness are other common congenital defects. *B,* Severe congenital glaucoma caused by rubella virus. Observe the dense corneal haze, enlarged corneal diameter, and deep anterior chamber. (*A,* Courtesy of Dr. Richard Bargy, Department of Ophthalmology, Cornell–New York Hospital. *B,* Courtesy of Dr. Daniel I Weiss, Department of Ophthalmology, New York University College of Medicine. From Cooper LA, et al: *Am J Dis Child 110:*416, 1965. Copyright 1965, American Medical Association.)

occurs during the first 4 to 5 weeks after fertilization because this period includes the most susceptible organogenetic periods of the eye, internal ear, heart, and brain (Fig. 8-15). The risk of anomalies from rubella infection during the second and third trimesters is low (about 10%), but functional defects of the CNS (mental retardation) and internal ear (hearing loss) may result if infection occurs during the late fetal period. There is no evidence of fetal anomalies after the fifth gestational month (Korones, 1986; Isada et al., 1990); however, infections may produce chronic disease and dysfunction of the eye, ear, and CNS (Behrman et al., 1996).

Cytomegalovirus (CMV). Infection with CMV is the most common viral infection of the human fetus. Because the disease seems to be fatal when it affects the embryo, it is believed that most pregnancies end in spontaneous abortion when the infection occurs during the first trimester. Newborn infants infected during the early fetal period usually show no clinical signs and are identified through screening programs (Williamson et al., 1990). Later in pregnancy, *CMV infection may result in IUGR, microphthalmia, chorioretinitis, blindness, microcephaly, cerebral calcification, mental retardation, deafness, cerebral palsy, and hepatosplenomegaly* (Reynolds et al., 1986; Riley, 1997). Of particular concern are cases of *asymptomatic CMV infection*, which are often associated with audiological, neurological, and neurobehavioral disturbances in infancy. See Embree (1994) for details.

Herpes Simplex Virus (HSV). It has been reported that maternal infection with HSV in early pregnancy increases the abortion rate by threefold, and infection after the twentieth week is associated with a higher rate of prematurity. Infection of the fetus with HSV usually occurs very late in pregnancy, probably most often during delivery. The congenital abnormalities that have been observed in newborns included typical cutaneous lesions and, in some cases, microcephaly, microphthalmia, spasticity, retinal dysplasia, and mental retardation (Gibbs and Sweet, 1989; Persaud, 1990; Behrman et al., 1996).

Varicella (Chickenpox). Varicella and herpes zoster (shingles) are caused by the same virus, *varicella-zoster virus* (Fuccillo, 1986). There is convincing evidence that maternal *varicella infection during the first 4 months of pregnancy causes congenital anomalies*—skin scarring, muscle atrophy, hypoplasia of the limb, rudimentary digits, eye and brain damage, and mental retardation (Gibbs and Sweet, 1989; Koren, 1995). There is about a 20% chance of these or other anomalies when the infection occurs during the critical period of development (Fig. 8-15). After 20 weeks of gestation, there is apparently no proven teratogenic risk.

Human Immunodeficiency Virus (HIV). This retrovirus causes acquired immunodeficiency syndrome (AIDS). HIV infection in pregnant women is now a prevalent and serious health problem. There is conflicting information on the fetal effects of in utero infection with HIV (Embree et al., 1989; Johnstone, 1996). Some of the congenital anomalies reported are growth failure, microcephaly, and specific craniofacial features (Parks, 1996). Most cases of transmission of the virus from mother to fetus probably occur at about the time of delivery. Breastfeeding increases the risk of transmitting the virus to the newborn. Preventing the transmission of the virus to women and their infants is of obvious importance because of the potential fetal and infantile effects (Johnstone, 1996; Parks, 1996).

Toxoplasmosis. *Toxoplasma gondii*, an intracellular parasite, occurs widely. It was named after the gondi, a North African rodent in which the organism was first detected. This parasite may be found in the blood stream, tissues, or reticuloendothelial cells, leukocytes, and epithelial cells. *Maternal infection* (Yokota, 1995; Lynfield and Eaton, 1995) is usually acquired by:

- eating raw or poorly cooked meat (usually pork or lamb containing *Toxoplasma* cysts)
- close contact with infected domestic animals (usually *cats*) or soil

It is thought that the soil and garden vegetables may become contaminated with infected cat feces carrying oocysts (the encysted or encapsulated zygote in the life cycle of sporozoan protozoa). **Oocysts** can also be transported to food by flies and cockroaches.

The *Toxoplasma gondii organism crosses the placental membrane and infects the fetus* (Figs. 8-24 and 8-25), causing destructive changes in the brain (intracranial calcifications) and eyes (chorioretinitis) that result in **mental deficiency**, microcephaly, microphthalmia, and hydrocephaly (Persaud, 1990; Yokota, 1995). Fetal death may follow infection, especially during the early stages of pregnancy. Mothers of congenitally defective infants are often unaware of having had **toxoplasmosis**, the disease caused by the parasitic organism. Because animals (cats, dogs, rabbits, and other domestic and wild animals) may be infected with this parasite, pregnant women should avoid them and the eating of raw or poorly cooked meat from them (e.g., rabbits). In addition, eggs of domestic fowl should be well cooked and unpasteurized milk should be avoided. For more details, see Lynfield and Eaton (1995) and McLeod and Remington (1996).

Congenital Syphilis. The incidence of congenital syphilis is steadily increasing with more cases now than in any of the past two decades. One in 10,000 liveborn infants in the United States is infected (Ricci et al., 1989). *Treponema pallidum*, the small, spiral microorganism that causes syphilis, rapidly crosses the placental membrane as early as 9 to 10 weeks of gestation. The fetus can become infected at any stage of the disease or at any stage of pregnancy (Azimi, 1996; Nathan et al., 1997). *Primary maternal infections* (acquired during pregnancy) nearly always cause serious fetal infection and congenital anomalies; however, adequate treatment of the mother kills the organism, thereby preventing it from crossing the placental membrane and infecting the fetus (Nathan et al., 1997). *Secondary maternal infections* (acquired before pregnancy) seldom result in fetal disease and anomalies. If the mother is untreated, stillbirths occur in about one-fourth of cases. Only 20% of all untreated pregnant women will deliver a normal infant at term. Early manifestations of untreated maternal syphilis are congenital deafness, abnormal teeth and bones, hydrocephalus, and mental retardation (Ingall and Musher, 1983; Persaud, 1990). Late manifestations of untreated congenital syphilis are destructive lesions of the palate and nasal septum, dental abnormalities (centrally notched, widely spaced peg-shaped upper central incisors—*Hutchinson's teeth*—and abnormal facies (frontal bossing, saddlenose, and poorly developed maxilla). For more information about these facial characteristics, see Ray (1995) and Azimi (1996).

RADIATION AS A TERATOGEN

Exposure to **high levels of ionizing radiation** may injure embryonic cells, resulting in cell death, chromosome injury, and retardation of mental development and physical growth. The severity of the embryonic damage is related to the absorbed dose, the dose rate, and the stage of embryonic or fetal development when

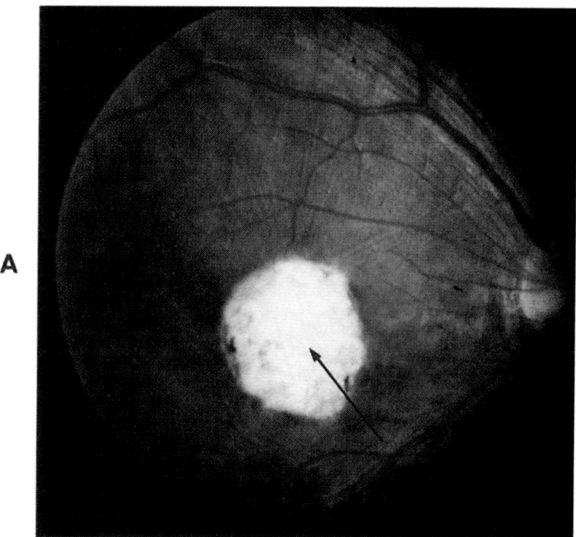

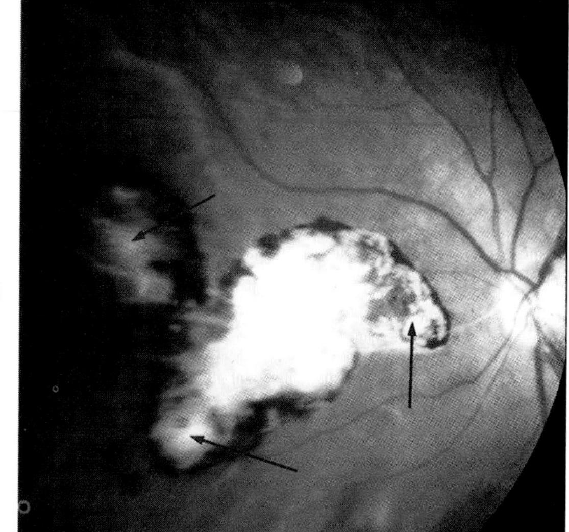

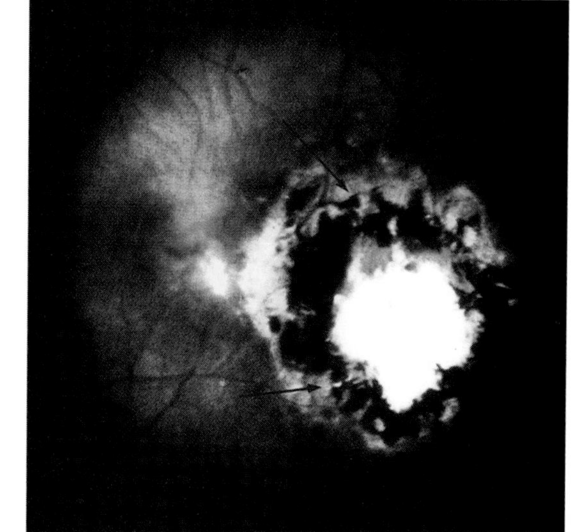

■ **Figure 8-24.** Chorioretinitis of congenital ocular toxoplasmosis induced by *Toxoplasma* infection. *A,* Necrotizing cicatricial lesion of the macula *(arrow)*. *B,* Satellite lesion around and adjacent to necrotizing cicatricial main lesion *(arrows)*. *C,* Recrudescent lesion adjacent to large necrotizing cicatricial main lesion *(arrows)*. (From Yokota K: *Congen Anom 35:*151, 1995.)

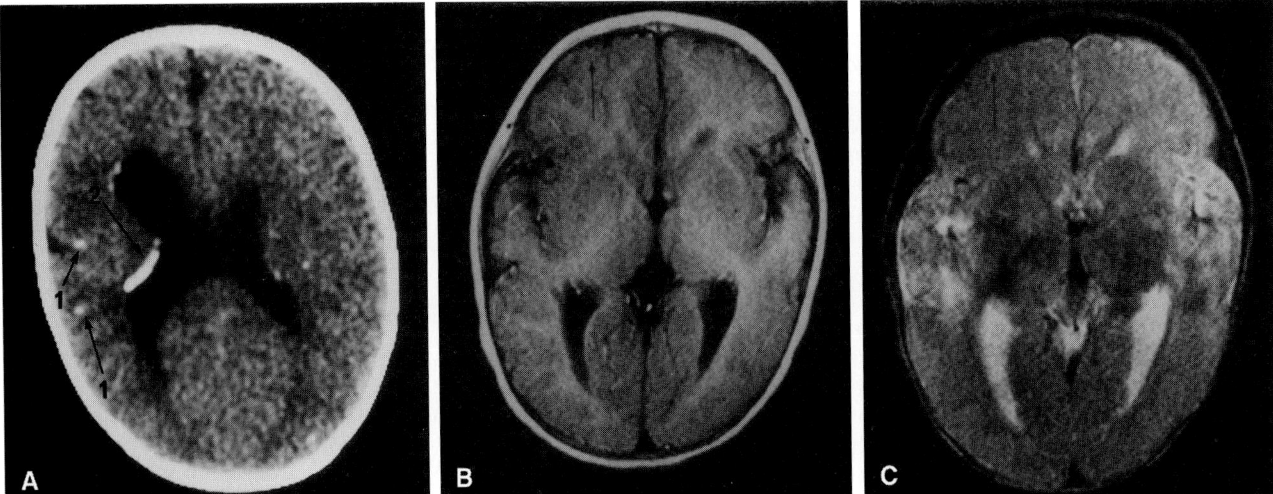

■ **Figure 8–25.** Congenital anomalies induced by *Toxoplasma* infection. The following diagnostic images were obtained at 2 years and 9 months of age. *A,* Plain CT. The lateral ventricles are moderately dilated. Multiple calcified foci are apparent in the brain parenchyma *(arrows 1)* and along the ventricular wall *(arrow 2)*. *B,* MRI, T_1WI, (400/22, 0.5T). The cortical gyri are widened on the left side and the cortex is thickened in the left frontal lobe *(arrow)* compared with corresponding structure on the right. *C,* MRI, T_2WI, (2,500/120, 0.5T). The left frontal lobe shows abnormal hypointensity *(arrow)*. (From Yokota K: *Congen Anom 35:*151, 1995.)

the exposure occurs. In the past, large amounts of ionizing radiation (hundreds to several thousand rads) were given inadvertently to embryos and fetuses of pregnant women who had cancer of the cervix. In all cases their embryos were severely malformed or killed. Growth retardation, microcephaly, spina bifida cystica (see Chapter 18), pigment changes in the retina, cataracts, cleft palate, skeletal and visceral abnormalities, and mental retardation have been observed in infants who survived after receiving high levels of ionizing radiation. Development of the central nervous system (CNS) was nearly always affected (Kriegel et al., 1986). Profound cellular changes have been experimentally induced in the brains of laboratory animals following in utero exposure to low-dose ionizing radiation (Ralcewicz and Persaud, 1995).

Observations of Japanese atomic bomb survivors and their children suggest that 8 to 16 weeks after fertilization (10 to 18 weeks after LNMP) is the period of greatest sensitivity for radiation damage to the brain, resulting in **severe mental retardation**. By the end of the sixteenth week, most neuronal proliferation is completed, after which the risk of mental retardation decreases. It is generally accepted that large doses of radiation (over 25,000 millirads) are harmful to the developing CNS (Schull, 1995). Accidental exposure of pregnant women to radiation is a common cause for anxiety (Brent 1986b; Bentur et al., 1991).

There is no conclusive proof that human congenital anomalies have been caused by diagnostic levels of radiation. Scattered radiation from an x-ray examination of a part of the body that is not near the uterus (e.g., the thorax, sinuses, teeth) produces a dose of only a few millirads, which is not teratogenic to the embryo. For example, a radiograph of the thorax of a pregnant women in the first trimester results in a whole-body dose to her embryo or fetus of approximately 1 millirad. If the embryonic radiation exposure is 5 rads or less, the radiation risks to the embryo are minuscule (Brent, 1986b; Bentur et al., 1991); however, it is prudent to be cautious during diagnostic examinations of the pelvic region in pregnant women (radiographical examinations and medical diagnostic tests using radioisotopes) because they result in exposure of the embryo to 0.3 to 2 rads. The recommended limit of maternal exposure of the whole body to radiation from all sources is 500 millirads for the entire gestational period.

Electromagnetic Fields. There is no evidence that there is an increased risk of IUGR or other developmental defects following maternal exposure to low-frequency electromagnetic fields (electric blankets, video display terminals, etc.; see Bracken et al., 1995; Robert, 1996).

Ultrasonic Waves. Ultrasonography is widely used during pregnancy for fetal diagnosis and prenatal care. A review of the safety of obstetrical ultrasonography (Reece et al., 1990) concluded that "current data indicate that there are no confirmed biological effects on patients and their fetuses from the use of diagnostic ultrasound evaluation and the benefits to patients exposed to prudent use of this modality outweigh the risks, if any." There is some concern about possible harmful effects (IUGR, delayed speech, etc.) of repeated ultrasound examinations of the fetus (Newnham et al., 1993; Campbell et al., 1993).

MATERNAL FACTORS AS TERATOGENS

Maternal diseases can sometimes lead to a higher risk of abnormalities in the offspring. Poorly controlled *diabetes mellitus* in the mother with persisting hyperglycemia and ketosis, particularly during embryogenesis, is associated with a two- to threefold higher incidence of birth defects (Reece and Eriksson, 1996). No specific diabetic embryopathic syndrome exists, but the infant of the diabetic mother is usually large (*macrosomia*), with prominent fat pads over the upper back and lower jaw. The common anomalies include *holoprosencephaly* (failure of the forebrain to divide into hemispheres), meroencephaly (partial absence of the brain), sacral agenesis, vertebral anomalies, congenital heart defects, and limb defects (Behrman et al., 1996; Tyrala, 1996). For details regarding the management of diabetes in pregnancy, see Hadden (1996).

If untreated, women who are homozygous for phenylalanine hydroxylase deficiency — **phenylketonuria** (PKU) — and those with hyperphenylalaninemia are at a higher risk of having an offspring with microcephaly, cardiac defects, mental retardation, and IUGR. The congenital anomalies can be prevented if the PKU mother is placed on a phenylalanine-restricted diet prior to and during the pregnancy (Levy and Ghavami, 1996). **Maternal PKU is a metabolic teratogen.**

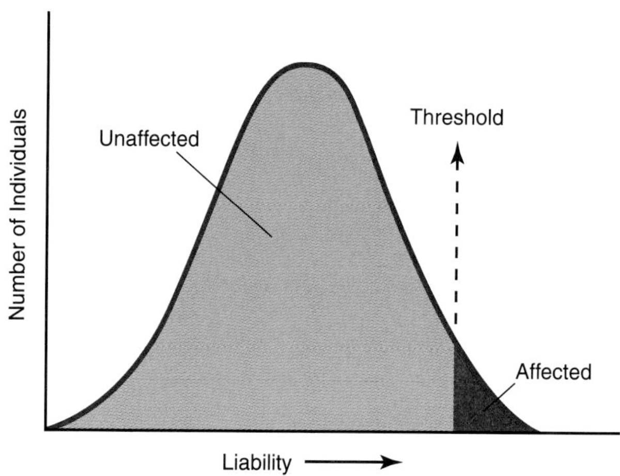

■ **Figure 8-26.** Multifactorial threshold model. Liability to a trait is distributed normally with a threshold dividing the population into unaffected and affected classes. (From Thompson MW, McInnes RR, Willard HF: *Thompson & Thompson Genetics in Medicine,* 5th ed. Philadelphia, WB Saunders, 1991.)

MECHANICAL FACTORS AS TERATOGENS

The significance of mechanical influences in the uterus on congenital postural deformities is still an open question. The amniotic fluid absorbs mechanical pressures, thereby protecting the embryo from most external trauma. It is generally accepted that congenital abnormalities caused by external injury to the mother are extremely rare, but possible (Hinden, 1965). *Congenital dislocation of the hip and clubfoot* may be caused by mechanical forces, particularly in a malformed uterus. Such deformations may be caused by any factor that restricts the mobility of the fetus, thereby causing prolonged compression in an abnormal posture (Connor and Ferguson-Smith, 1987). A significantly reduced quantity of amniotic fluid (*oligohydramnios*) may result in mechanically induced deformation of the limbs (see Chapter 7), e.g., hyperextension of the knee (Dunn, 1976). Intrauterine amputations or other anomalies caused by local constriction during fetal growth may result from *amniotic bands* — rings formed as a result of rupture of the amnion during early pregnancy (Behrman et al., 1996). For information on the pathogenesis of *amniotic band syndrome*, see Lockwood et al. (1989).

ANOMALIES CAUSED BY MULTIFACTORIAL INHERITANCE

Many common congenital anomalies (e.g., cleft lip with/without cleft palate) have familial distributions consistent with multifactorial inheritance (MFI) (Fig. 8-1). For a list of the characteristics of MFI, see Thompson et al. (1991). Multifactorial inheritance may be represented by a model in which "liability" to a disorder is a continuous variable determined by a combination of genetic and environmental factors, with a developmental threshold dividing individuals with the anomaly from those without it (Fig. 8-26). *Multifactorial traits are often single major anomalies*, such as cleft lip, isolated cleft palate, neural tube defects (e.g., meroanencephaly and spina bifida cystica), pyloric stenosis, and congenital dislocation of the hip. Some of these anomalies may also occur as part of the phenotype in syndromes determined by single-gene inheritance, chromosome abnormality, or an environmental teratogen. The *recurrence risks* used for genetic counseling of families having congenital anomalies determined by MFI are *empirical risks* based on the frequency of the anomaly in the general population and in different categories of relatives. In individual families, such estimates may be inaccurate because they are usually averages for the population rather than precise probabilities for the individual family. For further discussion of MFI and genetic counseling of families of patients with multifactorial traits, see Thompson et al. (1991).

SUMMARY OF HUMAN BIRTH DEFECTS

A congenital anomaly is a structural abnormality of any type that is present at birth. It may be macroscopic or microscopic, on the surface or within the body. There are four clinically significant types of anomalies: malformation, disruption, deformation, and dysplasia. Congenital anomalies may be induced by genetic factors or by environmental factors that cause derangements during prenatal development. Most common congenital anomalies, however, show the family patterns expected of *multifactorial inheritance* with a threshold and are determined by a combination of genetic and environmental factors.

About 3% of all liveborn infants have an obvious major anomaly. Additional anomalies are detected after birth; thus, the incidence is about 6% in 2-year-olds and 8% in 5-year-olds. Other anomalies (about 2%) are detected later in life (e.g., during surgery or autopsy).

Congenital anomalies may be single or multiple and of minor or major clinical significance. *Single minor anomalies are present in about 14% of newborns.* These anomalies are of no serious medical consequence, but they alert the clinician to the possible presence of an associated major anomaly; 90% of infants with multiple minor anomalies have one or more associated major anomalies. Of the 3% of infants born with a major congenital anomaly, 0.7% have multiple major anomalies.

Major anomalies are more common in early embryos (up to 15%) than they are in newborn infants (up to 3%). Most severely malformed embryos are usually spontaneously aborted during the first 6 to 8 weeks. Some congenital anomalies are caused by *genetic factors* (chromosome abnormalities and mutant genes). A few congenital abnormalities are caused by *environmental factors* (infectious agents, environmental chemicals, and drugs); however, most common anomalies result from a complex *interaction between genetic and environmental factors.* The cause of most congenital anomalies is unknown.

During the first 2 weeks of development, teratogenic agents usually kill the embryo or have no effect, rather than cause congenital anomalies. During the *organogenetic period,* teratogenic agents disrupt development and may cause *major congenital anomalies.* During the fetal period teratogens may produce morphological and functional abnormalities, particularly of the brain and eyes. *Mental retardation* may result from high levels of radiation and infectious agents.

CLINICALLY ORIENTED PROBLEMS

Case 8–1

A physician was concerned about the drugs a woman said she was taking when she first sought medical advice during her pregnancy.

- What percentage of congenital anomalies are caused by drugs, environmental chemicals, and infectious agents?
- Why may it be difficult for doctors to attribute specific congenital anomalies to specific drugs?
- What should pregnant women know about the use of drugs during pregnancy?

Case 8–2

During a pelvic examination, a 38-year-old woman learned that she was pregnant. The physician was concerned about her age inasmuch as it was her first pregnancy.

- Do women over the age of 35 have an increased risk of bearing malformed children?
- If a 38-year-old woman becomes pregnant, what prenatal diagnostic tests would likely be performed?
- What genetic abnormality might be detected?
- Can a 44-year-old woman have a normal baby?

Case 8–3

A pregnant woman asked her doctor, "Are any drugs considered safe during early pregnancy?"

- Can you name some commonly prescribed drugs that are safe to use?
- What commonly used drugs should be avoided?

Case 8–4

A 10-year-old girl contracted German measles and her mother was worried that the child might develop cataracts and heart defects.

- What would the physician likely tell the mother?

Case 8–5

A pregnant woman with two cats that often "spent the night out" was told by a friend that she should avoid them during her pregnancy. She was also told to avoid flies and cockroaches.

- When she consulted her physician, what would she likely be told?

Discussion of these problems appears at the back of the book.

REFERENCES AND SUGGESTED READING

Aase JM: Clinical recognition of FAS. Difficulties of detection and diagnosis. *Alcohol Health & Research World 18:*5, 1994.

Abel EL (ed): *Fetal Alcohol Syndrome. From Mechanism to Prevention.* Boca Raton, CRC Press, 1996.

Amin-Zaki L, Elhassani S, Majeed MA, et al: Intrauterine methylmercury poisoning in Iraq. *Pediatrics 54:*587, 1974.

Arnell H, Gustafsson J, Ivarsson SA, Anneren G: Growth and pubertal development in Down syndrome. *Acta Paediatr 85:*1102, 1996.

Azimi P: Spirochetal infections. *In* Behrman RE, Kliegman RM, Arvin AM (eds): *Nelson Textbook of Pediatrics,* 15th ed. Philadelphia, WB Saunders, 1996.

Baldwin CT, Hoth CF, Amos JA, et al: An exonic mutation in the *HuP2* paired domain gene causes Waardenburg's syndrome. *Nature 355:*637, 1992.

Barr HM, Streissguth AP: Caffeine use during pregnancy and child outcome: a 7-year prospective study. *Neurotoxicol Teratol 13:*441, 1991.

Barr Jr M: Teratogen update: Angiotensin-converting enzyme inhibitors. *Teratology 50:*399, 1994.

Beckman DA, Brent RL: Mechanisms of teratogenesis. *Annual Rev Pharmacol Toxicol 24:*483, 1984.

Behrman RE, Kliegman RM, Arvin AM (eds): *Nelson Textbook of Pediatrics,* 15th ed. Philadelphia, WB Saunders, 1996.

Bellinger D: Teratogen update: lead. *Teratology 50:*367, 1994.

Belloni E, Muenke M, Roessler E, et al: Identification of *Sonic hedgehog* as a candidate gene responsible for holoprosencephaly. *Nature Genet 14:*353, 1996.

Bennett R, Persaud TVN, Moore KL: Experimental studies on the effects of aluminum on pregnancy and fetal development. *Anat Anz 138:*365, 1975.

Bentur Y, Horlatsch N, Koren G: Exposure to ionizing radiation during pregnancy: perception of teratogenic risk and outcome. *Teratology 43:*109, 1991.

Bergsma D (ed): *Birth Defects Atlas and Compendium.* The National Foundation—March of Dimes. Birth Defects: Original Article Series. Baltimore, Williams & Wilkins, 1973.

Blancato JK, Eglinton G, George J, et al: Prenatal diagnosis of partial trisomy through *in situ* DNA probes. *J Reprod Med 40:*537, 1995.

Bracken MB, Belanger K, Hellenbrand K, et al: Exposure to electromagnetic fields during pregnancy with emphasis on electrically heated beds: association with birth weight and intrauterine growth retardation. *Epidemiology 6:*263, 1995.

Breg WR: Autosomal abnormalities. *In* Gardner LI (ed): *Endocrine and Genetic Diseases of Childhood and Adolescence,* 2nd ed. Philadelphia, WB Saunders, 1975.

Brent RL: The complexities of solving the problem of human malformation. *In* Sever JL, Brent RL (eds): *Teratogen Update: Environmentally Induced Birth Defect Risks.* New York, Alan R Liss, 1986a.

Brent RL: Radiation teratogenesis. *In* Sever JL, Brent RL (eds): *Teratogen Update: Environmentally Induced Birth Defect Risks.* New York, Alan R Liss, 1986b.

Brent RL, Beckman DA: Angiotensin-converting enzyme inhibitors, an embryopathic class of drugs with unique properties: information for clinical teratology counselors. *Teratology 43:*543, 1991.

Brent RL, Holmes LB; Clinical and basic science from the thalidomide tragedy; what have we learned about the causes of limb defects? *Teratology 38:*241,1988.

Briggs GG, Freeman RK, Yaffe SJ; *Drugs in Pregnancy and Lactation,* 4th ed. Baltimore, Williams & Wilkins, 1994.

Brunelli S, Faiella A, Capra V, et al: Germline mutations in the homeobox gene *EMX2* in patients with schizencephaly. *Nature Genet 12:*94, 1996.

Burbacher TM, Rodier PM, Weiss B: Methylmercury developmental neurotoxicity: a comparison of effects in humans and animals. *Neurotoxical Teratol 12:*191, 1990.

Callen PW (ed): *Ultrasonography in Obstetrics and Gynecology,* 3rd ed. Philadelphia, WB Saunders, 1994.

Campbell JD, Elford RW, Brant RF: Case-control study of prenatal ultrasonography exposure in children with delayed speech. *Can Med Assoc J 149:*1435, 1993.

Carlson BM: *Human Embryology and Developmental Biology.* St Louis, Mosby, 1994.

Carr DH, Blackwell RE (eds): *Textbook of Reproductive Medicine.* Norwalk, Appleton & Lange, 1993.

Carr DH: Chromosome studies in selected spontaneous abortions: polyploidy in man. *J Med Genet 8:*164, 1971.

Carr DH, Law EM, Ekins JG: Chromosome studies in selected spontaneous abortions. IV. Unusual cytogenetic disorders. *Teratology 5:* 49, 1972.

Caskey CT, Pizzuti A, Fu Y-H, et al: Triplet repeat mutations in human disease. *Science 256:*784, 1992.

Castella EE, Ashton-Prolla P, Barreda-Mejia E, et al: Thalidomide, a current teratogen in South America. *Teratology 54:*273, 1996.

Chambers CD, Johnson KA, Dick LM, et al: Birth outcomes in pregnant women taking fluoxetine. *New Engl J Med 335:*1010, 1996.

Chodirker BN, Chudley AE, Reed MH, Persaud TVN: Possible prenatal hydantoin effect in a child born to a nonepileptic mother. *Am J Med Genet 27:*373, 1987.

Chudley AE, Hagerman RJ: The fragile X syndrome. *J Pediatr 110:* 821, 1987.

Cohen MM Jr: *The Child with Multiple Birth Defects,* 2nd ed. New York, Oxford University Press, 1997.

Cohlan SQ: Tetracycline staining of teeth. *In* Sever JL, Brent RL (eds): *Teratogen Update: Environmentally Induced Birth Defect Risks.* New York, Alan R Liss, 1986.

Connor JM, Ferguson-Smith MA: *Essential Medical Genetics,* 2nd ed. Oxford, Blackwell Scientific Publications, 1987.

Corby DG: Aspirin in pregnancy: maternal and fetal effects. *Pediatrics 62:*930, 1978.

Crane JP: Ultrasound evaluation of fetal chromosome disorders. *In* Callen PW (ed): *Ultrasonography in Obstetrics and Gynecology,* 3rd ed. Philadelphia, WB Saunders, 1994.

Cummings MR: *Human Heredity. Principles and Issues,* 2nd ed. New York, West Publishing, 1991.

Czeizel AE, Rockenbauer M: Teratogenic study of doxycycline. *Obstet Gynecol 89:*524, 1997.

Dansky LV, Finnell RH: Parental epilepsy, anticonvulsant drugs, and reproductive outcome — epidemiologic and experimental findings spanning 3 decades. 2. Human studies. *Reprod Toxicol 5:*301, 1991.

Day N, Sambamoorthi V, Taylor P, et al: Prenatal marijuana use and neonatal outcome. *Neurotoxicol Teratol 13:*329, 1991.

Delaney-Black V, Covington C, Ostrea Jr E, et al: Prenatal cocaine and neonatal outcome: evaluation of dose-response relationship. *Pediatrics 98:*735, 1996.

DeLuca LM: Retinoids and their receptors in differentiation, embryogenesis, and neoplasia. *FASEB J 5:*2924, 1991.

di Maria H, Courpotin C, Rouzioux C, et al: Transplacental transmission of human immunodeficiency virus. *Lancet 2:*215, 1986.

Drose JA, Dennis Ma, Thickman D: Infection in utero: US findings in 19 cases. *Radiology 178:*369, 1991.

Embree JE: Congenital cytomegalovirus infection. *Contemp Ped 6:*9, 1994.

Embree JE, Braddick M, Datta P, et al: Lack of correlation of maternal human immunodeficiency virus infection with neonatal malformations. *Pediatr Infect Dis J 8:*700, 1989.

Ferguson-Smith MA: Sex chromatin, Klinefelter's syndrome and mental deficiency. *In* Moore KL (ed): *The Sex Chromatin.* Philadelphia, WB Saunders, 1966.

Fleischer AC, Romero R, Manning FA, et al (eds): *The Principles and Practice of Ultrasonography in Obstetrics and Gynecology,* 4th ed. Norwalk, Appleton & Lange, 1991.

Forrest DD, Fordyce RR: *Fam Plan Perspect 20:*112, 1988. (Cited in Djerassi C: The bitter pill. *Science 245:*356, 1989.)

Fortin CF, Lalonde AB: The bendectin affair (of legal and general interest). *J SOGC 17:*61, 1995.

Fraser FC: Liability thresholds, malformations, and syndromes. *Am J Med Genet 66:*75, 1996.

Fraser FC, Sajoo A: Teratogenic potential of corticosteroids in humans. *Teratology 51:*45, 1995.

Fuccillo D: Congenital varicella. *In* Sever JL, Brent RL (eds): *Teratogen Update: Environmentally Induced Birth Defect Risks.* New York, Alan R Liss, 1986.

Ganguin G, Rempt E: Streptomycinbehandlung in der Schwangerschaft und ihre Auswirkung auf des Gehör des Kindes. *Z Laryngol Rhinol Otol 49:*496, 1970.

Garber JE: Long-term follow-up of children exposed *in utero* to antineoplastic agents. *Seminar in Oncology 16:*437, 1989.

Gardner EJ, Simons MJ, Snustad DP: *Principles of Genetics,* 8th ed. New York, John Wiley & Sons, 1991.

Garza A, Cordero JF, Mulinare J: Epidemiology of the early amnion rupture spectrum of defects. *Am J Dis Child 142:*541, 1988.

Gibbs RS, Sweet RL: Maternal and fetal infections — Clinical disorders. *In* Creasy RK, Resnik R (eds): *Maternal-Fetal Medicine: Principles and Practice,* 2nd ed. Philadelphia, WB Saunders, 1989.

Gibert-Barness E: *Potter's Pathology of the Fetus and Infant.* 2 vols. Mosby, St Louis, 1997.

Golden NL, Sokol RJ, Rubin I: Angel dust: possible effects on the fetus. *Pediatrics 65:*18, 1980.

Goldman AS, Zackai EH, Yaffe SJ: Fetal trimethadione syndrome. *In* Sever JL, Brent RL (eds): *Teratogen Update: Environmentally Induced Birth Defect Risks.* New York, Alan R Liss, 1986.

Goodwin BA, Huether CA: Revised estimates and projections of Down syndrome births in the United States, and the effects of prenatal diagnosis utilization, 1970-2002. *Prenat Diagn 7:*261, 1987.

Greenough A, Osborne J, Sutherland S (eds): *Congenital, Prenatal and Neonatal Infections.* Edinburgh, Churchill Livingstone, 1992.

Gregg NM: Congenital cataract following German measles in the mother. *Trans Ophthalmol Soc Aust 3:*35, 1941.

Grose C: Viral infections of the fetus and newborn. *In* Behrman RE, Kliegman RM, Arvin AM (eds): *Nelson Textbook of Pediatrics,* 15th ed. Philadelphia, WB Saunders, 1996.

Gwinn M, Pappaioanou M, George JR, et al: Prevalence of HIV infection in childbearing women in the United States. *JAMA 265:* 1704, 1991.

Hadden DR: The management of diabetes in pregnancy. *Postgrad Med J 72:*525, 1996.

Hall JG: Chromosomal clinical abnormalities. *In* Behrman RE, Kliegman RM, Arvin AM (eds): *Nelson Textbook of Pediatrics,* 15th ed. Philadelphia, WB Saunders, 1996.

Hankin JR: FAS prevention strategies. *Alcohol Health & Research World 18:*62, 1994.

Hanson JW: Fetal hydantoin effects. *In* Sever JL, Brent RL (eds): *Teratogen Update: Environmentally Induced Birth Defect Risks.* New York, Alan R Liss, 1986.

Hanssens M, Keirse MJNC, Vankelecom F, Van Assche FA: Fetal and neonatal effects of treatment with angiotensin-converting enzyme inhibitors in pregnancy. *Obstet Gynecol 78:*128, 1991.

Harris LE, Stayura LA, Ramirez-Talavera PF, Annegers JF: Congenital and acquired abnormalities observed in live-born and stillborn neonates. *Mayo Clin Proc 50:*85, 1975.

Harrison MR, Adzick NS, Flake AW: Prenatal management of the fetus with a correctable defect. *In* Callen PW (ed): *Ultrasonography in Obstetrics and Gynecology,* 3rd ed. Philadelphia, WB Saunders, 1994.

Hart WR, Zaharrow I, Kaplan BJ, et al: Cytologic findings in stilbestrol-exposed females with emphasis on detection of vaginal adenosis. *Acta Cytol (Baltimore) 20:*7, 1976.

Heitz D, Rousseau F, Devys D, et al: Isolation of sequences that span the fragile X and identification of a fragile X-related CpG island. *Science 251:*1236, 1991.

Herbst AL, Robboy SJ, Scully RE, Poskanzer DC: Clear-cell adenocarcincoma of the vagina and cervix in girls. Analysis of 170 registry cases. *Am J Obstet Gynecol 119:*713, 1974.

Herbst ALH, Ulfelder H, Poskanzer DC: Adenocarcinoma of the vagina. *N Engl J Med 284:*878, 1971.

Hinden E: External injury causing fetal deformity. *Arch Dis Child 40:* 80, 1965.

Holmes KK: Syphilis. *In* Thor GW, Adams RD, Braunwald E, et al (eds): *Harrison's Principles of Internal Medicine,* 8th ed. New York, McGraw-Hill, 1977.

Holmes LB: Bendectin. *In* Sever JL, Brent RL (eds): *Teratogen Update: Environmentally Induced Birth Defect Risks.* New York, Alan R Liss, 1986.

Holmes LB: Hydroxamic acid: a potential human teratogen that could be recommended to treat ureaplasma. *Teratology 53:*227, 1996.

Holzgreve W, Carey JC, Hall BD: Warfarin-induced fetal abnormalities. *Lancet 2:*914, 1976.

Hook EB: Rates of chromosomal abnormalities at different maternal ages. *Obstet Gynecol 58:*282, 1981.

Hook EB, Cross PK, Jackson L, et al: Maternal age-specific rates of 47, +21 and other cytogenetic abnormalities diagnosed in the first trimester of pregnancy in chorionic villus biopsy specimens: comparison with rates expected from observations at amniocentesis. *Am J Hum Genet 42:*797, 1988.

Hook EB, Cross PK, Schreinemachers DM: Chromosomal abnormality rates at amniocentesis and in live-born infants. *JAMA 249:*2034, 1983.

Hook EB, Hamerton JL: The frequency of chromosome abnormalities detected in consecutive newborn studies—Differences between studies—Results by sex and by severity of phenotypic involvement. *In* Hook EB, Porter IH (eds): *Population Cytogenetics: Studies in Humans.* New York, Academic Press, 1977.

Hook EB, Warburton D: The distribution of chromosomal genotypes associated with Turner syndrome: livebirth prevalence rates and evidence for diminished fetal mortality and severity of genotypes associated with structural X abnormalities or mosaicism. *Human Genet 64:*24, 1983.

Hudson SP: Selected viral infections in pregnancy. *J SOGC 16:*1245, 1994.

Ingall D, Musher D: Syphilis. *In* Remington JS, Klein JO (eds): *Diseases of the Fetus and Newborn Infant,* 2nd ed. Philadelphia, WB Saunders, 1983.

Inouye M: Radiation-induced apoptosis and developmental disturbance of the brain. *Congen Anom 35:*1, 1995.

Isada N, Sever J, Larsen J: Rubella. *In* Quilligan EJ, Zuspan FP (eds): *Current Therapy in Obstetrics and Gynecology,* vol 3. Philadelphia, WB Saunders, 1990.

Jacobson CB, Berlin CM: Possible reproductive detriment in LSD users. *JAMA 222:*1367, 1972.

Johnstone FD: HIV and pregnancy. *Br J Obstet Gynaecol 103:*1184, 1996.

Jones KL: Dysmorphology: *In* Behrman RE, Kliegman RM, Arvin AM (eds): *Nelson Textbook of Pediatrics,* 15th ed. Philadelphia, WB Saunders, 1996.

Jones KL: Effects of chemical and environmental agents. *In* Creasy RK, Resnik R (eds): *Maternal-Fetal Medicine: Principles and Practice,* 2nd ed. Philadelphia, WB Saunders, 1989.

Jones KL: *Smith's Recognizable Patterns of Human Malformation,* 5th ed. Philadelphia, WB Saunders, 1997.

Jones KL, Smith DW, Streissguth AP, Myrianthopoulos NC: Outcome in offspring of chronic alcoholic women. *Lancet 1:*1076, 1974.

Kaltenbach KA, Finnegan LP: Prenatal narcotic exposure: perinatal and developmental effects. *Neurotoxicol 10:*597, 1989.

Kaufman MH: New insights into triploidy and tetraploidy, from an analysis of model systems for these conditions. *Hum Reprod 6:*8, 1991.

Kaufman RH: Consequence of in utero exposure to diethylstilbestrol. *In* Copelan LJ, Jarrell J, McGregor J (eds): *Textbook of Gynecology.* Philadelphia, WB Saunders, 1993.

Kendrick JS, Merritt RK: Woman and smoking: an update for the 1990s. *Am J Obstet Gynecol 175:*528, 1996.

Khoury MJ: Commentary: contributions of epidemiology to the study of birth defects in humans. *Teratology 52:*186, 1995.

King RA, Rotter JI, Motulsky AG: *The Genetic Basis of Common Diseases.* New York, Oxford University Press, 1992.

Kinnon C: Genes in diagnosis and therapy. *Br J Hosp Med 56:*132, 1996.

Kirkilionis AJ, Chudley AE, Gregory CA, Hamerton JL: Molecular and clinical overlap of Angelman and Prader-Willi syndrome phenotypes. *Am J Med Genet 40:*454, 1991.

Kliegman RM: Teratogens. *In* Behrman RE, Kliegman RM, Arvin AM (eds): *Nelson Textbook of Pediatrics,* 15th ed. Philadelphia, WB Saunders, 1996.

Knoll JHM, Nicholls RD, Magenis RE, et al: Angelman and Prader-Willi syndrome share a common chromosome 15 deletion but differ in parental origin of the deletion. *Am J Med Genet 32:*285, 1989.

Kochhar DM: Retinoids and retinoid receptors in teratogenesis. *Congen Anom 35:*55, 1995.

Koren G: Chickenpox during pregnancy. *Can Fam Physician 41:* 1477, 1995.

Koren G: Cocaine use by pregnant women in Toronto. *Can Fam Physician 42:*1677, 1996.

Koren G (ed): *Maternal-Fetal Toxicology: A Clinicians Guide.* New York, Marcel Dekker, 1990.

Korones SB: Congenital rubella—An encapsulated review. *In* Sever JL, Brent RL (eds): *Teratogen Update: Environmentally Induced Birth Defect Risks.* New York, Alan R Liss, 1986.

Kriegel H, Schmahl W, Gerber GB, Stieve FE: *Radiation Risks to the Developing Nervous System.* Stuttgart, Gustav Fischer, 1986.

Laegreid L, Olegard R, Walstrom J, Conradi N: Teratogenic effects of benzodiazepine use during pregnancy. *J Pediatr 114:*126, 1989.

Lammer EJ, Chen ET, Hoar RM, et al: Retinoic acid embryopathy. *New Engl J Med 313:*837, 1985.

Larson JW Jr: Congenital toxoplasmosis. *In* Sever JL, Brent RL (eds): *Teratogen Update: Environmentally Induced Birth Defect Risks.* New York, Alan R Liss, 1986.

Lenz W: A short history of thalidomide embryopathy. *Teratology 38:* 203, 1988.

Lenz W: Kindliche Missbildungen nach Medikament während der Gravidität? *Dtsch Med Wochenschr 86:*2555, 1961.

Levy HL, Ghavami M: Maternal phenylketonuria: a metabolic teratogen. *Teratology 53:*176, 1996.

Li D-Km, Mueller BA, Hickok DE, et al: Maternal smoking during pregnancy and the risk of congenital urinary tract anomalies. *Am J Public Health 86:*249, 1996.

Linden MG, Bender BG, Robinson A: Intrauterine diagnosis of sex chromosome aneuploidy. *Obstet Gynecol 87:*468, 1996.

Little BB, Wilson GN, Jackson G: Is there a cocaine syndrome? Dysmorphic and anthropometric assessment of infants exposed to cocaine. *Teratology 54:*145, 1996.

Lockwood C, Ghidini A, Romero R, Hobbins JC: Amniotic band syndrome: reevaluation of its pathogenesis. *Am J Obstet Gynecol 160:*1030, 1989.

Long SY: Does LSD induce chromosomal damage and malformations? A review of the literature. *Teratology 6:*75, 1972.

Lynfield R, Eaton RB: Teratogen update: congenital toxoplasmosis. *Teratology 52:*176, 1995.

Ma S, Kalousek DK, Yuen BH, et al: An improved technique for molecular cytogenetic analysis of human preimplantation embryos with fluorescence *in situ* hybridization. *J Reprod Med 41:*379, 1996.

Manuelidis L: Individual interphase chromosome domains revealed by *in situ* hybridization. *Hum Genet 71:*288, 1985.

Matsumoto HG, Goyo L, Takevchi T: Fetal minamata disease. A neuropathological study of two cases of intrauterine intoxication by a methyl mercury compound. *J Neuropathol Exp Neurol 24:*563, 1965.

Mattos TC, Giugliani R, Haase HB: Congenital malformations detected in 731 autopsies of children aged 0 to 14 years. *Teratology 35:*305, 1987.

McBride WG: Thalidomide and congenital abnormalities. *Lancet 2:* 1358, 1961.

McFarlin BL, Bottems, SF: Maternal syphilis; the next pregnancy. *Am J Perinatol 13:*513, 1996.

McKusick VA: *Mendelian Inheritance in Man. Catalogs of Autosomal Dominant, Autosomal Recessive, and X-linked Phenotypes.* Baltimore, The Johns Hopkins University Press, 1975.

McLeod R, Remington JS: Toxoplasmosis. *In* Behrman RE, Kliegman RM, Arrin AM (eds): *Nelson Textbook of Pediatrics,* 15th ed. Philadelphia, WB Saunders, 1996.

Medicodes' Hospital and Payer: International Classification of Diseases, 9th Revision. *Clinical Modification*, 4th ed, vols 1-3, Salt Lake City, Medicode, Inc., 1995.

Melkonian R, Baker D: Risks of industrial mercury exposure in pregnancy. *Obstet Gynecol Surv 43:*637, 1988.

Milberger S, Biederman J, Faraone SV, et al: Is maternal smoking during pregnancy a risk factor for attention deficit hyperactivity disorder in children? *Am J Psychiatry 153:*1138, 1996.

Miller E, Hare JW, Cloherty JP, et al: Elevated maternal hemoglobin A_1C in early pregnancy and major congenital anomalies in infants of diabetic mother. *N Engl J Med 304:*1331, 1981.

Milunsky A (ed): *Genetic Disorders and the Fetus,* 3rd ed. Baltimore, John Hopkins University Press, 1992.

Milunsky A, Graef JW, Gaynor MF Jr: Methotrexate-induced congenital malformations. *J Pediatr 72:*790, 1968.

Mittendorf R: Teratogen update: carcinogenesis and teratogenesis associated with exposure to diethylstilbestrol (DES) in utero. *Teratology 51:*435, 1995.

Moore KL (ed): *The Sex Chromatin.* Philadelphia, WB Saunders, 1966.

Moore KL: *Clinically Oriented Anatomy,* 3rd ed. Baltimore, Williams & Wilkins, 1992.

Moore KL, Barr ML: Smears from the oral mucosa in the detection of chromosomal sex. *Lancet 2:*57, 1955.

Muragaki Y, Mundlos S, Upton J, Olsen BR: Altered growth and branching patterns in synpolydactyly caused by mutations in HOXD 13. *Science 272:*548, 1996.

Nahas GG: Cannabis: toxicological properties and epidemiological aspects. *Med J Australia 145:*82, 1986.

Nahmias AJ, Visintine AM, Reimer CB, et al: Herpes simplex virus infection of the fetus and newborn. *In* Krugman S, Gershon AA (eds): *Infections of the Fetus and Newborn. Progress in Clinical and Biological Research,* vol 3. New York, Alan R Liss, 1975.

Nash JE, Persaud TVN: Embryopathic risks of cigarette smoking. *Exp Pathol 33:*65, 1988a.

Nash JE, Persaud TVN: Reproductive and teratological risks of caffeine. *Anat Anz 167:*265, 1988b.

Nathan L, Bohman VR, Sanchez PJ, et al: *In utero* infection with *Treponema pallidum* in early pregnancy. *Prenat Diagn 17:*119, 1997.

Nelson K, Holmes LB: Malformations due to presumed spontaneous mutations in newborn infants. *N Engl J Med 320:*19, 1989.

Nelson MM, Fofar JL: Associations between drugs administered during pregnancy and congenital abnormalities of the fetus. *Br Med J 1:*523, 1971.

Neu RL, Gardner LI: Abnormalities of the sex chromosomes. *In* Gardner LL (ed): *Endocrine and Genetic Diseases of Childhood and Adolescence,* 2nd ed. Philadelphia, WB Saunders, 1975.

Newman CGH: Clinical aspects of thalidomide embryopathy—A continuing preoccupation. *In* Sever JL, Brent RL (eds): *Teratogen Update: Enviornmentally Induced Birth Defect Risks.* New York, Alan R Liss, 1986a.

Newman CGH: The thalidomide syndrome: risks of exposure and spectrum of malformations. *Clin Perinatol 13:*555, 1986b.

Newnham JP, Evans SF, Michael CA, et al: Effects of frequent ultrasound during pregnancy; a randomised controlled trial. *Lancet 342:*887, 1993.

Nora AH, Nora JJ: A syndrome of multiple congenital anomalies associated with teratogenic exposure. *Arch Environ Health 30:*17, 1975.

Nurminen T, Rantala K, Kurppa K, Holmberg PC: Agricultural work during pregnancy and selected structural malformations in Finland. *Epidemiology 6:*23, 1995.

Nyberg DA, Mahony BS, Pretorius DH (eds): *Diagnostic Ultrasound of Fetal Anomalies.* Chicago, Year Book Medical Publishers, 1990.

Otake M, Schull WJ, Yoshimaru HL: Brain damage among the prenatally exposed. *J Rad Res 32(Suppl):*249, 1991.

Page EW, Villee CA, Villee DB: *Human Reproduction: Essentials of Reproductive and Perinatal Medicine,* 3rd ed. Philadelphia, WB Saunders, 1981.

Papavassiliou AG: Molecular medicine: transcription factors. *N Engl J Med 332:*45, 1995.

Parks W: Human immunodeficiency virus. *In* Behrman RE, Kliegman RM, Arvin AM (eds): *Nelson Textbook of Pediatrics,* 15th ed. Philadelphia, WB Saunders, 1996.

Patterson RM: Seizure disorders in pregnancy. *Med Clin North Am 73:*661, 1989.

Paulson G, Paulson RB: Seizure disorders in pregnancy. *In* Quilligan EJ, Zuspan FP: (eds): *Current Therapy in Obstetrics and Gynecology,* vol 3. Philadelphia, WB Saunders, 1990.

Pearson PL, Bobrow M, Vosa CG: Technique for identifying Y chromosomes in human interphase nuclei. *Nature 226:*78, 1970.

Persaud TVN: *Environmental Causes of Human Birth Defects.* Springfield, Charles C Thomas, 1990.

Persaud TVN: Fetal alcohol syndrome. *Critical Rev Anat Cell Biol 1:* 277, 1988.

Persaud TVN: Meromelia and other developmental abnormalities in experimental oligohydramnios. *Anat Anz 133:*499, 1973.

Persaud TVN: Pregnancy and the workplace. *Contemp Ob Gyn 4:*20, 1995.

Persaud TVN: *Problems of Birth Defects. From Hippocrates to Thalidomide and After.* Baltimore, University Park Press, 1977.

Persaud TVN: *Teratogenesis. Experimental Aspects and Clinical Implications.* Jena, Gustav Fischer Verlag, 1979.

Persaud TVN, Chudley AE, Skalko RG: *Basic Concepts in Teratology.* New York, Alan R Liss, 1985.

Persaud TVN, Ellington AC: Teratogenic activity of cannabis resin. *Lancet 2:*406, 1968.

Persaud TVN, Moore KL: Causes and prenatal diagnosis of congenital abnormalities. *J Obstet Gynecol Nursing 3:*40, 1974.

Pinkel D, Straume T, Gray JW: Cytogenic analysis using quantitative high sensitivity, fluorescence hybridization. *Proc Natl Acad Sci USA 83:*2934, 1986.

Ralcewicz TA, Persaud TVN: Effects of prenatal exposure to low dose ionizing radiation on the development of the cerebellar cortex in the rat. *Histol Histopathol 10:*371, 1995.

Randall T: Thalidomide's back in the news, but in more favorable circumstances. *JAMA 263:*1467, 1990.

Ray JG: Lues-lues: maternal and fetal considerations of syphilis. *Obstet Gynecol Surv 50:*845, 1995.

Reece EA, Assimakopoulos E, Zheng X-Z, et al: The safety of obstetric ultrasonography. Concern for the fetus. *Obstet Gynecol 6:*139, 1990.

Reece EA, Eriksson UJ: The pathogenesis of diabetes-associated congenital malformations. *Obstet Gynecol Clin North Am 23:*29, 1996.

Reece EA, Hobbins JC: Diabetic embryopathy: pathogenesis, prenatal diagnosis and prevention. *Obstet Gynecol Surv 41:*325, 1986.

Reece EA, Hobbins JC, Mahoney MJ, Petrie RH: *Handbook of Medicine of the Fetus & Mother.* Philadelphia, JB Lippincott, 1995.

Remington JS, Klein JO (eds): *Infectious Diseases of the Fetus and Newborn Infant,* 4th ed. Philadelphia, WB Saunders, 1995.

Rendle-Short TJ: Tetracycline in teeth and bone. *Lancet 1:*118, 1962.

Reynolds DW, Stagno S, Alford CA: Congenital cytomegalovirus infection. *In* Sever JL, Brent RL (eds): *Teratogen Update: Environmentally Induced Birth Defect Risks.* New York, Alan R Liss, 1986.

Ricci JM, Fojaco RM, O'Sullivan MJ: Congenital syphilis: The University of Miami/Jackson Memorial Medical Centre Experience, 1986-1988. *Obstet Gynecol 74:*687, 1989.

Riley Jr HD: History of the cytomegalovirus. *South Med J 90:*184, 1997.

Robert E: Teratogen update: electromagnetic fields. *Teratology* 54: 305, 1996.

Roessler E, Belloni E, Gaudenz K, et al: Mutations in the human *Sonic Hedgehog* gene cause holoprosencephaly. *Nature Genet 14:* 357, 1996.

Rogan WJ: PCBs and cola colored babies: Japan 1968 and Taiwan, 1979. *In* Sever JL, Brent RL (eds): *Teratogen Update: Environmentally Induced Birth Defect Risks*. New York, Alan R Liss, 1986.

Rosenberg AA, Galan HL: Fetal drug therapy. *Pediatr Clin North Am 44:*113, 1997.

Rosenberg RN: DNA-triplet repeats and neurological disease. *N Engl J Med 335:*1222, 1996.

Ross A, Raab GM, Mok J, et al: Maternal HIV infection, drug use, and growth of uninfected children in their first 3 years. *Arch Dis Child 73:*490, 1995.

Rothman KJ, Moore LL, Singer MR, et al: Teratogenicity of high vitamin A intake. *N Engl J Med 333:*1369, 1995.

Saenger P: Turner's syndrome. *N Engl J Med 335:*1749, 1996.

Sanders RC (ed): *Structural Fetal Abnormalities. The Total Picture*. St Louis, Mosby, 1996.

Schull WJ: *Effects of Atomic Radiation: A Half-Century of Studies from Hiroshima and Nagasaki*. Toronto, John Wiley and Sons, 1995.

Seeds JW, Azizkham RG: *Congenital Malformations. Antenatal Diagnosis, Perinatal Management, and Counseling*. Rockville, Aspen, 1990.

Seto A, Einarson T, Koren G: Pregnancy outcome following first trimester exposure to antihistamines: meta-analysis. *Am J Perinatal 14:*119, 1997.

Shepard TH: *Catalog of Teratogenic Agents,* 7th ed. Baltimore, The Johns Hopkins University Press, 1992.

Shepard TH: "Proof" of human teratogenicity. *Teratology 50:*97, 1994.

Shepard TH, Fantel AG, Fitzsimmons J: Congenital defect rates among spontaneous abortuses. Twenty years of monitoring. *Teratology 39:*325, 1989.

Shiota K, Uwabe C, Nishimura H: High prevalence of defective human embryos at the early postimplantation period. *Teratology 35:* 309, 1987.

Simpson JL, Elias S (eds): *Essentials of Prenatal Diagnosis*. New York, Churchill Livingstone, 1993.

Snyder RD: Congenital mercury poising. *N Engl J Med 284:*1014, 1971.

Sobell JL, Heston LL, Sommer SS: Delineation of genetic predisposition to multifactorial disease — A general approach on the threshold of feasibility. *Genomics 12:*1, 1992.

Spranger J, Benirschke K, Hall JG, et al: Errors of morphogenesis: concepts and terms. *J Pediatr 100:*160, 1982.

Stephens TD: Proposed mechanisms of action in thalidomide embryopathy. *Teratology 38:*229, 1988.

Stevenson RE, Hall JG, Goodman RM (eds): *Human Malformations and Related Anomalies,* vols I & II. New York, Oxford University Press, 1993.

Strauss RS: Effects of the intrauterine environment on childhood growth. *Br Med Bull 53:*81, 1997.

Swayze VW, Johnson VP, Hanson JW, et al: Magnetic resonance imaging of brain anomalies in fetal alcohol syndrome. *Pediatrics 99:*232, 1997.

Taeusch HW, Ballard RA, Avery ME (eds): *Schaffer and Avery's Diseases of the Newborn,* 6th ed. Philadelphia, WB Saunders, 1991.

Tanaka H: Functional damage in the developing brain induced by maternal environmental agents: ethanol, tobacco and low-copper level. *Congen Anom 35:*435, 1995.

Tassabehji M, Read AP, Newton VE, et al: Warrdenburg's syndrome patients have mutations in the human homologue of the *Pax-3* paired box gene. *Nature 355:*635, 1992.

Thiersch JB: Therapeutic abortions with a folic acid antagonists, 4-aminopteroylglutamic acid (4-amino-PGA), administered by the oral route. *Am J Obstet Gynecol 63:*1298, 1952.

Thompson MW, McInnes RR, Willard HF: *Thompson & Thompson Genetics in Medicine,* 5th ed. Philadelphia, WB Saunders, 1991.

Turrentine MA, Braems G, Ramirez MM: Use of thrombolytics for the treatment of thromboembolic disease during pregnancy. *Obstet Gynecol Surv 50:*534, 1995.

Tyrala EE: The infant of the diabetic mother. *Obstet Gynecol Clin North Am 23:*221, 1996.

Uchida IA: Radiation-induced nondisjunction. *Environ Health Perspect 31:*13, 1979.

Ulfelder H: DES — Transplacental teratogen — and possible carcinogen. *In* Sever JL, Brent RL (eds): *Teratogen Update: Environmentally Induced Birth Defect Risks*. New York, Alan R Liss, 1986.

Vorherr H, Vorherr UF, Mehta P, et al: Vaginal absorption of povidone-iodine. *JAMA 244:*2628, 1980.

Wald NJ, Cuckle HS: AFP screening in early pregnancy. *In* Spencer JAD (ed): *Fetal Monitoring*. Oxford, Oxford University Press, 1991.

Warkany J: Anti-tuberculous drugs. *In* Sever JL, Brent RL (eds): *Teratogen Update: Environmentally Induced Birth Defect Risks*. New York, Alan R Liss, 1986.

Warkany J: Teratogen update: lithium. *Teratology 38:*593, 1988.

Warkany J: Warfarin embryopathy. *Teratology 14:*205, 1976.

Wasserman CR, Shaw GM, O'Malley CD, et al: Parental cigarette smoking and risk of congenital anomalies of the heart, neural tube, or limb. *Teratology 53:*261, 1996.

Werler MM, Pober BR, Holmes LB: Smoking and Pregnancy. *In* Sever JL, Brent RL (eds): *Teratogen Update: Environmentally Induced Birth Defect Risks*. New York, Alan R Liss, 1986.

Wigglesworth JS: *Perinatal Pathology,* 2nd ed. Philadelphia, WB Saunders, 1996.

Wilcox AJ, Baird DD, Weinberg CR, et al: Fertility in men exposed prenatally to diethylstilbestrol. *N Engl J Med 332:*1441, 1995.

Wilkins L, Jones Jr HW, Holman GH, Stempfel RS Jr: Masculinization of the female fetus in association with administration of oral and intramuscular progestins during gestation; non-adrenal female pseudohermaphroditism. *J Clin Endocrinol Metab 18:*559, 1958.

Williamson WD, Percy AK, Yow MD, et al: Asymptomatic congenital cytomegalovirus infection. *Am J Dis Child 144:*1365, 1990.

Winston NJ, Braude PR, Pickering SJ, et al: The instance of abnormal morphology and nucleocytoplasmic ratios in 2-, 3- and 5-day human pre-embryos. *Human Reprod 6:*17, 1991.

Wynter HH, Persaud TVN: Results of a three-year study of birth defects in Jamaica. *Environ Child Health 18:*293, 1972.

Yokota K: Congenital anomalies induced by Toxoplasma infection. *Congen Anom 35:*151, 1995.

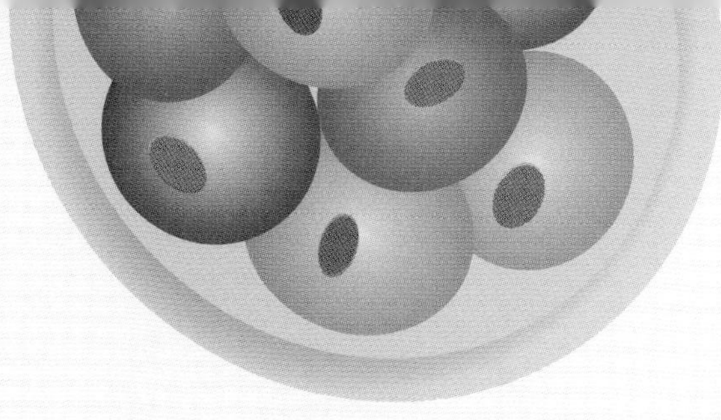

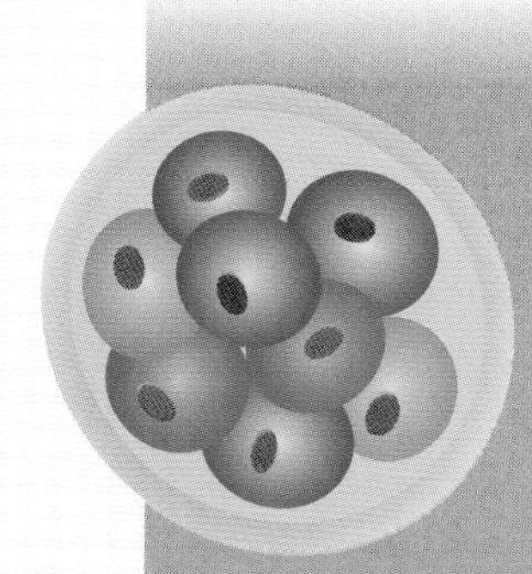

Body Cavities, Mesenteries, and Diaphragm

9

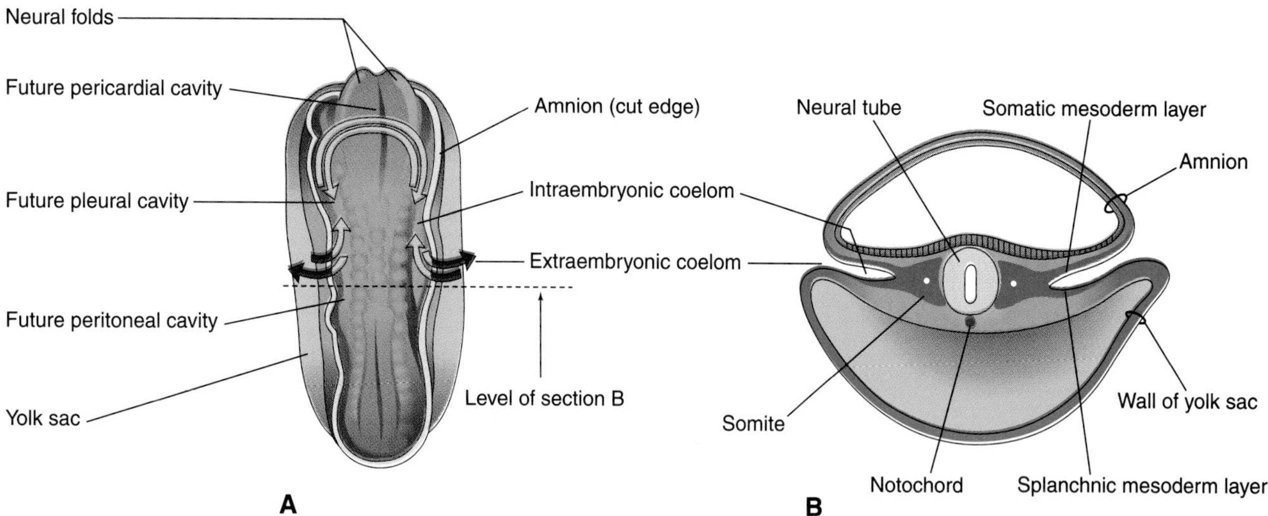

■ **Figure 9–1.** *A,* Drawing of a dorsal view of a 22-day-old embryo showing the outline of the horseshoe-shaped intraembryonic coelom. The amnion has been removed and the coelom is shown as if the embryo were translucent. The continuity of the intraembryonic coelom, as well as the communication of its right and left limbs with the extraembryonic coelom, is indicated by arrows. *B,* Transverse section through the embryo at the level shown in *A.*

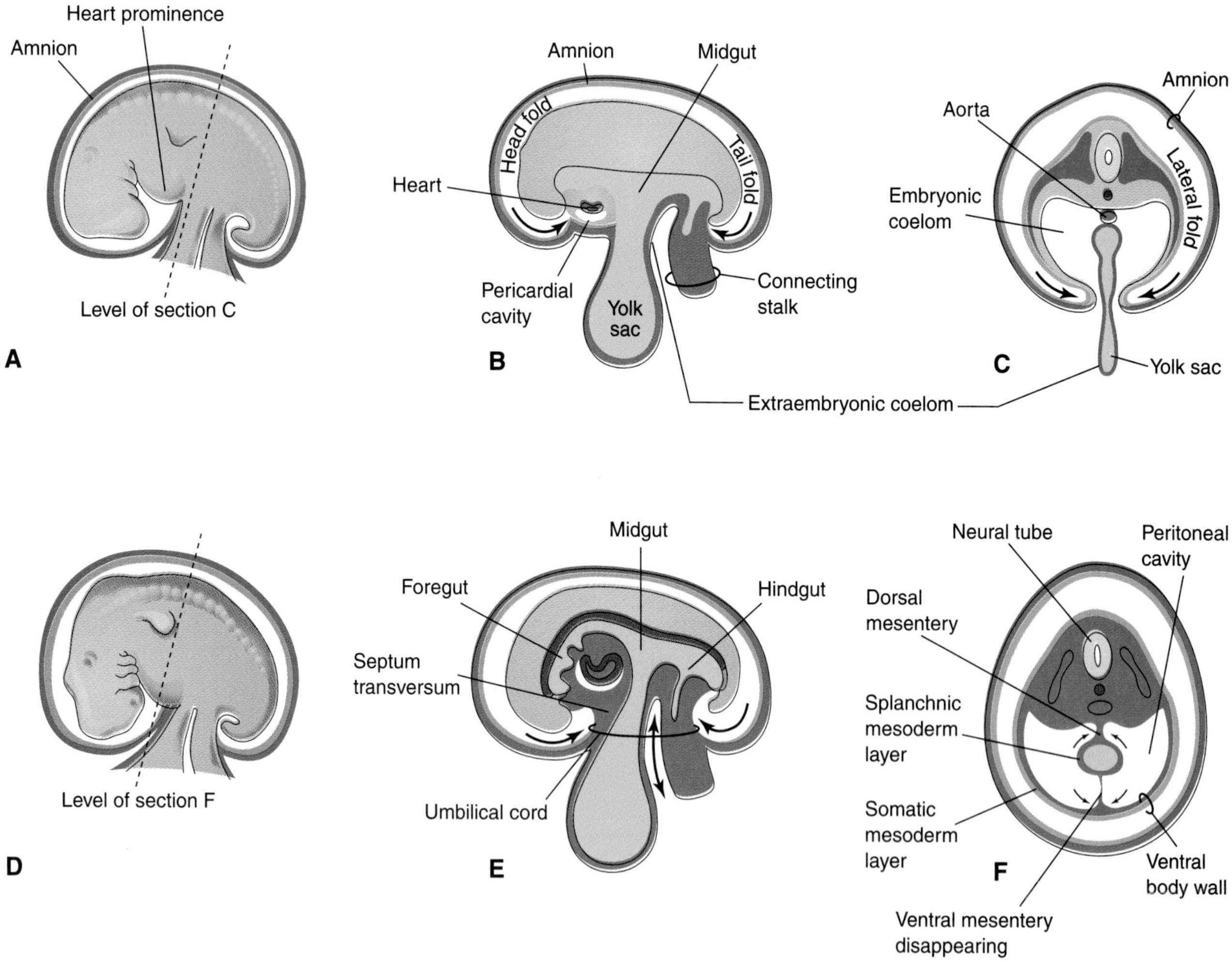

Heart prominence
Amnion
Level of section C
A
Amnion
Midgut
Head fold
Tail fold
Heart
Pericardial cavity
Yolk sac
Connecting stalk
B
Amnion
Aorta
Embryonic coelom
Lateral fold
C
Yolk sac
Extraembryonic coelom
Level of section F
D
Midgut
Foregut
Hindgut
Septum transversum
Umbilical cord
E
Neural tube
Peritoneal cavity
Dorsal mesentery
Splanchnic mesoderm layer
Somatic mesoderm layer
F
Ventral body wall
Ventral mesentery disappearing

■ **Figure 9–2.** Drawings illustrating embryonic folding and its effects on the intraembryonic coelom and other structures. *A,* Lateral view of an embryo (about 26 days). *B,* Schematic sagittal section of this embryo showing the head and tail folds. *C,* Transverse section at the level shown in *A,* indicating how fusion of the lateral folds gives the embryo a cylindrical form. *D,* Lateral view of an embryo (about 28 days). *E,* Schematic sagittal section of this embryo showing the reduced communication between the intraembryonic and extraembryonic coeloms *(double-headed arrow).* *F,* Transverse section as indicated in *D,* illustrating formation of the ventral body wall and disappearance of the ventral mesentery. The arrows indicate the junction of the somatic and splanchnic layers of mesoderm. The somatic mesoderm will become the parietal peritoneum lining the abdominal wall, and the splanchnic mesoderm will become the visceral peritoneum covering the organs (e.g., the stomach).

■ Early development of the intraembryonic coelom—primordium of the embryonic body cavities—is described in Chapter 4. Early in the fourth week, the **intraembryonic coelom** appears as a horseshoe-shaped cavity in the cardiogenic and lateral mesoderm (Fig. 9-1*A*). The curve or bend in this cavity at the cranial end of the embryo represents the future *pericardial cavity,* and its limbs (lateral extensions) indicate the future *pleural and peritoneal cavities.* The distal part of each limb of the intraembryonic coelom opens into the **extraembryonic coelom** at the lateral edges of the embryonic disc (Fig. 9-1*B*). This communication is important because most of the midgut normally herniates through this communication into the umbilical cord, where it develops into most of the small intestine and part of the large intestine (discussed in Chapter 12). In embryos of lower animal forms, the intraembryonic coelom provides short-term storage for excretory products. In human embryos, the coelom provides room for the organs to develop and move. During embryonic folding in the horizontal plane, the limbs of the intraembryonic coelom are brought together on the ventral aspect of the embryo (Fig. 9-2). The ventral mesentery degenerates in the region of the future peritoneal cavity, resulting in a large embryonic peritoneal cavity extending from the heart to the pelvic region (Figs. 9-2*F* and 9-3*E*).

THE EMBRYONIC BODY CAVITY

The intraembryonic coelom, or embryonic body cavity, gives rise to three well-defined coelomic or body cavities during the fourth week (Figs. 9-2 to 9-4):

- a *pericardial cavity*
- two *pericardioperitoneal canals* connecting the pericardial and peritoneal cavities
- a large *peritoneal cavity*

These body cavities have a parietal wall lined by mesothelium (major part of future parietal layer) derived from somatic mesoderm, and a visceral wall covered by mesothelium (future visceral layer) derived from splanchnic mesoderm (Fig. 9-3*E*). The peritoneal cavity (major part of intraembryonic coelom) is connected with the extraembryonic coelom at the umbilicus (Fig. 9-4*C* and *D*). The **peritoneal cavity** loses its connection with the extraembryonic coelom during the tenth week as the intestines return to the abdomen from the umbilical cord (see Chapter 12). During formation of the *head fold,* the heart and **pericardial cavity** move ventrocaudally, anterior to the foregut (Fig. 9-2*B*). As a result, the pericardial cavity opens into the pericardioperitoneal canals, which pass dorsal to the foregut (Fig. 9-4*B* and *D*). After embryonic folding, the caudal part of the foregut, the midgut, and the hindgut are suspended in the peritoneal cavity from the posterior abdominal wall by the *dorsal mesentery* (Figs. 9-2*F* and 9-3*C* to *E*).

Mesenteries

A mesentery is a double layer of peritoneum that begins as an extension of the visceral peritoneum covering an organ; *it connects the organ to the body wall and conveys vessels and nerves to it.* Transiently, the dorsal and ventral mesenteries divide the peritoneal cavity into right and left halves (Fig. 9-3*C*), but the ventral mesentery soon disappears (Fig. 9-3*E*), except where it is attached to the caudal part of the foregut (primordium of the stomach and proximal part of the duodenum). The peritoneal cavity then becomes a continuous space (Figs. 9-3 and 9-4). The arteries supplying the primitive gut—*celiac trunk* (foregut), *superior mesenteric artery* (midgut), and *inferior mesenteric artery* (hindgut)—pass between the layers of the dorsal mesentery (Fig. 9-3*C*).

Division of Embryonic Body Cavity

Each pericardioperitoneal canal lies lateral to the foregut (future esophagus) and dorsal to the **septum transversum**—a thick plate of mesodermal tissue that occupies the space between the thoracic cavity and yolk stalk (Fig. 9-4*A* and *B*). The septum transversum is the primordium of the **central tendon of the diaphragm**. Partitions form concurrently in each pericardioperitoneal canal that separate the pericardial cavity from the pleural cavities and the pleural cavities from the peritoneal cavity. Because of the *growth of the bronchial buds* (primordia of bronchi and lungs) into the pericardioperitoneal canals (Fig. 9-5*A*), a pair of membranous ridges is produced in the lateral wall of each canal:

- The cranial ridges—the *pleuropericardial folds*—are located superior to the developing lungs.
- The caudal ridges—the *pleuroperitoneal folds*—are located inferior to the lungs.

THE PLEUROPERICARDIAL MEMBRANES

As the pleuropericardial folds enlarge, they form partitions that separate the pericardial cavity from the pleural cavities. These partitions—*pleuropericardial membranes*—contain the **common cardinal veins** (Fig. 9-5*A* and *B*). These large veins drain the primordial venous system into the *sinus venosus* of the primordial heart (see Chapter 14). Initially the **bronchial buds** are small relative to the heart and pericardial cavity (Fig. 9-5*A*). They then grow laterally from the caudal end of the trachea into the pericardioperitoneal canals (future pleural canals). As the primordial **pleural cavities** expand ventrally around the heart, they extend into the body wall, splitting the mesenchyme into:

- an outer layer that becomes the thoracic wall
- an inner layer (the pleuropericardial membrane) that becomes the *fibrous pericardium,* the outer layer of the pericardial sac enclosing the heart (Fig. 9-5*C* and *D*)

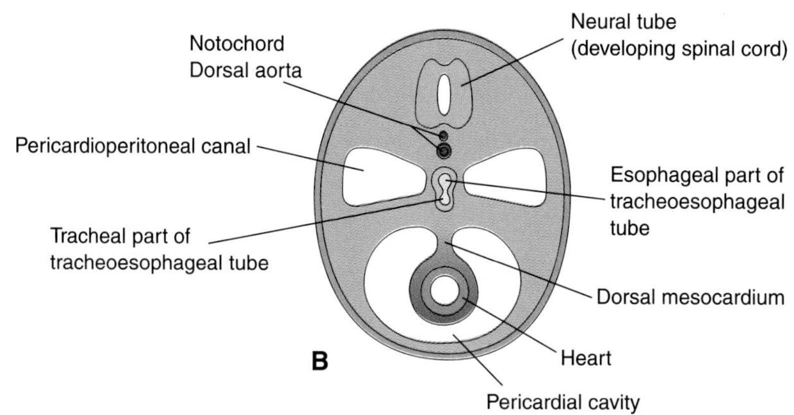

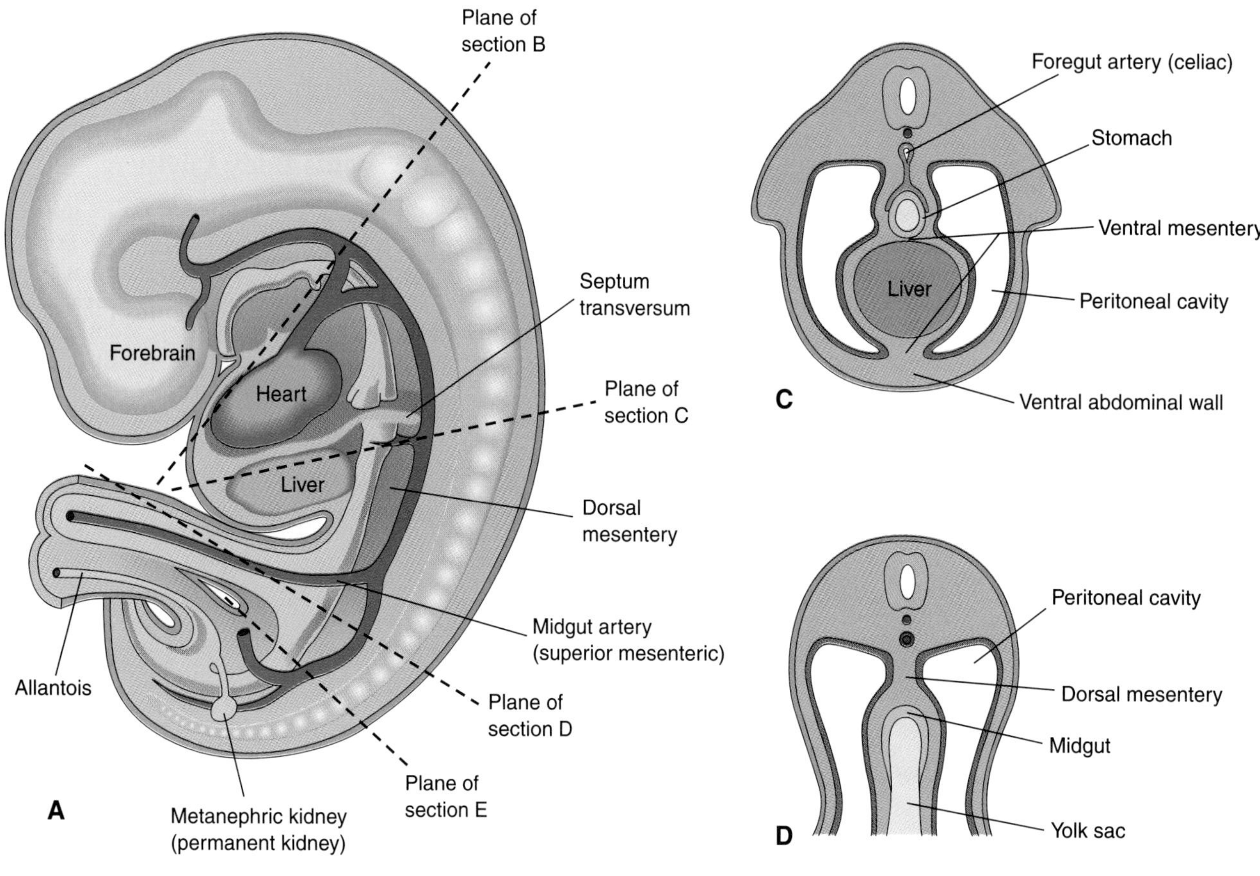

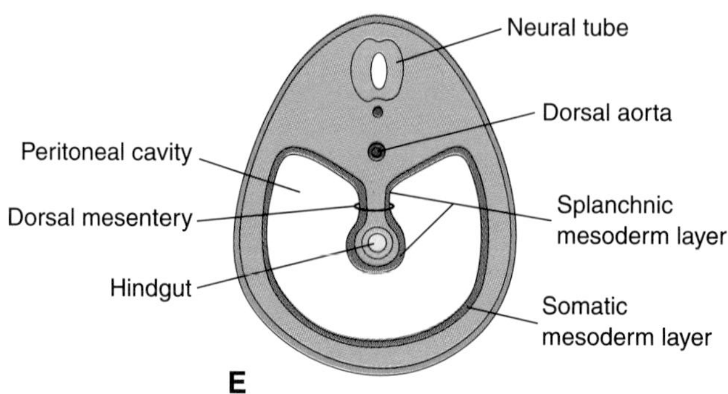

Figure 9–3. Diagrams illustrating the mesenteries at the beginning of the fifth week. *A,* Schematic sagittal section. Note that the dorsal mesentery serves as a pathway for the arteries supplying the developing gut. Nerves and lymphatics also pass between the layers of this mesentery. *B* to *E,* Transverse sections through the embryo at the levels indicated in *A.* The ventral mesentery disappears, except in the region of the terminal esophagus, stomach, and first part of the duodenum. Note that the right and left parts of the peritoneal cavity, separate in *C,* are continuous in *E.*

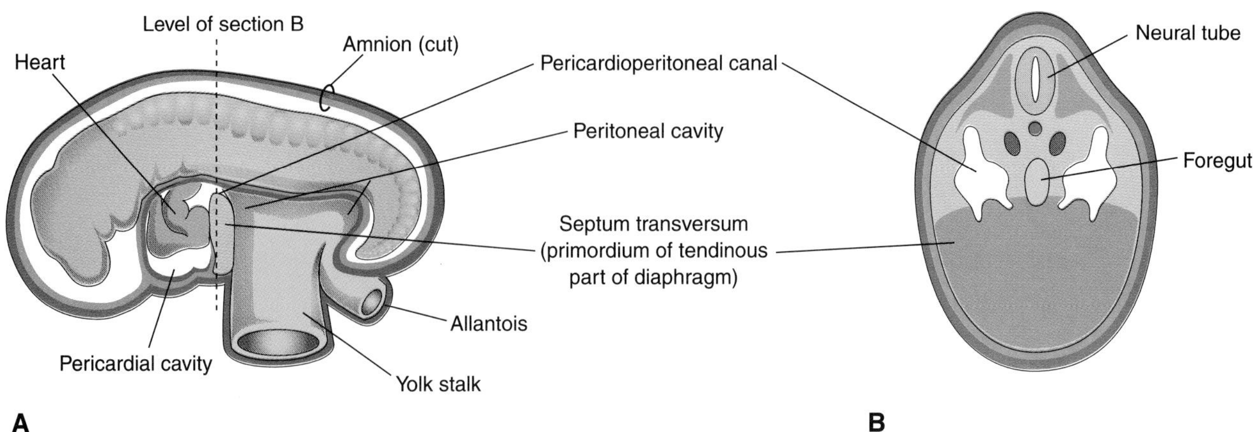

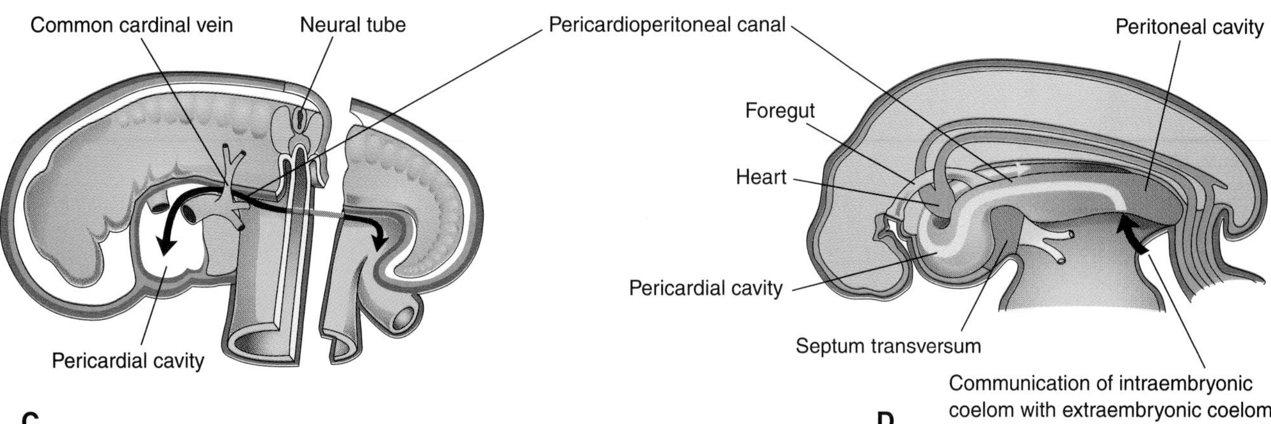

■ **Figure 9–4.** Schematic drawings of an embryo (about 24 days). *A,* The lateral wall of the pericardial cavity has been removed to show the primitive heart. *B,* Transverse section of the embryo illustrating the relationship of the pericardioperitoneal canals to the septum transversum (primordium of central tendon of diaphragm) and the foregut. *C,* Lateral view of the embryo with the heart removed. The embryo has also been sectioned transversely to show the continuity of the intraembryonic and extraembryonic coeloms. *D,* Sketch showing the pericardioperitoneal canals arising from the dorsal wall of the pericardial cavity and passing on each side of the foregut to join the peritoneal cavity. The arrow shows the communication of the extraembryonic coelom with the intraembryonic coelom and the continuity of the intraembryonic coelom at this stage.

The pleuropericardial membranes project into the cranial ends of the *pericardioperitoneal canals* (Fig. 9-5*B*). With subsequent growth of the common cardinal veins, descent of the heart, and expansion of the pleural cavities, the pleuropericardial membranes become mesenterylike folds extending from the lateral thoracic wall. By the seventh week the pleuropericardial membranes fuse with the mesenchyme ventral to the esophagus, forming the *primordial mediastinum* and separating the pericardial cavity from the pleural cavities (Fig. 9-5*C*). The **mediastinum** consists of a mass of mesenchyme (embryonic connective tissue) that extends from the sternum to the vertebral column, separating the developing lungs (Fig. 9-5*D*). The right pleuropericardial opening closes slightly earlier than the left one, probably because the right common cardinal vein is larger than the left one and produces a larger pleuropericardial membrane.

Congenital Pericardial Defects

Defective formation and/or fusion of the pleuropericardial membranes separating the pericardial and pleural cavities is an uncommon congenital anomaly. This abnormality results in a congenital defect of the pericardium, usually on the left side. Consequently, the pericardial cavity communicates with the pleural cavity. In very unusual cases, part of the left atrium herniates into the pleural cavity at each heartbeat.

THE PLEUROPERITONEAL MEMBRANES

As the *pleuroperitoneal folds* enlarge, they project into the pericardioperitoneal canals. Gradually the folds become membranous, forming the *pleuroperito-*

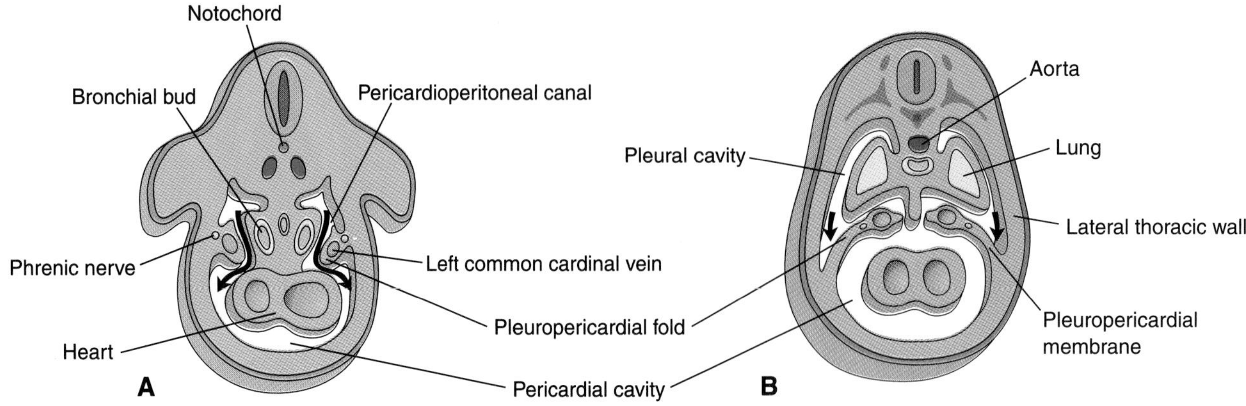

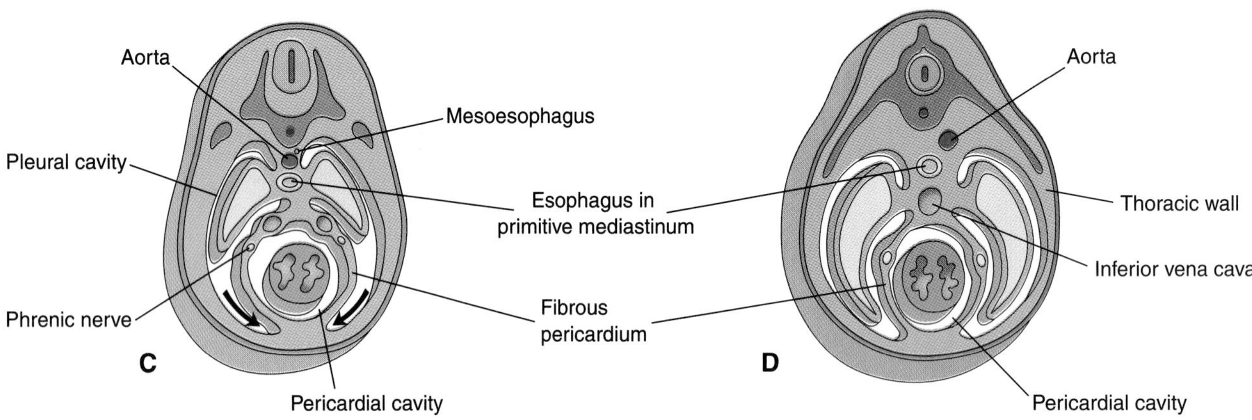

■ **Figure 9–5.** Schematic drawings of transverse sections through embryos cranial to the septum transversum, illustrating successive stages in the separation of the pleural cavities from the pericardial cavity. Growth and development of the lungs, expansion of the pleural cavities, and formation of the fibrous pericardium are also shown. *A,* 5 weeks. The arrows indicate the communications between the pericardioperitoneal canals and the pericardial cavity. *B,* 6 weeks. The arrows indicate development of the pleural cavities as they expand into the body wall. *C,* 7 weeks. Expansion of the pleural cavities ventrally around the heart is shown. The pleuropericardial membranes are now fused in the median plane with each other and with the mesoderm ventral to the esophagus. *D,* 8 weeks. Continued expansion of the lungs and pleural cavities and formation of the fibrous pericardium and thoracic wall are illustrated.

neal membranes (Figs. 9-6 and 9-7). Eventually these membranes will separate the pleural cavities from the peritoneal cavity. The pleuroperitoneal membranes are produced as the developing lungs and pleural cavities expand and invade the body wall. They are attached dorsolaterally to the abdominal wall and initially their crescentic free edges project into the caudal ends of the pericardioperitoneal canals. They become relatively more prominent as the lungs enlarge cranially and the liver expands caudally. During the sixth week the pleuroperitoneal membranes extend ventromedially until their free edges fuse with the dorsal mesentery of the esophagus and septum transversum (Fig. 9-7*C*). This separates the pleural cavities from the peritoneal cavity. *Closure of the pleuroperitoneal openings* is assisted by the migration of myoblasts (primitive muscle cells) into the pleuroperitoneal membranes (Fig. 9-7*E*). The pleuroperitoneal opening on the right side closes slightly before the left one. The reason for this is uncertain but it may be related to the relatively large size of the right lobe of the liver at this stage of development.

DEVELOPMENT OF THE DIAPHRAGM

The diaphragm is a composite structure that develops from four embryonic components (Fig. 9-7):

- septum transversum
- pleuroperitoneal membranes
- dorsal mesentery of esophagus
- muscular ingrowth from lateral body walls

The diaphragm is a dome-shaped, musculotendinous partition that separates the thoracic and abdominal cavities.

The Septum Transversum

The transverse septum, composed of mesodermal tissue, is the primordium of the **central tendon of the diaphragm** (Fig. 9-7*D* and *E*). The septum transversum grows dorsally from the ventrolateral body wall and forms a semicircular shelf, which separates the heart from the liver (Fig. 9-6). During its early development, a large part of the liver is embedded in the septum transversum. The septum transversum is located caudal to the pericardial cavity and partially separates it from the developing peritoneal cavity. The septum transversum is first identifiable at the end of the third week as a mass of mesodermal tissue cranial to the pericardial cavity (see Chapter 5). After the head folds ventrally during the fourth week, the septum transversum forms a thick incomplete partition between the pericardial and abdominal cavities (Fig. 9-4). The septum transversum does not separate the thoracic and abdominal cavities completely. There is a large opening, the **pericardioperitoneal canal**, on each side of the esophagus (Fig. 9-7*B*). The septum transversum expands and fuses with the mesenchyme ventral to the esophagus (primitive mediastinum) and the pleuroperitoneal membranes (Fig. 9-7*C*).

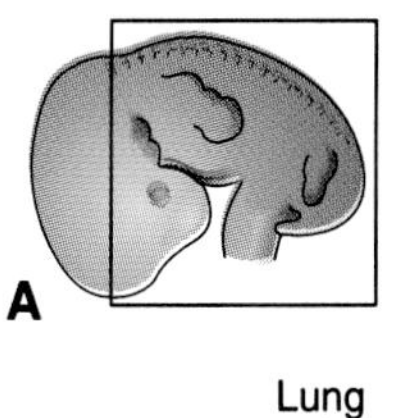

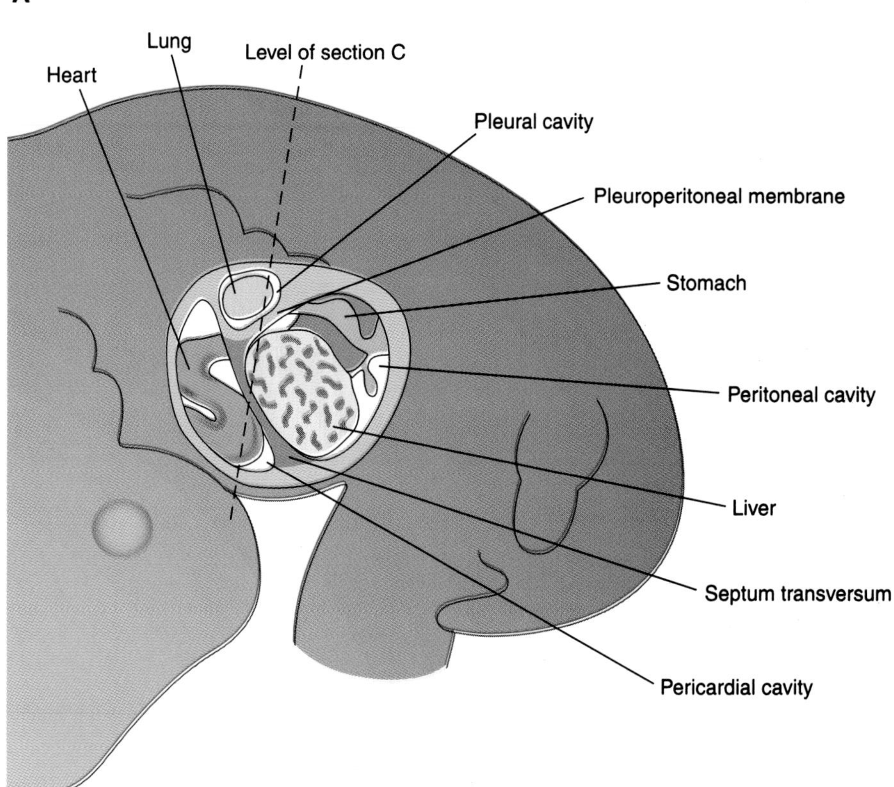

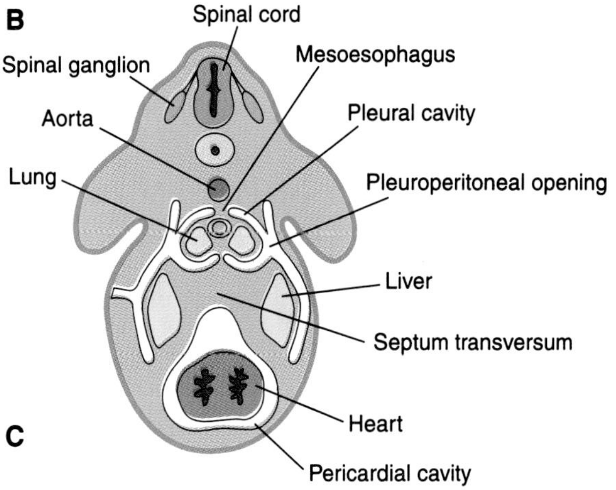

■ **Figure 9-6.** *A,* Sketch of a lateral view of an embryo (about 33 days). The rectangle indicates the area enlarged in *B*. *B,* The primordial body cavities are viewed from the left side after removal of the lateral body wall. *C,* Transverse section through the embryo at the level shown in *B*.

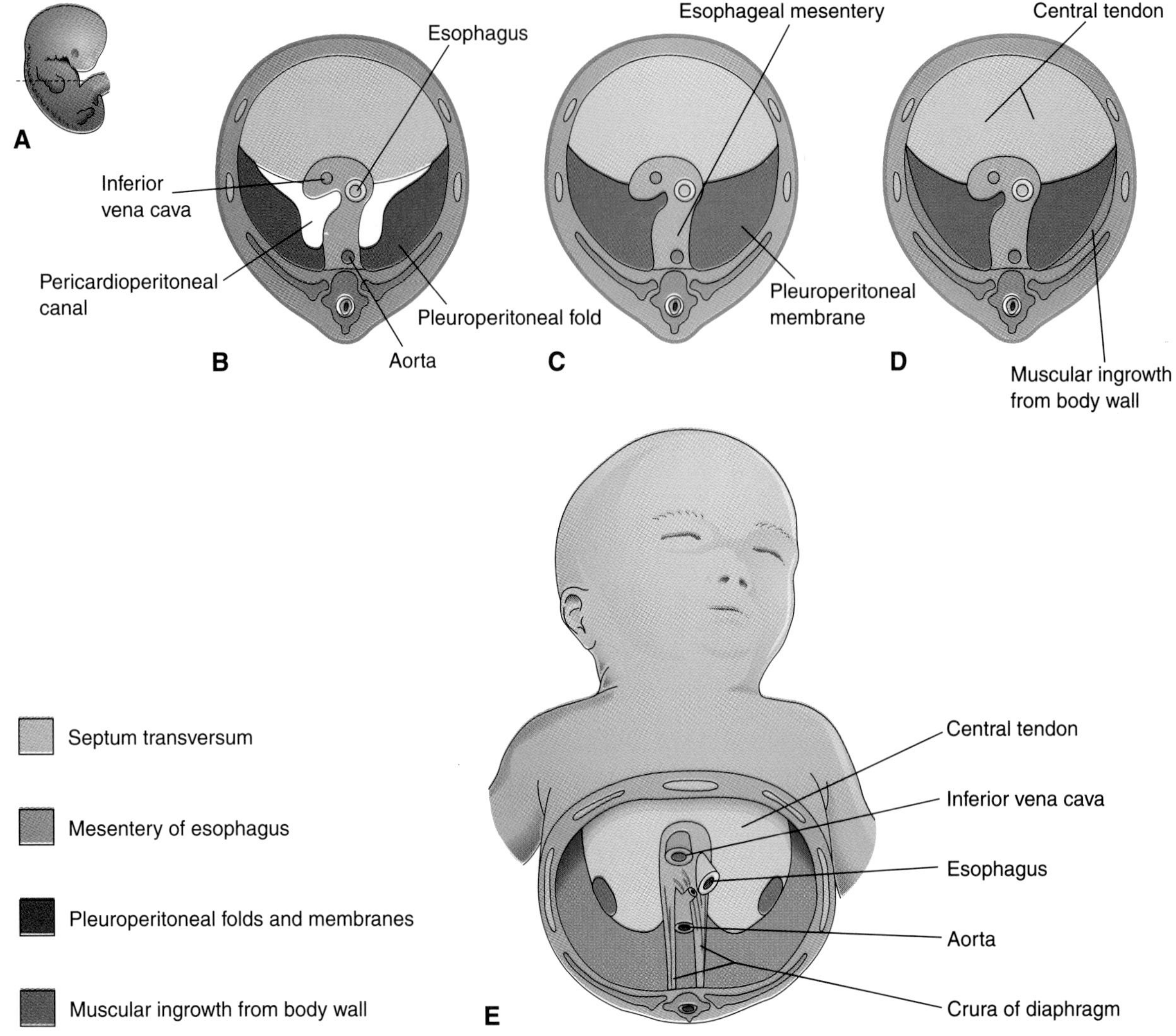

■ **Figure 9–7.** Drawings illustrating development of the diaphragm. *A,* Sketch of a lateral view of an embryo at the end of the fifth week (actual size), indicating the level of sections in *B* to *D*. *B* to *E* show the developing diaphragm as viewed inferiorly. *B,* Transverse section showing the unfused pleuroperitoneal membranes. *C,* Similar section at the end of the sixth week after fusion of the pleuroperitoneal membranes with the other two diaphragmatic components. *D,* Transverse section of a 12-week embryo after ingrowth of the fourth diaphragmatic component from the body wall. *E,* View of the diaphragm of a newborn infant, indicating the embryological origin of its components.

The Pleuroperitoneal Membranes

These membranes fuse with the dorsal mesentery of the esophagus and septum transversum (Fig. 9-7*C*). This completes the partition between the thoracic and abdominal cavities and forms the **primordial diaphragm**. Although the pleuroperitoneal membranes form large portions of the fetal diaphragm, they represent relatively small portions of the newborn infant's diaphragm (Fig. 9-7*E*).

The Dorsal Mesentery of the Esophagus

As previously described, the septum transversum and pleuroperitoneal membranes fuse with the dorsal mesentery of the esophagus. This mesentery constitutes the median portion of the diaphragm. The **crura of the diaphragm**—a leglike pair of diverging muscle bundles that cross in the median plane anterior to the aorta (Fig. 9-7*E*)—develop from myoblasts that grow into the dorsal mesentery of the esophagus.

The Muscular Ingrowth from the Lateral Body Walls

During the ninth to twelfth weeks the lungs and pleural cavities enlarge, "burrowing" into the lateral body walls (Fig. 9-5). During this excavation process the body-wall tissue is split into two layers:

- an external layer that becomes part of the definitive abdominal wall
- an internal layer that contributes muscle to peripheral portions of the diaphragm, external to the parts derived from the pleuroperitoneal membranes (Fig. 9-7*D* and *E*)

Further extension of the developing pleural cavities

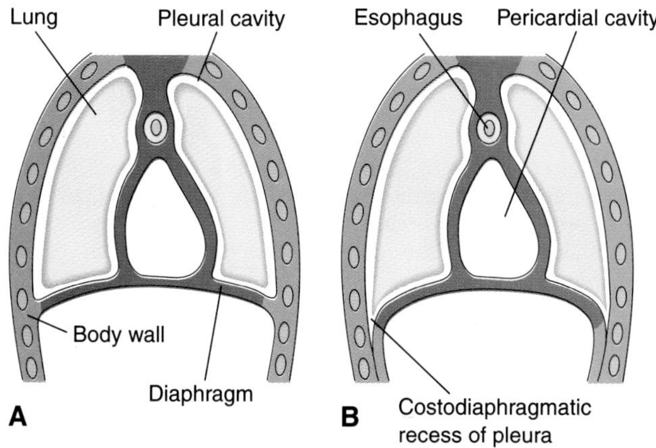

■ **Figure 9-8.** Diagrams illustrating extension of the pleural cavities into the body walls to form peripheral portions of the diaphragm, the costodiaphragmatic recesses, and the establishment of the characteristic dome-shaped configuration of the diaphragm. Note that body wall tissue is added peripherally to the diaphragm as the lungs and pleural cavities enlarge.

into the lateral body walls forms the right and left **costodiaphragmatic recesses** (Fig. 9-8), establishing the characteristic dome-shaped configuration of the diaphragm. After birth the costodiaphragmatic recesses become alternately smaller and larger as the lungs move in and out of them during inspiration and expiration.

Positional Changes and Innervation of the Diaphragm

During the fourth week of development the septum transversum, prior to its descent with the heart, lies opposite the third to fifth *cervical somites* (Fig. 9-9*A*). During the fifth week myoblasts (primitive muscles cells) from these somites migrate into the developing diaphragm, bringing their nerve fibers with them. Consequently, the **phrenic nerves** that supply motor innervation to the diaphragm arise from the ventral rami of the third, fourth, and fifth cervical spinal nerves. The three twigs on each side join together to form a phrenic nerve. The phrenic nerves also supply sensory fibers to the superior and inferior surfaces of the right and left domes of the diaphragm.

Rapid growth of the dorsal part of the embryo's body results in the *apparent descent of the diaphragm*. By the sixth week, the developing diaphragm is at the level of the thoracic somites (Fig. 9-9*B*). The phrenic nerves now have a descending course. As the diaphragm "moves" relatively farther caudally in the body, the nerves are correspondingly lengthened. By the beginning of the eighth week, the dorsal part of the diaphragm lies at the level of the first lumbar vertebra (Fig. 9-9*C*). Because of the embryonic origin of the phrenic nerves, they are about 30 cm long in adults (Moore, 1999). The embryonic phrenic nerves enter the diaphragm by passing through the pleuropericardial membranes. This explains why the phrenic nerves subsequently lie on the fibrous pericardium, the adult derivative of the pleuropericardial membranes (Fig. 9-5*C* and *D*).

As the four parts of the diaphragm fuse (Fig. 9-7), mesenchyme in the septum transversum extends into the other three parts. It forms myoblasts that differentiate into the skeletal muscle of the diaphragm; hence the motor nerve supply to the diaphragm is from the phrenic nerves. The sensory innervation of the diaphragm is also from the phrenic nerves, but its costal rim receives sensory fibers from the lower intercostal nerves because of the origin of the peripheral part of the diaphragm from the lateral body walls (Fig. 9-7*D* and *E*).

CONGENICAL DIAPHRAGMATIC HERNIA

The development of the diaphragm is a complex process; as a consequence, congenital defects may occur. A posterolateral defect of the diaphragm through which hernias occur is the most common anomaly. A congenital diaphragmatic hernia (CDH) is characterized by the presence of abdominal viscera in the thoracic cavity.

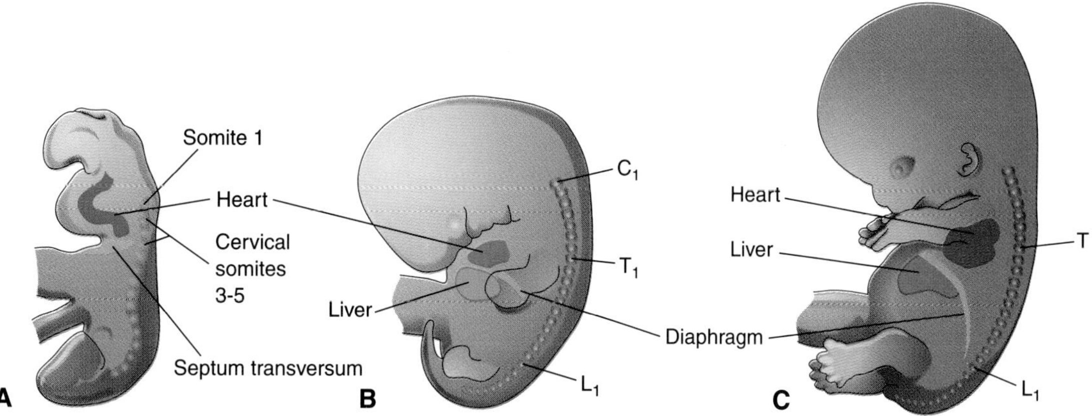

■ **Figure 9-9.** Diagrams illustrating positional changes of the developing diaphragm. *A,* About 24 days. The septum transversum is at the level of the third, fourth, and fifth cervical segments. *B,* About 41 days. *C,* About 52 days.

Posterolateral Defects of the Diaphragm

Posterolateral defect of the diaphragm is the only relatively common congenital anomaly of the diaphragm (Figs. 9-10*A* and *B*, and 9-11). This diaphragmatic defect occurs about once in 2200 newborn infants (Harrison, 1991) and is associated with **CDH** (herniation of abdominal contents into the thoracic cavity). Life-threatening breathing difficulties may be associated with CDH because of inhibition of development and inflation of lungs (Fig. 9-12). Moreover, fetal lung maturation may be delayed. *CDH is the most common cause of pulmonary hypoplasia* (Azarow et al, 1997; Wilson et al, 1997). **Polyhydramnios** (excess amniotic fluid) may also be present. CDH, usually unilateral, results from defective formation and/or fusion of the pleuroperitoneal membrane with the other three parts of the diaphragm (Fig. 9-7). This results in a large opening in the posterolateral region of the diaphragm. As a result, the peritoneal and pleural cavities are continuous with one another along the posterior body wall. The defect—sometimes referred to clinically as the foramen of Bochdalek—usually occurs on the left side in 85 to 90% of cases. The preponderance of left-sided defects is likely related to the earlier closure of the right pleuroperitoneal opening.

Prenatal diagnosis of CDH (Fig. 9-13) depends on the sonographic demonstration of abdominal organs in the thorax (Goldstein, 1994a). The diagnosis can also be confirmed by amniography (see Chapter 6)

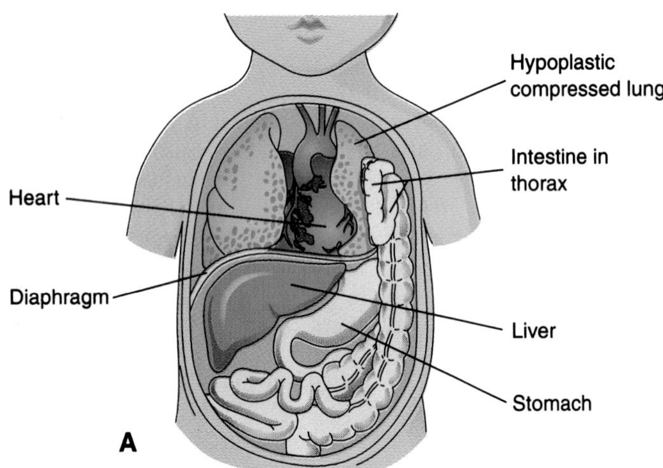

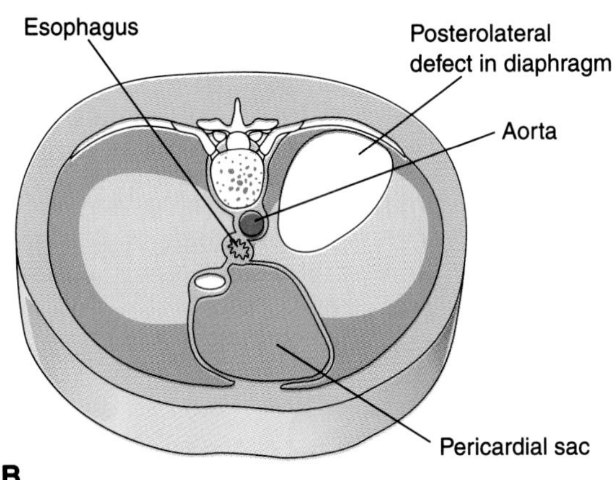

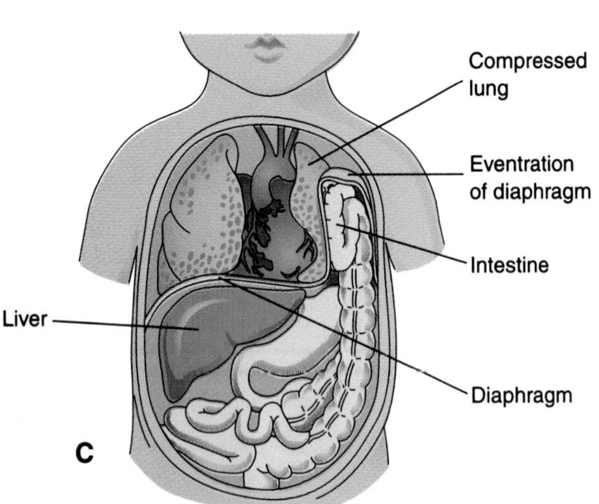

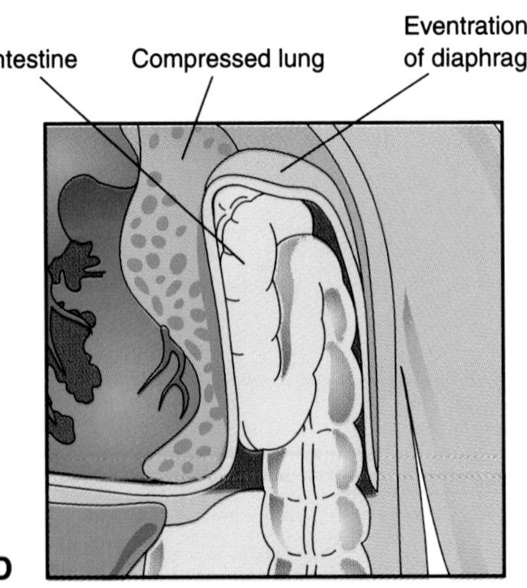

■ **Figure 9-10.** *A,* A "window" has been drawn on the thorax and abdomen to show the herniation of the intestine into the thorax through a posterolateral defect in the left side of the diaphragm. Note that the left lung is compressed and hypoplastic. *B,* Drawing of a diaphragm with a large posterolateral defect on the left side due to abnormal formation and/or fusion of the pleuroperitoneal membrane on the left side with the mesoesophagus and septum transversum. *C* and *D,* Eventration of the diaphragm resulting from defective muscular development of the diaphragm. The abdominal viscera are displaced into the thorax within a pouch of diaphragmatic tissue.

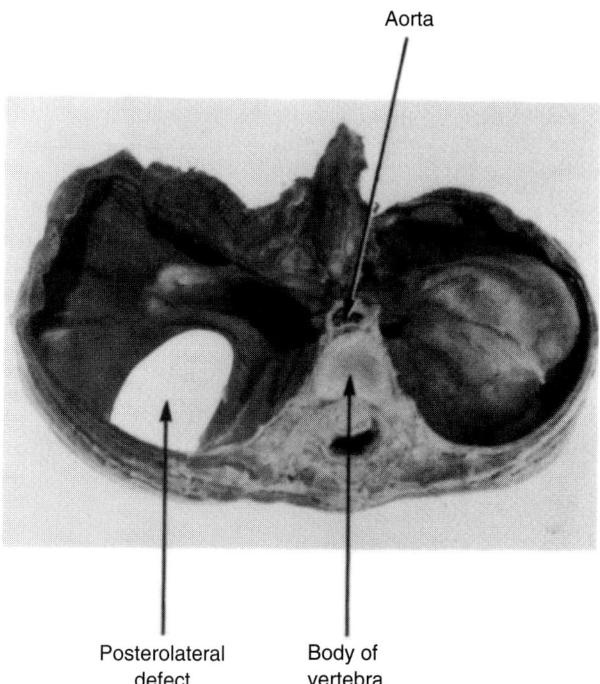

■ **Figure 9-11.** Photograph of a transverse section through the thoracic region of a stillborn infant, viewed from the thorax. Note the large left posterolateral defect of the diaphragm, which permitted the abdominal contents to pass into the thorax (CDH).

because the fetus swallows amniotic fluid, which can be observed in the thoracic cavity.

The pleuroperitoneal membranes normally fuse with the other three diaphragmatic components by the end of the sixth week (Fig. 9-7*C*). If a pleuroperitoneal canal is still open when the intestines return to the abdomen from the umbilical cord in the tenth week (see Chapter 12), some intestine and other viscera may pass into the thorax. The presence of abdominal viscera in the thorax pushes the lungs and heart anteriorly and compression of the lungs occurs (Goldstein, 1994b). Often the stomach, spleen, and most of the intestines herniate (Figs. 9-12 and 9-13). The abdominal viscera can usually move freely through the defect; consequently, they may be in the thoracic cavity when the infant is lying down and in the abdominal cavity when the infant is upright. Most babies born with CDH die not because there is a defect in the diaphragm or viscera in the chest, but because the lungs are hypoplastic because of compression of them during development (Harrison, 1991).

The severity of pulmonary developmental abnormalities depends on when and to what extent the abdominal viscera herniate into the thorax; i.e., on the timing and degree of compression of the fetal lungs. The effect on the ipsilateral (same side) lung is greater, but the contralateral lung also shows morphological changes (Harrison, 1991). If the abdominal viscera are in the thoracic cavity at birth, the initiation of respiration is likely to be impaired. The intestines dilate with swallowed air and compromise the functioning of the heart and lungs. Because the abdominal organs are most often in the left side of the thorax, the heart and mediastinum are usually displaced to the right.

The lungs in infants with CDH are often hypoplastic and greatly reduced in size. The growth retardation of the lungs results from lack of room for them to develop normally. The lungs are often aerated and achieve their normal size after reduction (repositioning) of the herniated viscera and repair of the defect in the diaphragm (Harrison, 1991); however, the mortality rate is high (approximately 76%). If there is severe **lung hypoplasia**, some primitive alveoli may rupture, causing air to enter the pleural cavity—*pneumothorax*. If necessary, CDH can be diagnosed and repaired prenatally between 22 and 28 weeks of gestation (20 to 26 weeks after fertilization), but this intervention carries considerable risk to the fetus and mother (Harrison, 1991).

Eventration of the Diaphragm

In this uncommon condition, half the diaphragm has defective musculature and balloons into the thoracic cavity as an aponeurotic (membranous) sheet, forming a diaphragmatic pouch (Fig. 9-10*C* and *D*). Consequently, there is superior displacement of abdominal viscera into the pocketlike outpouching of the diaphragm. This congenital anomaly results mainly from failure of muscular tissue from the body wall to extend into the pleuroperitoneal membrane on the affected side. *An eventration of the diaphragm is not a true diaphragmatic herniation*; it is a superior displacement of viscera into a saclike part of the diaphragm; however, the clinical manifestations of diaphragmatic eventration may simulate CDH (Hartman, 1996). During surgical repair, a muscular flap (e.g., from a back muscle such as the latissimus dorsi) or a prosthetic patch is used to strengthen the diaphragm.

Gastroschisis and Congenital Epigastric Hernia

This uncommon hernia occurs in the median plane between the xiphoid process and umbilicus. These defects are similar to umbilical hernias (see Chapter 12) except for their location. Gastroschisis and epigastric hernias result from failure of the lateral body folds to fuse completely when forming the anterior abdominal wall during folding in the fourth week (Fig. 9-2*C* and *F*). The small intestine herniates into the amniotic fluid and can be detected prenatally by ultrasonography (Langer and Harrison, 1991; Goldstein, 1994b).

Congenital Hiatal Hernia

There may be herniation of part of the fetal stomach through an excessively large **esophageal hiatus**—the opening in the diaphragm through which the esopha-

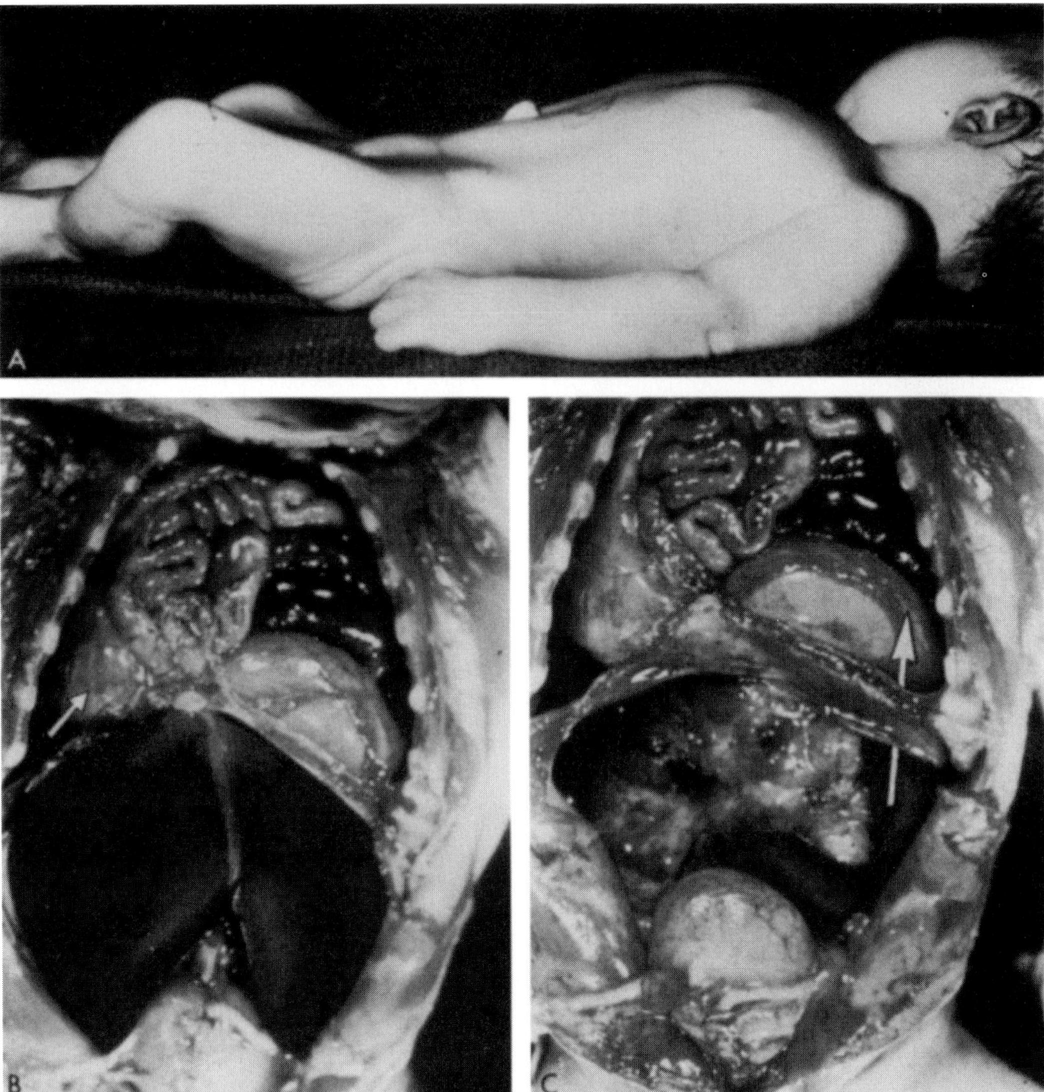

■ **Figure 9–12.** *A,* Photograph of an infant with CDH resulting from a large left posterolateral diaphragmatic defect similar to that shown in Figure 9–11. Note the relatively flat abdomen resulting from herniation of abdominal viscera into the thorax through the defect. *B,* The thoracic and abdominal cavities opened at autopsy to show the intestines and other viscera in the thoracic cavity. The arrow indicates the heart, which has been displaced to the right. *C,* The liver has been removed, showing that only attached parts of the intestine have remained in the abdominal cavity. The arrow passes through the diaphragmatic defect. (Courtesy of Dr. Jan Hoogstraten, Children's Hospital, Health Sciences Centre, Winnipeg, Manitoba, Canada.)

gus and vagus nerves pass; however, this is an uncommon congenital defect. Although hiatal hernia is usually an acquired lesion occurring during adult life (Moore, 1992), a congenitally enlarged esophageal hiatus may be the predisposing factor in some cases.

Retrosternal (Parasternal) Hernia

Herniations occur through the *sternocostal hiatus* (foramen of Morgagni), the opening for the superior epigastric vessels in the retrosternal area. This hiatus is located between the sternal and costal parts of the diaphragm (Moore, 1992). Herniation of intestine into the pericardial sac may occur (Hartman, 1996) or conversely, part of the heart may descend into the peritoneal cavity in the epigastric region. Large defects are commonly associated with body wall defects in the umbilical region (e.g., omphalocele; see Chapter 12). Radiologists and pathologists often observe *fatty herniations* through the sternocostal hiatus; however, they are usually of no clinical significance.

Accessory Diaphragm

More than 30 cases of this rare anomaly have been reported. It is often associated with lung hypoplasia and other respiratory complications. An accessory diaphragm can be diagnosed by magnetic resonance imag-

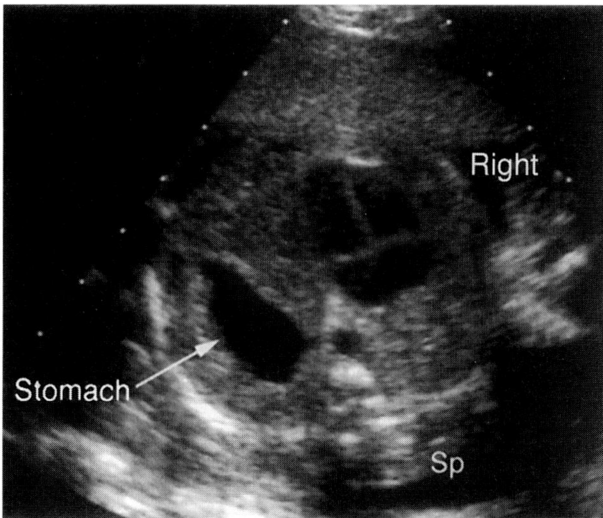

■ **Figure 9–13.** Ultrasound scan of the thorax showing the heart shifted to the right and the stomach on the left. The diaphragmatic hernia was detected at 23.4 weeks' gestation. The stomach has herniated through a posterolateral defect in the diaphragm (CDH). (Sp, vertebral column or spine.) (Courtesy of Dr. Wesley Lee, Division of Fetal Imaging, William Beaumont Hospital, Royal Oak, Michigan.)

ing (MRI) and computed tomography (CT) scanning, and is treated by surgical excision (Becmeur et al., 1995).

SUMMARY OF DEVELOPMENT OF BODY CAVITIES

The intraembryonic coelom, the primordium of the body cavities, begins to develop near the end of the third week. By the fourth week, it appears as a horseshoe-shaped cavity in the cardiogenic and lateral mesoderm. The curve of the "horseshoe" represents the future pericardial cavity and its lateral extensions represent the future pleural and peritoneal cavities.

During folding of the embryonic disc in the fourth week, lateral parts of the intraembryonic coelom move together on the ventral aspect of the embryo. When the caudal part of the ventral mesentery disappears, the right and left parts of the intraembryonic coelom merge to form the peritoneal cavity. As peritoneal parts of the intraembryonic coelom come together, the splanchnic layer of mesoderm encloses the primitive gut and suspends it from the dorsal body wall by a double-layered peritoneal membrane—the dorsal mesentery. The parietal layer of mesoderm lining the peritoneal, pleural, and pericardial cavities becomes the parietal peritoneum, parietal pleura, and serous pericardium, respectively.

Until the seventh week the embryonic pericardial cavity communicates with the peritoneal cavity through paired *pericardioperitoneal canals*. During the fifth and sixth weeks, folds (later membranes) form near the cranial and caudal ends of these canals. Fusion of the cranial *pleuropericardial membranes* with mesoderm ventral to the esophagus separates the pericardial cavity from the pleural cavities. Fusion of the caudal *pleuroperitoneal membranes* during formation of the diaphragm separates the pleural cavities from the peritoneal cavity.

The diaphragm develops from four structures:

- septum transversum
- pleuroperitoneal membranes
- dorsal mesentery of esophagus
- muscular ingrowth from lateral body walls

Clinically Oriented Problems

Case 9–1

A newborn infant suffered from severe respiratory distress. The abdomen was unusually flat and intestinal peristaltic movements were heard over the left side of the thorax.

- What congenital anomaly would you suspect?
- Explain the basis of the signs described above.
- How would the diagnosis likely be established?

Case 9–2

An ultrasound examination of an infant's thorax revealed intestine in the pericardial sac.

- What congenital anomaly could result in herniation of intestine into the pericardial cavity?
- What is the embryological basis of this defect?

Case 9–3

A CDH was diagnosed prenatally during an ultrasound examination.

- How common is posterolateral defect of the diaphragm?
- How do you think a newborn infant in whom this diagnosis is suspected should be positioned?
- Why would this positional treatment be given?
- Briefly describe surgical repair of CDH.
- Why do most newborns with CDH die?

Case 9–4

A baby was born with a hernia in the median plane, between the xiphoid process and umbilicus.

- Name this type of hernia.
- Is it common?
- What is the embryological basis of this congenital anomaly?

Discussion of these problems appears at the back of the book.

REFERENCES AND SUGGESTED READING

Azarow K, Messineo A, Pearl R, et al: Congenital diaphragmatic hernia—A tale of two cities: The Toronto experience. *J Pediatr Surg* 32:395, 1997.

Becmeur F, Horta P, Donato L, et al: Accessory diaphragm—review of 31 cases in the literature. *Eur J Pediatr Surg* 5:43, 1995.

Behrman RE, Kliegman RM, Arvin AM (eds): *Nelson Textbook of Pediatrics,* 15th ed. Philadelphia, WB Saunders, 1996.

Ellis K, Leeds NE, Himmelstein A: Congenital deficiencies in the parietal pericardium. A review with two new cases including successful diagnosis by plain roentgenography. *AJR Am J Roentgenol 82:*125, 1959.

Fosberg RG, Jakubiak JW, Delaney TB: Congenital partial absence of the pericardium. *Ann Thorac Surg 5:*171, 1968.

Gibbs DL, Rice HE, Farrell JA, et al: Familial diaphragmatic agenesis: An autosomal-recessive syndrome with a poor prognosis. *J Pediatr Surg 32:*366, 1997.

Glick PL, Irish MS, Holm BA (eds): New insights into the pathophysiology of congenital diaphragmatic hernia. *Clin Perinatol 23:*62, 1996.

Goldstein RB: Ultrasound evaluation of the fetal thorax. *In* Callen PW (ed): *Ultrasonography in Obstetrics and Gynecology,* 3rd ed. Philadelphia, WB Saunders, 1994a.

Goldstein RB: Ultrasound evaluation of the fetal abdomen. *In* Callen PW (ed): *Ultrasonography in Obstetrics and Gynecology,* 3rd ed. Philadelphia, WB Saunders, 1994b.

Harrison MR: The fetus with a diaphragmatic hernia: Pathophysiology, natural history, and surgical management. *In* Harrison MR, Golbus MS, Filly RA (eds): *The Unborn Patient. Prenatal Diagnosis and Treatment,* 2nd ed. Philadelphia, WB Saunders, 1991.

Hartman GE: Diaphragmatic hernia. *In* Behrman RE, Kliegman RM, Arvin AM (eds): *Nelson Textbook of Pediatrics,* 15th ed. Philadelphia, WB Saunders, 1996.

Kluth D, Tenbrinck R, von Ekesparre M, et al: The natural history of congenital diaphragmatic hernia and pulmonary hypoplasia in the embryo. *J Pediatr Surg 28:*456, 1993.

Langer JC, Harrison MR: The fetus with an abdominal wall defect. *In* Harrison MR, Golbus MS, Filly RA (eds): *The Unborn Patient. Prenatal Diagnosis and Treatment,* 2nd ed. Philadelphia, WB Saunders, 1991.

Laxdal OE, McDougall H, Mellen GW: Congenital eventration of the diaphragm. *N Engl J Med 250:*401, 1954.

McNamara JJ, Eraklis AJ, Gross RE: Congenital posterolateral diaphragmatic hernia in the newborn. *J Thorac Cardiovasc Surg 55:*55, 1968.

Moore KL: *Clinically Oriented Anatomy,* 3rd ed. Baltimore, Williams & Wilkins, 1992.

Moya FR, Thomas VL, Romaguera J, et al: Fetal lung maturation in congenital diaphragmatic hernia. *Am J Obstet Gynecol 173:*1401, 1995.

Skandalakis JE, Gray SW: *The Embryological Basis for the Treatment of Congenital Defects.* Baltimore, Williams & Wilkins, 1994.

Wells LJ: Development of the human diaphragm and pleural sacs. *Contr Embryol Carneg Instn 35:*107, 1954.

Wilson JM, Lund DP, Lillehei CW, Vacanti JP: Congenital diaphragmatic hernia—A tale of two cities: The Boston experience. *J Pediatr Surg 32:*401, 1997.

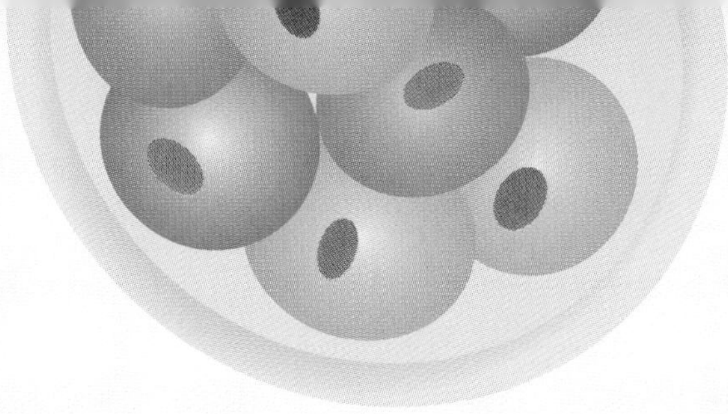

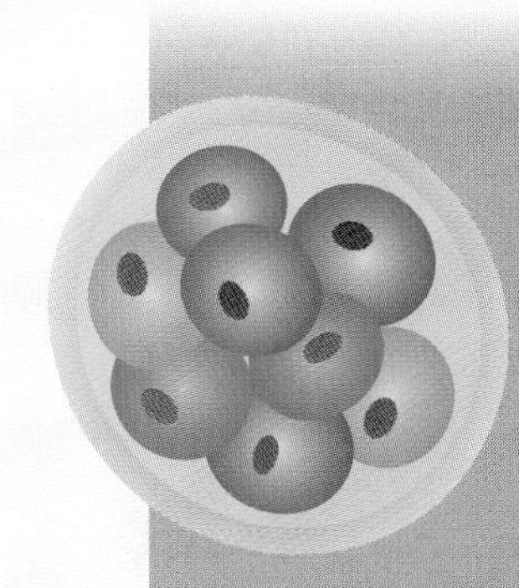

The Pharyngeal (Branchial) Apparatus

10

■ The head and neck regions of a 4-week-old human embryo somewhat resemble these regions of a fish embryo of a comparable stage of development. This explains the former use of the adjective *branchial*, which is derived from the Greek word *branchia*, gill. By the end of the embryonic period, these gill-like structures have either become rearranged and adapted to new functions or disappeared.

The **pharyngeal (branchial) apparatus** (Fig. 10–1) consists of:

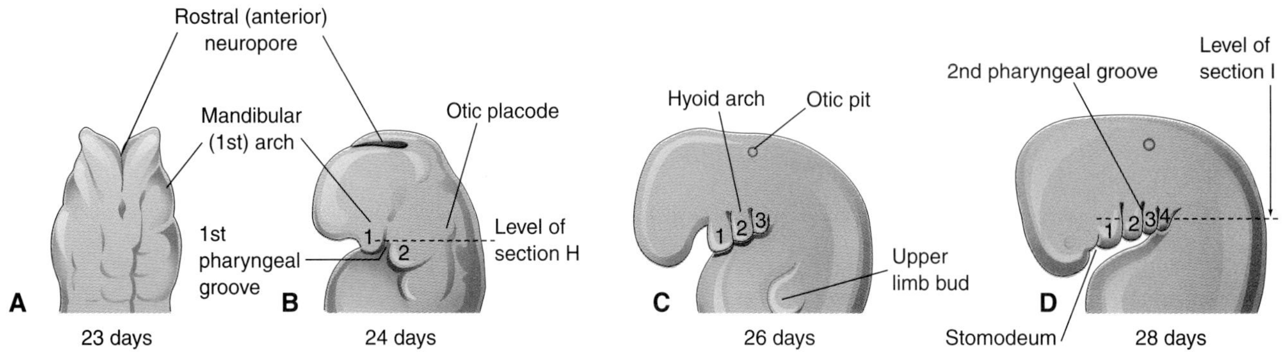

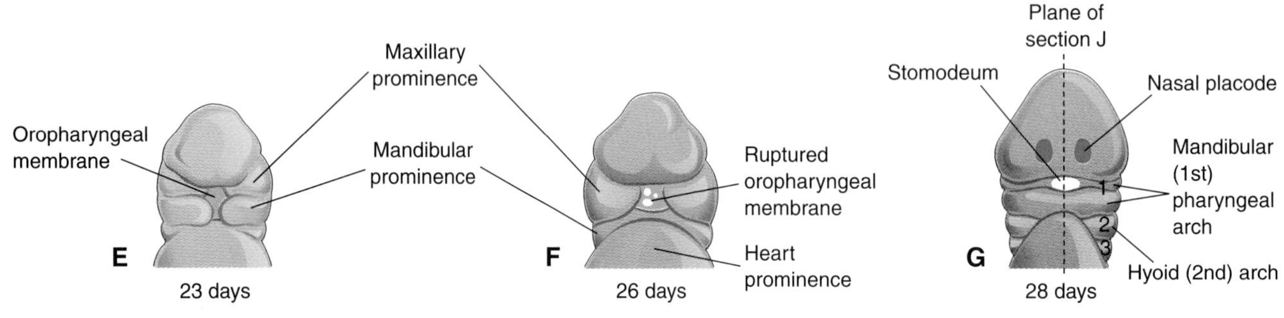

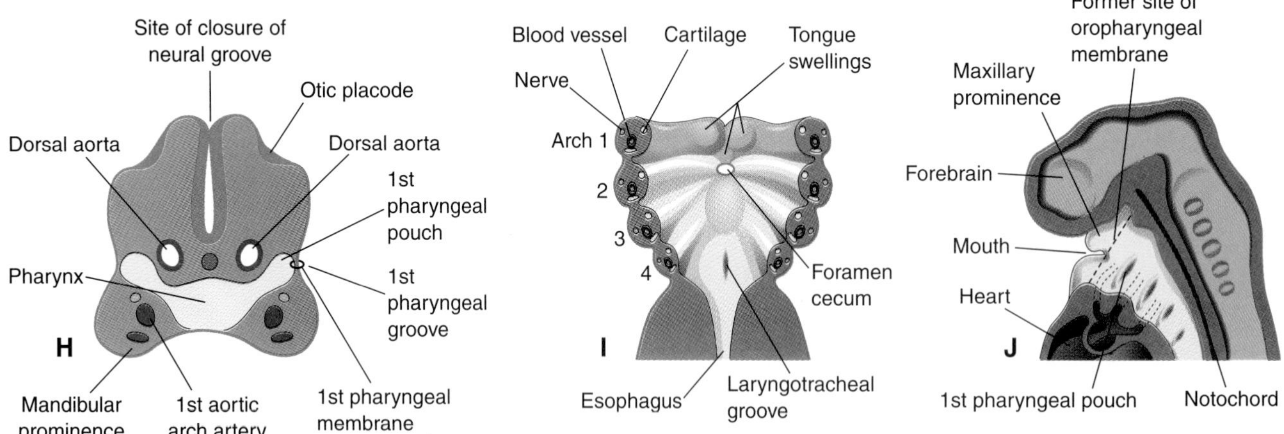

Germ Layer Derivatives

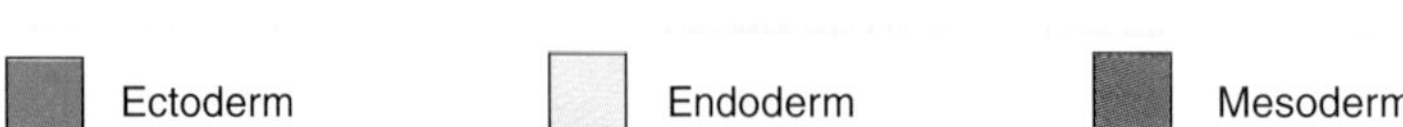

■ **Figure 10–1.** Drawings illustrating the human pharyngeal apparatus. *A,* Dorsal view of the cranial part of an early embryo. *B* to *D,* Lateral views showing later development of the pharyngeal arches. *E* to *G,* Ventral or facial views illustrating the relationship of the first pharyngeal arch to the stomodeum. *H,* Horizontal section through the cranial region of an embryo. *I,* Similar section illustrating the arch components and floor of the primordial pharynx. *J,* Sagittal section of the cranial region of an embryo, illustrating the openings of the pharyngeal pouches in the lateral wall of the primitive pharynx.

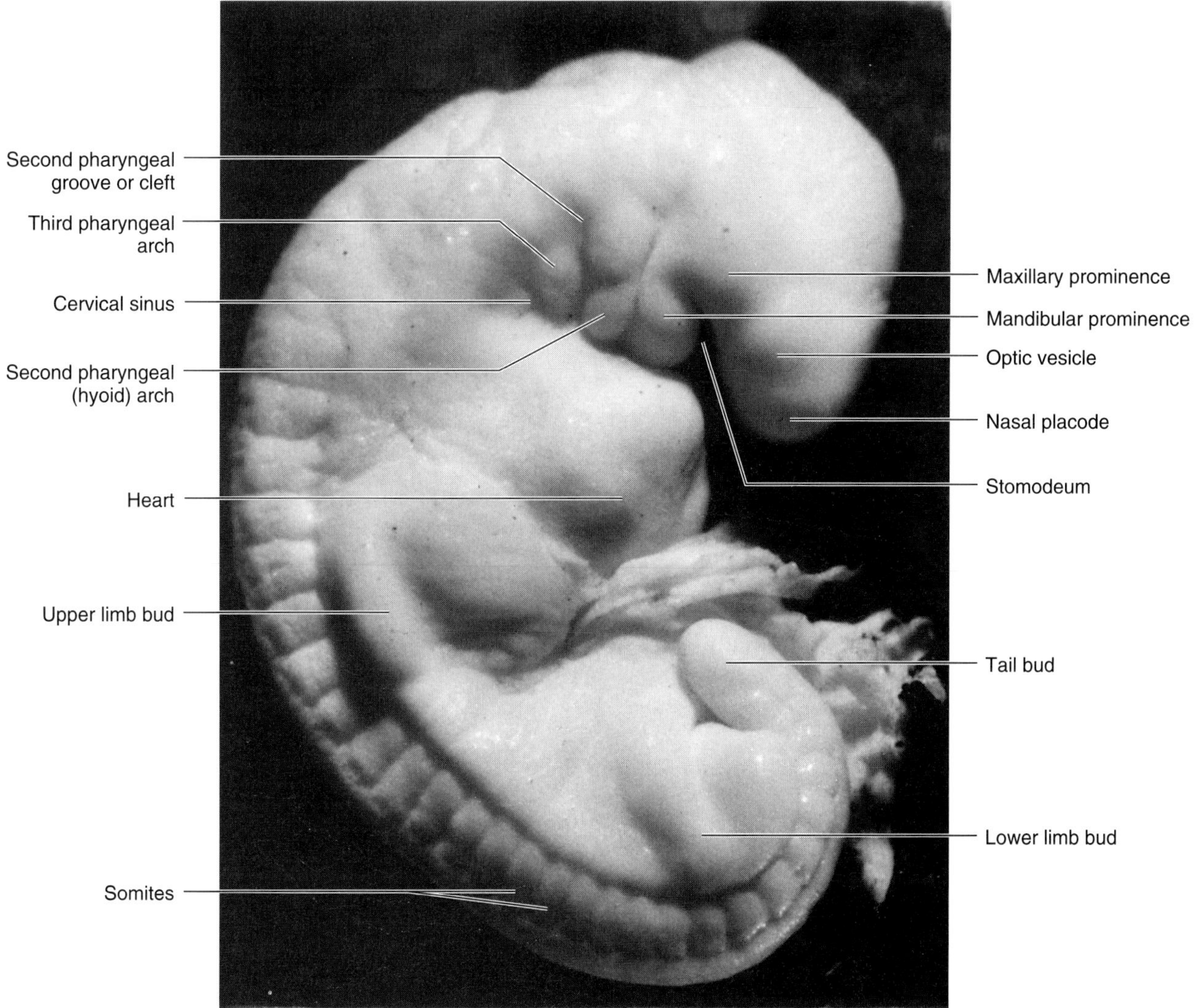

■ **Figure 10–2.** Macrophotograph of a stage 13, 4½-week-old human embryo. (Courtesy of Professor Emeritus Dr. KV Hinrichsen, Medizinische Fakultät, Institut für Anatomie, Ruhr-Universität Bochum, Germany.)

- pharyngeal arches
- pharyngeal pouches
- pharyngeal grooves
- pharyngeal membranes

These embryonic structures contribute greatly to the formation of the head and neck. Most congenital anomalies in these regions originate during transformation of the pharyngeal apparatus into its adult derivatives. **Branchial anomalies** result from persistence of parts of the pharyngeal apparatus that normally disappear. Study of the development and modification of the human pharyngeal apparatus during formation of the head and neck can be confusing if the function of the branchial apparatus in lower forms is not understood. In fish and larval amphibians, the branchial apparatus forms a system of gills for exchanging oxygen and carbon dioxide between the blood and water. The branchial arches support the gills. A primordial branchial or pharyngeal apparatus develops in human embryos; however, no gills form. Consequently, the term **pharyngeal arch** is now used instead of branchial arch when describing the development of the head and neck regions of human embryos.

PHARYNGEAL ARCHES

The pharyngeal arches begin to develop early in the fourth week as **neural crest cells** migrate into the future head and neck regions (see Chapter 5). Laboratory studies in avian and mammalian embryos have contributed only partly to our understanding of the migration and distribution pattern of neural crest cells in relation to the pharyngeal arches (Noden, 1991; Kuratani and Aizawa, 1995). The first pair of pharyngeal arches, the primordium of the jaws, appears as surface elevations lateral to the developing pharynx (Fig. 10-1*A* and *B*). Soon other arches appear as obliquely disposed, rounded ridges on each side of the future head and neck regions (Fig. 10-1*C* and *D*). By the end of the fourth week, four well-defined pairs of pharyngeal arches are visible externally (Fig. 10-2). The fifth and sixth arches are rudimentary and are not

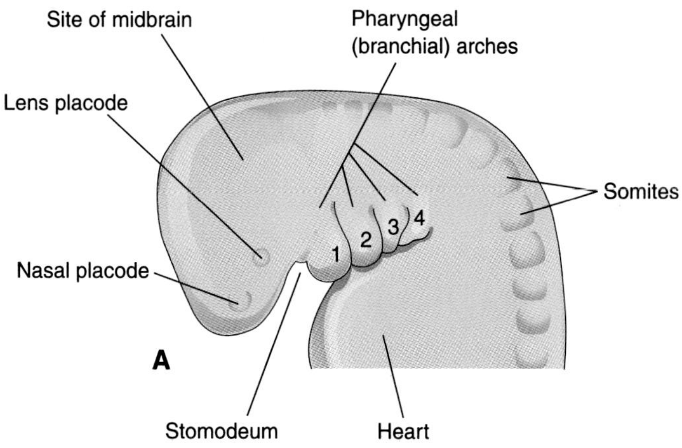

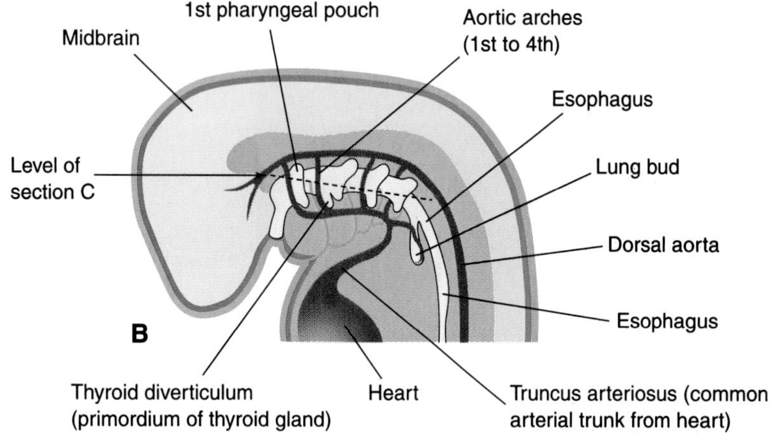

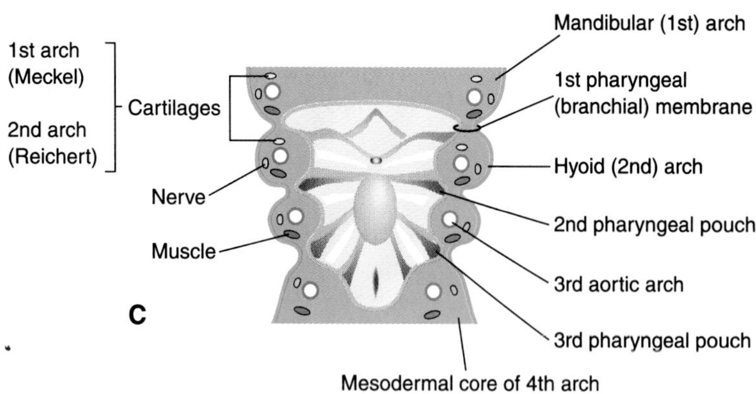

■ **Figure 10–3.** *A,* Drawing of the head, neck, and thoracic regions of a human embryo (about 28 days), illustrating the pharyngeal apparatus. *B,* Schematic drawing showing the pharyngeal pouches and aortic arches. *C,* Horizontal section through the embryo showing the floor of the primordial pharynx and illustrating the germ layer of origin of the pharyngeal arch components.

visible on the surface of the embryo. The arches are separated from each other by prominent fissures—the **pharyngeal grooves** (clefts). Like the pharyngeal arches, the grooves are numbered in a craniocaudal sequence.

The **first pharyngeal arch** (mandibular arch), develops two prominences: (Figs. 10-1*E* and *F* and 10-2).

- The smaller **maxillary prominence** (process) gives rise to the maxilla (upper jaw), zygomatic bone, and squamous part of the temporal bone.
- The larger **mandibular prominence** (process) forms the mandible (lower jaw).

Consequently, the first pair of pharyngeal arches plays a major role in facial development.

The **second pharyngeal arch** (hyoid arch) makes a major contribution to the formation of the hyoid bone. The pharyngeal arches caudal to the second arch are referred to by number only. The pharyngeal arches support the lateral walls of the primordial pharynx, which is derived from the cranial part of the foregut. The primordial mouth or **stomodeum** initially appears as a slight depression of the surface ectoderm (Fig. 10-1*D* and *E*). It is separated from the cavity of the primordial pharynx by a bilaminar membrane—the **oropharyngeal membrane**—which formed during the third week (see Chapter 4). It is composed of ectoderm externally and endoderm internally. The oropharyngeal membrane ruptures at about 26 days, bringing the primordial pharynx and foregut into communication with the amniotic cavity (Fig. 10-1*F* and *G*).

Pharyngeal Arch Components

Initially, each pharyngeal arch consists of a core of mesenchyme (embryonic connective tissue) and is covered externally by ectoderm and internally by endoderm (Fig. 10-1*H* and *I*). The original mesenchyme is derived from mesoderm in the third week. During the fourth week, most of the mesenchyme is derived from **neural crest cells** that migrate into the pharyngeal arches. It is the migration of neural crest cells into the arches and their differentiation into mesenchyme that produces the maxillary and mandibular prominences of the first arch (Fig. 10-2). Neural crest cells are unique in that, despite their neuroectodermal origin, they make a major contribution to mesenchyme in the head and neck as well as to structures in many other regions (see Chapter 5). Skeletal musculature and vascular endothelia, however, are derived from the original mesenchyme in the pharyngeal arches (Kirby and Bockman, 1984; Stricker et al., 1990; Noden, 1991; Graveson, 1993; Sulik, 1996).

Fate of the Pharyngeal Arches

The pharyngeal arches contribute extensively to the formation of the face, nasal cavities, mouth, larynx, pharynx, and neck (Figs. 10-3 and 10-4). During the fifth week, the second pharyngeal arch enlarges and overgrows the third and fourth arches, forming an ectodermal depression—the **cervical sinus** (Figs. 10-2 and 10-4*A* to *D*). By the end of the seventh week, the second to fourth pharyngeal grooves and the cervical sinus have disappeared, giving the neck a smooth contour.

A typical pharyngeal arch contains:

- an *aortic arch*, an artery that arises from the truncus arteriosus of the primordial heart (Fig. 10-3*B*) and runs around the primordial pharynx to enter the dorsal aorta
- a *cartilaginous rod* that forms the skeleton of the arch
- a *muscular component* that forms muscles in the head and neck
- a *nerve* that supplies the mucosa and muscles derived from the arch

The nerves that grow into the arches are derived from neuroectoderm of the primordial brain.

DERIVATIVES OF THE AORTIC ARCHES (PHARYNGEAL ARCH ARTERIES)

The transformation of the aortic arches into the adult arterial pattern of the head and neck is described with the cardiovascular system in Chapter 14. In fish these arteries supply blood to the capillary network of the gills. In human embryos the blood in the aortic arches supplies the arches and then enters the dorsal aorta.

DERIVATIVES OF THE PHARYNGEAL ARCH CARTILAGES

The dorsal end of the **first arch cartilage** (Meckel cartilage) is closely related to the developing ear and becomes ossified to form two middle ear bones, the **malleus** and **incus** (Fig. 10-5; Table 10-1). The middle part of the cartilage regresses, but its perichondrium forms the *anterior ligament of the malleus and the sphenomandibular ligament*. Ventral parts of the first arch cartilages form the horseshoe-shaped primordium of the mandible and, by keeping pace with its growth, guide its early morphogenesis (Hall, 1982). Each half of the mandible forms lateral to and in close association with its cartilage. The cartilage disappears as the mandible develops around it by intramembranous ossification (Fig. 10-5*B*). For details on the development of the mandible, see Sperber (1993).

The dorsal end of the **second arch cartilage** (Reichert cartilage), also closely related to the developing ear, ossifies to form the **stapes** of the middle ear and the **styloid process** of the temporal bone (Fig. 10-5*B*). The part of cartilage between the styloid process and hyoid bone regresses; its perichondrium forms the *stylohyoid ligament*. The ventral end of the second arch cartilage ossifies to form the lesser cornu (L., horn) and the superior part of the body of the *hyoid bone* (Fig. 10-5*B*).

The **third arch cartilage**, located in the ventral part of the arch, ossifies to form the greater cornu and

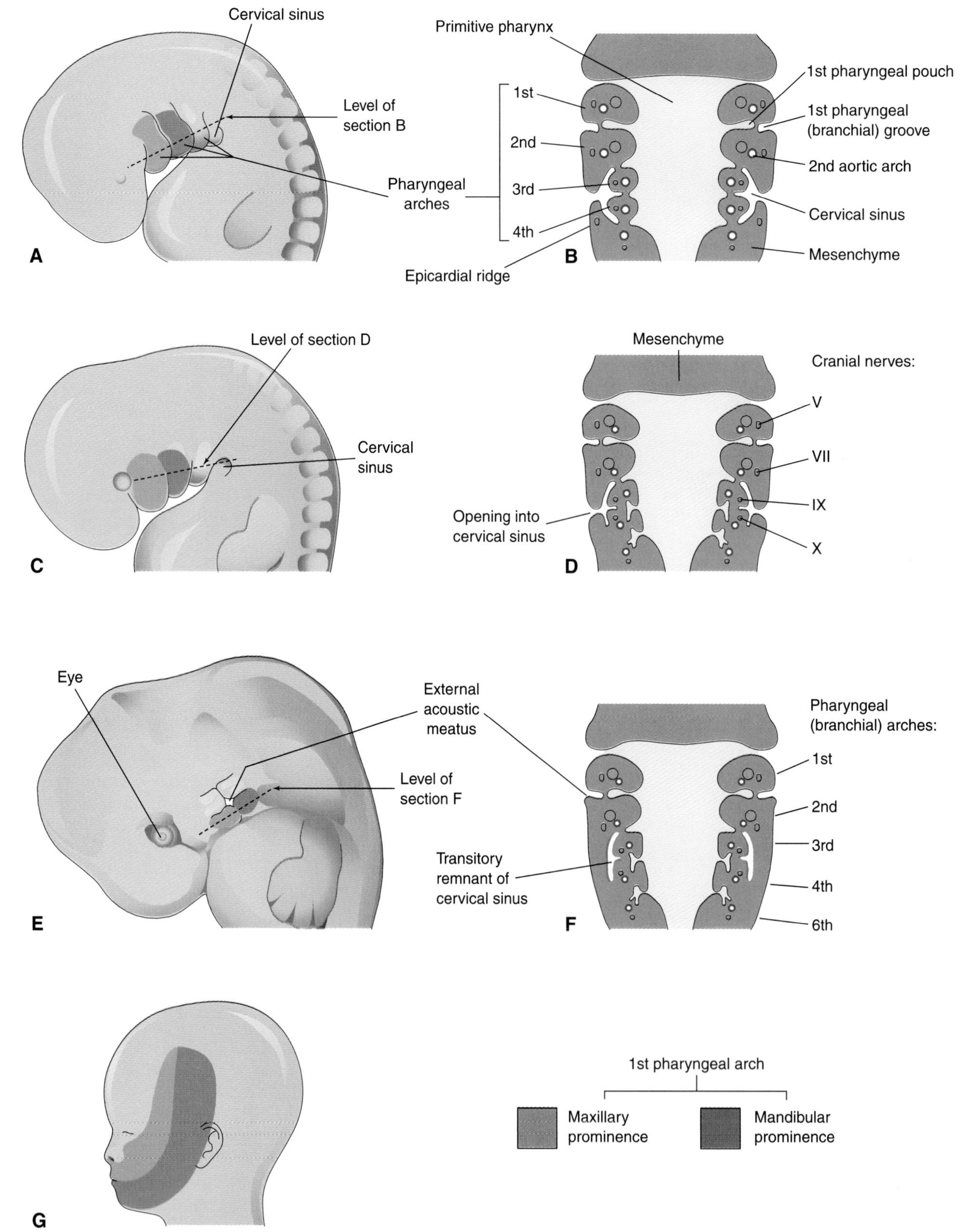

■ **Figure 10–4.** *A,* Lateral view of the head, neck, and thoracic regions of an embryo (about 32 days), showing the pharyngeal arches and cervical sinus. *B,* Diagrammatic section through the embryo at the level shown in *A,* illustrating growth of the second arch over the third and fourth arches. *C,* An embryo of about 33 days. *D,* Section of the embryo at the level shown in *C,* illustrating early closure of the cervical sinus. *E,* An embryo of about 41 days, *F,* Section of the embryo at the level shown in *E,* showing the transitory cystic remnant of the cervical sinus. *G,* Drawing of a 20-week fetus illustrating the area of the face derived from the first pair of pharyngeal arches.

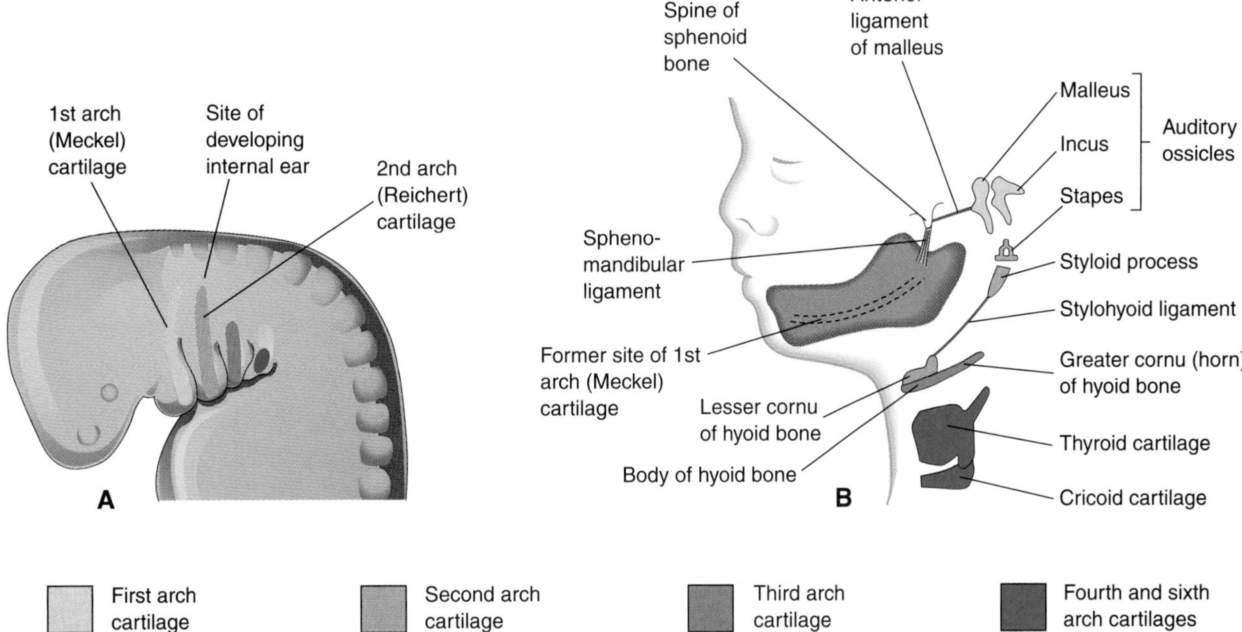

■ **Figure 10-5.** *A,* Schematic lateral view of the head, neck, and thoracic regions of a 4-week embryo, illustrating the location of the cartilages in the pharyngeal arches. *B,* Similar view of a 24-week fetus illustrating the adult derivatives of the arch cartilages. Note that the mandible is formed by membranous ossification of mesenchymal tissue surrounding the first arch (Meckel) cartilage. This cartilage acts as a template for development of the mandible, but does not contribute directly to the formation of it. Occasionally ossification of the second arch cartilage may extend from the styloid process along the stylohyoid ligament. When this occurs, it may cause pain in the region of the palatine tonsil.

the inferior part of the body of the hyoid bone. The **fourth and sixth arch cartilages** fuse to form the *laryngeal cartilages* (Fig. 10-5*B*; Table 10-1), except for the epiglottis. The cartilage of the epiglottis develops from mesenchyme in the *hypobranchial eminence* (see Fig. 10-24*A*), a prominence in the floor of the embryonic pharynx that is derived from the third and fourth pharyngeal arches.

Table 10-1 ■ Structures Derived From Pharyngeal Arch Components*

Arch	Nerve	Muscles	Skeletal Structures	Ligaments
First (mandibular)	Trigeminal†(CN V)	Muscles of mastication‡ Mylohyoid and anterior belly of digastric Tensor tympani Tensor veli palatini	Malleus Incus	Anterior ligament of malleus Sphenomandibular ligament
Second (hyoid)	Facial (CN VII)	Muscles of facial expression§ Stapedius Stylohyoid Posterior belly of digastric	Stapes Styloid process Lesser cornu of hyoid Upper part of body of hyoid bone	Stylohyoid ligament
Third	Glossopharyngeal (CN IX)	Stylopharyngeus	Greater cornu of hyoid Lower part of body of hyoid bone	
Fourth and sixth‖	Superior laryngeal branch of vagus (CN X) Recurrent laryngeal branch of vagus (CN X)	Cricothyroid Levator veli palatini Constrictors of pharynx Intrinsic muscles of larynx Striated muscles of esophagus	Thyroid cartilage Cricoid cartilage Arytenoid cartilage Corniculate cartilage Cuneiform cartilage	

* The derivatives of the aortic arch arteries are described in Chapter 14.
† The ophthalmic division does not supply any pharyngeal arch components.
‡ Temporalis, masseter, medial and lateral pterygoids.
§ Buccinator, auricularis, frontalis, platysma, orbicularis oris and orbicularis oculi.
‖ The fifth pharyngeal arch is often absent. When present, it is rudimentary and usually has no recognizable cartilage bar. The cartilaginous components of the fourth and sixth arches fuse to form the cartilages of the larynx.

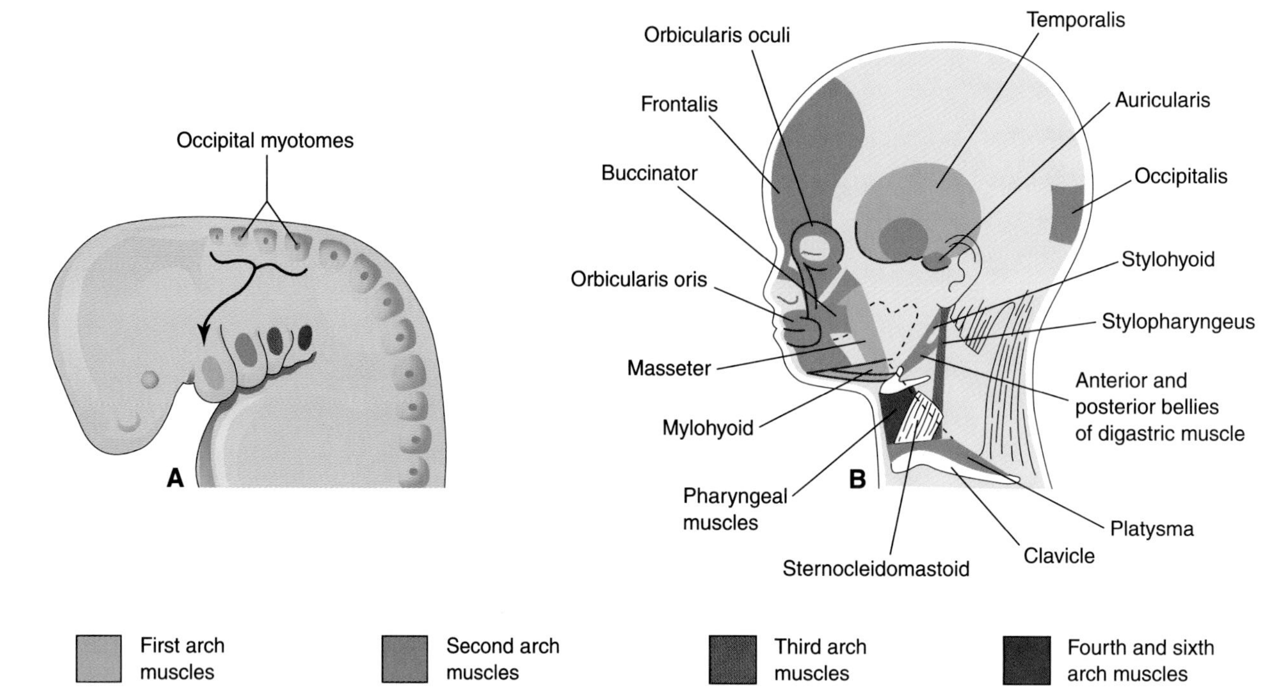

■ **Figure 10–6.** *A,* Sketch of lateral view of the head, neck, and thoracic regions of a 4-week embryo showing the muscles derived from the pharyngeal arches. The arrow shows the pathway taken by myoblasts from the occipital myotomes to form the tongue musculature. *B,* Sketch of the head and neck regions of a 20-week fetus, dissected to show the muscles derived from the pharyngeal arches. Parts of the platysma and sternocleidomastoid muscles have been removed to show the deeper muscles. Note that myoblasts from the second arch migrate from the neck to the head, where they give rise to the muscles of facial expression. These muscles are supplied by the facial nerve (CN, VII), the nerve of the second pharyngeal arch.

DERIVATIVES OF THE PHARYNGEAL ARCH MUSCLES

The muscular components of the arches form various striated muscles in the head and neck; for example, the musculature of the first pharyngeal arch forms the **muscles of mastication** and other muscles (Fig. 10-6; Table 10-1).

DERIVATIVES OF THE PHARYNGEAL ARCH NERVES

Each arch is supplied by its own cranial nerve (CN). The *special visceral efferent (branchial) components* of the cranial nerves supply muscles derived from the pharyngeal arches (Fig. 10-7; Table 10-1). Because mesenchyme from the pharyngeal arches contributes to the dermis and mucous membranes of the head and neck, these areas are supplied with *special visceral afferent nerves.*

The facial skin is supplied by the fifth cranial nerve—the **trigeminal nerve** (CN V). However, only its caudal two branches (*maxillary* and *mandibular*) supply derivatives of the first pharyngeal arch (Fig. 10-7*B*). CN V is the principal sensory nerve of the head and neck and is the motor nerve for the muscles of mastication (Table 10-1). Its sensory branches innervate the face, teeth, and mucous membranes of the nasal cavities, palate, mouth, and tongue (Fig. 10-7*C*).

The seventh cranial nerve (the **facial nerve** [CN VII]), the ninth cranial nerve (the **glossopharyngeal nerve** [CN IX]), and the tenth cranial nerve (the **vagus nerve** [CN X]) supply the second, third, and caudal (fourth to sixth) arches, respectively. The fourth arch is supplied by the superior laryngeal branch of the vagus (CN X) and the sixth arch by its recurrent laryngeal branch. The nerves of the second to sixth pharyngeal arches have little cutaneous distribution (Fig. 10-7*C*); however, they innervate the mucous membranes of the tongue, pharynx, and larynx.

PHARYNGEAL POUCHES

The *primordial pharynx,* derived from the foregut, widens cranially where it joins the primordial mouth or *stomodeum* (Figs. 10-3*A* and *B* and 10-4*B*), and narrows caudally where it joins the *esophagus.* The endoderm of the pharynx lines the internal aspects of the pharyngeal arches and passes into balloonlike diverticula—the **pharyngeal pouches** (Figs. 10-1*H* to *J* and 10-3*B* and *C*). The pairs of pouches develop in a craniocaudal sequence between the arches. The first pair of pouches, for example, lies between the first and second pharyngeal arches. There are four well-defined pairs of pharyngeal pouches; the fifth pair is absent or rudimentary. The endoderm of the pouches contacts the ectoderm of the pharyngeal grooves and together they form the double-layered **pharyngeal membranes** that separate the pharyngeal pouches from the pharyngeal grooves (Figs. 10-1*H* and 10-3*C*).

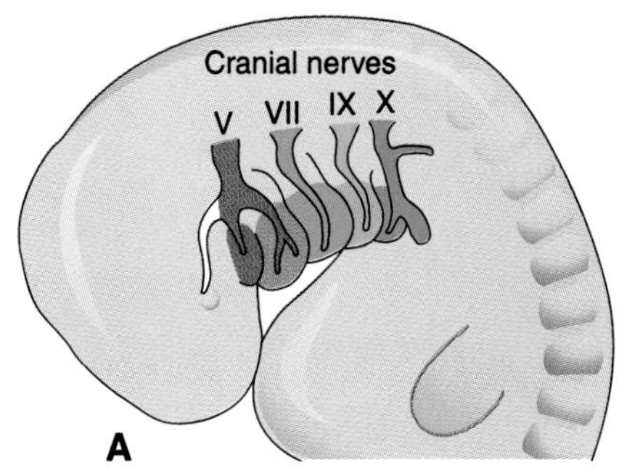

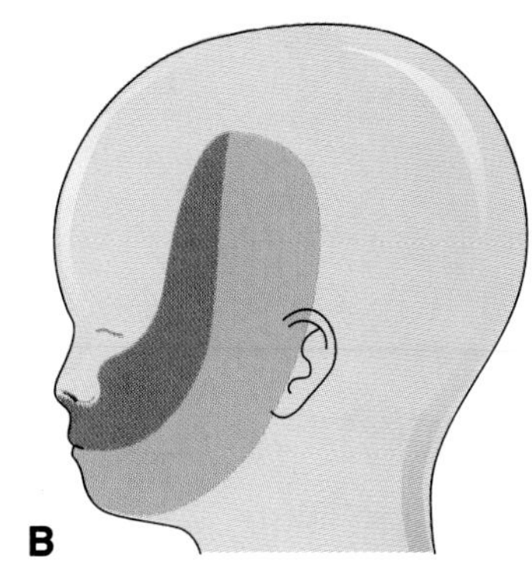

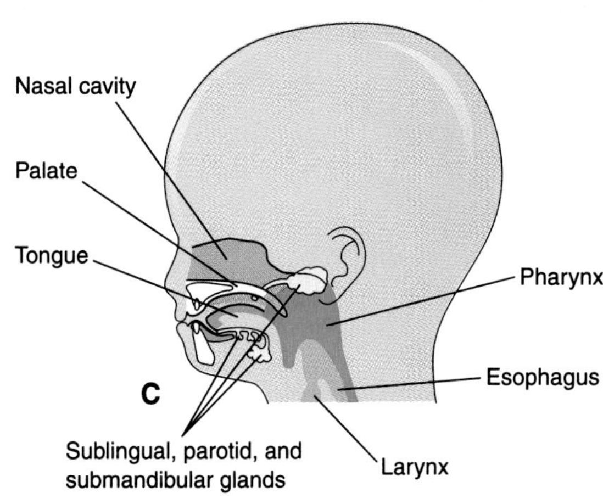

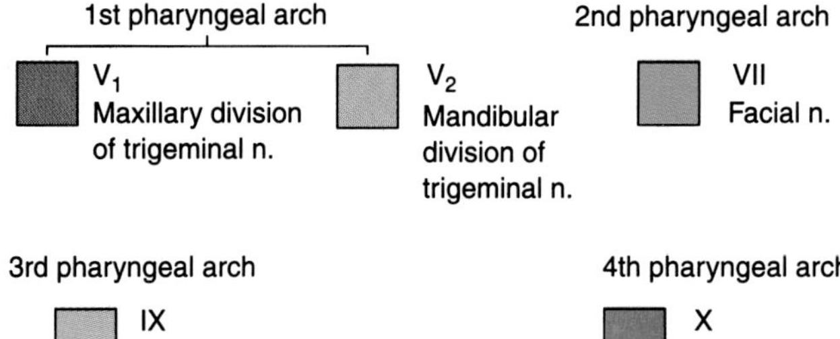

■ **Figure 10–7.** *A,* Lateral view of the head, neck, and thoracic regions of a 4-week embryo showing the cranial nerves supplying the pharyngeal arches. *B,* Sketch of the head and neck regions of a 20-week fetus showing the superficial distribution of the two caudal branches of the first arch nerve (CN V). *C,* Sagittal section of the fetal head and neck, showing the deep distribution of sensory fibers of the nerves to the teeth and mucosa of the tongue, pharynx, nasal cavity, palate, and larynx.

Derivatives of the Pharyngeal Pouches

The endodermal epithelial lining of the pharyngeal pouches gives rise to important organs in the head and neck.

THE FIRST PHARYNGEAL POUCH

The first pharyngeal pouch expands into an elongate *tubotympanic recess* (Fig. 10-8*B*). The expanded distal part of this recess contacts the first pharyngeal groove, where it later contributes to the formation of the **tympanic membrane** (eardrum). The cavity of the tubotympanic recess gives rise to the **tympanic cavity** and **mastoid antrum**. The connection of the tubotympanic recess with the pharynx gradually elongates to form the **pharyngotympanic tube** (auditory tube, eustachian tube). More details about the developing ear are given in Chapter 19.

THE SECOND PHARYNGEAL POUCH

Although the second pharyngeal pouch is largely obliterated as the **palatine tonsil** develops, part of the cavity of this pouch remains as the **tonsillar sinus** or fossa (Figs. 10-8*C* and 10-9). The endoderm of the second pouch proliferates and grows into the underlying mesenchyme. The central parts of these buds break down, forming crypts (pitlike depressions). The pouch endoderm forms the surface epithelium and lining of the **tonsillar crypts**. At about 20 weeks the mesenchyme around the crypts differentiates into lymphoid tissue, which soon organizes into the *lymphatic nodules* of the palatine tonsil.

THE THIRD PHARYNGEAL POUCH

The third pharyngeal pouch expands and develops a solid, dorsal bulbar part and a hollow, elongate ventral part (Fig. 10-8*B*). Its connection with the pharynx is reduced to a narrow duct that soon degenerates. By the sixth week the epithelium of each dorsal bulbar part begins to differentiate into an **inferior parathyroid gland** (parathyroid III). The epithelium of the elongate ventral parts of the third pair of pouches proliferates, obliterating their cavities. These bilateral primordia of the thymus come together in the median plane to form the bilobed **thymus**, which descends into the superior mediastinum. The bilobed form of this lymphatic organ remains throughout life, discretely encapsulated; each lobe has its own blood supply, lymphatic drainage, and nerve supply. For a discussion of the histological appearance of the thymus in adults, see Cormack (1993) and Gartner and Hiatt (1997). The primordia of the thymus and parathyroid glands lose their connections with the pharynx and migrate into the neck. Later the parathyroid glands separate from the thymus and come to lie on the dorsal surface of the thyroid gland (Figs. 10-8*C* and 10-9).

Histogenesis of the Thymus. This gland develops from epithelial cells derived from endoderm of the

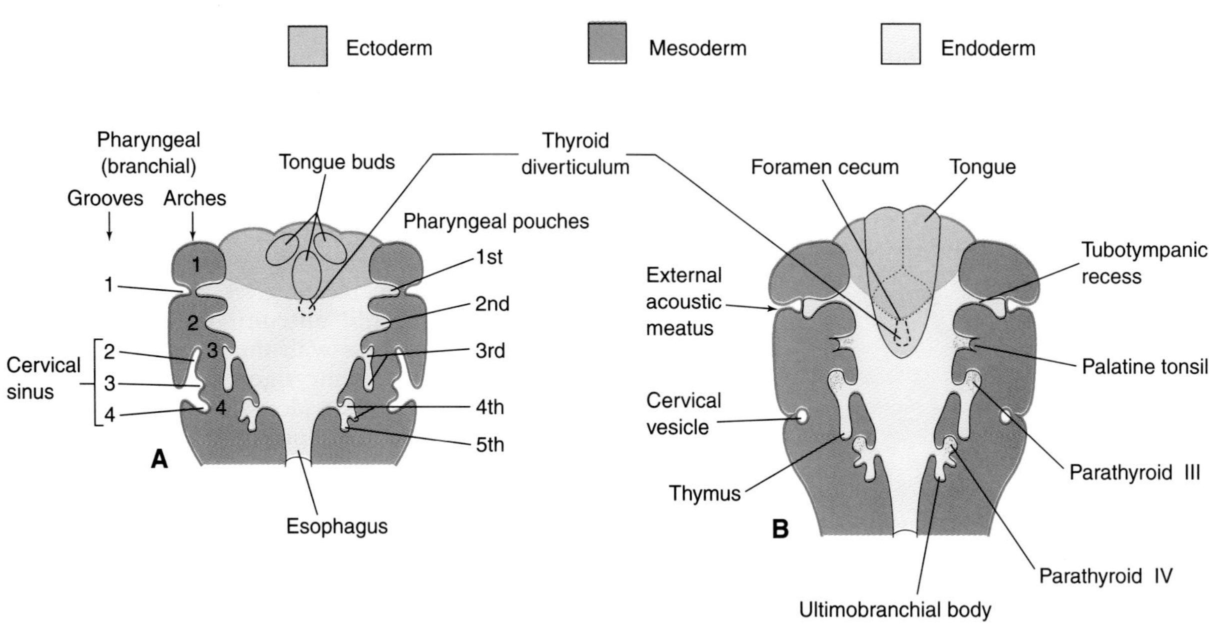

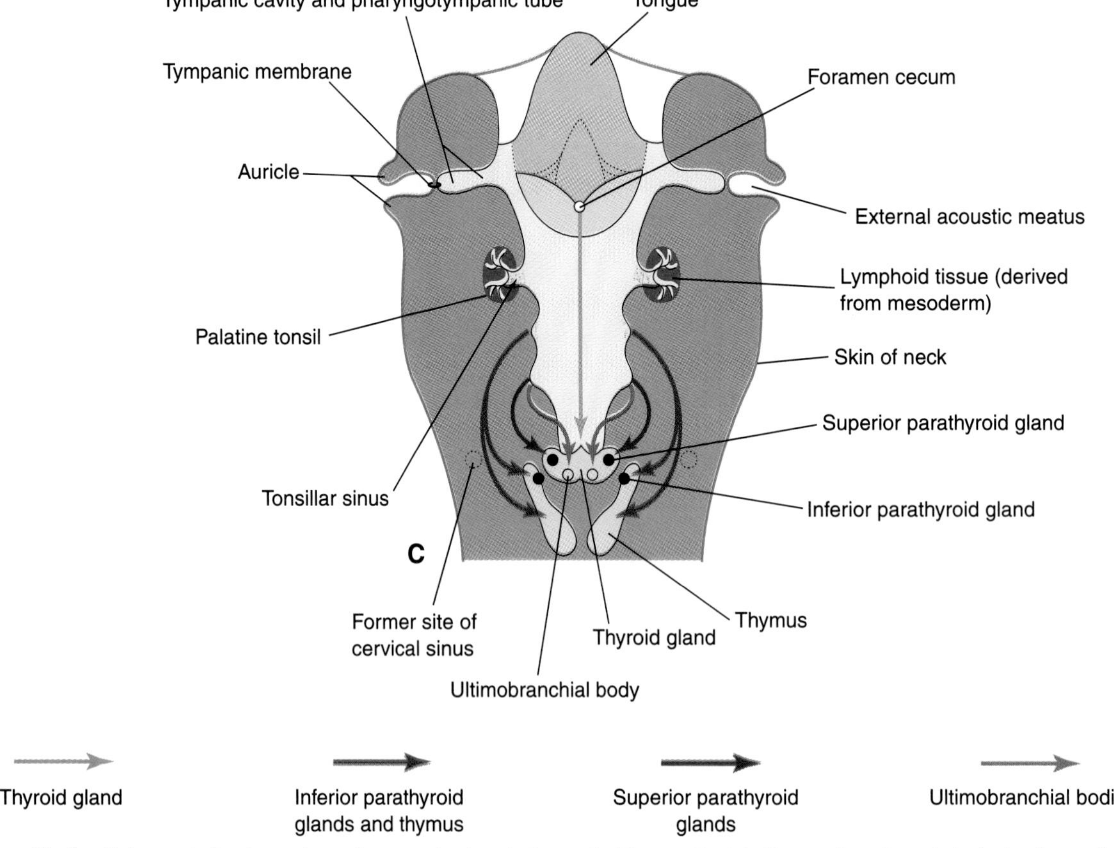

■ **Figure 10–8.** Schematic horizontal sections at the level shown in Figure 10–4*A*, illustrating the adult derivatives of the pharyngeal pouches. *A*, 5 weeks. Note that the second pharyngeal arch grows over the third and fourth arches, burying the second to fourth pharyngeal grooves in the cervical sinus. *B*, 6 weeks. *C*, 7 weeks. Note the migration of the developing thymus, parathyroid, and thyroid glands into the neck.

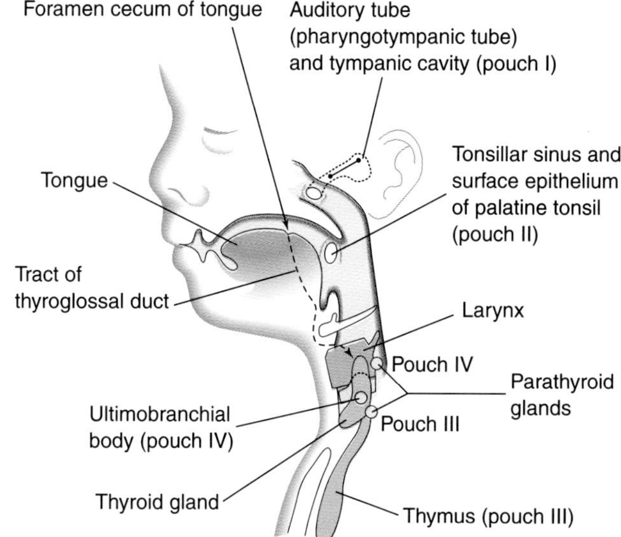

■ **Figure 10-9.** Schematic sagittal section of the head, neck, and upper thoracic regions of a 20-week fetus, showing the adult derivatives of the pharyngeal pouches and the descent of the thyroid gland into the neck.

third pair of pharyngeal pouches and from mesenchyme into which tubes of epithelial cells grow. The epithelial tubes soon become solid cords that proliferate and give rise to side branches. Each side branch becomes the core of a lobule of the thymus. Some cells of the epithelial cords become arranged around a central point, forming small groups of cells—the **thymic corpuscles** (Hassall corpuscles). Other cells of the epithelial cords spread apart but retain connections with each other to form an *epithelial reticulum*. The mesenchyme between the epithelial cords forms thin incomplete septa between the lobules. *Lymphocytes* soon appear and fill the interstices between the epithelial cells. The lymphocytes are derived from *hematopoietic stem cells,* which form blood cells.

The thymic primordium is surrounded by a thin layer of mesenchyme that is essential for its development. This mesenchyme, as well as certain epithelial cells in the thymus and a peculiar muscle cell in the medulla of the gland, is derived from *neural crest cells*. Extirpation (removal) of these cells in animal experiments produces a wide range of developmental defects, including some in the thymus (Bockman and Kirby, 1984). Growth and development of the thymus are not complete at birth. It is a relatively large organ during the perinatal period and may extend superiorly through the superior aperture of the thorax into the root of the neck. During late childhood, as puberty is reached, the thymus begins to diminish in relative size (i.e., undergoes involution). By adulthood it is often scarcely recognizable because of fat infiltrating the cortex of the gland (Steinman, 1986); however it is still functional and important for the maintenance of health. In addition to secreting thymic hormones, the adult thymus primes thymocytes before releasing them to the periphery (Kendall, 1991).

THE FOURTH PHARYNGEAL POUCH

The fourth pharyngeal pouch also expands into dorsal bulbar and elongate ventral parts (Figs. 10-8 and 10-9). Its connection with the pharynx is reduced to a narrow duct that soon degenerates. By the sixth week, each dorsal part develops into a **superior parathyroid gland** (parathyroid IV), which lies on the dorsal surface of the thyroid gland. As described, the parathyroid glands derived from the third pouches descend with the thymus and are carried to a more inferior position than the parathyroid glands derived from the fourth pouches. This explains why the parathyroid glands derived from the third pair of pouches are located inferior to those from the fourth pouches (Fig. 10-9).

Histogenesis of the Parathyroid Glands. The epithelium of the dorsal parts of the third and fourth pouches proliferates during the fifth week and forms small nodules on the dorsal aspect of each pouch. Vascular mesenchyme soon grows into these nodules, forming a capillary network. The chief or **principal cells** differentiate during the embryonic period and are believed to become functionally active in regulating fetal calcium metabolism. The **oxyphil cells** differentiate 5 to 7 years after birth.

The elongated ventral part of each fourth pouch develops into an **ultimobranchial body**, which received its name because it is the last of the series of structures derived from the pharyngeal pouches. The ultimobranchial body fuses with the thyroid gland and its cells disseminate within it, giving rise to the **parafollicular cells** of the thyroid gland; they are also called **C cells** to indicate that they produce *calcitonin*, a hormone that is involved in the regulation of the normal calcium level in body fluids (Gartner and Hiatt, 1997). *C cells differentiate from neural crest cells* that migrate from the pharyngeal arches into the fourth pair of pharyngeal pouches.

THE FIFTH PHARYNGEAL POUCH

When it develops, this rudimentary pouch becomes part of the fourth pharyngeal pouch and helps to form the ultimobranchial body.

PHARYNGEAL GROOVES

The head and neck regions of the human embryo exhibit four pharyngeal grooves (clefts) on each side during the fourth and fifth weeks (Fig. 10-1*B* to *D*). These grooves separate the pharyngeal arches externally. Only one pair of grooves contributes to adult structures; the first pair persists as the **external acoustic meatus** (Fig. 10-8*C*). The other grooves lie in a slitlike depression—the **cervical sinus**—and are normally obliterated with the sinus as the neck develops (Fig. 10-4*B*, *D*, and *F*).

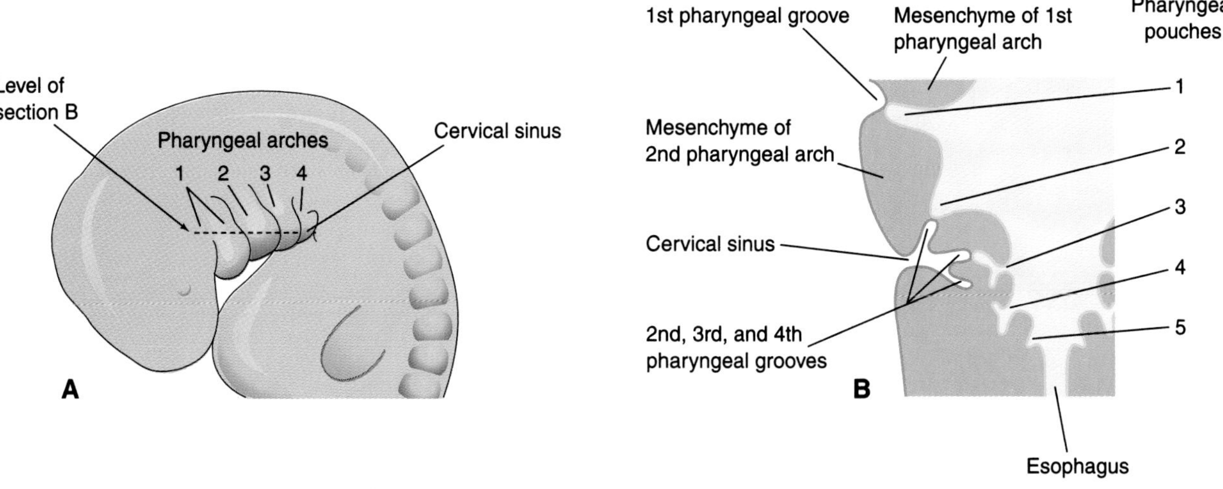

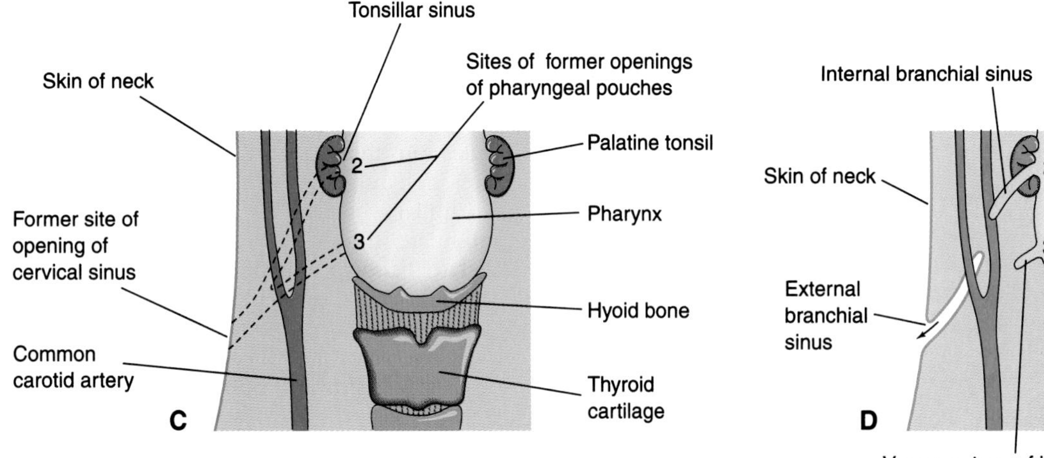

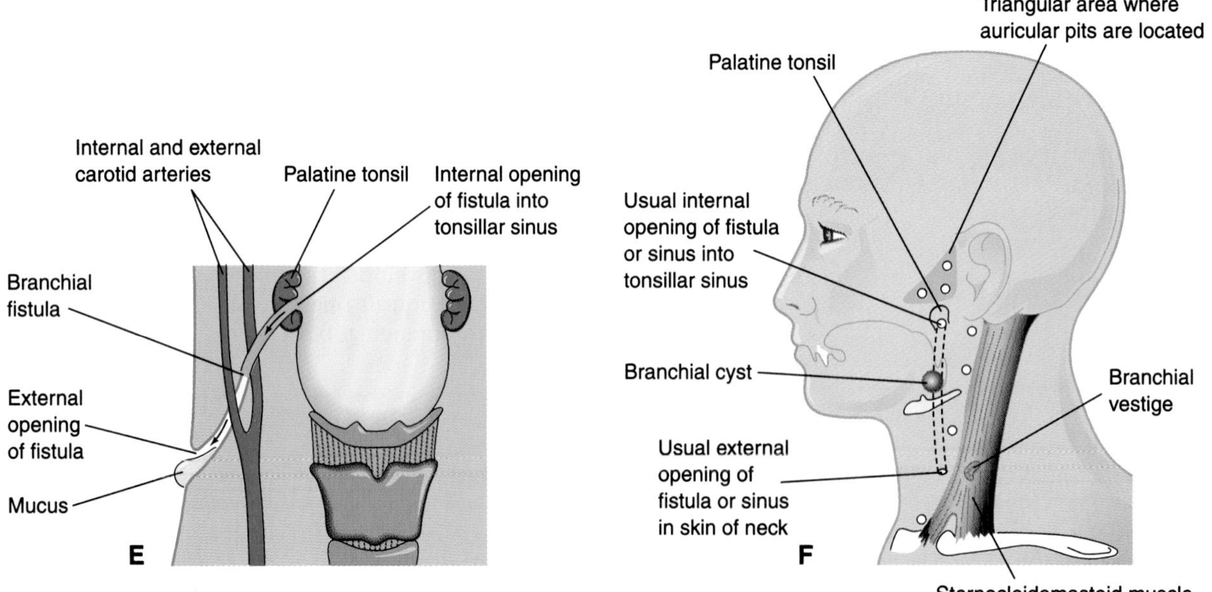

■ **Figure 10–10.** *A,* Drawing of the head, neck, and thoracic regions of a 5-week embryo, showing the cervical sinus that is normally present at this stage. *B,* Horizontal section of the embryo, at the level shown in *A,* illustrating the relationship of the cervical sinus to the pharyngeal arches and pouches. *C,* Diagrammatic sketch of the adult pharyngeal and neck regions, indicating the former sites of openings of the cervical sinus and pharyngeal pouches. The *broken lines* indicate possible courses of branchial fistulas. *D,* Similar sketch showing the embryological basis of various types of branchial sinus. *E,* Drawing of a branchial fistula resulting from persistence of parts of the second pharyngeal groove and second pharyngeal pouch. *F,* Sketch showing possible sites of branchial cysts and openings of branchial sinuses and fistulas. A branchial vestige is also illustrated (see also Fig. 10–14).

PHARYNGEAL MEMBRANES

The pharyngeal membranes appear in the floors of the pharyngeal grooves on each side of the head and neck regions of the human embryo during the fourth week (Figs. 10-1*H* and 10-3*C*). These membranes form where the epithelia of a groove and a pouch approach each other. The endoderm of the pouches and the ectoderm of the grooves are soon separated by mesenchyme. Only one pair of membranes contributes to the formation of adult structures; the *first pharyngeal membrane*, along with the intervening layer of mesenchyme, becomes the **tympanic membrane** (Fig. 10-8*C*).

Anomalies of the Head and Neck

Most congenital anomalies of the head and neck originate during transformation of the pharyngeal apparatus into adult structures. Most defects represent remnants of the pharyngeal apparatus that normally disappear as the adult structures develop (Stricker et al., 1990).

Congenital Auricular Sinuses and Cysts

Small auricular sinuses (pits) and cysts are usually found in a triangular area of skin anterior to the auricle of the external ear (Fig. 10-10*F*); however, they may occur in other sites around the auricle or in its lobule (earlobe). Although some sinuses and cysts are remnants of the first pharyngeal groove, others represent ectodermal folds sequestered during formation of the auricle from the auricular hillocks (swellings that form the auricle). These small sinuses and cysts are classified as minor anomalies that are of no serious medical consequence.

Branchial Sinuses

Branchial sinuses are uncommon and almost all that open externally on the side of the neck result from failure of the second pharyngeal groove and the cervical sinus to obliterate (Figs. 10-10*D* and 10-11*A* and *B*). The blind pit or sinus typically opens along the anterior border of the sternocleidomastoid muscle in the inferior third of the neck. Anomalies of the other pharyngeal grooves (first, third, or fourth) occur in about 5% of cases (Cote and Giandi, 1996).

External branchial sinuses are commonly detected during infancy because of the discharge of mucous material from their orifices in the neck (Fig. 10-11*A*). These *lateral cervical sinuses* are bilateral in about 10% of cases and are commonly associated with auricular sinuses.

Internal branchial sinuses open into the pharynx and are very rare. Because they usually open into the tonsillar sinus or near the palatopharyngeal arch (Fig. 10-10*D* and *F*), almost all these sinuses result from persistence of the proximal part of the second pharyngeal pouch. Normally this pouch disappears as the palatine tonsil develops; its normal remnant is the tonsillar sinus.

Branchial Fistula

An abnormal canal that opens internally into the tonsillar sinus and externally in the side of the neck is a *branchial fistula*, which results from persistence of parts of the second pharyngeal groove and second pharyngeal pouch (Figs. 10-10*E* and *F* and 10-11*C* and *D*). The fistula ascends from its opening in the neck through the subcutaneous tissue and platysma muscle to reach the carotid sheath (Moore, 1992). The fistula then passes between the internal and external carotid arteries and opens into the tonsillar sinus. In older patients there may be a disagreeable taste in the mouth because of the discharge of material into the oropharynx from the fistula.

Piriform Sinus Fistula

A piriform sinus fistula is thought to result from persistence of remnants of the ultimobranchial body (Miyauchi et al., 1992); the fistula traces the migration path of this embryonic body to the thyroid gland (Fig. 10-8*C*).

Branchial Cysts

The third and fourth pharyngeal arches are buried in the *cervical sinus* (Fig. 10-10*B*). Remnants of parts of the cervical sinus and/or the second pharyngeal groove may persist and form a spherical or elongate cyst (Fig. 10-10*F*). Although they may be associated with branchial sinuses and drain through them, branchial cysts often lie free in the neck just inferior to the angle of the mandible. They may, however, develop anywhere along the anterior border of the sternocleidomastoid muscle. Branchial cysts often do not become apparent until late childhood or early adulthood, when they produce a slowly enlarging, painless swelling in the neck (Fig. 10-12). The cysts enlarge because of the accumulation of fluid and cellular debris derived from desquamation of their epithelial linings (Fig. 10-13). Branchial cysts have been observed in the parathyroid glands and may arise from cystic degeneration and accumulation of secretions in embryological remnants that normally disappear (Chetty and Forder, 1991).

Branchial Vestiges

Normally the pharyngeal cartilages disappear, except for parts that form ligaments or bones; however, in unusual cases cartilaginous or bony remnants of pharyngeal arch cartilages appear under the skin in the side of the neck (Fig. 10-14). These are usually found anterior to the inferior third of the sternocleidomastoid muscle (Fig. 10-10*F*).

First Arch Syndrome

Abnormal development of the components of the first pharyngeal arch results in various congenital anomalies of the eyes, ears, mandible, and palate that together constitute the first arch syndrome (Fig. 10-15). This

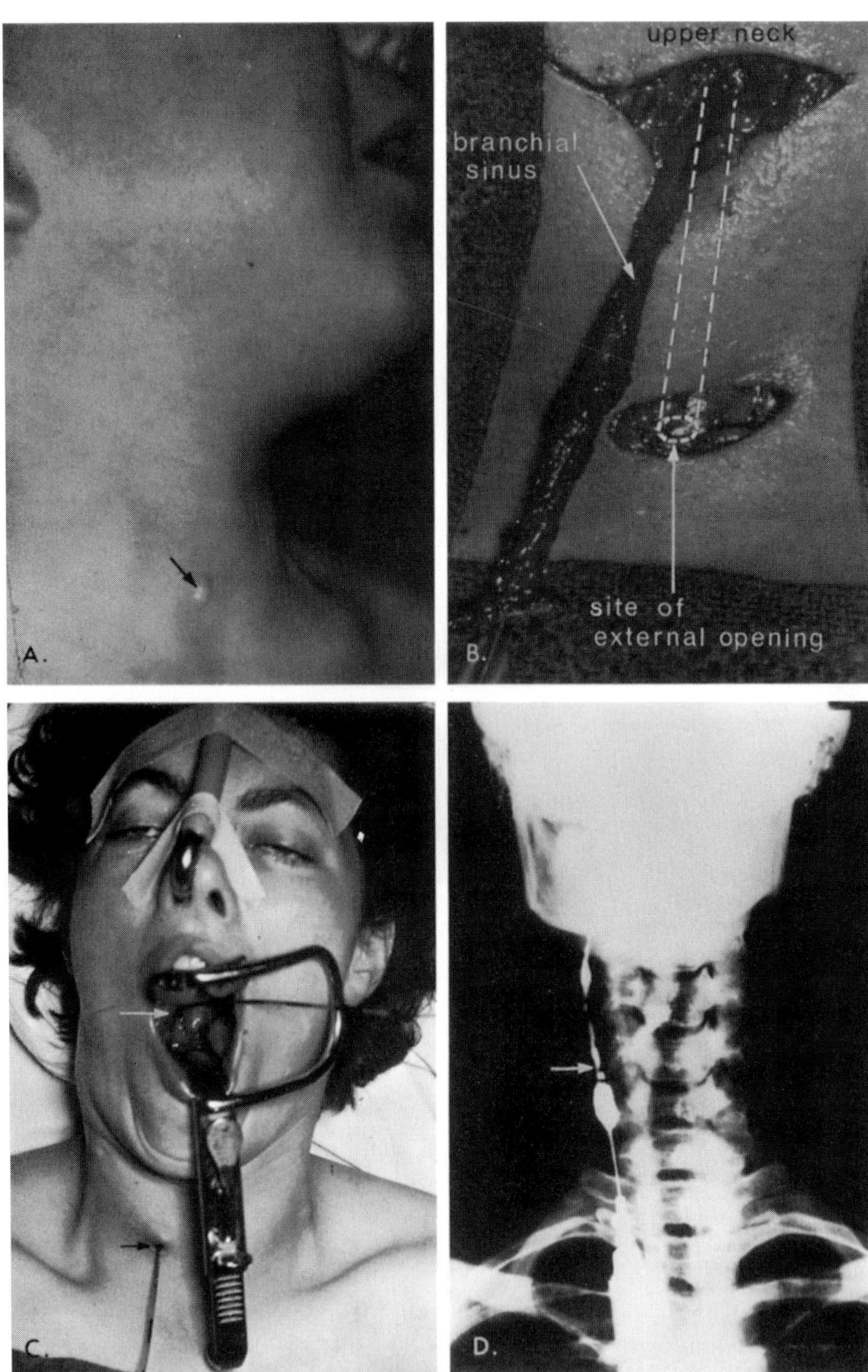

■ **Figure 10–11.** *A,* Photograph of a child's head and neck showing mucus oozing from the external opening of a branchial sinus *(arrow),* which is located just anterior to the sternocleidomastoid muscle. *B,* Photograph of a branchial sinus taken during its excision. Its external opening in the skin of the neck and the original course of the sinus in the subcutaneous tissue are indicated by broken lines. (From Swenson O: *Pediatric Surgery,* 1958. Courtesy of Appleton-Century-Crofts.) *C,* Photograph illustrating a branchial fistula in an adult female. The catheter enters the internal opening in the tonsillar sinus *(white arrow),* passes through the fistula, and leaves through the opening in the neck *(black arrow). D,* Radiograph taken after injection of a contrast medium, showing the course of the fistula *(arrow)* through the neck. (Courtesy of Dr. DA Kernahan, The Children's Memorial Hospital, Chicago.)

set of symptoms is believed to result from insufficient migration of neural crest cells into the first arch during the fourth week. *There are two main manifestations of the first arch syndrome* (Gorlin et al., 1990; van der Meulen et al., 1990; Behrman et al., 1996; Sulik, 1996):

- In the **Treacher Collins syndrome** (mandibulofacial dysostosis), caused by an autosomal dominant gene, there is malar hypoplasia (underdevelchopment of the zygomatic bones of the face) with downslanting palpebral fissures, defects of the lower eyelids, deformed external ears, and sometimes abnormalities of the middle and internal ears.
- In the **Pierre Robin syndrome**, hypoplasia of the mandible, cleft palate, and defects of the eye and ear are observed. Many cases of this syndrome are sporadic; however, some appear to have a genetic basis. In the *Robin morphogenetic complex,* the initiating defect is a small mandible (micrognathia), which results in posterior displacement of the tongue and obstruction to full

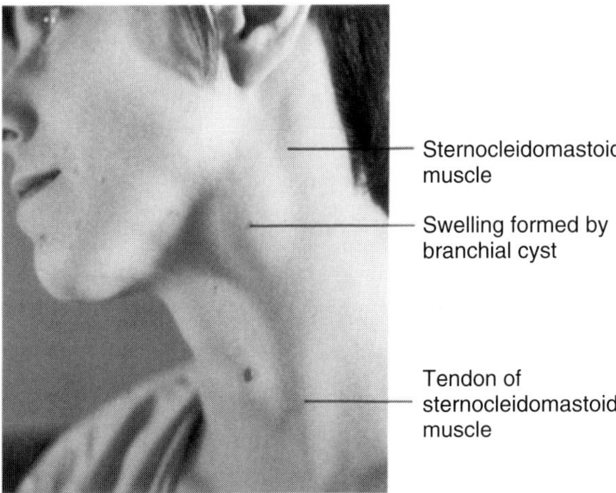

■ **Figure 10–12.** Photograph of the head, neck, and upper thoracic regions of a 27-year-old woman showing the swelling produced by a branchial cyst just anterior to her sternocleidomastoid muscle. The cyst was not visible at birth but developed slowly during her mid-twenties. The cyst was successfully excised. (From Moore KL: *Clinically Oriented Anatomy,* 3rd ed. Williams & Wilkins, Baltimore, 1995.)

closure of the palatine processes, resulting in a bilateral cleft palate.

DiGeorge Syndrome: Congenital Thymic Aplasia and Absence of Parathyroid Glands

Infants with these anomalies are born without a thymus and parathyroid glands; in some cases, ectopic glandular tissue has been found. The disease is characterized by *congenital hypoparathyroidism*, increased susceptibility to infections, anomalies of the mouth (shortened philtrum of lip [fish-mouth deformity]), low-set notched ears, nasal clefts, *thyroid hypoplasia*, and cardiac abnormalities (defects of the arch of the aorta and heart). The *DiGeorge syndrome* occurs be-

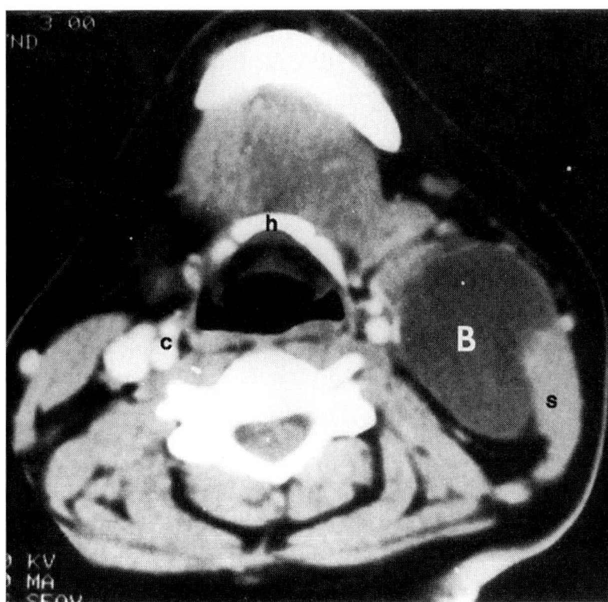

■ **Figure 10–13.** Branchial cleft cyst (B). This is a computed tomographic (CT) image of the neck region of a woman who presented with a "lump" in the neck, similar to that shown in Figure 10–12. The low-density cyst is anterior to the right sternocleidomastoid muscle **(s)** at the level of the hyoid bone **(h)**. The normal appearance of the carotid sheath **(c)** is shown for comparison with the compressed sheath on the right side. (From McNab T, McLennan MK, Margolis M: Radiology rounds. *Can Fam Physician 41:*1673, 1995.)

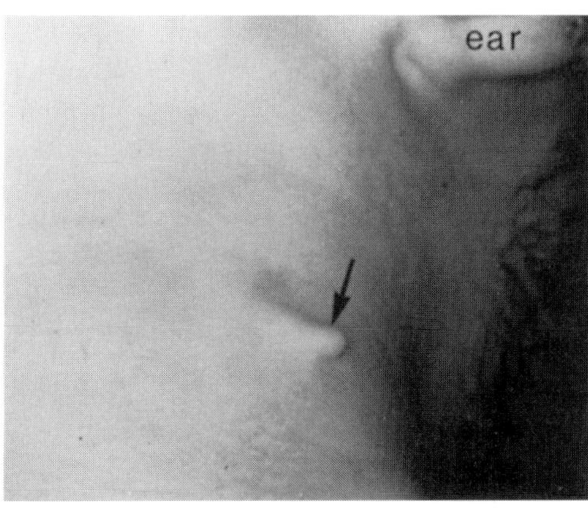

■ **Figure 10–14.** Photograph of a cartilaginous branchial vestige under the skin of a child's neck. (From Raffensperger JG: *Swenson's Pediatric Surgery,* 5th ed. 1990. Courtesy of Appleton-Century-Crofts.)

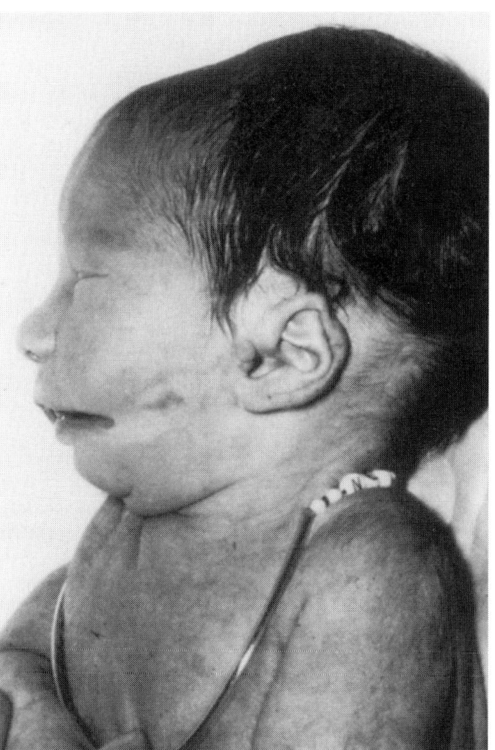

■ **Figure 10–15.** Photograph of an infant with the first arch syndrome, a pattern of anomalies resulting from insufficient migration of neural crest cells into the first pharyngeal arch. Note the following: deformed auricle of the external ear, preauricular appendage, defect in cheek between the auricle and the mouth, hypoplasia of the mandible, and macrostomia (large mouth).

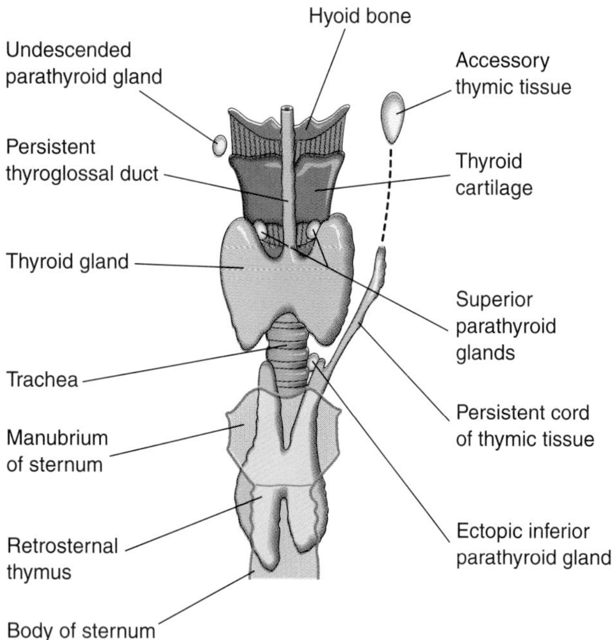

■ **Figure 10-16.** Drawing of an anterior view of the thyroid gland, thymus, and parathyroid glands, illustrating various congenital anomalies that may occur.

cause the third and fourth pharyngeal pouches fail to differentiate into the thymus and parathyroid glands. The facial abnormalities result primarily from abnormal development of the first arch components during formation of the face and ears. The DiGeorge syndrome usually results from a deletion (loss of a chromosome segment; Thompson et al., 1991). The syndrome may also result from a teratogen acting during the fourth to sixth weeks when the pharyngeal arches are transforming into adult derivatives.

Accessory Thymic Tissue

An isolated mass of thymic tissue may persist in the neck, often close to an inferior parathyroid gland (Fig. 10-16). This tissue breaks free from the developing thymus as it migrates caudally in the neck.

Variations in the Thymus

Variations in the shape of the thymus occur but they are not clinically significant. It may exhibit slender cords or prolongations into the neck on each side, anterolateral to the trachea. These processes may be connected to the inferior parathyroid glands by fibrous strands.

Ectopic Parathyroid Glands

The parathyroids are highly variable in number (two to six) and location. They may be found anywhere near or within the thyroid glands or thymus. The superior glands are more constant in position than the inferior ones (Moore, 1992). Occasionally an inferior parathyroid gland fails to descend and remains near the bifurcation of the common carotid artery. In other cases it may accompany the thymus into the thorax.

Abnormal Number of Parathyroid Glands

Uncommonly there are more than four parathyroid glands. Supernumerary parathyroid glands probably result from division of the primordia of the original glands. Absence of a parathyroid gland results from failure of one of the primordia to differentiate or from atrophy of a gland early in development.

DEVELOPMENT OF THE THYROID GLAND

The thyroid gland is the first endocrine gland to develop in the embryo. It begins to form about 24 days after fertilization from a median endodermal thickening in the floor of the primordial pharynx (Fig. 10-17). This thickening soon forms a small outpouching —the **thyroid diverticulum**. As the embryo and tongue grow, the developing thyroid gland descends in the neck, passing ventral to the developing hyoid bone and laryngeal cartilages. For a short time the developing thyroid gland is connected to the tongue by a narrow tube, the **thyroglossal duct** (Fig. 10-17*B* and *C*).

At first the thyroid diverticulum is hollow but it soon becomes solid and divides into right and left lobes, which are connected by the *isthmus of the thyroid gland,* which lies anterior to the developing second and third tracheal rings. By seven weeks the thyroid gland has assumed its definitive shape and has usually reached its final site in the neck (Fig. 10-17*D*). By this time the thyroglossal duct has normally degenerated and disappeared. The proximal opening of the thyroglossal duct persists as a small blind pit, the **foramen cecum of the tongue**. A pyramidal lobe extends superiorly from the isthmus in about 50% of people. The **pyramidal lobe** may be attached to the hyoid bone by fibrous and/or some smooth muscle— the *levator glandulae thyroideae*. A pyramidal lobe and the associated smooth muscle represent a persistent part of the distal end of the thyroglossal duct (Fig. 10-18).

Histogenesis of the Thyroid Gland

The thyroid primordium consists of a solid mass of endodermal cells. This cellular aggregation later breaks up into a network of epithelial cords because of the invasion of the surrounding vascular mesenchyme (embryonic connective tissue). By the tenth week the cords have divided into small cellular groups. A lumen soon forms in each cell cluster and the cells become arranged in a single layer around a lumen. During the eleventh week colloid begins to appear in these structures—**thyroid follicles**—thereafter, iodine concentration and the synthesis of *thyroid hormones* can be demonstrated. For a detailed account of the histogenesis of the thyroid gland, see Shepard (1975). Studies have shown that an insulin-like **epidermal growth factor**, as well as other related factors, are involved in the replication and growth of the thyroid follicular cells (Fisher and Polk, 1989).

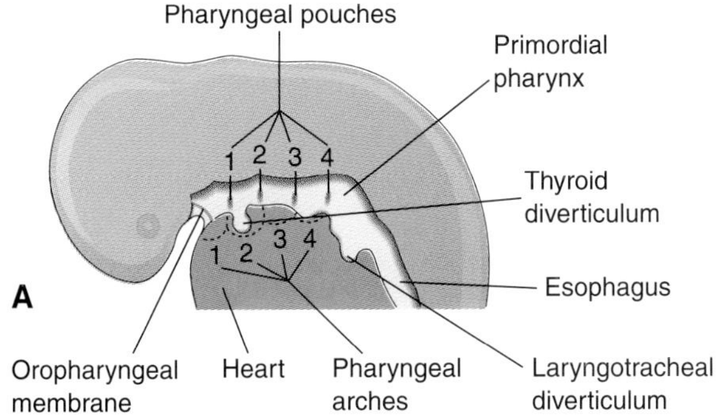

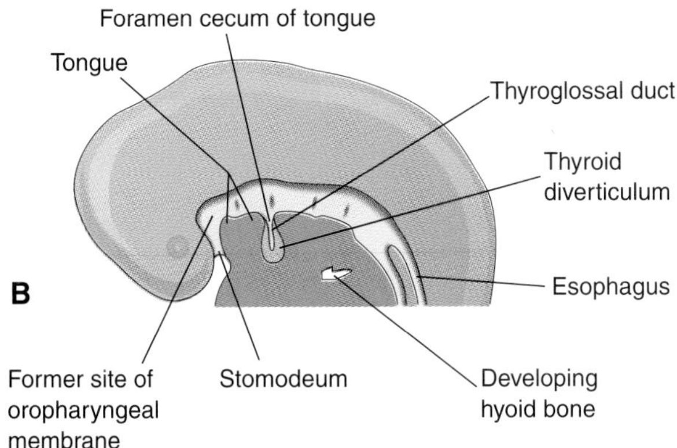

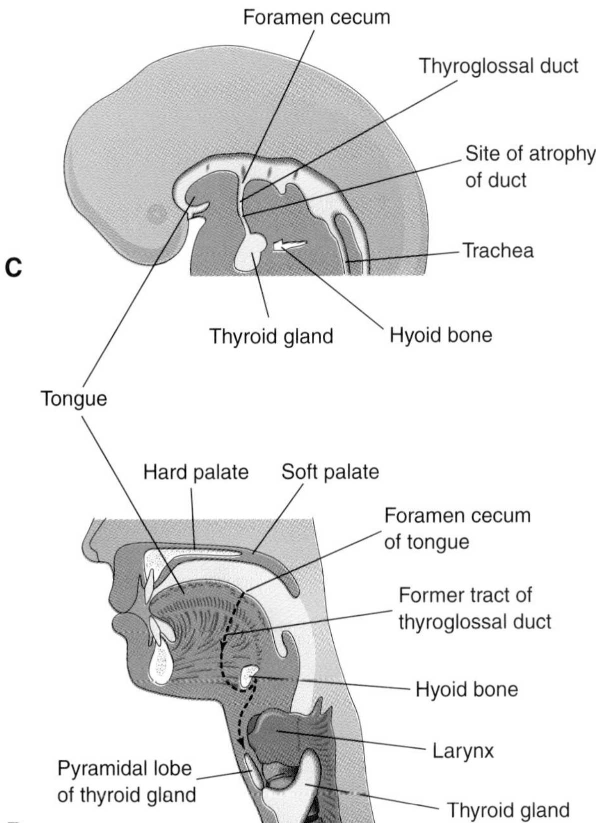

■ **Figure 10–17.** Development of the thyroid gland. *A, B,* and *C,* Schematic sagittal sections of the head and neck regions of embryos at 4, 5, and 6 weeks, illustrating successive stages in the development of the thyroid gland. *D,* Similar section of an adult head and neck showing the path taken by the thyroid gland during its embryonic descent (indicated by the former tract of the thyroglossal duct).

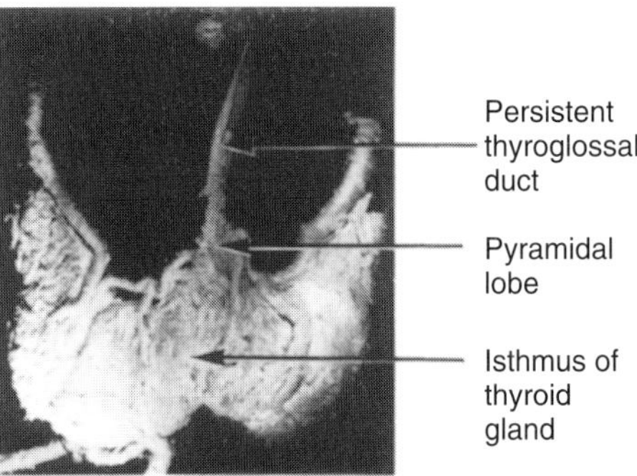

■ **Figure 10–18.** Photograph of the anterior surface of a dissected adult thyroid gland, showing persistence of the thyroglossal duct. Observe the pyramidal lobe ascending from the superior border of the isthmus. It represents a persistent portion of the inferior end of the thyroglossal duct.

Congenital Hypothyroidism

The primary cause of congenital hypothyroidism is a derangement in the development of the thyroid gland, rather than central causes related to the hypothalamic-pituitary axis (Miculan et al., 1993).

Thyroglossal Duct Cysts and Sinuses

Cysts may form anywhere along the course followed by the thyroglossal duct during descent of the thyroid gland from the tongue (Fig. 10–19). Normally the thyroglossal duct atrophies and disappears, but a remnant of it may persist and form a cyst in the tongue (Urao et al., 1996) or in the anterior part of the neck, usually just inferior to the hyoid bone (Fig. 10–20). Most thyroglossal duct cysts are observed by the age of 5 years. Unless the lesions become infected, most of them are asymptomatic. The swelling produced by a *thyroglossal duct cyst* usually develops as a painless, progressively enlarging, movable mass (Fig. 10–21). The cyst may contain some thyroid tissue (Johnson et al., 1996). Following infection of a cyst, a perforation of the skin occurs in some cases, forming a **thyroglossal duct sinus** that usually opens in the median plane of the neck, anterior to the laryngeal cartilages (Fig. 10–19*A*).

Ectopic Thyroid Gland

An ectopic thyroid gland is an infrequent congenital anomaly and is usually located along the normal route-

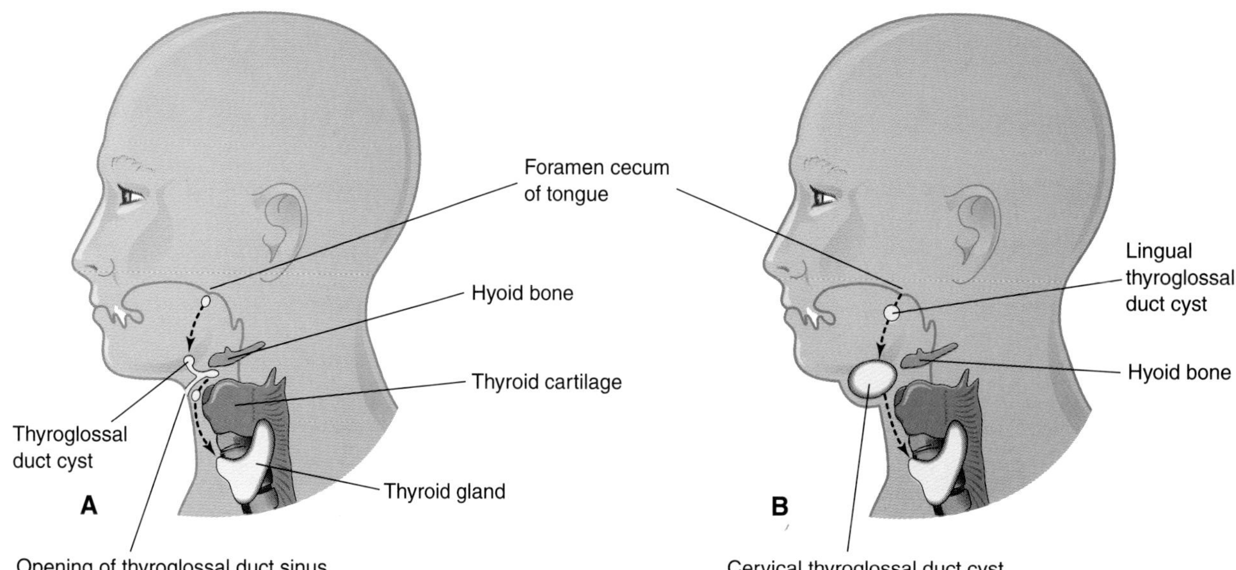

■ **Figure 10–19.** *A,* Diagrammatic sketch of the head and neck showing the possible locations of thyroglossal duct cysts. A thyroglossal duct sinus is also illustrated. The *broken line* indicates the course taken by the thyroglossal duct during descent of the developing thyroid gland from the foramen cecum to its final position in the anterior part of the neck. *B,* Similar sketch illustrating lingual and cervical thyroglossal duct cysts. Most thyroglossal duct cysts are located just inferior to the hyoid bone.

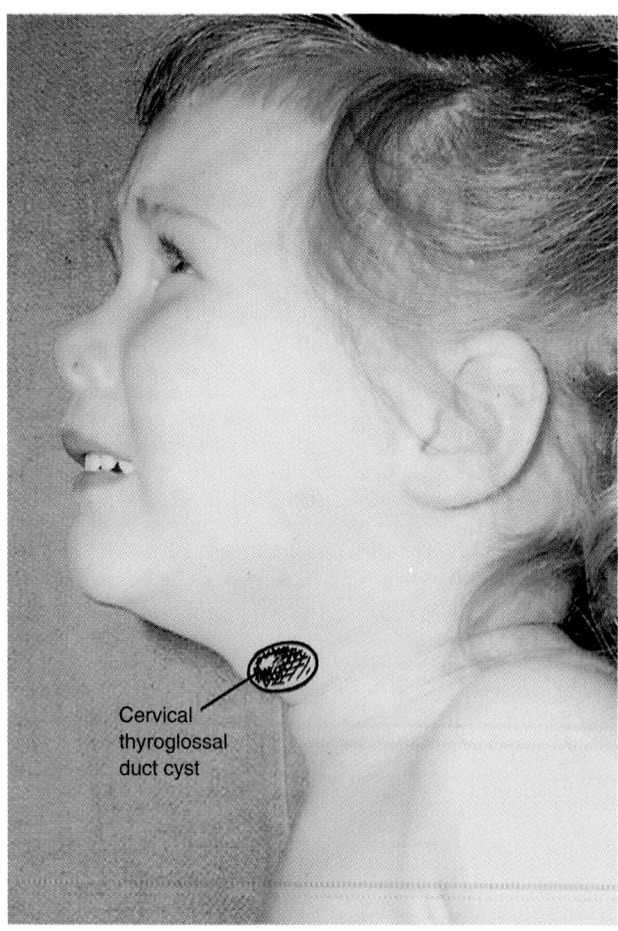

■ **Figure 10–20.** Typical thyroglossal duct cyst in a female child. The round, firm mass (indicated by the sketch) produced a swelling in the median plane of the neck just inferior to the hyoid bone.

of its descent from the tongue (Fig. 10–17*C*). **Lingual thyroid glandular tissue** is the most common of ectopic thyroid tissues; intralingual thyroid masses are found in as many as 10% of autopsies, although they are clinically relevant in only 1 in 4000 patients with thyroid disease (Spinner et al., 1994). Incomplete descent of the thyroid gland results in the **sublingual thyroid gland** appearing high in the neck, at or just inferior to the hyoid bone (Figs. 10–22 and 10–23). As a rule, an ectopic sublingual thyroid gland in the neck is the only thyroid tissue present. It is clinically important to differentiate an ectopic thyroid gland from a thyroglossal duct cyst or an accessory thyroid gland in order to prevent *inadvertent surgical removal of the thyroid gland* (Leung et al., 1995), because this may be the only thyroid tissue present. Failure to do so may leave the person permanently dependent on thyroid medication.

Accessory Thyroid Gland Tissue

Accessory thyroid gland tissue may also appear in the thymus superior to the thyroid gland. Although this tissue may be functional, it is often of insufficient size to maintain normal function if the thyroid gland is removed. An *accessory thyroid gland* may develop in the neck lateral to the thyroid cartilage. It usually lies on the thyrohyoid muscle. Accessory thyroid glandular tissue originates from remnants of the thyroglossal duct.

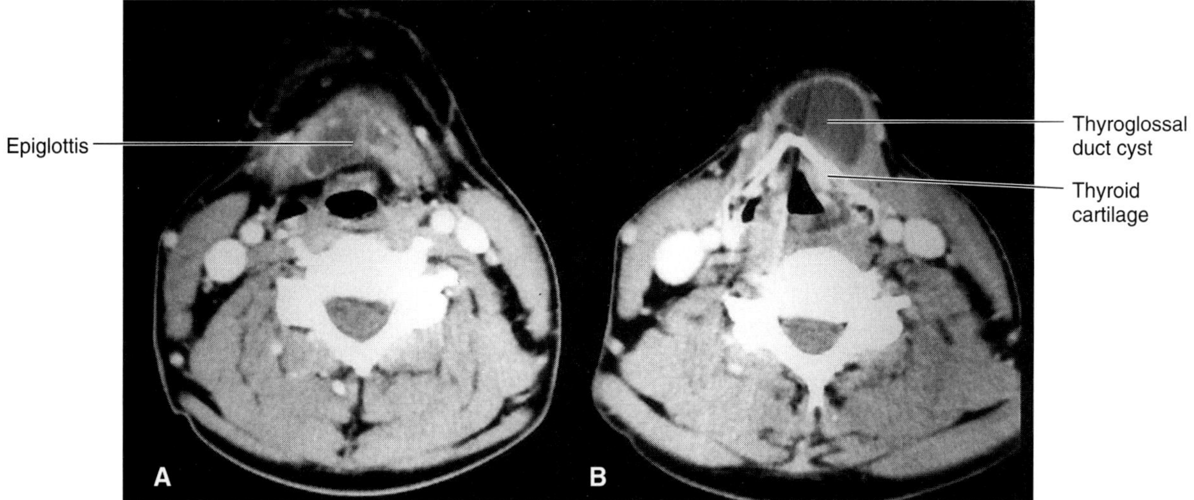

■ **Figure 10–21.** Computed tomographic (CT) images. *A,* Level of the thyrohyoid membrane and base of the epiglottis. *B,* Level of thyroid cartilage, which is calcified. The thyroglossal duct cyst extends cranially to the margin of the hyoid bone. (Courtesy of Dr. Gerald S. Smyser, Altru Health System, Grand Forks, North Dakota.)

Agenesis of the Thyroid Gland

Absence of the thyroid gland, one or both lobes, is a rare anomaly. In cases of thyroid hemiagenesis (unilateral failure of formation), the left lobe is more commonly absent.

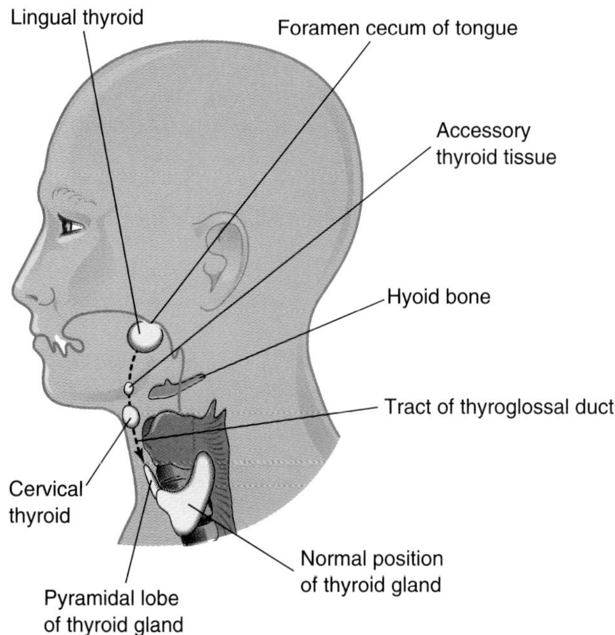

■ **Figure 10–22.** Diagrammatic sketch of the head and neck, showing the usual sites of ectopic thyroid tissue. The *broken line* indicates the path followed by the thyroid gland during its descent and the former tract of the thyroglossal duct.

DEVELOPMENT OF THE TONGUE

Near the end of the fourth week, a median triangular elevation appears in the floor of the primordial pharynx, just rostral to the foramen cecum (Fig. 10-24*A*). This swelling—the **median tongue bud** (tuberculum impar)—is the first indication of tongue development. Soon, two oval **distal tongue buds** (lateral lingual swellings) develop on each side of the median tongue bud. The three lingual buds result from the proliferation of mesenchyme in ventromedial parts of the first pair of pharyngeal arches. The distal tongue buds rapidly increase in size, merge with each other, and overgrow the median tongue bud. *The merged distal tongue buds form the anterior two-thirds (oral part) of the tongue* (Fig. 10-24*C*). The plane of fusion of the distal tongue buds is indicated superficially by the *median sulcus of the tongue* and internally by the fibrous *lingual septum* (Moore, 1992). The median tongue bud forms no recognizable part of the adult tongue.

Formation of the posterior third (pharyngeal part) of the tongue is indicated by two elevations that develop caudal to the foramen cecum (Fig. 10-24*A*):

- The *copula* (L., bond, tie) forms by fusion of the ventromedial parts of the second pair of pharyngeal arches.
- The *hypobranchial eminence* develops caudal to the copula from mesenchyme in the ventromedial parts of the third and fourth pairs of arches.

As the tongue develops the copula is gradually overgrown by the hypobranchial eminence and disappears (Fig. 10-24*B* and *C*). As a result, the pharyngeal part of the tongue develops from the rostral part of the hypobranchial eminence, a derivative of the third pair of pharyngeal arches.

The line of fusion of the anterior and posterior parts

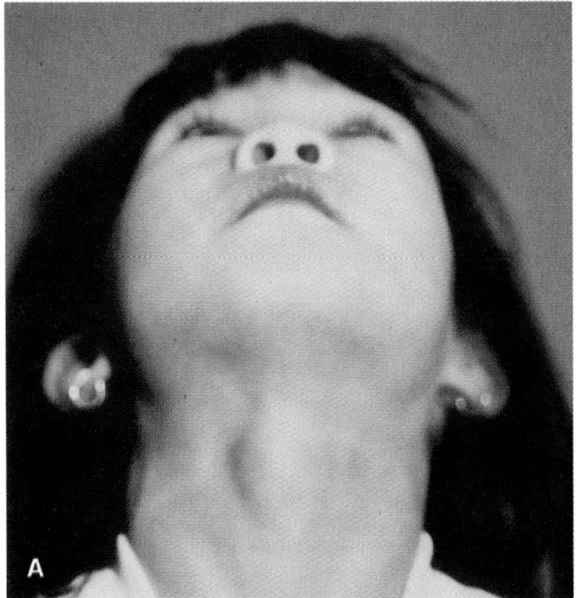

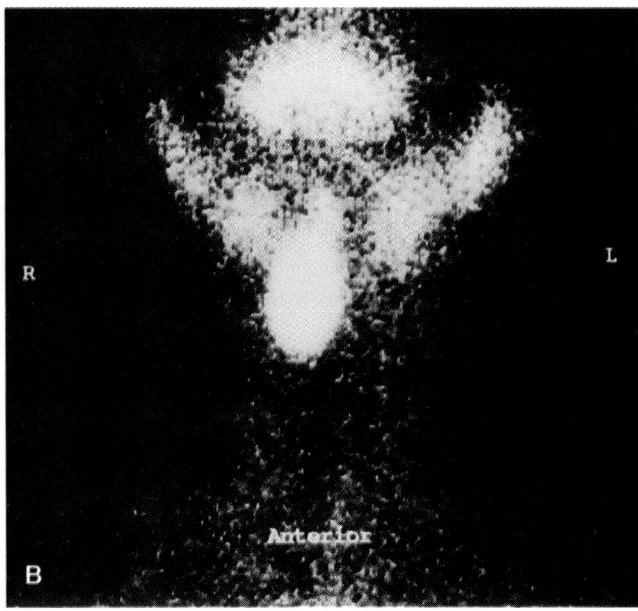

■ **Figure 10–23.** *A,* Photograph of a sublingual thyroid mass in a 5-year-old girl. *B,* Technetium-99m pertechnetate scan showing a sublingual thyroid without evidence of functioning thyroid tissue in lower neck. (From Leung AKC, Wong AL, Robson WLLM: Ectopic thyroid gland simulating a thyroglossal duct cyst. *Can J Surg 38:*87, 1995.)

of the tongue is roughly indicated by a V-shaped groove—the **terminal sulcus** (Figs. 10-24*C* and 10-25). Pharyngeal arch mesenchyme forms the connective tissue and vasculature of the tongue. Most of the *tongue muscles* are derived from myoblasts that migrate from the occipital myotomes (Fig. 10-6*A*). The *hypoglossal nerve* (CN XII) accompanies the myoblasts during their migration and innervates the tongue muscles as they develop. The entire tongue is within the mouth at birth; its posterior third descends into the oropharynx by 4 years of age (Sperber, 1993).

Papillae and Taste Buds of the Tongue

The lingual papillae appear toward the end of the eighth week. The *vallate* and *foliate papillae* appear first, close to terminal branches of the glossopharyngeal nerve (CN IX). The *fungiform papillae* appear later near terminations of the chorda tympani branch of the facial nerve (CN VII). The most common lingual papillae, known as *filiform papillae* because of their threadlike shape (L. *filum*, thread), develop during the early fetal period (10 to 11 weeks). They contain afferent nerve endings that are *sensitive to touch*. For histological and anatomical details of the lingual papillae and taste buds, see Cormack (1993) and Gartner and Hiatt (1997).

Taste buds develop during weeks 11 to 13 by inductive interaction between the epithelial cells of the tongue and invading gustatory nerve cells from the chorda tympani, glossopharyngeal, and vagus nerves (Sperber, 1993; Gartner and Hiatt, 1997). Most taste buds form on the dorsal surface of the tongue and some develop on the palatoglossal arches, palate, posterior surface of the epiglottis, and the posterior wall of the oropharynx. The injection of saccharin into the amniotic cavity results in increased swallowing by the fetus (Sperber, 1993). Fetal responses in the face can be induced by bitter-tasting substances at 26 to 28 weeks, indicating that reflex pathways between taste buds and facial muscles are established by this stage.

Nerve Supply of the Tongue

The development of the tongue explains its nerve supply. The sensory nerve supply to the mucosa of almost the entire *anterior two-thirds of the tongue* (oral part) is from the lingual branch of the mandibular division of the *trigeminal nerve* (CN V), the nerve of the first pharyngeal arch. This arch forms the median and distal tongue buds (Fig. 10-24). Although the facial nerve is the nerve of the second pharyngeal arch, its chorda tympani branch supplies the taste buds in the anterior two-thirds of the tongue, except for the vallate papillae. Because the second arch component, the copula, is overgrown by the third arch, the facial nerve (CN VII) does not supply any of the tongue mucosa, except for the taste buds in the oral part of the tongue. The *vallate papillae* in the oral part of the tongue are innervated by the *glossopharyngeal nerve* (CN IX) of the third pharyngeal arch (Fig. 10-24*C*). The reason usually given for this is that the mucosa of the posterior third of the tongue is pulled slightly anteriorly as the tongue develops. The *posterior third of the tongue* (pharyngeal part) is innervated mainly by the *glossopharyngeal nerve* of the third pharyngeal arch. The superior laryngeal branch of the vagus nerve (CN X) of the fourth arch supplies a small area of the tongue anterior to the epiglottis (Fig. 10-24*C*). All **muscles of the tongue** are supplied by the *hypoglossal nerve* (CN XII), except for the palatoglossus, which is supplied from the pharyngeal plexus by fibers arising from the *vagus nerve* (CN X).

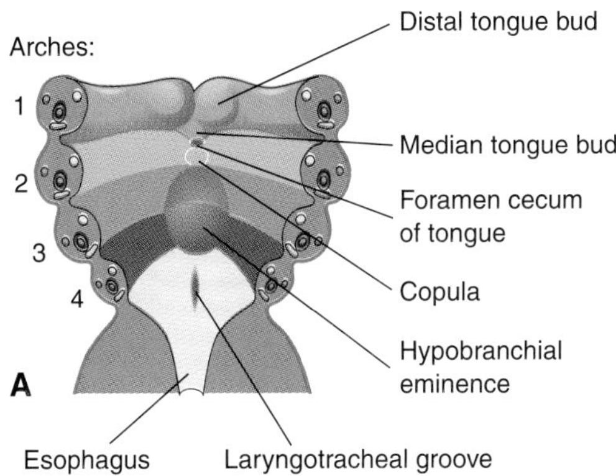

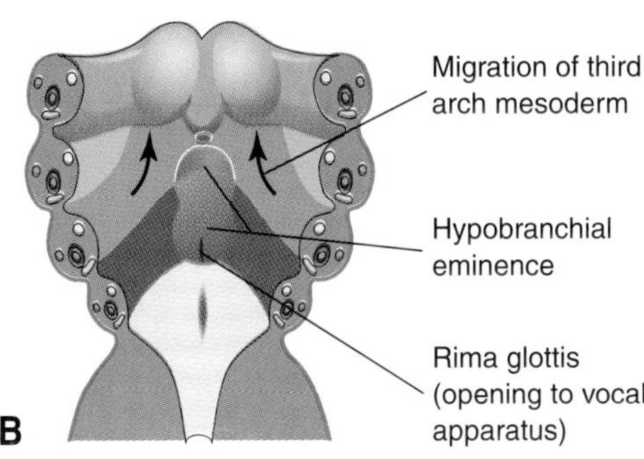

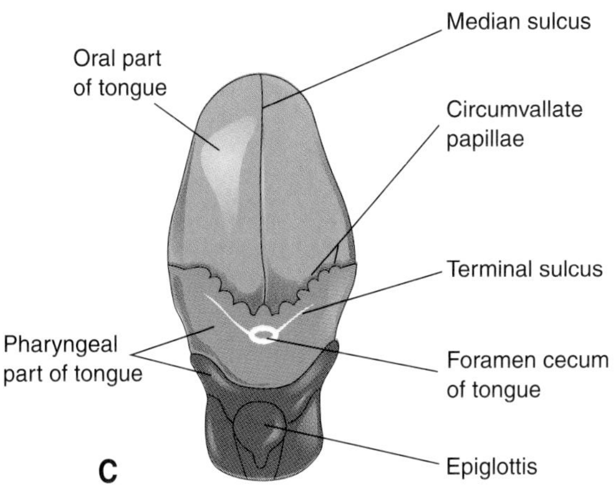

Arch Derivatives of Tongue

1st pharyngeal arch (CN V-mandibular division)
2nd pharyngeal arch (CN VII-chorda tympani)
3rd pharyngeal arch (CN IX-glossopharyngeal)
4th pharyngeal arch (CN X-vagus)

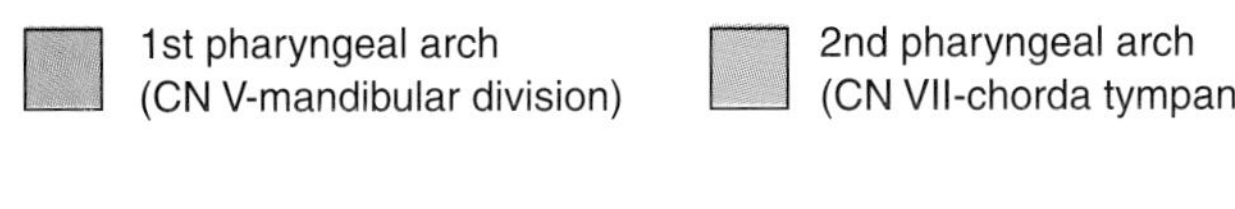

■ **Figure 10–24.** *A* and *B*, Schematic horizontal sections through the pharynx at the level shown in Figure 10–4*A*, showing successive stages in the development of the tongue during the fourth and fifth weeks. *C*, Drawing of the adult tongue showing the pharyngeal arch derivation of the nerve supply of its mucosa.

Congenital Anomalies of the Tongue

Abnormalities of the tongue (Gr. *glōssa*) are uncommon, except for fissuring of the tongue and hypertrophy of the lingual papillae, which are characteristics of infants with Down syndrome (see Chapter 8).

Congenital Lingual Cysts and Fistulas

Cysts in the tongue may be derived from remnants of the thyroglossal duct (Fig. 10-19). They may enlarge and produce symptoms of pharyngeal discomfort and/or *dysphagia* (difficulty in swallowing). Fistulas are also derived from persistence of lingual parts of the thyroglossal duct; they open through the *foramen cecum* into the oral cavity.

Ankyloglossia (Tongue-Tie)

The lingual frenulum normally connects the inferior surface of the tongue to the floor of the mouth (Moore, 1992). Sometimes the frenulum is short and extends to the tip of the tongue. This interferes with its free protrusion and may make breast-feeding difficult. Tongue-tie occurs in about one in 300 North American infants but is usually of no functional significance (Behrman et al., 1996). A short frenulum usually stretches with time, making surgical correction of the anomaly unnecessary. Ankyloglossia is often found in combination with other craniofacial anomalies (van der Meulen et al., 1990).

Macroglossia

An excessively large tongue is not common (Severtson and Petruzzelli, 1996). It results from generalized hypertrophy of the tongue, usually resulting from lymphangioma (a lymph tumor) or muscular hypertrophy. For a list of syndromes featuring macrostomia, see Jones (1997).

Microglossia

An abnormally small tongue is extremely rare and is usually associated with *micrognathia* (underdeveloped mandible and recession of the chin) and limb defects (*Hanhart syndrome*). For a list of syndromes featuring microstomia, see Jones (1997).

Bifid or Cleft Tongue (Glossoschisis)

Incomplete fusion of the distal tongue buds results in a deep median sulcus or groove in the tongue; usually this cleft does not extend to the tip of the tongue. This is a very uncommon anomaly.

DEVELOPMENT OF THE SALIVARY GLANDS

During the sixth and seventh weeks, the salivary glands begin as solid epithelial buds from the primordial oral cavity (Fig. 10-7*C*). The club-shaped ends of these epithelial buds grow into the underlying mesenchyme. The connective tissue in the glands is derived

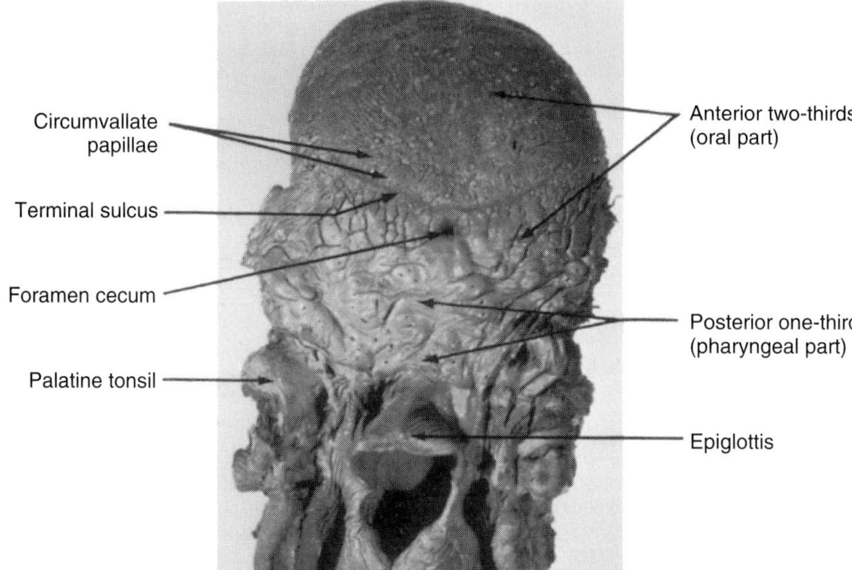

■ **Figure 10–25.** Photograph of the dorsum of an adult tongue (cadaveric specimen). The foramen cecum indicates the site of origin of the thyroid diverticulum and thyroglossal duct in the embryo. The terminal sulcus demarcates the developmentally different pharyngeal and oral parts of the tongue.

from neural crest cells. All parenchymal (secretory) tissue arises by proliferation of the oral epithelium.

The **parotid glands** are the first to appear (early in the sixth week). They develop from buds that arise from the oral ectodermal lining near the angles of the stomodeum. The buds grow toward the ears and branch to form solid cords with rounded ends. Later the cords canalize — develop lumina — and become ducts by about 10 weeks. The rounded ends of the cords differentiate into acini. Secretions commence at 18 weeks (Sperber, 1993). The capsule and connective tissue develop from the surrounding mesenchyme.

The **submandibular glands** appear late in the sixth week. They develop from endodermal buds in the floor of the stomodeum. Solid cellular processes grow posteriorly, lateral to the developing tongue. Later they branch and differentiate. Acini begin to form at 12 weeks and secretory activity begins at 16 weeks (Sperber, 1993). Growth of the submandibular glands continues after birth with the formation of mucous acini. Lateral to the tongue, a linear groove forms that soon closes over to form the *submandibular duct*.

The **sublingual glands** appear in the eighth week, about 2 weeks later than the other salivary glands. They develop from multiple endodermal epithelial buds in the paralingual sulcus (Fig. 10-7*C*). These buds branch and canalize to form 10 to 12 ducts that open independently into the floor of the mouth.

DEVELOPMENT OF THE FACE

The facial primordia begin to appear early in the fourth week around the large *stomodeum* (Fig. 10-26*A* and *B*). Facial development depends upon the inductive influence of the prosencephalic and rhombencephalic organizing centers (Sperber, 1993). The **prosencephalic organizing center**, derived from prechordal mesoderm that migrates from the primitive streak, is located rostral to the notochord and ventral to the prosencephalon or forebrain (see Chapter 18). The **rhombencephalic organizing center** is ventral to the rhombencephalon (hindbrain).

The **five facial primordia** appear as prominences around the stomodeum (Fig. 10-26*A*):

- the single frontonasal prominence
- the paired maxillary prominences
- the paired mandibular prominences

The paired facial prominences are derivatives of the first pair of pharyngeal arches. The prominences are produced predominantly by the proliferation of **neural crest cells** that migrate from the lower mesencephalon and upper rhombencephalon regions of the neural folds into the arches during the fourth week. These cells are the major source of connective tissue components, including cartilage, bone, and ligaments in the facial and oral regions. The results of experimental studies in chick and mouse embryos indicate that myoblasts, originating from paraxial and prechordal mesoderm, contribute to the craniofacial voluntary muscles (Noden, 1991; Sulik, 1996).

The **frontonasal prominence** (FNP) surrounds the ventrolateral part of the forebrain, which gives rise to the *optic vesicles* that form the eyes (Figs. 10-26*C* and 10-27). The frontal portion of the FNP forms the forehead; the nasal part of the FNP forms the rostral boundary of the stomodeum and nose. The paired **maxillary prominences** form the lateral boundaries of the stomodeum and the paired **mandibular prominences** constitute the caudal boundary of the primitive mouth (Fig. 10-27). The five facial prominences are active **centers of growth** in the underlying mesenchyme. This embryonic connective tissue is continuous from one prominence to the other. Facial development occurs mainly between the fourth and eighth

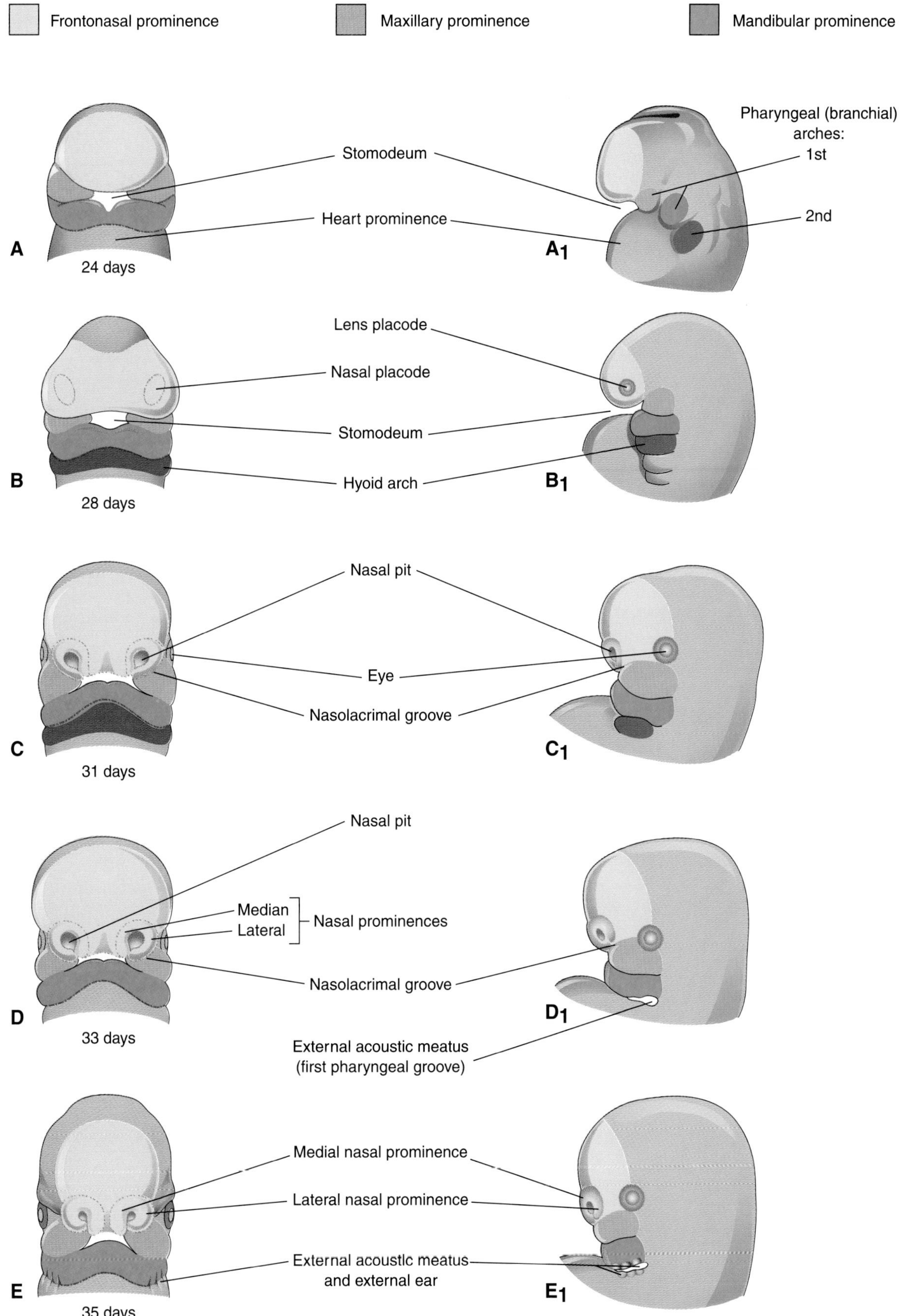

■ **Figure 10–26.** Diagrams illustrating progressive stages in the development of the human face.

Illustration continued on following page

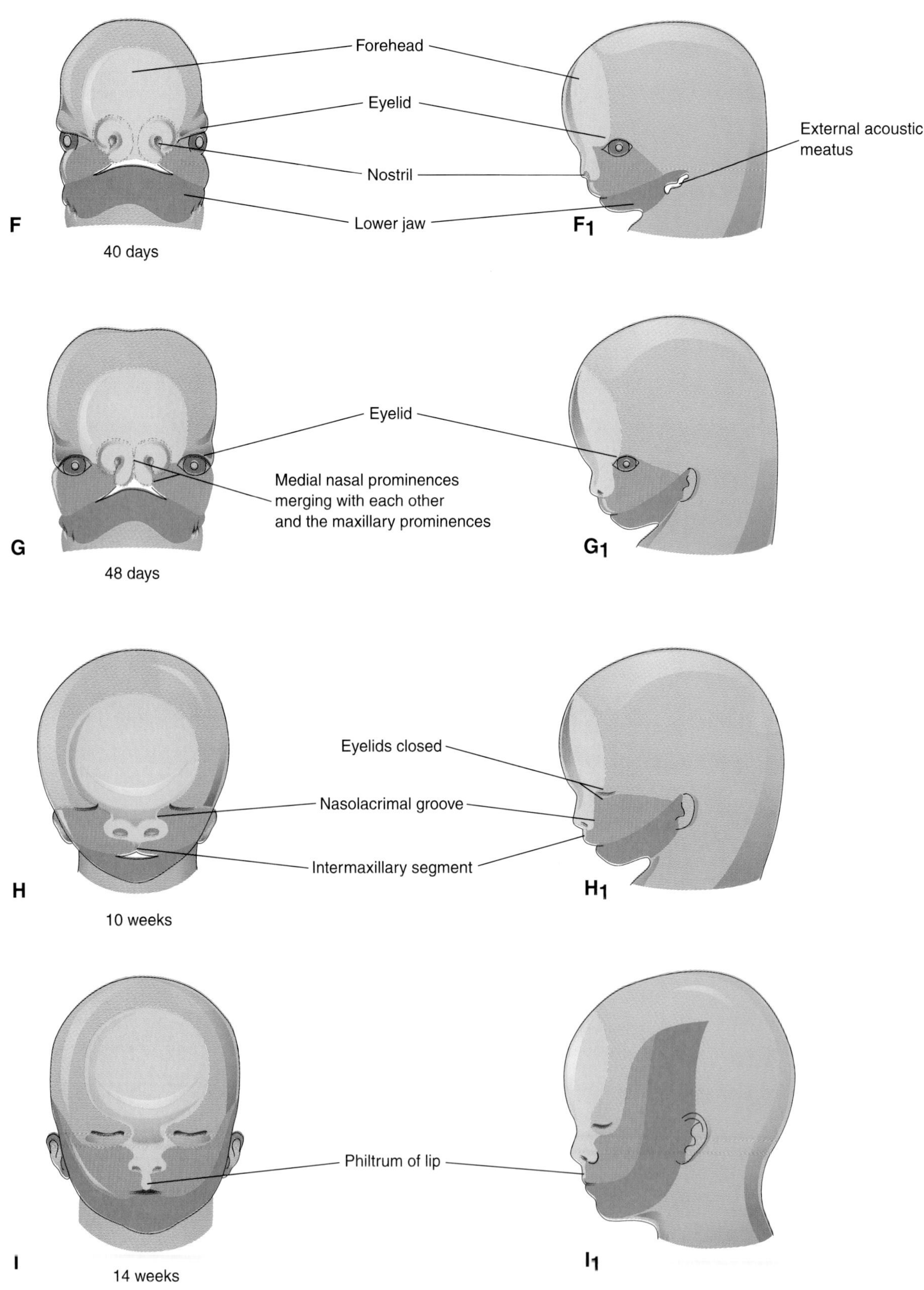

■ **Figure 10–26.** *Continued*

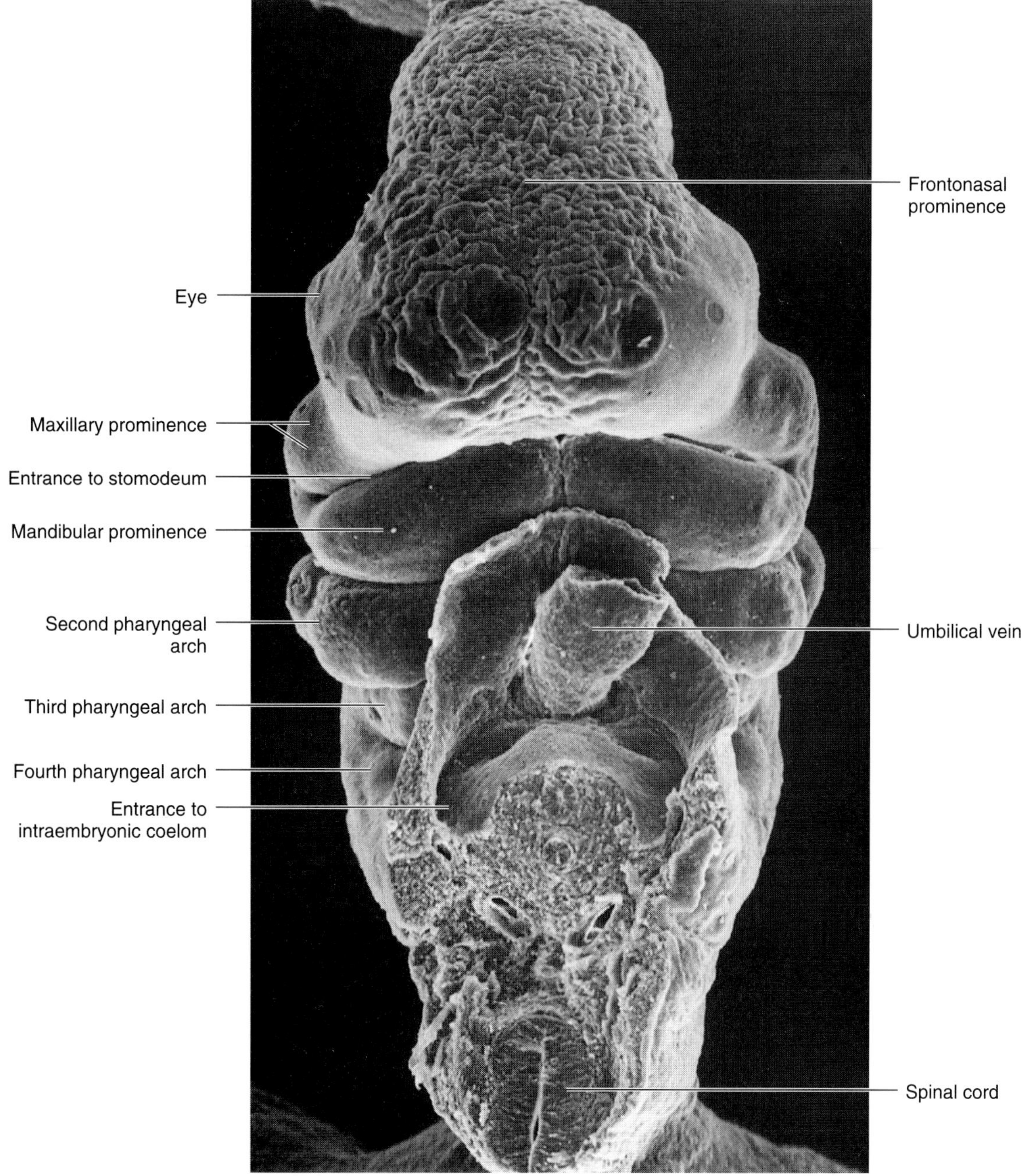

■ **Figure 10–27.** Scanning electron micrograph of a ventral view of a stage 14 embryo (30–32 days old). (Courtesy of Professor Emeritus Dr. KV Hinrichsen, Medizinische Fakultät, Institut für Anatomie, Ruhr-Universität Bochum, Germany.)

weeks (Fig. 10-26*A* to *G*). By the end of the embryonic period, the face has an unquestionably human appearance. Facial proportions develop during the fetal period (Fig. 10-26*H* and *I*). The lower jaw and lower lip are the first parts of the face to form. They result from merging of the medial ends of the mandibular prominences in the median plane.

By the end of the fourth week, bilateral oval thickenings of the surface ectoderm — **nasal placodes** — the primordia of the nose and nasal cavities, have developed on the inferolateral parts of the FNP (Figs. 10-28 and 10-29*A* and *B*). Initially these placodes are convex, but later they are stretched to produce a flat depression in each placode (Hinrichsen, 1985). Mesenchyme in the margins of the placodes proliferates, producing horseshoe-shaped elevations — the **medial and lateral nasal prominences**. As a result, the nasal placodes lie in depressions — the **nasal pits** (Fig. 10-29*C* and *D*). These pits are the primordia of the anterior nares (nostrils) and nasal cavities (Fig. 10-29*E*).

Proliferation of mesenchyme in the maxillary prominences causes them to enlarge and grow medially toward each other and the nasal prominences (Figs. 10-26*D* to *G*, 10-27, and 10-28). The medial migration of the maxillary prominences moves the medial nasal prominences toward the median plane and each other. Each lateral nasal prominence is separated from the maxillary prominence by a cleft called the **nasolacrimal groove** (Figs. 10-26*C* and *D*).

By the end of the fifth week, the *primordia of the auricles* of the external ears have begun to develop (Figs. 10-26*E* and 10-30). Six **auricular hillocks** (small mesenchymal swellings) form around the first pharyngeal groove (three on each side), the primordia of the auricle and external acoustic meatus (canal), respectively. Initially the external ears are located in the neck region (Fig. 10-31); however, as the mandible develops they ascend to the side of the head at the level of the eyes (Fig. 10-26*H*). By the end of the sixth week, each maxillary prominence has begun to merge with the lateral nasal prominence along the line of the **nasolacrimal groove** (Figs. 10-32 and 10-33). This establishes continuity between the side of the nose, formed by the lateral nasal prominence, and the cheek region formed by the maxillary prominence.

The **nasolacrimal duct** develops from a rodlike thickening of ectoderm in the floor of the nasolacrimal groove. This thickening gives rise to a solid epithelial

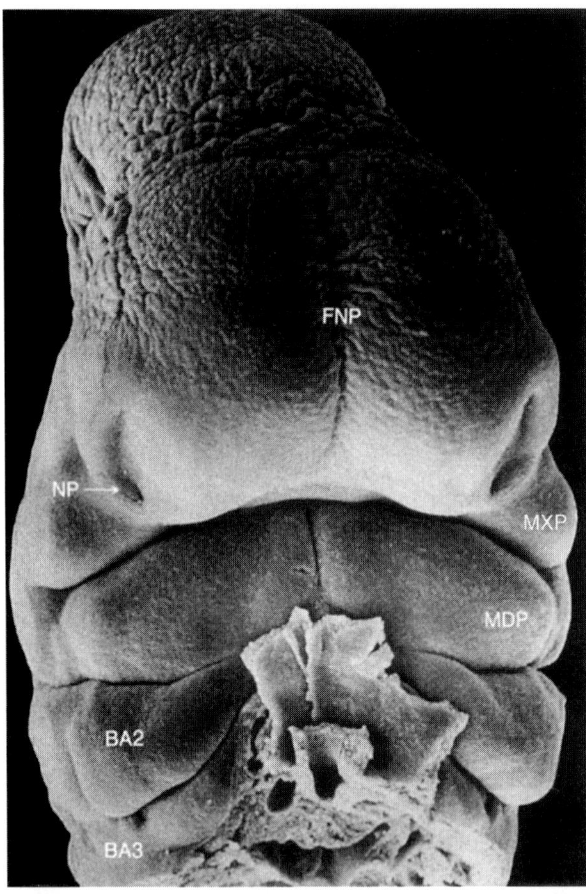

■ **Figure 10-28.** Scanning electron micrograph of a ventral view of a human embryo of about 33 days (stage 15, crown-rump length [CRL] 8 mm). Observe the prominent frontonasal process (FNP) surrounding the telencephalon (forebrain). Also observe the nasal pits (NP) located in the ventrolateral regions of the frontonasal prominence. Medial and lateral nasal prominences surround these pits. The cuneiform, wedge-shaped maxillary prominences (MXP) form the lateral boundaries of the stomodeum. The fusing mandibular prominences (MDP) are located just caudal to the stomodeum. The second pharyngeal arch (BA2) is clearly visible and shows overhanging margins (opercula). The third pharyngeal arch (BA3) is also clearly visible. (From Hinrichsen K: The early development of morphology and patterns of the face in the human embryo. *Adv Anat Embryol Cell Biol 98*:1–79, 1985.)

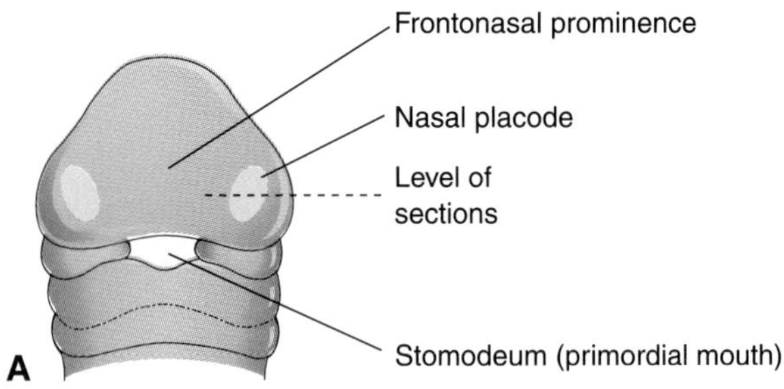

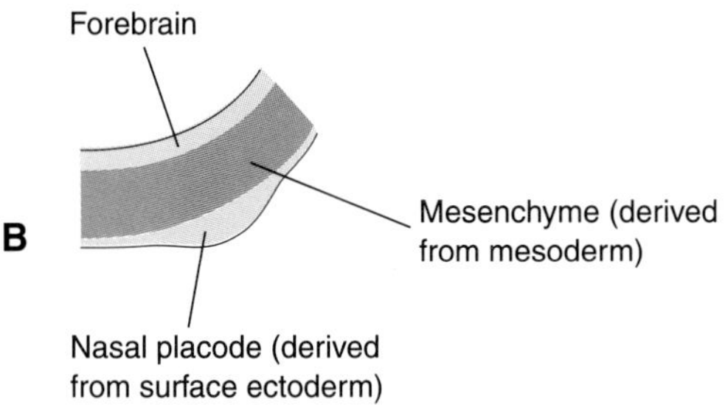

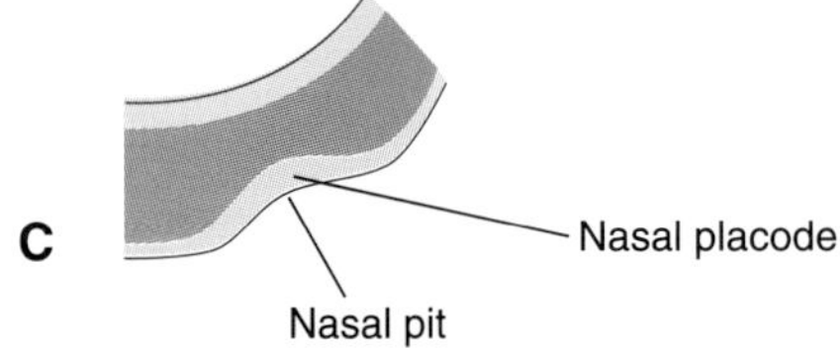

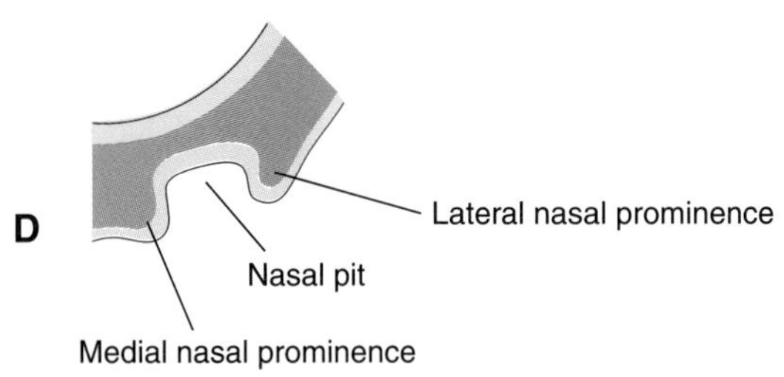

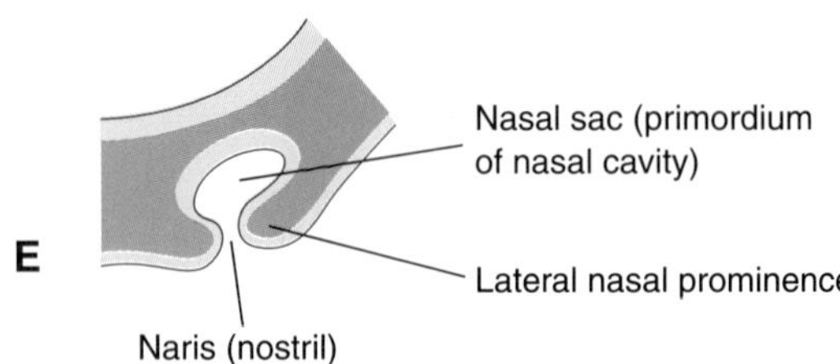

■ **Figure 10-29.** Progressive stages in the development of a human nasal sac (future nasal cavity). *A*, Ventral view of embryo of about 28 days. *B* to *E*, transverse sections through the left side of the developing nasal sac.

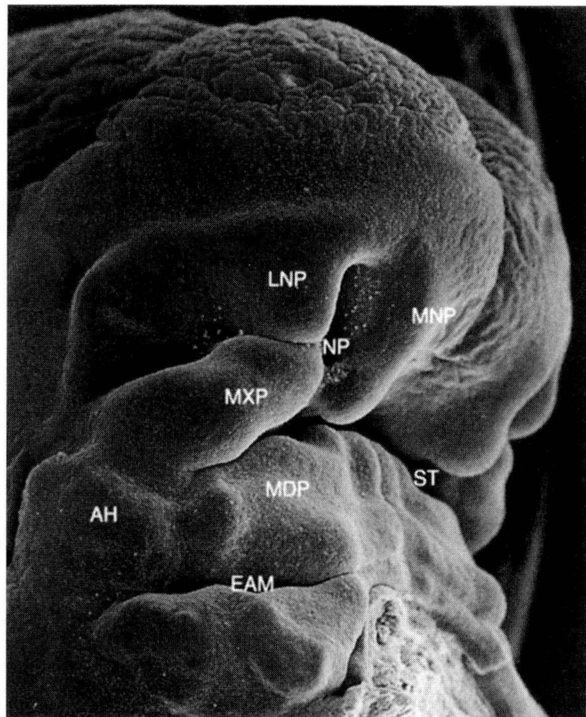

■ **Figure 10–30.** Scanning electron micrograph of the craniofacial region of a human embryo of about 41 days (stage 16, crown-rump length [CRL] 10.8 mm) viewed obliquely. The maxillary prominence (MXP) appears puffed up laterally and wedged between the lateral (LNP) and medial (MNP) nasal prominences surrounding the nasal pit (NP). The auricular hillocks (AH) can be seen on both sides of the pharyngeal groove between the 1st (mandibular) and 2nd (hyoid) arches, which will form the external acoustic meatus (EAM). (ST, stomodeum; MDP, mandibular prominence.) (From Hinrichsen K: The early development of morphology and patterns of the face in the human embryo. *Adv Anat Embryol Cell Biol 98*:1–79, 1985.)

cord that separates from the ectoderm and sinks into the mesenchyme. Later, as a result of cell degeneration, this epithelial cord canalizes to form the nasolacrimal duct. The cranial end of this duct expands to form the **lacrimal sac**. By the late fetal period, the nasolacrimal duct drains into the inferior meatus in the lateral wall of the nasal cavity (Moore, 1992). The duct usually becomes completely patent only after birth. Part of the nasolacrimal duct occasionally fails to canalize, resulting in a congenital anomaly—*atresia of the nasolacrimal duct*. (For more details, see Ogawa and Gonnering, 1991.) Obstruction of the nasolacrimal duct with clinical symptoms occurs in about 6% of newborn infants.

During the seventh week there is a shift in the blood supply of the face from the internal to the external carotid artery (Sperber, 1993). This change is related to transformation of the primordial aortic arch pattern into the postnatal arterial arrangement. Between the seventh and tenth weeks, the medial nasal prominences merge with each other and with the maxillary and lateral nasal prominences (Fig. 10-26*H* and *G*). Merging of these prominences requires disintegration of their contacting surface epithelia. This results in intermingling of the underlying mesenchymal cells. Merging of the medial nasal and maxillary prominences results in continuity of the upper jaw and lip and separation of the nasal pits from the stomodeum.

As the medial nasal prominences merge, they form an intermaxillary segment (Figs. 10-26*H* and 10-33*E* and *F*). The **intermaxillary segment** gives rise to:

- the middle part or philtrum of the upper lip
- the premaxillary part of the maxilla and its associated gingiva (gum)
- the primary palate

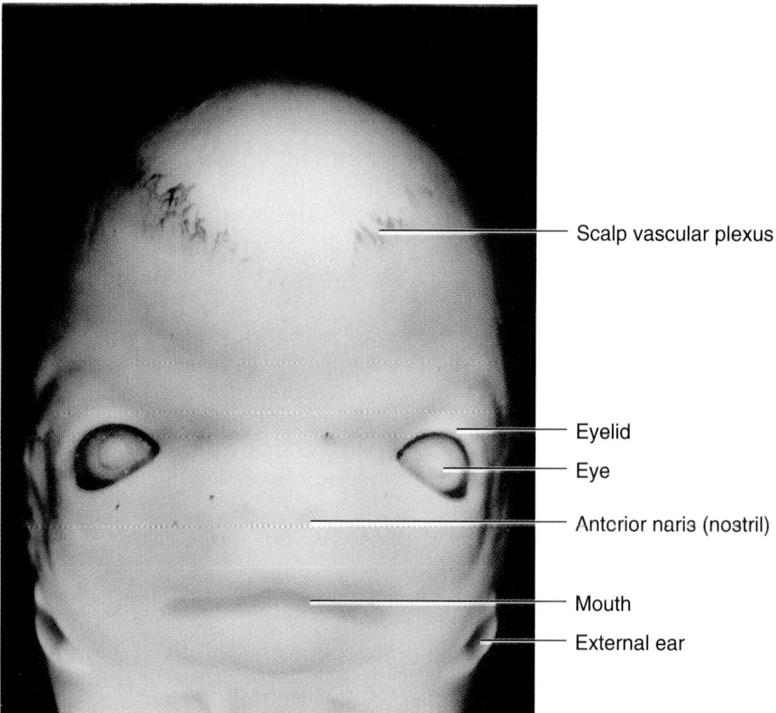

■ **Figure 10–31.** Ventral view of the face of an embryo at Carnegie stage 22, about 54 days. Observe that the eyes are widely separated and the ears low-set at this stage. (From Nishimura H et al: *Prenatal Development of the Human With Special Reference to Craniofacial Structures: An Atlas.* Bethesda, US Department of Health, Education, and Welfare, NIH, 1977.)

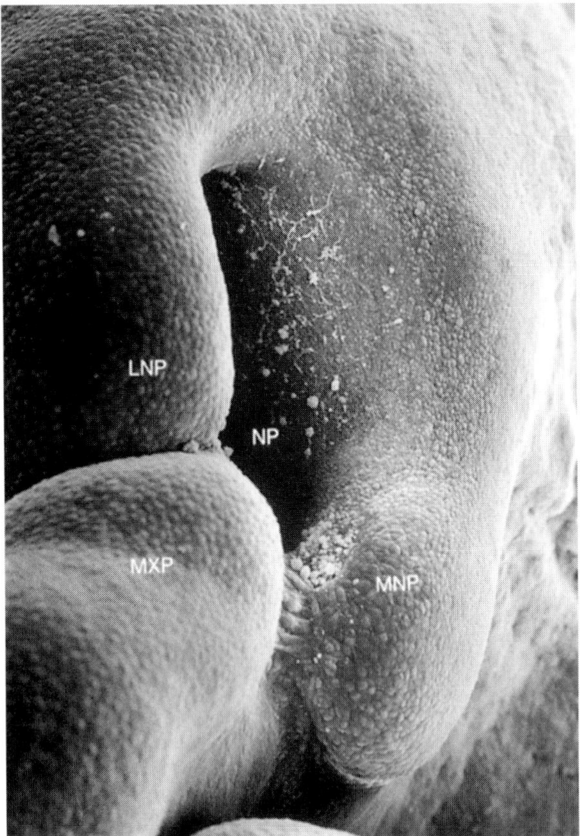

■ **Figure 10–32.** Scanning electron micrograph of the right nasal region of a human embryo of about 41 days (stage 17, crown-rump length [CRL] 10.8 mm) showing the maxillary prominence (MXP) fusing with the medial nasal prominence (MNP). Observe the large nasal pit (NP). Epithelial bridges can be seen between these prominences. Observe the furrow representing the nasolacrimal groove between the MXP and the lateral nasal prominence (LNP). (From Hinrichsen K: The early development of morphology and patterns of the face in the human embryo. *Adv Anat Embryol Cell Biol 98*:1–79, 1985.)

Lateral parts of the upper lip, most of the maxilla, and the secondary palate form from the maxillary prominences (Fig. 10-26*H*). These prominences merge laterally with the mandibular prominences. The primitive lips and cheeks are invaded by mesenchyme from the second pair of pharyngeal arches, which differentiates into the facial muscles (Fig. 10-6; Table 10-1). These *muscles of facial expression* are supplied by the facial nerve (CN VII), the nerve of the second arch. The mesenchyme in the first pair of arches differentiates into the *muscles of mastication* and a few others, all of which are innervated by the trigeminal nerves (CN V), which supply the first pair of arches.

Summary of facial development (Fig. 10-26):

- The FNP forms the forehead and the dorsum and apex of the nose.
- The lateral nasal prominences form the sides (alae) of the nose.
- The medial nasal prominences form the nasal septum.
- The maxillary prominences form the upper cheek regions and most of the upper lip.
- The mandibular prominences give rise to the chin, lower lip, and lower cheek regions.

In addition to these fleshy derivatives, various bones are derived from the mesenchyme in the facial prominences. Until the end of the sixth week the primitive jaws are composed of masses of mesenchymal tissue. The lips and *gingivae* (gums) begin to develop when a linear thickening of the ectoderm, the *labiogingival lamina*, grows into the underlying mesenchyme (see Fig. 10-37*B*). Gradually, most of the lamina degenerates, leaving a *labiogingival groove* between the lips and the gingivae (see Fig. 10-37*H*). A small area of the labiogingival lamina persists in the median plane to form the *frenulum of the upper lip*, which attaches the lip to the gingiva.

Final development of the face occurs slowly during the fetal period and results mainly from changes in the proportion and relative positions of the facial components. During the early fetal period the nose is flat and the mandible is underdeveloped (Fig. 10-26*H*); they obtain their characteristic form as facial development is completed (Fig. 10-26*I*). As the brain enlarges, a prominent forehead is created and the eyes move medially. As the mandible and head enlarge, the auricles of the external ears rise to the level of the eyes.

The smallness of the face prenatally results from:

- the rudimentary upper and lower jaws
- the unerupted primary teeth
- the small size of the nasal cavities and maxillary sinuses (Sandham and Nelson, 1985; Vermeij-Keers, 1990)

DEVELOPMENT OF THE NASAL CAVITIES

As the face develops, the *nasal placodes* become depressed, forming *nasal pits* (Figs. 10-28, 10-29, and 10-32). Proliferation of the surrounding mesenchyme forms the medial and lateral **nasal prominences**, which results in deepening of the nasal pits and formation of **primordial nasal sacs**. Each nasal sac grows dorsally, ventral to the developing forebrain (Fig. 10-34*A*). At first the nasal sacs are separated from the oral cavity by the **oronasal membrane.** This membrane ruptures by the end of the sixth week bringing the nasal and oral cavities into communication (Fig. 10-34*C*). A temporary epithelial plug is formed in the nasal cavity from proliferation of the cells lining it. Between 13 to 15 weeks the nasal plug disappears following its resorption (Nishimura, 1993). The regions of continuity between the nasal and oral cavities are the **primordial choanae**, which lie posterior to the primary palate. After the *secondary palate* develops, the choanae are located at the junction of the nasal cavity and pharynx (Fig. 10-34*D*). While these changes are occurring, the *superior, middle, and inferior* **conchae** develop as elevations of the lateral walls of the nasal cavities (Fig. 10-34*D*). Concurrently the ectodermal epithelium in the roof of each nasal cavity becomes specialized to form the **olfactory epithelium**. Some epithelial cells differentiate into *olfactory receptor cells* (neurons). The axons of these cells constitute the **olfactory nerves**, which grow into the *olfactory bulbs* of the brain (Fig. 10-34*C* and *D*).

The Paranasal Sinuses

Some paranasal (air) sinuses begin to develop during late fetal life, such as the **maxillary sinuses;** the remainder of them develop after birth. They form from outgrowths or diverticula of the walls of the nasal cavities and become pneumatic (air-filled) extensions of the nasal cavities in the adjacent bones, such as the maxillary sinuses in the maxillae and the frontal sinuses in the frontal bones. The original openings of the diverticula persist as the orifices of the adult sinuses.

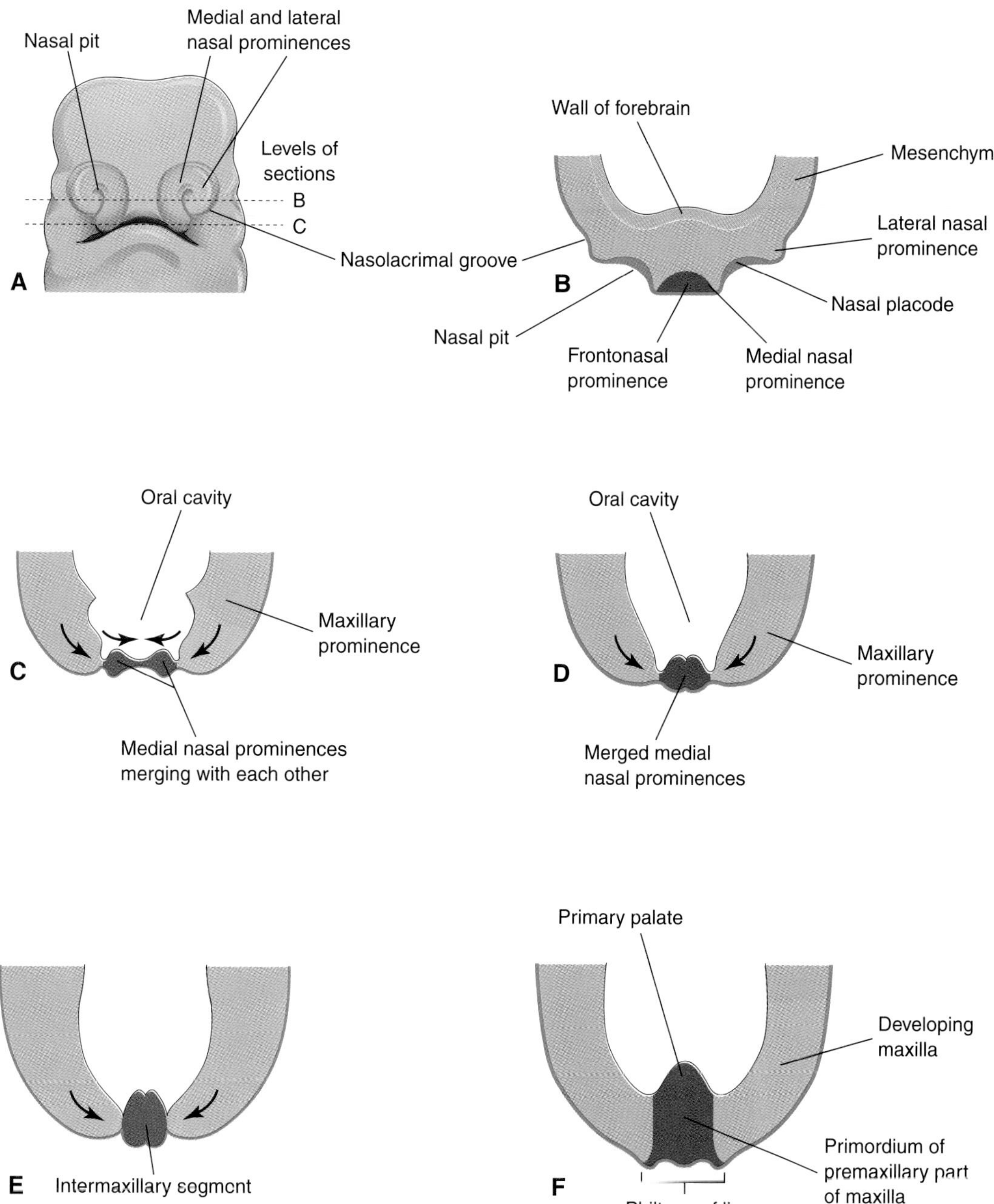

■ **Figure 10-33.** Diagrams illustrating early development of the maxilla, palate, and upper lip. *A,* Facial view of a 5-week embryo. *B* and *C,* Sketches of horizontal sections at the levels shown in *A*. The arrows in *C* indicate subsequent growth of the maxillary and medial nasal prominences toward the median plane and merging of the prominences with each other. *D* to *F,* Similar sections of older embryos illustrating merging of the medial nasal prominences with each other and the maxillary prominences to form the upper lip.

Paranasal Sinuses in the Newborn and Postnatal Development

Most of the paranasal sinuses are rudimentary or absent in newborn infants. The **maxillary sinuses** are small at birth (3 to 4 mm in diameter). These sinuses grow slowly until puberty and are not fully developed until all the permanent teeth have erupted in early adulthood. *No frontal or sphenoidal sinuses are present at birth.* The ethmoidal cells (sinuses) are small before the age of 2 years and they do not begin to grow rapidly until 6 to 8 years of age. Around the age of 2 years, the two most anterior ethmoidal cells grow into the frontal bone, forming a frontal sinus on each side. Usually the **frontal sinuses** are visible in radiographs by the seventh year. The two most posterior ethmoidal cells grow into the sphenoid bone at about the age of 2 years, forming two **sphenoidal sinuses**. Growth of the paranasal sinuses is important in altering the size and shape of the face during infancy and childhood, and in adding resonance to the voice during adolescence.

From the sixth to the eighth weeks, the nasal epithelium invaginates the nasal septum, just superior to the primitive palate, to form bilateral diverticula—the *vomeronasal organs* (of Jacobson). These vestigial chemosensory structures form blind pouches that reach their greatest development by the twenty-fifth week (Fig. 10-35). A *vomeronasal cartilage* develops ventral to each of these organs. The vomeronasal organs are lined by neurosensory epithelium similar to the olfactory epithelium. A vomeronasal nerve projects to a small accessory olfactory bulb. During late fetal life the vomeronasal organs begin to regress and usually disappear along with their nerves and accessory bulbs. The *vomeronasal cartilages* are usually the only adult remnants of these vestigial organs. These narrow strips of cartilage are located between the inferior edge of the cartilage of the nasal septum and the vomer (Moore, 1992).

Remnants of Vomeronasal Organs

Remnants of one or both vomeronasal organs may give rise to cysts that present wide orifices opening into the nasal vestibule on each side of the nasal septum. The remnants usually remain undetected and asymptomatic; however, in some cases they have been linked with various pathological conditions (Gabriele, 1967). Although *atavistic remnants* in humans, the vomeronasal organs are well developed in other mammals and are olfactory chemoreceptor organs that aid the sense of smell (Bhatnagar, 1991).

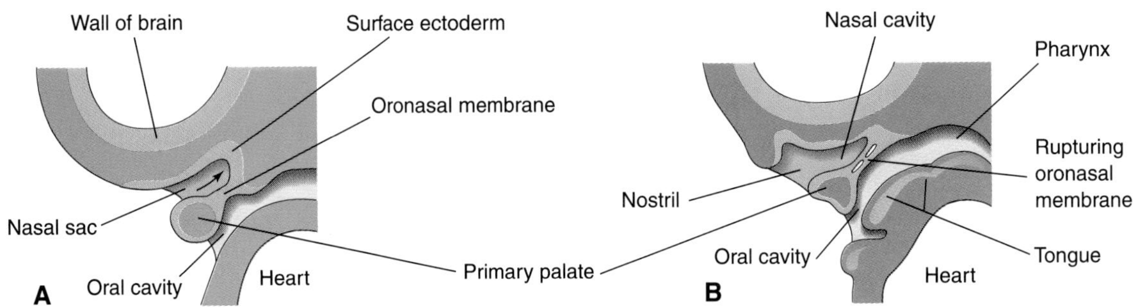

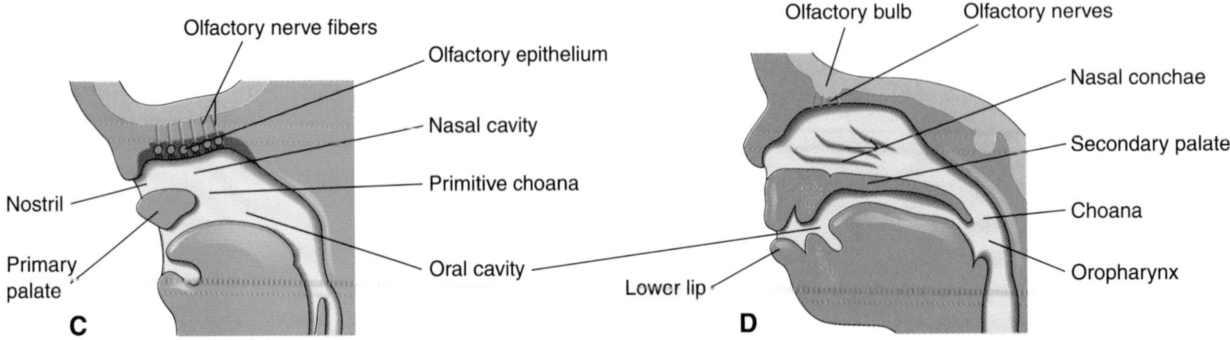

■ **Figure 10-34.** Drawings of sagittal sections of the head showing development of the nasal cavities. The nasal septum has been removed. *A,* 5 weeks. *B,* 6 weeks, showing breakdown of the oronasal membrane. *C,* 7 weeks, showing the nasal cavity communicating with the oral cavity and development of the olfactory epithelium. *D,* 12 weeks, showing the palate and the lateral wall of the nasal cavity.

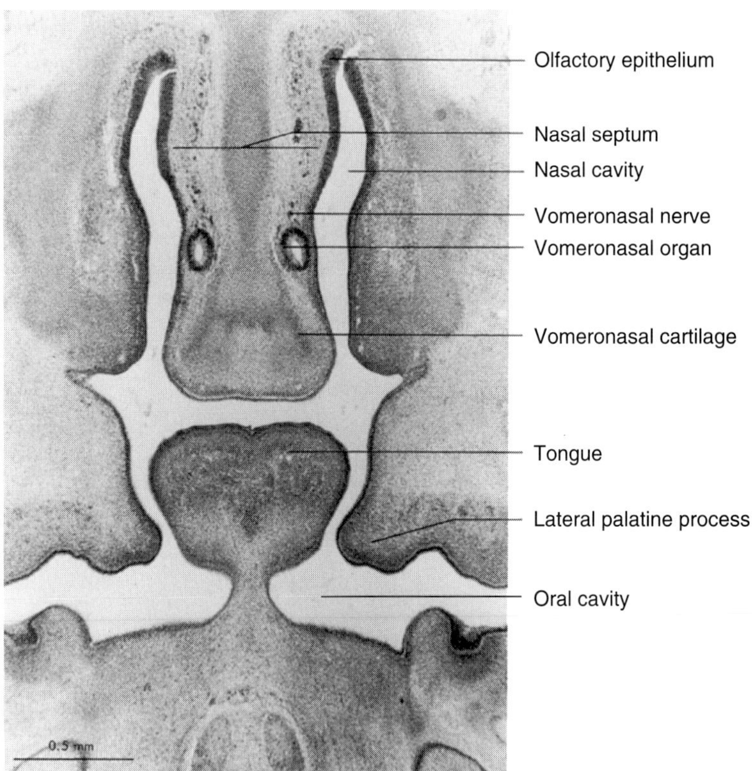

■ **Figure 10–35.** Photomicrograph of a frontal section through the developing mouth and nasal regions of a 22-mm human embryo of about 54 days. (Courtesy of Dr. Kunwar Bhatnagar, Professor of Anatomy, School of Medicine, University of Louisville, Louisville, Kentucky.)

DEVELOPMENT OF THE PALATE

The palate develops from two primordia:

- the primary palate
- the secondary palate

Palatogenesis begins at the end of the fifth week; however, development of the palate is not completed until the twelfth week. The *most critical period of development of the palate* is from the end of the sixth week until the beginning of the ninth week.

The Primary Palate

Early in the sixth week the primary palate — **median palatine process** — begins to develop from the deep part of the *intermaxillary segment of the maxilla* (Figs. 10-33*F* and 10-34). Initially this segment, formed by merging of the medial nasal prominences, is a wedge-shaped mass of mesenchyme between the internal surfaces of the maxillary prominences of the developing maxillae. The primary palate forms the *premaxillary part of the maxilla* (Fig. 10-36). It repre-

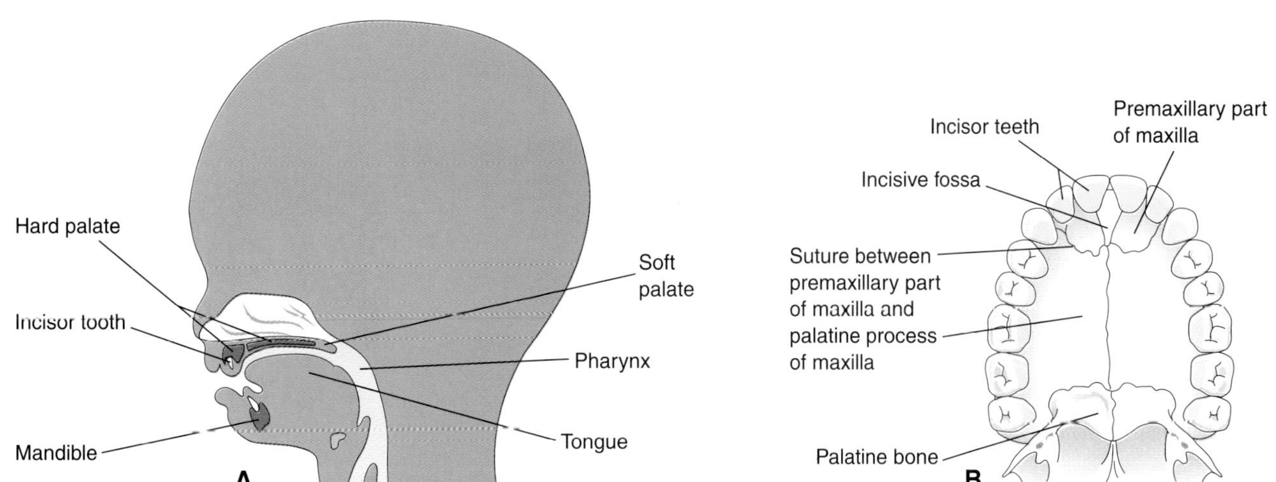

■ **Figure 10–36.** *A,* Drawing of a sagittal section of the head of 20-week fetus illustrating the location of the palate. *B,* The bony palate and alveolar arch of a young adult. The suture between the premaxillary part of the maxilla and the fused palatine processes of the maxillae is usually visible in skulls of young persons. It is not visible in the hard palates of most dried skulls because they are usually from old adults.

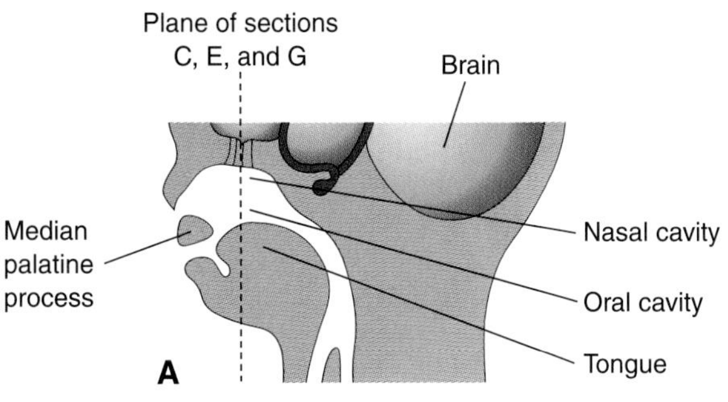

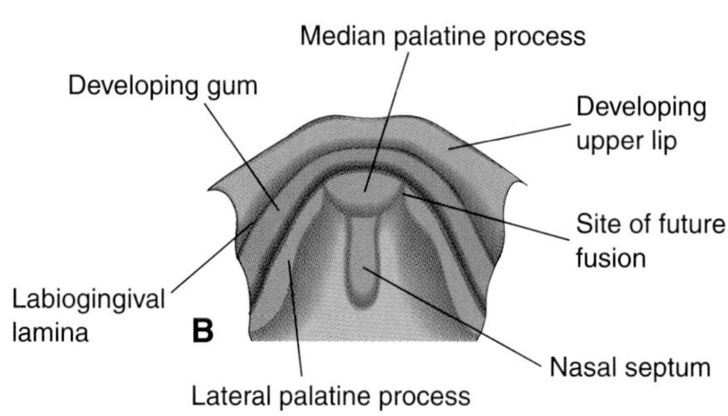

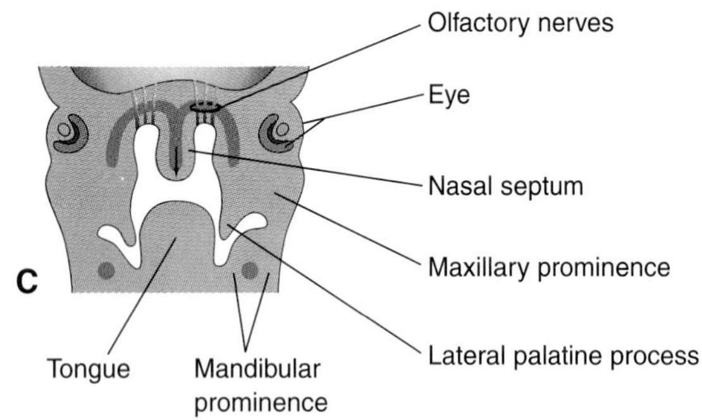

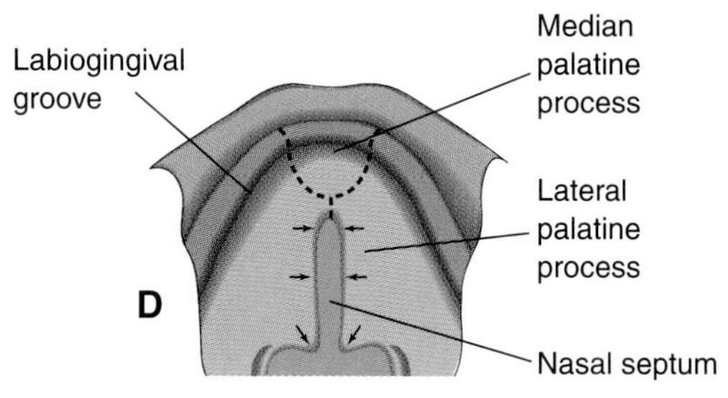

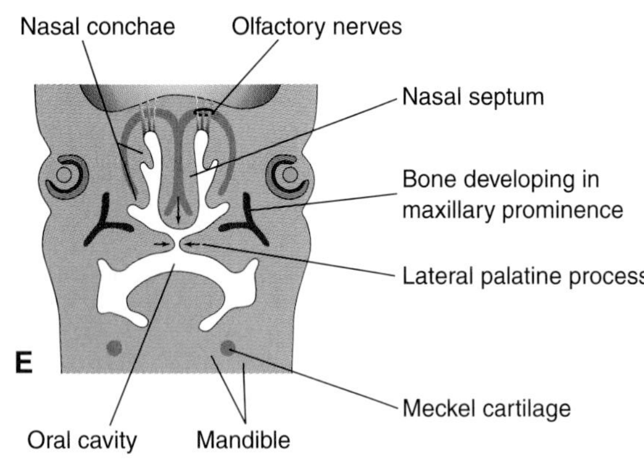

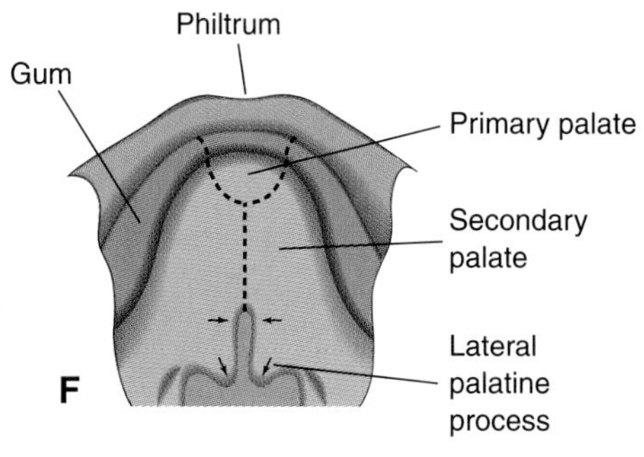

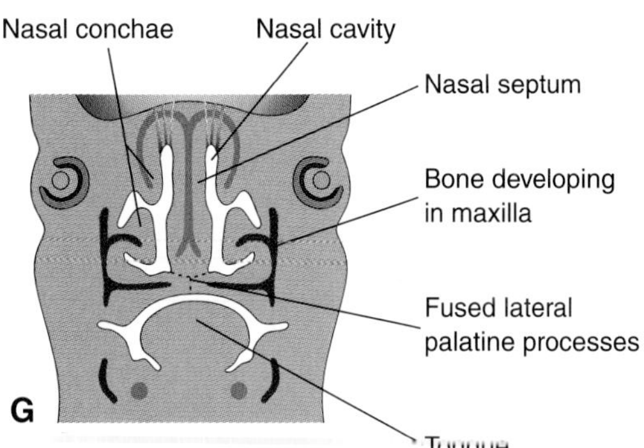

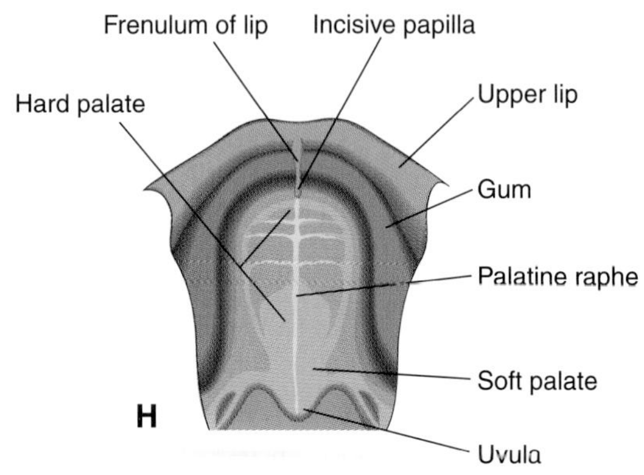

■ **Figure 10–37.** *A,* Sketch of a sagittal section of the embryonic head at the end of the sixth week showing the median palatine process or primary palate. *B, D, F,* and *H,* Drawings of the roof of the mouth from the sixth to twelfth weeks illustrating development of the palate. The broken lines in *D* and *F* indicate sites of fusion of the palatine processes. The arrows indicate medial and posterior growth of the lateral palatine processes. *C, E,* and *G,* Drawings of frontal sections of the head illustrating fusion of the lateral palatine processes with each other and the nasal septum, and separation of the nasal and oral cavities.

sents only a small part of the adult hard palate (i.e., anterior to the incisive fossa).

The Secondary Palate

The secondary palate is the primordium of the hard and soft parts of the palate that extend posteriorly from the incisive fossa (Fig. 10-36). The secondary palate begins to develop early in the sixth week from two mesenchymal projections that extend from the internal aspects of the maxillary prominences. Initially these structures — the **lateral palatine processes** or palatal shelves — project inferomedially on each side of the tongue (Figs. 10-37*B* and 10-38*A* and *B*). As the jaws develop, the tongue becomes relatively smaller and moves inferiorly. During the seventh and eighth weeks, the lateral palatine processes elongate and ascend to a horizontal position superior to the tongue (Sandham, 1985a and c). Gradually the processes (shelves) approach each other and fuse in the median plane (Figs. 10-37*E* to *H* and 10-38*C*). They also fuse with the nasal septum and the posterior part of the primary palate. Elevation of the palatal processes or shelves to the horizontal position is believed to be caused by an intrinsic *shelf elevating force* that is generated by the hydration of hyaluronic acid in the mesenchymal cells within the palatal processes (Ferguson, 1988).

The **nasal septum** develops as a downgrowth from internal parts of the merged medial nasal prominences (Figs. 10-37 and 10-38). The fusion between the nasal septum and the palatine processes begins anteriorly during the ninth week and is completed posteriorly by the twelfth week, superior to the primordium of the hard palate.

Bone gradually develops in the primary palate, forming the premaxillary part of the maxilla, which lodges the incisor teeth (Fig. 10-36*B*). Concurrently, bone extends from the maxillae and palatine bones into the lateral palatine processes (palatal shelves) to form the **hard palate** (Fig. 10-37*E* and *G*). The posterior parts of these processes do not become ossified. They extend posteriorly beyond the nasal septum and fuse to form the **soft palate**, including its soft conical projection — the **uvula** (Fig. 10-37*D*, *F*, and *H*). The *median palatine raphe* indicates the line of fusion of the lateral palatine processes.

A small **nasopalatine canal** persists in the median plane of the palate between the premaxillary part of the maxilla and the palatine processes of the maxillae. This canal is represented in the adult hard palate by the **incisive fossa** (Fig. 10-36*B*), which is the common opening for the small right and left *incisive canals* (Moore, 1992). An irregular suture runs from the incisive fossa to the alveolar process of the maxilla, between the lateral incisor and canine teeth on each side (Fig. 10-36*B*). It is visible in the anterior region of the palates of young persons. This suture indicates where the embryonic primary and secondary palates fused.

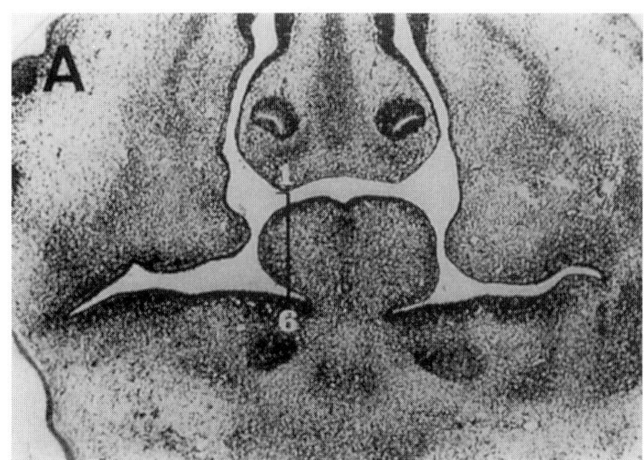

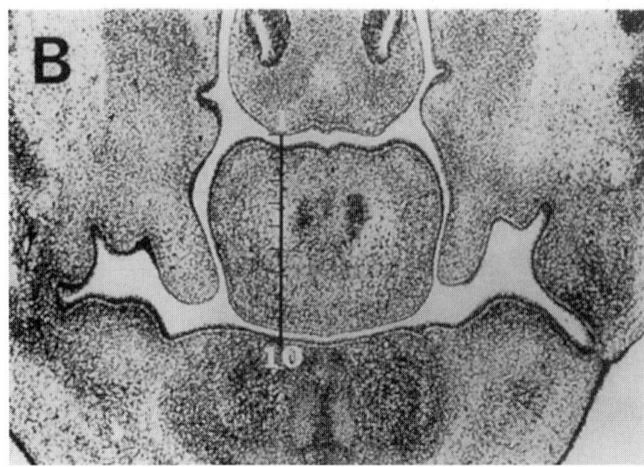

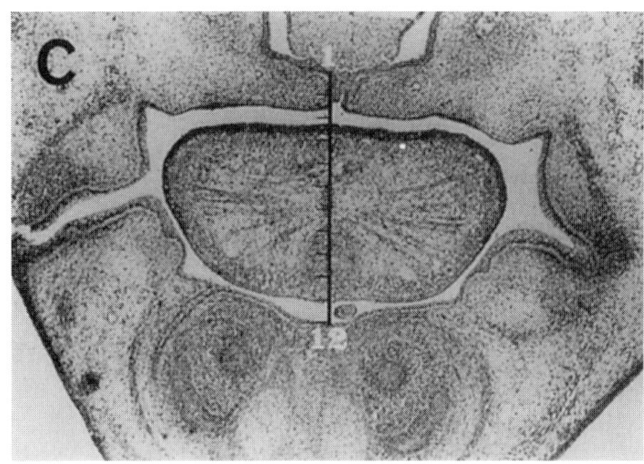

■ **Figure 10-38.** Coronal sections of human embryonic heads showing palatal process (shelf) development during the eighth week. *A,* Embryo with a crown-rump length (CRL) of 24 mm. This section shows early development of the palatine processes. The scale shows 6 units from the lowest point of the nasal septum to the floor of the oral cavity. *B,* Embryo with a CRL of 27 mm. This section shows the palate just prior to palatal process elevation. The scale shows 10 units from the lowest point of the nasal septum to the floor of the oral cavity. *C,* Embryo with a CRL of 29 mm (near the end of the eighth week). The palatine processes are elevated and fused. The scale shows 12 units from the lowest point of the nasal septum to the floor of the oral cavity. (From Sandham A: Embryonic facial vertical dimension and its relationship to palatal shelf elevation. *Early Hum Dev 12:*241, 1985).

Cleft Lip and Palate

Clefts of the upper lip and palate are common (Thompson et al., 1991; Behrman et al., 1996). The defects are usually classified according to developmental criteria, with the incisive fossa as a reference landmark. Cleft lip and palate are especially conspicuous because they result in an abnormal facial appearance and defective speech. There are *two major groups of cleft lip and palate* (Figs. 10-39 to 10-41):

- clefts involving the upper lip and anterior part of the maxilla, with or without involvement of parts of the remaining hard and soft regions of the palate
- clefts involving the hard and soft regions of the palate

Anterior cleft anomalies include cleft lip, with or without cleft of the alveolar part of the maxilla. A complete anterior cleft anomaly is one in which the cleft extends through the lip and the alveolar part of the maxilla to the incisive fossa, separating the anterior and posterior parts of the palate (Fig. 10-40*E* and *F*). Anterior cleft anomalies result from a deficiency of mesenchyme in the maxillary prominence(s) and the intermaxillary segment (Fig. 10-33*E*).

Posterior cleft anomalies include clefts of the secondary or posterior palate that extend through the soft and hard regions of the palate to the incisive fossa, separating the anterior and posterior parts of the palate (Fig. 10-40*G* and *H*). Posterior cleft anomalies are caused by defective development of the secondary palate and result from growth distortions of the lateral palatine processes, which prevent their medial migration and fusion.

Clefts involving the upper lip, with or without cleft palate, occur about once in 1000 births; however, their frequency varies widely among ethnic groups (Thompson et al., 1991); 60 to 80% of affected infants are males. The clefts vary from small notches of the vermilion border of the lip (Fig. 10-41*B*) to larger ones that extend into the floor of the nostril and through the alveolar part of the maxilla (Figs. 10-39 and 10-41*A*, *C*, and *D*). Cleft lip can be unilateral or bilateral.

Unilateral cleft lip (Figs. 10-39, 10-41*A*, and 10-42) results from failure of the maxillary prominence on the affected side to unite with the merged medial nasal prominences. This is the consequence of failure of the mesenchymal masses to merge and the mesenchyme to proliferate and smooth out the overlying epithelium. This results in a *persistent labial groove* (Fig. 10-43*D*). In addition the epithelium in the labial groove becomes stretched and the tissues in the floor of the persistent groove break down. As a result, the lip is divided into medial and lateral parts (Fig. 10-43*G* and *H*). Sometimes a bridge of tissue, a **Simonart band**, joins the parts of the incomplete cleft lip (Fig. 10-41*B*).

Bilateral cleft lip (Figs. 10-41*C* and *D* and 10-44*B*) results from failure of the mesenchymal masses in the maxillary prominences to meet and unite with the merged medial nasal prominences. The epithelium in both labial grooves becomes stretched and breaks down. In bilateral cases the defects may be dissimilar, with varying degrees of defect on each side. When there is a complete bilateral cleft of the lip and alveolar part of the maxilla, the intermaxillary segment hangs free and projects anteriorly. These defects are especially deforming because of the loss of continuity of the *orbicularis oris muscle*, which closes the mouth and purses the lips as occurs when whistling (Moore, 1992).

Median cleft of the upper lip is an extremely rare defect (see Fig. 10-45*A*). It results from a mesenchymal deficiency, which causes partial or complete failure of the medial nasal prominences to merge and form the intermaxillary segment. A median cleft of the lip is a characteristic feature of the *Mohr syndrome*, which is transmitted as an autosomal recessive trait (Gorlin et al., 1990). **Median cleft of the lower lip** is also very rare and is caused by failure of the mesenchymal masses in the mandibular prominences to merge completely and smooth out the embryonic cleft between them (Fig. 10-26*A*).

A **complete cleft palate** indicates the maximum degree of clefting of any particular type; for example, a *complete cleft of the posterior palate* is an anomaly in which the cleft extends through the soft palate and anteriorly to the incisive fossa. The landmark for distinguishing anterior from posterior cleft anomalies is the *incisive fossa*. Anterior and posterior cleft anomalies are embryologically distinct.

Cleft palate, with or without cleft lip, occurs about once in 2500 births and is more common in females than in males. The cleft may involve only the uvula, giving it a fishtail appearance (Fig. 10-40*B*), or it may extend through the soft and hard regions of the palate (Figs. 10-40*C* and *D* and 10-44*C* and *D*). In severe cases associated with cleft lip, the cleft in the palate

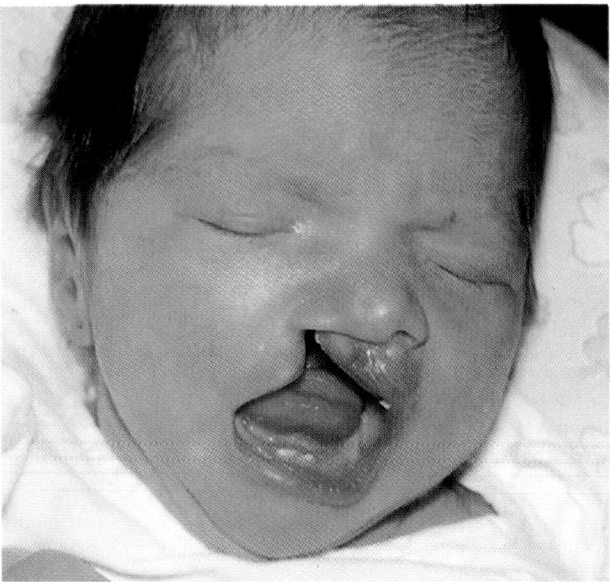

■ **Figure 10-39.** Infant with unilateral cleft lip and palate. Clefts of the lip, with or without cleft palate, occur about once in 1000 births; 60 to 80% of affected infants are males. (Courtesy of Dr. AE Chudley, Professor of Pediatrics and Child Health, Children's Hospital and University of Manitoba, Winnipeg, Manitoba, Canada.)

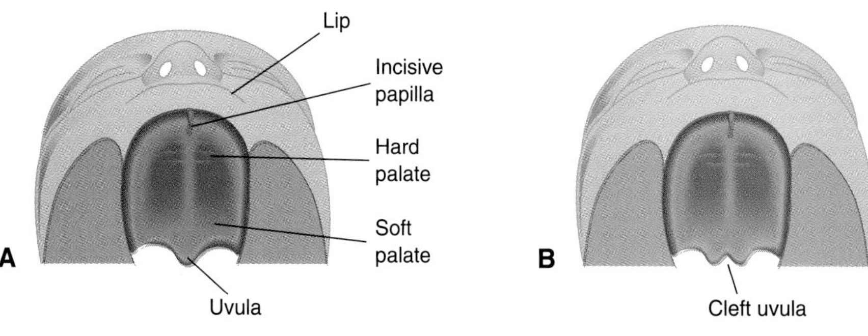

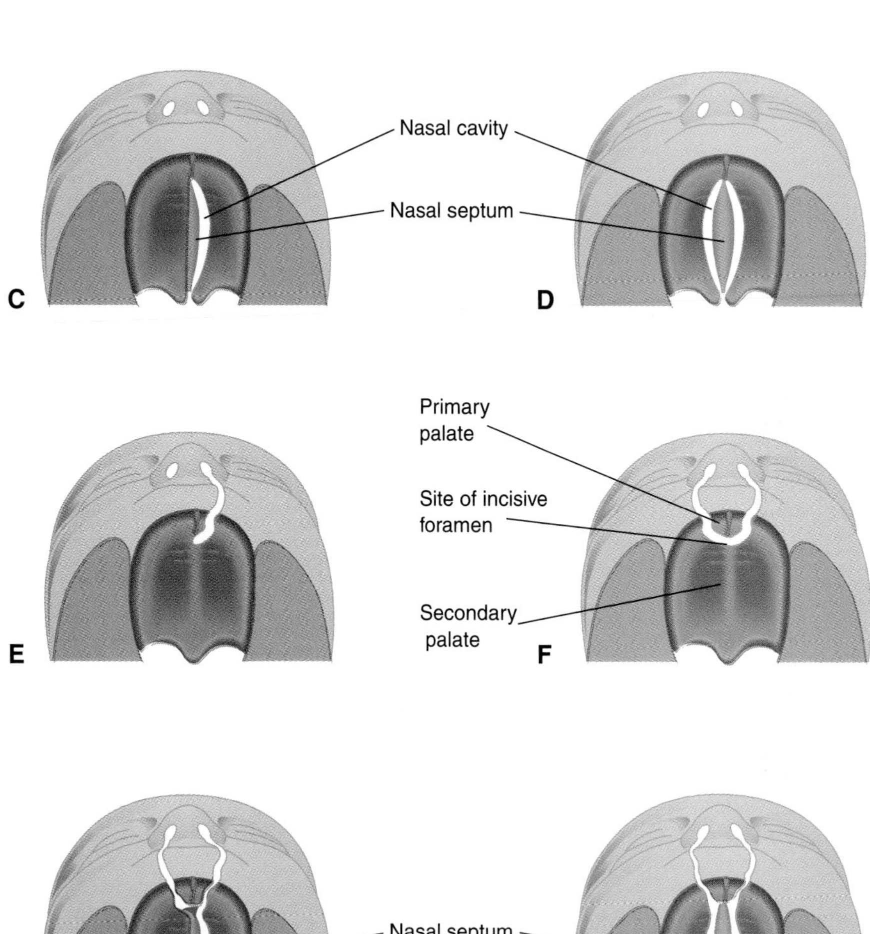

■ **Figure 10–40.** Drawings illustrating various types of cleft lip and palate. *A,* Normal lip and palate. *B,* Cleft uvula. *C,* Unilateral cleft of the posterior or secondary palate. *D,* Bilateral cleft of the posterior palate. *E,* Complete unilateral cleft of the lip and alveolar process of the maxilla with a unilateral cleft of the anterior or primary palate. *F,* Complete bilateral cleft of the lip and alveolar processes of the maxillae with bilateral cleft of the anterior palate. *G,* Complete bilateral cleft of the lip and alveolar processes of the maxillae with bilateral cleft of the anterior palate and unilateral cleft of the posterior palate. *H,* Complete bilateral cleft of the lip and alveolar processes of the maxillae with complete bilateral cleft of the anterior and posterior palate.

extends through the alveolar part of the maxilla and the lips on both sides (Figs. 10–40*G* and *H* and 10–44*B*).

The embryological basis of cleft palate is failure of the mesenchymal masses in the lateral palatine processes to meet and fuse with each other, with the nasal septum, and/or with the posterior margin of the median palatine process (Figs. 10–33*D* and 10–40). Unilateral and bilateral clefts in the palate are classified into three groups:

- *Clefts of the anterior (primary) palate* (i.e., clefts anterior to the incisive fossa) result from failure of mesenchymal masses in the lateral palatine processes (palatine shelves) to meet and fuse with the mesenchyme in the primary palate (Fig. 10–40*E* and *F*).
- *Clefts of the posterior (secondary) palate* (i.e., clefts posterior to the incisive fossa) result from failure of mesenchymal masses in the lateral palatine processes to meet and fuse with each other and the nasal septum (Fig. 10–40*B*, C, and *D*).
- *Clefts of the anterior and posterior parts of the palate* (i.e., clefts of the primary and secondary palates) result from failure of the mesenchymal masses in the lateral palatine processes to meet and fuse with mesenchyme in the primary palate,

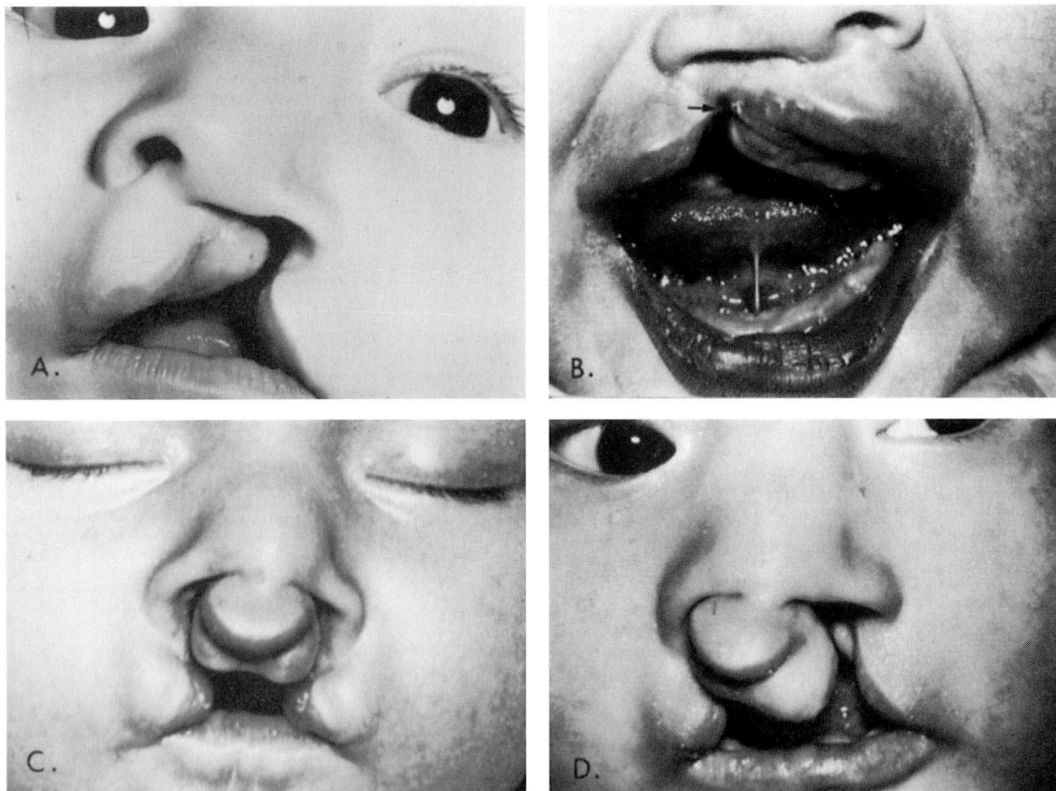

■ **Figure 10–41.** Photographs illustrating various types of cleft lip. *A* and *B,* Unilateral cleft lip. The cleft in *B* is incomplete; the arrow indicates a band of tissue (Simonart band) connecting the cleft parts of the lip. *C* and *D,* Bilateral cleft lip. (Courtesy of Dr. D. A. Kernahan, The Children's Memorial Hospital, Chicago.)

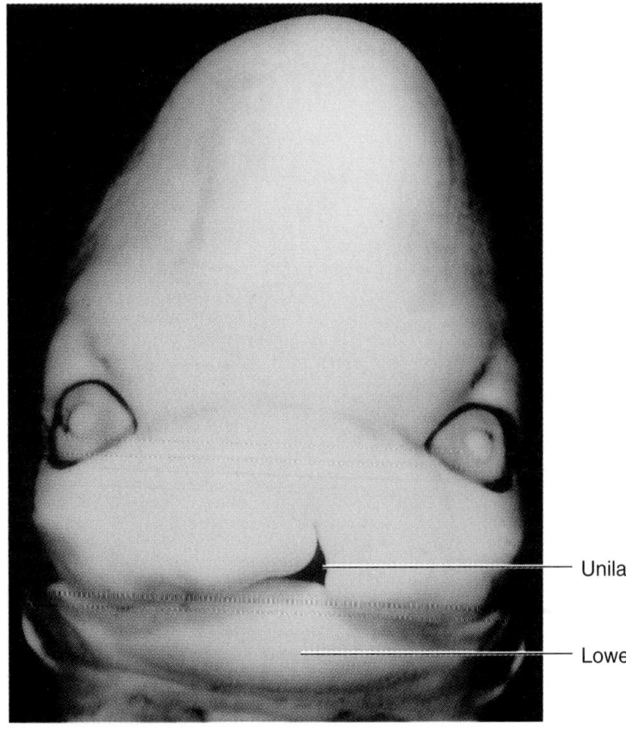

■ **Figure 10–42.** Ventral view of the face of an embryo at Carnegie stage 20 (about 51 days) with a unilateral cleft lip. (From Nishimura H et al: *Prenatal Development of the Human With Special Reference to Craniofacial Structures: An Atlas.* Bethesda, US Department of Health, Education, and Welfare, NIH, 1977.)

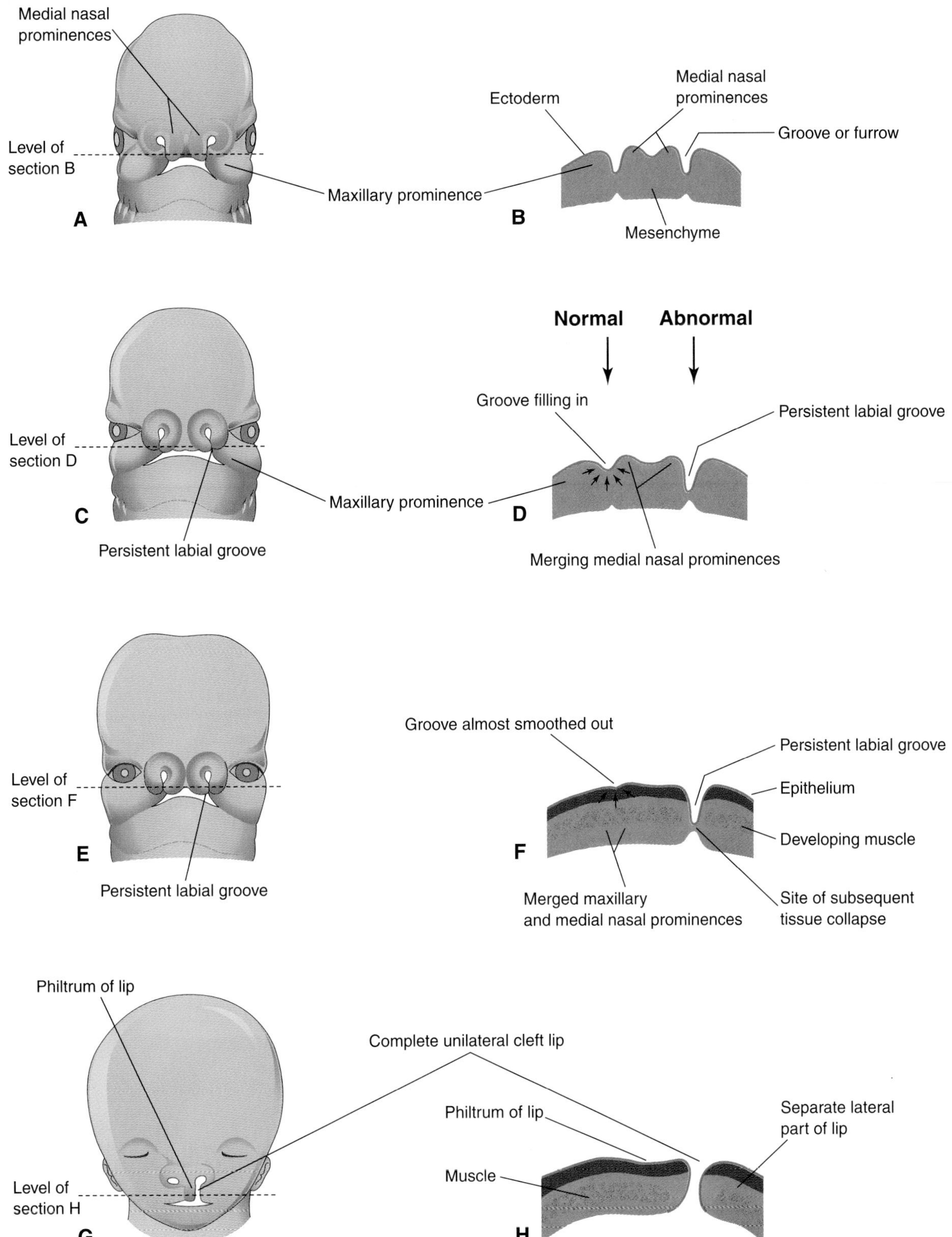

■ **Figure 10–43.** Drawings illustrating the embryological basis of complete unilateral cleft lip. *A,* 5-week embryo. *B,* Horizontal section through the head illustrating the grooves between the maxillary prominences and the merging medial nasal prominences. *C,* 6-week embryo showing a persistent labial groove on the left side. *D,* Horizontal section through the head showing the groove gradually filling in on the right side following proliferation of mesenchyme *(arrows). E,* Seven-week embryo. *F,* Horizontal section through the head showing that the epithelium on the right has almost been pushed out of the groove between the maxillary and medial nasal prominences. *G,* 10-week fetus with a complete unilateral cleft lip. *H,* Horizontal section through the head after stretching of the epithelium and breakdown of the tissues in the floor of the persistent labial groove on the left side, forming a complete unilateral cleft lip.

with each other, and the nasal septum (Fig. 10-40*G* and *H*).

Most clefts of the lip and palate result from multiple factors (**multifactorial inheritance**; see Chapter 8): genetic and nongenetic, each causing a minor developmental disturbance (Vanderas, 1987; Niermeyer and Van der Meulen, 1990; Thompson et al., 1991; Behrman et al., 1996). How teratogenic factors induce cleft lip and palate is still unknown. Experimental studies have given us some insight into the cellular and molecular basis of these defects (Greene, 1989; Schubert et al., 1990; Sulik, 1996). Based on experimental findings and limited clinical experience, it has been suggested that vitamin B complex given prophylactically to pregnant women who are at risk for cleft lip and palate might decrease the occurrence of facial clefting (Schubert et al., 1990).

Some clefts of the lip and/or palate appear as part of syndromes determined by single mutant genes (Thompson et al., 1991). Other clefts are parts of chromosomal syndromes, especially **trisomy 13** (see Chapter 8). A few cases of cleft lip and/or palate appear to have been caused by teratogenic agents (e.g., anticonvulsant drugs [Hanson, 1980]). Studies of twins indicate that genetic factors are of more importance in cleft lip, with or without cleft palate, than in cleft palate alone. A sibling of a child with a cleft palate has an elevated risk of having a cleft palate, but no increased risk of having a cleft lip. A cleft of the lip and alveolar process of the maxilla that continues through the palate is usually transmitted through a male sex-linked gene. When neither parent is affected, the *recurrence risk* in subsequent siblings (brother or sister) is about 4%. For further discussion of recurrence risks, see Thompson et al. (1991). The fact that the palatine processes fuse about a week later in females may explain why isolated cleft palate is more common in females than in males.

Facial Clefts

Various types of facial cleft may occur but they are all extremely rare. Severe clefts are usually associated with gross anomalies of the head. ***Oblique facial clefts*** (orbitofacial fissures) are often bilateral and extend from the upper lip to the medial margin of the orbit (Fig. 10-45*C*). When this occurs the nasolacrimal ducts are open grooves (persistent nasolacrimal grooves). Oblique facial clefts associated with cleft lip result from failure of the mesenchymal masses in the maxillary prominences to merge with the lateral and medial nasal prominences. Lateral or transverse facial clefts run from the mouth toward the ear. Bilateral clefts result in a very large mouth, a condition called *macrostomia* (Fig. 10-45*D*). In severe cases the clefts in the cheeks extend almost to the ears.

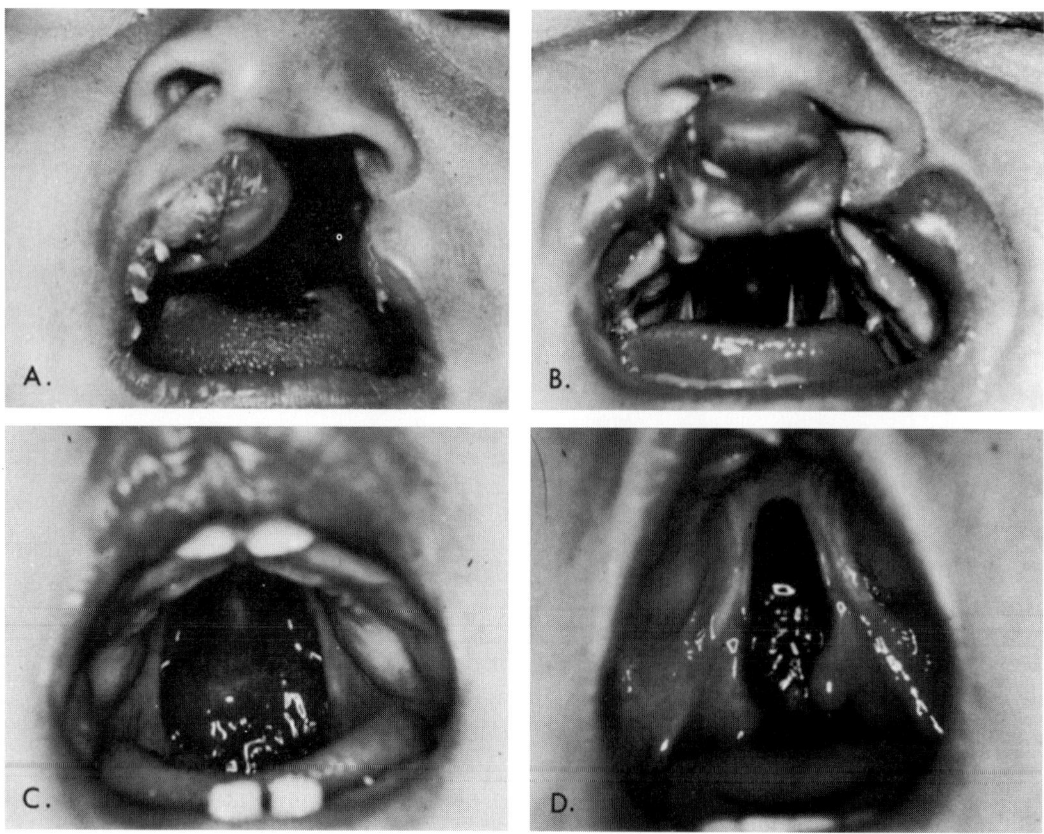

■ **Figure 10-44.** Photographs illustrating congenital anomalies of the lip and palate. *A,* Complete unilateral cleft of the lip and alveolar process. *B,* Complete bilateral cleft of the lip and alveolar process with bilateral cleft of the anterior palate. *C* and *D,* Bilateral cleft of the posterior or secondary palate; the lip is normal.

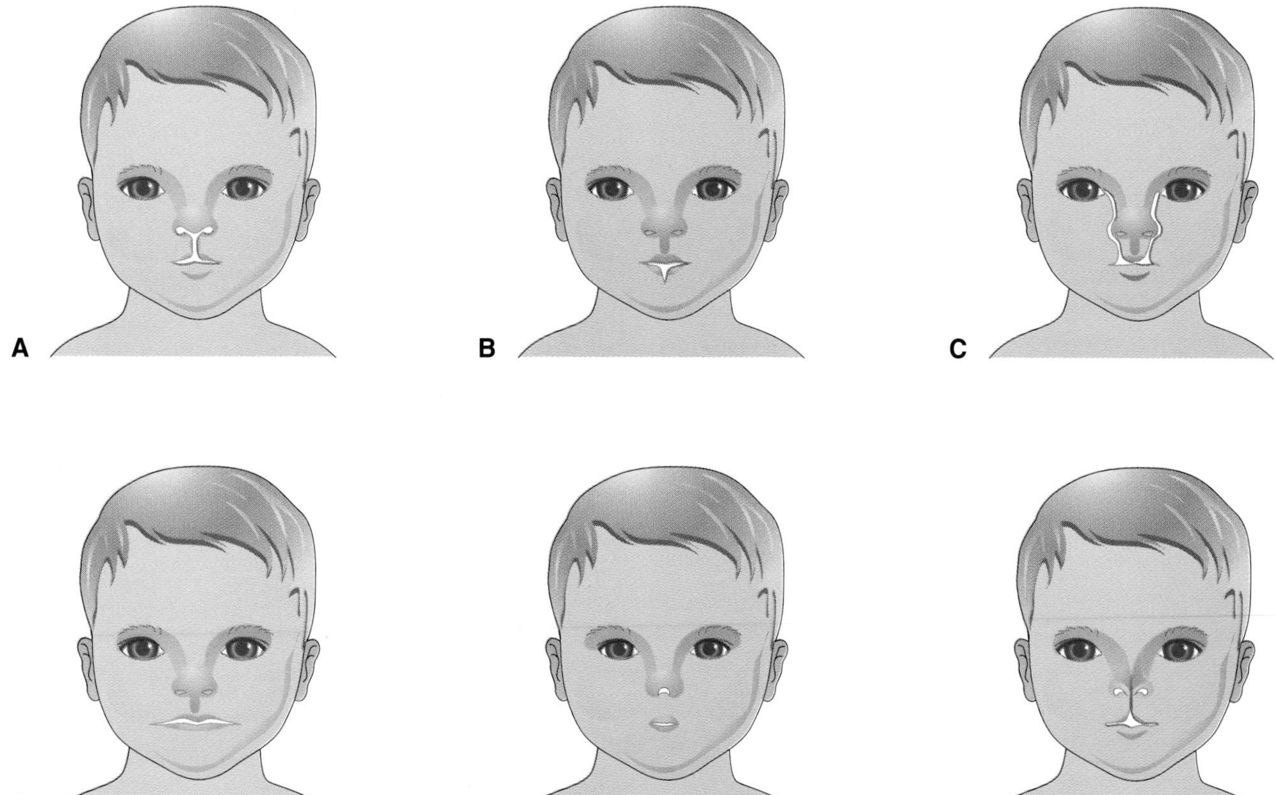

■ **Figure 10–45.** Drawings of unusual congenital anomalies of the face. *A,* Median cleft of the upper lip. *B,* Median cleft of the lower lip. *C,* Bilateral oblique facial clefts with complete bilateral cleft lip. *D,* Macrostomia. *E,* Single nostril and microstomia; these anomalies are not usually associated. *F,* Bifid nose and incomplete median cleft lip.

Other Facial Anomalies

Congenital *microstomia* (small mouth) results from excessive merging of the mesenchymal masses in the maxillary and mandibular prominences of the first arch (Fig. 10-45*E*). In severe cases the abnormality may be associated with underdevelopment (hypoplasia) of the mandible. *Absence of the nose* occurs when no nasal placodes form. A *single nostril* results when only one nasal placode forms (Fig. 10-45*E*). *Bifid nose* results when the medial nasal prominences do not merge completely; the nostrils are widely separated and the nasal bridge is bifid (Fig. 10-45*F*). In mild forms of bifid nose, there is a groove in the tip of the nose.

By the beginning of the second trimester (Fig. 10-26*I*), features of the fetal face can be identified sonographically. Using this imaging technique (Fig. 10-46), fetal facial anomalies are readily recognizable (Benacerraf, 1994).

SUMMARY OF THE PHARYNGEAL APPARATUS

During the fourth and fifth weeks the primitive pharynx is bounded laterally by **pharyngeal arches**. Each arch consists of a core of mesenchyme covered externally by ectoderm and internally by endoderm. The original mesenchyme of each arch is derived from mesoderm; later, **neural crest cells** migrate into the arches and are the major source of their connective tissue components, including cartilage, bone, and ligaments in the oral and facial regions. Each pharyngeal arch contains an artery, a cartilage rod, a nerve, and a muscular component. Externally the pharyngeal arches are separated by **pharyngeal grooves** (clefts). Internally the arches are separated by evaginations of the pharynx—**pharyngeal pouches**. Where the ectoderm of a groove contacts the endoderm of a pouch, **pharyngeal membranes** are formed. The arches, pouches, grooves, and membranes make up the pharyngeal apparatus. Development of the tongue, face, lips, jaws, palate, pharynx, and neck largely involves transformation of the pharyngeal apparatus into adult structures. The adult derivatives of the various pharyngeal arch components are summarized in Table 10-1 and the derivatives of the pouches are illustrated in Figure 10-8.

The *pharyngeal grooves* disappear except for the first pair, which persists as the *external acoustic meatus*. The pharyngeal membranes also disappear, except for the first pair, which becomes the *tympanic membranes*. The first pharyngeal pouch gives rise to the

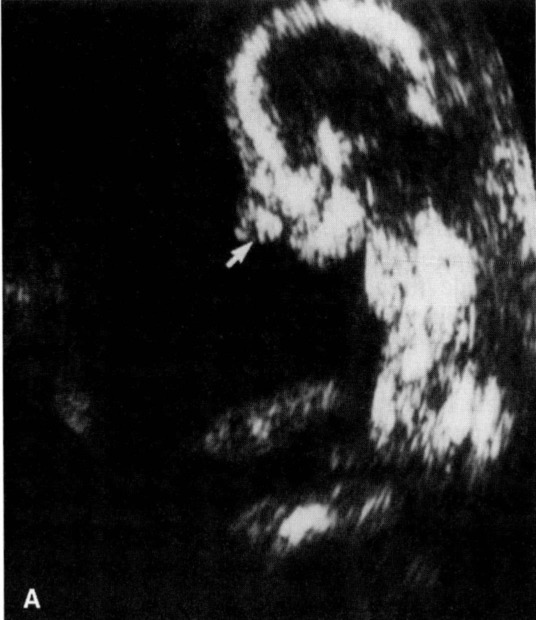

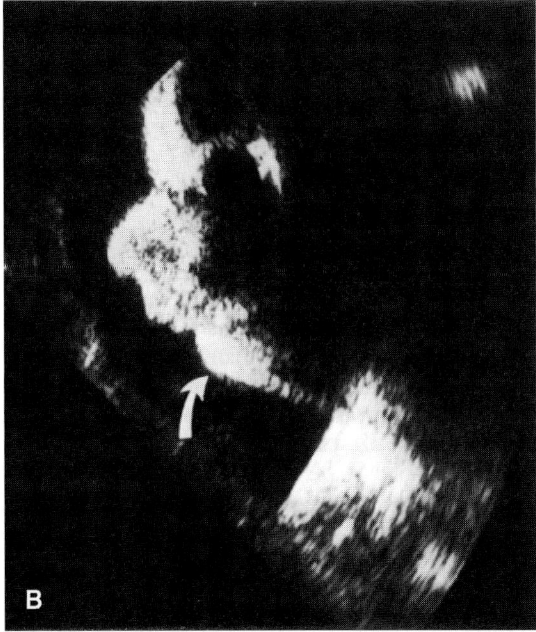

■ **Figure 10–46.** Ultrasound images of the head. *A,* Sagittal view of an early second-trimester fetus with complete bilateral cleft lip and palate showing anterior displacement of the intermaxillary part of the upper lip *(arrow).* (From Benacerraf BR: Ultrasound evaluation of the fetal face. *In* Callen PW [ed]: *Ultrasonography in Obstetrics and Gynecology,* 3rd ed. Philadelphia, WB Saunders, 1994.) *B,* Sagittal view of the profile of a third-trimester fetus with trisomy 13, showing severe micrognathia *(arrow).* (From Benacerraf BR, Miller W, Frigoletto F: Sonographic detection of fetuses with trisomy 13 and 18: Accuracy and limitations. *Am J Obstet Gynecol 158:*404, 1988.)

tympanic cavity, mastoid antrum, and pharyngotympanic tube. The second pharyngeal pouch is associated with the development of the palatine tonsil. The *thymus* is derived from the third pair of pharyngeal pouches, and the *parathyroid glands* are formed from the third and fourth pairs of pharyngeal pouches.

The **thyroid gland** develops from a downgrowth from the floor of the primitive pharynx in the region where the tongue develops. The parafollicular (C) cells in the thyroid gland are derived from the *ultimobranchial bodies*, which are derived mainly from the fourth pair of pharyngeal pouches.

Most congenital anomalies of the head and the neck originate during transformation of the pharyngeal apparatus into adult structures. Branchial cysts, sinuses, and fistulas may develop from parts of the second pharyngeal groove, the cervical sinus, or the second pharyngeal pouch that fail to obliterate.

An *ectopic thyroid gland* results when the thyroid gland fails to descend completely from its site of origin in the tongue. The thyroglossal duct may persist or remnants of it may give rise to *thyroglossal duct cysts and ectopic thyroid tissue masses*. Infected cysts may perforate the skin and form *thyroglossal duct sinuses* that open anteriorly in the median plane of the neck.

Because of the complicated development of the face and palate, congenital anomalies of the face and palate are common. Anomalies result from *maldevelopment of neural crest tissue* that gives rise to the skeletal and connective tissue primordia of the face. Neural crest cells may be deficient in number, may not complete their migration to the face, or they may fail in their inductive capacity. Anomalies of the face and palate result from an arrest of development and/or a failure of fusion of the facial prominences and palatal processes involved.

Cleft lip is a common congenital anomaly. Although frequently associated with cleft palate, *cleft lip and palate are etiologically distinct anomalies* that involve different developmental processes occurring at different times. Cleft lip results from failure of mesenchymal masses in the medial nasal and maxillary prominences to merge, whereas **cleft palate** results from failure of mesenchymal masses in the palatine processes (palatal shelves) to meet and fuse. Most cases of cleft lip, with or without cleft palate, are caused by a combination of genetic and environmental factors (*multifactorial inheritance*). These factors interfere with the migration of *neural crest cells* into the maxillary prominences of the first pharyngeal arch. If the number of cells is insufficient, clefting of the lip and/or palate may occur. Other cellular and molecular mechanisms may be involved.

Clinically Oriented Problems

Case 10–1

The mother of a two-year-old boy consulted her pediatrician about an intermittent discharge of mucoid material from a small opening in the side of his neck. There was also extensive redness and swelling in the inferior third of the neck, just anterior to the sternocleidomastoid muscle.

- What is the most likely diagnosis?
- What is the probable embryological basis of this intermittent mucoid discharge?
- Discuss the etiology of this congenital anomaly.

Case 10–2

During a subtotal thyroidectomy a surgeon could locate only one inferior parathyroid gland.

- Where might the other one be located?
- What is the embryological basis for the ectopic location of this gland?

Case 10–3

A young woman consulted her physician about a swelling in the anterior part of her neck, just inferior to the hyoid bone.

- What kind of a cyst might be present?
- Are they always in the median plane?
- Discuss the embryological basis of these cysts.
- With what might such a swelling be confused?

Case 10–4

A male infant was born with a unilateral cleft lip extending into the floor of his nose and through the alveolar process of his maxilla.

- What is the embryological basis of these anomalies?
- Neither parent had a cleft lip or cleft palate. Are genetic factors likely involved?
- Are these anomalies more common in males?
- What is the chance that the next child will have a cleft lip?

Case 10–5

An epileptic mother who was treated with an anticonvulsant drug during pregnancy gave birth to a child with cleft lip and palate.

- Is there any evidence indicating that these drugs increase the incidence of these anomalies?
- Discuss the respective etiologies of these two birth defects.

Discussion of these problems appears at the back of the book.

REFERENCES AND SUGGESTED READING

Arreola GA, Serna NP, Parra RH, Salinas MGA: Morphogenesis of the lateral nasal wall from 6 to 36 weeks. *Otolaryngol Head Neck Surg 114:*54, 1996.

Behrman RE, Kliegman RM, Arvin AM (eds): *Nelson Textbook of Pediatrics,* 15th ed. Philadelphia, WB Saunders, 1996.

Benacerraf BR: Ultrasound evaluation of the fetal face. *In* Callen PW (ed): *Ultrasonography in Obstetrics and Gynecology,* 3rd ed. Philadelphia, WB Saunders, 1994

Bhatnagar K: Personal communication, University of Louisville, Louisville, Kentucky, 1991.

Bockman DE, Kirby ML: Dependence of thymus development on derivatives of the neural crest. *Science 223:*498, 1984.

Chetty R, Forder MD: Parathyroiditis associated with hyperthyroidism and branchial cysts. *Am J Clin Pathol 96:*348, 1991.

Connor JM, Ferguson-Smith MA: *Essential Medical Genetics,* 2nd ed. Oxford, Blackwell Scientific Publications, 1987.

Cormack DH: *Essential Histology*. Philadelpha, JB Lippincott, 1993.

Cote DN, Giandi GJ: Fourth branchial cleft cysts. *Otolaryngol Head Neck Surg 114:*95, 1996.

Crelin ES: Development of the upper respiratory system. *Clin Symp 28:*3–30, 1976.

Farkas LG, Deutsch CK; Anthropometric determination of craniofacial morphology. *Am J Med Genet 65:*1, 1996.

Ferguson MWJ: Palate development. *Development 103(Suppl):*41, 1988.

Fisher DA, Polk DH: Development of the thyroid. *Bailliere's Clin Endocrin Metabol 3:*627, 1989.

Gabriele OF: Persistent vomeronasal organ. *Am J Roentgenol 99:*697, 1967.

Gartner LP, Hiatt JL: *Color Textbook of Histology*. Philadelphia, WB Saunders, 1997.

Gasser RF, Shigihara S, Shimada K: Three-dimensional development of the facial nerve path through the ear region in human embryos. *Am Otol Rhinol Laryngol 103:*395, 1994.

Gilbert-Barness E (ed): *Potter's Pathology of The Fetus and Infant*. 2 vols. St Louis, Mosby, 1997.

Gorlin RJ, Cohen MM Jr, Levin LS: *Syndromes of the Head and Neck,* 3rd ed. New York, Oxford University Press, 1990.

Graveson AC: Neural crest contributions to the development of the vertebrate head. *Am Zool 33:*424, 1993.

Greene RM: Signal transduction during craniofacial development. *Crit Rev Toxicol 20:*153, 1989.

Hall BK: How is mandibular growth controlled during development and evolution. *J Craniofac Genet Dev Biol 2:*45, 1982.

Hall BK: Mechanisms of craniofacial development. *In* Vig KWL, Burdi AR (eds): *Craniofacial Morphogenesis and Dysmorphogenesis*. Ann Arbor, The University of Michigan, 1988.

Hall BK: Evolutionary aspects of craniofacial structures and development. *Cleft Palate Craniofac J 32:*520, 1995.

Hall BK, Miyake T: Divide, accumulate, differentiate: cell condensation in skeletal development revisited. *Int J Dev Biol 39:*881, 1995.

Hanson JW: Patterns of abnormal human craniofacial development. *In* Pratt RM, Christiansen RL (eds): *Current Research Trends in Prenatal Craniofacial Development*. New York, Elsevier North-Holland, 1980.

Hayden GD, Arnold GG: The ear. *In* Kendig EL, Jr, Chernick V (eds): *Disorders of the Respiratory Tract in Children,* 4th ed. Philadelphia, WB Saunders, 1983.

Hinrichsen K: The early development of morphology and patterns of the face in the human embryo. *Adv Anat Embryol Cell Biol 98:*1–79, 1985.

Jaffee BF: The branchial arches. *In* Ferguson CF, Kendig EL Jr (eds): *Disorders of the Respiratory Tract in Children,* Vol II: *Pediatric Otolaryngology,* 2nd ed. Philadelphia, WB Saunders, 1972.

Johnson IJM, Smith I, Akintunde MO, et al: Assessment of pre-operative investigations of thyroglossal cysts. *J R Coll Surg Edinb 41:*48, 1996.

Jones KL: *Smith's Recognizable Patterns of Human Malformation,* 5th ed. Philadelphia, WB Saunders, 1997.

Källén B, Harris J, Robert E: The epidemiology of orofacial clefts. 2 associated malformations. *J Craniofac Genet Dev Biol 16:*242, 1996.

Karmody CS: Autosomal dominant first and second arch syndrome. *In* Bergsma D (ed): *Malformation Syndromes,* vol 10. New York, International Medical Book Corp, 1974.

Kendall MD: Functional anatomy of the thymic microenvironment. *J Anat 177:*1, 1991.

Kirby MF, Bockman DE: Neural crest and normal development: a new perspective. *Anat Rec 209:*1, 1984.

Koppe T, Yamamoto T, Tanaka O, Nagai H: Investigations on the growth pattern of the maxillary sinus in Japanese human fetuses. *Okajmas Folia Anat Jpn 71:*311, 1994.

Kuratani S, Aizawa S: Patterning of the cranial nerves in the chick embryo is dependent on cranial mesoderm and rhombomeric metamerism. *Develop Growth Differ 37:*717, 1995.

Leung AKC, Wong AL, Robson WLLM: Ectopic thyroid gland simulating a thyroglossal duct cyst: a case report. *Can J Surg 38:*87, 1995.

Martins AG: Lateral cervical sinus and pre-auricular sinuses. *Br Med J 5*:255, 1961.

McKenzie J: The first arch syndrome. *Dev Med Child Neurol 8*:55, 1966.

Melsen B: Palatal growth studies on human autopsy material. *Am J Orthod 68*:42, 1975.

Miculan J, Turner S, Paes BA: Congenital hypothyroidism: diagnosis and management. *Neonatal Netw 12*:25, 1993.

Miyake T, Cameron AM, Hall BK: Stage-specific onset of condensation and matrix deposition for Meckel's and first arch cartilages in inbred C57BL/6 mice. *J Craniofac Dev Biol 16*:32, 1996.

Miyauchi A, Matsuzuka F, Kima K, Katayama S: Piriform sinus fistula and the ultimobrachial body. *Histopathology 20*:227, 1992.

Moore KL: *Clinically Oriented Anatomy,* 3rd ed. Baltimore, Williams & Wilkins, 1992.

Morris HL, Bardach J: Cleft lip and palate and related disorders: issues for future research of high priority. *Cleft Palate J 26*:141, 1989.

Müller TS, Ebensperger C, Neubüser A, et al: Expression of avian *Pax* 1 and *Pax* 9 is intrinsically regulated in the pharyngeal endoderm, but depends on environmental influences in the paraxial mesoderm. *Dev Biol 178*:403, 1996.

Niermeyer MF, Van der Meulen JC: Genetics of craniofacial malformation. *In* Stricker M, Van der Meulen JC, Raphael B, Mazzola R (eds): *Craniofacial Malformations*. Edinburgh, Churchill Livingstone, 1990.

Nishimura Y: Embryological study of nasal cavity development in human embryos with reference to congenital nostril atresia. *Acta Anat 147*:140, 1993.

Noden DM: Interactions and fates of avian craniofacial mesenchyme. *Development 103(Suppl)*:121, 1988.

Noden DM: Cell movements and control of patterned tissue assembly during craniofacial development. *J Craniofac Genet Dev Biol 11*:192, 1991.

Noden DM: Vertebrate craniofacial development:novel approaches and new dilemmas. *Curr Opin Genet Dev 2*:576, 1992.

Ogawa GSH, Gonnering RS: Congenital nasolacrimal duct obstruction. *J Pediatr 119*:12, 1991.

Ohta Y, Suwa F, Yang L, et al: Development and histology of fibrous architecture of the fetal temporomandibular joint. *Okajimas Folia Anat Jpn 70*:1, 1993.

Pleifer G (ed): *Craniofacial Abnormalities and Clefts of the Lip, Alveolus and Palate*. New York, Greorg Thieme Verlag, 1991.

Poswillo D: The aetiology and pathogenesis of craniofacial deformity. *Development 103(Suppl)*:213, 1988.

Raffensperger JG (ed): *Swenson's Pediatric Surgery,* 5th ed. Philadelphia, WB Saunders, 1990.

Robert E, Källén B, Harris J: The epidemiology of orofacial clefts. I. Some general epidemiological characteristics. *J Craniofac Genet Dev Biol 16*:234, 1996.

Ross RB, Johnston MC: *Cleft Lip and Palate*. Baltimore, Williams & Wilkins, 1972.

Sandham A: Embryonic head posture and palatal shelf elevation. *Early Hum Dev 11*:69, 1985a.

Sandham A: Classification of clefting deformity. *Early Hum Dev 12*: 81, 1985b.

Sandham A: Embryonic facial vertical dimension and its relationship to palatal shelf elevation. *Early Hum Dev 12*:241, 1985c.

Sandham A, Nelson R: Embryology of the middle third of the face. *Early Hum Dev 10*:313, 1985.

Sata I, Ishikawa H, Shimada K, et al: Morphology and analysis of the development of the human temporomandibular joint and masticatory muscle. *Acta Anat 149*:55, 1994.

Schubert J, Schmidt R, Raupach H-W: New findings explaining the mode of action in prevention of facial clefting and first clinical experience. *J Craniomaxillofac Surg 18*:343, 1990.

Severtson M, Petruzzelli GJ: Macroglossia. *Otolaryngol Head Neck Surg 114*:501, 1996.

Shepard TH: Development of the thyroid gland. *In* Gardner LI (ed): *Endocrine and Genetic Diseases of Childhood and Adolescence,* 2nd ed. Philadelphia, WB Saunders, 1975.

Sheridan MF, Bruns AD, Burgess LPA: Hemiagenesis of the thyroid gland. *Otolaryngol Head Neck Surg 112*:621, 1995.

Sivan E, Chan L, Mallozzi-Eberle A: Sonographic imaging of the fetal face and the establishment of normative dimensions for chin length and upper lip width. *Am J Perinatol 14*:191, 1997.

Sperber GH: *Craniofacial Embryology,* 4th ed. (revised reprint). London, Butterworths, 1993.

Spinner RJ, Moore KL, Gottfried MR, et al: Thoracic intrathymic thyroid. *Ann Surg 220*:91, 1994.

Steinman GG: Changes of the human thymus during ageing. *In* Müller-Hermelink HK (ed): The Human Thymus. Histophysiology and Pathology. *Current Topics in Pathology*. 75:43, 1986.

Stricker M, Raphael B, Van der Meulen J, Mazzola R: Craniofacial growth and development. *In* Stricker M, Van der Meulen JC, Raphael B, Mazzola R (eds): *Craniofacial Malformations.* Edinburgh, Churchill Livingstone, 1990.

Sulik KK: Craniofacial development. *In* Turvey TA, Vig KWL, Fonseca RJ (eds): *Facial Clefts and Craniosynostosis. Principles and Management*. Philadephia, WB Saunders, 1996.

Taeusch HW, Ballard RB, Avery ME (eds): *Schaffer & Avery's Diseases of the Newborn,* 6th ed. Philadelphia, WB Saunders, 1991.

Thompson MW, McInnes RR, Willard HF: *Thompson & Thompson Genetics in Medicine,* 5th ed. Philadelphia, WB Saunders Co, 1991.

Urao M, Teitelbaum DH, Miyano T: Lingual thyroglossal duct cyst: a unique surgical approach. *J Pediatr Surg 31*:1574, 1996.

Vanderas AP: Incidence of cleft lip, cleft palate, and cleft lip and palate among races: a review. *Cleft Palate J 24*:216, 1987.

van der Meulen J, Mozzola B, Stricker M, Raphael B: Classification of craniofacial malformations. *In* Stricker M, Van der Meulen JC, Raphael B, Mazzola R (eds): *Craniofacial Malformations*. Edinburgh, Churchill Livingstone, 1990.

Vermeij-Keers C: Craniofacial embryology and morphogenesis: normal and abnormal. *In* Stricker M, Van der Meulen JC, Raphael B, Mazzola R (eds): *Craniofacial Malformations.* Edinburgh, Churchill Livingstone, 1990.

Warwick R: *Nomina Embryologica,* 3rd ed. Edinburgh, Churchill Livingstone, 1989.

Wedden SE, Ralphs JR, Tickle C: Pattern formation in the facial primordia. *Development 103(suppl)*:31, 1988.

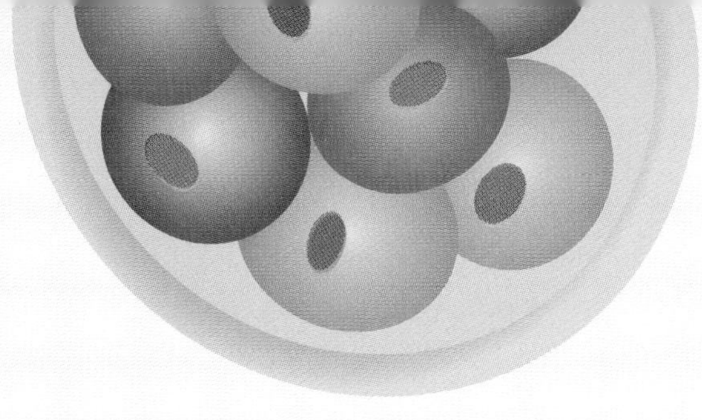
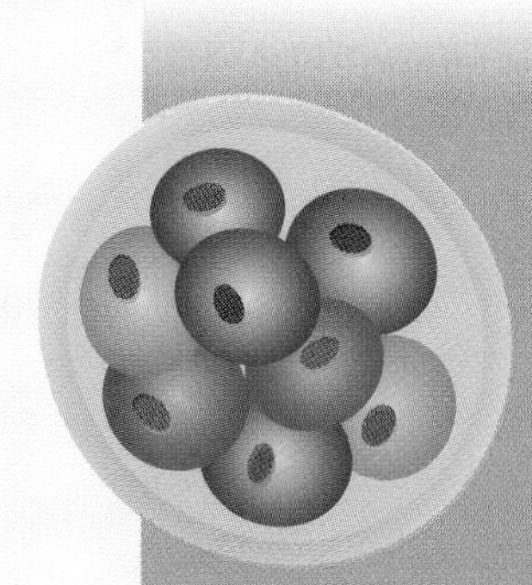

The Respiratory System

11

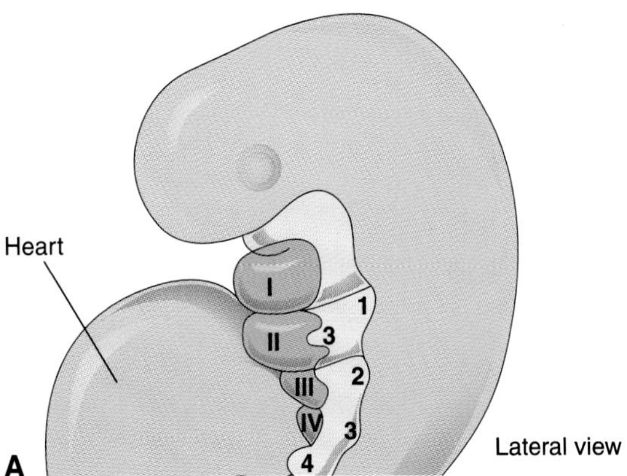

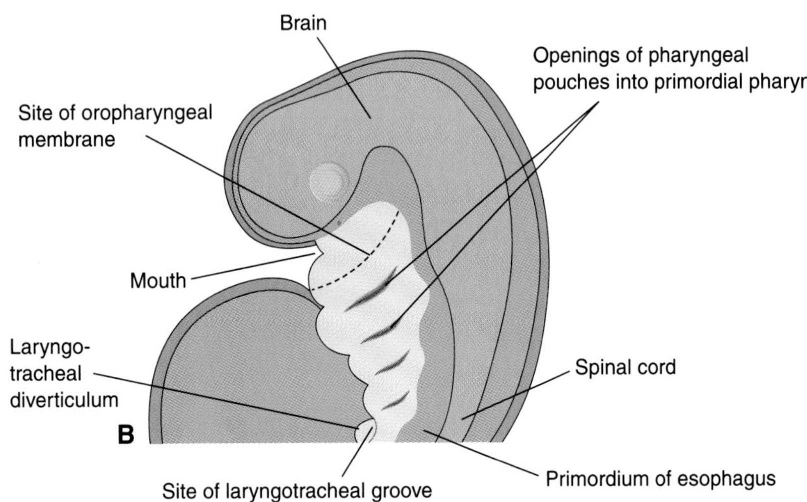

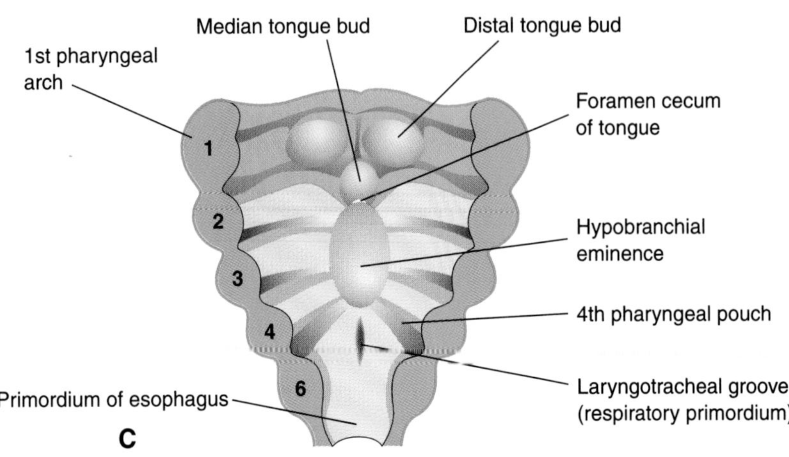

■ **Figure 11–1.** *A*, Drawing of a lateral view of a 4-week-old embryo, illustrating the relationship of the pharyngeal apparatus to the developing respiratory system. *B*, Diagrammatic sagittal section of the cranial half of the embryo. *C*, Horizontal section of the embryo, illustrating the floor of the primordial pharynx and the location of the laryngotracheal groove.

■ Development of the upper respiratory organs — the nasal cavities, for example — is described in Chapter 10. The **lower respiratory organs** (larynx, trachea, bronchi, and lungs) begin to form during the fourth week of development. The **respiratory primordium** is indicated at 26 to 27 days by a median outgrowth from the caudal end of the ventral wall of the primordial pharynx — the **laryngotracheal groove** (Fig. 11-1). This rudiment of the tracheobronchial tree develops caudal to the fourth pair of pharyngeal pouches. The endoderm lining the laryngotracheal groove gives rise to the epithelium and glands of the larynx, trachea, bronchi, and the pulmonary epithelium. The connective tissue, cartilage, and smooth muscle in these structures develop from the splanchnic mesenchyme surrounding the foregut (see Fig. 11-4). By the end of the fourth week, the laryngotracheal groove has evaginated to form a pouchlike **laryngotracheal diverticulum** (respiratory diverticulum), which is located ventral to the caudal part of the foregut (Figs. 11-1*B* and 11-2*A*). As this diverticulum elongates, it is invested with splanchnic mesenchyme and its distal end enlarges to form a globular **lung bud** (Fig. 11-2*B*).

The laryngotracheal diverticulum soon separates from the **primordial pharynx**; however, it maintains communication with it through the *primordial laryngeal inlet* (Fig. 11-2*C*). Longitudinal **tracheoesophageal folds** (ridges) develop in the laryngotracheal diverticulum, approach each other, and fuse to form a partition — the **tracheoesophageal septum** (Fig. 11-2*D* and *E*). This septum divides the cranial part of the foregut into a ventral portion, the **laryngotracheal tube** (primordium of the larynx, trachea, bronchi, and lungs), and a dorsal portion (primordium of the oropharynx and esophagus (Fig. 11-2*F*). The opening of the laryngotracheal tube into the pharynx becomes the **laryngeal inlet** (Figs. 11-2*C* and 11-3*C*).

DEVELOPMENT OF THE LARYNX

The epithelial lining of the larynx develops from the endoderm of the cranial end of the laryngotracheal tube. The cartilages of the larynx develop from the cartilages in the fourth and sixth pairs of pharyngeal arches (see Chapter 10). The laryngeal cartilages develop from mesenchyme that is derived from *neural crest cells.* The mesenchyme at the cranial end of the laryngotracheal tube proliferates rapidly, producing paired **arytenoid swellings** (Fig. 11-3*B*). These swellings grow toward the tongue, converting the slitlike aperture — the *primordial glottis* — into a T-shaped **laryngeal inlet** and reducing the developing laryngeal lumen to a narrow slit. The laryngeal epithelium proliferates rapidly, resulting in *temporary occlusion of the laryngeal lumen.* Recanalization of the larynx occurs by the tenth week. The *laryngeal ventricles* form during this recanalization process. These recesses are bounded by folds of mucous membrane that become the *vocal folds* (cords) and *vestibular folds* (Sañudo and Domenech-Mateu, 1990).

The **epiglottis** develops from the caudal part of the

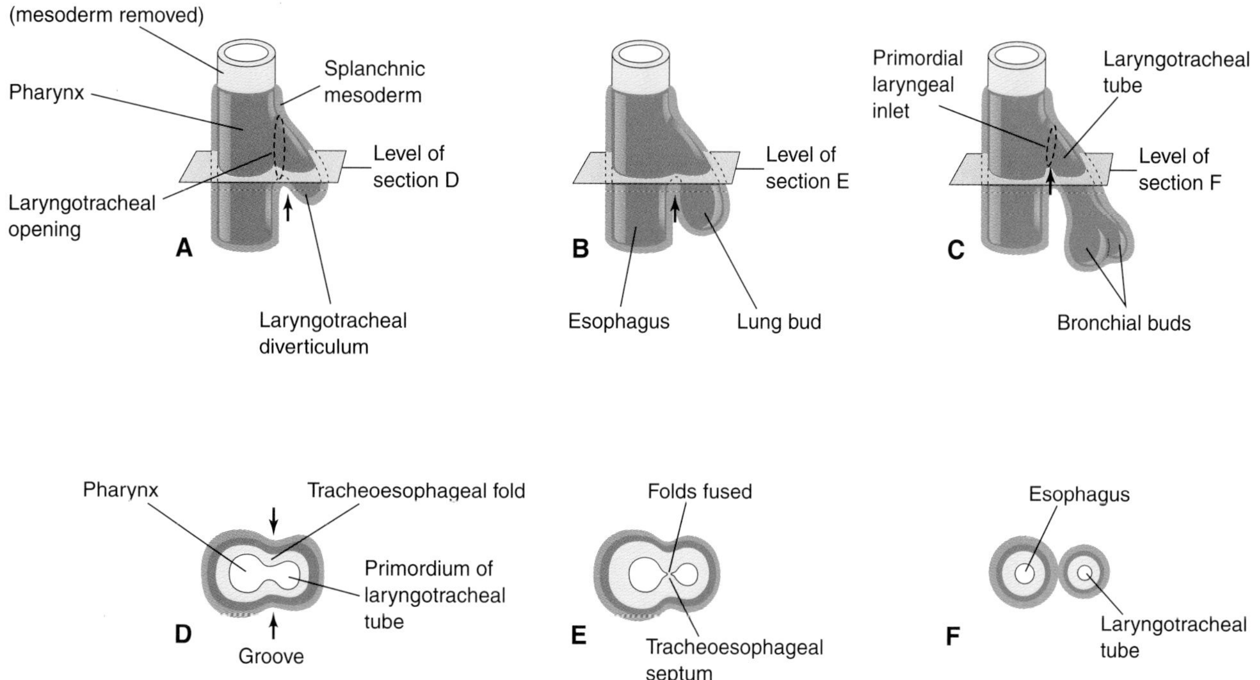

■ **Figure 11–2.** Drawings illustrating successive stages in the development of the tracheoesophageal septum during the fourth and fifth weeks. *A, B,* and *C,* Lateral views of the caudal part of the primordial pharynx showing the laryngotracheal diverticulum and partitioning of the foregut into the esophagus and laryngotracheal tube. *D, E,* and *F,* Transverse sections illustrating formation of the tracheoesophageal septum and showing how it separates the foregut into the laryngotracheal tube and esophagus.

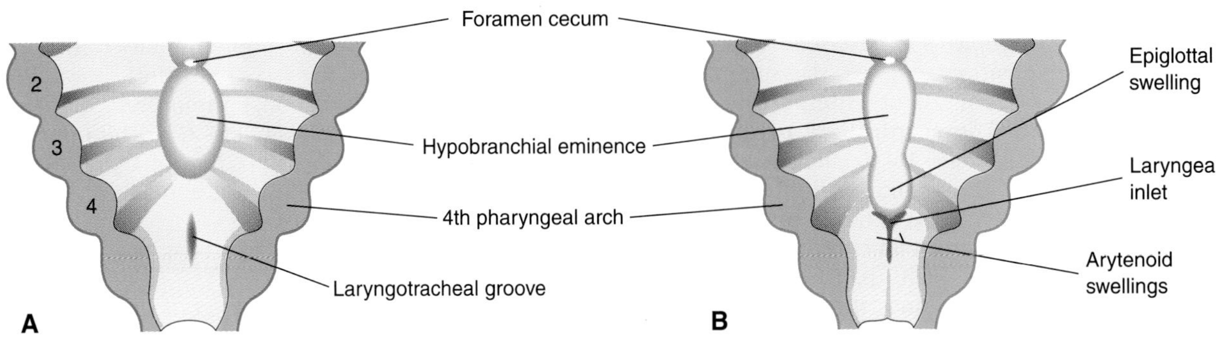

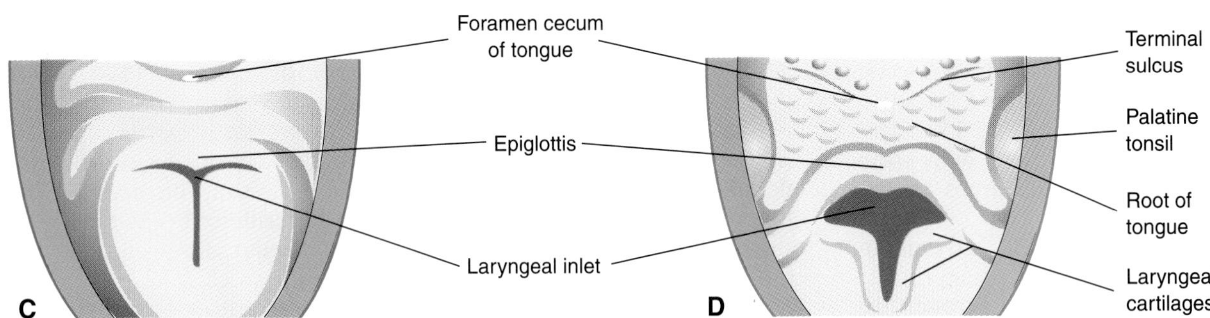

■ **Figure 11–3.** Drawings illustrating successive stages in the development of the larynx. *A,* 4 weeks. *B,* 5 weeks. *C,* 6 weeks. *D,* 10 weeks. The epithelium lining the larynx is of endodermal origin. The cartilages and muscles of the larynx arise from mesenchyme in the fourth and sixth pairs of pharyngeal arches. Note that the laryngeal inlet or aditus changes in shape from a slitlike opening to a T-shaped inlet as the mesenchyme surrounding the developing larynx proliferates.

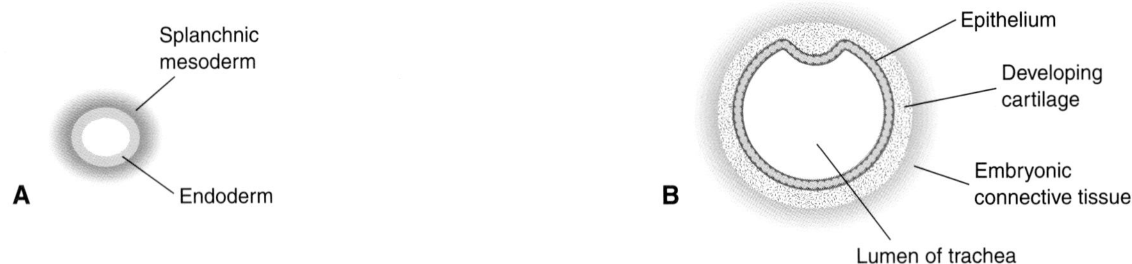

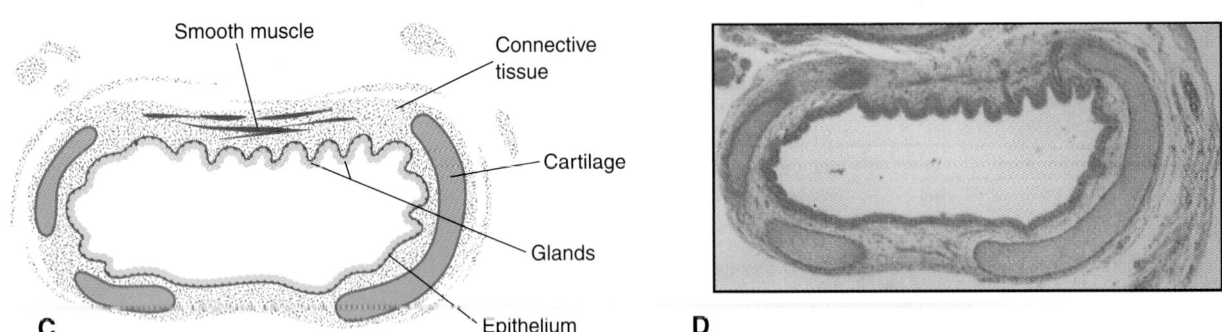

■ **Figure 11–4.** Drawings of transverse sections through the laryngotracheal tube illustrating progressive stages in the development of the trachea. *A,* 4 weeks. *B,* 10 weeks. *C,* 11 weeks. Note that endoderm of the tube gives rise to the epithelium and glands of the trachea and that mesenchyme surrounding the tube forms the connective tissue, muscle, and cartilage. *D,* Photomicrograph of a transverse section of the developing trachea at 14 weeks. (*D,* from Moore KL, Persaud TVN, Shiota K: *Color Atlas of Clinical Embryology.* Philadelphia, WB Saunders, 1994.)

hypobranchial eminence, a prominence produced by proliferation of mesenchyme in the ventral ends of the third and fourth pharyngeal arches (Fig. 11-3*B* to *D*). The rostral part of this eminence forms the posterior third or pharyngeal part of the tongue (see Chapter 10). Because the *laryngeal muscles* develop from myoblasts in the fourth and sixth pairs of pharyngeal arches, they are innervated by the laryngeal branches of the vagus nerves (CN X) that supply these arches (see Table 10-1). Growth of the larynx and epiglottis is rapid during the first three years after birth. By this time the epiglottis has reached its adult form (De Vries and De Vries, 1991).

Laryngeal Atresia

This rare anomaly results in obstruction of the upper fetal airway—**congenital high airway obstruction syndrome** (CHAOS). Distal to the atresia (blockage) or stenosis (narrowing), the airways become dilated, the lungs are enlarged and echogenic (capable of producing echoes), the diaphragm is either flattened or inverted, and there is fetal ascites and/or hydrops (accumulation of serous fluid). Prenatal ultrasonography permits diagnosis of these anomalies (Hedrick et al., 1994).

Laryngeal Web

This uncommon anomaly results from incomplete recanalization of the larynx during the tenth week. A membranous web forms at the level of the vocal folds, partially obstructing the airway.

DEVELOPMENT OF THE TRACHEA

The endodermal lining of the laryngotracheal tube distal to the larynx differentiates into the epithelium and glands of the trachea and the pulmonary epithelium. The cartilage, connective tissue, and muscles of the trachea are derived from the splanchnic mesenchyme surrounding the laryngotracheal tube (Fig. 11-4).

Tracheoesophageal Fistula

A **fistula** (abnormal communication) between the trachea and esophagus occurs about once in 3000 to 4500 live births (Fig. 11-5); most affected infants are males. In more than 85% of cases, the fistula is associated with **esophageal atresia** (Herbst, 1996; Behrman et al., 1996). Tracheoesophageal fistula results from incomplete division of the cranial part of the foregut into respiratory and esophageal parts during the fourth week. Incomplete fusion of the tracheoesophageal folds results in a **defective tracheoesophageal septum** and an abnormal communication between the trachea and esophagus.

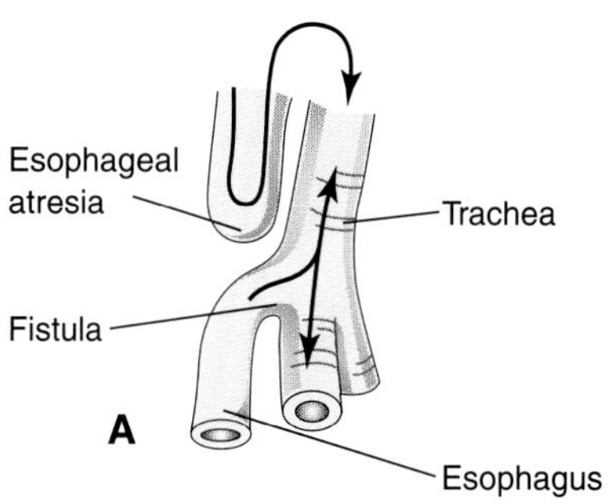

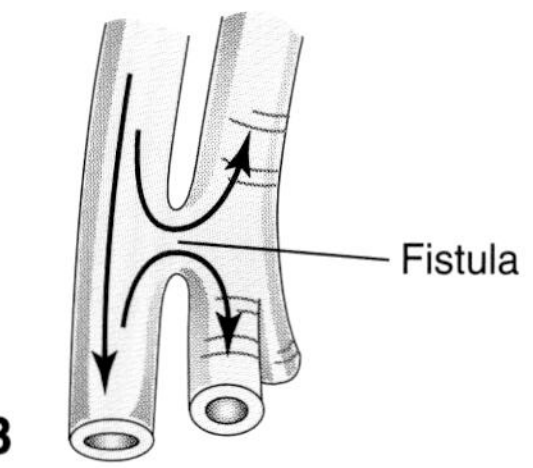

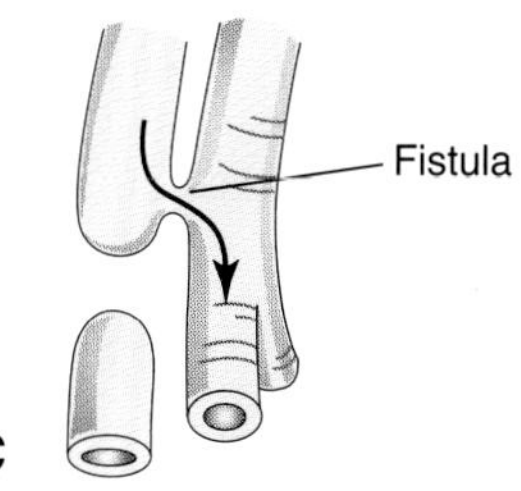

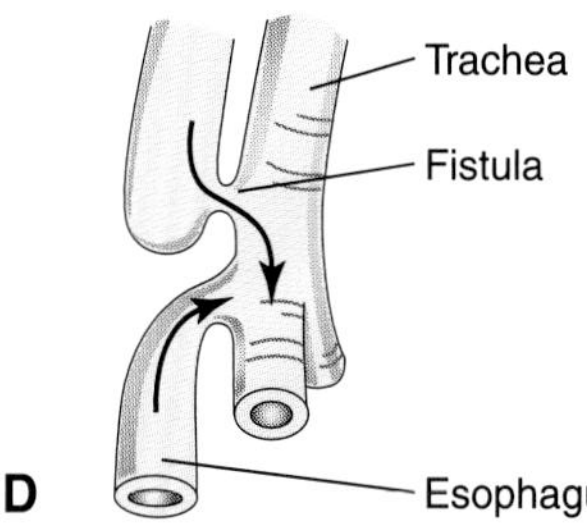

■ **Figure 11–5.** Sketches illustrating the four main varieties of tracheoesophageal fistula. Possible directions of the flow of the contents are indicated by arrows. Esophageal atresia, as illustrated in *A*, is associated with tracheoesophageal fistula in more than 85% of cases. The abdomen rapidly becomes distended as the stomach and intestines fill with air. *B*, Fistula between the trachea and esophagus. In *C*, air cannot enter the distal esophagus and stomach. Air can enter the distal esophagus and stomach in *D*, and the esophageal and gastric contents may enter the trachea and lungs.

Tracheoesophageal fistula is the most common anomaly of the lower respiratory tract. Four main varieties of tracheoesophageal fistula may develop (Fig. 11-5). The most common anomaly is for the superior part of the esophagus to end blindly (*esophageal atresia*) and for the inferior part to join the trachea near its bifurcation (Fig. 11-5*A*). Other varieties of this anomaly are illustrated in Figure 11-5*B* to *D*. Infants with the common type of tracheoesophageal fistula and esophageal atresia cough and choke when swallowing because of the accumulation of excessive amounts of saliva in the mouth and upper respiratory tract. When the infant attempts to swallow milk, it rapidly fills the esophageal pouch and is regurgitated. Gastric contents may also reflux from the stomach through the fistula into the trachea and lungs (Vos and Ekkelkamp, 1996). This causes choking and may result in pneumonia or *pneumonitis* (inflammation of the lungs). **Polyhydramnios** (see Chapter 7) is often associated with esophageal atresia and tracheoesophageal fistula. The excess amniotic fluid develops because fluid cannot pass to the stomach and intestines for absorption and subsequent transfer through the placenta to the mother's blood for disposal.

Laryngotracheoesophageal Cleft

Uncommonly, the larynx and upper trachea may fail to separate completely from the esophagus for a variable distance (Behrman et al., 1996). Symptoms of this congenital anomaly are similar to those of tracheoesophageal fistula, but *aphonia* (absence of voice) is a distinguishing feature.

Tracheal Stenosis and Atresia

Narrowing (stenosis) and obstruction (atresia) of the trachea are uncommon anomalies that are usually associated with one of the varieties of tracheoesophageal fistula. Stenoses and atresias probably result from unequal partitioning of the foregut into the esophagus and trachea. Sometimes there is a web of tissue obstructing airflow (*incomplete tracheal atresia*).

Tracheal Diverticulum

This extremely rare anomaly consists of a blind, bronchus-like projection from the trachea. The outgrowth may terminate in normal-appearing lung tissue, forming a *tracheal lobe* of the lung.

DEVELOPMENT OF THE BRONCHI AND LUNGS

The lung bud that developed at the caudal end of the laryngotracheal tube during the fourth week (Fig. 11-2*B*) soon divides into two outpouchings—the **bronchial buds** (Figs. 11-2*C* and 11-6*A*). These endodermal buds grow laterally into the pericardioperitoneal canals, the primordia of the pleural cavities (Fig. 11-6*B*). Together with the surrounding splanchnic mesenchyme, the bronchial buds differentiate into the bronchi and their ramifications in the lungs. Early in the fifth week the connection of each bronchial bud with the trachea enlarges to form the primordium of a **primary** or **main bronchus** (Fig. 11-7). The embryonic right main bronchus is slightly larger than the left one and is oriented more vertically. This embryonic relationship persists in the adult; consequently a foreign body is more liable to enter the right main bronchus than the left one. The primary or main bronchi subdivide into **secondary** or **stem bronchi** (Fig. 11-7). On the right the superior secondary bronchus will supply the upper or superior lobe of the lung, whereas the inferior secondary bronchus subdivides into two bronchi, one to the middle lobe of the right lung and the other to the lower or inferior lobe. On the left the two secondary bronchi supply the upper and lower lobes of the lung. Each secondary bronchus undergoes progressive branching.

Tertiary or **segmental bronchi**, ten in the right lung and eight or nine in the left lung, begin to form by the seventh week. As this occurs, the surrounding mesenchyme also divides. Each segmental bronchus with its surrounding mass of mesenchyme is the primordium of a **bronchopulmonary segment**. For a description of the adult anatomy of these clinically important segments, see Moore (1992). By 24 weeks, about 17 orders of branches have formed and **respiratory bronchioles** have developed (Fig. 11-8*B*). An additional seven orders of airways develop after birth.

As the bronchi develop, cartilaginous plates develop from the surrounding splanchnic mesenchyme. The bronchial smooth musculature and connective tissue and the pulmonary connective tissue and capillaries are also derived from this mesenchyme. As the lungs develop they acquire a layer of *visceral pleura* from

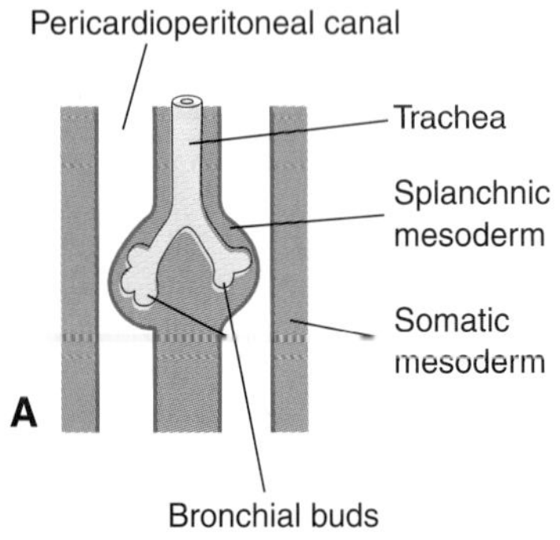

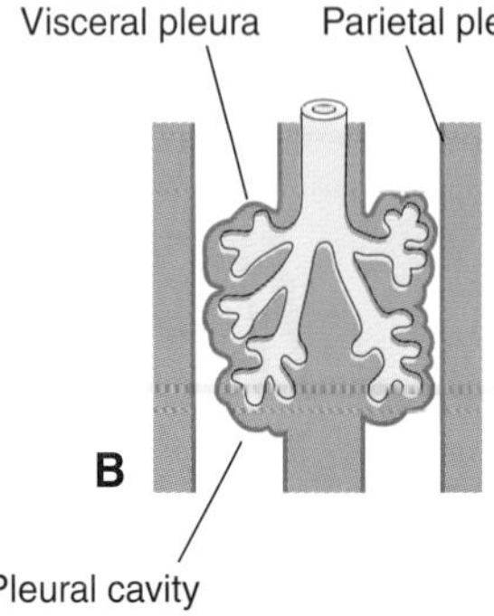

■ **Figure 11-6.** Diagrams illustrating growth of the developing lungs into the splanchnic mesenchyme adjacent to the medial walls of the pericardioperitoneal canals (primordial pleural cavities). Development of the layers of the pleura is also shown. *A*, 5 weeks. *B*, 6 weeks.

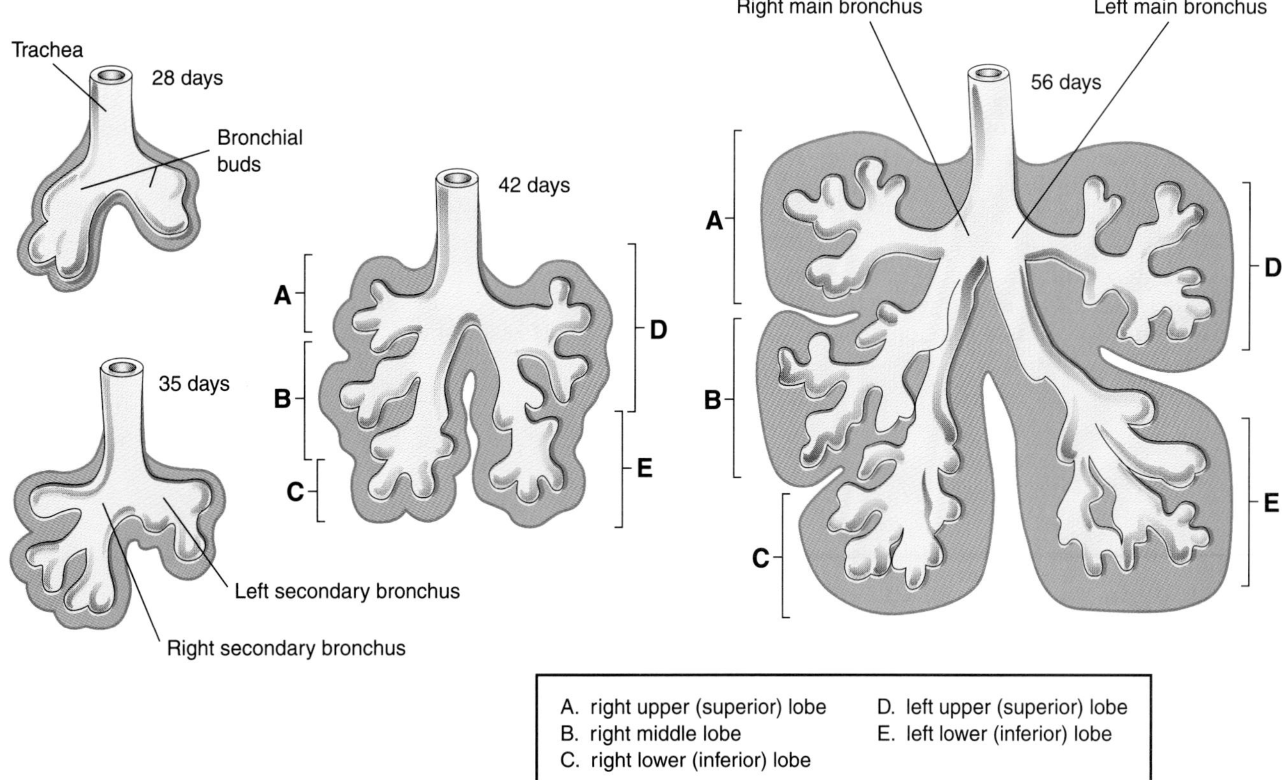

A. right upper (superior) lobe	D. left upper (superior) lobe
B. right middle lobe	E. left lower (inferior) lobe
C. right lower (inferior) lobe	

■ **Figure 11–7.** Successive stages in the development of the bronchi and lungs.

the splanchnic mesenchyme. With expansion, the lungs and pleural cavities grow caudally into the mesenchyme of the body wall and soon lie close to the heart. The thoracic body wall becomes lined by a layer of *parietal pleura*, derived from the somatic mesoderm (Fig. 11-6*B*).

Maturation of the Lungs

Maturation of the lungs is divided into four periods:

- pseudoglandular period
- canalicular period
- terminal sac period
- alveolar period

For information on the regulation of normal lung growth and the hormonal control of lung maturation, see Ballard (1989), Scarpelli (1990), Thurlbeck (1995), and Adamson (1997).

PSEUDOGLANDULAR PERIOD (5 TO 17 WEEKS)

The developing lung somewhat resembles an exocrine gland during this period (Figs. 11-8*A* and 11-9*A*). By 17 weeks all major elements of the lung have formed, except those involved with gas exchange. Respiration is not possible; hence, *fetuses born during this period are unable to survive*.

CANALICULAR PERIOD (16 TO 25 WEEKS)

This period overlaps the pseudoglandular period because cranial segments of the lungs mature faster than caudal ones. During the canalicular period the lumina of the bronchi and terminal bronchioles become larger, and the lung tissue becomes highly vascular (Figs. 11-8*B* and 11-9*B*). By 24 weeks, each terminal bronchiole has given rise to two or more **respiratory bronchioles**, each of which then divides into three to six tubular passages — the **alveolar ducts**. Respiration is possible toward the end of the canalicular period because some thin-walled *terminal sacs* (primordial alveoli) have developed at the ends of the respiratory bronchioles, and *the lung tissue is well vascularized*. Although a fetus born toward the end of this period may survive if given intensive care, it often dies because its respiratory and other systems are still relatively immature.

TERMINAL SAC PERIOD (24 WEEKS TO BIRTH)

During this period many more terminal sacs develop (Figs. 11-8*C* and 11-9*C*), and *their epithelium becomes very thin*. Capillaries begin to bulge into these developing alveoli. The intimate contact between epithelial and endothelial cells establishes the **blood-air barrier**, which permits adequate gas exchange for survival of the fetus if it is born prematurely. By 24 weeks, the terminal sacs are lined mainly by squamous epithelial cells of endodermal origin—**type I alveolar cells** or pneumocytes—across which gas exchange occurs. The capillary network proliferates rapidly in the mesenchyme around the developing alveoli and there is concurrent active development of lymphatic capillaries. Scattered among the squamous epithelial cells are rounded secretory epithelial cells—**type II alveolar cells** or pneumocytes—*which secrete pulmonary surfactant,* a complex mixture of phospholipids. **Surfactant** forms as a monomolecular film over the internal walls of the terminal sacs, lowering surface tension at the air-alveolar interface (Whitsett, 1991). The maturation of alveolar type II cells and surfactant production varies widely in fetuses of different gestational ages (Chernick and Kryger, 1990). The production of surfactant increases during the terminal stages of pregnancy, particularly during the last 2 weeks before birth.

Surfactant counteracts surface tension forces and facilitates expansion of the terminal sacs (primitive alveoli). Consequently, fetuses born prematurely at 24 to 26 weeks after fertilization may survive if given intensive care; however, they may suffer from respiratory distress because of *surfactant deficiency.*

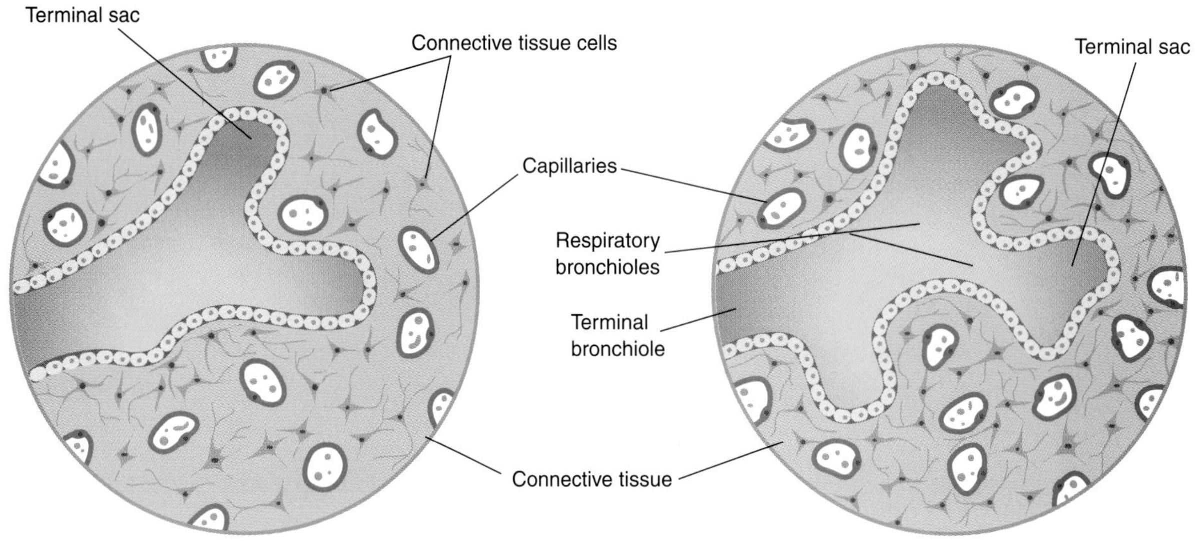

■ **Figure 11–8.** Diagrammatic sketches of histological sections, illustrating progressive stages of lung development. In *C* and *D*, note that the alveolocapillary membrane is thin and that some capillaries bulge into the terminal sacs (future alveoli).

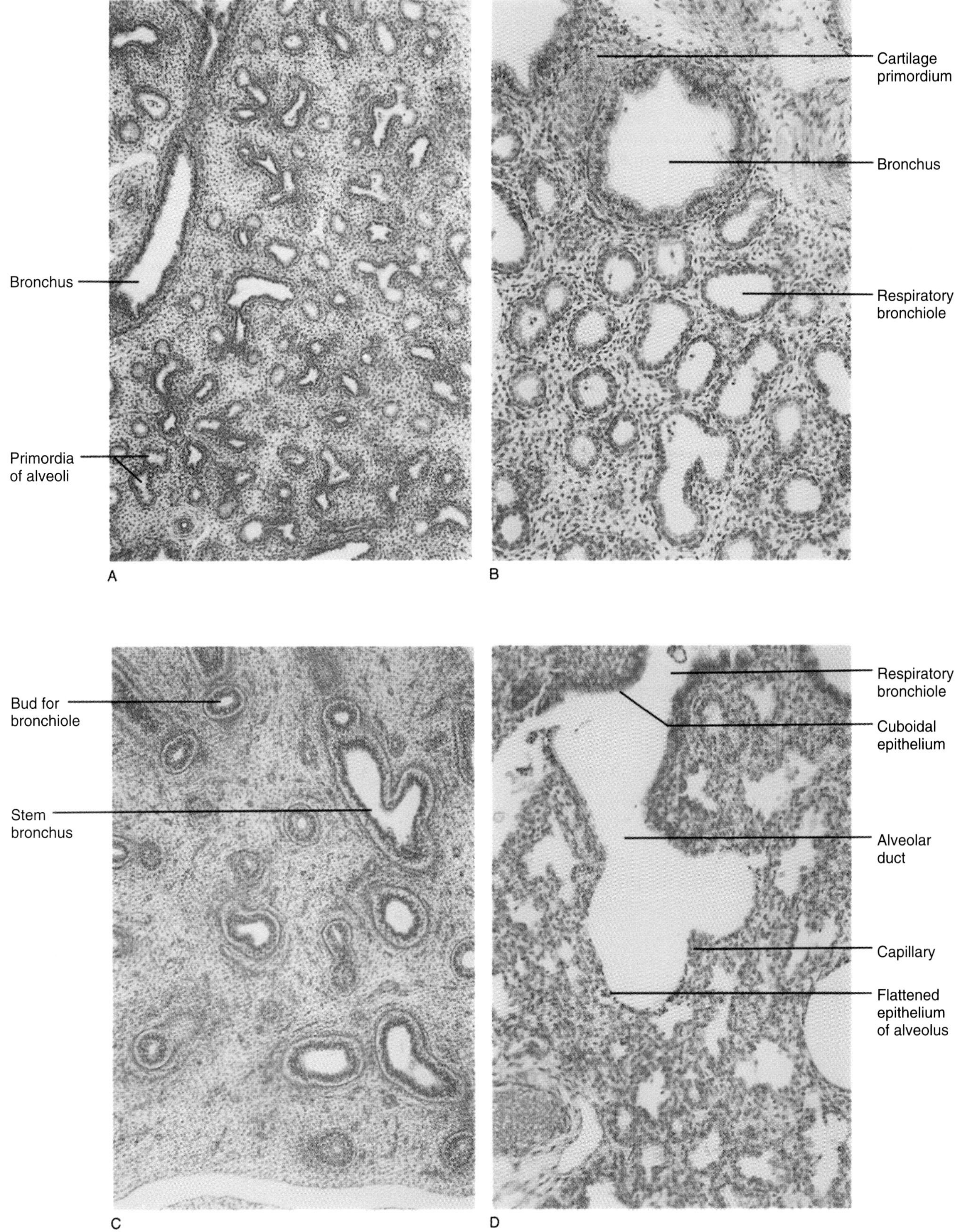

■ **Figure 11–9.** Photomicrographs of sections of developing human lungs. *A,* Pseudoglandular period, 8 weeks. Note the "glandular" appearance of the lung at this stage. *B,* Canalicular period, 16 weeks. The lumina of the bronchi and terminal bronchioles are enlarging. *C,* Canalicular period, 18 weeks. Note that many blood vessels are developing in the mesenchyme surrounding the sections of bronchi and terminal bronchioles. *D,* Terminal sac period, 24 weeks. Observe the thin-walled terminal sacs (primordial alveoli) that have developed at the ends of the respiratory bronchioles. Also observe that the number of blood vessels has increased and that some of them are closely associated with the developing alveoli. (From Moore KL, Persaud TVN, Shiota K: *Color Atlas of Clinical Embryology.* Philadelphia, WB Saunders, 1994.)

Surfactant production begins by 20 weeks but it is present in only small amounts in premature infants; it does not reach adequate levels until the late fetal period. By 26 to 28 weeks after fertilization the fetus usually weighs about 1000 gm and sufficient terminal sacs and surfactant are present to permit survival of a prematurely born infant. Before this, the lungs are usually incapable of providing adequate gas exchange, partly because the alveolar surface area is insufficient and the vascularity underdeveloped. It is not the presence of thin terminal sacs or a primordial alveolar epithelium so much as the development of an adequate pulmonary vasculature and sufficient surfactant that is critical to the survival of premature infants.

ALVEOLAR PERIOD (LATE FETAL PERIOD TO CHILDHOOD)

Exactly when the terminal sac period ends and the alveolar period begins depends on the definition of the term **alveolus** (Behrman et al., 1996). Structures analogous to alveoli are present at 32 weeks of gestation. The epithelial lining of the terminal sacs attenuates to an extremely thin squamous epithelial layer. The type I alveolar cells become so thin that the adjacent capillaries bulge into the terminal sacs (Figs. 11-8*D* and 11-9*D*). By the late fetal period, the lungs are capable of respiration because the **alveolocapillary membrane** (pulmonary diffusion barrier or respiratory membrane) is sufficiently thin to allow gas exchange. Although the lungs do not begin to perform this vital function until birth, they must be well developed so that they are capable of functioning as soon as the baby is born. At the beginning of the alveolar period, each respiratory bronchiole terminates in a cluster of thin-walled terminal sacs, separated from one another by loose connective tissue. These terminal sacs represent future alveolar ducts. The transition from dependence on the placenta for gas exchange to autonomous gas exchange requires the following adaptive changes in the lungs (Behrman et al., 1996):

- production of adequate surfactant in the alveoli
- transformation of the lungs from secretory into gas exchanging organs
- establishment of parallel pulmonary and systemic circulations

For more information about adaptation of the newborn to air-breathing, see Behrman et al. (1996).

Characteristic mature alveoli do not form until after birth; about 95% of alveoli develop postnatally. Before birth the immature alveoli appear as small bulges on the walls of respiratory bronchioles and terminal sacs (future alveolar ducts). After birth the primordial alveoli enlarge as the lungs expand, but most increase in the size of the lungs results from an increase in the number of respiratory bronchioles and primordial alveoli rather than from an increase in the size of the alveoli. From the third to the eighth year or so, the number of immature alveoli continues to increase (Thurlbeck, 1995). Unlike mature alveoli, immature alveoli have the potential for forming additional primordial alveoli. As these alveoli increase in size, they become mature alveoli. The major mechanism for increasing the number of alveoli is the formation of secondary connective tissue septa that subdivide existing primordial alveoli. Initially the septa are relatively thick, but they are soon transformed into mature thin septa that are capable of gas exchange.

Lung development during the first few months after birth is characterized by an exponential increase in the surface of the air-blood barrier (Behrman et al., 1996). This increase is accomplished by the multiplication of pulmonary alveoli and capillaries. About 50 million alveoli, one-sixth of the adult number, are present in the lungs of a full-term newborn infant. On chest radiographs, therefore, the lungs of newborn infants are denser than adult lungs. By about the eighth year, the adult complement of 300 million alveoli is present (Ballard, 1989). Molecular studies have led to the recognition of several regulatory substances that participate in mesenchymal-epithelial interactions and in lung development. For example, *keratinocyte growth factor*, a member of the family of fibroblast growth factors, was shown to be involved in lung morphogenesis by influencing branching, epithelial growth differentiation, and patterning of rat lung explants in culture (Shiratori et al., 1996).

Breathing movements occur before birth, exerting sufficient force to cause aspiration of some amniotic fluid into the lungs. These fetal breathing movements, which can be detected by real-time ultrasonography, are not continuous, but they are essential for normal lung development. The pattern of fetal breathing movements is widely used in the diagnosis of labor and as a predictor of fetal outcome in preterm delivery. By birth the fetus has had the advantage of several months of breathing exercise. *Fetal breathing movements*, which increase as the time of delivery approaches, probably condition the respiratory muscles. In addition these movements stimulate lung development, possibly by creating a pressure gradient between the lungs and the amniotic fluid (Behrman et al., 1996).

At birth the lungs are about half-filled with fluid derived from the amniotic cavity, lungs, and tracheal glands. Aeration of the lungs at birth is not so much the inflation of empty collapsed organs but rather the rapid replacement of intra-alveolar fluid by air. *The fluid in the lungs is cleared at birth by three routes:*

- through the mouth and nose by pressure on the thorax during delivery
- into the pulmonary capillaries
- into the lymphatics and pulmonary arteries and veins

In the fetus near term, the pulmonary lymphatic vessels are relatively larger and more numerous than in the adult (Crelin, 1976). Lymph flow is rapid during the first few hours after birth and then diminishes. *Three factors are important for normal lung development* (Goldstein, 1994):

- adequate thoracic space for lung growth
- fetal breathing movements
- adequate amniotic fluid volume

Oligohydramnios and Lung Development

The fluid in the lungs is an important stimulus for lung development. When oligohydramnios (an insufficient amount of amniotic fluid) is severe and chronic because of amniotic fluid leakage, for example, lung development is retarded and severe pulmonary hypoplasia results (Goldstein, 1994).

Lungs of a Newborn

Fresh healthy lungs always contain some air; consequently, pulmonary tissue removed from them will float in water. A diseased lung, partly filled with fluid, may not float. Of medicolegal significance is the fact that the lungs of a stillborn infant are firm and sink when placed in water because they contain fluid, not air.

Respiratory Distress Syndrome

This disease affects about 2% of live newborn infants, and those born prematurely are most susceptible. These infants develop rapid, labored breathing shortly after birth. Respiratory distress syndrome (RDS) is also known as *hyaline membrane disease* (Verma, 1995; Behrman et al., 1996). An estimated 30% of all neonatal disease results from hyaline membrane disease (HMD) or its complications. For more information about HMD, see Behrman et al. (1996).

Surfactant deficiency is a major cause of RDS or HMD. The lungs are underinflated and the alveoli contain a fluid of high protein content that resembles a glassy or *hyaline membrane*. This membrane is believed to be derived from a combination of substances in the circulation and from the injured pulmonary epithelium. It has been suggested that prolonged *intrauterine asphyxia* may produce irreversible changes in the type II alveolar cells, making them incapable of producing surfactant. There appear to be other causes for absence or deficiency of surfactant in premature and full-term infants (Toki et al., 1995). All the growth factors and hormones controlling surfactant production have not been identified (Ballard, 1989), but *thyroxine* is a potent stimulator of surfactant production.

Glucocorticoid treatment during pregnancy accelerates fetal lung development and surfactant production. This finding has led to the routine clinical use of corticosteroids (betamethasone) for the *prevention of RDS*. In addition, clinical trials with exogenous surfactant (**surfactant replacement therapy**) are in progress in many centers.

Pleural Effusion

Pleural effusion (fluid in the pleural cavity) can be detected sonographically (Goldstein, 1994). **Chylothorax**—an accumulation of chyle (lymph and triglyceride fat) in the pleural cavity—is the most frequent cause of isolated pleural effusion resulting in respiratory distress. In severe cases, the pleural effusion causes the lungs to collapse (Fig. 11-10). Fluid can be drained from the pleural cavity of the fetus through a catheter to permit better lung expansion and lung growth. The catheter drains the fluid in the pleural cavity into the amniotic sac.

Lobe of Azygos Vein

This lobe appears in the right lung in about 1% of people. It develops when the apical bronchus grows superiorly, medial to the arch of the azygos vein, instead of lateral to it. As a result, the vein comes to lie at the bottom of a fissure in the superior lobe (Moore, 1992), which produces a linear marking on a radiograph of the lungs.

Congenital Lung Cysts

Cysts (filled with fluid or air) are thought to be formed by the dilation of terminal bronchi (Salzberg, 1983). They probably result from a disturbance in bronchial

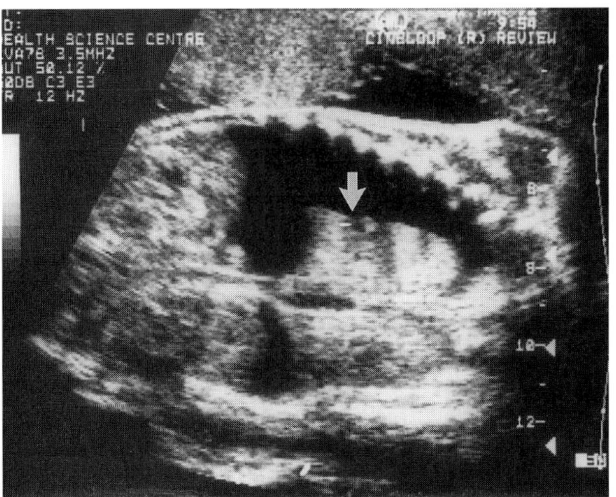

■ **Figure 11–10.** Ultrasound image of a fetus (24 weeks' gestation) with large bilateral pleural effusions. The collapsed left lung (arrow) is clearly outlined by the larger left pleural effusion. This fetus had severe upper body edema and required intrauterine treatment by insertion of a pleural-amniotic shunt to reach term in good condition. (Courtesy of Dr. C. R. Harman, Department of Obstetrics, Gynecology and Reproductive Sciences, Women's Hospital and University of Manitoba, Winnipeg, Manitoba, Canada.)

development during late fetal life. If several cysts are present, the lungs have a honeycomb appearance on radiographs. Congenital lung cysts are usually located at the periphery of the lung. Other cystic conditions in the fetal lung, with highly variable outcome, have been described (MacGillivray et al., 1993).

Agenesis of the Lungs

Absence of the lungs results from failure of the bronchial buds to develop. Agenesis of one lung is more common than bilateral agenesis, but both conditions are rare. *Unilateral pulmonary agenesis* is compatible with life. The heart and other mediastinal structures are shifted to the affected side and the existing lung is hyperexpanded.

Lung Hypoplasia

In infants with congenital diaphragmatic hernia, or congenital heart disease (CHD) (see Chapter 9), the lung is unable to develop normally because it is compressed by the abnormally positioned abdominal viscera. Lung hypoplasia is characterized by a markedly reduced lung volume (Lee et al., 1996). Most infants with CHD die of pulmonary insufficiency, despite optimal postnatal care, because their lungs are too hypoplastic to support extrauterine life (Harrison, 1991).

Accessory Lung

A small accessory lung (*pulmonary sequestration*) is very uncommon. It is almost always located at the base of the left lung. It does not communicate with the tracheobronchial tree and its blood supply is usually systemic rather than pulmonary in origin.

SUMMARY OF THE RESPIRATORY SYSTEM

The lower respiratory system begins to develop around the middle of the fourth week from a median **laryngotracheal groove** in the floor of the primordial pharynx. The groove deepens to produce a **laryngotracheal diverticulum**, which soon becomes separated from the foregut by tracheoesophageal folds that fuse to form a **tracheoesophageal septum**. This septum results in the formation of the esophagus and laryngotracheal tube. The endoderm of the **laryngotracheal tube** gives rise to the epithelium of the lower respiratory organs and the tracheobronchial glands. The splanchnic mesenchyme surrounding the laryngotracheal tube forms the connective tissue, cartilage, muscle, and blood and lymphatic vessels of these organs.

Pharyngeal arch mesenchyme contributes to formation of the epiglottis and connective tissue of the larynx. The **laryngeal muscles** are derived from mesenchyme in the caudal pharyngeal arches. The **laryngeal cartilages** are derived from the cartilaginous bars in the fourth and sixth pairs of pharyngeal arches, which are derived from *neural crest cells* (see Table 10-1).

During the fourth week the laryngotracheal tube develops a lung bud at its distal end, which divides into two **bronchial buds** during the early part of the fifth week. Each bronchial bud soon enlarges to form a **primary** or **main bronchus,** and then each primary bronchus gives rise to two new bronchial buds, which develop into **secondary bronchi**. The right inferior secondary bronchus soon divides into two bronchi. The secondary bronchi supply the lobes of the developing lungs. Each bronchus undergoes progressive branching to form **segmental bronchi**. Each segmental bronchus, with its surrounding mesenchyme, is the primordium of a **bronchopulmonary segment**. Branching continues until about 17 orders of branches have formed. Additional airways are formed after birth, until about 24 orders of branches are present.

Lung development is divided into four periods. During the **pseudoglandular period** (5 to 17 weeks), the bronchi and terminal bronchioles form. During the **canalicular period** (16 to 25 weeks), the lumina of the bronchi and terminal bronchioles enlarge, the respiratory bronchioles and alveolar ducts develop, and the lung tissue becomes highly vascular. During the **terminal sac period** (24 weeks to birth), the alveolar ducts give rise to terminal sacs (primordial alveoli). The terminal sacs are initially lined with cuboidal epithelium that begins to attenuate to squamous epithelium at about 26 weeks. By this time, capillary networks have proliferated close to the alveolar epithelium and the lungs are usually sufficiently well developed to permit survival of the fetus if it is born prematurely. The **alveolar period**, the final stage of lung development, occurs from the late fetal period to about 8 years of age, as the lungs mature. The number of respiratory bronchioles and primitive alveoli increases.

The respiratory system develops so that it is capable of immediate function at birth. To be capable of respiration, the lungs must acquire an **alveolocapillary membrane** that is sufficiently thin, and an adequate amount of *surfactant* must be present. A deficiency of surfactant appears to be responsible for the failure of primordial alveoli to remain open, resulting in **RDS.** Growth of the lungs after birth results mainly from an increase in the number of respiratory bronchioles and alveoli. New alveoli form for at least 8 years after birth.

Major congenital anomalies of the lower respiratory system are uncommon, except for **tracheoesophageal fistula**, which is usually associated with *esophageal atresia*. These anomalies result from faulty partitioning of the foregut into the esophagus and trachea during the fourth and fifth weeks.

Clinically Oriented Problems

Case 11–1

Choking and continuous coughing were observed in a newborn infant. There was an excessive amount of mucus secretion and saliva in the infant's mouth and the infant experienced considerable difficulty in breathing. The pediatrician was unable to pass a catheter through the esophagus into the stomach.

- What congenital anomalies would be suspected?
- Discuss the embryological basis of these defects.
- What kind of an examination do you think would be used to confirm the tentative diagnosis?

Case 11–2

A premature infant developed rapid, shallow respiration shortly after birth. A diagnosis of *respiratory distress syndrome* (RDS) was made.

- How do you think the infant might attempt to overcome his or her inadequate exchange of oxygen and carbon dioxide?
- What usually causes RDS?
- What treatment is currently used clinically to prevent RDS?
- A deficiency of what substance is associated with RDS?

Case 11–3

The parents of a newborn infant were told that their son had a fistula between his trachea and esophagus.

- What is the most common type of tracheoesophageal fistula?
- What is its embryological basis?
- What anomaly of the digestive tract is frequently associated with this abnormality?

Case 11–4

A newborn infant with esophageal atresia experienced respiratory distress with cyanosis shortly after birth. Radiographs demonstrated air in the infant's stomach.

- How did the air enter the stomach?
- What other problem might result in an infant with this fairly common type of congenital anomaly?

Discussion of these problems is given at the back of the book.

REFERENCES AND SUGGESTED READING

Achiron R, Strauss S, Seidman DS, et al: Fetal lung hyperechogenicity: prenatal ultrasonographic diagnosis, natural history and neonatal outcome. *Ultrasound Obstet Gynecol 6*:40, 1995.

Adamson IYR: Development of lung structure. *In* Crystal RG, West JB, Weibel ER (eds): *The Lung: Scientific Foundations,* 2nd ed. Philadelphia, Lippincott-Raven Publishers, 1997.

Ballard PL: Hormonal control of lung maturation. *Bailliere's Clin Endocrin Metabol 3*:723, 1989.

Behrman RE, Kliegman RM, Arvin AM (eds): *Nelson Textbook of Pediatrics,* 15th ed. Philadelphia, WB Saunders, 1996.

Boyden EA: Development and growth of the airways. *In* Hodson WA (ed): *Development of the Lung*. New York, Marcel Deckker, 1977.

Broers JL, de Leij L, ter Haar A, et al: Expression of intermediate filament proteins in fetal and adult human lung tissues. *Differentiation 40*:119, 1989.

Bucher U, Reid L: Development of the intrasegmental bronchial tree: The pattern of branching and development of cartilage at various stages of intrauterine life. *Thorax 16*:207, 1961.

Chernick V, Kryger MH: Pediatric lung disease. *In* Kryger MH (ed): *Introduction to Respiratory Medicine,* 2nd ed. New York, Churchill Livingstone, 1990.

Chernick V, Mellins RB (eds): *Basic Mechanisms of Pediatric Respiratory Disease: Cellular and Integrative*. Philadelphia, BC Decker, 1991.

Cooke IR, Berger PJ: Precursor of respiratory pattern in the early gestation mammalian fetus. *Brain Res 522*:333, 1990.

Cormack DH: *Ham's Histology,* 9th ed. Philadelphia, JB Lippincott, 1987.

Crelin ES: Development of the upper respiratory system. *Clin Symp 28*:3, 1976.

De Vries PA, De Vries CR: Embryology and development. *In* Othersen HB Jr (ed): *The Pediatric Airway*. Philadelphia, WB Saunders, 1991.

Endo H, Oka T: An immunohistochemical study of bronchial cells producing surfactant protein A in the developing human fetal lung. *Early Human Develop 25*:149, 1991.

Fowler CL, Pokorny WJ, Wagner ML, Kessler MS: Review of bronchopulmonary foregut malformations. *J Pediatr Surg 23*:793, 1988.

Godfrey S: Growth and development of the respiratory system—functional development. *In* Davis JA, Dobbing J (eds): *Scientific Foundations of Paediatrics*. Philadelphia, WB Saunders, 1974.

Goldstein RB: Ultrasound evaluation of the fetal thorax. *In* Callen PW (ed): *Ultrasonography in Obstetrics and Gynecology,* 3rd ed. Philadelphia, WB Saunders, 1994.

Hadlock FP: Sonographic prediction of fetal lung maturity. *In* Callen PW (ed): *Ultrasonography in Obstetrics and Gynecology,* 3rd ed. Philadelphia, WB Saunders, 1994.

Harrison MR: The fetus with a diaphragmatic hernia: pathology, natural history, and surgical management. *In* Harrison MR, Golbus MS, Filly RA (eds): *The Unborn Patient. Prenatal Diagnosis and Treatment,* 2nd ed. Philadelphia, WB Saunders, 1991.

Hedrick MH, Ferro MM, Filly RA, et al: Congenital high airway obstruction syndrome (CHAOS): a potential for perinatal intervention. *J Pediatr Surg 29*:271, 1994.

Herbst JL: The esophagus. *In* Behrman RE (ed): *Nelson Textbook of Pediatrics,* 15th ed. Philadelphia, WB Saunders, 1996.

Hislop A, Reid L: Growth and development of the respiratory system—anatomical development. *In* Davis JA, Dobbing J (eds): *Scientific Foundations of Paediatrics*. Philadelphia, WB Saunders, 1974.

Hodson WA (Ed): *Development of the Lung*. New York, Marcel Dekker, 1977.

Hollinger PH, Johnson KC, Schiller F: Congenital anomalies of the larynx. *Ann Otol 63*:581, 1954.

Hume R: Fetal lung development. *In* Hillier SG, Kitchener HC, Neilson JP (eds): *Scientific Essentials of Reproductive Medicine*. Philadelphia, WB Saunders, 1996.

Kozuma S, Nemoto A, Okai T, Mizuno M: Maturational sequence of fetal breathing movements. *Biol Neonate 60(Suppl 1)*:36, 1991.

Landing BH: Pathogenetic considerations of respiratory tract malformations in humans. *In* Persaud TVN (ed): *Advances in the Study of Birth Defects. Cardiovascular, Respiratory, Gastrointestinal and Genitourinary Malformations,* vol 6. New York, Alan R Liss, 1982.

Lauria MR, Gonik B, Romero R: Pulmonary hypoplasia: pathogenesis, diagnosis and antenatal prediction. *Obstet Gynecol 86*:466, 1995.

Lee A, Kratochwil A, Stümpflen I, et al: Fetal lung volume determination by three-dimensional ultrasonography. *Am J Obstet Gynecol 175*:588, 1996.

Moore KL: *Clinically Oriented Anatomy,* 3rd ed. Baltimore, Williams & Wilkins, 1992.

MacGillivray TE, Harrison MR, Goldstein RB, Adzick NS: Disappearing fetal lung lesions. *J Pediatr Surg 28*:1321, 1993.

O'Rahilly R, Boyden E: The timing and sequence of events in the development of the human respiratory system during the embryonic period proper. *Z Anat Entwicklungsgesch 141*:237, 1973.

O'Rahilly R, Tucker JA: The early development of the larynx in staged human embryos. Part 1. Embryos of the first five weeks (to stage 15). *Ann Otol Rhinol Laryngol 82(Suppl 7)*:1, 1973.

Patrick J, Gagnon R: Fetal breathing and body movement. *In* Creasy RK, Resnik R (eds): *Maternal-Fetal Medicine. Principles and Practice,* 2nd ed. Philadelphia, WB Saunders, 1989.

Ramenofsky ML: Bronchogenic cyst. *In* Creasy RK, Resnik R (eds): *Maternal-Fetal Medicine. Principles and Practice,* 2nd ed. Philadelphia, WB Saunders, 1989.

Salzberg AM: Congenital malformations of the lower respiratory tract. *In* Kendig EL Jr, Chernick V (eds): *Disorders of the Respiratory Tract in Children,* 4th ed. Philadelphia, WB Saunders, 1983.

Sañudo JR, Domenech-Mateu JM: The laryngeal primordium and epithelial lamina. A new interpretation. *J Anat 171*:207, 1990.

Scarpelli EM (ed): *Pulmonary Physiology: Fetus, Newborn, Child and Adolescent,* 2nd ed. Philadelphia, Lea and Febiger, 1990.

Schwartz MZ, Ramachandran P: Congenital malformations of the lung and mediastinum—a quarter century of experience from a single institution. *J Pediatr Surg 32*:44, 1997.

Shiratori M, Oshika E, Ung LP, et al: Keratinocyte growth factor and embryonic rat lung morphogenesis. *Am J Respir Cell Mol Biol 15*: 328, 1996.

Smith EI: The early development of the trachea and oesophagus in relation to atresia of the oesophagus and tracheo-oesophageal fistula. *Contr Embryol Carneg Instn 245*:36, 1957.

Thrane EV, Becher R, Lag M, et al: Differential distribution and increased levels of RAS proteins during lung development. *Lung Research 23*:35, 1997.

Thurlbeck WM: Lung growth and development. *In* Thurlbeck WM, Churg AM (eds): *Pathology of the Lung,* 2nd ed. New York, Thieme Medical Publishers, 1995.

Toki N, Sueishi K, Minamitani M, et al: Immunohistochemical distribution of surfactant apoproteins in hypoplastic lungs of nonimmunologic hydrops fetalis. *Hum Pathol 26*:1252, 1995.

Tooley WH: Lung disease and lung development. *In* Hodson WA (ed): *Development of the Lung*. New York, Marcel Dekker, 1977.

Verma RP: Respiratory distress syndrome of the newborn infant. *Obstet Gynecol Surv 50*:542, 1995.

Vos A, Ekkelkamp S: Congenital tracheoesophageal fistula: preventing recurrence. *J Pediatr Surg 31*:936, 1996.

Wells LJ, Boyden EA: The development of the bronchopulmonary segments in human embryos of horizons XVII and XIX. *Am J Anat 95*:163, 1954.

Whitsett JA: Molecular aspects of the pulmonary surfactant system in the newborn. *In* Chernick V, Mellins RB (eds): *Basic Mechanisms of Pediatric Respiratory Disease: Cellular and Integrative*. Philadelphia, BC Decker, 1991.

Wiseman NE, Macpherson RI: Pulmonary sequestration. *In* Persaud TVN (ed): *Advances in the Study of Birth Defects. Cardiovascular, Respiratory, Gastrointestinal and Genitourinary Malformations,* vol 6. New York, Alan R Liss, 1982.

Wolfson VP, Laitman JT: Ultrasound investigation of fetal human upper respiratory anatomy. *Anat Rec 227*:363, 1990.

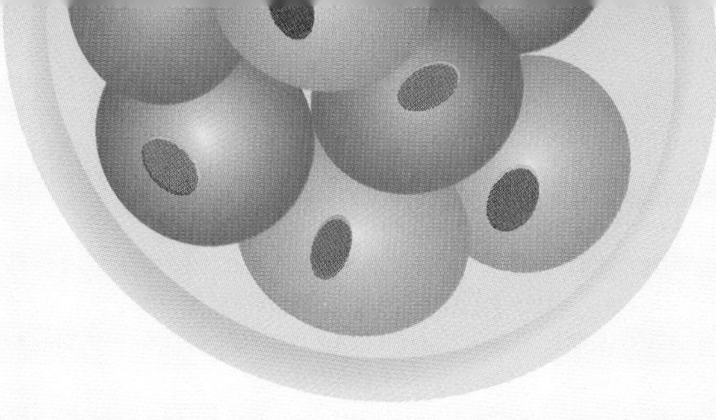

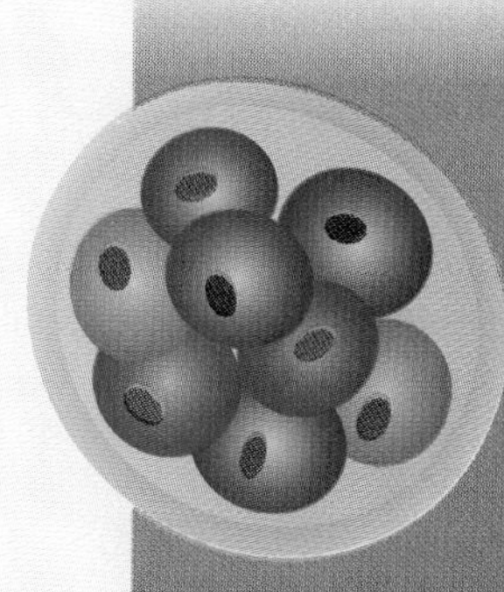

The Digestive System

12

■ The **primordial (primitive) gut** at the beginning of the fourth week is closed at its cranial end by the **oropharyngeal membrane** (see Fig. 10-1) and at its caudal end by the **cloacal membrane** (Fig. 12-1*B*). The primordial gut forms during the fourth week as the head, tail, and lateral folds incorporate the dorsal part of the yolk sac into the embryo (see Chapter 5). The endoderm of the primordial gut gives rise to most of the epithelium and glands of the digestive tract. The epithelium at the cranial and caudal extremities of the tract is derived from ectoderm of the **stomodeum** (primordial mouth) and **proctodeum** (anal pit), respectively (Fig. 12-1*A* and *B*). The muscular, connective tissue, and other layers of the wall of the digestive tract are derived from the splanchnic mesenchyme surrounding the primordial gut. For descriptive purposes the primordial gut is divided into three parts: foregut, midgut, and hindgut.

THE FOREGUT

The derivatives of the foregut are:

- the *primordial pharynx* and its derivatives (oral cavity, pharynx, tongue, tonsils, salivary glands, and upper respiratory system), which are discussed in Chapter 10
- the *lower respiratory system* (described in Chapter 11)
- the *esophagus and stomach*
- the *duodenum*, proximal to the opening of the bile duct
- the *liver, biliary apparatus* (hepatic ducts, gallbladder, and bile duct), and *pancreas*

All these foregut derivatives, *except* the pharynx, respiratory tract, and most of the esophagus, are supplied by the *celiac artery*, the artery of the foregut (Fig. 12-1*B*).

Development of the Esophagus

The esophagus develops from the foregut immediately caudal to the primordial pharynx (Fig. 12-1*B*). The partitioning of the trachea from the esophagus by the **tracheoesophageal septum** is described in Chapter 11. Initially, the esophagus is short but it elongates rapidly, mainly because of the growth and descent of the heart and lungs. The esophagus reaches its final relative length by the seventh week. Its epithelium and glands are derived from endoderm. The epithelium proliferates and partly or completely obliterates the lumen; however, recanalization of the esophagus normally occurs by the end of the embryonic period. The striated muscle constituting the muscularis externa of the superior third of the esophagus is derived from mesenchyme in the caudal pharyngeal arches. The smooth muscle, mainly in the inferior third of the esophagus, develops from the surrounding splanchnic mesenchyme (Gemonov and Kolesnikov, 1990). Both types of muscle are innervated by branches of the vagus nerves (CN X), which supply the caudal pharyngeal arches (see Table 10-1).

Esophageal Atresia

Blockage of the esophagus occurs with an incidence of 1 in 3000 to 4500 live births (Herbst, 1996). About one-third of affected infants are born prematurely. Esophageal atresia is associated with **tracheoesophageal fistula** in more than 85% of cases (see Fig. 11-5). It may occur as a separate anomaly, but this is less common. Esophageal atresia results from deviation of the *tracheoesophageal septum* in a posterior direction (see Fig. 11-2); as a result, there is incomplete separation of the esophagus from the laryngotracheal tube. Isolated esophageal atresia may be associated with

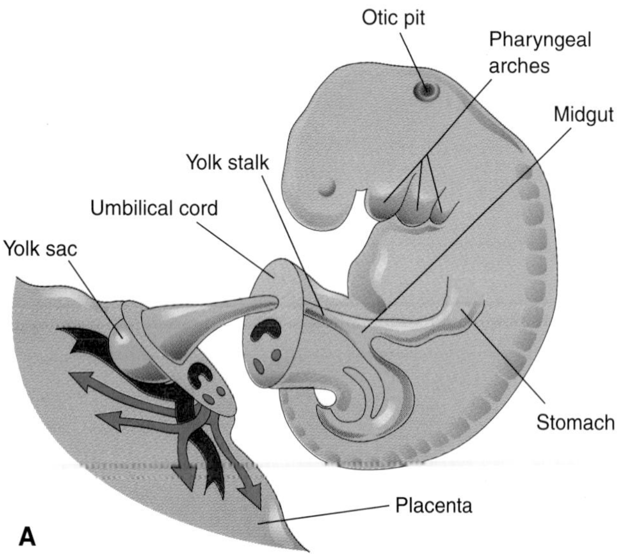

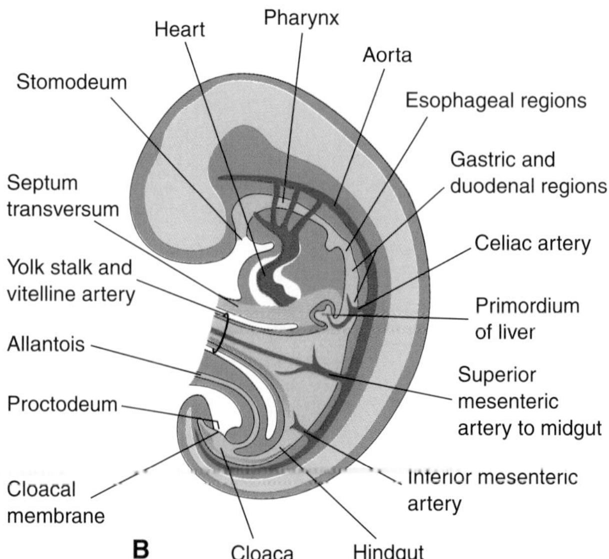

■ **Figure 12-1.** *A*, Lateral view of a 4-week-old embryo showing the relationship of the primordial gut to yolk sac. *B*, Drawing of a median section of the embryo showing the early digestive system and its blood supply. The primordial gut is a long tube extending the length of the embryo. Its blood vessels are derived from the vessels that supplied the yolk sac.

other congenital anomalies, e.g., *anorectal atresia* and anomalies of the urogenital system. In these cases the atresia results from *failure of recanalization of the esophagus* during the eighth week of development. The cause of this arrest of development is thought to result from defective growth of endodermal cells (Herbst, 1996).

A fetus with esophageal atresia is unable to swallow amniotic fluid; consequently, this fluid cannot pass to the intestine for absorption and transfer through the placenta to the maternal blood for disposal. This results in **polyhydramnios**, the accumulation of an excessive amount of amniotic fluid. Newborn infants with esophageal atresia usually appear healthy, and their first swallows are normal. Suddenly, fluid returns through the nose and mouth and *respiratory distress* occurs. Inability to pass a catheter through the esophagus into the stomach strongly suggests esophageal atresia. A radiographic examination demonstrates the anomaly by imaging the nasogastric tube arrested in the proximal esophageal pouch. Surgical repair of esophageal atresia now results in survival rates of more than 85%.

Esophageal Stenosis

Narrowing of the lumen of the esophagus can exist anywhere, but it usually occurs in its distal third, either as a web or a long segment of esophagus with a threadlike lumen. Esophageal stenosis usually results from incomplete recanalization of the esophagus during the eighth week of development, but it may result from a failure of esophageal blood vessels to develop in the affected area. As a result, atrophy of a segment of the esophageal wall occurs.

Short Esophagus

Initially the esophagus is very short. If it fails to elongate sufficiently as the neck and thorax develop, part of the stomach may be displaced superiorly through the esophageal hiatus into the thorax—**congenital hiatal hernia**. Most hiatal hernias occur long after birth, usually in middle-aged people, and result from weakening and widening of the esophageal hiatus in the diaphragm (Moore, 1992).

Development of the Stomach

The distal part of the foregut is initially a simple tubular structure (Fig. 12-1*B*). Around the middle of the fourth week, a slight dilation indicates the site of the future stomach. It first appears as a fusiform enlargement of the caudal part of the foregut and is initially oriented in the median plane (Figs. 12-1 and 12-2*B*). This primordium soon enlarges and broadens ventrodorsally. During the next 2 weeks the dorsal border of the primitive stomach grows faster than its ventral border; this demarcates the **greater curvature of the stomach** (Fig. 12-2*D*). For an account of the kinetics of cell proliferation during morphogenesis of the stomach, see Menard and Arsenault (1990).

ROTATION OF THE STOMACH

As the stomach enlarges and acquires its adult shape, it slowly rotates 90 degrees in a clockwise direction around its longitudinal axis. The effects of rotation on the stomach are (Figs. 12-2 and 12-3):

- The ventral border (lesser curvature) moves to the right and the dorsal border (greater curvature) moves to the left.
- The original left side becomes the ventral surface and the original right side becomes the dorsal surface.
- Before rotation, the cranial and caudal ends of the stomach are in the median plane (Fig. 12-2*B*). During rotation and growth of the stomach, its cranial region moves to the left and slightly inferiorly, and its caudal region moves to the right and superiorly.
- After rotation, the stomach assumes its final position with its long axis almost transverse to the long axis of the body (Fig. 12-2*E*). The rotation and growth of the stomach explain why the left vagus nerve supplies the anterior wall of the adult stomach and the right vagus nerve innervates its posterior wall.

MESENTERIES OF THE STOMACH

The stomach is suspended from the dorsal wall of the abdominal cavity by a dorsal mesentery—the **dorsal mesogastrium** (Fig. 12-3*A*). This mesentery is originally in the median plane but it is carried to the left during rotation of the stomach and formation of the *omental bursa* or lesser sac of peritoneum (Fig. 12-3*A* to *C*). A ventral mesentery or **ventral mesogastrium** attaches the stomach and duodenum to the liver and the ventral abdominal wall (Fig. 12-2*C*).

The Omental Bursa (Lesser Peritoneal Sac)

Isolated clefts (cavities) develop in the mesenchyme forming the thick dorsal mesogastrium (Fig. 12-3*A* and *B*). The clefts soon coalesce to form a single cavity—the **omental bursa** or lesser peritoneal sac (Fig. 12-3*C* and *D*). Rotation of the stomach is thought to pull the dorsal mesogastrium to the left, thereby enlarging the bursa, a large recess of the peritoneal cavity. The omental bursa expands transversely and cranially and soon lies between the stomach and the posterior abdominal wall. This pouchlike bursa (L., purse) facilitates movements of the stomach.

The superior part of the omental bursa is cut off as the diaphragm develops, forming a closed space—the *infracardiac bursa*. If it persists, it usually lies medial to the base of the right lung. The inferior portion of the superior part of the omental bursa persists as the

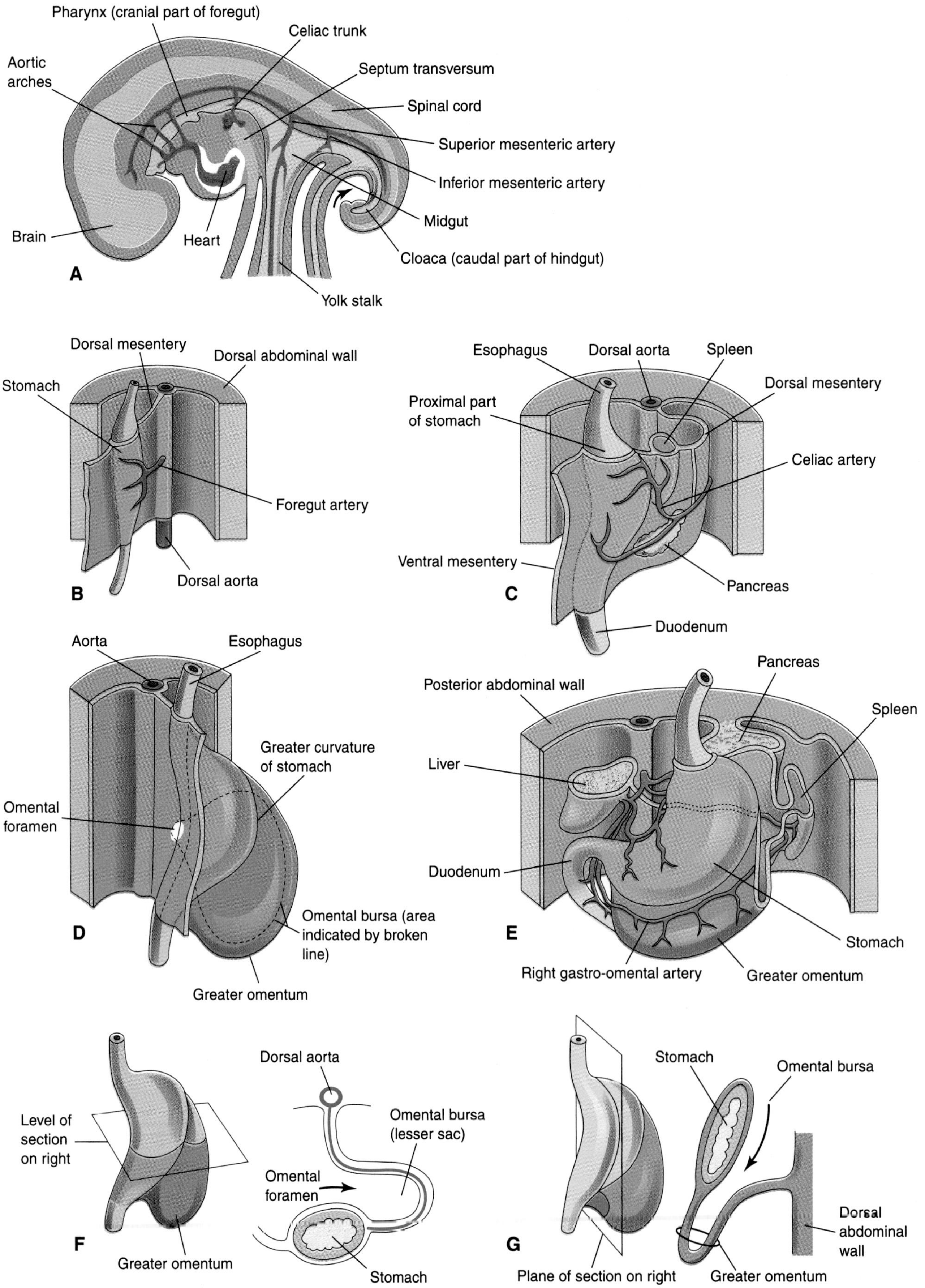

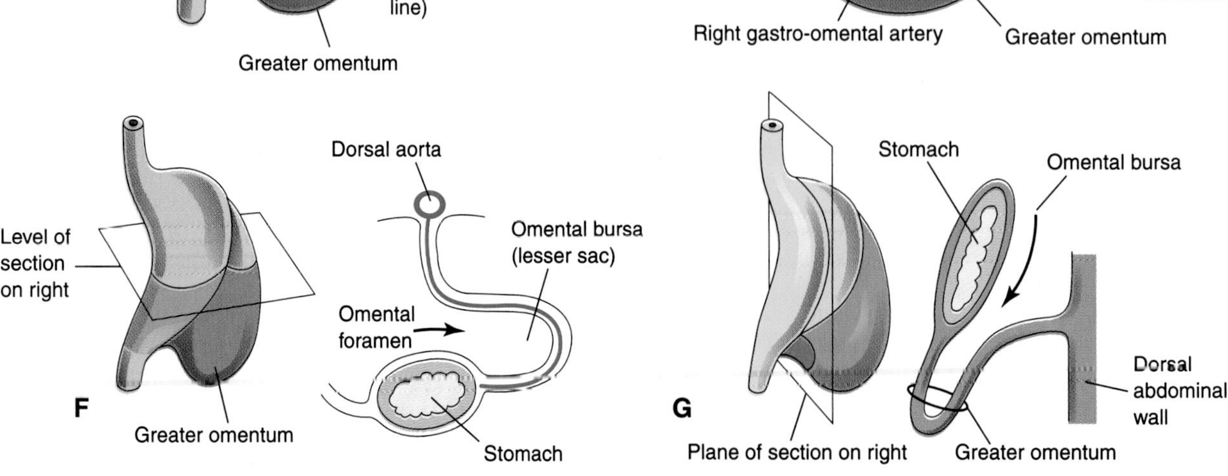

■ **Figure 12–2.** Drawings illustrating development and rotation of the stomach and formation of the omental bursa (lesser sac) and greater omentum. *A*, Drawing of a median section of a 28-day-old embryo. *B*, Anterolateral view of a 28-day-old embryo. *C*, Embryo about 35 days. *D*, Embryo about 40 days. *E*, Embryo about 48 days. *F*, Lateral view of the stomach and greater omentum of an embryo at about 52 days. The transverse section shows the omental foramen and omental bursa. *G*, Sagittal section showing the omental bursa and greater omentum.

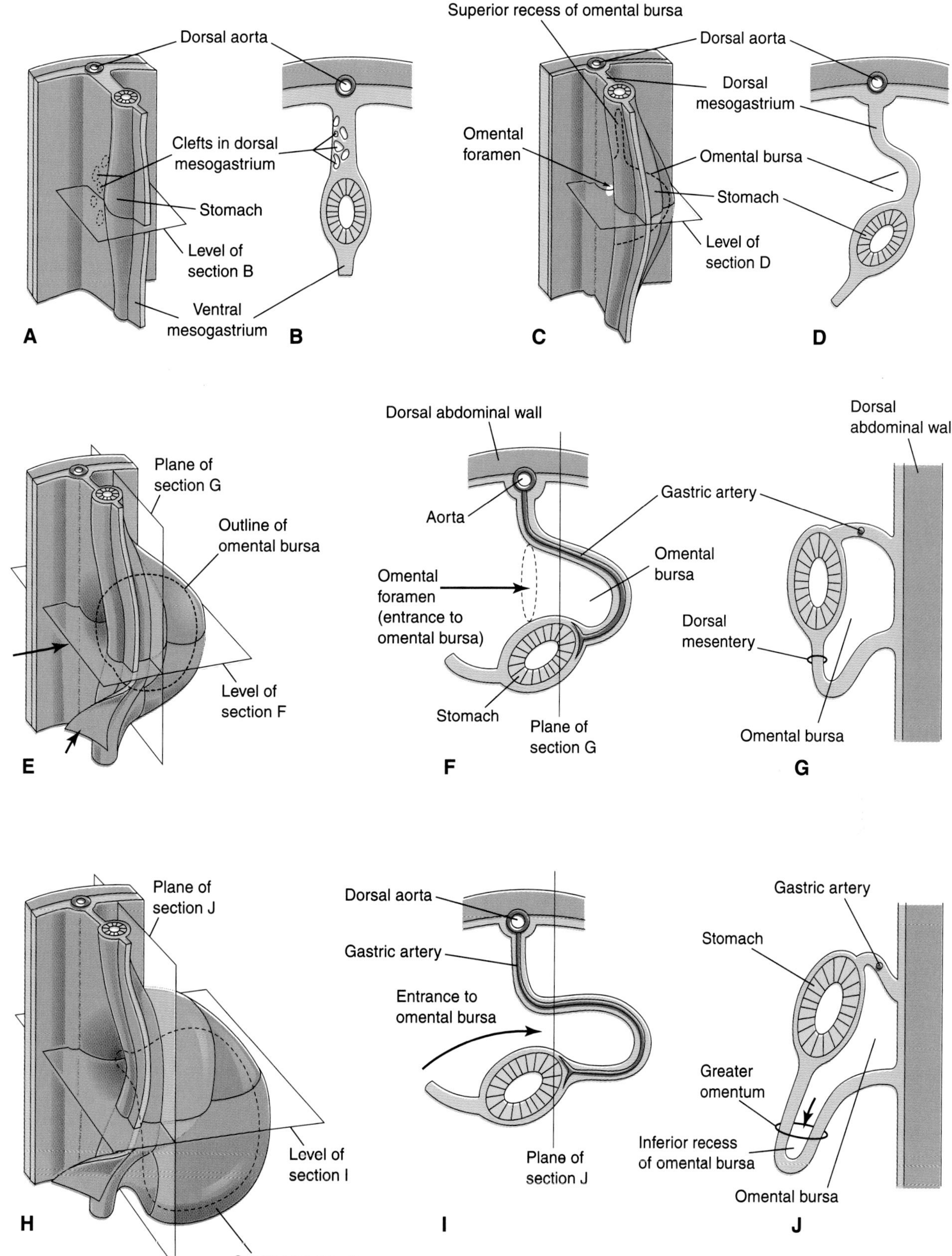

■ **Figure 12–3.** Drawings illustrating development of the stomach and its mesenteries, and formation of the omental bursa (lesser sac). *A*, 5 weeks. *B*, Transverse section showing clefts in the dorsal mesogastrium. *C*, Later stage after coalescence of the clefts to form the omental bursa. *D*, Transverse section showing the initial appearance of the omental bursa. *E*, The dorsal mesentery has elongated and the omental bursa has enlarged. *F* and *G*, Transverse and sagittal sections, respectively, showing elongation of the dorsal mesogastrium and expansion of the omental bursa. *H*, 6 weeks, showing the greater omentum and expansion of the omental bursa. *I* and *J*, Transverse and sagittal sections, respectively, showing the inferior recess of the omental bursa and the omental foramen.

superior recess of the omental bursa (Moore, 1992). As the stomach enlarges, the omental bursa expands and acquires an **inferior recess of the omental bursa** between the layers of the elongated dorsal mesogastrium—the **greater omentum** (L., fat skin). This four-layered membrane overhangs the developing intestines (Fig. 12-3*J*). The inferior recess disappears as the layers of the greater omentum fuse (see Fig. 12-15*F*). The omental bursa communicates with the main part of the peritoneal cavity through a small opening—the **omental (epiploic) foramen** (Figs. 12-2*D* and *F* and 12-3*E* and *F*). In the adult, this foramen is located posterior to the free edge of the lesser omentum (Moore, 1992).

Congenital Hypertrophic Pyloric Stenosis

Anomalies of the stomach are uncommon except for hypertrophic pyloric stenosis (Wyllie, 1996). This anomaly affects one in every 150 males and one in every 750 females. In infants with this abnormality, there is a marked **thickening of the pylorus**, the distal sphincteric region of the stomach (Fig. 12-4). The circular and, to a lesser degree, the longitudinal muscles in the pyloric region are hypertrophied. This results in severe *stenosis (narrowing) of the pyloric canal* and obstruction to the passage of food. As a result, the stomach becomes markedly distended and the infant expels the stomach's contents with considerable force (**projectile vomiting**). Surgical relief of the pyloric obstruction is the usual treatment. The cause of congenital pyloric stenosis is unknown, but the high incidence of the condition in both infants of monozygotic twins suggests the involvement of genetic factors. Multifactorial inheritance of this disorder is likely (Wyllie, 1996). For a discussion of the inheritance of congenital pyloric stenosis, see Thompson et al. (1991).

Development of the Duodenum

Early in the fourth week the duodenum begins to develop from the caudal part of the foregut, the cranial part of the midgut, and the splanchnic mesenchyme associated with these endodermal parts of the primordial gut (Fig. 12-5*A*). The junction of the two parts of the duodenum is just distal to the origin of the bile duct (common bile duct). The developing duodenum grows rapidly, forming a C-shaped loop that projects ventrally (Fig. 12-5*B* to *D*). As the stomach rotates, the duodenal loop rotates to the right and comes to lie retroperitoneally (external to the peritoneum). Because of its derivation from the foregut and midgut, the duodenum is supplied by branches of the celiac and superior mesenteric arteries that supply these parts of the primitive gut (Fig. 12-1). During the fifth and sixth weeks, the lumen of the duodenum becomes progressively smaller and is temporarily obliterated because of the proliferation of its epithelial cells. Normally vacuolation occurs because of degeneration of the epithelial cells; as a result, the duodenum normally becomes recanalized by the end of the embry-

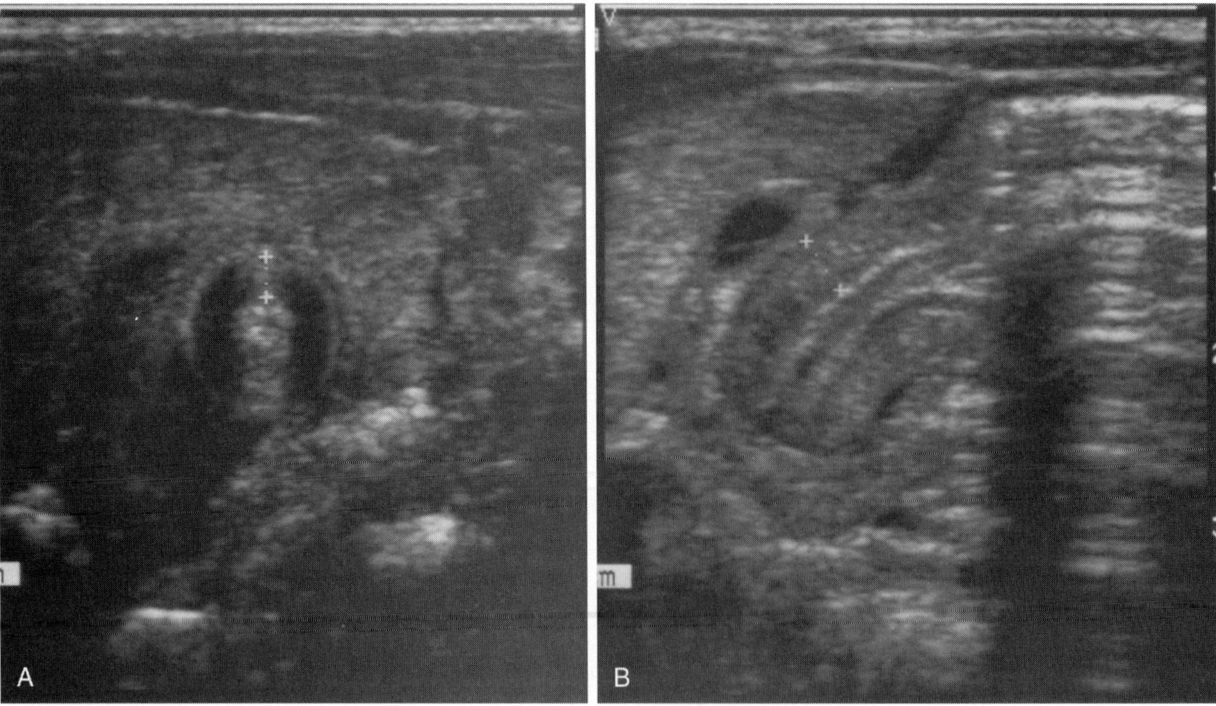

■ **Figure 12-4.** *A*, Transverse abdominal sonogram demonstrating a pyloric muscle wall thickness of greater than 4 mm (distance between crosses). *B*, Horizontal image demonstrating a pyloric channel length greater than 14 mm (wall thickness outlined between crosses) in an infant with hypertrophic pyloric stenosis. (From Wyllie R: Pyloric stenosis and other congenital anomalies of the stomach. *In* Behrman RE, Kliegman RM, Arvin AM [eds]: *Nelson Textbook of Pediatrics,* 15th ed. Philadelphia, WB Saunders, 1996.)

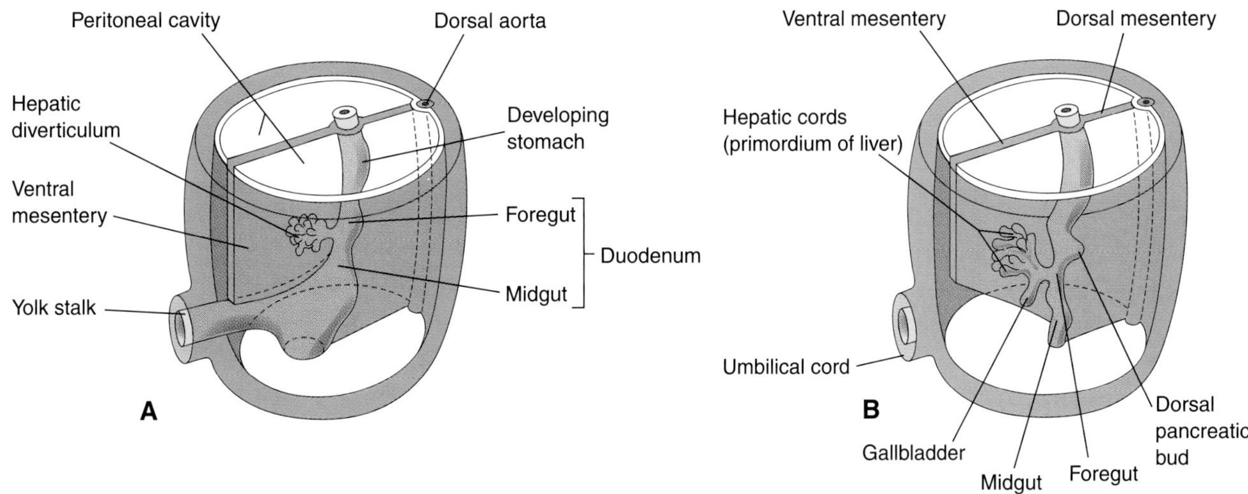

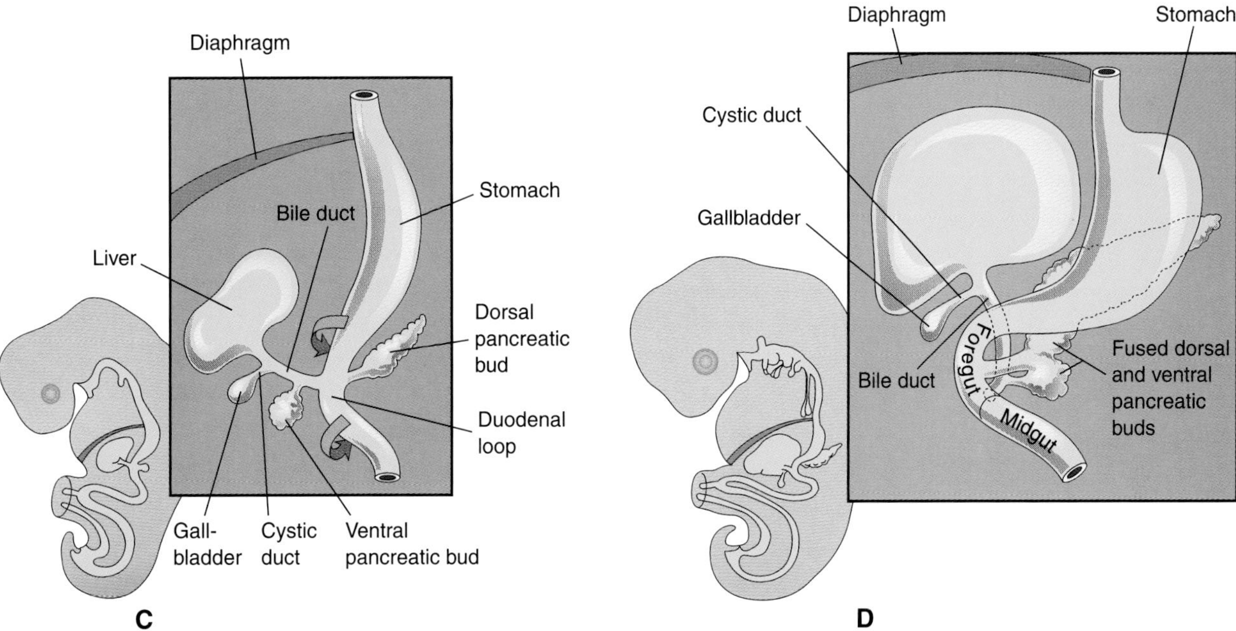

■ **Figure 12–5.** Drawings illustrating progressive stages in the development of the duodenum, liver, pancreas, and extrahepatic biliary apparatus. *A*, 4 weeks. *B* and *C*, 5 weeks. *D*, 6 weeks. The pancreas develops from dorsal and ventral buds that fuse to form the pancreas. Note that the entrance of the bile duct into the duodenum gradually shifts from its initial position to a posterior one. This explains why the bile duct in the adult passes posterior to the duodenum and the head of the pancreas.

onic period (Fig. 12-6*C* and *D*). By this time most of the ventral mesentery of the duodenum has disappeared.

Duodenal Stenosis

Partial occlusion of the duodenal lumen—duodenal stenosis (Fig. 12-6*A*)—usually results from incomplete recanalization of the duodenum resulting from defective vacuolization (Fig. 12-6E_3). Most stenoses involve the horizontal (third) and/or ascending (fourth) parts of the duodenum. Because of the occlusion, the stomach's contents (usually containing bile) are often expelled.

Duodenal Atresia

Complete occlusion of the lumen of the duodenum—duodenal atresia (Fig. 12-6*B*)—is not common. Twenty to 30% of affected infants have Down syndrome and an additional 20% are premature (Wyllie, 1996). In about 20% of cases, the bile duct enters the duodenum just distal to the opening of the hepatopancreatic ampulla (Moore, 1992). During duodenal development, the lumen is completely occluded by epithelial cells. If reformation of the lumen fails to occur (Fig. 12-6D_3), a short segment of the duodenum is occluded (Fig. 12-6F_2). Investigation of families with *familial duodenal atresia* suggests an autosomal recessive inheritance (Best et al., 1989). Most atresias involve the descending

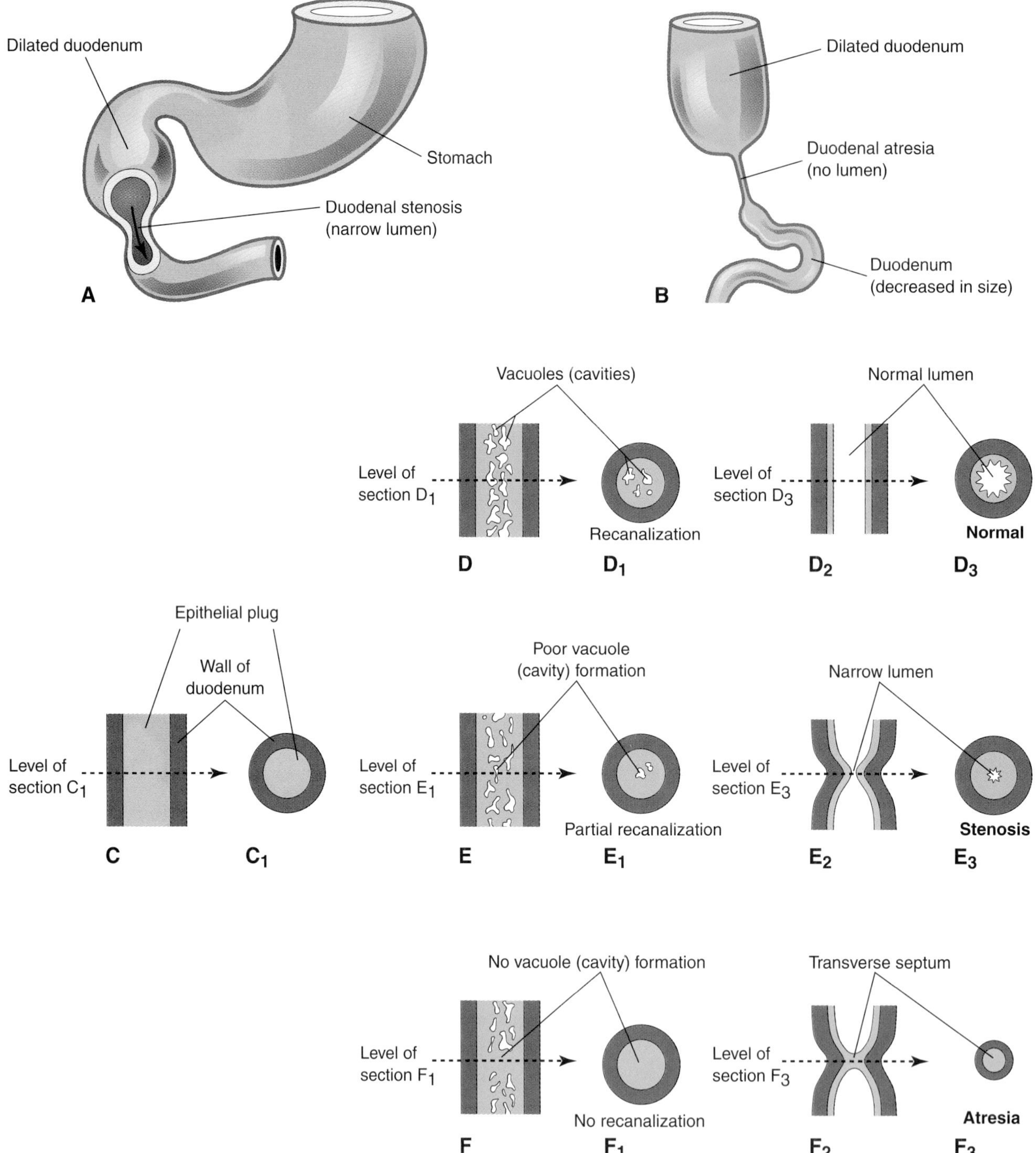

■ **Figure 12–6.** Diagrams illustrating the embryological basis of the two common types of congenital intestinal obstruction. *A*, Duodenal stenosis. *B*, Duodenal atresia. *C* to *F*, Diagrammatic longitudinal and transverse sections of the duodenum showing (1) normal recanalization (*D* to D_3), (2) stenosis (*E* to E_3), and atresia (*F* to F_3). Most duodenal atresias occur in the descending (second) and horizontal (third) parts of the duodenum.

(second) and horizontal (third) parts of the duodenum and are located distal to the opening of the bile duct.

In infants with duodenal atresia, vomiting begins within a few hours of birth. The vomitus almost always contains bile; often, there is *distention of the epigastrium*—the upper central area of the abdomen—resulting from an overfilled stomach and superior part of the duodenum. Duodenal atresia may occur as an isolated anomaly, but other severe congenital anomalies are often associated with it; e.g, Down syndrome, anular pancreas, cardiovascular abnormalities, and anorectal anomalies. **Polyhydramnios** also occurs because duodenal atresia prevents normal absorption of amniotic fluid by the intestines. The diagnosis of duodenal atresia is suggested by the presence of a "double bubble sign" on plain radiographs or ultrasound scans (Fig. 12–7). The double bubble appearance is caused by a distended, gas-filled stomach and proximal duodenum.

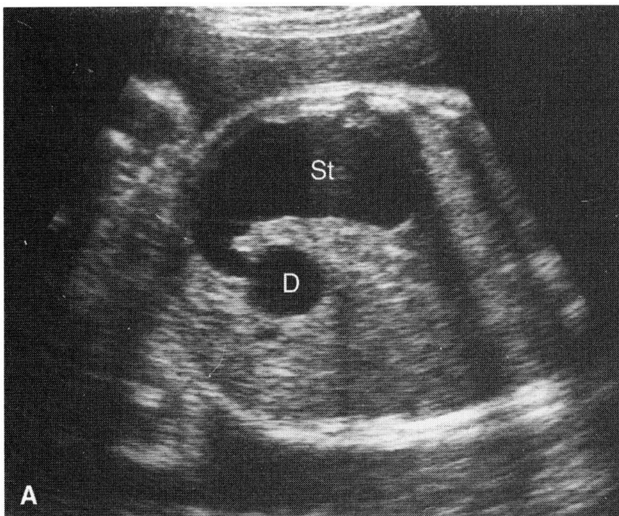

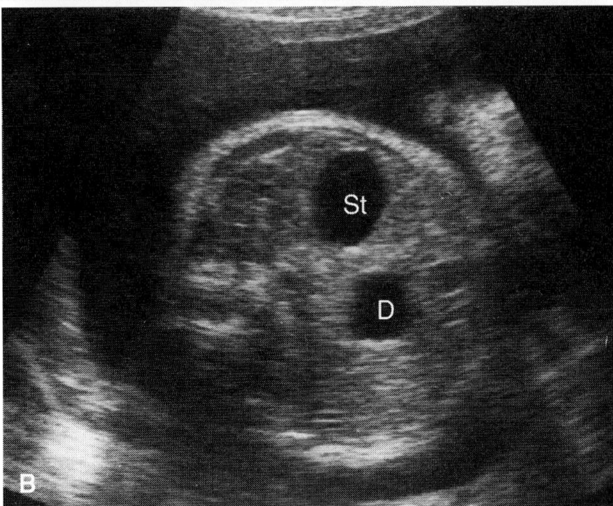

■ **Figure 12–7.** Ultrasound scans of a fetus at 33 weeks of gestation (31 weeks after fertilization) showing duodenal atresia. *A*, An oblique scan showing the dilated, fluid-filled stomach **(St)** entering the proximal duodenum **(D)**, which is also enlarged because of the atresia (blockage) distal to it. *B*, Transverse scan illustrating the characteristic "double bubble" appearance of the stomach and duodenum when there is duodenal atresia. (Courtesy of Dr. Lyndon M. Hill, Magee-Women's Hospital, Pittsburgh, Pennsylvania.)

Development of the Liver and Biliary Apparatus

The liver, gallbladder, and biliary duct system arise as a ventral outgrowth from the caudal part of the foregut early in the fourth week (Figs. 12-5*A* and 12-8*A*). The **hepatic diverticulum** (liver bud) extends into the septum transversum, a mass of splanchnic mesoderm between the developing heart and midgut. The septum transversum forms the central tendon of the diaphragm (see Chapter 9) and the ventral mesentery in this region. The hepatic diverticulum enlarges rapidly and divides into two parts as it grows between the layers of the *ventral mesentery* (Fig. 12-5*A*). The larger cranial part of the hepatic diverticulum is the **primordium of the liver**. The proliferating endodermal cells give rise to interlacing cords of hepatic cells and to the epithelial lining of the intrahepatic portion of the biliary apparatus. The *hepatic cords* anastomose around endothelium-lined spaces, the primordia of the *hepatic sinusoids*. The fibrous and *hematopoietic tissue* and *Kupffer cells* of the liver are derived from mesenchyme in the septum transversum.

The liver grows rapidly and, from the fifth to tenth weeks, fills a large part of the abdominal cavity (Fig. 12-8*C* and *D*). The quantity of oxygenated blood flowing from the umbilical vein into the liver determines the development and functional segmentation of the liver (Champetier et al., 1989b). Initially, the right and left lobes are about the same size, but the right lobe soon becomes larger. *Hematopoiesis begins during the sixth week*, giving the liver a bright reddish appearance. This hemopoietic activity (formation of various types of blood cells and other formed elements) is mainly responsible for the relatively large size of the liver between the seventh and ninth weeks of development. By the ninth week, the liver accounts for about 10% of the total weight of the fetus. *Bile formation* by the hepatic cells begins during the twelfth week.

The small caudal part of the hepatic diverticulum becomes the **gallbladder**, and the stalk of the diverticulum forms the **cystic duct** (Fig. 12-5*C*). Initially, the extrahepatic biliary apparatus is occluded with epithelial cells, but it is later canalized because of vacuolation resulting from degeneration of these cells. The stalk connecting the hepatic and cystic ducts to the duodenum becomes the **bile duct** (common bile duct). Initially, this duct attaches to the ventral aspect of the duodenal loop; however, as the duodenum grows and rotates, the entrance of the bile duct is carried to the dorsal aspect of the duodenum (Fig. 12-5*C* and *D*). The bile entering the duodenum through the bile duct after the thirteenth week gives the **meconium** (intestinal contents) a dark green color.

THE VENTRAL MESENTERY

This thin, double-layered membrane gives rise to:

- the *lesser omentum*, passing from the liver to the lesser curvature of the stomach (*hepatogastric ligament*) and from the liver to the duodenum (*hepatoduodenal ligament*)
- the *falciform ligament*, extending from the liver to the ventral abdominal wall

The *umbilical vein* passes in the free border of the falciform ligament on its way from the umbilical cord to the liver. The ventral mesentery also forms the *visceral peritoneum of the liver*. The liver is covered by peritoneum except for the *bare area* that is in direct contact with the diaphragm.

Anomalies of the Liver

Minor variations of liver lobulation are common but congenital anomalies of the liver are rare. Variations of the hepatic ducts, bile duct, and cystic duct are common and clinically significant (Moore, 1992). *Accessory hepatic ducts* may be present, and awareness of their possible presence is of surgical importance. These accessory ducts are narrow channels running from the right lobe of the liver into the anterior surface of the body of the gallbladder. In some cases, the cystic duct opens into an accessory hepatic duct rather than into the common hepatic duct.

Extrahepatic Biliary Atresia

This is the most serious anomaly of the extrahepatic biliary system and occurs in 1:10,000 to 15,000 live births (Balistreri, 1996). The most common form of extrahepatic biliary atresia (present in 85% of cases) is obstruction of the ducts at or superior to the *porta hepatis*—a deep transverse fissure on the visceral surface of the liver, about 5 cm long in adults (Moore, 1992). Failure of the bile ducts to canalize often results from persistence of the solid stage of duct development. Biliary atresia could also result from liver infection during late fetal development. *Jaundice* occurs soon after birth. When biliary atresia cannot be corrected surgically, the child may die if a liver transplant is not performed (Karrer and Raffensperger, 1990).

Development of the Pancreas

The pancreas develops between the layers of the mesentery from dorsal and ventral **pancreatic buds of endodermal cells** that arise from the caudal part of the foregut that is developing into the proximal part of the duodenum (Figs. 12-9 and 12-10*A* and *B*). Most of the pancreas is derived from the dorsal pan-

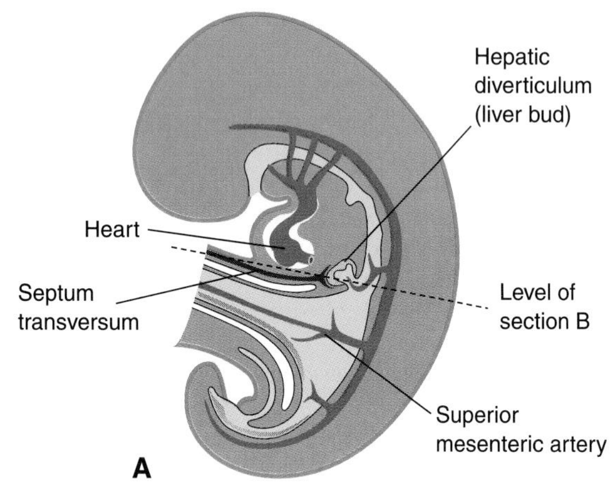

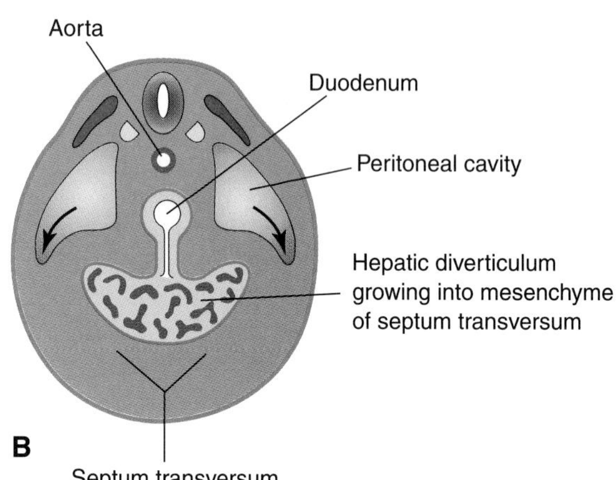

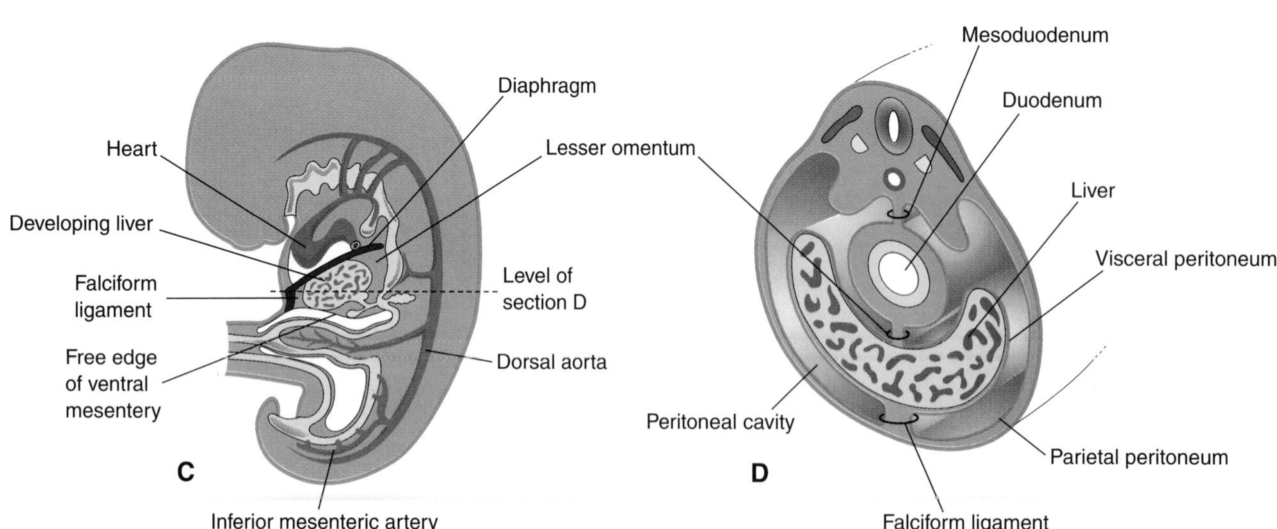

■ **Figure 12–8.** Drawings illustrating how the caudal part of the septum transversum becomes stretched and membranous as it forms the ventral mesentery. *A*, Median section of a 4-week embryo. *B*, Transverse section of the embryo showing expansion of the peritoneal cavity (arrows). *C*, Sagittal section of a 5-week embryo. *D*, Transverse section of the embryo after formation of the dorsal and ventral mesenteries. Note that the liver is joined to the ventral abdominal wall and to the stomach and the duodenum by the falciform ligament and lesser omentum, respectively.

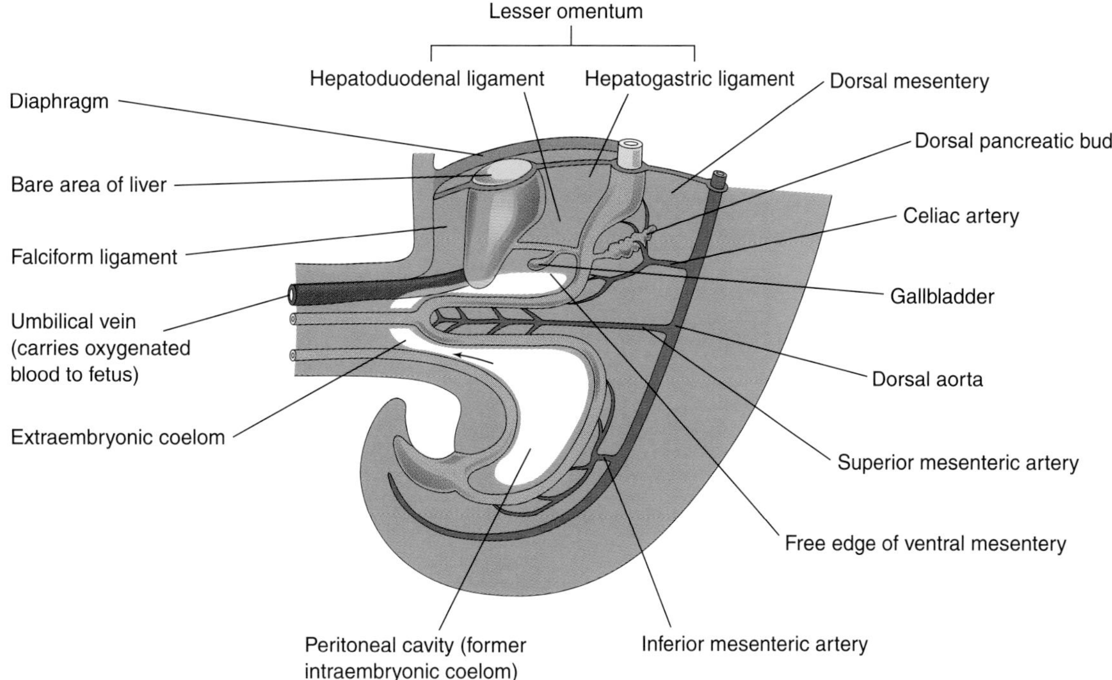

■ **Figure 12–9.** Diagrammatic sketch of a median section of the caudal half of an embryo at the end of the fifth week showing the liver and its associated ligaments. The arrow indicates the communication of the peritoneal cavity with the extraembryonic coelom. Because of the rapid growth of the liver and the midgut loop, the abdominal cavity temporarily becomes too small to contain the developing intestines; consequently, they enter the extraembryonic coelom in the proximal part of the umbilical cord.

creatic bud. The larger **dorsal pancreatic bud** appears first and develops a slight distance cranial to the ventral bud. It grows rapidly between the layers of the dorsal mesentery. The **ventral pancreatic bud** develops near the entry of the bile duct into the duodenum and grows between the layers of the ventral mesentery. As the duodenum rotates to the right and becomes C-shaped, the ventral pancreatic bud is carried dorsally with the bile duct (Fig. 12-10*C* to *G*). It soon lies posterior to the dorsal pancreatic bud and later fuses with it.

The ventral pancreatic bud forms the *uncinate process* and part of the head of the pancreas. As the stomach, duodenum, and ventral mesentery rotate, the pancreas comes to lie along the dorsal abdominal wall. As the pancreatic buds fuse, their ducts anastomose. The **main pancreatic duct** forms from the duct of the ventral bud and the distal part of the duct of the dorsal bud (Fig. 12-10*G*). The proximal part of the duct of the dorsal bud often persists as an *accessory pancreatic duct* that opens into the *minor duodenal papilla*, located about 2 cm cranial to the main duct. The two ducts often communicate with each other. In about 9% of people, the pancreatic duct systems fail to fuse and the original two ducts persist (Moore, 1992).

HISTOGENESIS OF THE PANCREAS

The parenchyma of the pancreas is derived from the endoderm of the pancreatic buds, which forms a network of tubules. Early in the fetal period, acini begin to develop from cell clusters around the ends of these tubules (primordial ducts). The **pancreatic islets** develop from groups of cells that separate from the tubules and soon come to lie between the acini. **Insulin secretion** begins during the early fetal period (10 weeks [von Dorsche, 1990]). The *glucagon-* and *somatostatin*-containing cells develop before differentiation of the insulin-secreting cells. Glucagon has been detected in fetal plasma at 15 weeks (von Dorsche, 1990). With increasing fetal age, the total pancreatic insulin and glucagon content also increases. The connective tissue sheath and interlobular septa of the pancreas develop from the surrounding splanchnic mesenchyme. When there is *maternal diabetes mellitus*, the insulin-secreting beta cells in the fetal pancreas are chronically exposed to high levels of glucose. As a result, these cells undergo hypertrophy in order to increase the rate of insulin secretion (Carr, 1988).

Accessory Pancreatic Tissue

Accessory pancreatic tissue is most often located in the wall of the stomach or duodenum, or in an ileal (Meckel) diverticulum.

Anular Pancreas

Although anular (annular) pancreas is uncommon, the anomaly warrants description because it may cause duodenal obstruction (Fig. 12-11*C*). The ringlike or anular part of the pancreas consists of a thin, flat band of pancreatic tissue surrounding the descending or second part of the duodenum. An anular pancreas may cause obstruction of the duodenum shortly after birth or much later. Blockage of the duodenum develops if inflammation or malignant disease develops in an anular pancreas. An increased incidence of pancreatitis and peptic ulcer have been detected in patients with this abnormal pancreas. Males are affected much more frequently than females. Anular pancreas probably results from the growth of a bifid ventral pancreatic bud around the duodenum (Fig. 12-11*A* to *C*). The parts of the bifid ventral bud then fuse with the dorsal bud, forming a pancreatic ring (L. *anulus*).

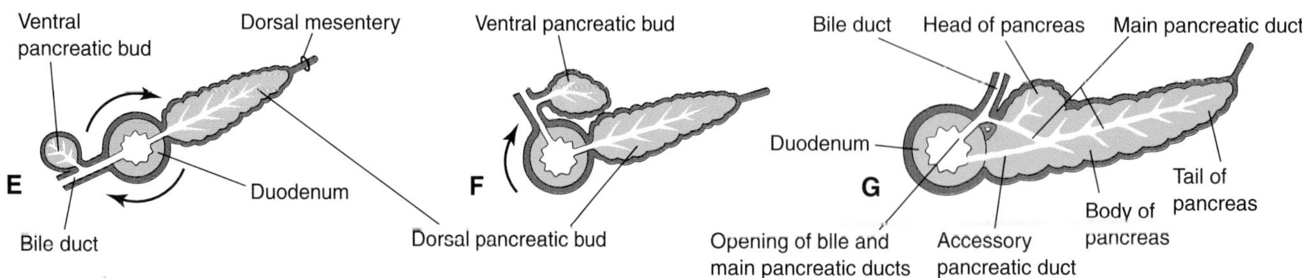

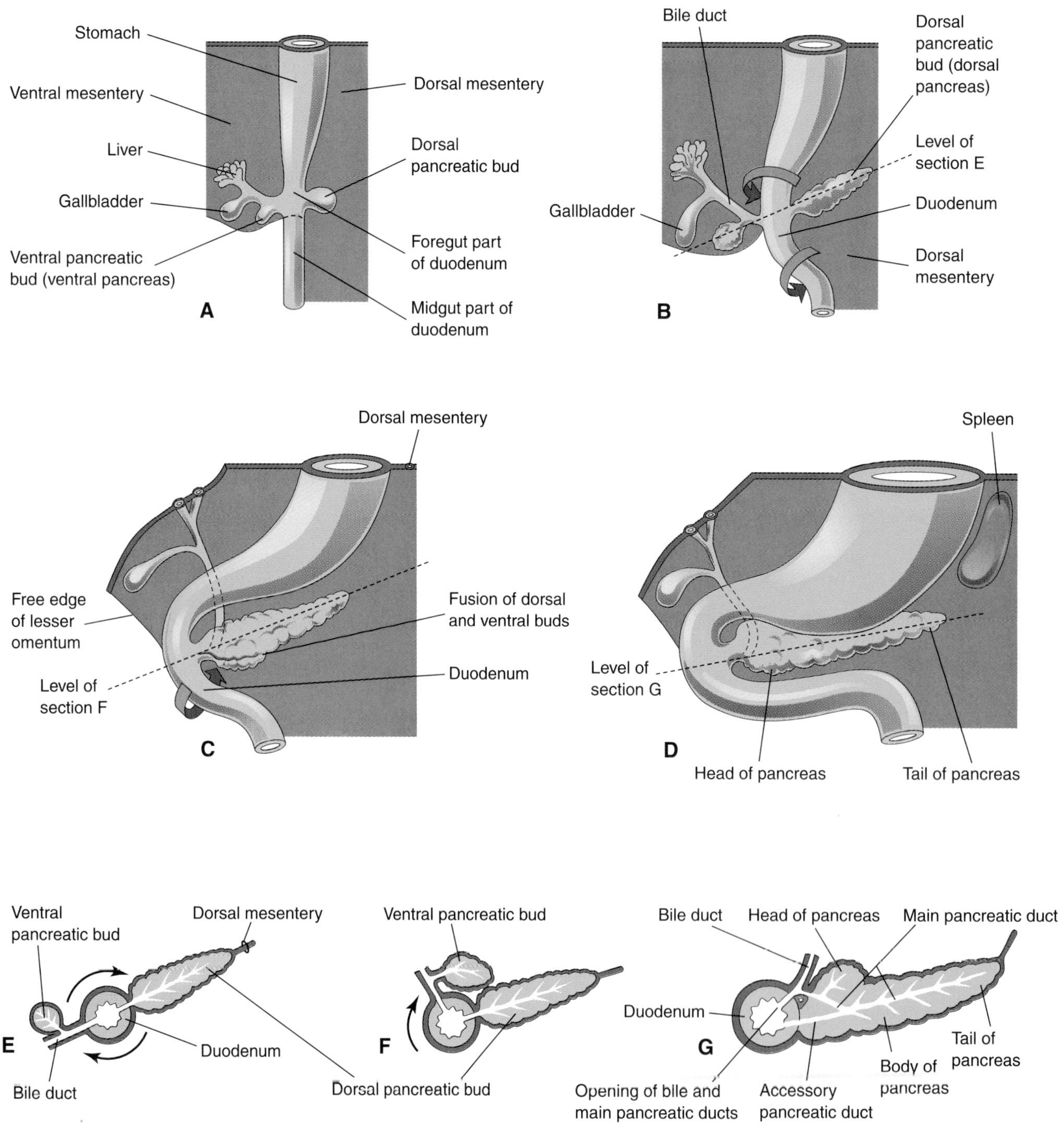

■ **Figure 12-10.** *A* to *D*, Schematic drawings showing successive stages in the development of the pancreas from the fifth to the eighth weeks. *E* to *G*, Diagrammatic transverse sections through the duodenum and developing pancreas. Growth and rotation (arrows) of the duodenum bring the ventral pancreatic bud toward the dorsal bud; they subsequently fuse. Note that the bile duct initially attaches to the ventral aspect of the duodenum and is carried around to the dorsal aspect as the duodenum rotates. The main pancreatic duct is formed by the union of the distal part of the dorsal pancreatic duct and the entire ventral pancreatic duct. The proximal part of the dorsal pancreatic duct usually obliterates, but it may persist as an accessory pancreatic duct.

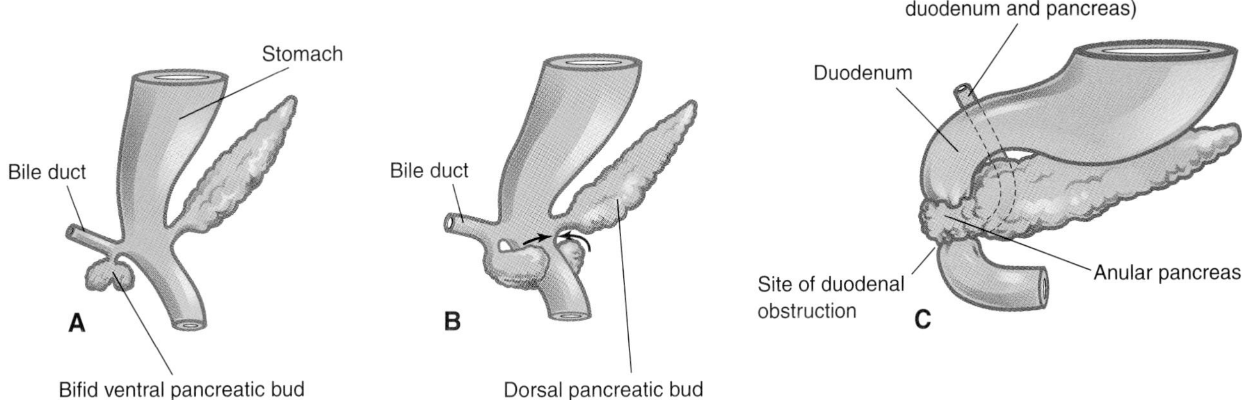

■ **Figure 12–11.** *A* and *B*, Drawings illustrating the probable embryological basis of an anular (annular) pancreas. *C*, An anular pancreas encircling the duodenum. This anomaly sometimes produces complete obstruction (atresia) or partial obstruction (stenosis) of the duodenum. In most cases the anular pancreas encircles the second part of the duodenum, distal to the hepatopancreatic ampulla; see Moore (1992) for a discussion of the clinical anatomy of this ampulla.

DEVELOPMENT OF THE SPLEEN

Development of the spleen is described with the digestive system because this organ is derived from a mass of mesenchymal cells located between the layers of the dorsal mesogastrium (Fig. 12-12). The spleen, a large vascular lymphatic organ, begins to develop during the fifth week but does not acquire its characteristic shape until early in the fetal period. The spleen is lobulated in the fetus but the lobules normally disappear before birth. The notches in the superior border of the adult spleen are remnants of the grooves that separated the fetal lobules (Moore, 1992). As the stomach rotates, the left surface of the mesogastrium fuses with the peritoneum over the left kidney. This fusion explains the dorsal attachment of the *splenorenal ligament* (lienorenal ligament) and why the adult splenic artery, the largest branch of the celiac trunk, follows a tortuous course posterior to the omental bursa and anterior to the left kidney (Fig. 12-12*C*).

Histogenesis of the Spleen

The mesenchymal cells in the splenic primordium differentiate to form the capsule, connective tissue framework, and parenchyma of the spleen. The spleen functions as a hematopoietic center until late fetal life, but it retains its potential for blood cell formation even in adult life.

Accessory Spleen

One or more small splenic masses may develop in one of the peritoneal folds, commonly near the hilum of the spleen or adjacent to the tail of the pancreas. An accessory spleen occurs in about 10% of people and is usually about 1 cm in diameter. An accessory spleen may be embedded partly or wholly in the tail of the pancreas or within the gastrosplenic ligament.

THE MIDGUT

The derivatives of the midgut are:

- the small intestine, including most of the duodenum
- the cecum, vermiform appendix, ascending colon, and the right half to two thirds of the transverse colon

All these midgut derivatives are supplied by the **superior mesenteric artery**, the artery of the midgut (Fig. 12-1). The midgut loop is suspended from the dorsal abdominal wall by an elongated mesentery (Fig. 12-13*A*). As the midgut elongates, it forms a ventral, U-shaped loop of gut—the **midgut loop**—which projects into the remains of the extraembryonic coelom in the proximal part of the umbilical cord. At this stage, the intraembryonic coelom communicates with extraembryonic coelom at the umbilicus (Fig. 12-9). This movement of the intestine is a **physiological umbilical herniation**. It occurs at the beginning of the sixth week and is the normal migration of the midgut into the umbilical cord (Figs. 12-13 and 12-14). The midgut loop communicates with the yolk sac through the narrow *yolk stalk* until the tenth week. Umbilical herniation occurs because there is not enough room in the abdomen for the rapidly growing midgut. The shortage of space is caused mainly by the relatively massive liver and the two sets of kidneys that exist during this period of development.

The midgut loop has a cranial limb and a caudal limb. The *yolk stalk* is attached to the apex of the midgut loop where the two limbs join (Fig. 12-13*A*). The cranial limb grows rapidly and forms small intestinal loops, but the caudal limb undergoes very little change except for development of the **cecal diverticulum**, the primordium of the cecum and appendix (Fig. 12-13*C*).

Rotation of the Midgut Loop

While it is in the umbilical cord, the midgut loop rotates 90 degrees counterclockwise around the axis

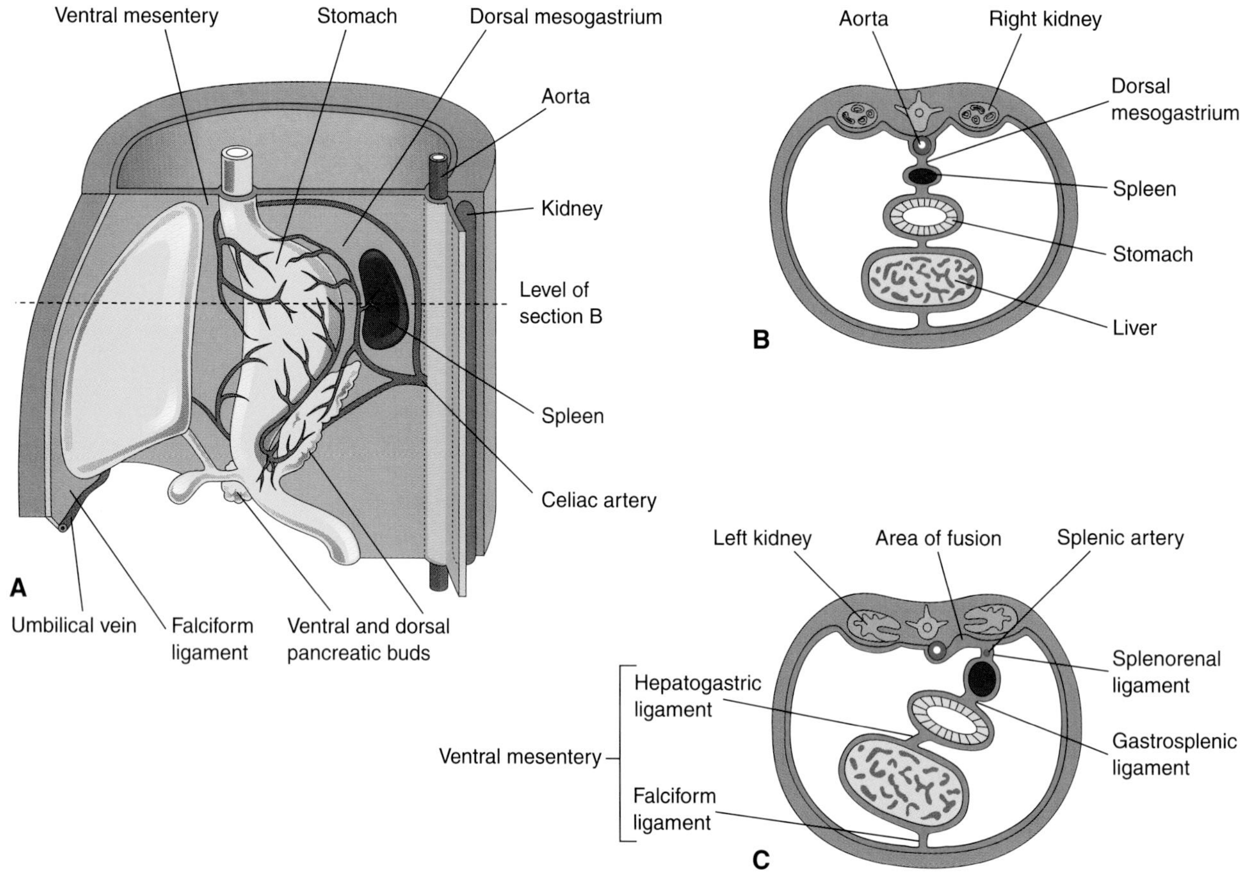

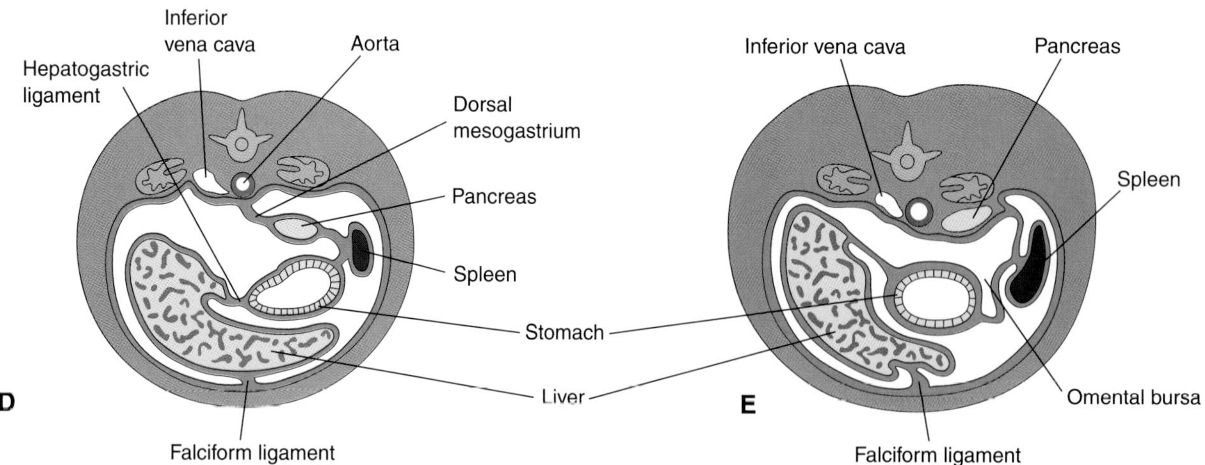

■ **Figure 12–12.** *A*, Drawing of the left side of the stomach and associated structures at the end of the fifth week. Note that the pancreas, spleen, and celiac artery are between the layers of the dorsal mesogastrium. *B*, Transverse section of the liver, stomach, and spleen at the level shown in *A*, illustrating their relationship to the dorsal and ventral mesenteries. *C*, Transverse section of a fetus showing fusion of the dorsal mesogastrium with the peritoneum on the posterior abdominal wall. *D* and *E*, Similar sections showing movement of the liver to the right and rotation of the stomach. Observe the fusion of the dorsal mesogastrium to the dorsal abdominal wall. As a result, the pancreas becomes retroperitoneal.

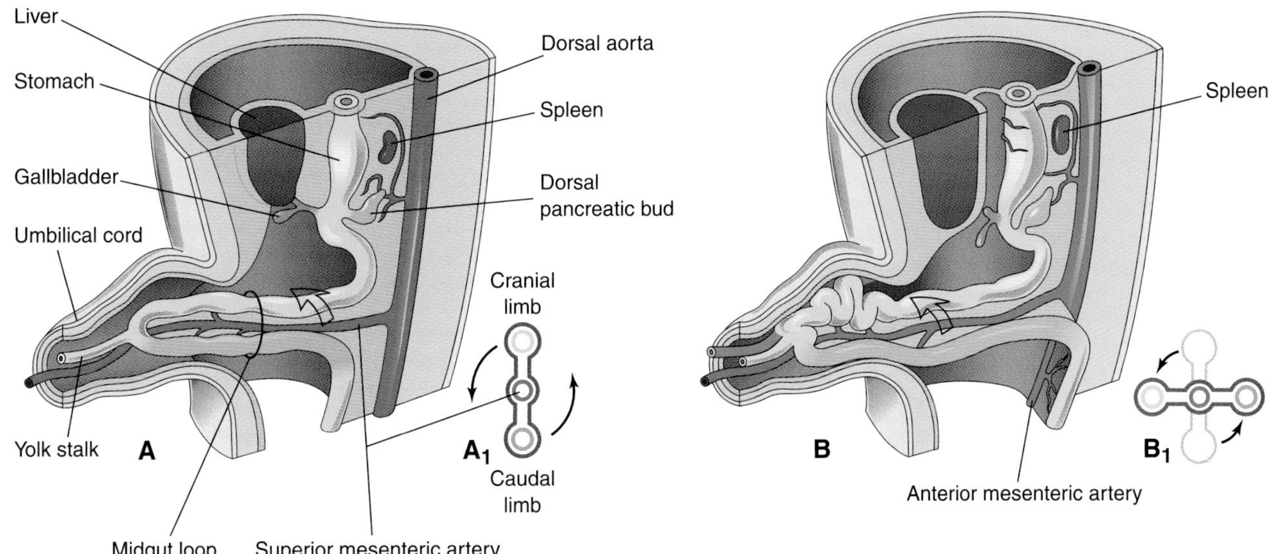

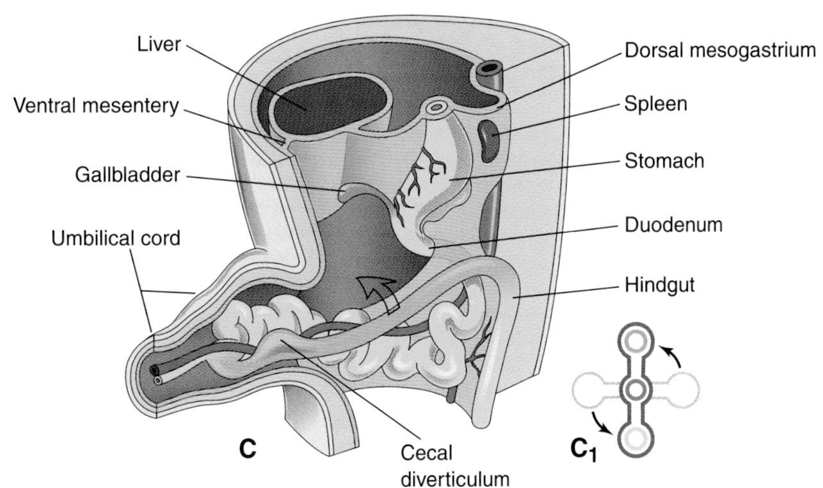

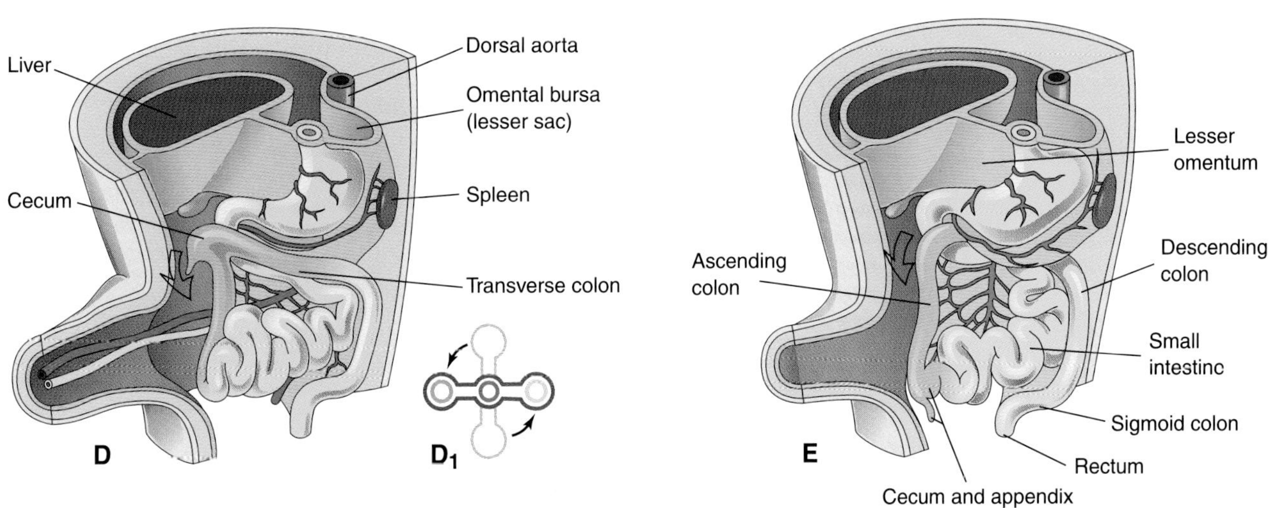

■ **Figure 12–13.** Schematic drawings illustrating the rotation of the midgut, as seen from the left. *A*, Around the beginning of the sixth week, showing the midgut loop in the proximal part of the umbilical cord. *A*, Transverse section through the midgut loop, illustrating the initial relationship of the limbs of the midgut loop to the artery. *B*, Later stage showing the beginning of midgut rotation. B_1, Illustration of the 90-degree counterclockwise rotation that carries the cranial limb of the midgut to the right. *C*, About 10 weeks, showing the intestines returning to the abdomen. C_1, Illustration of a further rotation of 90 degrees. *D*, About 11 weeks, after return of intestines to the abdomen. D_1, illustration of a further 90-degree rotation of the gut, for a total of 270 degrees. *E*, Later fetal period, showing the cecum rotating to its normal position in the lower right quadrant of the abdomen.

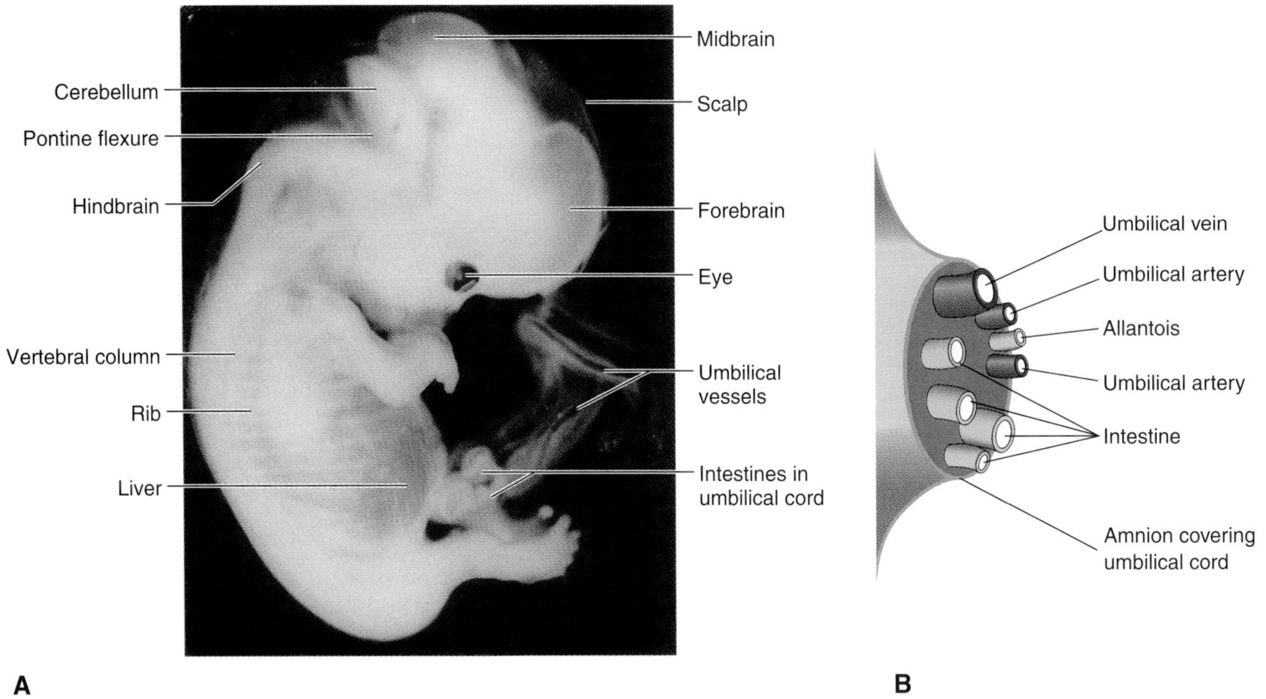

■ **Figure 12–14.** *A*, Photograph of a 28-mm human embryo (about 56 days). Note the herniated intestine derived from the midgut loop in the proximal part of the umbilical cord. Also note the umbilical blood vessels. Observe also the cartilaginous ribs, the prominent eye, the large liver, and the relatively well developed brain. (Courtesy of Dr. Bruce Fraser, formerly Associate Professor of Anatomy, Faculty of Medicine, Memorial University, St. John's, Newfoundland.) *B*, Schematic drawing showing the structures in the proximal part of the umbilical cord.

of the *superior mesenteric artery* (Fig. 12-13*B*). This brings the cranial limb of the midgut loop to the right and the caudal limb to the left. During rotation the midgut elongates and forms loops of small bowel (jejunum and ileum).

RETURN OF THE MIDGUT TO THE ABDOMEN

During the tenth week the intestines return to the abdomen (Fig. 12-13*C* and *D*). It is not known what causes the intestine to return, but the decrease in the size of the liver and kidneys and the enlargement of the abdominal cavity are important factors. This process has been called *reduction of the physiological midgut hernia*. The small intestine (formed from the cranial limb) returns first, passing posterior to the superior mesenteric artery and occupying the central part of the abdomen. As the large intestine returns, it undergoes a further 180-degree counterclockwise rotation (Fig. 12-13C_1 and D_1). Later it comes to occupy the right side of the abdomen. The ascending colon becomes recognizable as the posterior abdominal wall progressively elongates (Fig. 12-13*E*).

FIXATION OF THE INTESTINES

Rotation of the stomach and duodenum causes the duodenum and pancreas to fall to the right, where they are pressed against the posterior abdominal wall by the colon. The adjacent layers of peritoneum fuse and subsequently disappear (Fig. 12-15*C* and *F*); consequently, most of the duodenum and the head of the pancreas become retroperitoneal (posterior to the peritoneum). The attachment of the dorsal mesentery to the posterior abdominal wall is greatly modified after the intestines return to the abdominal cavity. At first the dorsal mesentery is in the median plane. As the intestines enlarge, lengthen, and assume their final positions, their mesenteries are pressed against the posterior abdominal wall. The mesentery of the ascending colon fuses with the parietal peritoneum on this wall and disappears; consequently, the ascending colon also becomes retroperitoneal (Fig. 12-15*B* and *E*).

The enlarged colon presses the duodenum against the posterior abdominal wall; as a result, most of the duodenal mesentery is absorbed (Fig. 12-15*C*, *D*, and *F*). Consequently, the duodenum, except for about the first 2.5 cm (derived from the foregut), has no mesentery and lies retroperitoneally. Other derivatives of the midgut loop (e.g., the jejunum and ileum) retain their mesenteries. The mesentery is at first attached to the median plane of the posterior abdominal wall (Fig. 12-13*B* and *C*). After the mesentery of the ascending colon disappears, the fan-shaped mesentery of the small intestines acquires a new line of attachment that passes from the duodenojejunal junction inferolaterally to the ileocecal junction (Fig. 12-15*D*).

The Cecum and Vermiform Appendix

The primordium of the cecum and wormlike (L. *vermiform*) appendix—the **cecal diverticulum**—appears in the sixth week as a swelling on the antimesenteric border of the caudal limb of the midgut loop (Fig. 12-13*C* and 12-16*A*). The apex of the cecal diverticulum does not grow as rapidly as the rest of it; thus, the appendix is initially a small diverticulum of the cecum (Fig. 12-16*B*). The appendix increases rapidly in length so that at birth it is a relatively long, worm-shaped tube arising from the distal end of the cecum (Fig. 12-16*D*). After birth the wall of the cecum grows unequally, with the result that the appendix comes to enter its medial side (Fig. 12-16*E*). The appendix is subject to considerable variation in position. As the ascending colon elongates, the appendix may pass posterior to the cecum (*retrocecal appendix*) or colon (*retrocolic appendix*). It may also descend over the brim of the pelvis (*pelvic appendix*). *In about 64% of people, the appendix is located retrocecally* (Moore, 1992).

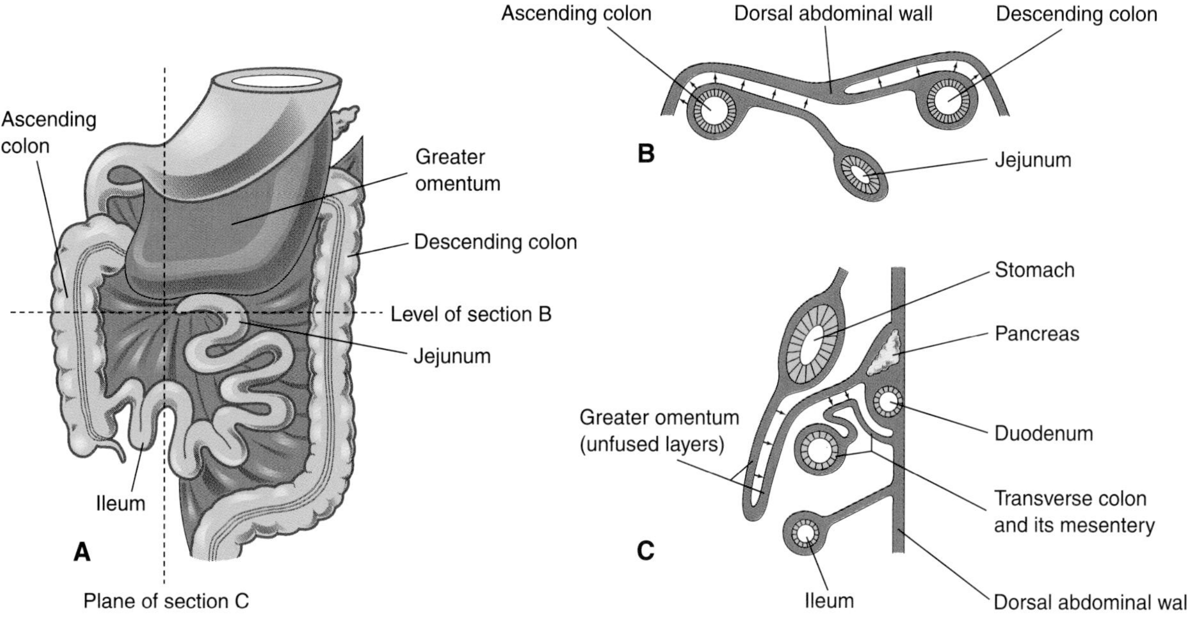

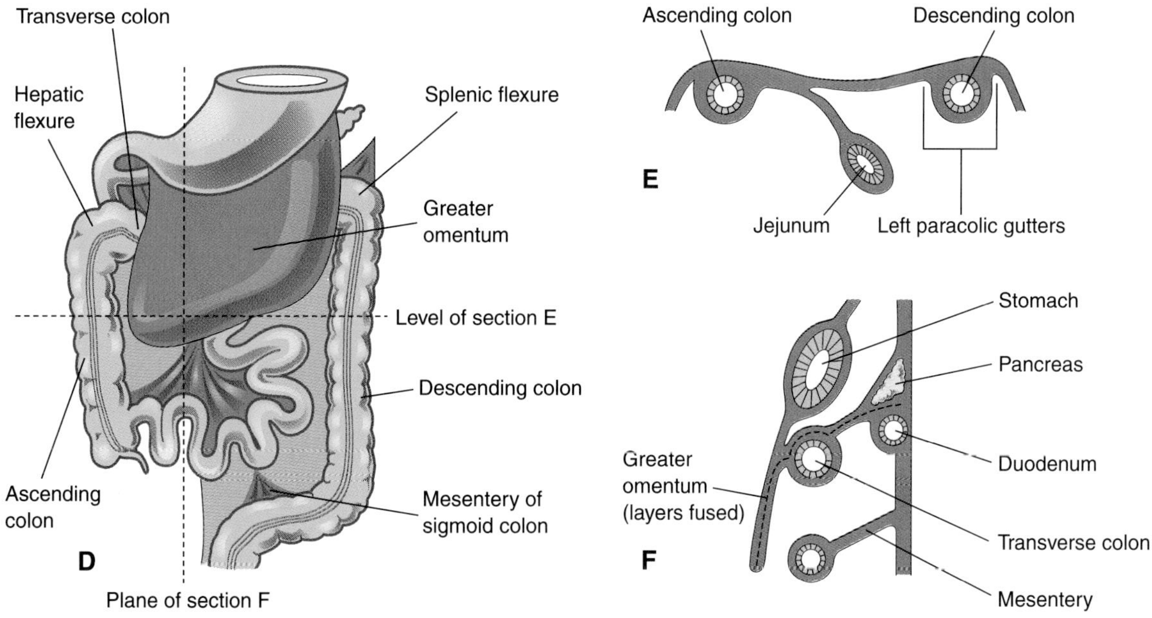

■ **Figure 12-15.** Fixation of the intestines. *A*, Ventral view of the intestines prior to their fixation. *B*, Transverse section at the level shown in *A*. The arrows indicate areas of subsequent fusion. *C*, Sagittal section at the plane shown in *A*, illustrating the greater omentum overhanging the transverse colon. The arrows indicate areas of subsequent fusion. *D*, Ventral view of the intestines after their fixation. *E*, Transverse section at the level shown in *D* after disappearance of the mesentery of the ascending and descending colon. *F*, Sagittal section at the plane shown in *D*, illustrating fusion of the greater omentum with the mesentery of the transverse colon and fusion of the layers of the greater omentum.

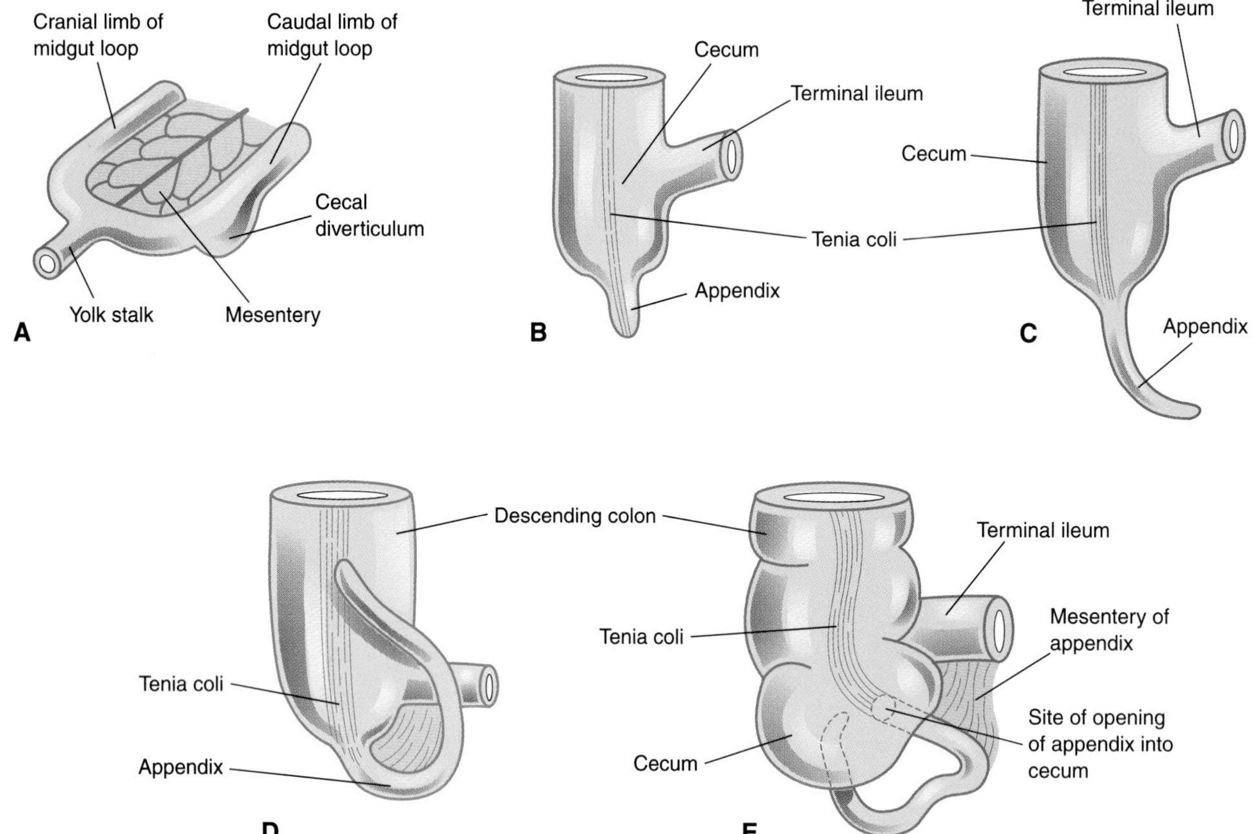

■ **Figure 12–16.** Drawings showing successive stages in the development of the cecum and vermiform appendix. *A*, 6 weeks. *B*, 8 weeks. *C*, 12 weeks. *D*, At birth. Note that the appendix is relatively long and is continuous with the apex of the cecum. *E*, Adult. Note the appendix is now relatively short and lies on the medial side of the cecum. In about 64% of people, the appendix is located posterior to the cecum (retrocecal). In about 32% of people, it appears as illustrated in *E*. The tenia coli is a thickened band of longitudinal muscle in the wall of the colon, which ends at the base of the appendix.

Anomalies of the Midgut

Congenital abnormalities of the intestine are common; most of them are anomalies of gut rotation—**malrotation of the gut**—that result from incomplete rotation and/or fixation of the intestines.

Congenital Omphalocele

This anomaly is a persistence of the herniation of abdominal contents into the proximal part of the umbilical cord (Figs. 12-17 and 12-18). Herniation of intestines into the cord occurs in about 1 of 5000 births and herniation of liver and intestines in 1 of about 10,000 births (Kleigman, 1996). The size of the hernia depends on its contents. The abdominal cavity is proportionately small when there is an omphalocele because the impetus for it to grow is absent. Immediate surgical repair is required (Behrman et al., 1996). Omphalocele results from failure of the intestines to return to the abdominal cavity during the tenth week. The covering of the hernial sac is the epithelium of the umbilical cord, a derivative of the amnion.

Umbilical Hernia

When the intestines return to the abdominal cavity during the tenth week and then herniate through an imperfectly closed umbilicus, an umbilical hernia forms. This common type of hernia is different from an omphalocele. In umbilical hernia, the protruding mass (usually the greater omentum and some of the small intestine) is covered by subcutaneous tissue and skin. The hernia usually does not reach its maximum size until the end of the first month after birth. It usually ranges from 1 to 5 cm. The defect through which the hernia occurs is in the linea alba (Moore, 1992). The hernia protrudes during crying, straining, or coughing and can be easily reduced through the fibrous ring at the umbilicus. Surgery is not usually performed unless the hernia persists to the age of 3 to 5 years (Kleigman, 1996).

Gastroschisis

This anomaly is among the more common of congenital abdominal wall defects (Fig. 12-19). Gastroschisis results from a defect near the median plane of the ventral abdominal wall. The linear defect permits extrusion of the abdominal viscera without involving the umbilical cord. The viscera protrude into the amniotic cavity and are bathed by amniotic fluid. The term *gastroschisis*, which literally means a "split or open stomach," is a misnomer because it is the anterior abdominal wall that is split, not the stomach. The defect usually occurs on the right side near the median plane and is more common in males than females. The anomaly results from incomplete closure of the lateral folds during the fourth week (see Chapter 5). Exposure to environmental drugs and chemicals might be involved in the etiology of gastroschisis.

Nonrotation of the Midgut

This relatively common condition, sometimes called *left-sided colon*, is generally asymptomatic, but twisting of the intestines (*volvulus*) may occur (Fig. 12–20*A*). Nonrotation occurs when the midgut loop does not rotate as it reenters the abdomen. As a result, the caudal limb of the loop returns to the abdomen first, and the small intestine lies on the right side of the abdomen and the entire large intestine on the left. When volvulus occurs, the superior mesenteric artery may be obstructed, resulting in infarction and gangrene of the bowel supplied by it.

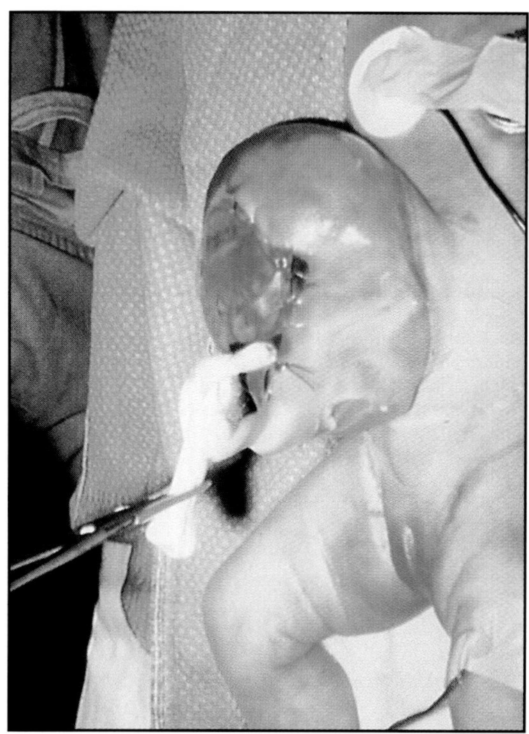

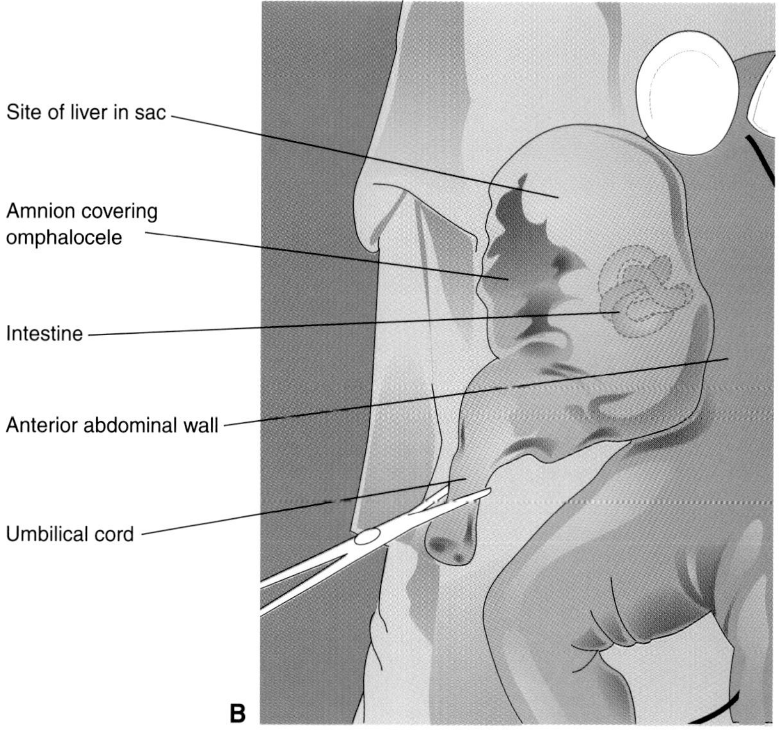

■ **Figure 12–17.** *A,* Photograph of an infant with an omphalocele. (Courtesy of Dr. N. E. Wiseman, Pediatric Surgeon, Children's Hospital, Winnipeg, Manitoba, Canada.) *B,* Drawing of the same infant with a large omphalocele resulting from a median defect of the abdominal muscles, fascia, and skin at the umbilicus that resulted in the herniation of intra-abdominal structures (liver and intestine) into the proximal end of the umbilical cord. It is covered by a membrane composed of peritoneum and amnion. In some cases, an omphalocele may be a persistence of the normal embryonic stage of umbilical herniation.

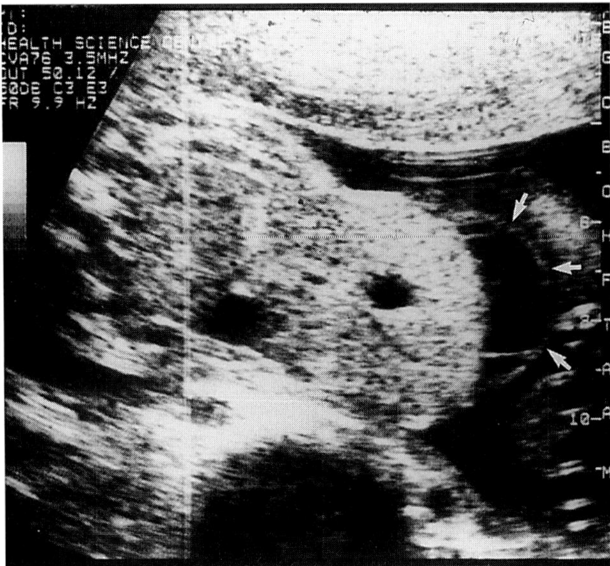

■ **Figure 12–18.** Sonogram of the abdomen of a fetus (28 weeks' gestation) showing a large omphalocele, with much of the liver protruding from the abdomen. The mass also contained a small membrane-covered sac (small arrows). The umbilical cord was integrally involved in the anomaly. (Courtesy of Dr. C. R. Harman, Department of Obstetrics, Gynecology and Reproductive Sciences, Women's Hospital and University of Manitoba, Winnipeg, Manitoba, Canada.)

Mixed Rotation and Volvulus

In this condition, the cecum lies just inferior to the pylorus of the stomach and is fixed to the posterior abdominal wall by peritoneal bands that pass over the duodenum (Fig. 12-20*B*). These bands and the volvulus of the intestines cause **duodenal obstruction**. This type of malrotation results from failure of the midgut loop to complete the final 90 degrees of rotation (Fig. 12-13*D*); consequently, the terminal part of the ileum returns to the abdomen first.

Reversed Rotation

In very unusual cases, the midgut loop rotates in a clockwise rather than a counterclockwise direction (Fig. 12-20*C*). As a result, the duodenum lies anterior to the superior mesenteric artery (SMA) rather than posterior to it, and the transverse colon lies posterior to the SMA instead of anterior to it. In these infants, the transverse colon may be obstructed by pressure from the SMA. In very rare cases, the small intestine lies on the left side of the abdomen and the large intestine lies on the right side, with the cecum in the center. This unusual situation results from malrotation of the midgut followed by failure of fixation of the intestines (Valioulis et al., 1997).

Subhepatic Cecum and Appendix

If the cecum adheres to the inferior surface of the liver when it returns to the abdomen (Fig. 12-13*D*), it will be drawn superiorly as the liver diminishes in size; as a result, the cecum remains in its fetal position (Fig. 12-20*D*). Subhepatic cecum and appendix are more common in males and occur in about 6% of fetuses. Subhepatic cecum is not common in adults; however, when it occurs, it may create a problem in the diagnosis of appendicitis and during the surgical removal of the appendix (*appendectomy*).

Mobile Cecum

In about 10% of people the cecum has an unusual amount of freedom. *In very unusual cases* it may herniate into the right inguinal canal. A mobile cecum results from incomplete fixation of the ascending colon. This condition is clinically significant because of the possible variations in position of the appendix (Moore, 1992) and because twisting or volvulus of the cecum may occur.

Internal Hernia

In this anomaly, the small intestine passes into the mesentery of the midgut loop during the return of the intestines to the abdomen (Fig. 12-20*E*). As a result, a hernialike sac forms. This very uncommon condition usually does not produce symptoms and is often detected at autopsy or during an anatomical dissection.

Midgut Volvulus

In this anomaly the small intestine fails to enter the abdominal cavity normally and the mesenteries fail to undergo normal fixation; as a result, twisting of the intestines occurs (Fig. 12-20*F*). Only two parts of the intestine are attached to the posterior abdominal wall, the duodenum and proximal colon. The small intestine hangs by a narrow stalk that contains the superior mesenteric artery and vein. These vessels are usually twisted in this stalk and become obstructed at or near the duodenojejunal junction. The circulation to the twisted segment is often restricted; if the vessels are completely obstructed, gangrene will develop.

Stenosis and Atresia of the Intestine

Partial occlusion (stenosis) and complete occlusion (atresia) of the intestinal lumen (Fig. 12-6) account for about one-third of cases of intestinal obstruction (Wyllie, 1996). The obstructive lesion occurs most often in the duodenum (25%) and ileum (50%). The length of the area affected varies. These anomalies result from failure of an adequate number of vacuoles to form during recanalization of the intestine (Fig. 12-6). In some cases a transverse diaphragm forms, producing a **diaphragmatic atresia** (Fig. 12-6F_2). Another possible cause of stenoses and atresias is interruption of the blood supply to a loop of fetal intestine resulting from a **fetal vascular accident**; for example, an excessively mobile loop of intestine may become twisted, thereby interrupting its blood supply and leading to necrosis of the section of bowel involved. This necrotic segment later becomes a fibrous cord connecting the proximal and distal ends of normal intestine. Most atresias of the ileum are probably caused by infarction of the fetal bowel as the result of impairment of its blood supply resulting from volvulus. This impairment most likely occurs during the tenth week as the intestines return to the abdomen. Malfixation of the gut predisposes it to volvulus, strangulation, and impairment of its blood supply.

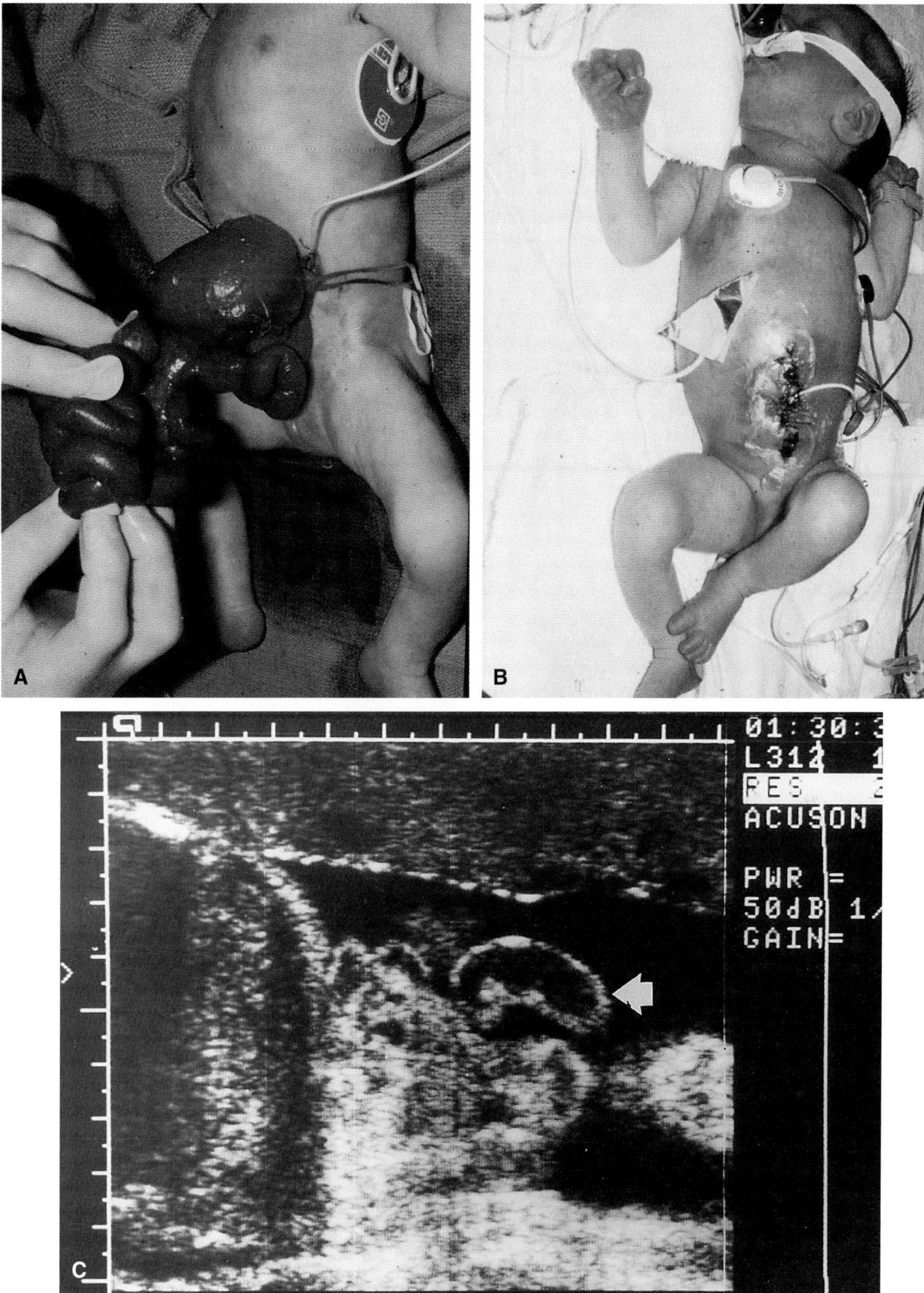

■ **Figure 12–19.** *A,* Photograph of a newborn infant with an anterior abdominal wall defect—gastroschisis. The defect was relatively small (2 to 4 cm) and involved all layers of the abdominal wall. It was located to the right of the umbilicus. *B,* Photograph of the infant after the viscera were returned to the abdomen and the defect was surgically closed. *C,* Sonogram of fetus (20 weeks' gestation) with gastroschisis. Loops of small bowel can be seen floating freely in the amniotic fluid (arrow), anterior to the fetal abdomen (left). *A* and *B,* courtesy of Dr. A. E. Chudley, Section of Genetics and Metabolism, Department of Pediatrics and Child Health, Children's Hospital, Winnipeg, Manitoba, Canada. *C,* courtesy of Dr. C. R. Harman, Department of Obstetrics, Gynecology and Reproductive Services, Women's Hospital and University of Manitoba, Winnipeg, Manitoba, Canada.)

Ileal Diverticulum and Other Yolk Stalk Remnants

This outpouching is one of the most common anomalies of the digestive tract (Fig. 12-21). A congenital ileal diverticulum (Meckel diverticulum) occurs in 2 to 4% of people (Moore, 1992) and is three to five times more prevalent in males than females. *An ileal diverticulum is of clinical significance* because it sometimes becomes inflamed and causes symptoms that mimic appendicitis. The wall of the diverticulum contains all layers of the ileum and may contain small patches of gastric and pancreatic tissues. The gastric mucosa often secretes acid, producing ulceration and bleeding (Fig. 12-22*A*). An ileal diverticulum is the remnant of the proximal portion of the yolk stalk. It typically appears as a fingerlike pouch about 3 to 6 cm long that *arises from the antimesenteric border of the ileum* (Fig. 12-21), 40 to 50 cm from the ileocecal junction. An ileal diverticulum may be connected to the umbilicus by a fibrous cord or a **umbilicoileal fistula** (Figs. 12-22*B* and 12-23*B*); other possible remnants of the yolk stalk are illustrated in Fig. 12-22*D* to *F*).

In rare instances there is abnormal reconstruction of the endodermal roof of the yolk sac during notochord formation (see Chapter 4). This results in the endoderm being attached to the notochord. When the dorsal part of the yolk sac is incorporated into the embryo as the primordial gut, a cord of endodermal cells passes from the gut to the vertebral column, which develops around the notochord. This endodermal cord may give rise to a giant diverticulum on the mesenteric side of the intestinal tract.

Duplication of the Intestine

Most intestinal duplications are cystic or tubular duplications. *Cystic duplications* are more common (Fig. 12-24*A* and *B*). Tubular duplications usually communicate with the intestinal lumen (Fig. 12-24*C*). Almost all duplications are caused by failure of normal recanalization; as a result, two lumina form (Fig. 12-24*H* and *I*). The duplicated segment of the bowel lies on the mesenteric side of the intestine.

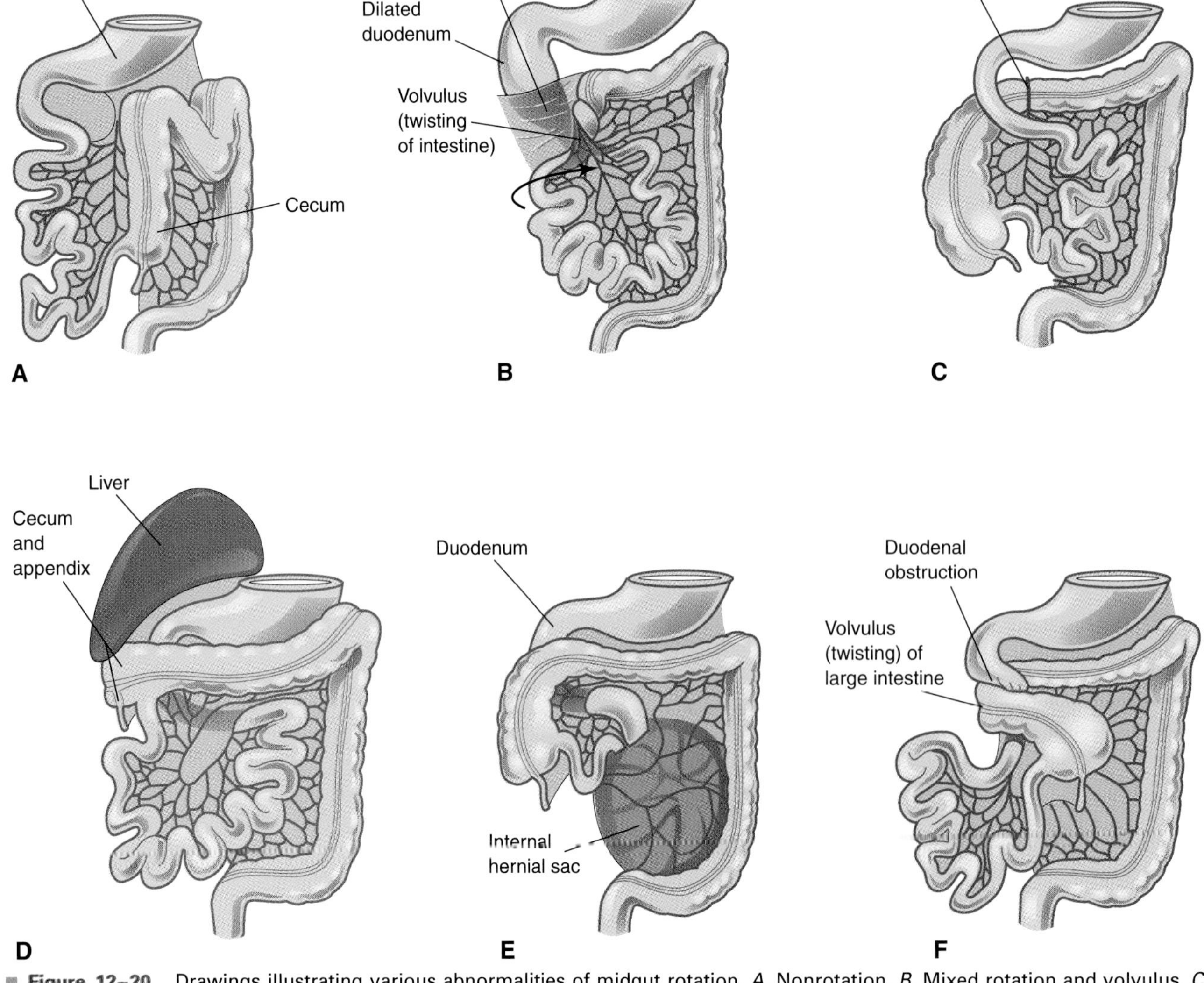

■ **Figure 12-20.** Drawings illustrating various abnormalities of midgut rotation. *A*, Nonrotation. *B*, Mixed rotation and volvulus. *C*, Reversed rotation. *D*, Subhepatic cecum and appendix. *E*, Internal hernia. *F*, Midgut volvulus.

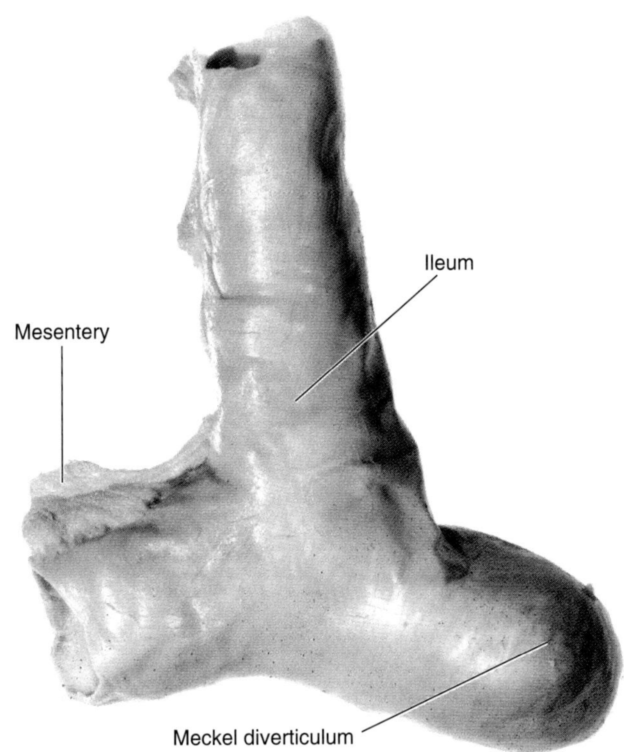

■ **Figure 12–21.** Photograph of a typical ileal diverticulum, commonly referred to clinically as a Meckel diverticulum. This is a cadaveric specimen. Only a small percentage of these diverticula produce symptoms. Ileal diverticula are one of the most common anomalies of the digestive tract. They occur in 2 to 4% of people and are three to four times more prevalent in males than females. (From Moore KL, Persaud TVN, Shiota K: Color Atlas of Clinical Embryology. Philadelphia, WB Saunders, 1994.)

THE HINDGUT

The derivatives of the hindgut are:

- the left one-third to one-half of the transverse colon; the descending colon and sigmoid colon; the rectum and the superior part of the anal canal
- The epithelium of the urinary bladder and most of the urethra (see Chapter 13)

All these hindgut derivatives are supplied by the *inferior mesenteric artery*, the artery of the hindgut. The junction between the segment of transverse colon derived from the midgut and that originating from the hindgut is indicated by the change in blood supply from a branch of the superior mesenteric artery (midgut artery) to a branch of the inferior mesenteric artery (hindgut artery). The descending colon becomes retroperitoneal as its mesentery fuses with the peritoneum on the left posterior abdominal wall and then disappears (Fig. 12-15). The mesentery of the sigmoid colon is retained, but it is shorter than in the embryo.

The Cloaca

This terminal portion of the hindgut is an endoderm-lined cavity that is in contact with the surface ectoderm at the **cloacal membrane** (Fig. 12-25*A* and *B*). This membrane is composed of endoderm of the cloaca and ectoderm of the **proctodeum** or anal pit (Fig. 12-25*D*). The cloaca, the expanded terminal part of the hindgut, receives the *allantois* ventrally (Fig. 12-25*A*), which is a fingerlike diverticulum of the yolk sac. For a description of this rudimentary structure, see Chapter 4.

PARTITIONING OF THE CLOACA

The cloaca is divided into dorsal and ventral parts by a wedge of mesenchyme — the **urorectal septum** — which develops in the angle between the allantois and hindgut. As the septum grows toward the cloacal membrane, it develops forklike extensions that produce infoldings of the lateral walls of the cloaca (Fig. 12-25B_1). These folds grow toward each other and fuse, forming a partition that divides the cloaca into two parts (Fig. 12-25D_1 and F_1):

- the *rectum* and cranial part of the *anal canal* dorsally
- the *urogenital sinus* ventrally

By the seventh week, the urorectal septum has fused with the cloacal membrane, dividing it into a dorsal **anal membrane** and a larger ventral **urogenital membrane** (Fig. 12-25*E* and *F*). The area of fusion of the urorectal septum with the cloacal membrane is represented in the adult by the **perineal body**, the tendinous center of the perineum (Moore, 1992). This fibromuscular node is the *landmark of the perineum* where several muscles converge and attach. The urorectal septum also divides the **cloacal sphincter** into anterior and posterior parts. The posterior part becomes the *external anal sphincter*, and the anterior part develops into the superficial transverse perineal, bulbospongiosus, and ischiocavernosus muscles (Moore, 1992). This developmental fact explains why one nerve, the **pudendal nerve**, supplies all these muscles. Mesenchymal proliferations produce elevations of the surface ectoderm around the **anal membrane**. As a result, this membrane is soon located at the bottom of an ectodermal depression — the **proctodeum** or anal pit (Fig. 12-25*E*). The anal membrane usually ruptures at the end of the eighth week, bringing the distal part of the digestive tract (anal canal) into communication with the amniotic cavity.

THE ANAL CANAL

The superior two-thirds (about 25 mm) of the adult anal canal are derived from the *hindgut*; the inferior one third (about 13 mm) develops from the **proctodeum** (Fig. 12-26). The junction of the epithelium derived from the ectoderm of the proctodeum and the endoderm of the hindgut is roughly indicated by the irregular **pectinate line**, located at the inferior limit of the anal valves (Moore, 1992). This line indicates the approximate former site of the anal membrane. About

2 cm superior to the anus is an **anocutaneous line** ("white line"). This is approximately where the composition of the anal epithelium changes from columnar to stratified squamous cells. At the anus, the epithelium is keratinized and continuous with the skin around the anus. The other layers of the wall of the anal canal are derived from splanchnic mesenchyme. There is scanty information on the morphological differentiation of the anal sphincter muscles (Bourdelat et al., 1990).

Because of its hindgut origin, the superior two-thirds of the anal canal are mainly supplied by the *superior rectal artery*, the continuation of the inferior mesenteric artery (hindgut artery). The venous drainage of this superior part is mainly via the *superior rectal vein*, a tributary of the inferior mesenteric vein. The lymphatic drainage of the superior part is eventually to the *inferior mesenteric lymph nodes*. Its nerves are from the autonomic nervous system. Because of its origin from the proctodeum, the inferior one-third of the anal canal is supplied mainly by the *inferior rectal arteries*, branches of the internal pudendal artery. The venous drainage is through the *inferior rectal vein*, a tributary of the internal pudendal vein that drains into the internal iliac vein. The lymphatic drainage of the inferior part of the anal canal is to the *superficial inguinal lymph nodes*. Its nerve supply is from the *inferior rectal nerve*; hence, it is sensitive to pain, temperature, touch, and pressure.

The differences in blood supply, nerve supply, and venous and lymphatic drainage of the anal canal are important clinically (Moore, 1992); e.g., when considering the metastasis (spread) of tumor cells. The characteristics of carcinomas in the two parts also differ. Tumors in the superior part are painless and arise from columnar epithelium, whereas those in the inferior part are painful and arise from stratified squamous epithelium.

Anomalies of the Hindgut

Most anomalies of the hindgut are located in the anorectal region and result from abnormal development of

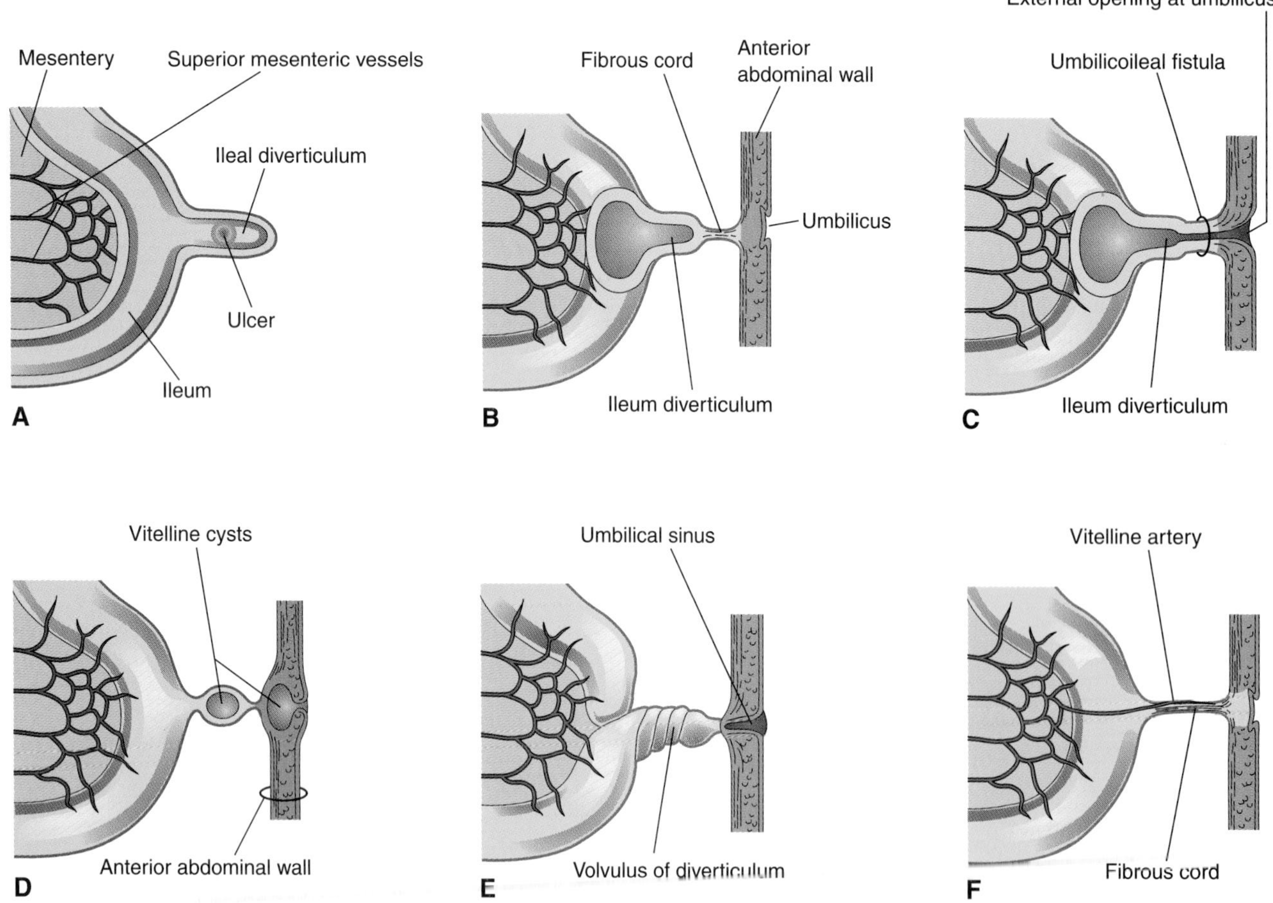

■ **Figure 12–22.** Drawings illustrating ileal (Meckel) diverticula and other remnants of the yolk stalk. *A*, Section of the ileum and a diverticulum with an ulcer. *B*, A diverticulum connected to the umbilicus by a fibrous cord. *C*, Umbilicoileal fistual resulting from persistence of the entire intra-abdominal portion of the yolk stalk. *D*, Vitelline cysts at the umbilicus and in a fibrous remnant of the yolk stalk. *E*, Umbilical sinus resulting from the persistence of the yolk stalk near the umbilicus. *F*, The yolk stalk has persisted as a fibrous cord connecting the ileum with the umbilicus. A persistent vitelline artery extends along the fibrous cord to the umbilicus.

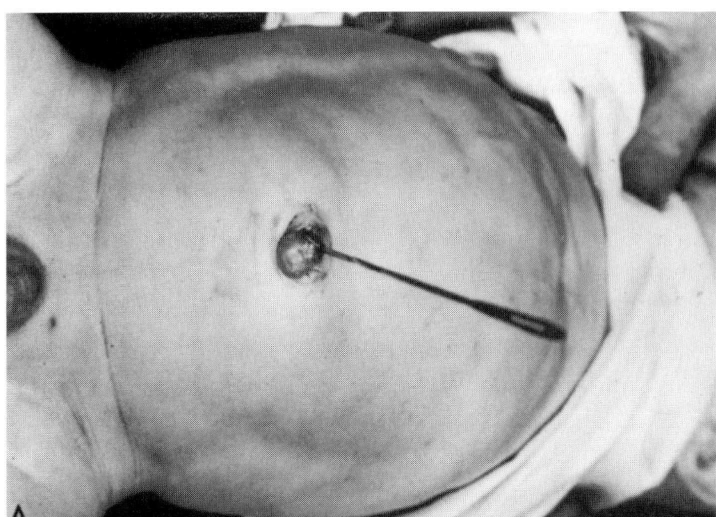

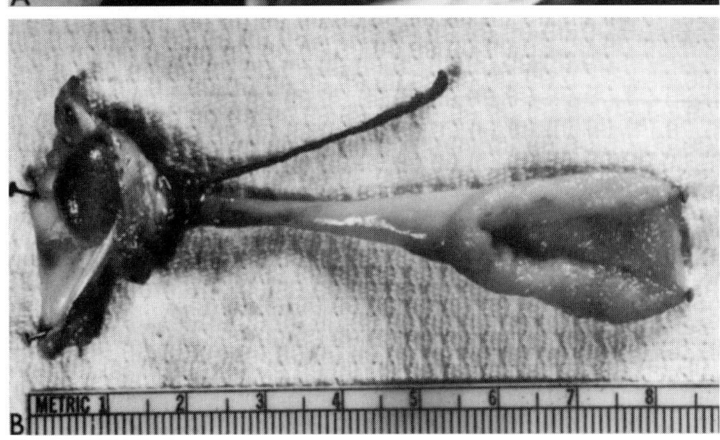

■ **Figure 12–23.** *A,* Photograph of the abdomen of an infant with an umbilicoileal fistula. A probe has been inserted into the fistula. It extends from the umbilicus to the ileum (a distance of about 5 cm). *B,* The excised fistula with a granulomatous-looking bulge at the ileal end. (From Ballard RB, Avery ME, Taeusch HW: *Schaffer's Diseases of the Newborn,* 6th ed. Philadelphia, WB Saunders, 1984, p 383.)

the urorectal septum. Clinically, they are divided into high and low anomalies depending on whether the rectum terminates superior or inferior to the *puborectal sling* formed by the puborectalis, a part of the levator ani muscle (Moore, 1992).

Congenital Megacolon

In infants with congenital megacolon or **Hirschsprung disease** (Fig. 12-27), a part of the colon is dilated because of the *absence of autonomic ganglion cells* in the myenteric plexus distal to the dilated segment of colon. The enlarged colon—**megacolon** (Gr. *megas,* big)—has the normal number of ganglion cells. The dilation results from failure of peristalsis in the aganglionic segment, which prevents movement of the intestinal contents. In most cases only the rectum and sigmoid colon are involved, but occasionally ganglia are also absent from more proximal parts of the colon. Congenital megacolon is the most common cause of neonatal obstruction of the colon and accounts for 33% of all neonatal obstructions; males are affected more often than females (4:1). Congenital megacolon results from failure of neural crest cells to migrate into the wall of the colon during the fifth to seventh weeks. This results in failure of parasympathetic ganglion cells to develop in the *Auerbach and Meissner plexuses.* The cause of failure of some neural crest cells to complete their migration is unknown.

Imperforate Anus and Anorectal Anomalies

Imperforate anus occurs about once in every 5000 newborn infants and is more common in males (Figs. 12-28 and 12-29*C*). *Most anorectal anomalies result from abnormal development of the urorectal septum,* resulting in incomplete separation of the cloaca into urogenital and anorectal portions (Fig. 12-29*A*). There is normally a temporary communication between the rectum and anal canal dorsally from the bladder and urethra ventrally (Fig. 12-25*C*), but it closes when the urorectal septum fuses with the cloacal membrane (Fig. 12-25*E*). Lesions are classified as "low" or "high" depending on whether the rectum ends superior or inferior to the puborectalis muscle (Moore, 1992). The following are low anomalies of the anorectal region.

Anal Agenesis, With or Without a Fistula

The anal canal may end blindly or there may be an ectopic opening (**ectopic anus**) or an **anoperineal**

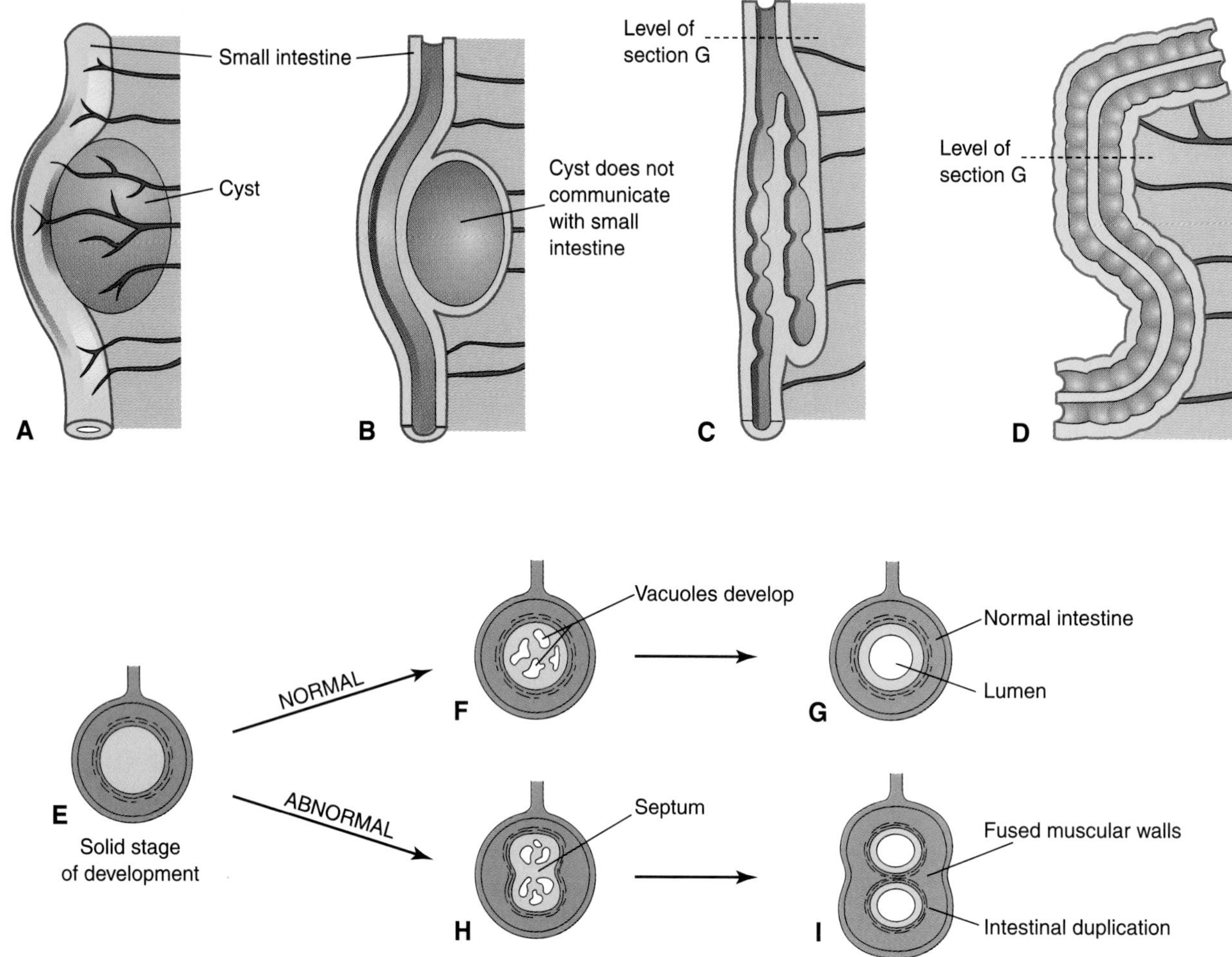

■ **Figure 12–24.** *A,* Cystic duplication of the small intestine. Note that it is on the mesenteric side and receives branches from the arteries supplying the intestine. *B,* Longitudinal section of the duplication shown in *A.* It does not communicate with the intestine, but its musculature is continuous with the gut wall. *C,* A short tubular duplication of the small intestine. *D,* A long duplication of the small intestine showing a partition consisting of the fused muscular wall. *E,* Transverse section of the intestine during the solid stage. *F,* Normal vacuole formation. *G,* Coalescence of the vacuoles and reformation of the lumen. *H,* Two groups of vacuoles have formed. *I,* Coalescence of the vacuoles illustrated in *H* results in intestinal duplication.

fistula that commonly opens into the perineum (Fig. 12-29*D* and *E*). The abnormal canal may, however, open into the vagina in females or the urethra in males (Figs. 12-29*F* and *G*). More than 90% of low anorectal anomalies are associated with an external fistula. **Anal agenesis with a fistula** results from incomplete separation of the cloaca by the urorectal septum.

Anal Stenosis

The anus is in the normal position but the anus and anal canal are narrow (Fig. 12-29*B*). This anomaly is probably caused by a slight dorsal deviation of the urorectal septum as it grows caudally to fuse with the cloacal membrane. As a result, the anal canal and anal membrane are small. Sometimes only a small probe can be inserted into the anal canal.

Membranous Atresia of the Anus

The anus is in the normal position, but a thin layer of tissue separates the anal canal from the exterior (Figs. 12-28 and 12-29*C*). The membrane is thin enough to bulge on straining and appears blue from the presence of meconium superior to it. This anomaly results from failure of the anal membrane to perforate at the end of the eighth week.

Anorectal Agenesis, With or Without a Fistula

This anomaly and those that follow are classified as high anomalies of the anorectal region. The rectum ends superior to the puborectalis muscle when there is anorectal agenesis. This is the most common type of anorectal anomaly, which accounts for about two-thirds of anorectal defects. Although the rectum ends blindly, there is usually a fistula to the bladder (*recto-vesical fistula*) or urethra (*rectourethral fistula*) in males, or to the vagina (*rectovaginal fistula*) or the vestibule of the vagina (*rectovestibular fistula*) in females (Fig. 12-29*F* and *G*). Passage of meconium or flatus (gas) in the urine is diagnostic of a rectourinary fistula. *Anorectal agenesis with a fistula* is the result of incomplete separation of the cloaca by the urorectal

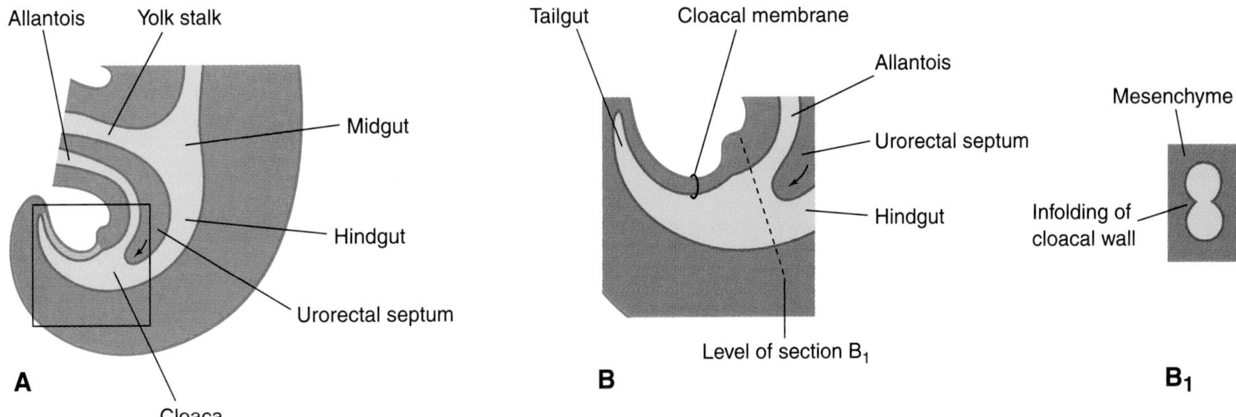

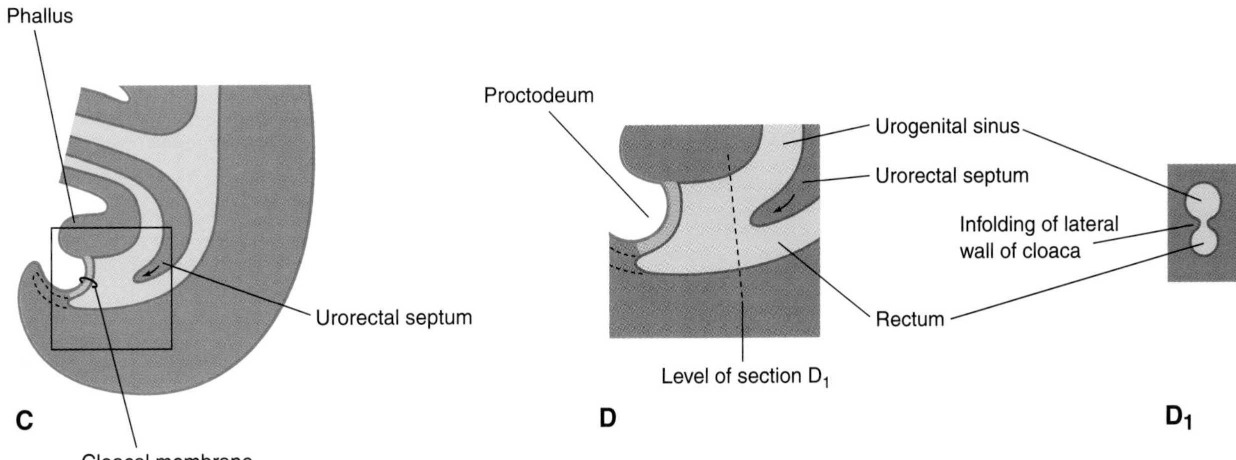

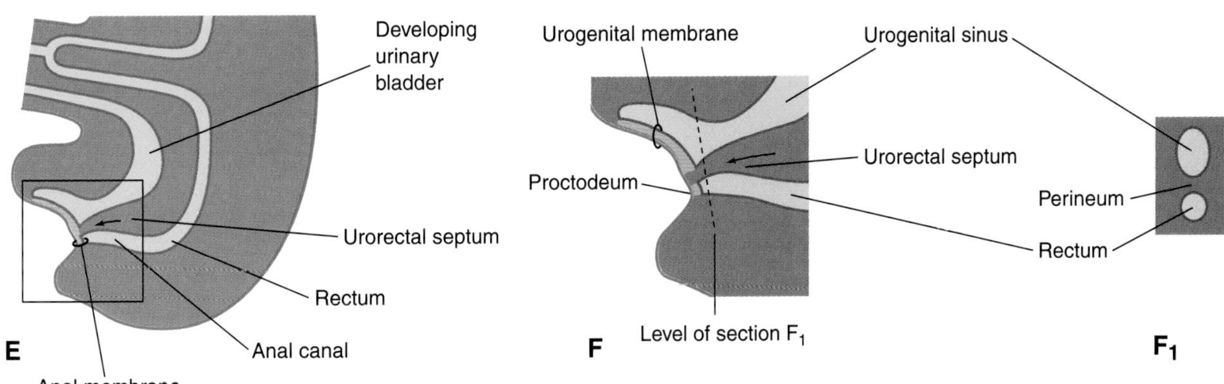

■ **Figure 12–25.** Drawings illustrating successive stages in the partitioning of the cloaca into the rectum and urogenital sinus by the urorectal septum. *A, C,* and *E,* Views from the left side at 4, 6, and 7 weeks respectively. *B, D,* and *F,* Enlargements of the cloacal region. B_1, D_1, and F_1, Transverse sections of the cloaca at the levels shown in *B,D,* and *F,* respectively. Note that the tailgut (shown in *B*) degenerates and disappears as the rectum forms from the dorsal part of the cloaca (shown in *C*).

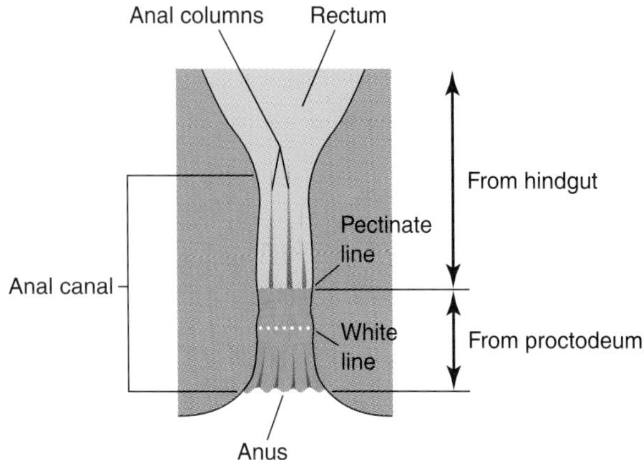

■ **Figure 12–26.** Sketch of the rectum and anal canal showing their developmental origins. Note that the superior two-thirds of the anal canal are derived from the hindgut and are endodermal in origin, whereas the inferior one-third of the anal canal is derived from the proctodeum and is ectodermal in origin. Because of their different embryological origins, the superior and inferior parts of the anal canal are supplied by different arteries and nerves and have different venous and lymphatic drainages.

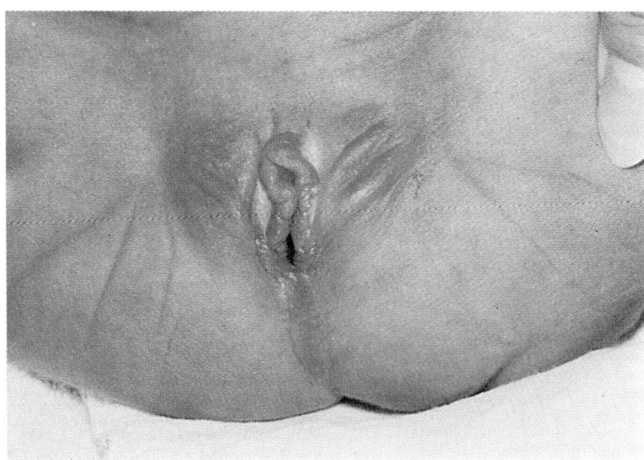

■ **Figure 12–28.** Female neonate with membranous anal atresia (imperforate anus). A tracheoesophageal fistula was also present. In most cases of anal atresia, a thin layer of tissue separates the anal canal from the exterior. This anomaly results from failure of the anal membrane to perforate at the end of the eighth week. Some form of imperforate anus occurs about once in every 5000 neonates; it is more common in males. (Courtesy of Dr. A. E. Chudley, Section of Genetics and Metabolism, Department of Pediatrics and Child Health, Children's Hospital, Winnipeg, Manitoba, Canada.)

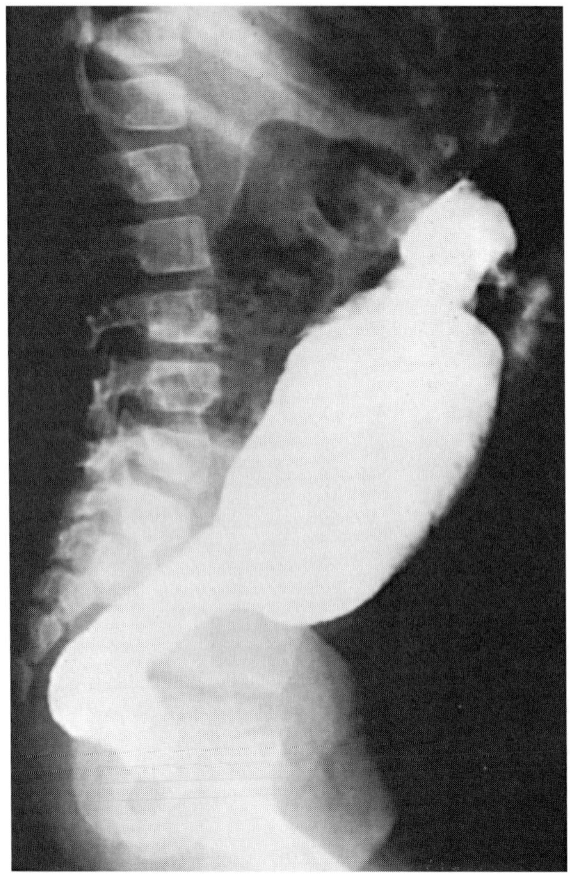

■ **Figure 12–27.** Lateral radiographic view of the colon after a barium enema in a 3-year-old girl with Hirschsprung disease. The aganglionic distal segment is narrow, with distended normal ganglionic bowel above it. (From Wyllie R: Congenital aganglionic megacolon [Hirschsprung disease]. *In* Behrman RE, Kliegman RM, Arvin AM [eds]: *Nelson Textbook of Pediatrics,* 15th ed. Philadelphia, WB Saunders, 1996.)

septum. In newborn males with this condition, *meconium* (feces) may be observed in the urine; whereas fistulas in females result in the presence of meconium in the vestibule of the vagina.

Rectal Atresia

The anal canal and rectum are present but they are separated (Fig. 12-29*H* and *I*). Sometimes the two segments of bowel are connected by a fibrous cord, the remnant of the atretic portion of the rectum. The cause of rectal atresia may be abnormal recanalization of the colon or more likely defective blood supply, as discussed with atresia of the small intestine. For more information on atresia and stenosis at different levels of the gastrointestinal tract, see Harris et al. (1995).

SUMMARY OF THE DIGESTIVE SYSTEM

The **primordial gut** forms during the fourth week from the part of the yolk sac that is incorporated into the embryo. The endoderm of the primordial gut gives rise to the epithelial lining of most of the digestive tract and biliary passages together with the parenchyma of its glands, including the liver and pancreas. The epithelium at the cranial and caudal extremities of the digestive tract is derived from the ectoderm of the stomodeum and proctodeum, respectively. The muscular and connective tissue components of the digestive tract are derived from the splanchnic mesenchyme surrounding the primordial gut.

The **foregut** gives rise to the pharynx, lower respiratory system, esophagus, stomach, duodenum (proxi-

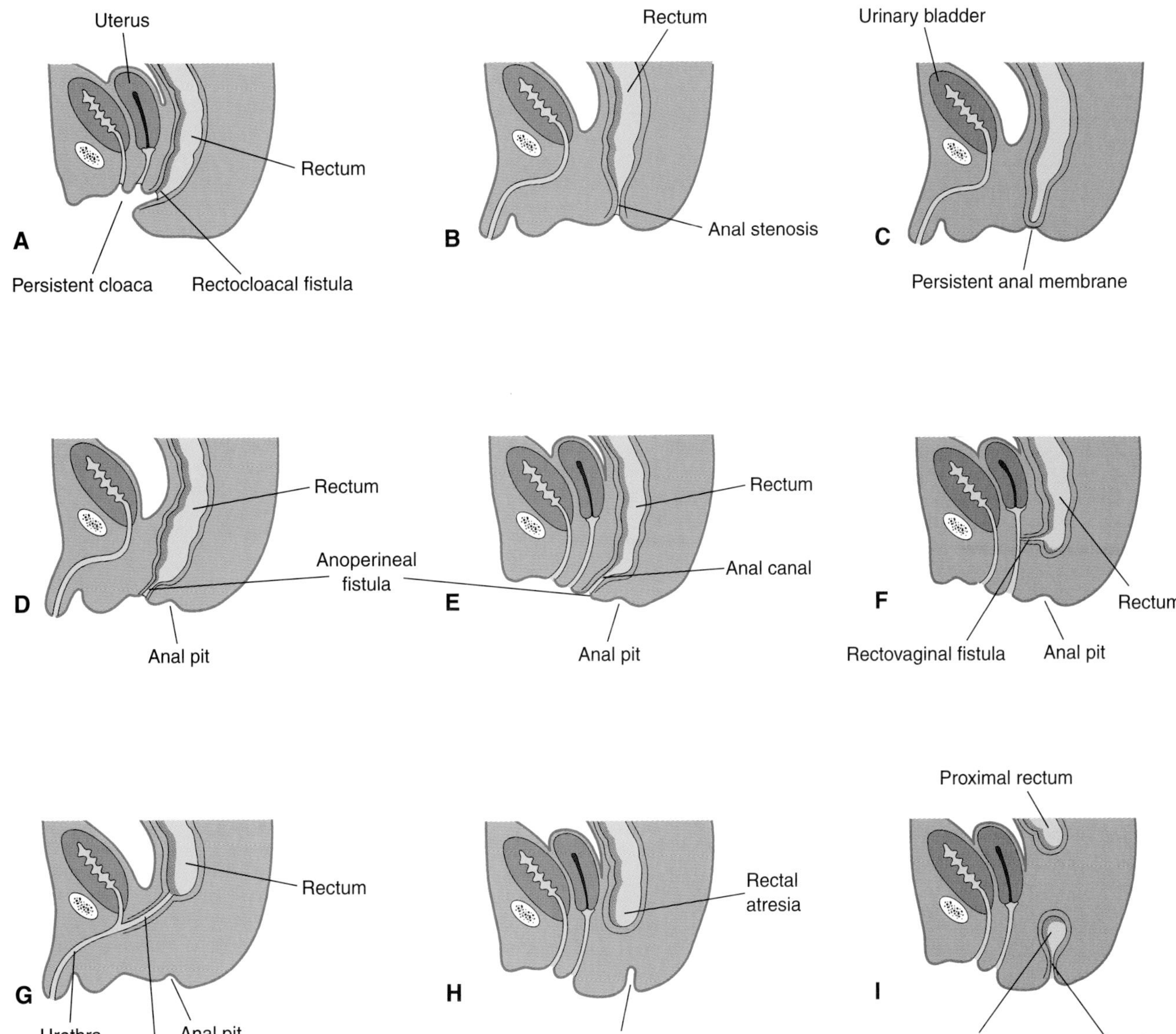

■ **Figure 12–29.** Drawings illustrating various types of anorectal anomaly. *A*, Persistent cloaca. Note the common outlet for the intestinal, urinary, and reproductive tracts. *B*, Anal stenosis. *C*, Membranous anal atresia (covered anus). *D* and *E*, Anal agenesis with a perineal fistula. *F*, Anorectal agenesis with a rectovaginal fistula. *G*, Anorectal agenesis with a rectourethral fistula. *H* and *I*, Rectal atresia.

mal to the opening of the bile duct), liver, pancreas, and biliary apparatus. Because the trachea and esophagus have a common origin from the foregut (see Chapter 11), incomplete partitioning by the tracheoesophageal septum results in stenoses or atresias, with or without fistulas between them.

The **hepatic diverticulum**, the primordium of the liver, gallbladder, and biliary duct system, is an outgrowth of the endodermal epithelial lining of the foregut. The epithelial liver cords and primordia of the **biliary system**, which develop from the hepatic diverticulum, grow into the septum transversum. Between the layers of the *ventral mesentery* derived from the septum transversum, these primordial cells differentiate into the *parenchyma of the liver* and the lining of the ducts of the biliary system.

Congenital duodenal atresia results from failure of the vacuolization and recanalization process to occur following the normal solid stage of the duodenum. Usually the epithelial cells degenerate and the lumen of the duodenum is restored. Obstruction of the duodenum can also be caused by an *anular pancreas.*

The **pancreas** develops from dorsal and ventral *pancreatic buds* that originate from the endodermal lining of the foregut. When the duodenum rotates to the right, the ventral pancreatic bud moves dorsally and fuses with the dorsal pancreatic bud. The **ventral pancreatic bud** forms most of the head of the pancreas, including the uncinate process. The **dorsal pancreatic bud** forms the remainder of the pancreas. In some fetuses the duct systems of the two buds fail to fuse, and an *accessory pancreatic duct* forms.

The **midgut** gives rise to the duodenum (distal to the bile duct), jejunum, ileum, cecum, vermiform appendix, ascending colon, and the right half to two-thirds of the transverse colon. The midgut forms a U-shaped intestinal loop that herniates into the umbilical cord during the sixth week because there is no room for it in the abdomen. While in the umbilical cord, the **midgut loop** rotates counterclockwise through 90 degrees. During the tenth week, the intestines rapidly return to the abdomen, rotating a further 180 degrees during this process.

Omphaloceles, malrotations, and abnormal fixation of the gut result from failure of return or abnormal rotation of the intestine in the abdomen. Because the gut is normally occluded during the fifth and sixth weeks due to rapid mitotic activity of its epithelium, *stenosis* (partial obstruction), *atresia* (complete obstruction), and *duplications* result if recanalization fails to occur or occurs abnormally. Various remnants of the yolk stalk may persist. *Ileal (Meckel) diverticula* are common; however, only a few of them become inflamed and produce pain.

The **hindgut** gives rise to the left one-third to one-half of the transverse colon, the descending and sigmoid colon, the rectum, and the superior part of the anal canal. The inferior part of the anal canal develops from the proctodeum. The caudal part of the hindgut, known as the *cloaca*, is divided by the *urorectal septum* into the urogenital sinus and rectum. The urogenital sinus mainly gives rise to the urinary bladder and urethra (see Chapter 13). At first the rectum and the superior part of the anal canal are separated from the exterior by the *anal membrane*, but this membrane normally breaks down by the end of the eighth week.

Most **anorectal anomalies** result from abnormal partitioning of the cloaca by the urorectal septum into the rectum and anal canal posteriorly and the urinary bladder and urethra anteriorly. Arrested growth and/or deviation of the urorectal septum in a dorsal direction cause most anorectal abnormalities, such as rectal atresia and abnormal connections (fistulas) between the rectum and the urethra, urinary bladder, or vagina.

Clinically Oriented Problems

Case 12–1

A female infant was born prematurely at 32 weeks' gestation to a 39-year-old woman whose pregnancy was complicated by *polyhydramnios*. Amniocentesis at 16 weeks showed that the infant had trisomy 21. The baby began to vomit within a few hours after birth. Marked dilation of the epigastrium was noted. Radiographs of the abdomen showed gas in the stomach and the superior part of the duodenum, but no other intestinal gas was observed. A *diagnosis of duodenal atresia* was made.

- Where does obstruction of the duodenum usually occur?
- What is the embryological basis of this congenital anomaly?
- What caused distention of the infant's epigastrium?
- Is duodenal atresia commonly associated with malformations such as the Down syndrome?
- What is the embryological basis of the *polyhydramnios* in this case?

Case 12–2

The umbilicus of a newborn infant failed to heal normally. It was swollen and there was a persistent discharge from the umbilical stump. After probing, a *sinus tract* was outlined with radiopaque oil during fluoroscopy. The tract was resected on the ninth day after birth and its distal end was found to terminate in a *diverticulum of the ileum*.

- What is the embryological basis of the sinus tract?
- What is the usual clinical name given to this type of ileal diverticulum?
- Is this anomaly common?

Case 12–3

A female infant was born with a small dimple where the anus should have been. Examination of the infant's vagina revealed meconium and an opening of a sinus tract in the posterior wall of the vagina. Radiographic examination using a contrast medium injected through a tiny catheter inserted into the opening revealed a fistulous connection with the lower bowel.

- With which part of the lower bowel would the fistula probably be connected?
- Name this anomaly.
- What is the embryological basis of this condition?

Case 12–4

A newborn infant was born with a light gray, shiny mass measuring the size of an orange and protruding from the umbilical region. The mass was covered by a thin transparent membrane.

- What is this congenital anomaly called?
- What is the origin of the membrane covering the mass?
- What would be the composition of the mass?
- What is the embryological basis of this protrusion?

Case 12–5

A newborn infant appeared normal at birth; however, excessive vomiting and abdominal distention developed after a few hours. The vomitus contained bile, and only a little meconium was passed. Radiographic examination showed a gas-filled stomach and dilated, gas-filled loops of small bowel, but no air was present in the large intestine. This indicated a congenital obstruction of the small bowel.

- What part of the small bowel was probably obstructed?

- What would the condition be called?
- Why was only a little meconium passed?
- What would likely be observed at operation?
- What was the probable embryological basis of the condition?

Discussion of these problems appears at the back of the book.

REFERENCES AND SUGGESTED READING

Ackerman P: Congenital defects of the abdominal wall. *In* Huffstadt AJC (ed): *Congenital Malformations*. Amsterdam, Excerpta Medica, 1980.

Balistreri WF: Liver and biliary atresia. *In* Behrman RE, Kliegman RM, Arvin AM (eds): *Nelson Textbook of Pediatrics,* 15th ed. Philadelphia, WB Saunders, 1996.

Bear JC: Infantile hypertrophic pyloric stenosis: approaches to liability. *In* Persaud TVN (ed): *Advances in the Study of Birth Defects. Cardiovascular, Respiratory, Gastrointestinal and Genitourinary Malformations,* vol 6. New York, Alan R Liss, 1982.

Beasley SW, Myers NA, Auldist AW (eds): *Oesophageal Atresia*. London, Chapman and Hall, 1991.

Behrman RE, Kliegman RM, Arvin AM (eds): *Nelson Textbook of Pediatrics,* 15th ed. Philadelphia, WB Saunders, 1996.

Best LG, Wiseman NE, Chudley AE: Familial duodenal atresia: a report of two families and review. *Am J Med Genet 34:*442, 1989.

Bissett WM: Development of intestinal motility. *Arch Dis Child 66:*3, 1991.

Bourdelat D, Barbet JP, Hidden G: The morphological differentiation of the internal sphincter muscle of the anus in the human embryo and fetus. *Surg Radiol Anat 12:*151, 1990.

Brassett C, Ellis H: Transposition of the viscera. *Clin Anat 4:*139, 1991.

Carr BR: Fertilization, implantation, and endocrinology of pregnancy. *In* Griffin JE, Ojeda SR (eds): *Textbook of Endocrine Physiology*. New York, Oxford University Press, 1988.

Champetier J, Letoublon C, Arvieux C, et al: Les variations de division des voies biliares extrahepatiques: signification et origine, consequences chirurgicales. *J Chir (Paris) 126:*147, 1989a.

Champetier J, Yver R, Tomasella T: Functional anatomy of the liver of the human fetus: applications to ultrasonography. *Surg Radiol Anat 11:*53, 1989b.

Cobb RA, Williamson RCN: Embryology and development abnormalities of the large intestine. *In* Phillips SF, Pemberton JH, Shorter RG (eds): *The Large Intestine; Physiology, Pathophysiology, and Disease*. New York, Raven, 1991.

Cockburn F, Carachi R, Goel KN, Young DG: *Children's Medicine and Surgery*. London, Arnold, 1996.

Cywes S, Davies MRQ, Rode H: Congenital jejuno-ileal atresia and stenosis. *In* Persaud TVN (ed): *Advances in the Study of Birth Defects. Cardiovascular, Respiratory, Gastrointestinal and Genitourinary Malformations,* vol 6. New York, Alan R Liss, 1982.

Dillon PW, Cilley RE: Newborn surgical emergencies-gastrointestinal anomalies, abdominal wall defects. *Pediatr Clin North Am 40:* 1289, 1993.

Drongowski RA, Smith RK Jr, Coran AG, Klein MD: Contribution of demographic and environmental factors to the etiology of gastroschisis: a hypothesis. *Fetal Diagn Ther 6:*14, 1991.

Estrada RL: *Anomalies of Intestinal Rotation and Fixation*. Springfield, Charles C Thomas, 1968.

Fallin LT: The development and cytodifferentiation of the islets of Langerhans in human embryos and foetuses. *Acta Anat 68:*147, 1967.

Filly RA: Sonographic anatomy of the normal fetus. *In* Harrison MR, Golbus MS, Filly RA (eds): *The Unborn Patient: Prenatal Diagnosis and Treatment,* 2nd ed. Philadelphia, WB Saunders, 1991.

Fitzgerald MJT, Nolan JP, O'Neil MN: The position of the human caecum in fetal life. *J Anat 109:*71, 1971.

Gemonov VV, Kolesnikov LL: Development of oesophageal tissue structures in human embryogenesis. *Anat Anz 171:*13, 1990.

Gilbert-Barnes E (ed): *Pathology of the Fetus and Infant.* 2 vols. St Louis, Mosby, 1997.

Grand RJ, Watkins JB, Torti FM: Progress in gastroenterology: development of the human gastrointestinal tract. A review. *Gastroenterology 70:*790, 1976.

Harris J, Källén B, Robert E: Descriptive epidemiology of alimentary tract anomalies. *Teratology 52:*15, 1995.

Herbst JJ: The esophagus. *In* Behrman RE et al (eds): *Nelson Textbook of Pediatrics,* 15th ed. Philadelphia, WB Saunders, 1996.

Karrer FM, Raffensperger JG: Biliary atresia. *In* Raffensperger JG (ed): *Swenson's Pediatric Surgery,* 5th ed. Norwalk, Appleton & Lange, 1990.

Kirillova IA, Novikova IV, Bragina ZN: Pathology of developmental defects of the digestive system in human embryos (in Russian). *Arkh Patol 52:*14, 1990.

Kliegman RM: The umbilicus. *In* Behrman RE, Kliegman RM, Arvin AM (eds): *Nelson Textbook of Pediatrics,* 15th ed. Philadelphia, WB Saunders, 1996.

Kluth MWD, Lambrecht W: Anorectal malformation: a new anatomic variant resembling an H-type fistula. *J Pediatr Surg 31:*1682, 1996.

Lebenthal E, Leung YK: Feeding the premature and compromised infant: gastrointestinal consideration. *Pediatr Clin North Am 35:* 215, 1988.

Martinez NS, Morlach CG, Dockerty B, et al: Heterotopic pancreatic tissue involving the stomach. *Am Surg 147:*1, 1958.

McLean JM: Embryology of the pancreas. *In* Howat HT, Sarles H (eds): *The Exocrine Pancreas*. Philadelphia, WB Saunders, 1979.

Meizner I, Levy A, Barnhard Y: Cloacal exstrophy sequence: an exceptional ultrasound diagnosis. *Obstet Gynecol 86:*446, 1995.

Menard D, Arsenault P: Cell proliferation in developing human stomach. *Anat Embryol (Berl) 182:*509, 1990.

Moore KL: *Clinically Oriented Anatomy,* 3rd ed. Baltimore, Williams & Wilkins, 1992.

Noordijk JA: Omphalocele and gastroschisis. *In* Persaud TVN (ed): *Advances in the Study of Birth Defects. Cardiovascular, Respiratory, Gastrointestinal and Genitourinary Malformations,* vol 6. New York, Alan R Liss, 1982.

Pena A: Total urogenital mobilization—an easier way to repair cloacas. *J Pediatr Surg 32:*263, 1997.

Phelps S, Fisher R, Partington A, Dykes E: Prenatal ultrasound diagnosis of gastrointestinal malformations. *J Pediatr Surg 32:*438, 1997.

Raffensperger JF (ed): *Swenson's Pediatric Surgery*. Norwalk, Appleton & Lange, 1990.

Rawdon BB, Andrew W: Comment on "Do the pancreatic primordial buds in embryogenesis have the potential to provide all pancreatic endocrine cells?" *Medical Hypotheses 35:*275, 1991.

Severn CB: A morphoglocial study of the development of the human liver. I. Development of the hepatic diverticulum *Am J Anat 131:* 133, 1971.

Severn CB: A morphological study of the development of the human liver. II. Establishment of liver parenchyma, extrahepatic ducts, and associated venous channels. *Am J Anat 133:*85, 1972.

Taeusch HW, Ballard RB, Avery ME (eds) *Schaffer and Avery's Diseases of the Newborn,* 6th ed. Philadelphia, WB Saunders, 1991.

Thompson JC: *Atlas of Surgery of the Stomach, Duodenum, and Small Bowel*. St Louis, Mosby Year Book, 1992.

Thompson MW, McInnes RR, Willard HF: *Thompson & Thompson Genetics in Medicine,* 5th ed. Philadelphia, WB Saunders, 1991.

Ulshen M: Stomach and intestines. *In* Behrman RE, Kliegman RM, Arvin AM (eds): *Nelson Textbook of Pediatrics,* 15th ed. Philadelphia, WB Saunders, 1996.

Valioulis I, Anagnostopoulos D, Sfougaris D: Reversed midgut rotation in a neonate: case report with a brief review of the literature. *J Pediatr Surg 32:*643, 1997.

Vaos GC: Quantitative assessment of the stage of neuronal maturation in the human fetal gut—a new dimension in the pathogenesis of developmental anomalies of the myenteric plexus. *J Pediatr Surg 24:*920, 1989.

von Dorsche HH: Inselorgan. *In* Hinrichsen KV (ed): *Humanembryologie*. Berlin, Springer-Verlag, 1990.

Wolf-Coote SA, Louw J, Poerstamper HM, Du Toit DF: Do the pancreatic primordial buds in embryogenesis have potential to provide all pancreatic endocrine cells? *Medical Hypotheses 31*:313, 1990.

Wyllie R: Pyloric stenosis and other congenital anomalies of the stomach; intestinal atresia, stenosis, and malformations; intestinal duplications, Meckel diverticulum, and other remnants of the omphalomesenteric duct. *In* Behrman RE, Kliegman RM, Arvin AM (eds): *Nelson Textbook of Pediatrics,* 15th ed. Philadelphia, WB Saunders, 1996.

Yoon PW, Bresee JS, Olney RS, et al: Epidemiology of biliary atresia: a population-based study. *Pediatrics 99*:376, 1997.

Zona JZ: Umbilical anomalies. *In* Raffensperger JG (ed): *Swenson's Pediatric Surgery,* 5th ed. Norwalk, Appleton & Lange, 1990.

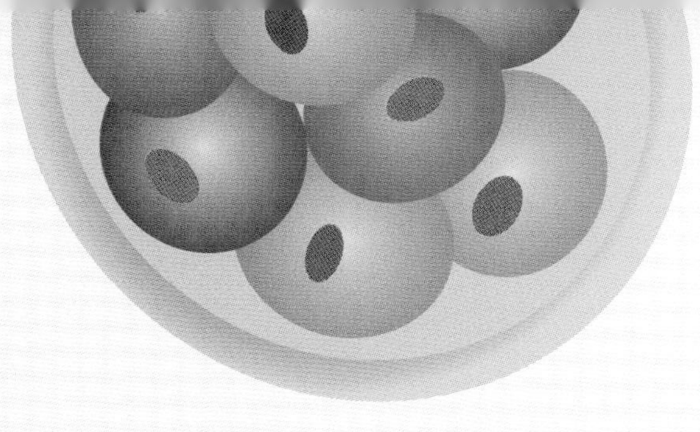

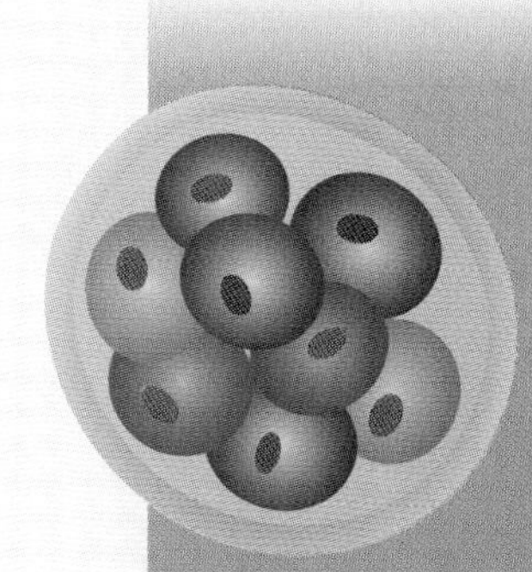

The Urogenital System

13

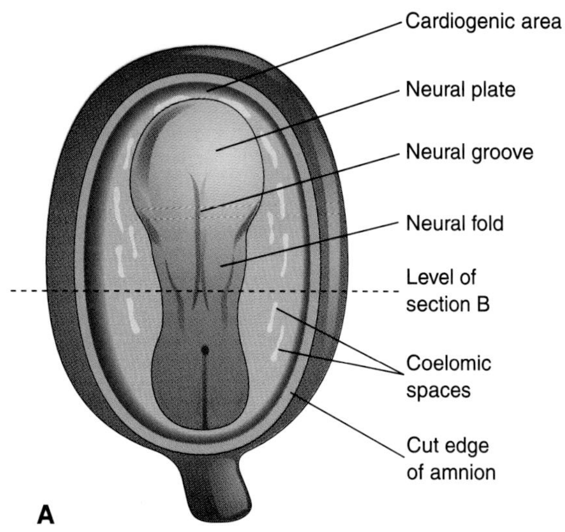

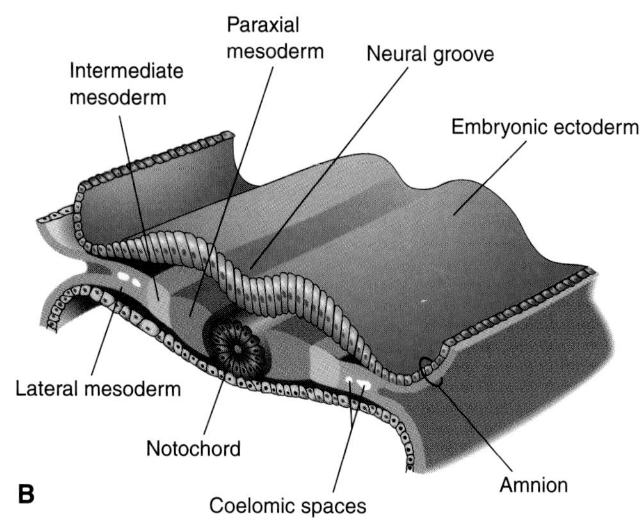

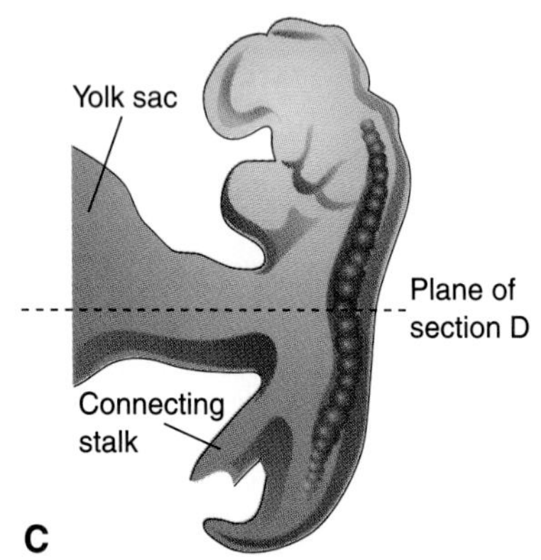

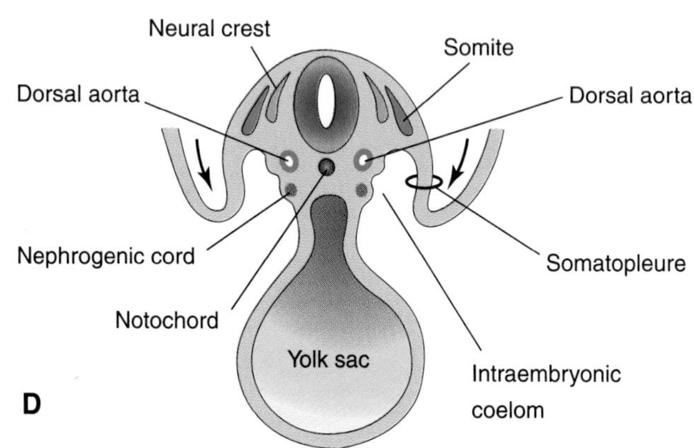

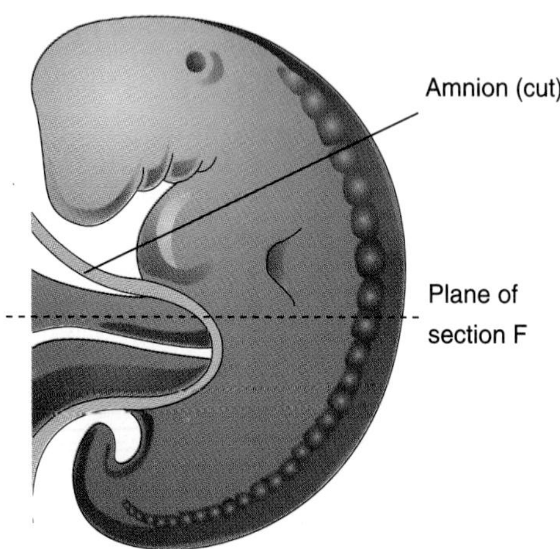

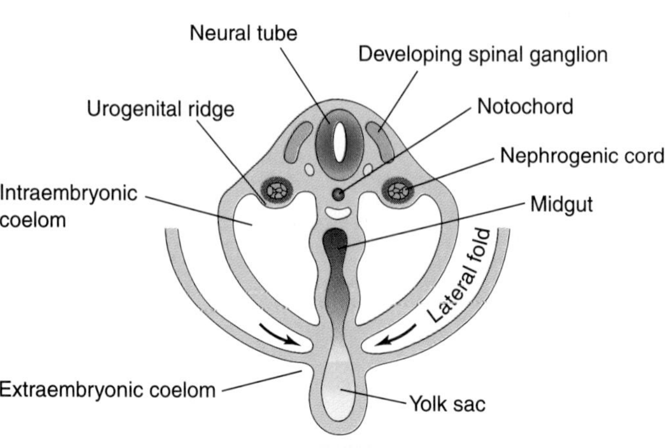

■ **Figure 13–1.** *A,* Dorsal view of an embryo during the third week (about 18 days). *B,* Transverse section of the embryo showing the position of the intermediate mesoderm before lateral folding of the embryo. *C,* Lateral view of an embryo during the fourth week (about 24 days). *D,* Transverse section of the embryo after the commencement of folding, showing the nephrogenic cords of mesoderm. *E,* Lateral view of an embryo later in the fourth week (about 26 days). *F,* Transverse section of the embryo showing the lateral folds meeting each other ventrally. Observe the position of the urogenital ridges and nephrogenic cords.

■ The urogenital system can be divided functionally into the *urinary (excretory) system* and the *genital (reproductive) system*. Embryologically these systems are closely associated. They are also closely associated anatomically especially in adult males; e.g., the urethra conveys both urine and semen. Although these systems are separate in normal adult females, the urethra and vagina open into a common space or cavity — the vestibule of the vagina — between the labia minora (Moore, 1992).

Development of the *suprarenal (adrenal) glands* is described in this chapter for two reasons:

- They are closely related to the superior poles of the kidneys.
- *Congenital adrenal hyperplasia* (CAH) causes virilization (masculinization) of female external genitalia; e.g., enlargement of the clitoris.

The urogenital system develops from the intermediate mesoderm, which extends along the dorsal body wall of the embryo (Fig. 13-1*A* and *B*). During folding of the embryo in the horizontal plane (see Chapter 5), this mesoderm is carried ventrally and loses its connection with the somites (Fig. 13-1*C*). A longitudinal elevation of mesoderm — the **urogenital ridge** —forms on each side of the dorsal aorta (Fig. 13-1*D*). It gives rise to parts of the urinary and genital systems. The part of the urogenital ridge giving rise to the urinary system is the **nephrogenic cord** or ridge (Fig. 13-1*C* to *F*); the part giving rise to the genital system is the **genital** or **gonadal ridge**.

DEVELOPMENT OF THE URINARY SYSTEM

The urinary system begins to develop before the genital system. The urinary system consists of:

- the *kidneys*, which excrete urine
- the *ureters*, which convey urine from the kidneys to the bladder
- the *urinary bladder*, which stores urine temporarily
- the *urethra*, which carries urine from the bladder to the exterior

Development of the Kidneys and Ureters

Three sets of excretory organs or kidneys develop in human embryos:

- the *pronephros*
- the *mesonephros*
- the *metanephros*

The first set of kidneys — the *pronephroi* (plural of pronephros) — are rudimentary and nonfunctional. They are analogous to the kidneys in primitive fishes. The second set of kidneys — the *mesonephroi* — are well developed and function briefly; they are analogous to the kidneys of amphibians. The third set of kidneys — the *metanephroi* — become the permanent kidneys.

PRONEPHROI

These transitory, nonfunctional structures appear in human embryos early in the fourth week. They are represented by a few cell clusters and tortuous tubular structures in the neck region (Fig. 13-2*A*). The pronephric ducts run caudally and open into the cloaca (Fig. 13-2*B*). The rudimentary pronephroi soon degenerate; however, most of the pronephric ducts persist and are utilized by the next set of kidneys.

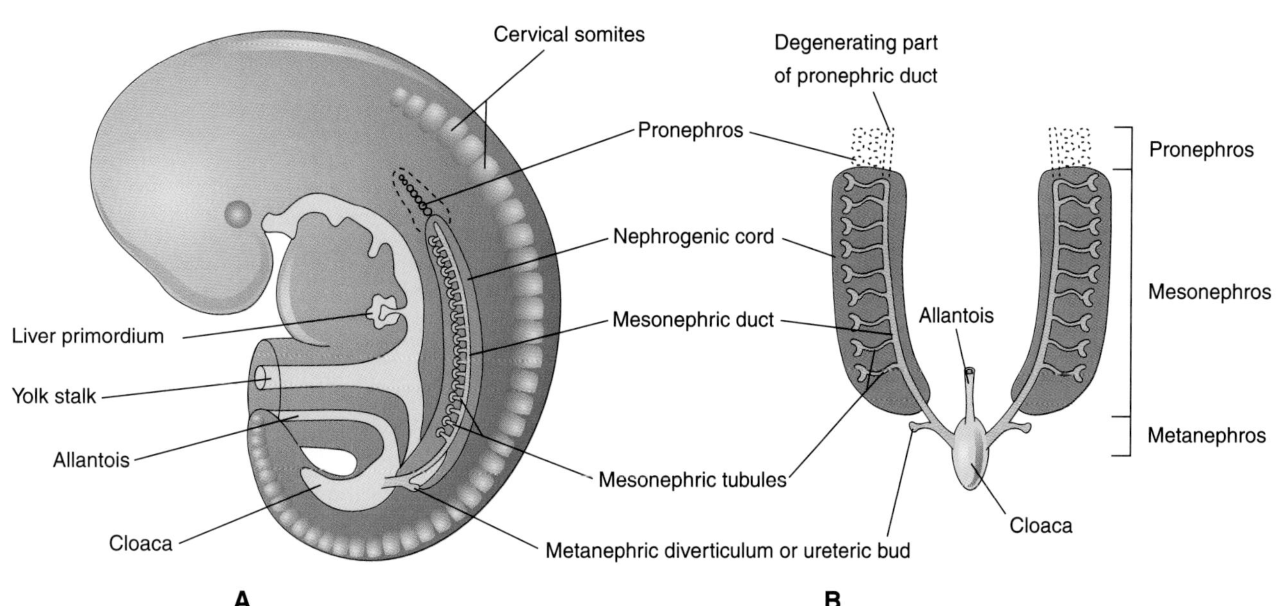

■ **Figure 13–2.** Diagrammatic sketches illustrating the three sets of excretory systems in an embryo during the fifth week. *A*, Lateral view. *B*, Ventral view. The mesonephric tubules have been pulled laterally; their normal position is shown in *A*.

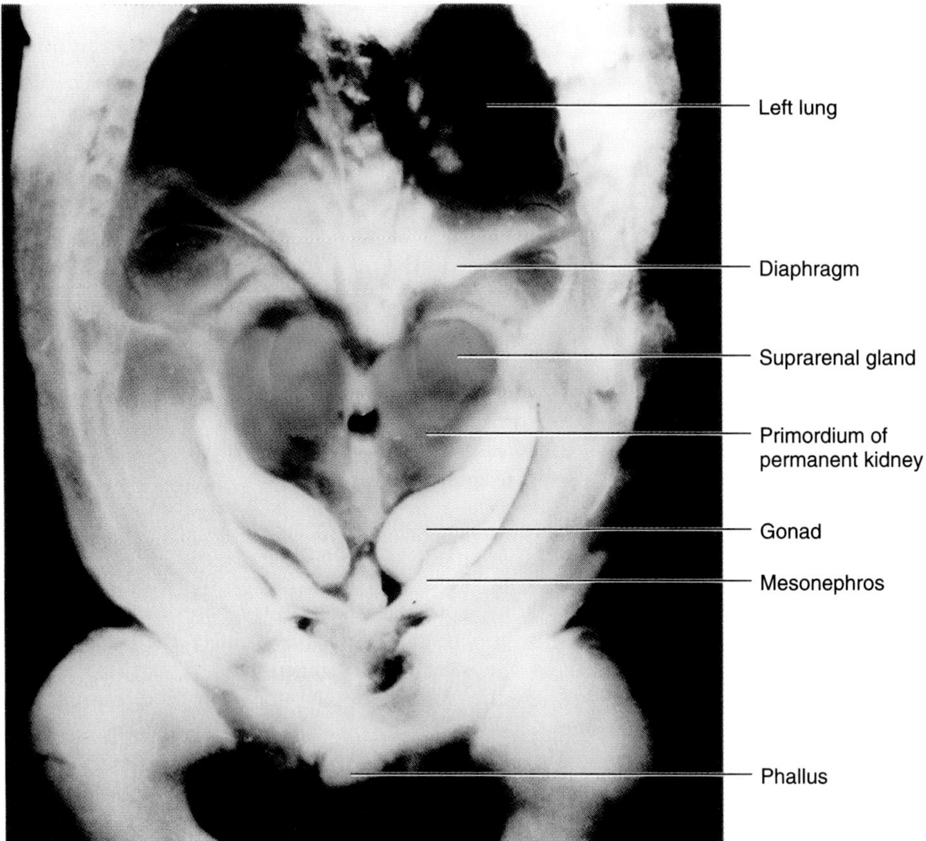

■ **Figure 13–3.** Dissection of the thorax, abdomen, and pelvis of an embryo at Carnegie stage 22, about 54 days. Observe the large suprarenal (adrenal) glands and the elongated mesonephroi (mesonephric kidneys). Also observe the gonads (testes or ovaries). The sex of these glands is not obvious in an external view such as this. External evidence of sex is not recognizable either. The phallus will develop into a penis or a clitoris depending on the genetic sex of the embryo. (From Nishimura H [ed]: *Atlas of Human Prenatal Histology.* Tokyo, Igaku-Shoin, 1983.)

MESONEPHROI

These large, elongated, excretory organs appear late in the fourth week, caudal to the rudimentary pronephroi (Fig. 13-2). They are well developed and function as ***interim kidneys*** until the permanent kidneys develop (Fig. 13-3). The mesonephric kidneys consist of glomeruli and mesonephric tubules (Figs. 13-3 to 13-5). The tubules open into the **mesonephric duct**, which was originally the pronephric duct. The meso-

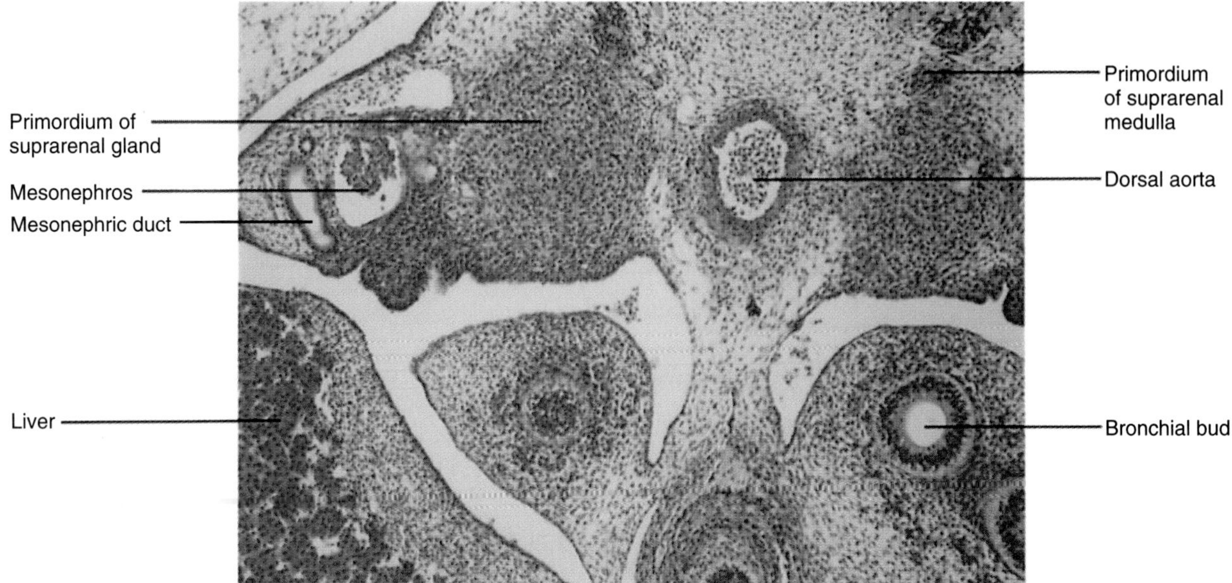

■ **Figure 13–4.** Photomicrograph of a transverse section of an embryo at Carnegie stage 17, about 42 days, primarily to show the mesonephros and developing suprarenal (adrenal) glands. Observe that the developing cortex of each gland is large, whereas the small medulla lies dorsal to the cortex. Observe that the mesonephros extends into the thorax at this stage (see also Fig. 13–5*A*). (From Moore KL, Persaud TVN, Shiota K: *Color Atlas of Clinical Embryology.* Philadelphia, WB Saunders, 1994.)

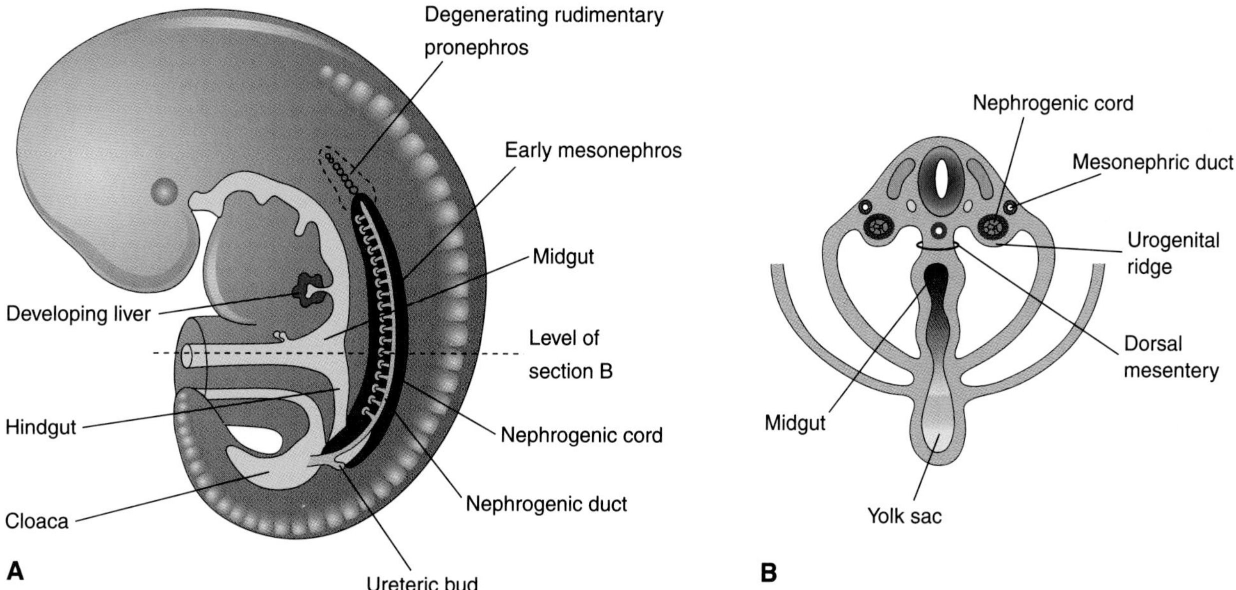

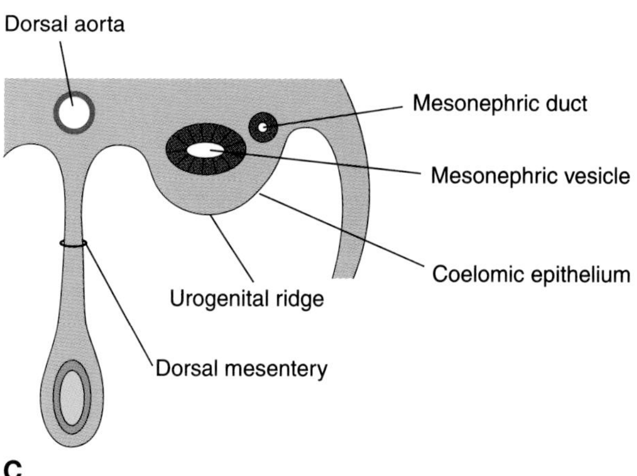

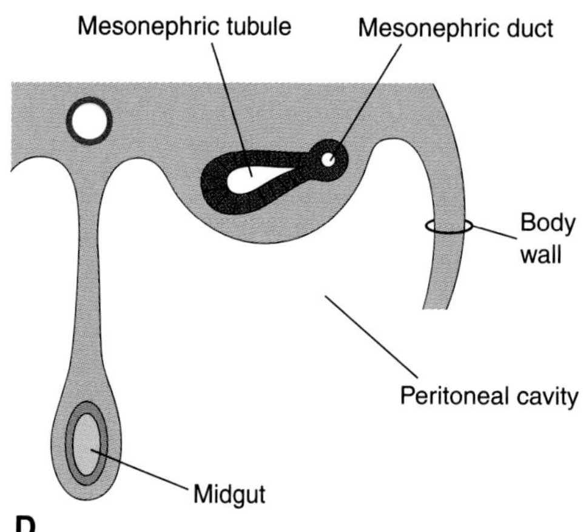

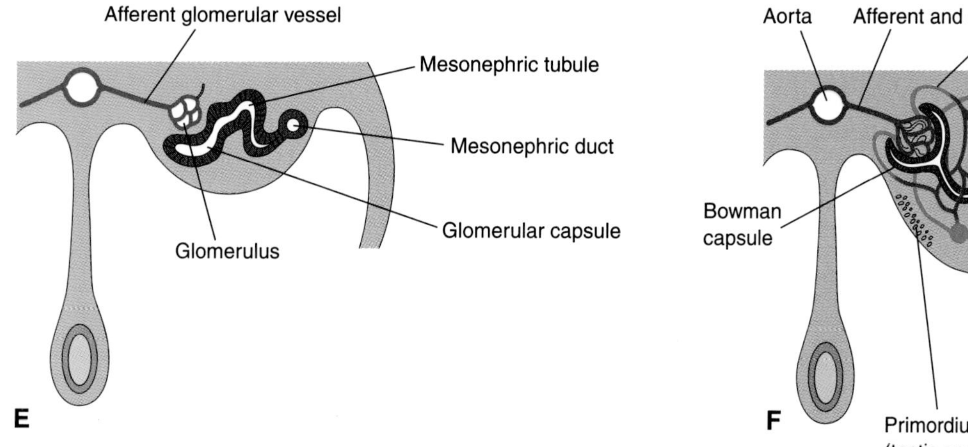

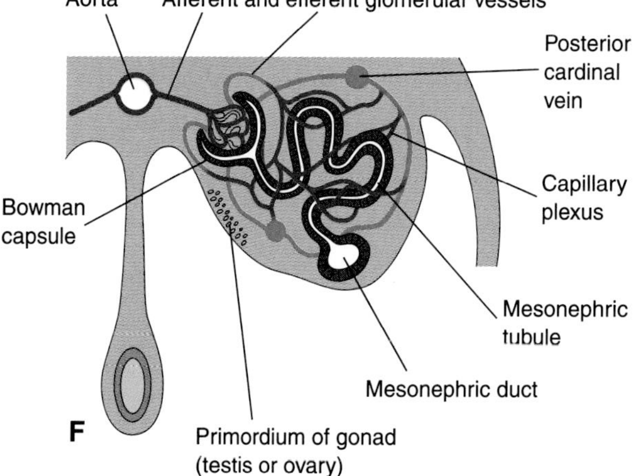

■ **Figure 13–5.** *A,* Sketch of a lateral view of a 5-week embryo showing the extent of the mesonephros and the primordium of the metanephros or permanent kidney. *B,* Transverse section of the embryo showing the nephrogenic cords from which the mesonephric tubules develop. *C* to *F,* Sketches of transverse sections showing successive stages in the development of a mesonephric tubule between the fifth and eleventh weeks. Note that the mesenchymal cell cluster in the nephrogenic cord develops a lumen, thereby forming a mesonephric vesicle. The vesicle soon becomes an S-shaped mesonephric tubule and extends laterally to join the pronephric duct, now renamed the mesonephric duct. The expanded medial end of the mesonephric tubule is invaginated by blood vessels to form a glomerular capsule (Bowman capsule). The cluster of capillaries projecting into this capsule is the glomerulus.

nephric duct opens into the cloaca. The mesonephroi degenerate toward the end of the first trimester; however, their tubules become the efferent ductules of the testes and the mesonephric ducts have several adult derivatives in the male.

METANEPHROI

The metanephroi or **permanent kidneys** begin to develop early in the fifth week and start to function about 4 weeks later (Behrman et al., 1996). *Urine formation* continues throughout fetal life. Urine is excreted into the amniotic cavity and mixes with the amniotic fluid. A mature fetus swallows several hundred milliliters of amniotic fluid each day, which is absorbed by the intestine. The waste products are transferred through the placental membrane into the maternal blood for elimination. The permanent kidneys develop from two sources:

- the *metanephric diverticulum* or ureteric bud
- the *metanephric mass of intermediate mesoderm* (metanephrogenic blastema)

The metanephric diverticulum is an outgrowth from the mesonephric duct near its entrance into the cloaca, and the metanephric mesoderm is derived from the caudal part of the nephrogenic cord (Fig. 13-6). Both primordia of the metanephros are of mesodermal origin. See Bard (1996) for information regarding molecular mechanisms in kidney morphogenesis. The expression pattern of more than 200 genes associated with the kidneys has been reported, but their function is largely unknown. The expression of two genes, WT1 and BF-2, are of particular interest in the early development of the mouse kidney. The relevance of gene *knockout* studies in mice with respect to the human kidney is uncertain; however, the findings should provide a better understanding of kidney development and renal anomalies.

The **metanephric diverticulum,** or **ureteric bud,** is the primordium of the *ureter, renal pelvis, calices,* and *collecting tubules* (Fig. 13-6*C* to *E*). As it elongates the metanephric diverticulum penetrates the metanephric mesoderm, inducing the formation of a **metanephric mass of intermediate mesoderm** over its expanded end (Fig. 13-6*B*). Cell surface N-linked oligosaccharides appear to be important for this inductive interaction between the ureteric bud and the metanephric mesoderm (Fleming, 1990). The stalk of the metanephric diverticulum becomes the **ureter** and its expanded cranial end forms the *renal pelvis.*

The straight **collecting tubules** undergo repeated

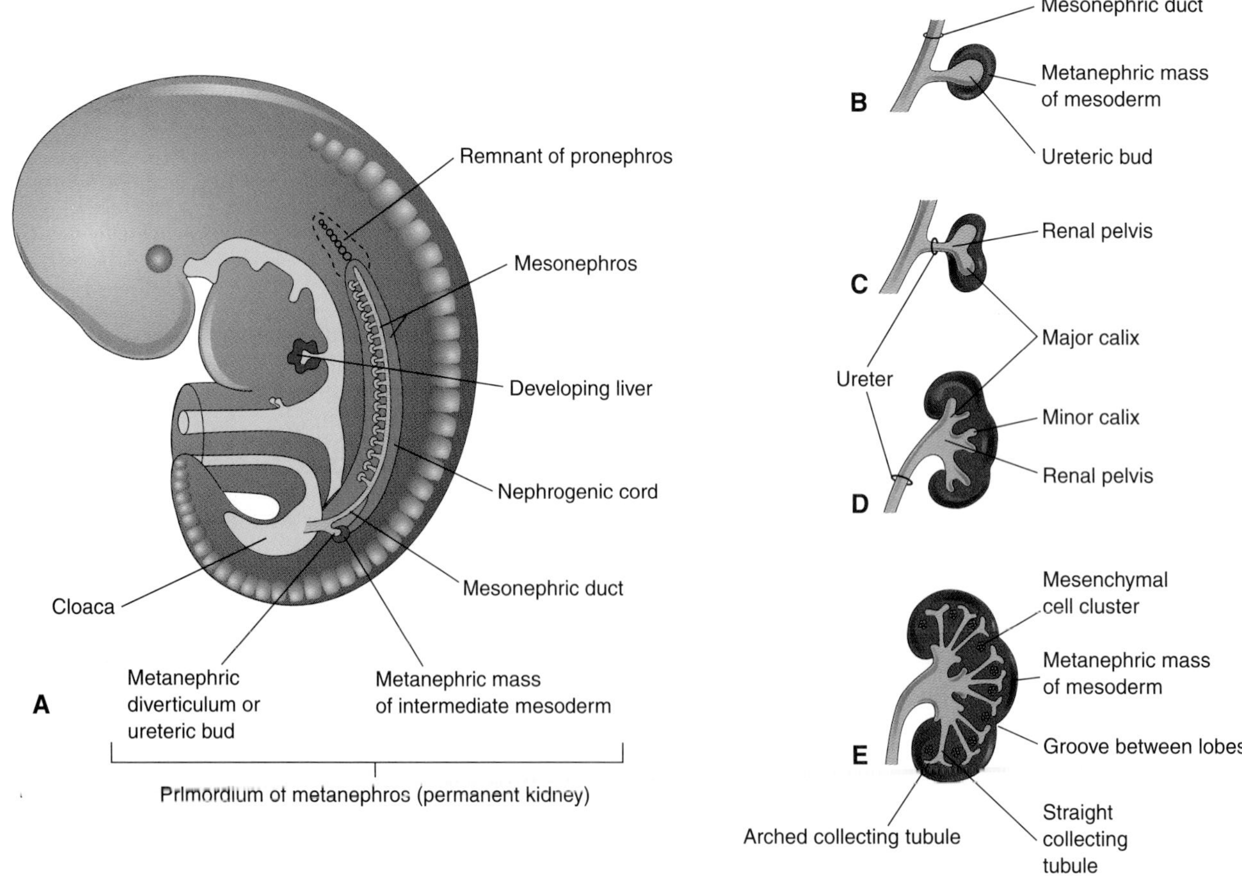

■ **Figure 13-6.** Development of the metanephros or permanent kidney. *A,* Sketch of a lateral view of a 5-week embryo, showing the primordium of the metanephros. *B* to *E,* Sketches showing successive stages in the development of the metanephric diverticulum or ureteric bud (fifth to eighth weeks). Observe the development of the ureter, renal pelvis, calices, and collecting tubules.

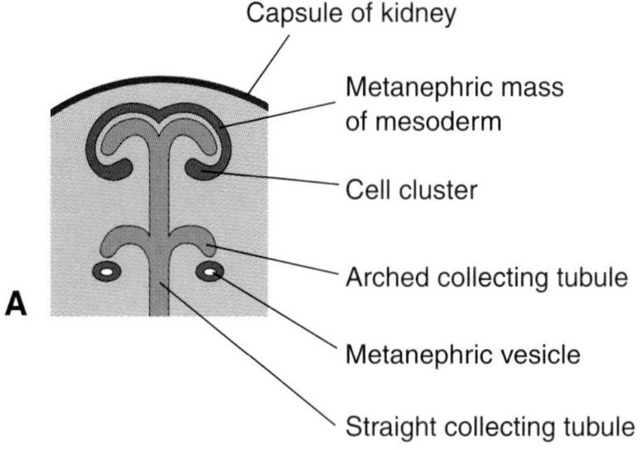

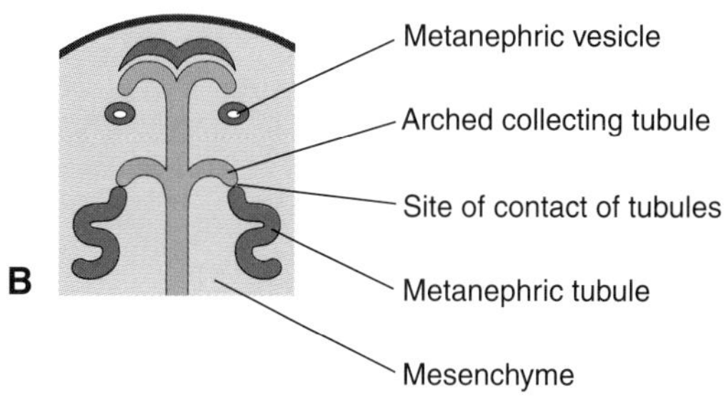

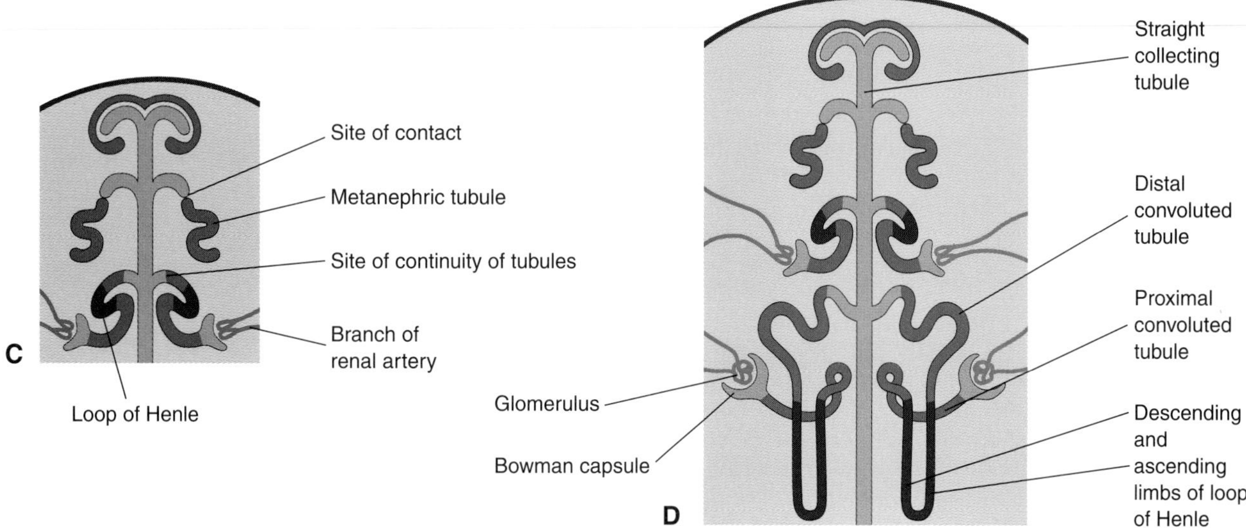

■ **Figure 13–7.** Diagrammatic sketches illustrating stages in nephrogenesis—the development of nephrons. *A*, Nephrogenesis commences around the beginning of the eighth week. *B* and *C*, Note that the metanephric tubules, the primordia of the nephrons, become continuous with the collecting tubules to form uriniferous tubules. *D*, The number of nephrons more than doubles from 20 weeks to 38 weeks. Observe that nephrons are derived from the metanephric mass of mesoderm and that the collecting tubules are derived from the metanephric diverticulum.

branching, forming successive generations of collecting tubules. The first four generations of tubules enlarge and become confluent to form the **major calices** (Fig. 13-6*C* to *E*), and the second four generations coalesce to form the **minor calices**. The remaining generations of tubules form the collecting tubules. The end of each arched collecting tubule induces clusters of mesenchymal cells in the metanephric mass of mesoderm to form small **metanephric vesicles** (Fig. 13-7*A*). These vesicles elongate and become **metanephric tubules** (Fig. 13-7*B* and *C*). As these renal tubules develop, their proximal ends are invaginated by glomeruli. The **renal corpuscle** (glomerulus and Bowman capsule) and its proximal convoluted tubule, loop of Henle, and distal convoluted tubule constitute a **nephron** (Fig. 13-7*D*). Each distal convoluted tubule contacts an arched collecting tubule and the tubules become confluent. Between the tenth and eighteenth weeks of gestation, the number of glomeruli increases gradually, then they increase rapidly until the thirty-second week, when an upper limit is reached (Gasser et al., 1993).

A **uriniferous tubule** consists of two embryologically different parts (Figs. 13-6 and 13-7):

- a *nephron* derived from the metanephric mass of mesoderm
- a *collecting tubule* derived from the metanephric diverticulum

Tissue culture studies have shown that branching of the metanephric diverticulum is dependent upon induction by the metanephric mesoderm and that differ-

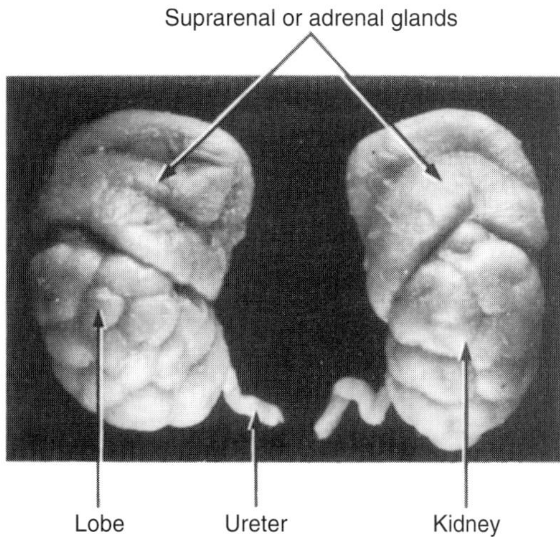

■ **Figure 13–8.** Photograph of the kidneys and suprarenal glands of a 28-week fetus (×2). The external evidence of the lobes usually disappears by the end of the first postnatal year. Note the large size of the suprarenal glands at this age. During the first 2 weeks after birth, these glands reduce to about half this size.

entiation of the nephrons depends upon induction by the collecting tubules. It has been suggested that a member (Wnt-2) of the Wnt family of genes may participate in renal morphogenesis, especially in the development of the nephron (Herzlinger et al., 1994). Expression of the nerve growth factor receptor in the developing nephrogenic tissue is required for formation of the kidney tubules (Sariola et al., 1991).

The **fetal kidneys** are subdivided into lobes that are visible externally (Fig. 13-8). This lobulation diminishes toward the end of the fetal period, but the lobes are still indicated in the kidneys of a newborn infant. The lobulation usually disappears during infancy as the nephrons increase and grow. The lobulated character of the kidneys is obscured in adults; however, in very rare cases the lobes are recognizable externally, as they are in certain animals (e.g., cattle). At term, each kidney contains 800,000 to 1,000,000 nephrons. The increase in kidney size after birth results mainly from the elongation of the proximal convoluted tubules of Henle, as well as an increase of interstitial tissue. It is now believed that nephron formation is complete at birth (Behrman et al., 1996), except in premature infants. Functional maturation of the kidneys occurs after birth. Glomerular filtration begins around the ninth fetal week and the rate of filtration increases after birth (Arant, 1987; Behrman et al., 1996).

POSITIONAL CHANGES OF THE KIDNEYS

Initially the permanent or metanephric kidneys lie close to each other in the pelvis, ventral to the sacrum (Fig. 13-9*A*). As the abdomen and pelvis grow, the kidneys gradually come to lie in the abdomen and move farther apart (Fig. 13-9*B* and *C*). They attain their adult position by the ninth week (Fig. 13-9*D*). This "migration" (relative ascent) results mainly from the growth of the embryo's body caudal to the kidneys. In effect, the caudal part of the embryo grows away from the kidneys so that they progressively occupy more cranial levels. Eventually they are retroperitoneal (external or posterior to the peritoneum) on the posterior abdominal wall. Initially the hilum of the kidney, where vessels and nerves enter and leave, faces ventrally; however, as the kidney "ascends," it rotates medially almost 90 degrees. By the ninth week the hilum is directed anteromedially (Figs. 13-3 and 13-9*C* and *D*).

CHANGES IN THE BLOOD SUPPLY OF THE KIDNEYS

As the kidneys "ascend" from the pelvis, they receive their blood supply from vessels that are close to them.

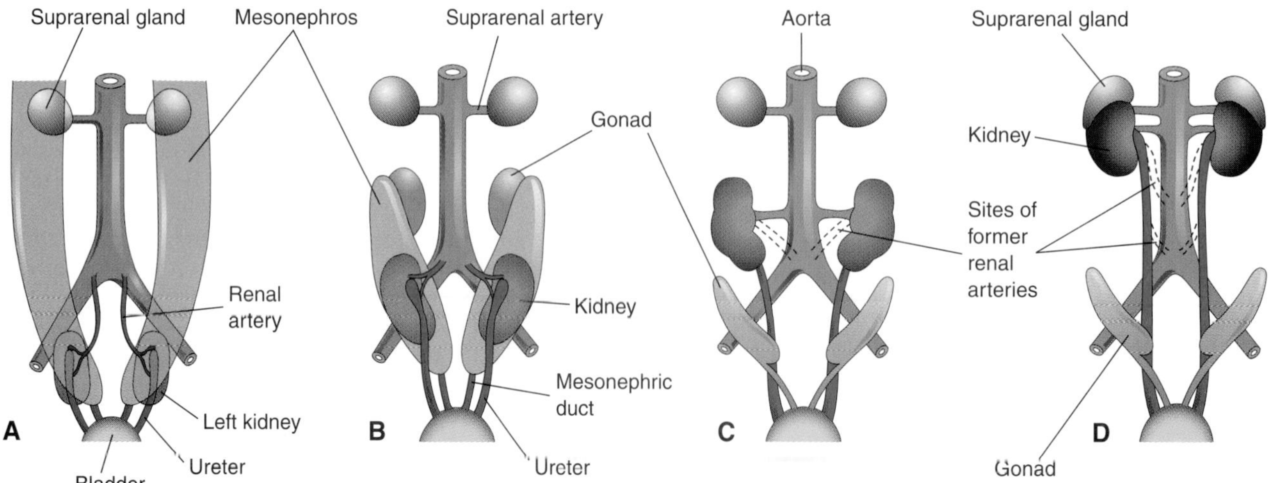

■ **Figure 13–9.** *A* to *D*, Diagrammatic ventral views of the abdominopelvic region of embryos and fetuses (sixth to ninth weeks) showing medial rotation and "ascent" of the kidneys from the pelvis to the abdomen. *A* and *B*, Observe also the size regression of the mesonephroi. *C* and *D*, Note that as the kidneys "ascend," they are supplied by arteries at successively higher levels and that the hilum of the kidney (where the vessels and nerves enter) is eventually directed anteromedially.

Initially the renal arteries are branches of the common iliac arteries (Fig. 13-9A and *B*). As they "ascend" further, the kidneys receive their blood supply from the distal end of the aorta. When they reach a higher level, they receive new branches from the aorta (Fig. 13-9*C* and *D*). Normally the caudal branches undergo involution and disappear. When the kidneys come into contact with the *suprarenal glands* in the ninth week; their "ascent" stops. The kidneys receive their most cranial arterial branches from the abdominal aorta; these branches become the permanent **renal arteries**. The right renal artery is longer and often more superior.

Accessory Renal Arteries

The relatively common variations in the blood supply to the kidneys reflect the manner in which the blood supply continually changed during embryonic and early fetal life (Fig. 13-9). A single renal artery to each kidney is present in about 70% of people. About 25% of adult kidneys have two to four renal arteries (Moore, 1992). Accessory (supernumerary) renal arteries usually arise from the aorta superior or inferior to the main renal artery and follow it to the hilum (Fig. 13-10*A*, *C*, and *D*). Accessory renal arteries may enter the kidneys directly, usually into the superior or inferior poles. An accessory artery to the inferior pole may cross anterior to the ureter and obstruct it, causing **hydronephrosis**—distention of the pelvis and calices with urine (Fig. 13-10*B*). If the artery enters the inferior pole of the right kidney, it usually crosses anterior to the inferior vena cava and ureter. It is important to be aware that accessory renal arteries are end arteries; consequently, if an accessory artery is damaged or ligated, the part of the kidney supplied by it is likely to become ischemic. Accessory arteries are about twice as common as accessory veins.

Congenital Anomalies of the Kidneys and Ureters

Some abnormality of the kidneys and ureters occurs in 3 to 4% of the newborn infants. Anomalies in shape and position are most common. Many fetal urinary tract abnormalities can be detected before birth by ultrasonography (Daneman and Alton, 1991; Fine, 1992; Mahony, 1994).

Renal Agenesis

Unilateral renal agenesis is relatively common, occurring about once in every 1000 newborn infants

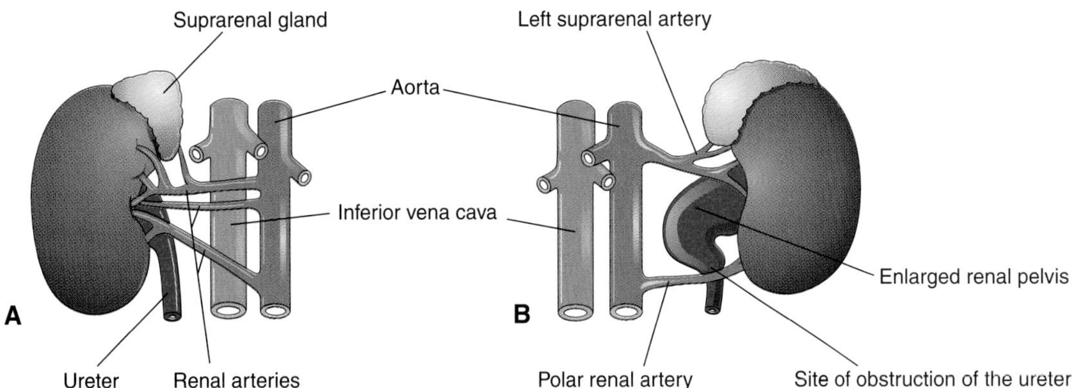

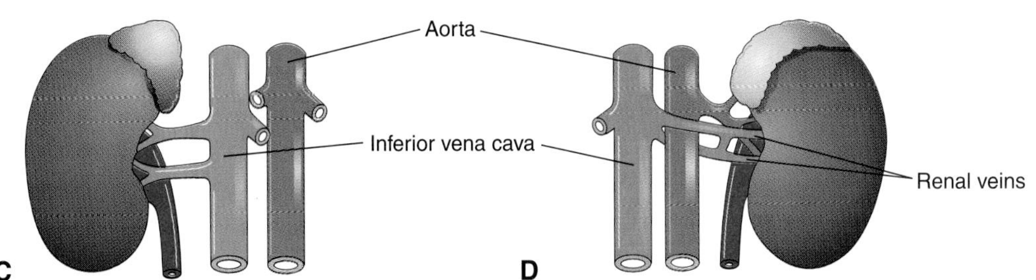

■ **Figure 13-10.** Drawings illustrating common variations of renal vessels. *A* and *B*, Multiple renal arteries. Note the accessory vessels entering the poles of the kidney. The polar renal artery, illustrated in *B*, has obstructed the ureter and produced an enlarged renal pelvis. *C* and *D*, Multiple renal veins are less common than supernumerary arteries.

(Fig. 13-12*A*). Males are affected more often than females, and the left kidney is usually the one that is absent (Fig. 13-11). Unilateral absence of a kidney often causes no symptoms and is usually not discovered during infancy because the other kidney usually undergoes compensatory hypertrophy and performs the function of the missing kidney. Unilateral renal agenesis should be suspected in infants with a *single umbilical artery* (see Chapter 7). If discovered during infancy, agenesis is usually detected during the course of evaluation for other congenital anomalies or because of urinary tract symptoms (Mahony, 1994).

Bilateral renal agenesis *is associated with oligohydramnios* (see Chapter 7) because little or no urine is excreted into the amniotic cavity (Peipert and Donnenfeld, 1991). Decreased amniotic fluid volume in the absence of other causative factors, such as rupture of the fetal membranes, alerts the sonographer to search for urinary tract anomalies (Mahony, 1994). Bilateral absence of the kidneys occurs about once in 3000 births and is incompatible with postnatal life. These infants have a characteristic facial appearance: the eyes are widely separated and have epicanthic folds; the ears are low set; the nose is broad and flat; the chin is receding, and there are limb defects. Fetal electrolyte stability is not impaired because it is controlled by exchange through the placental membrane (see Chapter 7). Most infants with bilateral renal agenesis die shortly after birth or during the first months of life.

Absence of kidneys results when the metanephric diverticula fail to develop or the ureteric primordia degenerate. Failure of the metanephric diverticulum to penetrate the metanephric mesoderm results in absence of kidney development because no nephrons are induced by the collecting tubules to develop from the metanephric mass of mesoderm. Renal agenesis probably has a multifactorial etiology. There is clinical evidence that complete in utero involution of multicystic kidneys could lead to renal agenesis with a blind ending ureter on the same side (Mesrobian et al., 1993).

Malrotation of the Kidneys

If a kidney fails to rotate, the hilum faces anteriorly, that is, the fetal kidney retains its embryonic position (Figs. 13-9*A* and 13-12*C*). If the hilum faces posteriorly, rotation of the kidney proceeded too far; if it faces laterally, lateral instead of medial rotation occurred. Abnormal rotation of the kidneys is often associated with ectopic kidneys.

Ectopic Kidneys

One or both kidneys may be in an abnormal position (Fig. 13-12*B*, *E*, and *F*). Usually they are more inferior than usual and have not rotated; consequently, the hilum faces anteriorly. Most ectopic kidneys are located in the pelvis (Fig. 13-13), but some lie in the inferior part of the abdomen. **Pelvic kidneys** and other forms of ectopia result from failure of the kidneys to "ascend." Pelvic kidneys are close to each other and may fuse to form a discoid or *pancake kidney* (Fig. 13-12*E*). Ectopic kidneys receive their blood supply from blood vessels near them (internal or external iliac arteries and/or aorta). They are often supplied by multiple vessels. Sometimes a kidney crosses to the other side resulting in **crossed renal ectopia** with or without fusion. An unusual type of abnormal kidney is *unilateral fused kidney* (Fig. 13-12*D*). The developing kidneys fuse while they are in the pelvis, and one kidney "ascends" to its normal position, carrying the other one with it.

Horseshoe Kidney

In 1 in about 500 persons, the poles of the kidneys are fused; usually it is the inferior poles that fuse. About 7% of persons with Turner syndrome have horseshoe kidneys (Behrman et al., 1996). The large U-shaped kidney usually lies in the hypogastrium, anterior to the inferior lumbar vertebrae (Fig. 13-14). Normal ascent of the fused kidneys is prevented because they are caught by the root of the inferior mesenteric artery. *A horseshoe kidney usually produces no symptoms* because its collecting system develops normally and the ureters enter the bladder. If urinary flow is impeded, signs and symptoms of obstruction and/or infection may appear. *Wilms tumors* are two to eight times more frequent in children with horseshoe kidney than in the general population (Behrman et al., 1996).

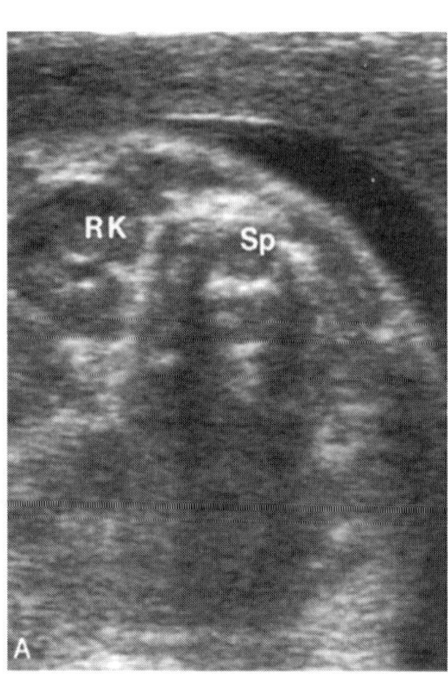

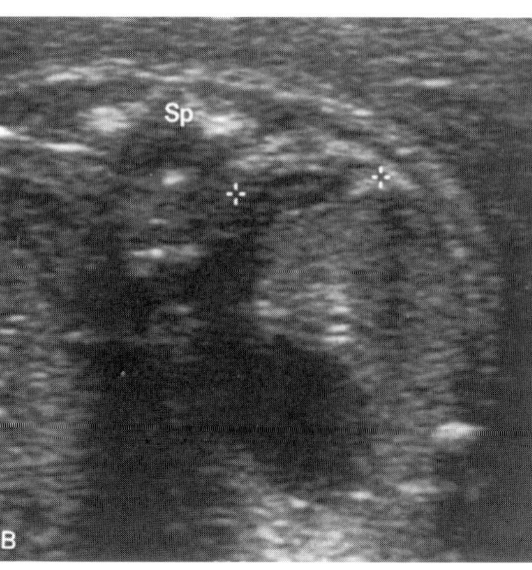

■ **Figure 13-11.** Sonograms of a fetus with unilateral renal agenesis. *A,* Transverse scan at the level of the lumbar region of the vertebral column or spine **(Sp)** showing the right kidney **(RK)** but not the left kidney. *B,* Transverse scan at a slightly higher level, showing the left suprarenal gland *(between cursors)* within the left renal fossa. (From Mahony BS: Ultrasound evaluation of the fetal genitourinary system. *In* Callen PW [ed]: *Ultrasonography in Obstetrics and Gynecology,* 3rd ed. Philadelphia, WB Saunders, 1994.)

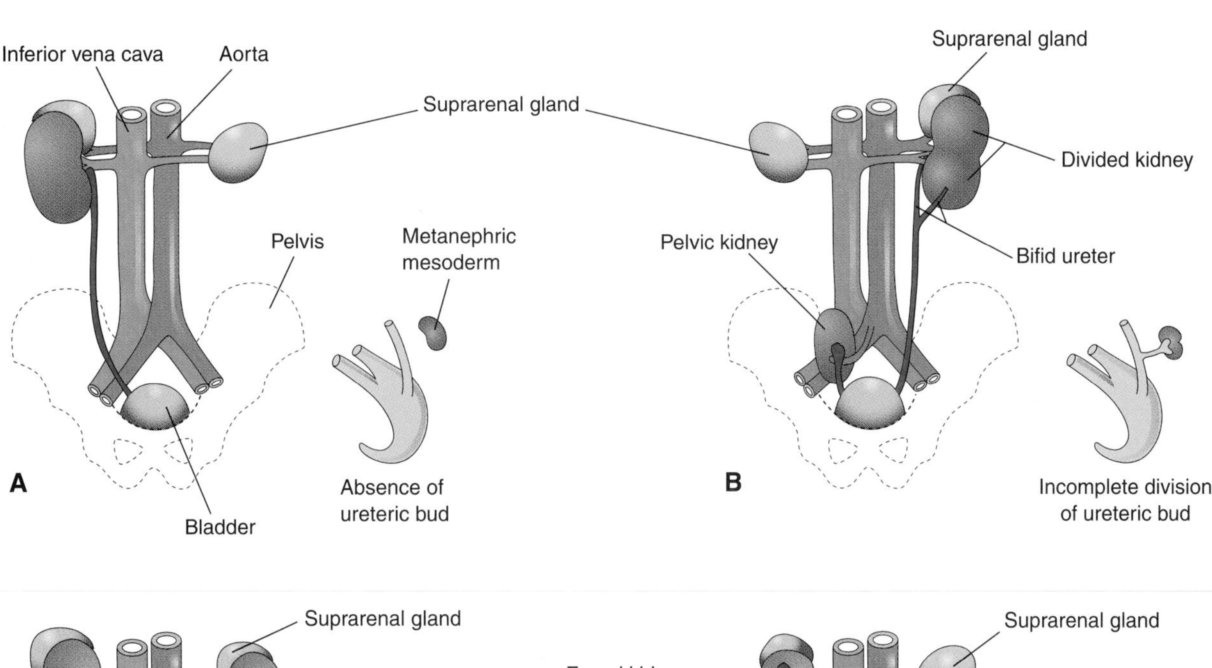

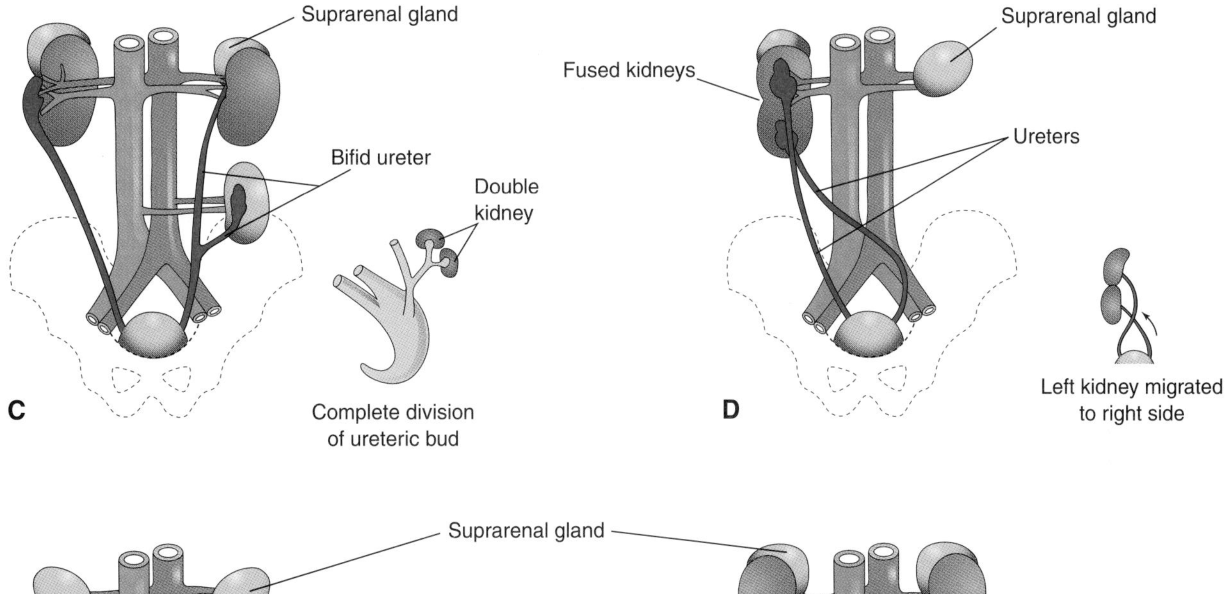

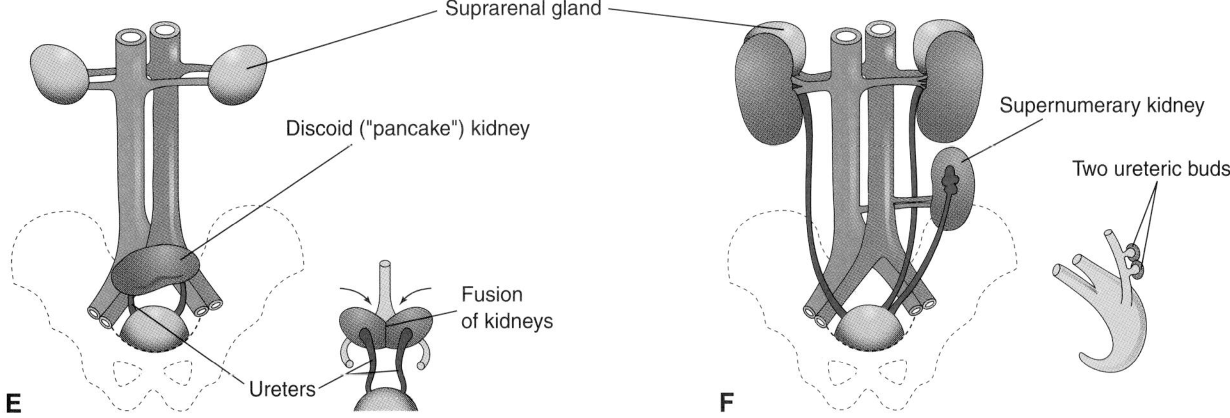

■ **Figure 13–12.** Drawings illustrating various anomalies of the urinary system. The small sketch to the lower right of each drawing illustrates the probable embryological basis of the anomaly. *A,* Unilateral renal agenesis. *B,* Right side, pelvic kidney; left side, divided kidney with a bifid ureter. *C,* Right side, malrotation of the kidney; left side, bifid ureter and supernumerary kidney. *D,* Crossed renal ectopia. The left kidney crossed to the right side and fused with the right kidney. *E,* Discoid kidney resulting from fusion of the kidneys while they were in the pelvis. *F,* Supernumerary left kidney resulting from the development of two ureteric buds.

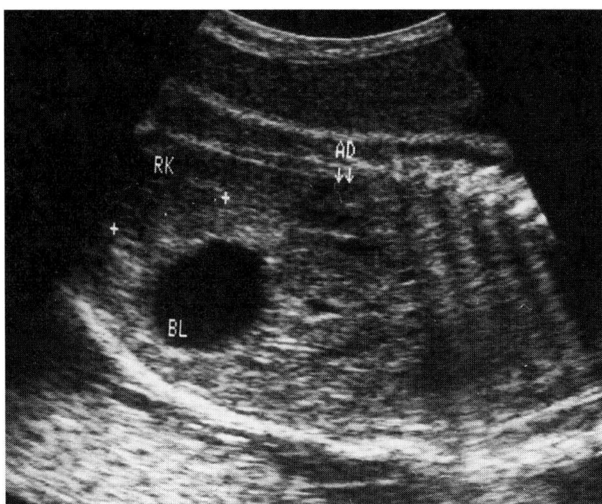

■ **Figure 13–13.** Sonogram of the pelvis of a fetus at 31 weeks of gestation (29 weeks after fertilization). Observe the abnormally low position of the right kidney **(RK)** near the urinary bladder **(BL)**. This pelvic kidney resulted from its failure to "ascend" during the sixth to ninth weeks. Also observe the normal location of the suprarenal or adrenal gland **(AD)**, which develops separately from the kidney. When the kidneys "ascend" into the abdomen, the suprarenal glands lie at their superior poles. (Courtesy of Dr. Lyndon M. Hill, Director of Ultrasound, Magee-Women's Hospital, Pittsburgh, Pennsylvania.)

Duplications of the Urinary Tract

Duplications of the abdominal part of the ureter and the renal pelvis are common, but a **supernumerary kidney** is rare (Fig. 13-12*F*). These anomalies result from division of the metanephric diverticulum (ureteric bud). The extent of the duplication depends on how complete the division of the diverticulum was. Incomplete division of the ureteric primordium results in a divided kidney with a bifid ureter (Fig. 13-12*B*). Complete division results in a double kidney with a bifid ureter (Fig. 13-12*B*) or separate ureters (Fig. 13-15). A supernumerary kidney with its own ureter probably results from the formation of two ureteric diverticula.

Ectopic Ureter

An ectopic ureter opens anywhere except into the urinary bladder. In males ectopic ureters usually open into the neck of the bladder or into the prostatic part of the urethra (Moore, 1992), but they may enter the ductus deferens, prostatic utricle, or seminal vesicle (Behrman et al., 1996). In females, ectopic ureteric orifices may be in the bladder neck, urethra, vagina, or vestibule of the vagina (Fig. 13-16). *Incontinence* is the common complaint resulting from an ectopic ureteric orifice because the urine flowing from the orifice does not enter the bladder; instead it continually dribbles from the urethra in males and the urethra and/or vagina in females.

Ureteric ectopia results when the ureter is not incorporated into the posterior part of the urinary bladder; instead it is carried caudally with the mesonephric duct and is incorporated into the caudal portion of the vesical part of the urogenital sinus. Because this part of the sinus becomes the prostatic urethra in males and the urethra in females, the common location of ectopic ureteric orifices is understandable. When two ureters form on one side, (Fig. 13-15), they usually open into the urinary bladder (Fig. 13-12*F*). In some males the extra ureter is carried caudally and drains into the neck of the bladder or into the prostatic part of the urethra.

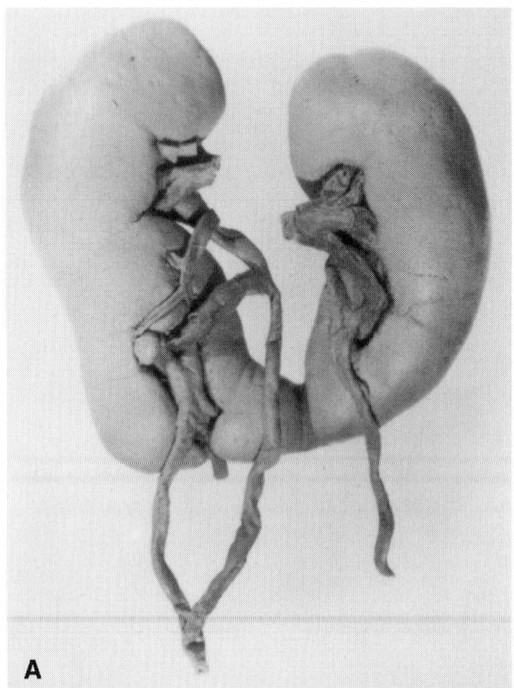

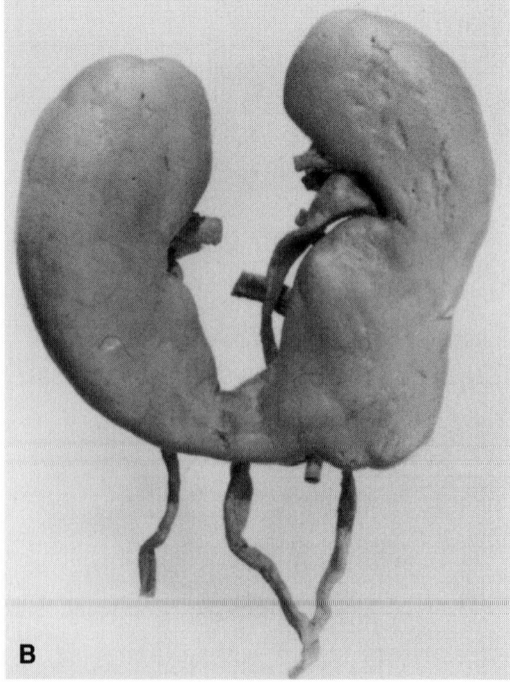

■ **Figure 13–14.** Photographs of a horseshoe kidney resulting from fusion of the inferior poles of the kidneys while they were in the pelvis. *A,* Anterior view. *B,* Posterior view. The larger right kidney has a bifid ureter.

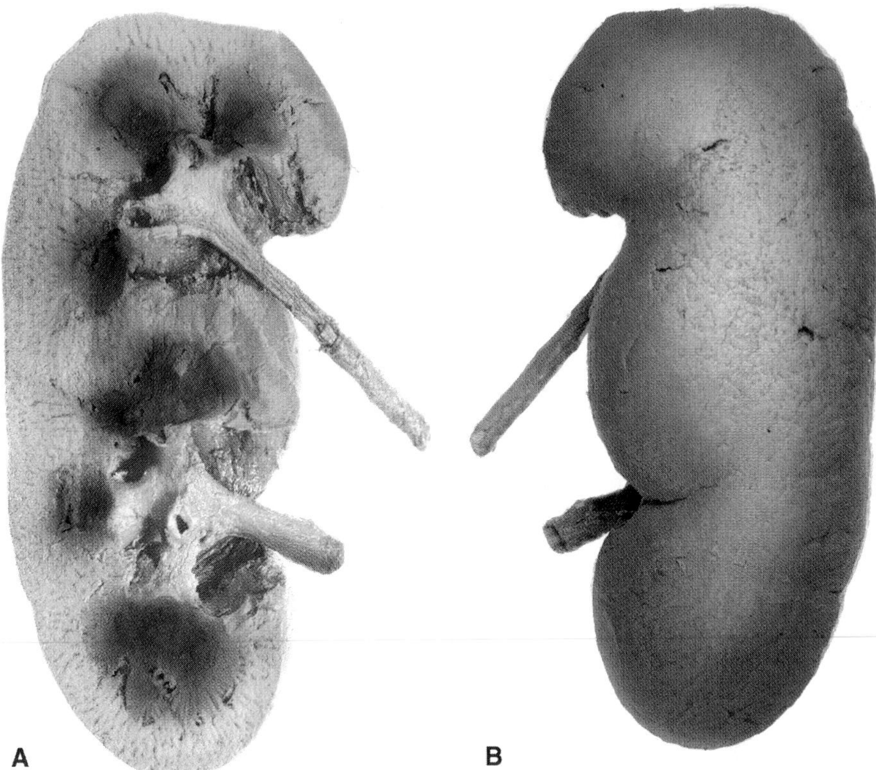

■ **Figure 13–15.** Photographs of a duplex kidney with two ureters and renal pelves. This congenital anomaly results from incomplete division of the metanephric diverticulum or ureteric bud. *A,* Longitudinal section through the kidney showing two renal pelves and calices. *B,* Anterior surface of the kidney.

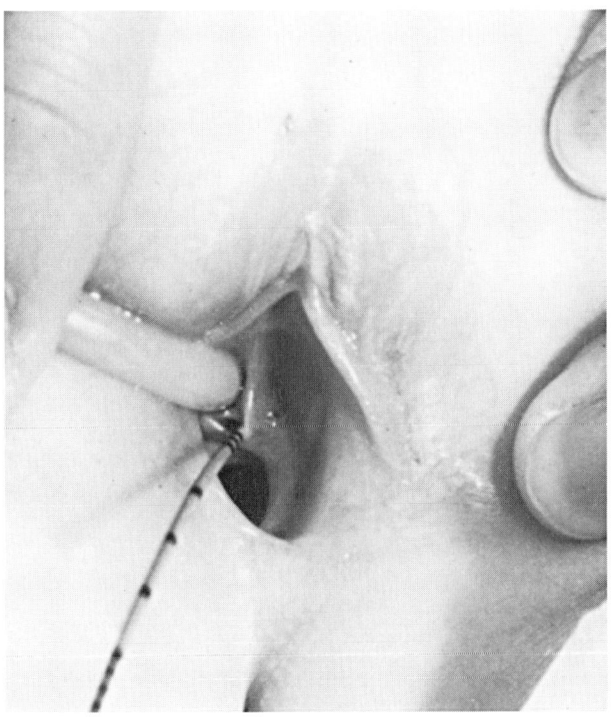

■ **Figure 13–16.** Ectopic ureter. This girl has an ectopic ureter entering the vestibule of the vagina near the external urethral orifice. The thin ureteral catheter with transverse marks has been introduced through the ureteric orifice into the ectopic ureter. This girl had a normal voiding pattern and constant urinary dribbling. (From Behrman RE, Kliegman RM, Arvin AM [eds]: *Nelson Textbook of Pediatrics,* 15th ed. Philadelphia, WB Saunders, 1996.)

Multicystic Dysplastic Kidney (MCDK)

The congenital form of this disease is relatively common. Death usually occurs shortly after birth; however, an increasing number of these infants are surviving because of hemodialysis and kidney transplants. The kidneys contain multiple small to large cysts (Fig. 13-17), which cause severe renal insufficiency. About 90% of dysplastic kidneys result from urinary tract obstruction during kidney formation (Mahony, 1994). Several hypotheses have been proposed for the congenital form of the disease. For many years it was thought that the cysts were the result of failure of the ureteric bud derivatives to join the tubules derived from the metanephric mesoderm. It is now believed that the cystlike formations are wide dilations of parts of otherwise continuous nephrons, particularly of the loops of Henle (Moffatt, 1982).

Development of the Urinary Bladder

Division of the cloaca by the **urorectal septum** (Fig. 13-18*A*) into a dorsal rectum and a ventral urogenital sinus was described in Chapter 12. For descriptive purposes, the **urogenital sinus** is divided into three parts (Fig. 13-18*C*):

- a cranial *vesical part* that is continuous with the allantois
- a middle *pelvic part* that becomes the urethra in the bladder neck and the prostatic part of

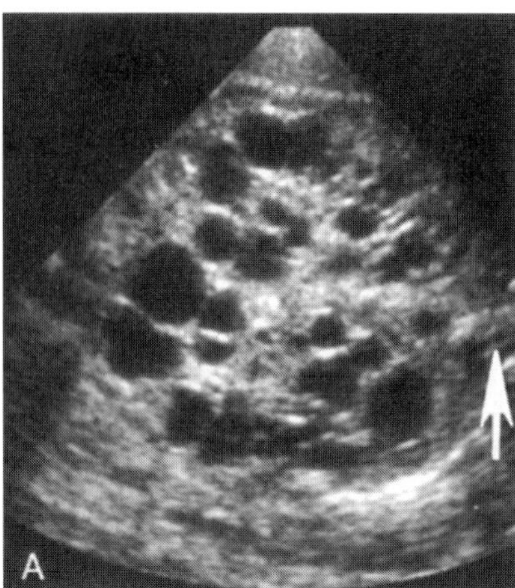

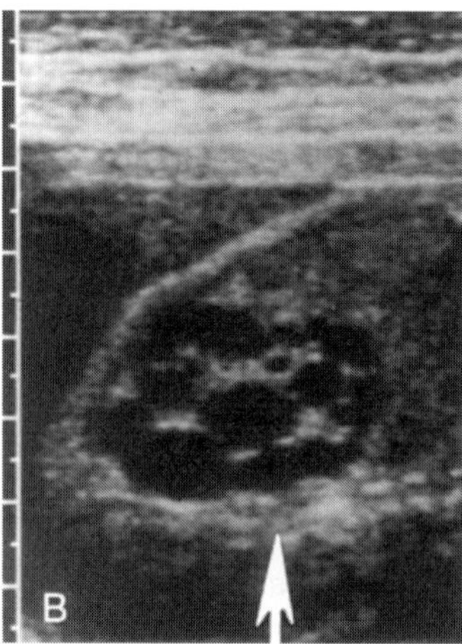

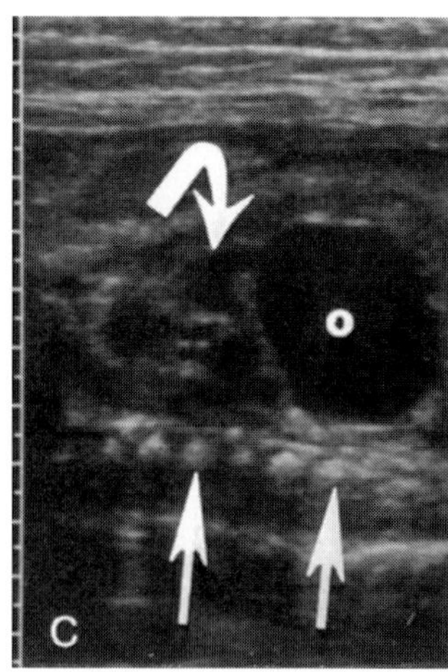

■ **Figure 13–17.** *A,* Bilateral multicystic dysplastic kidneys associated with profound oligohydramnios. Observe the multiple cysts of varying sizes without demonstrable communication or anatomical arrangement. *B,* Unilateral disease with a normal amount of amniotic fluid presumes a functioning contralateral kidney. In this case, the renal contour is relatively well preserved. *C,* Segmental disease occurs with atresia of one of the ureters leading from a duplex kidney—one that has two pelvicocaliceal systems (Fig. 13–15). The straight arrows indicate the vertebral column and the curved arrow indicates the multicystic dysplastic lower pole of the duplex kidney. **O,** obstructed upper pole moiety (part). (From Mahony BS: Ultrasound evaluation of the fetal genitourinary system. *In* Callen PW (ed): *Ultrasonography in Obstetrics and Gynecology,* 3rd ed. Philadelphia, WB Saunders, 1994.)

the urethra in males and the entire urethra in females

- a caudal *phallic part* that grows toward the genital tubercle

The bladder develops mainly from the vesical part of the urogenital sinus, but its trigone region is derived from the caudal ends of the mesonephric ducts (Fig. 13-18*A*). The epithelium of the bladder is derived from the endoderm of the vesical part of the urogenital sinus. The other layers of its wall develop from adjacent splanchnic mesenchyme. Initially the bladder is continuous with the **allantois**, a vestigial structure (Fig. 13-18*C*). The allantois soon constricts and becomes a thick fibrous cord, the **urachus**. It extends from the apex of the bladder to the umbilicus (Figs. 13-18*G* and 13-19). In the adult the urachus is represented by the *median umbilical ligament* (Moore, 1992).

As the bladder enlarges, distal portions of the mesonephric ducts are incorporated into its dorsal wall (Fig. 13-18*B* to *H*). These ducts contribute to the formation of the connective tissue in the *trigone of the bladder*, but the epithelium of the entire bladder is derived from the endoderm of the urogenital sinus. As the mesonephric ducts are absorbed, the ureters come to open separately into the urinary bladder (Fig. 13-18*C* to *H*). Partly because of traction exerted by the kidneys during their "ascent," the orifices of the ureters move superolaterally and the ureters enter obliquely through the base of the bladder. The orifices of the mesonephric ducts move close together and enter the prostatic part of the urethra as the caudal ends of these ducts become the *ejaculatory ducts*. The distal ends of the mesonephric ducts in females degenerate.

In infants and children the urinary bladder, even when empty, is in the abdomen. It begins to enter the pelvis major at about 6 years of age, but it does not enter the pelvis minor and become a pelvic organ until after puberty (Moore, 1992). The apex of the urinary bladder in adults is continuous with the **median umbilical ligament**, which extends posteriorly along the posterior surface of the anterior abdominal wall; this ligament is the fibrous remnant of the urachus. The *median umbilical ligament* lies between the *medial umbilical ligaments*, which are the fibrous remnants of the umbilical arteries (see Chapter 14).

Urachal Anomalies

A remnant of the lumen usually persists in the inferior part of the urachus in infants; in about 50% of cases, the lumen is continuous with the cavity of the bladder. Remnants of the epithelial lining of the urachus may give rise to **urachal cysts** (Fig. 13-20*A*). Small cysts can be observed in about one-third of cadavers, but urachal cysts are not usually detected in living persons unless they become infected and enlarge. The patent inferior end of the urachus may dilate to form a **urachal sinus** that opens into the bladder. The lumen in the superior part of the urachus may also remain patent and form a urachal sinus that opens at the umbilicus (Fig. 13-20*B*). Very rarely the entire urachus remains patent and forms a **urachal fistula** that allows urine to escape from its umbilical orifice (Fig. 13-20*C*).

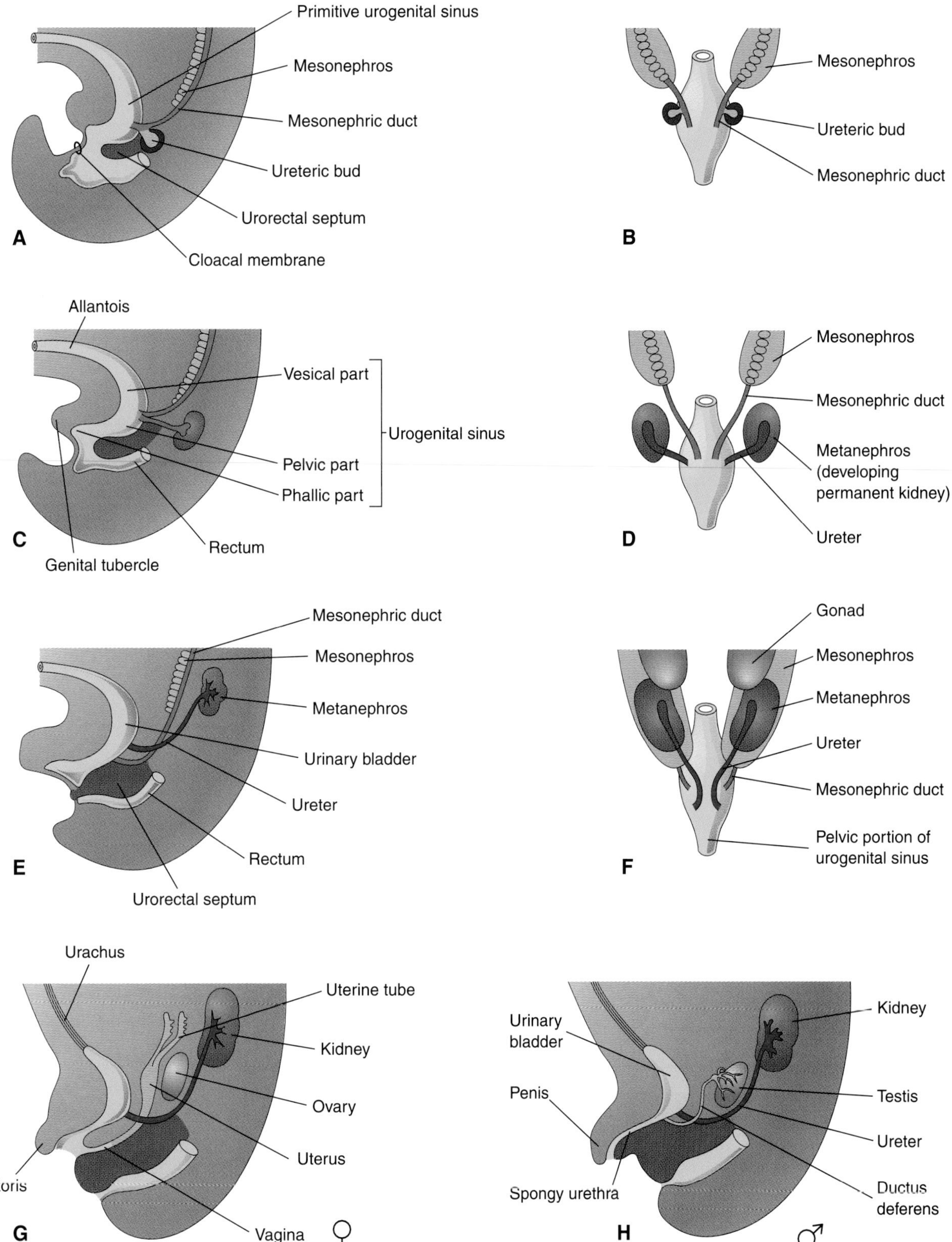

■ **Figure 13–18.** Diagrams showing division of the cloaca into the urogenital sinus and rectum; absorption of the mesonephric ducts; development of the urinary bladder, urethra, and urachus, and changes in the location of the ureters. *A,* Lateral view of the caudal half of a 5-week embryo. *B, D,* and *F,* Dorsal views. *C, E, G,* and *H,* Lateral views. The stages shown in *G* and *H* are reached by the twelfth week.

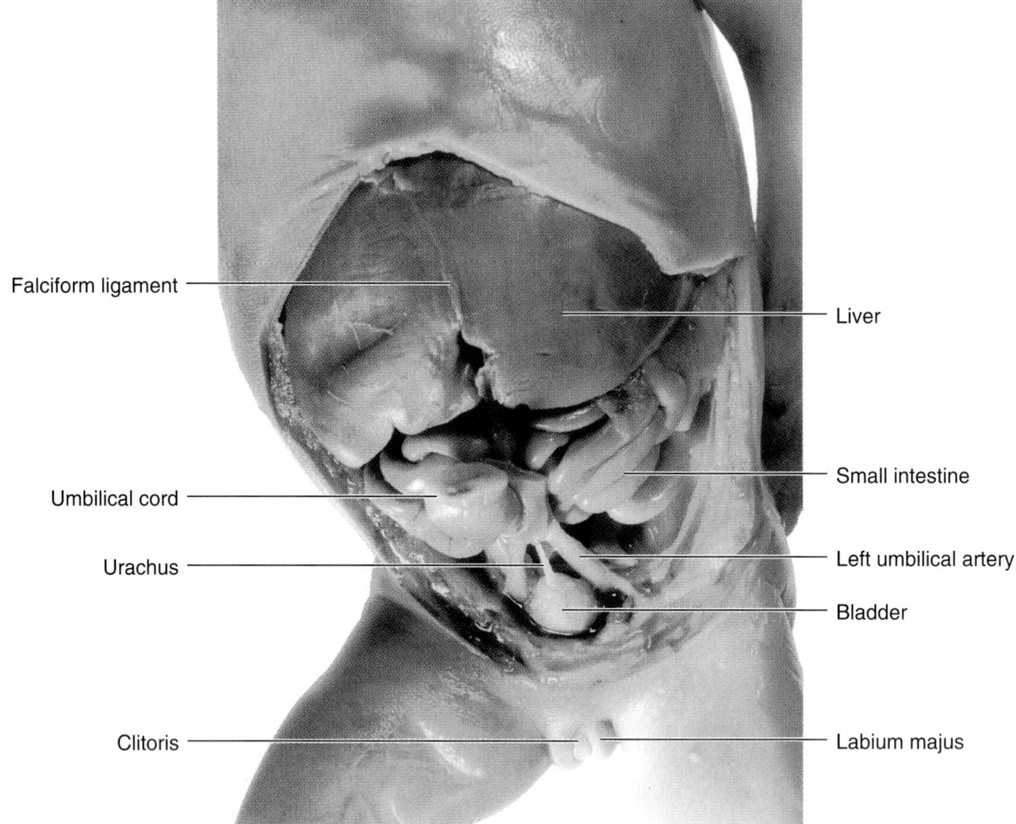

■ **Figure 13–19.** Photograph of a dissection of the abdomen and pelvis of an 18-week-old female fetus, showing the relation of the urachus to the urinary bladder and umbilical arteries. Note that the clitoris is relatively large at this stage.

Congenital Megacystis

A pathological large bladder—**megacystis** or megalocystis—may result from a congenital disorder of the ureteric bud, which may be associated with dilation of the renal pelvis and blunting of the calices. The large bladder may result from posterior urethral valves (Fig. 13-21). Absolute renal failure and pulmonary hypoplasia of lethal degree are the consequences of this anomaly, unless intrauterine treatment is effected.

Exstrophy of the Bladder

This severe anomaly occurs about once in every 10,000 to 40,000 births (Behrman et al., 1996). Exstrophy of the bladder (Fig. 13-22*A* and *B*) occurs chiefly in males. Exposure and *protrusion of the posterior wall of the bladder* characterize this congenital anomaly. The trigone of the bladder and the ureteric orifices are exposed and urine dribbles intermittently from the everted bladder. **Epispadias** and wide separation of the pubic bones are associated with complete exstrophy of the bladder. In some cases the penis is divided into two parts and the halves of the scrotum are widely separated (Fig. 13-23).

Exstrophy of the bladder is caused by incomplete median closure of the inferior part of the anterior abdominal wall (Fig. 13-24). The defect involves the anterior abdominal wall and the anterior wall of the urinary bladder. The anomaly is the result of failure of mesenchymal cells to migrate between the ectoderm of the abdomen and cloaca during the fourth week (Fig. 13-24*B* and *C*). As a result, the inferior parts of the rectus muscles are absent and the external and internal oblique and the transversus abdominis muscles are deficient. No muscle and connective tissue form in the anterior abdominal wall over the urinary bladder (Bruch et al., 1996). Later, the thin epidermis and anterior wall of the bladder rupture, causing wide communication between the exterior and the mucous membrane of the bladder. There are many variants of bladder exstrophy, ranging from the presence of an intravesical septum to complete bladder duplication, with exstrophy of one or both bladders (Fouda-Neel et al., 1996).

Development of the Urethra

The epithelium of most of the male urethra and the entire female urethra is derived from endoderm of the urogenital sinus (Figs. 13-18 and 13-25). The distal part of the urethra in the male is derived from the

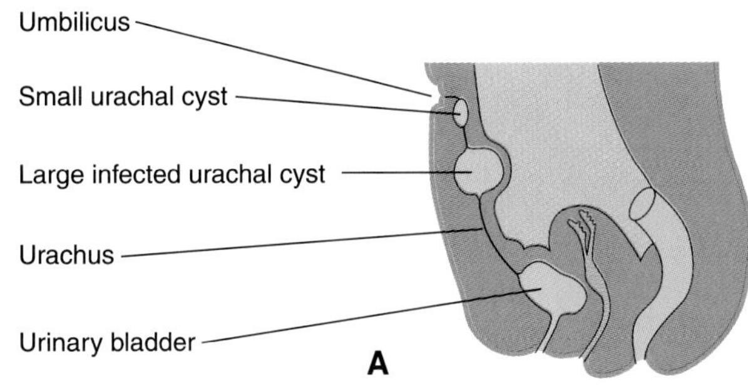

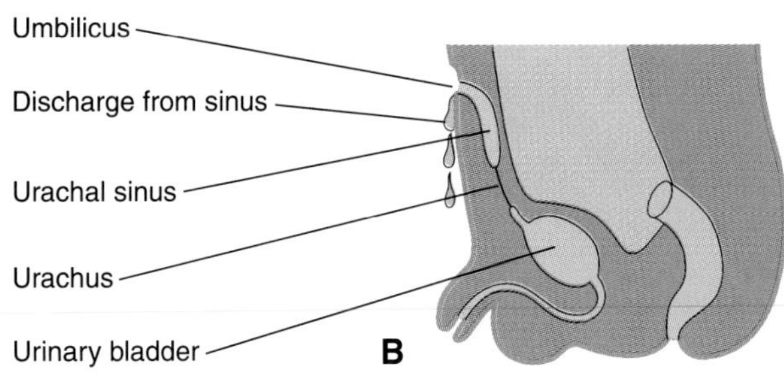

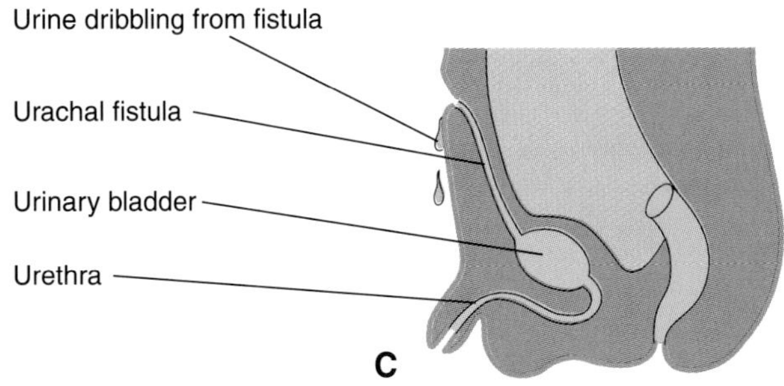

■ **Figure 13–20.** Diagrams illustrating urachal anomalies. *A,* Urachal cysts. The most common site is in the superior end of the urachus just inferior to the umbilicus. *B,* Two types of urachal sinus are illustrated: One opens into the bladder; the other opens at the umbilicus. *C,* Patent urachus or urachal fistula connecting the bladder and umbilicus.

glandular (urethral) plate. This ectodermal plate grows from the tip of the glans penis to meet the part of the spongy urethra derived from the phallic part of the urogenital sinus (Fig. 13-25*A* to *C*). The glandular plate becomes canalized and joins the rest of the spongy urethra; consequently, the epithelium of the terminal part of the urethra is derived from surface ectoderm. The connective tissue and smooth muscle of the urethra in both sexes is derived from the adjacent splanchnic mesenchyme.

DEVELOPMENT OF THE SUPRARENAL GLANDS

The cortex and medulla of the suprarenal (adrenal) glands have different origins (Fig. 13-26). The **cortex** develops from mesoderm and the **medulla** differentiates from **neural crest cells**. The cortex is first indicated during the sixth week by an aggregation of mesenchymal cells on each side, between the root of the dorsal mesentery and the developing gonad (see Fig. 13-28*C*). The cells that form the *fetal cortex* are derived from the mesothelium lining the posterior abdominal wall. The cells that form the medulla are derived from an adjacent *sympathetic ganglion*, which is derived from the neural crest. Initially the neural crest cells form a mass on the medial side of the fetal cortex (Fig. 13-26*B*). As they are surrounded by the fetal cortex, these cells differentiate into the *secretory cells* of the suprarenal medulla.

Later more mesenchymal cells arise from the mesothelium and enclose the fetal cortex. These cells give rise to the permanent cortex (Fig. 13-26*C*). Differentiation of the characteristic suprarenal cortical zones begins during the late fetal period. The zona glomerulosa and zona fasciculata are present at birth, but the zona reticularis is not recognizable until the end of the third year (Fig. 13-26*H*). The suprarenal glands of the human fetus are 10 to 20 times larger than the adult glands relative to body weight, and are large compared with the kidneys (Fig. 13-8). These large glands result from the extensive size of the fetal cortex. The suprarenal medulla remains relatively small until after birth. The suprarenal glands rapidly become smaller as the fetal cortex regresses during the first year. The glands lose about one-third of their weight during the first 2 or 3 weeks after birth and do not regain their original weight until the end of the second year. For a review of the regulation of fetal suprarenal growth, differentiation, maturation, and subcellular mechanisms controlling fetal suprarenal function, see Pepe and Albrecht, 1990.

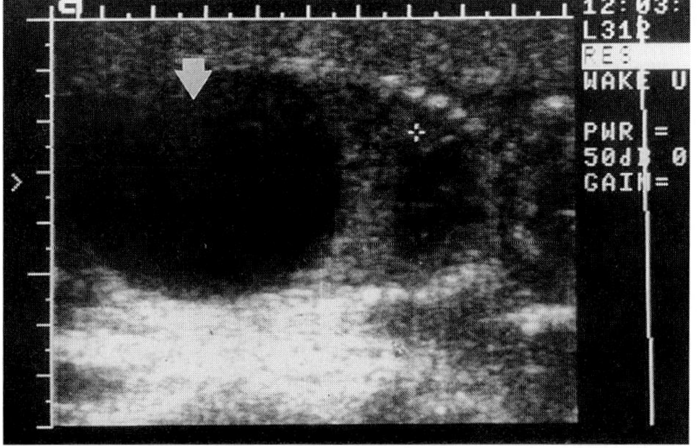

■ **Figure 13–21.** Sonogram of a male fetus of 18 weeks of gestation with megacystis (enlarged bladder) caused by posterior urethral valves. The cross is placed on the fourth intercostal space, the level to which the diaphragm has been elevated by this very large (black = urine) fetal bladder *(arrow).* Absolute renal failure and pulmonary hypoplasia of a lethal degree are consequences of this presentation, unless intrauterine treatment is effected. In this case, the fetus survived because of the placement of a pigtail catheter within the fetal bladder, allowing drainage of urine into the amniotic cavity. (Courtesy of Dr. C. R. Harman, Department of Obstetrics, Gynecology and Reproductive Sciences, Women's Hospital and University of Manitoba, Winnipeg, Manitoba, Canada.)

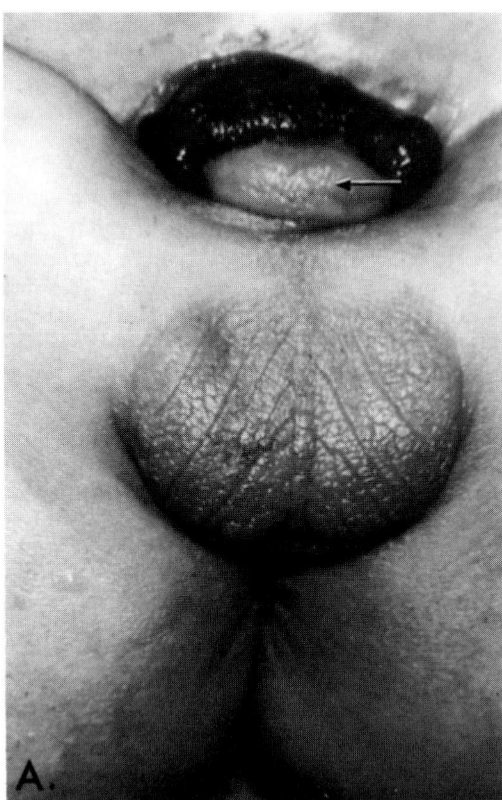

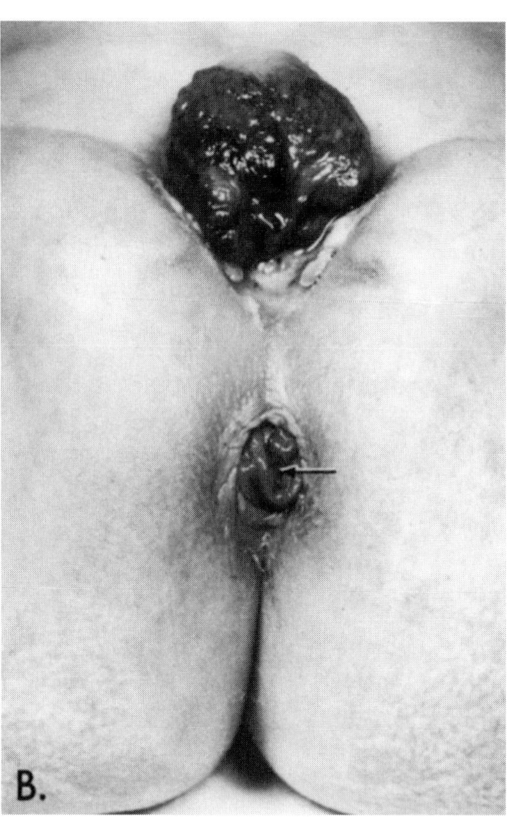

■ **Figure 13–22.** Photographs of infants with exstrophy of the bladder. Because of defective closure of the inferior part of the anterior abdominal wall and the anterior wall of the bladder, the urinary bladder appears as an everted bulging mass inferior to the umbilicus. *A,* Male. Epispadias is also present and the penis *(arrow)* is small and flattened. (Courtesy of Dr. C. C. Ferguson, Children's Hospital, Winnipeg, Manitoba, Canada.) *B,* Female with bladder exstrophy and a slight prolapse *(arrow)* of the rectum. (Courtesy of Mr. Innes Williams, Genitourinary Surgeon, The Hospital for Sick Children, Great Ormond Street, London, England.)

Congenital Adrenal Hyperplasia (CAH)

An abnormal increase in the cells of the suprarenal cortex results in excessive androgen production during the fetal period. In females this usually causes masculinization of the external genitalia and enlargement of the clitoris, for example (Fig. 13-27). Affected male infants have normal external genitalia and may go undetected in early infancy. Later in childhood in both sexes, androgen excess leads to rapid growth and accelerated skeletal maturation (Thompson et al., 1991). The **adrenogenital syndrome** associated with CAH manifests itself in various clinical forms that can be correlated with enzymatic deficiencies of cortisol biosynthesis. CAH is a group of *autosomal recessive disorders* that result in virilization of female fetuses. CAH

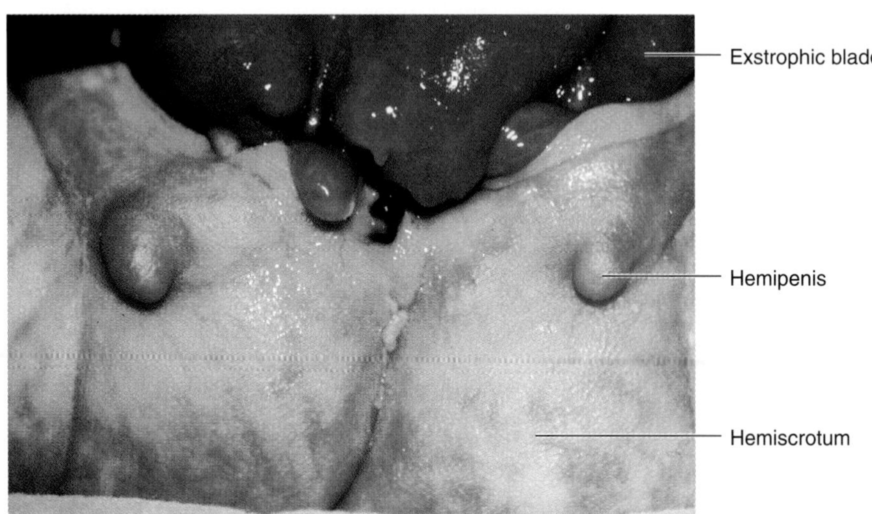

■ **Figure 13–23.** Exstrophy of the bladder in a male infant. The bladder mucosa is visible and the halves of the penis and scrotum are widely separated. (Courtesy of Dr. A. E. Chudley, Section of Genetics and Metabolism, Department of Pediatrics and Child Health, Children's Hospital and University of Manitoba, Winnipeg, Manitoba, Canada.)

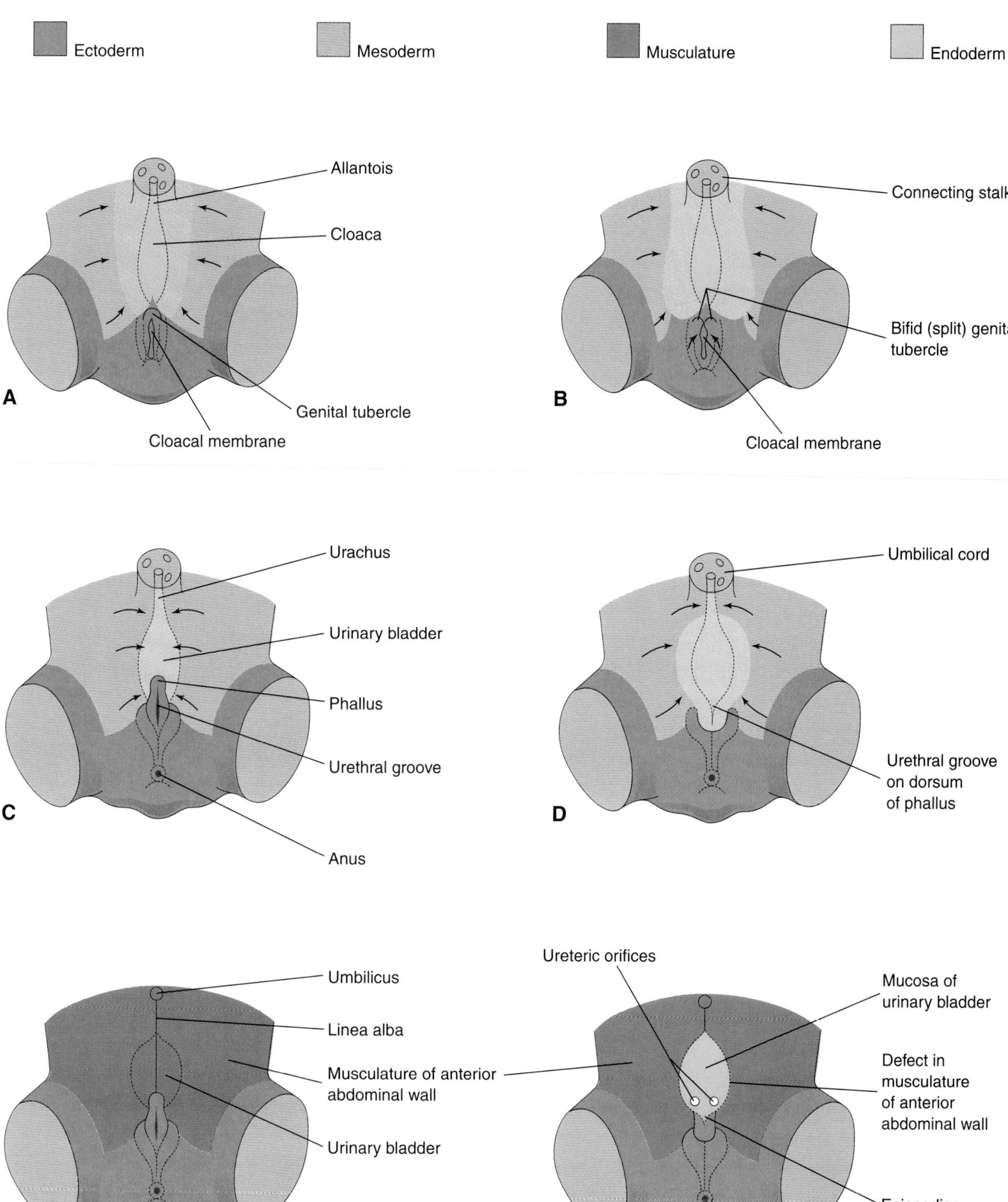

■ **Figure 13–24.** *A, C,* and *E,* Normal stages in the development of the infraumbilical abdominal wall and the penis during the fourth to eighth weeks. Note that mesoderm and later muscle reinforce the ectoderm of the developing anterior abdominal wall. *B, D,* and *F,* Probable stages in the development of exstrophy of the bladder and epispadias. In *B* and *D,* note that the mesenchyme (embryonic connective tissue) falls to extend into the anterior abdominal wall anterior to the urinary bladder. Also note that the genital tubercle is located in a more caudal position than usual, and that the urethral groove has formed on the dorsal surface of the penis. In *F,* the surface ectoderm and anterior wall of the bladder have ruptured, resulting in exposure of the posterior wall of the bladder. Note that the musculature of the anterior abdominal wall is present on each side of the defect. (Based on Patten BM, Barry A: The genesis of exstrophy of the bladder and epispadias. *Am J Anat 90:*35, 1952.)

Spongy urethra
Coronary groove
Glans penis
Ectoderm
A
Body of penis
Glandular plate

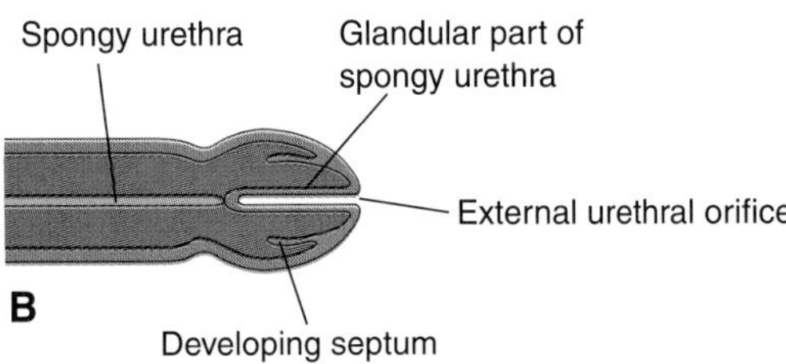

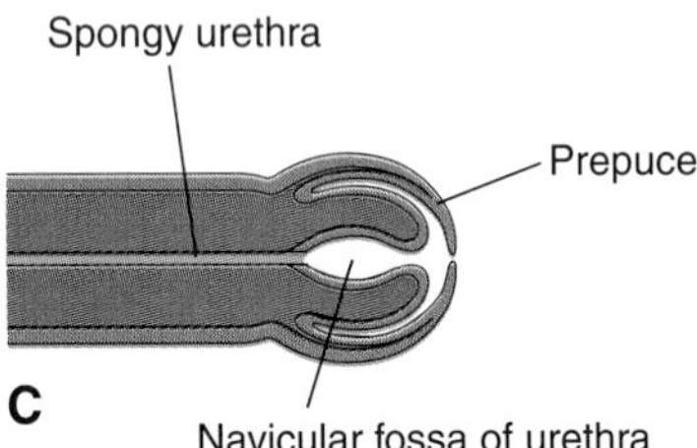

■ **Figure 13–25.** Schematic longitudinal sections of the distal part of the developing penis, illustrating development of the prepuce (foreskin) and the glandular part of the spongy urethra. *A,* 11 weeks. *B,* 12 weeks. *C,* 14 weeks. The epithelium of the spongy urethra has a dual origin; most of it is derived from endoderm of the phallic part of the urogenital sinus. The distal part of the urethra lining the navicular fossa is derived from surface ectoderm.

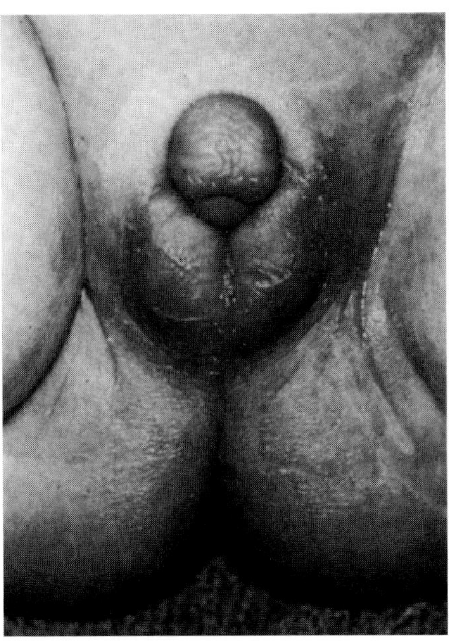

■ **Figure 13–27.** Masculinized external genitalia of a female infant with congenital adrenal hyperplasia (CAH). The virilization was caused by excessive androgens produced by the suprarenal (adrenal) glands during the fetal period.

is caused by a genetically determined mutation in the cytochrome P450c21-steroid 21-hydroxylase gene, which causes a deficiency of adrenal cortical enzymes that are necessary for the biosynthesis of various steroid hormones. The reduced hormone output results in an increased release of adrenocorticotropic hormone (ACTH), which causes adrenal hyperplasia and overproduction of androgens by the hyperplastic suprarenal glands. For details about the adrenal hyperplasias and their genetic basis, see New et al. (1989); Thompson et al. (1991); Speiser and New (1994).

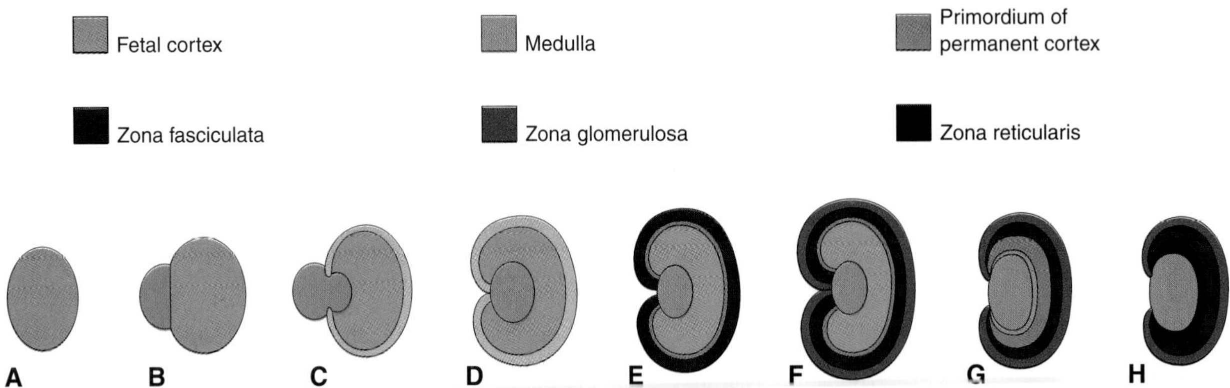

■ **Figure 13–26.** Schematic drawings illustrating development of the suprarenal (adrenal) glands. *A,* 6 weeks, showing the mesodermal primordium of the fetal cortex. *B,* 7 weeks, showing the addition of neural crest cells. *C,* 8 weeks, showing the fetal cortex and the early permanent cortex beginning to encapsulate the medulla. *D* and *E,* Later stages of encapsulation of the medulla by the cortex. *F,* Newborn, showing the fetal cortex and two zones of the permanent cortex. *G,* 1 year; the fetal cortex has almost disappeared. *H,* 4 years, showing the adult pattern of cortical zones. Note that the fetal cortex has disappeared and that the gland is smaller than it was at birth *(F).*

DEVELOPMENT OF THE GENITAL SYSTEM

Although the chromosomal and genetic sex of an embryo is determined at fertilization by the kind of sperm that fertilizes the ovum (see Chapter 2), male and female morphological characteristics do not begin to develop until the seventh week. The early genital systems in the two sexes are similar; therefore the initial period of genital development is referred to as the *indifferent stage of sexual development*.

Development of the Gonads

The gonads (testes and ovaries) are derived from three sources (Fig. 13-28):

- the *mesothelium* (mesodermal epithelium) lining the posterior abdominal wall
- the underlying *mesenchyme* (embryonic connective tissue)
- the *primordial germ cells*

THE INDIFFERENT GONADS

The initial stages of gonadal development occur during the fifth week when a thickened area of mesothelium develops on the medial side of the mesonephros (Fig. 13-28). Proliferation of this epithelium and the underlying mesenchyme produces a bulge on the medial side of the mesonephros—the **gonadal (genital) ridge** (Fig. 13-29). Fingerlike epithelial cords—the **pri-**

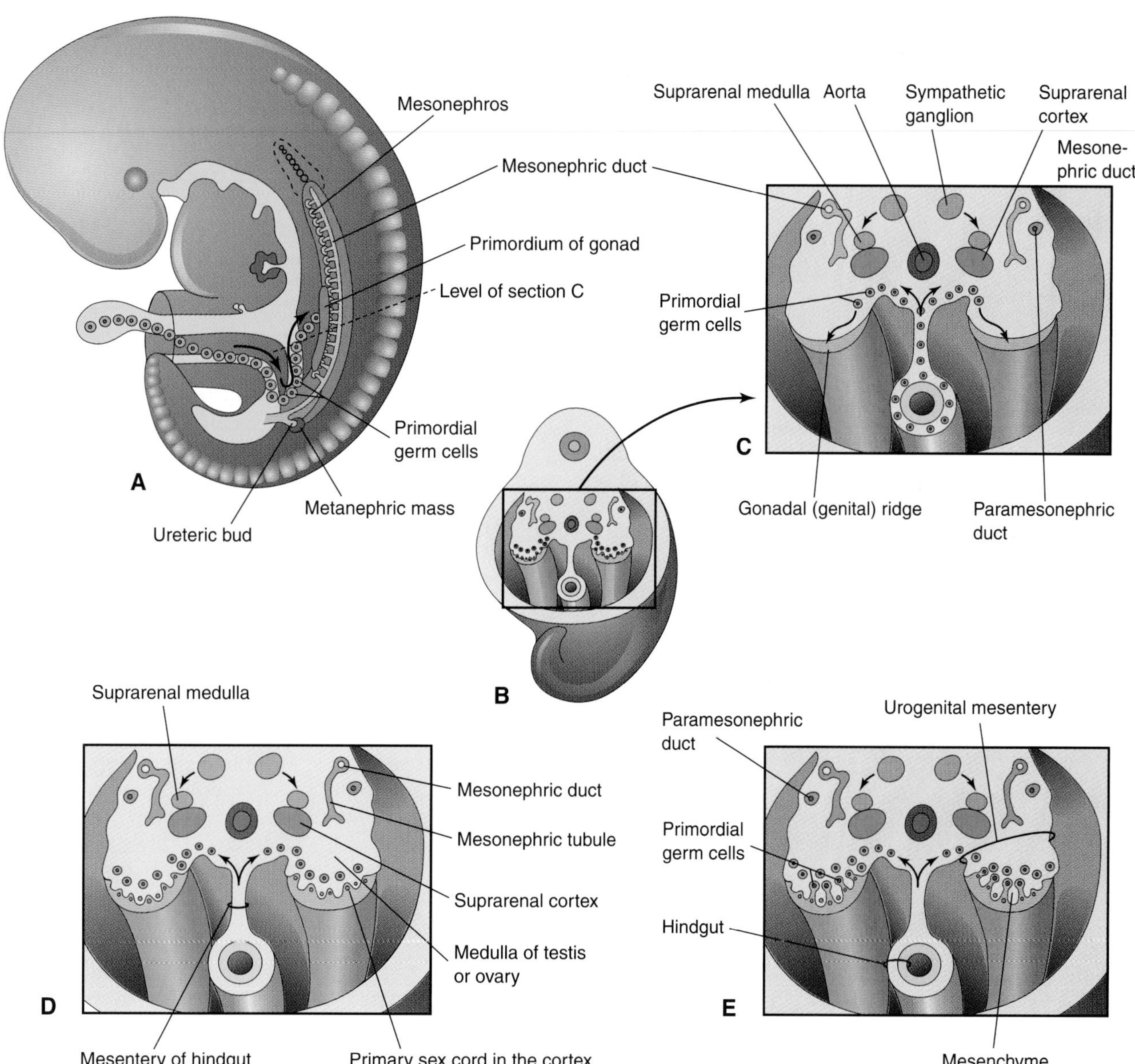

■ **Figure 13-28.** *A,* Sketch of a 5-week embryo illustrating the migration of primordial germ cells from the yolk sac into the embryo. *B,* Three-dimensional sketch of the caudal region of a 5-week embryo, showing the location and extent of the gonadal ridges. *C,* Transverse section showing the primordium of the suprarenal (adrenal) glands, the gonadal (genital) ridges, and the migration of primordial germ cells into the developing gonads. *D,* Transverse section of a 6-week embryo showing the primary sex cords. *E,* Similar section at a later stage showing the indifferent gonads and paramesonephric ducts.

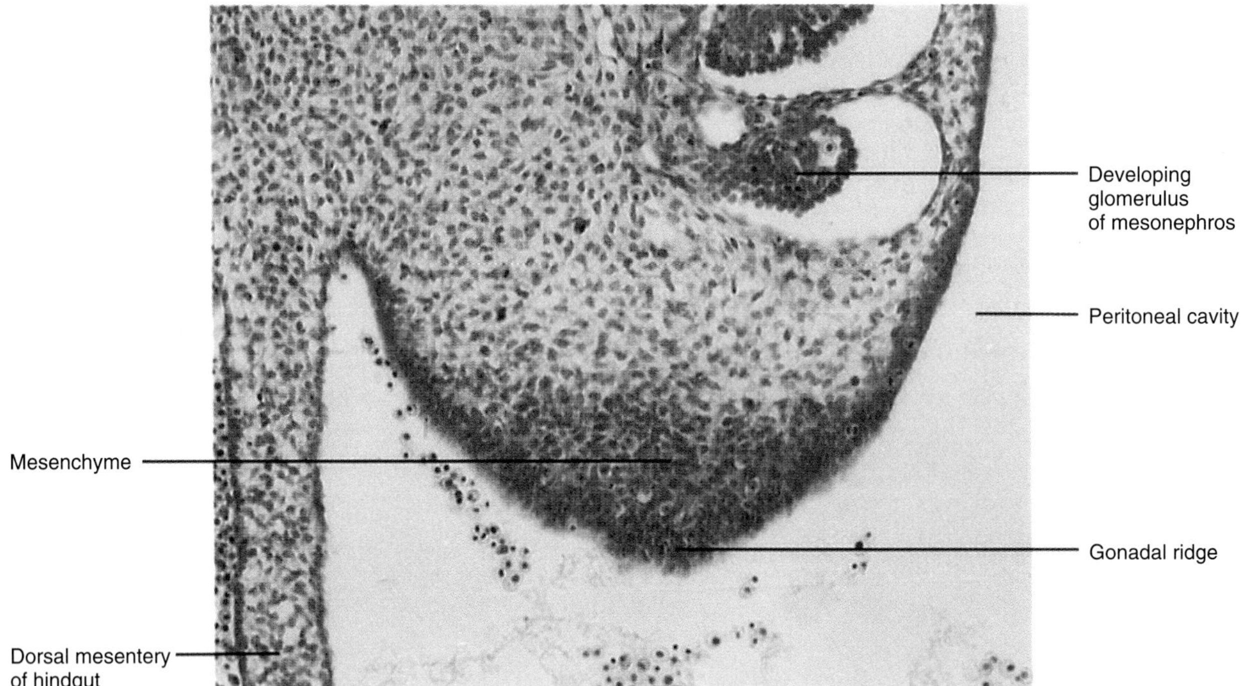

■ **Figure 13–29.** Photomicrograph of a transverse section of the abdomen of an embryo at Carnegie stage 16, about 40 days, showing the gonadal (genital) ridge, which will develop into a testis or an ovary depending on the genetic sex of the embryo. Most of the developing gonad is composed of mesenchyme derived from the coelomic epithelium of the gonadal ridge. The large round cells in the gonad are primordial germ cells. (From Moore KL, Persaud TVN, Shiota K: *Color Atlas of Clinical Embryology*. Philadelphia, WB Saunders, 1994.)

mary sex cords—soon grow into the underlying mesenchyme (Fig. 13-28*D*). The indifferent gonad now consists of an external *cortex* and an internal *medulla*. In embryos with an XX sex chromosome complex, the cortex of the **indifferent gonad** differentiates into an ovary and the medulla regresses. In embryos with an XY sex chromosome complex, the medulla differentiates into a testis and the cortex regresses, except for vestigial remnants (see Table 13-1).

PRIMORDIAL GERM CELLS

These large, spherical primitive sex cells are visible early in the fourth week among the endodermal cells of the yolk sac near the origin of the allantois. During folding of the embryo (see Chapter 5), the dorsal part of the yolk sac is incorporated into the embryo. As this occurs, the primordial germ cells migrate along the dorsal mesentery of the hindgut to the gonadal ridges (Fig. 13-28*A*). During the sixth week the primordial germ cells enter the underlying mesenchyme and are incorporated in the *primary sex cords* (Fig. 13-28*E*).

SEX DETERMINATION

Chromosomal and genetic sex is established at fertilization and depends upon whether an X-bearing sperm or a Y-bearing sperm fertilizes the X-bearing ovum. The type of gonads that develop is determined by the sex chromosome complex (XX or XY). Before the seventh week the gonads of the two sexes are identical in appearance and are called **indifferent gonads** (Fig. 13-29). Development of the male phenotype requires a Y chromosome, but only the short arm of this chromosome is critical for sex determination. The SRY gene for a *testis-determining factor* (TDF) has been localized in the "sex-determining region of the Y chromosome" (Berta et al., 1990; Thompson et al., 1991). Two X chromosomes are required for the development of the female phenotype. A number of genes and regions of the X chromosome have special roles in sex determination.

The Y chromosome has a testis-determining effect on the medulla of the indifferent gonad. It is the TDF regulated by the Y chromosome that determines testicular differentiation. Under the influence of this organizing factor, the primary sex cords differentiate into seminiferous tubules (Fig. 13-30). The absence of a Y chromosome (i.e., an XX sex chromosome complement), results in the formation of an ovary. Consequently, the type of sex chromosome complex established at fertilization determines the type of gonad that differentiates from the indifferent gonad (Mittwoch, 1992). The type of gonads present then determines the type of sexual differentiation that occurs in the genital ducts and external genitalia. It is the androgen **testosterone**, produced by the fetal testes, that determines maleness. Primary female sexual differentiation in the fetus does not depend on hormones; it occurs even if the ovaries are absent and apparently is not under hormonal influence.

Abnormal Sex Chromosome Complexes

In embryos with abnormal sex chromosome complexes, such as XXX or XXY, the number of X chromosomes appears to be unimportant in sex determination. If a *normal* Y chromosome is present, the embryo develops as a male. If no Y chromosome is present, or the testis-determining region of the Y chromosome has been lost, female development occurs. The loss of an X chromosome does not appear to interfere with the migration of primordial germ cells to the gonadal ridges, because some germ cells have been observed in the fetal gonads of 45, X females with Turner syndrome. Two X chromosomes are needed, however, to bring about complete ovarian development.

The seminiferous tubules remain solid (i.e., no lumina) until puberty, at which time lumina begin to develop. The walls of the seminiferous tubules are composed of two kinds of cell (Fig. 13-30):

- *Sertoli cells*, supporting cells derived from the surface epithelium of the testis
- spermatogonia, primordial sperm cells derived from the primordial germ cells

Sertoli cells constitute most of the seminiferous epithelium in the fetal testis (Figs. 13-30 and 13-31*C*). During later development the surface epithelium of the testis flattens to form the mesothelium on the external surface of the adult testis. The **rete testis** becomes continuous with 15 to 20 mesonephric tubules that become **efferent ductules** (ductuli efferentes). These ductules are connected with the mesonephric duct, which becomes the **ductus epididymis** (Figs. 13-30 and 13-32*A*).

DEVELOPMENT OF TESTES

Embryos with a Y chromosome in their sex chromosome complement usually develop testes. A coordinated sequence of genes induces the development of testes (Thompson et al., 1991). The SRY gene for TDF on the short arm of the Y chromosome acts as the switch that directs development of the indifferent gonad into a testis (Berta et al., 1990; DiGeorge, 1996). TDF induces the primary sex cords to condense and extend into the medulla of the indifferent gonad, where they branch and anastomose to form the **rete testis**. The connection of the sex cords—**seminiferous (testicular) cords**—with the surface epithelium is lost when a thick fibrous capsule, the tunica albuginea, develops (Fig. 13-30). The development of the dense **tunica albuginea** is the characteristic and diagnostic feature of testicular development in the fetus. Gradually the enlarging testis separates from the degenerating mesonephros and becomes suspended by its own mesentery, the **mesorchium**. The seminiferous cords develop into the seminiferous tubules, tubuli recti, and rete testis.

The **seminiferous tubules** become separated by mesenchyme that gives rise to the **interstitial cells** (of Leydig). By about the eighth week, these cells begin to secrete androgenic hormones—*testosterone* and *androstenedione*, which induce masculine differentiation of the mesonephric ducts and the external genitalia. Testosterone production is stimulated by human chorionic gonadotrophin (hCG), which reaches peak amounts during the 8- to 12-week period (DiGeorge, 1996). In addition to testosterone, the fetal testes produces a glycoprotein known as **antimüllerian hormone** (AMH) or *müllerian inhibiting substance* (MIS). AMH is produced by the sustentacular cells (of Sertoli), which continues to puberty, after which the levels of AMH decrease. AMH suppresses development of the paramesonephric (müllerian) ducts.

DEVELOPMENT OF OVARIES

Gonadal development occurs slowly in female embryos. The X chromosomes bear genes for ovarian development, and an autosomal gene also appears to play a role in ovarian organogenesis (DiGeorge, 1996). The ovary is not identifiable histologically until about the tenth week. **Primary sex cords** do not become prominent but they extend into the medulla and form a rudimentary *rete ovarii*. This structure and the primary sex cords normally degenerate and disappear (Fig. 13-30). **Secondary sex cords** (cortical cords) extend from the surface epithelium of the developing ovary into the underlying mesenchyme during the early fetal period. This epithelium is derived from the mesothelium. As the cortical cords increase in size, **primordial germ cells** are incorporated into them. At about 16 weeks these cords begin to break up into isolated cell clusters—**primordial follicles**—each of which consists of an **oogonium**, derived from a primordial germ cell, surrounded by a single layer of flattened follicular cells derived from the sex cord (Fig. 13-30). Active mitosis of oogonia occurs during fetal life producing thousands of these primordial follicles (Fig. 13-31*D*).

No oogonia form postnatally. Although many oogonia degenerate before birth, the two million or so that remain enlarge to become primary oocytes before birth. After birth the surface epithelium of the ovary flattens to a single layer of cells continuous with the mesothelium of the peritoneum at the hilum of the ovary. The surface epithelium was formerly called the "germinal epithelium," which is inappropriate because it is now well established that the germ cells differentiate from the primordial germ cells (Fig. 13-30). The surface epithelium becomes separated from the follicles in the cortex by a thin fibrous capsule, the **tunica albuginea**. As the ovary separates from the regressing mesonephros, it is suspended by the **mesovarium**, which is its mesentery (Fig. 13-30).

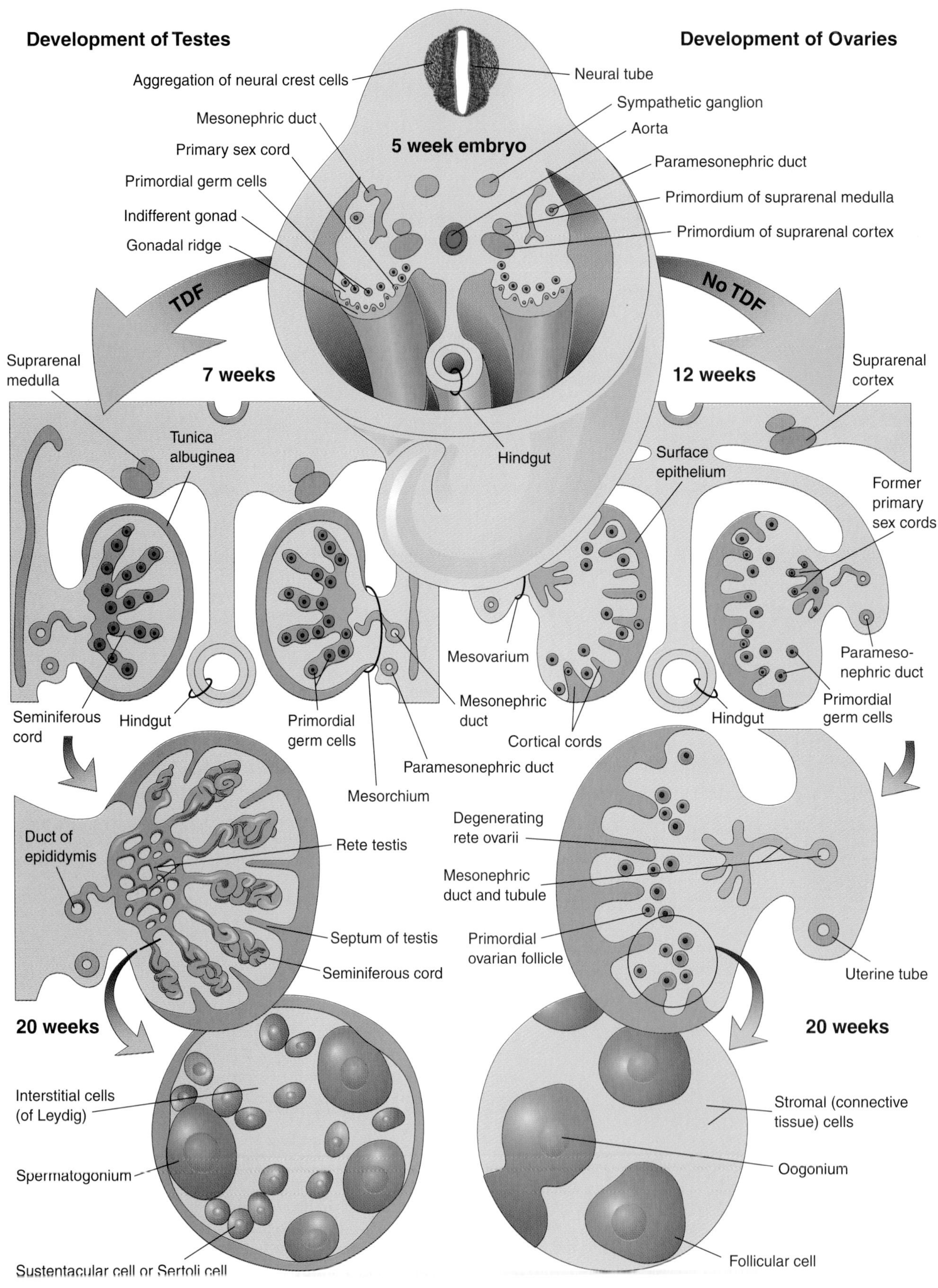

■ **Figure 13–30.** *See legend on the opposite page*

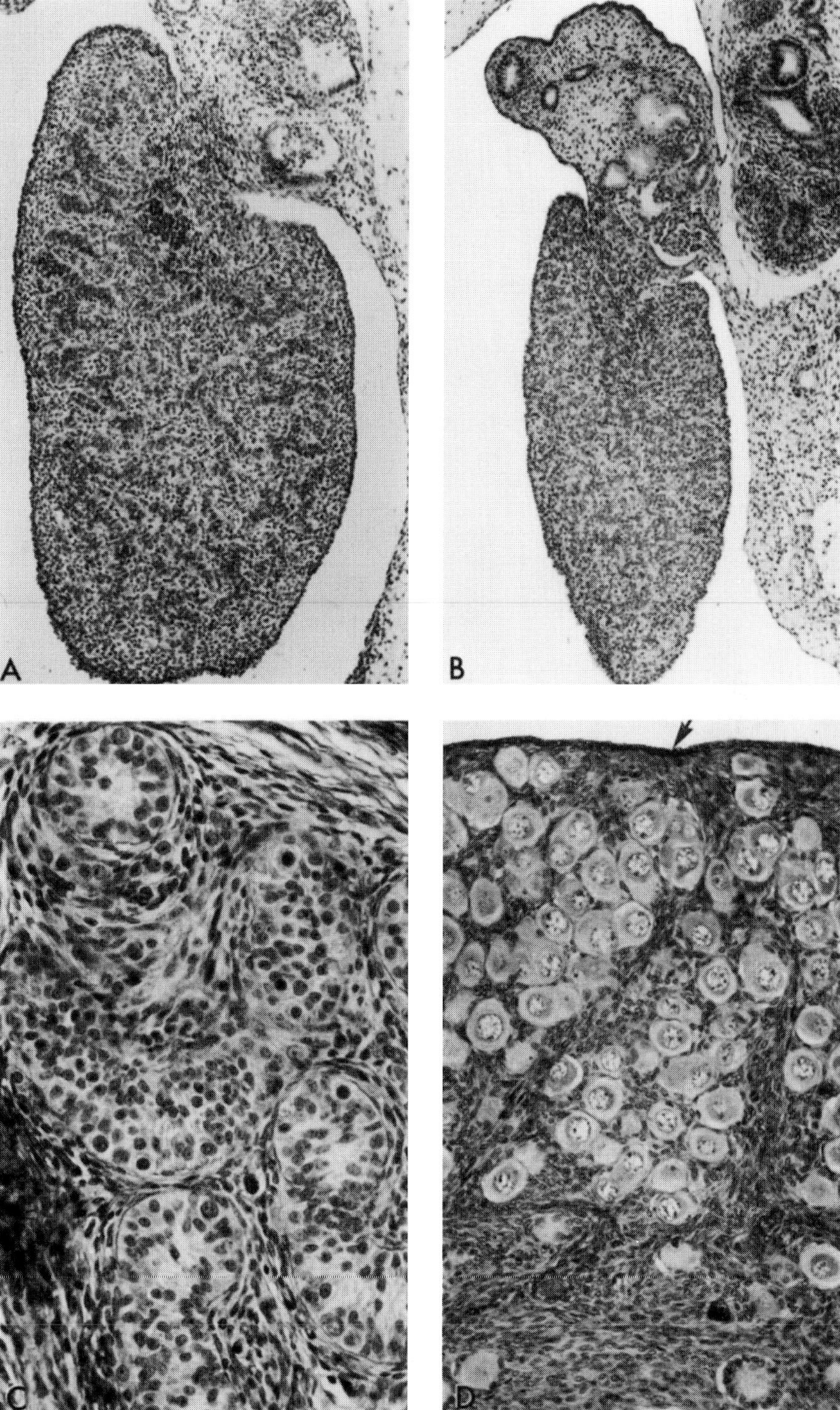

■ **Figure 13–31.** Transverse sections of gonads of human embryos and fetuses. *A,* Testis from an embryo of about 43 days, showing prominent seminiferous cords (×175). *B,* From an embryo of about the same age, a gonad that may be assumed to be an ovary because of the absence of primary sex cords (×125). *C,* Section of a testis from a male fetus born prematurely at 21 weeks, showing seminiferous tubules composed mostly of sustentacular or Sertoli cells. A few large spermatogonia are visible (×475). *D,* Section of an ovary from a 14-day-old female infant showing numerous primordial follicles in the cortex, each of which contains a primary oocyte. The arrow indicates the relatively thin surface epithelium of the ovary (×275). (From van Wagenen G, Simpson ME: *Embryology of the Ovary and Testis. Homo sapiens and Macaca mulatta.* 1965. Courtesy of Yale University Press.)

■ **Figure 13–30.** Schematic illustrations showing differentiation of the indifferent gonads of a 5-week embryo (top) into ovaries or testes. Left side shows the development of testes resulting from the effects of the testis-determining factor (TDF) located on the Y chromosome. Note that the primary sex cords become seminiferous cords, the primordia of the seminiferous tubules. The parts of the primary sex cords that enter the medulla of the testis form the rete testis. In the section of the testis at the bottom left, observe that there are two kinds of cells, spermatogonia, derived from the primordial germ cells and sustentacular or Sertoli cells derived from mesenchyme. Right side shows the development of ovaries in the absence of TDF. Cortical cords have extended from the surface epithelium of the gonad and primordial germ cells have entered them. They are the primordia of the oogonia. Follicular cells are derived from the mesenchyme (primitive connective tissue) separating the oogonia.

Urogenital sinus
Mesonephric duct
Paramesonephric duct

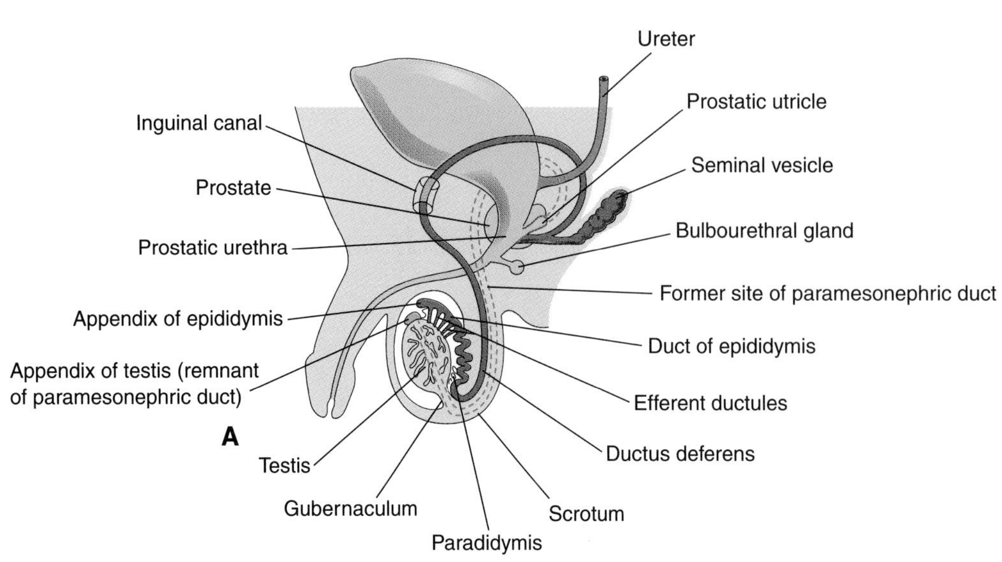

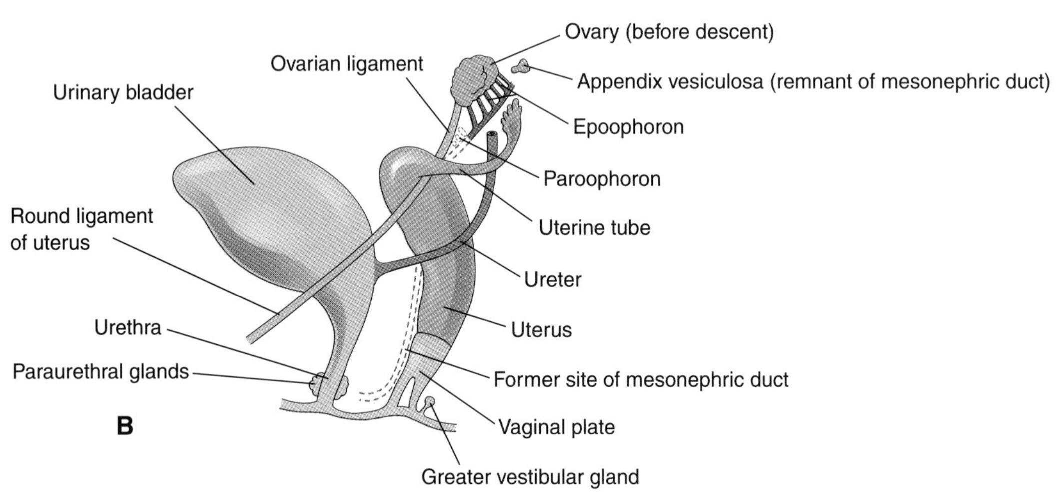

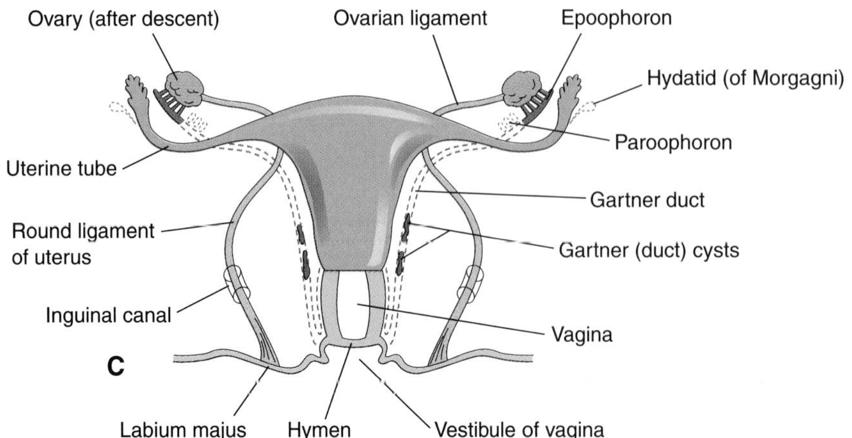

■ **Figure 13–32.** Schematic drawings illustrating development of the male and female reproductive systems from the genital ducts and urogenital sinus. Vestigial structures are also shown. *A,* Reproductive system in a newborn male. *B,* Female reproductive system in a 12-week fetus. *C,* Reproductive system in a newborn female.

Development of Genital Ducts

Both male and female embryos have two pairs of genital ducts. The mesonephric (wolffian) ducts play an important part in the development of the male reproductive system, and the paramesonephric (müllerian) ducts have a leading role in the development of the female reproductive system. During the fifth and sixth weeks, the genital system is in an **indifferent stage**, when both pairs of genital ducts are present.

The **mesonephric ducts**, which drained urine from the mesonephric kidneys, play an essential role in the development of the **male reproductive system** (Fig. 13-32*A*). Under the influence of testosterone produced by the fetal testes in the eighth week, the proximal part of each mesonephric duct becomes highly convoluted to form the **epididymis**. The remainder of this duct forms the **ductus deferens** and **ejaculatory duct**. In female fetuses the mesonephric ducts almost completely disappear; only a few nonfunctional remnants persist (Fig. 13-32*B* and *C*; see Table 13-1).

The **paramesonephric ducts** develop lateral to the gonads and mesonephric ducts (Fig. 13-30) and play an essential role in the development of the **female reproductive system**. The paramesonephric ducts form on each side from longitudinal invaginations of the mesothelium on the lateral aspects of the mesonephroi. The edges of these invaginations approach each other and fuse to form the paramesonephric ducts (Fig. 13-28*C* and *E*). The funnel-shaped cranial ends of these ducts open into the peritoneal cavity (Fig. 13-32*B* and *C*). The paramesonephric ducts pass caudally, parallel to the mesonephric ducts, until they reach the future pelvic region of the embryo. Here they cross ventral to the mesonephric ducts, approach each other in the median plane, and fuse to form a Y-shaped **uterovaginal primordium** (Fig. 13-33*A*). This tubular structure projects into the dorsal wall of the urogenital sinus and produces an elevation—the **sinus (müllerian) tubercle** (Fig. 13-33*B*).

DEVELOPMENT OF MALE GENITAL DUCTS AND GLANDS

The Sertoli cells of the fetal testes produce *masculinizing hormones* (e.g., testosterone) and a *müllerian inhibiting substance* (MIS). The Sertoli cells begin to produce MIS at 6 to 7 weeks. The interstitial cells begin producing testosterone in the eighth week (DiGeorge, 1996). **Testosterone**, the production of which is stimulated by hCG, stimulates the mesonephric ducts to form male genital ducts, whereas MIS causes the paramesonephric ducts to disappear by epithelial-mesenchymal transformation (Hay, 1990). As the mesonephros degenerates, some mesonephric tubules persist and are transformed into **efferent ductules** (Fig. 13-32*A*). These ductules open into the mesonephric duct, which has transformed into the duct of the epididymis—the **ductus epididymis**—in this region. Distal to the epididymis, the mesonephric duct acquires a thick investment of smooth muscle and becomes the **ductus deferens**. A lateral outgrowth from the caudal end of each mesonephric duct gives rise to the **seminal vesicle**. This pair of glands produces a secretion that nourishes the sperms. The part of the mesonephric duct between the duct of this gland and the urethra becomes the **ejaculatory duct**.

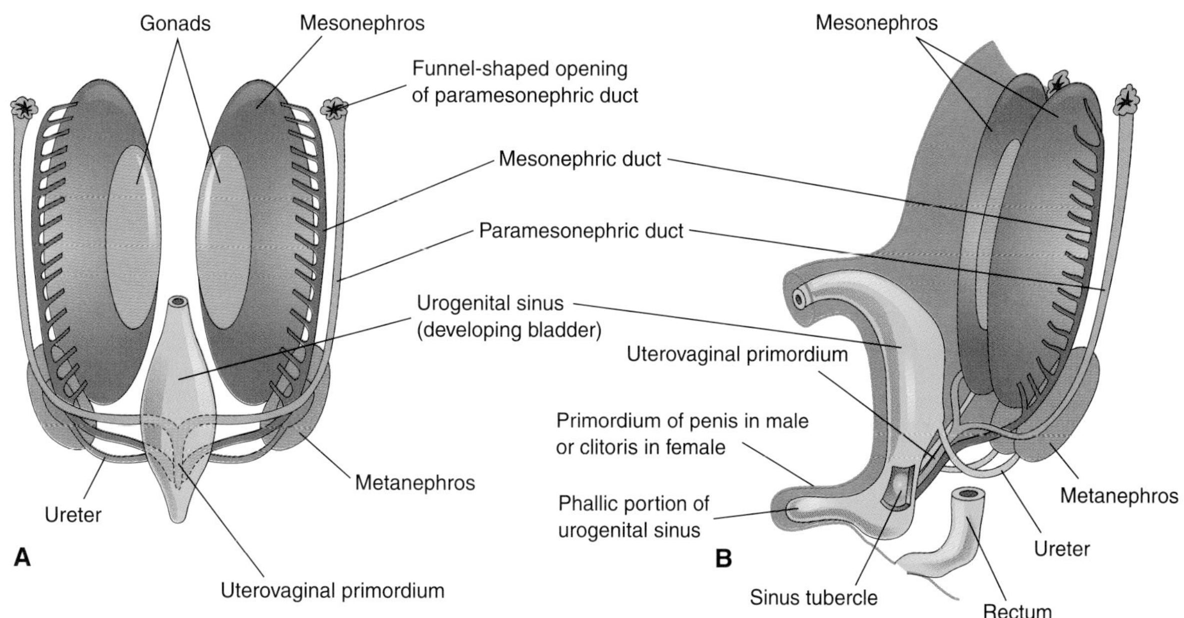

■ **Figure 13–33.** *A,* Sketch of a ventral view of the posterior abdominal wall of a 7-week embryo showing the two pairs of genital ducts present during the indifferent stage of sexual development. *B,* Lateral view of a 9-week fetus showing the sinus tubercle (müllerian tubercle) on the posterior wall of the urogenital sinus. It becomes the hymen in females and the seminal colliculus in males. The colliculus is an elevated part of the urethral crest on the posterior wall of the prostatic urethra.

Prostate

Multiple endodermal outgrowths arise from the prostatic part of the urethra and grow into the surrounding mesenchyme (Fig. 13-34*A* to *C*). The glandular epithelium of the prostate differentiates from these endodermal cells, and the associated mesenchyme differentiates into the dense stroma and smooth muscle of the prostate.

Bulbourethral Glands

These pea-sized structures develop from paired outgrowths from the spongy part of the urethra (Fig. 13-32*A*). The smooth muscle fibers and the stroma differentiate from the adjacent mesenchyme. The secretions of these glands contribute to the semen.

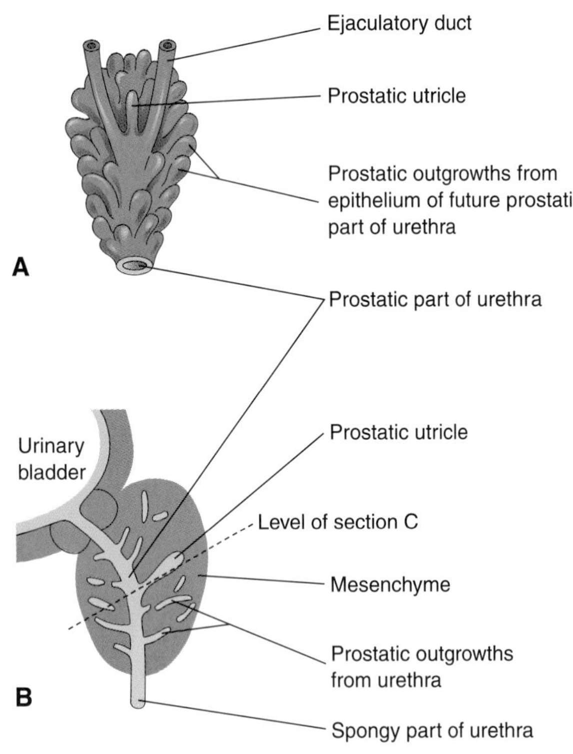

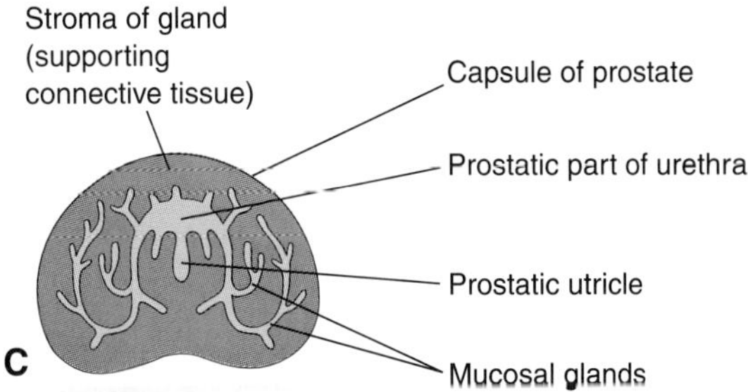

■ **Figure 13-34.** *A*, Dorsal view of the developing prostate in an 11-week fetus. *B*, Sketch of a median section of the developing urethra and prostate, showing numerous endodermal outgrowths from the prostatic urethra. The vestigial prostatic utricle is also shown. *C*, Section of the prostate (16 weeks) at the level shown in *B*.

DEVELOPMENT OF FEMALE GENITAL DUCTS AND GLANDS

In embryos with ovaries, the mesonephric ducts regress because of the absence of testosterone, and the paramesonephric ducts develop because of the absence of MIS. Although testosterone is essential for the stimulation of male sexual development, female sexual development does not depend on the presence of ovaries or hormones. The paramesonephric ducts form most of the female genital tract. The **uterine tubes** develop from the unfused cranial parts of the paramesonephric ducts (Fig. 13-32*B* and *C*). The caudal fused portions of these ducts form the **uterovaginal primordium**. As the name of this structure indicates, it gives rise to the uterus and vagina (superior part). The endometrial stroma and myometrium are derived from the adjacent splanchnic mesenchyme.

Female Ducts in Males

Similar development of the paramesonephric ducts occurs in males if testes fail to develop (**agonadal males**) because of the absence of MIS. When the testes are removed in animals before the initiation of differentiation of the genital ducts, the female duct system also develops. Removal of the ovaries of female embryos, however, has no effect on fetal sexual development. This indicates that the testes induce masculinity and repress femininity and that the ovaries are not necessary for primary sexual development.

Fusion of the paramesonephric ducts also brings together two peritoneal folds that form the right and left **broad ligaments**, and two peritoneal compartments—the **rectouterine pouch** and the **vesicouterine pouch** (Fig. 13-35*A* to *D*). Along the sides of the uterus, between the layers of the broad ligament, the mesenchyme proliferates and differentiates into cellular tissue—the **parametrium**—which is composed of loose connective tissue and smooth muscle.

DEVELOPMENT OF THE VAGINA

The vaginal epithelium is derived from the endoderm of the urogenital sinus and the fibromuscular wall of the vagina develops from the surrounding mesenchyme. Contact of the uterovaginal primordium with the urogenital sinus, forming the **sinus tubercle** (Fig. 13-33*B*), induces the formation of paired endodermal outgrowths—the **sinovaginal bulbs** (Fig. 13-35*A*). They extend from the urogenital sinus to the caudal end of the uterovaginal primordium. The sinovaginal bulbs fuse to form a **vaginal plate** (Fig. 13-32*B*). Later the central cells of this plate break down, forming the lumen of the vagina. The peripheral cells form the vaginal epithelium (Fig. 13-32*C*). There is a difference of opinion concerning the origin of the lining of the vagina. Some authorities consider the superior third of the vaginal epithelium to be derived from the

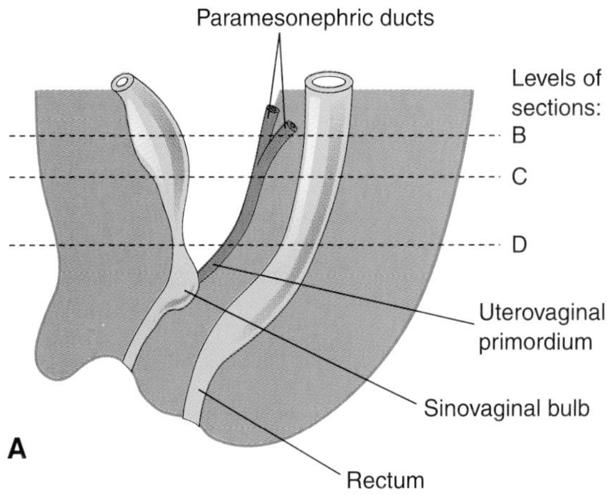

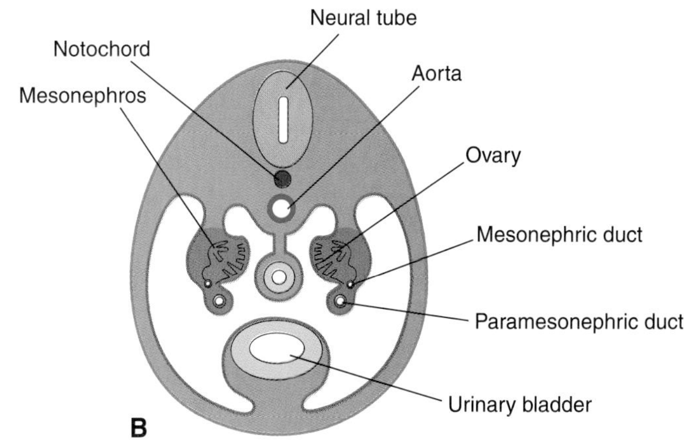

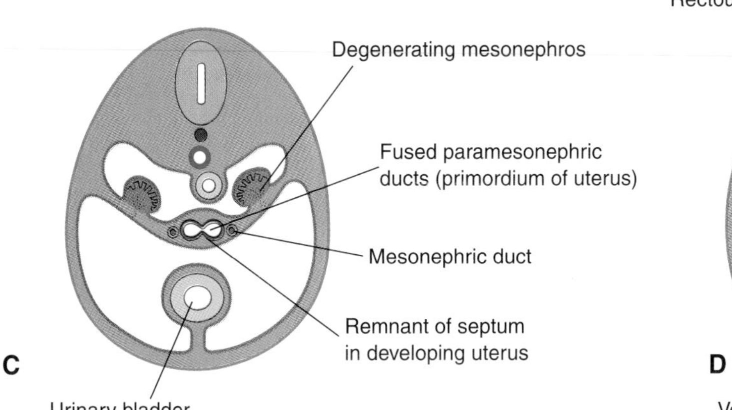

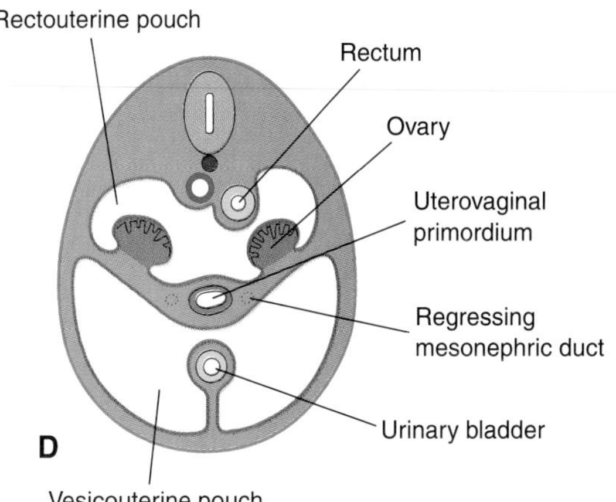

■ **Figure 13–35.** Early development of the ovaries and uterus. *A,* Schematic drawing of a sagittal section of the caudal region of an 8-week female embryo. *B,* Transverse section showing the paramesonephric ducts approaching each other. *C,* Similar section at a more caudal level illustrating fusion of the paramesonephric ducts. A remnant of the septum that initially separates them is shown. *D,* Similar section showing the uterovaginal primordium, broad ligament, and pouches in the pelvic cavity. Note that the mesonephric ducts have regressed.

uterovaginal primordium and the inferior two-thirds to arise from the urogenital sinus. Most investigators believe that the lining of the entire vagina is derived from the vaginal plate (Minh et al., 1989; Persaud, 1993).

Until late fetal life, the lumen of the vagina is separated from the cavity of the urogenital sinus by a membrane—the **hymen** (Figs. 13-32*C* and 13-36*H*). The hymen is formed by invagination of the posterior wall of the urogenital sinus, resulting from expansion of the caudal end of the vagina. The hymen usually ruptures during the perinatal period and remains as a thin fold of mucous membrane just within the vaginal orifice.

AUXILIARY GENITAL GLANDS IN THE FEMALE

Buds grow from the urethra into the surrounding mesenchyme and form **urethral glands** and **paraurethral glands** (of Skene). These glands correspond to the prostate gland in the male. Outgrowths from the urogenital sinus form the **greater vestibular glands** (of Bartholin), which are homologous to the bulbourethral glands in the male (Table 13-1).

VESTIGIAL STRUCTURES DERIVED FROM EMBRYONIC GENITAL DUCTS

During conversion of the mesonephric and paramesonephric ducts into adult structures, parts of them remain as vestigial structures. These vestiges are rarely seen unless pathological changes develop in them.

Mesonephric Remnants in Males

The cranial end of the mesonephric duct may persist as an *appendix of the epididymis,* which is usually attached to the head of the epididymis (Fig. 13-32*A*). Caudal to the efferent ductules, some mesonephric tubules may persist as a small body, the *paradidymis.*

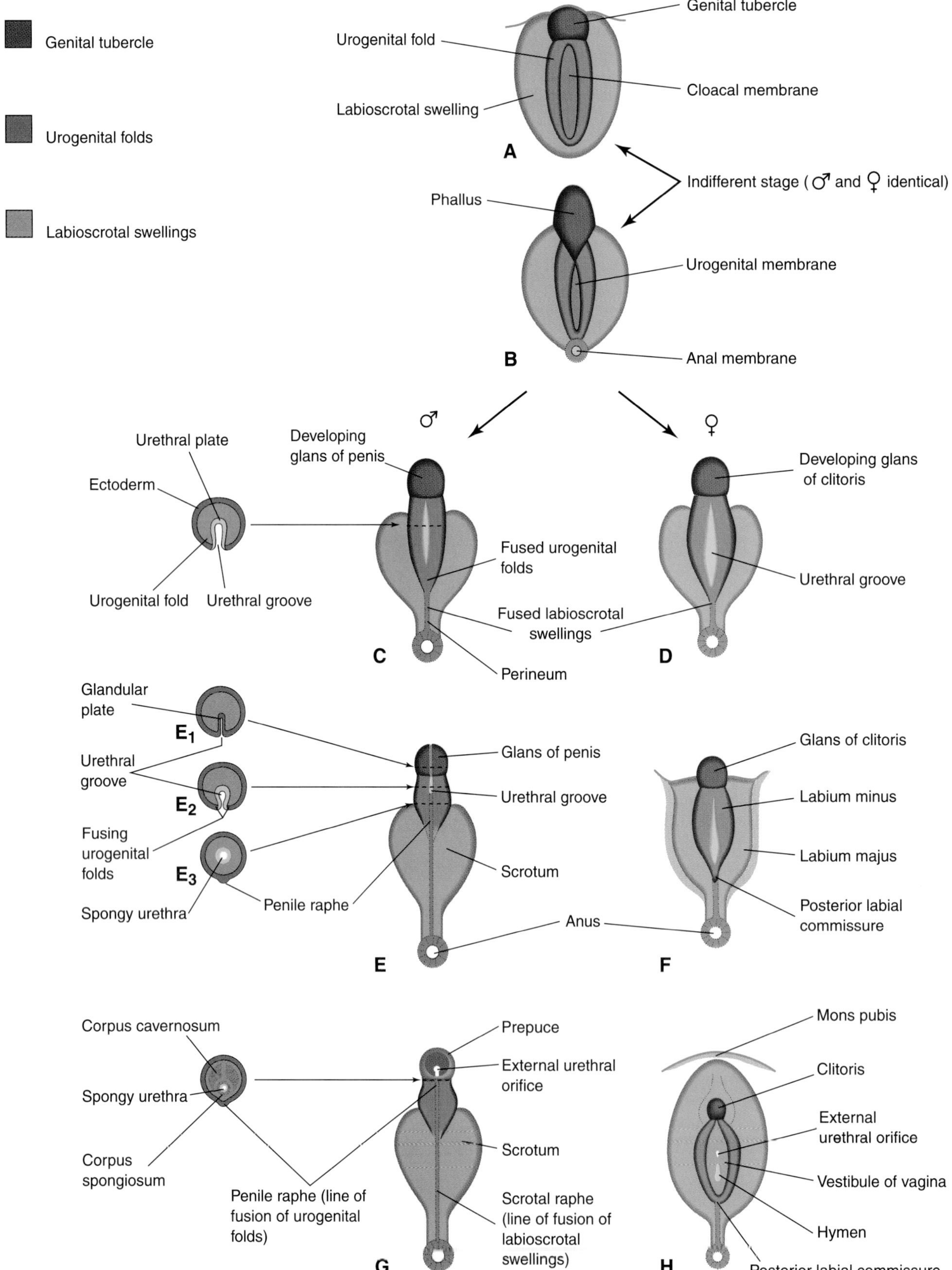

■ **Figure 13–36.** Development of the external genitalia. *A* and *B,* Diagrams illustrating the appearance of the genitalia during the indifferent stage (fourth to seventh weeks). *C, E,* and *G,* Stages in the development of male external genitalia at 9, 11, and 12 weeks, respectively. To the left are schematic transverse sections of the developing penis, illustrating formation of the spongy urethra. *D, F,* and *H,* Stages in the development of female external genitalia at 9, 11, and 12 weeks, respectively.

Table 13–1 ■ **Adult Derivatives and Vestigial Remains of Embryonic Urogenital Structures***

Male	Embryonic Structure	Female
Testis	***Indifferent gonad***	*Ovary*
Seminiferous tubules	***Cortex***	*Ovarian follicles*
Rete testis	***Medulla***	Rete ovarii
Gubernaculum testis	***Gubernaculum***	*Ovarian ligament*
		Round ligament of uterus
Ductuli efferentes	***Mesonephric tubules***	Epoophoron
Paradidymis		Paroophoron
Appendix of epididymis	***Mesonephric duct***	Appendix vesiculosa
Duct of epididymis		Duct of epoophoron
Ductus deferens		Duct of Gartner
Ureter, pelvis, calices and collecting tubules		*Ureter, pelvis, calices and collecting tubules*
Ejaculatory duct and seminal vesicle		
Appendix of testis	***Paramesonephric duct***	Hydatid (of Morgagni)
		Uterine tube
		Uterus
Urinary bladder	***Urogenital sinus***	*Urinary bladder*
Urethra (except *navicular fossa)*		*Urethra*
Prostatic utricle		*Vagina*
Prostate gland		*Urethral and paraurethral glands*
Bulbourethral glands		*Greater vestibular glands*
Seminal colliculus	***Sinus tubercle***	Hymen
Penis	***Phallus***	*Clitoris*
Glans penis		*Glans clitoridis*
Corpora cavernosa penis		*Corpora cavernosa clitoridis*
Corpus spongiosum penis		*Bulb of the vestibule*
Ventral aspect of penis	***Urogenital folds***	*Labia minora*
Scrotum	***Labioscrotal swellings***	*Labia majora*

* Functional derivatives are in *italics*.

Mesonephric Remnants in Females

The cranial end of the mesonephric duct may persist as an *appendix vesiculosa* (Fig. 13-32*B*). A few blind tubules and a duct, the *epoophoron*, correspond to the efferent ductules and duct of the epididymis in the male. The epoophoron may persist in the mesovarium between the ovary and uterine tube (Fig. 13-32*B* and *C*). Closer to the uterus some rudimentary tubules may persist as the *paroophoron*. Parts of the mesonephric duct, corresponding to the ductus deferens and ejaculatory duct, may persist as the *duct of Gartner* between the layers of the broad ligament along the lateral wall of the uterus or in the wall of the vagina. These mesonephric duct remnants may give rise to *Gartner duct cysts* (Fig. 13-32*C*).

Paramesonephric Remnants in Males

The cranial end of the paramesonephric duct may persist as a vesicular *appendix of the testis,* which is attached to the superior pole of the testis (Fig. 13-32*A*). The *prostatic utricle*, a small saclike structure that opens into the prostatic urethra, is homologous to the vagina. The lining of the prostatic utricle is derived from the epithelium of the urogenital sinus. Within its epithelium, endocrine cells containing neuron-specific enolase and serotonin have been detected (Wernert et al., 1990). The *seminal colliculus*, a small elevation in the posterior wall of the prostatic urethra (Moore, 1992), is the adult derivative of the sinus tubercle (Fig. 13-33*B*). It is homologous to the hymen in the female (Table 13-1).

Paramesonephric Remnants in Females

Part of the cranial end of the paramesonephric duct that does not contribute to the infundibulum of the uterine tube may persist as a vesicular appendage (Fig. 13-32*C*), a *hydatid (of Morgagni)*.

Development of External Genitalia

Up to the seventh week of development the external genitalia are similar in both sexes. Distinguishing sexual characteristics begin to appear during the ninth week, but the external genitalia are not fully differentiated until the twelfth week. From the fourth to the early part of the seventh week, the external genitalia are sexually undifferentiated (Fig. 13-36*A* and *B*). Early in the fourth week, proliferating mesenchyme produces a **genital tubercle** in both sexes at the cranial end of the cloacal membrane. **Labioscrotal swellings** (genital swellings) and **urogenital folds** (urethral folds) soon develop on each side of the cloacal membrane. The genital tubercle soon elongates to form a **phallus**. When the urorectal septum fuses with the cloacal membrane at the end of the sixth week, it divides the cloacal membrane into a dorsal anal membrane and a ventral urogenital membrane (Fig. 13-36*B*). The **urogenital membrane** lies in the floor of a median cleft, the **urogenital groove**, which is bounded by the urogenital folds. The anal and urogenital membranes rupture a week or so later forming the **anus** and **urogenital orifice**, respectively. In the female fetus the urethra and vagina open into a common cavity, the **vestibule of the vagina**.

DEVELOPMENT OF MALE EXTERNAL GENITALIA

Masculinization of the indifferent external genitalia is induced by **testosterone** produced by the fetal testes (Fig. 13-36*C*, *E*, and *G*). As the phallus enlarges and elongates to become the penis, the urogenital folds form the lateral walls of the **urethral groove** on the ventral surface of the penis (Fig. 13-37*A* and *B*). This groove is lined by a proliferation of endodermal cells, the **urethral plate**, which extends from the phallic portion of the urogenital sinus. The **urogenital folds** fuse with each other along the ventral surface of the penis to form the *spongy urethra* (Fig. 13-36E_1 to E_3). The surface ectoderm fuses in the median plane of the penis, forming the **penile raphe** and enclosing the spongy urethra within the penis. At the tip of the glans penis an ectodermal ingrowth forms a cellular cord, the **glandular (urethral) plate**, which grows toward the root of the penis to meet the spongy urethra (Fig. 13-25*A*). This plate canalizes and joins the previously formed spongy urethra. This completes the terminal part of the urethra and moves the external urethral orifice to the tip of the glans penis (Fig. 13-25*C*).

During the twelfth week a circular ingrowth of ectoderm occurs at the periphery of the glans penis (Fig. 13-25*B*). When this ingrowth breaks down, it forms the **prepuce** (foreskin)—a covering fold of skin (Fig. 13-25*C*). For some time the prepuce is adherent to the glans and is usually not retractable at birth. Breakdown of the adherent surfaces normally occurs during infancy. The *corpora cavernosa penis* and *corpus spongiosum penis* develop from mesenchyme in the phallus. The **labioscrotal swellings** grow toward each other and fuse to form the scrotum (Fig. 13-36*E* and *G*). The line of fusion of these folds is clearly visible as the **scrotal raphe** (Figs. 13-36*G* and 13-37*C*). Two cases of *agenesis of the scrotum*, an extremely rare anomaly, have been reported (Verga and Avolio, 1996).

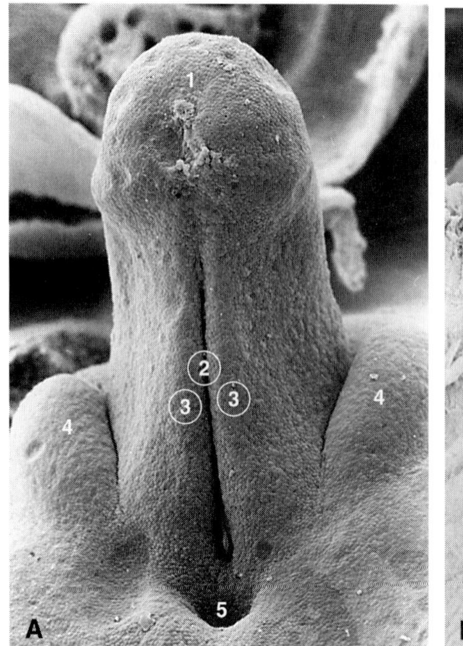

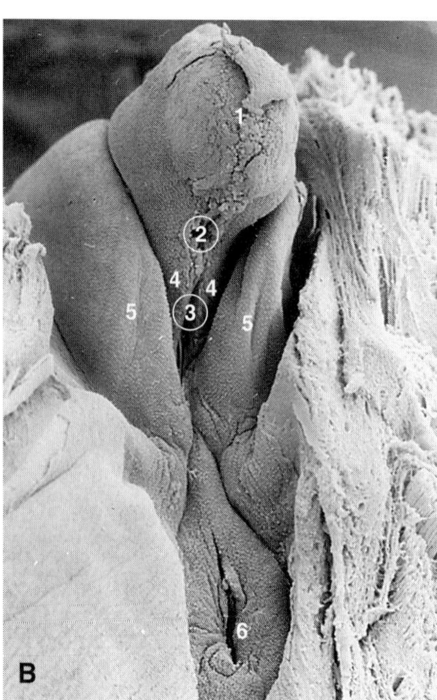

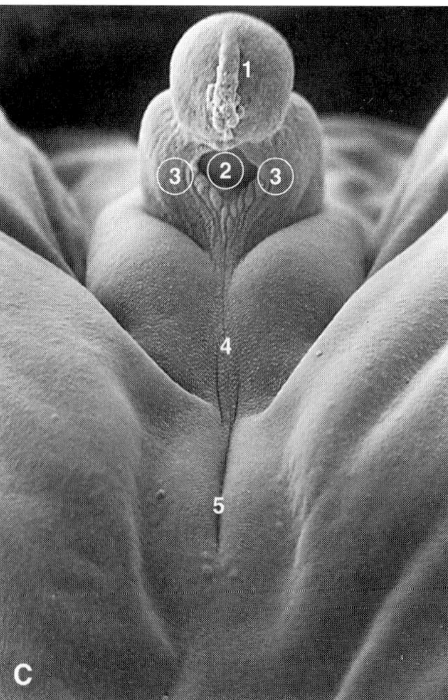

■ **Figure 13-37.** Scanning electron micrographs (SEMs) of the developing male external genitalia. *A,* SEM of the perineum during the indifferent stage of a 17-mm, 7-week-old embryo (×100). **1,** Developing glans penis with the glandular (urethral) plate. **2,** Urethral groove continuous with the urogenital sinus. **3,** Urogenital or urethral folds. **4,** Labioscrotal swellings. **5,** Anus. *B,* External genitalia of a 7.2-cm, 10-week-old fetus (×45). **1,** Glans clitoridis with glandular (urethral) plate. **2,** External urethral orifice. **3,** Opening into urogenital sinus. **4,** Urogenital fold (labium minus). **5,** Labioscrotal swelling (labium majus). **6,** Anus. *C,* SEM of the external genitalia of a 5.5-cm, 10-week-old male fetus (×40). **1,** Glans penis with glandular (urethral) plate. **2,** Remains of urethral groove. **3,** Urogenital (urethral) folds in the process of closing. **4,** Labioscrotal swellings fusing to form the scrotum. **5,** Anus. (From Hinrichsen KV: Embryologische Grundlagen. *In* Sohn C, Holzgreve W [eds]: *Ultraschall in Gynäkologie und Geburtshilfe.* New York, Georg Thieme Verlag, 1995.)

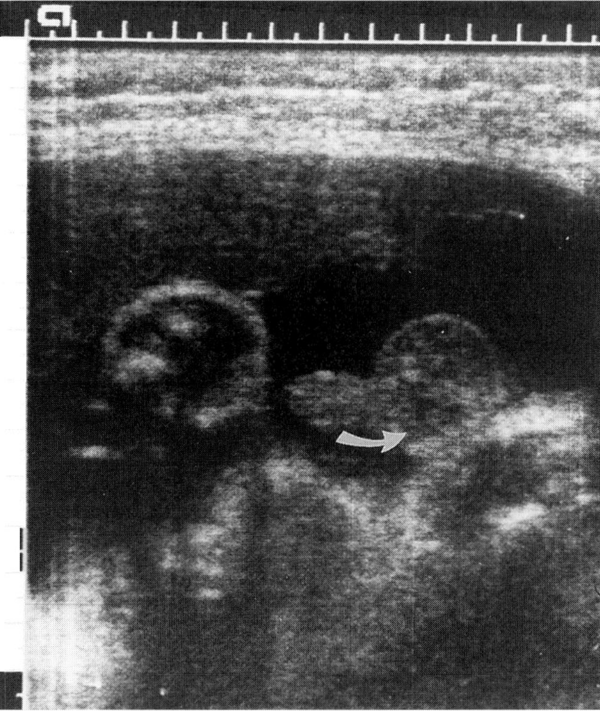

■ **Figure 13–38.** Sonogram of a male fetus (22 weeks' gestation) showing normal external genitalia. Observe the penis and scrotum. *Curved arrow,* testis. (Courtesy of Dr. C. R. Harman, Department of Obstetrics, Gynecology and Reproductive Sciences, Women's Hospital and University of Manitoba, Winnipeg, Manitoba, Canada.)

DEVELOPMENT OF FEMALE EXTERNAL GENITALIA

Feminization of the indifferent external genitalia is not clearly understood, but estrogens produced by the placenta and fetal ovaries appear to be involved (Fig. 13-36*D*, *F*, and *H*). Growth of the phallus gradually ceases and it becomes the **clitoris**, a very sensitive sexual organ. The clitoris, still relatively large at 18 weeks (Fig. 13-19), develops like the penis but the urogenital folds do not fuse, except posteriorly, where they join to form the *frenulum of the labia minora* (Moore, 1992). The unfused parts of the urogenital folds form the **labia minora**. The labioscrotal folds fuse posteriorly to form the *posterior labial commissure* and anteriorly to form the *anterior labial commissure* and *mons pubis* (Fig 13-36*H*). Most parts of the **labioscrotal folds** remain unfused and form two large folds of skin, the **labia majora**, which are homologous to the scrotum.

Determination of Fetal Sex

Visualization of the external genitalia during ultrasonography (Fig. 13-38) is clinically important for several reasons, such as detection of fetuses at risk for severe X-linked disorders (Thompson et al., 1991; Mahony, 1994). Careful examination of the perineum may detect **ambiguous genitalia** (Fig. 13-39). Only documentation of testes in the scrotum provides 100% gender determination, which is not possible in utero until 28 to 38 menstrual weeks (Mahony, 1994). Unfortunately, fetal position prevents good visualization of the perineum in 30% of fetuses.

When there is normal sexual differentiation, the appearance of the external and internal genitalia is consistent with the sex chromosome complement (i.e., XX or XY). Because early embryos have the potential to develop as either males or females, errors in sex determination and differentiation result in various degrees of intermediate sex—**intersexuality** or **hermaphroditism**. Hermaphroditism implies a discrepancy between the morphology of the gonads (testes/ovaries) and the appearance of the external genitalia. A person with ambiguous external genitalia is an **intersex** or **hermaphrodite**. Intersexual conditions are classified according to the histological appearance of the gonads:

- *True hermaphrodites* have ovarian and testicular tissue either in the same or in opposite gonads.
- *Female pseudohermaphrodites* have ovaries.
- *Male pseudohermaphrodites* have testes.

True Hermaphroditism

Persons with this *extremely rare intersexual condition* usually have chromatin-positive nuclei (contain sex chromatin) and 70% of them have a 46, XX chromosome constitution; about 20% have 46, XX / 46, XY mosaicism, and about 10% have a 46, XY chromosome

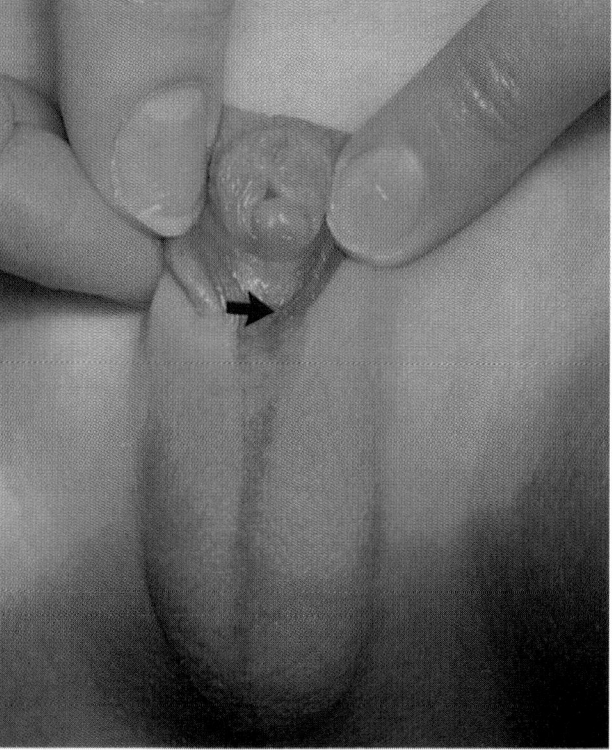

■ **Figure 13–39.** External genitalia of a 6-year-old girl showing an enlarged clitoris and fused labia majora that have formed a scrotumlike structure. The arrow indicates the opening into the urogenital sinus. This extreme masculinization is the result of congenital adrenal hyperplasia (CAH).

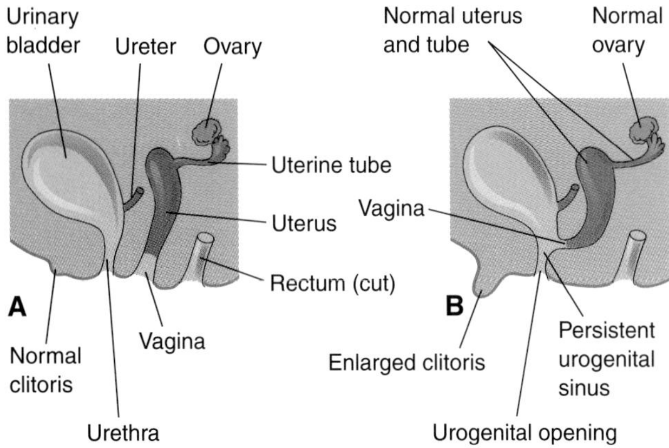

■ **Figure 13-40.** Schematic lateral views of the female urogenital system. *A*, Normal. *B*, Female pseudohermaphrodite caused by congenital adrenal hyperplasia (CAH). Note the enlarged clitoris and persistent urogenital sinus that were induced by androgens produced by the hyperplastic suprarenal glands.

constitution. The causes of true hermaphroditism are still poorly understood (DiGeorge, 1996). Most true hermaphrodites are reared as females (Behrman et al., 1996) and have both testicular and ovarian tissue (e.g., an ovary and a testis, or an ovotestis). These tissues are not usually functional. *True hermaphroditism results from an error in sex determination*. The phenotype may be male or female but the external genitalia are ambiguous. *Ovotestes* form if both the medulla and cortex of the indifferent gonads develop.

Female Pseudohermaphroditism

Persons with this intersexual condition have *chromatin-positive nuclei* and a 46, XX chromosome constitution. This anomaly results from exposure of the female fetus to excessive androgens, and the effects are principally virilization of the external genitalia (clitoral enlargement and labial fusion [Figs. 13-27 and 13-39]). The common cause of female pseudohermaphroditism is congenital adrenal hyperplasia (CAH). There is no ovarian abnormality, but the excessive production of androgens by the fetal suprarenal glands causes masculinization of the external genitalia, varying from enlargement of the clitoris to almost masculine genitalia. Commonly there is clitoral hypertrophy, partial fusion of the labia majora, and a persistent urogenital sinus (Fig. 13-40). In very unusual cases the masculinization may be so intense that a complete *clitoral urethra* results (DiGeorge, 1996). Female pseudohermaphrodites who do not have CAH are very rare. The administration of *androgenic agents* to women during pregnancy may cause similar anomalies of the fetal external genitalia (see Chapter 8). Most cases have resulted from the use of certain progestational compounds for the treatment of threatened abortion. *Masculinizing maternal tumors* can also cause virilization of female fetuses (e.g., benign adrenal adenoma and ovarian tumors, especially *arrhenoblastoma*).

Male Pseudohermaphroditism

Persons with this intersexual condition have *chromatin-negative nuclei* (do not contain sex chromatin) and a 46, XY chromosome constitution. The external and internal genitalia are variable, owing to varying degrees of development of the external genitalia and paramesonephric ducts. These anomalies are caused by inadequate production of testosterone and MIF by the fetal testes. Testicular development in these males ranges from rudimentary to normal (Meacham et al., 1991). Five genetic defects have been described in the enzymatic synthesis of testosterone by the fetal testes, and a defect in Leydig cell differentiation has been described (DiGeorge, 1996). These defects produce male pseudohermaphroditism through inadequate virilization of the male fetus.

Androgen Insensitivity Syndrome (AIS)

Persons with AIS—also called the **testicular feminization syndrome**—(1 in 20,000 live births) are normal-appearing females, despite the presence of testes and a 46, XY chromosome constitution (Fig. 13-41). The external genitalia are female but the vagina usually ends blindly in a pouch and the uterus and uterine tubes are absent or rudimentary. At puberty there is normal development of breasts and female characteristics, but menstruation does not occur and pubic hair is scanty or absent. The psychosexual orientation of women with AIS is entirely female and medically, legally, and socially, they are females. The testes are usually in the abdomen or the inguinal canals, but they may descend into the labia majora. The failure of masculinization to occur in these individuals results from a resistance to the action of testosterone at the cellular level in the genital tubercle and labioscrotal and urogenital folds.

Patients with **partial AIS** exhibit some masculinization at birth, such as ambiguous external genitalia, and may have an enlarged clitoris. The vagina ends blindly and the uterus is absent. Testes are in the inguinal canals or the labia majora. These patients usually have point mutations in the sequence that codes for the androgen receptor (Behrman et al., 1996).

The AIS results from a defect in the androgen receptor mechanism. Embryologically these females represent an extreme form of male pseudohermaphroditism, but they are not intersexes because they usually have normal external genitalia. Usually the testes are removed as soon as they are discovered because, in about one-third of these women, malignant tumors develop by 50 years of age (Behrman et al., 1996). AIS follows X-linked recessive inheritance, and the gene encoding the androgen receptor has been localized (DiGeorge, 1996). For details on the genetics of this condition, see Thompson et al. (1991).

Mixed Gonadal Dysgenesis

Persons with this very rare condition usually have chromatin-negative nuclei, a testis on one side, and an undifferentiated gonad on the other side. The internal genitalia are female, but male derivatives of the mesonephric ducts are sometimes present. The external genitalia range from normal female, through intermediate states, to normal male. At puberty neither breast development nor menstruation occurs, but varying degrees of virilization are common (McDonough, 1990).

Hypospadias

Hypospadias is the most common anomaly of the penis. In one of every 300 male infants, the external urethral orifice is on the ventral surface of the glans penis (**glandular hypospadias**), or on the ventral surface of the body of the penis (**penile hypospadias**). Usually the penis is underdeveloped and curved ventrally—**chordee**. There are four types of hypospadias (Fig. 13-42):

- glandular hypospadias
- penile hypospadias
- penoscrotal hypospadias
- perineal hypospadias.

The glandular and penile types of hypospadias constitute about 80% of cases (Fig. 13-42*A* and *B*). In **penoscrotal hypospadias** the urethral orifice is at the junction of the penis and scrotum (Fig. 13-42*C*). In **perineal hypospadias** the labioscrotal folds fail to fuse and the external urethral orifice is located between the unfused halves of the scrotum. Because the external genitalia in this severe type of hypospadias are ambiguous, persons with perineal hypospadias and cryptorchidism (undescended testes) are sometimes diagnosed as male pseudohermaphrodites.

Hypospadias results from inadequate production of androgens by the fetal testes and/or inadequate receptor sites for the hormones. These defects result in failure of canalization of the glandular plate and/or failure of fusion of the urogenital folds; as a consequence, there is incomplete formation of the spongy (penile) urethra. Differences in the timing and degree of hormonal failure, and/or in the failure of the development of receptor sites, account for the different types of hypospadias.

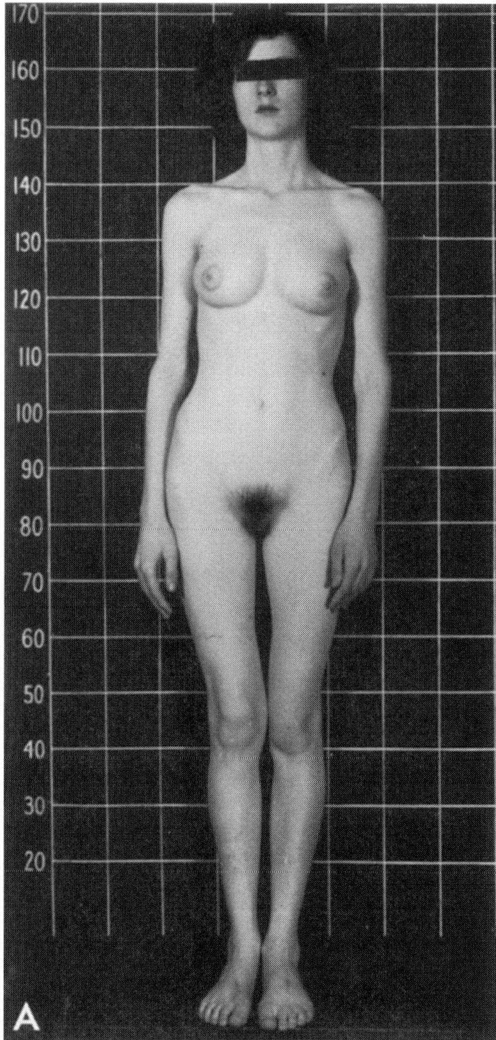

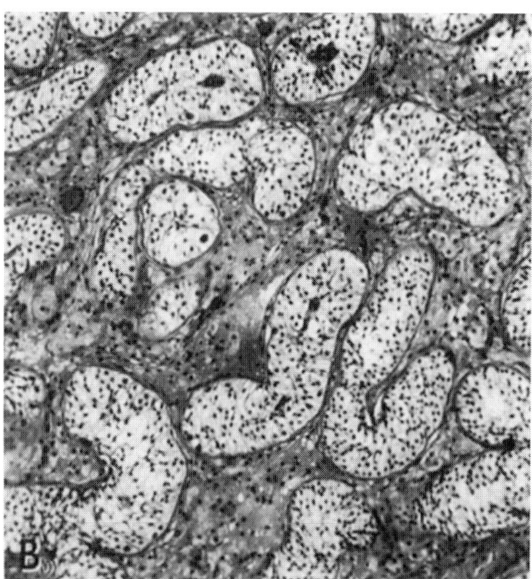

■ **Figure 13-41.** *A,* Photograph of a 17-year-old woman with androgen insensitivity syndrome (testicular feminization syndrome). The external genitalia are female but the patient has a 46, XY karyotype and testes. *B,* Photomicrograph of a section through a testis removed from the inguinal region of this woman, showing seminiferous tubules lined by Sertoli cells. There are no germ cells and the interstitial cells are hypoplastic. Medically, legally, and socially, these individuals are females. (From Jones HW, Scott WW: *Hermaphroditism, Genital Anomalies and Related Endocrine Disorders.* 1958. Courtesy of Williams & Wilkins, Baltimore.)

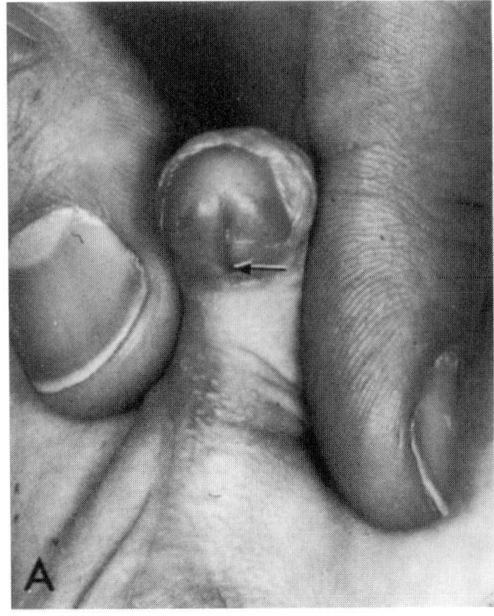

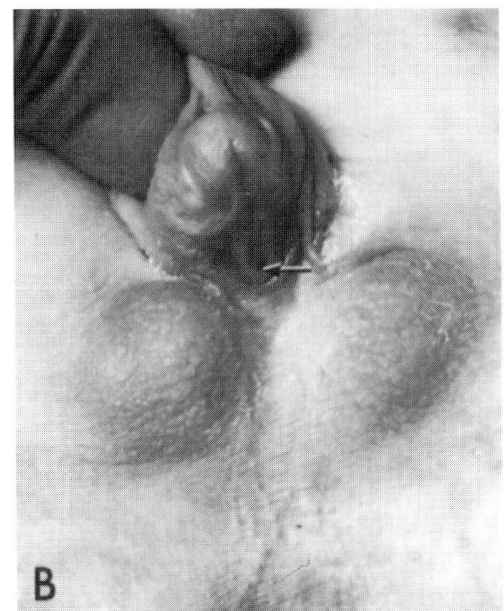

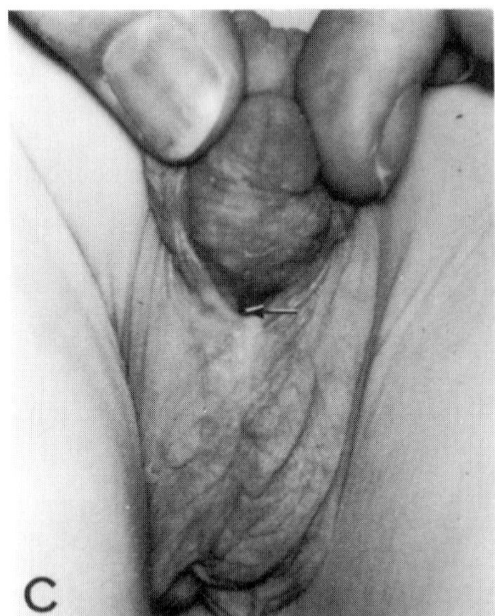

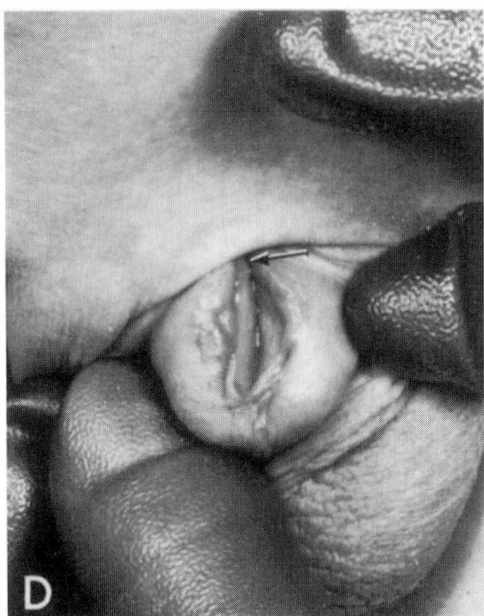

■ **Figure 13–42.** Photographs of penile anomalies. *A,* Glandular hypospadias. This is the most common form of hypospadias. The external urethral orifice (meatus) is on the ventral aspect of the glans *(arrow).* There is a shallow pit in the glans penis at the usual site of the urethral orifice. Note that there is a moderate degree of chordee, causing the penis to curve ventrally. (From Jolly H: *Diseases of Children,* 2nd ed. 1968. Courtesy of Blackwell Scientific Publications.) *B,* Penile hypospadias. The penis is short and curved (chordee). The external urethral orifice *(arrow)* is near the penoscrotal junction. *C,* Penoscrotal hypospadias. The external urethral orifice *(arrow)* is located at the penoscrotal junction. *D,* Epispadias. The external urethral orifice *(arrow)* is on the dorsal surface of the penis. (Courtesy of Mr. Innes Williams, Genitourinary Surgeon, The Hospital for Sick Children, Great Ormond Street, London, England.)

Epispadias

In one of every 30,000 male infants, the urethra opens on the dorsal surface of the penis (Fig. 13-42*D*). Although epispadias may occur as a separate entity, it is *often associated with exstrophy of the bladder* (Figs. 13-22 and 13-23). Epispadias may result from inadequate ectodermal-mesenchymal interactions during development of the genital tubercle. As a consequence, the genital tubercle develops more dorsally than in normal embryos. Consequently, when the urogenital membrane ruptures, the urogenital sinus opens on the dorsal surface of the penis. Urine is expelled at the root of the malformed penis.

Agenesis of External Genitalia

Congenital absence of the penis or clitoris is an extremely rare condition (Fig. 13-43). Failure of the genital tubercle to develop may result from inadequate ectodermal-mesenchymal interactions during the seventh week. The urethra usually opens into the perineum near the anus.

Bifid Penis and Double Penis

These anomalies are very rare and are usually associated with exstrophy of the bladder (Fig. 13-22*A*; see

Fouda-Neel et al., 1996). It may also be associated with urinary tract abnormalities and imperforate anus. Bifid penis results when two genital tubercles develop.

Micropenis

The penis is so small that it is almost hidden by the suprapubic pad of fat. This condition results from a fetal testicular failure and is commonly associated with hypopituitarism.

Anomalies of the Uterine Tubes, Uterus, and Vagina

Anomalies of the uterine tubes occur infrequently and only a few types have been reported. These include hydatid cysts, accessory ostia, complete and segmental absence, duplication of the tube, lack of the muscular layer, and failure of the tube to canalize.

Various types of uterine duplication and vaginal anomalies result from arrests of development of the uterovaginal primordium during the eighth week (Fig. 13-44):

- incomplete fusion of the paramesonephric ducts
- incomplete development of a paramesonephric duct
- failure of parts of one or both paramesonephric ducts to develop
- incomplete canalization of the vaginal plate to form the vagina

Abnormal Development of the Uterus

Double uterus (uterus didelphys) results from failure of fusion of the inferior parts of the paramesonephric ducts. It may be associated with a double or a single vagina (Fig. 13-44*A* to *C*). In some cases the uterus appears normal externally but is divided internally by a thin septum (Fig. 13-44*F*). If the duplication involves only the superior part of the body of the uterus, the condition is called **bicornuate uterus** (Fig. 13-44*D* and *E*). If one paramesonephric duct is retarded in its growth and does not fuse with the other one, a **bicornuate uterus with a rudimentary horn** (cornu) develops (Fig. 13-44*E*). The rudimentary horn may not communicate with the cavity of the uterus. A **unicornuate uterus** develops when one paramesonephric duct fails to develop; this results in a uterus with one uterine tube (Fig. 13-44*G*).

Absence of the Vagina and Uterus

Once in about every 4000 to 5000 female births, absence of the vagina occurs. This results from failure of the sinovaginal bulbs to develop and form the vaginal plate (Fig. 13-32*B*). When the vagina is absent, the uterus is usually absent also because the developing uterus (uterovaginal primordium) induces the formation of sinovaginal bulbs, which fuse to form the vaginal plate. Other anomalies involving the urogenital tract and the skeletal system may also be present (Mayer-Rokitansky-Küster-Hauser syndrome).

Vaginal Atresia

Failure of canalization of the vaginal plate results in blockage of the vagina. A transverse vaginal septum occurs in approximately 1 in 80,000 women (Reid, 1993). Usually the septum is located at the junction of the middle and superior thirds of the vagina. Failure of the inferior end of the vaginal plate to perforate results in an **imperforate hymen**. Variations in the appearance of the hymen are common (Muram, 1993). The vaginal orifice varies in diameter from very small to large, and there may be more than one orifice (Fig. 13-45).

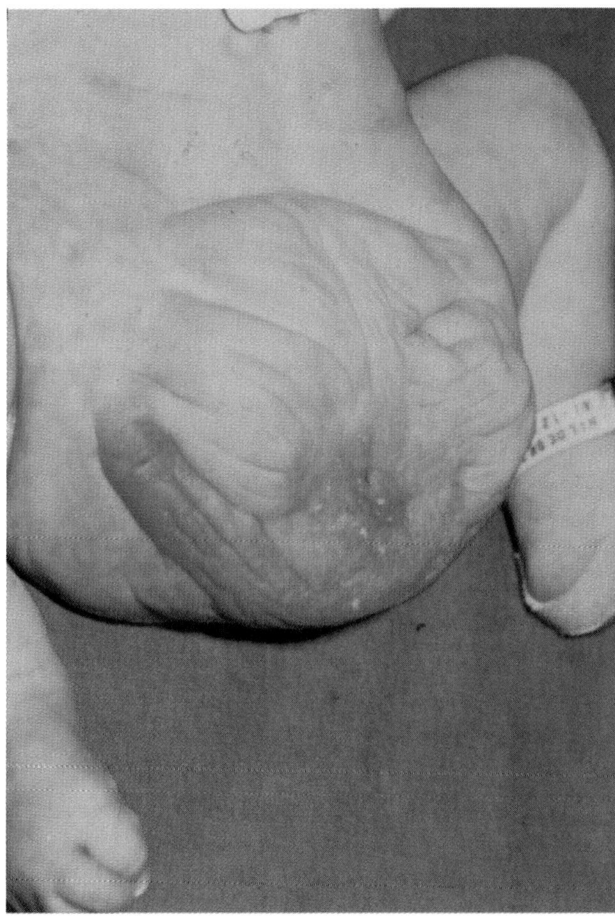

■ **Figure 13-43.** Ventral view of the perineum of an infant. No external genitalia are present. (Courtesy of Dr. A. E. Chudley, Section of Genetics and Metabolism, Department of Pediatrics and Child Health, Children's Hospital and University of Manitoba, Winnipeg, Manitoba, Canada.)

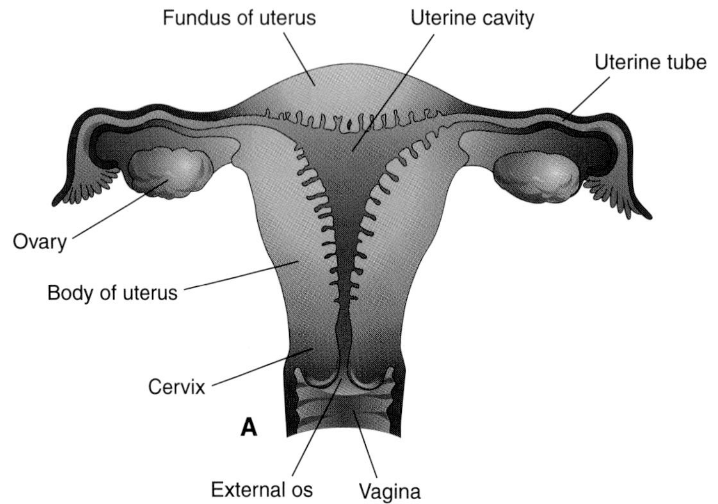

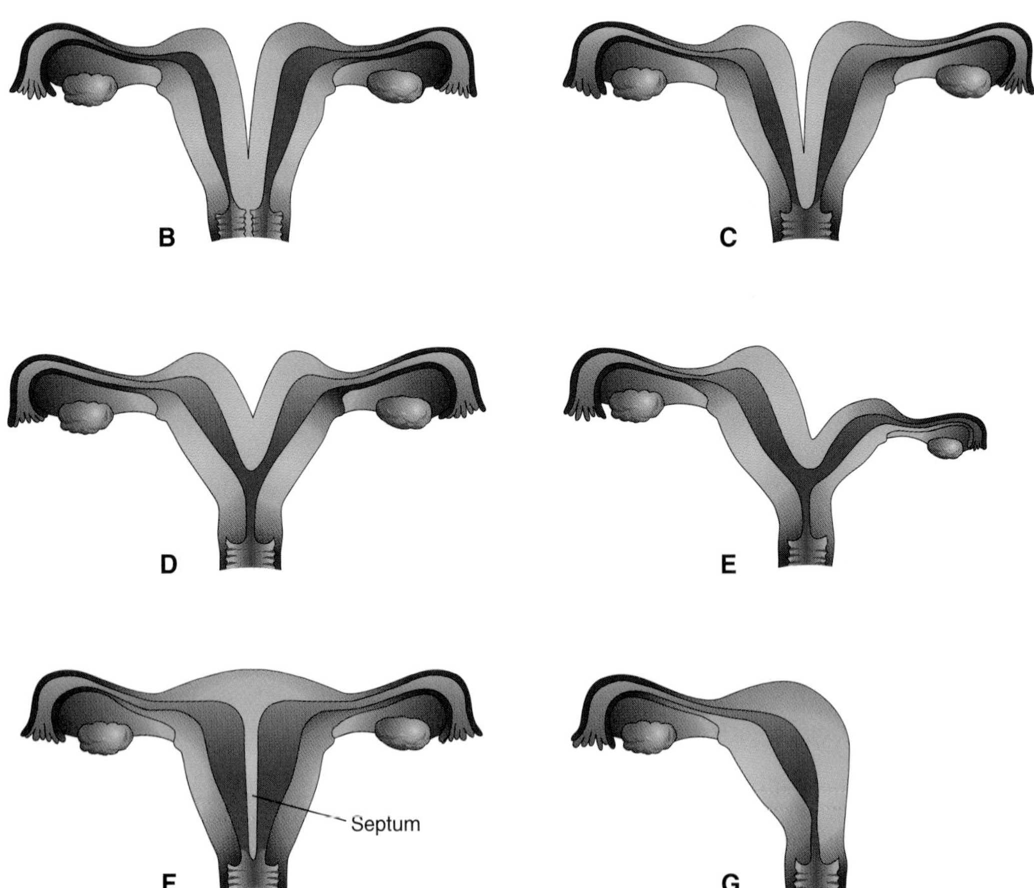

■ **Figure 13–44.** Drawings illustrating various types of uterine anomaly. *A,* Normal uterus and vagina. *B,* Double uterus (uterus didelphys) and double vagina. *C,* Double uterus with single vagina. *D,* Bicornuate uterus. *E,* Bicornuate uterus with a rudimentary left horn. *F,* Septate uterus. *G,* Unicornuate uterus.

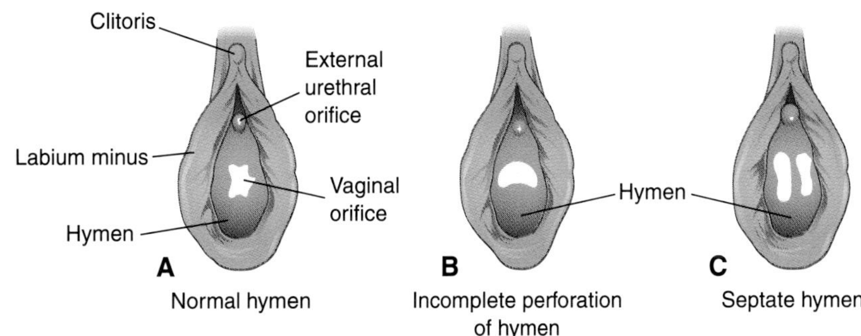

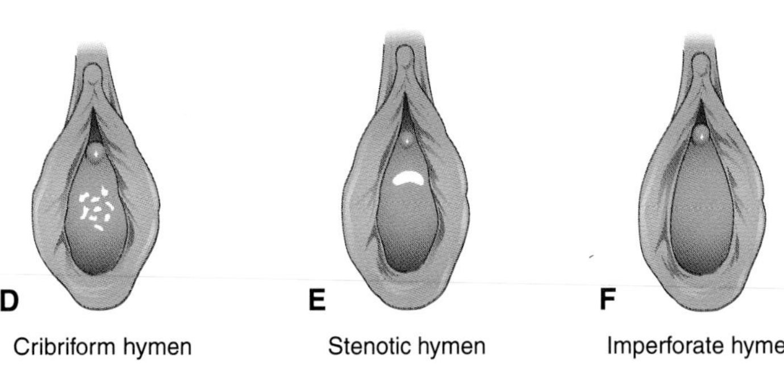

■ **Figure 13–45.** Congenital anomalies of the hymen. The normal appearance of the hymen is illustrated in *A*.

DEVELOPMENT OF THE INGUINAL CANALS

The inguinal canals form pathways for the testes to descend from their intra-abdominal position through the anterior abdominal wall into the scrotum. *Inguinal canals develop in both sexes* because of the morphologically indifferent stage of sexual development. As the mesonephros degenerates, a ligament—the **gubernaculum**—descends on each side of the abdomen from the inferior pole of the gonad (Fig. 13-46*A*). The gubernaculum passes obliquely through the developing anterior abdominal wall at the site of the future inguinal canal (Fig. 13-46*B* to *D*). The gubernaculum attaches caudally to the internal surface of the *labioscrotal swellings* (future halves of the scrotum or labia majora).

The **processus vaginalis** or vaginal process, an evagination of peritoneum, develops ventral to the gubernaculum and herniates through the abdominal wall along the path formed by the gubernaculum (Fig. 13-46*B*). The vaginal processus carries extensions of the layers of the abdominal wall before it, which form the walls of the inguinal canal. In males these layers also form the coverings of the spermatic cord and testis (Fig. 13-46*D* to *F*). The opening in the transversalis fascia produced by the vaginal process becomes the **deep inguinal ring**, and the opening created in the external oblique aponeurosis forms the **superficial inguinal ring** (Moore, 1992).

Descent of the Testes

Testicular descent is associated with:

- Enlargement of the testes and atrophy of the mesonephroi (mesonephric kidneys), which allow movement of the testes caudally along the posterior abdominal wall.
- Atrophy of the paramesonephric ducts induced by the MIS enables the testes to move transabdominally to the deep inguinal rings.
- Enlargement of the processus vaginalis guides the testis through the inguinal canal into the scrotum.

By 26 weeks the testes have descended retroperitoneally (external to the peritoneum) from the posterior abdominal wall to the deep inguinal rings (Fig. 13-46*B* and *C*). This change in position occurs as the fetal pelvis enlarges and the trunk of the embryo elongates. Transabdominal movement of the testes is largely a relative movement that results from growth of the cranial part of the abdomen away from the caudal part (future pelvic region).

Little is known about the cause of testicular descent through the inguinal canals into the scrotum but the process is controlled by androgens (e.g., testosterone) produced by the fetal testes (Wensing, 1988). The role of the gubernaculum in testicular descent is uncertain. Initially it forms a path through the anterior abdominal wall for the processus vaginalis to follow during formation of the inguinal canal. The gubernaculum also anchors the testis to the scrotum and appears to guide its descent into the scrotum. Passage of the testis through the inguinal canal may also be aided by the increase in intra-abdominal pressure resulting from the growth of abdominal viscera. Descent of the testes through the inguinal canals into the scrotum usually begins during the twenty-sixth week and takes 2 or 3 days. The testes pass external to the peritoneum and processus vaginalis. After the testes enter the scrotum, the inguinal canal contracts around the spermatic cord. More than 97% of full-term newborn boys have

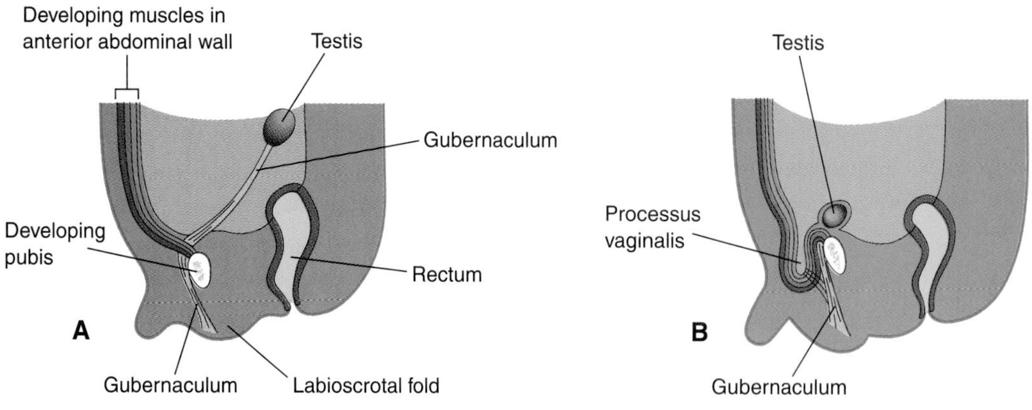

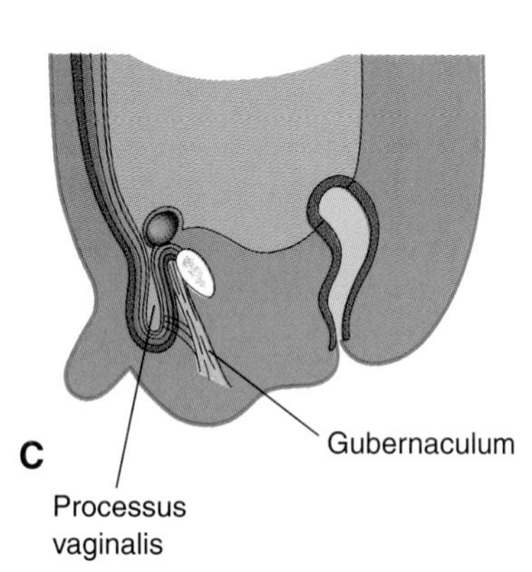

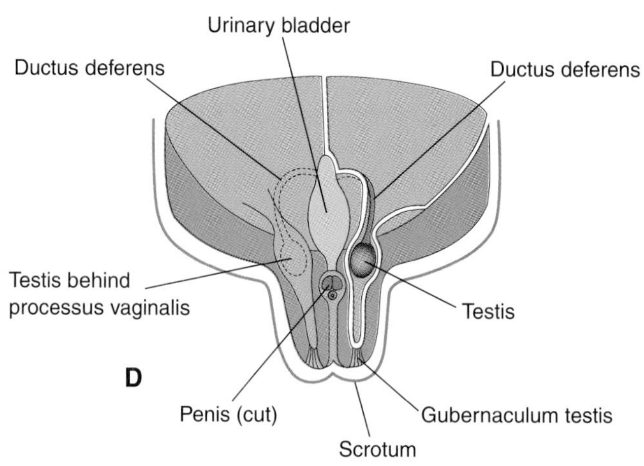

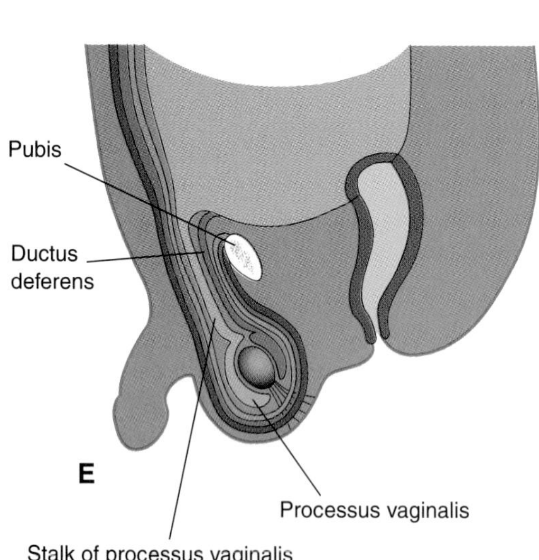

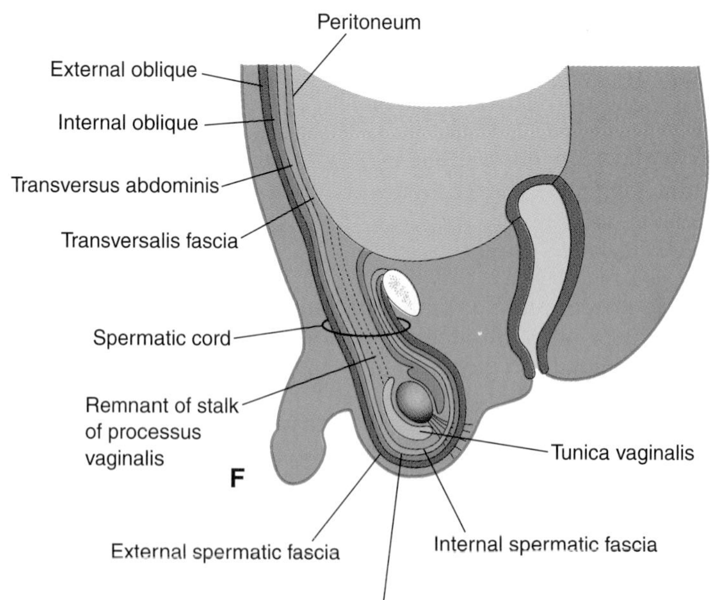

■ **Figure 13–46.** Schematic diagrams illustrating formation of the inguinal canals and descent of the testes. *A,* Sagittal section of a 7-week embryo showing the testis before its descent from the dorsal abdominal wall. *B* and *C,* Similar sections at about 28 weeks showing the processus vaginalis and the testis beginning to pass through the inguinal canal. Note that the processus vaginalis carries fascial layers of the abdominal wall before it. *D,* Frontal section of a fetus about 3 days later illustrating descent of the testis posterior to the processus vaginalis. The processus vaginalis has been cut away on the left side to show the testis and ductus deferens. *E,* Sagittal section of a newborn infant showing the processus vaginalis communicating with the peritoneal cavity by a narrow stalk. *F,* Similar section of a 1-month-old infant after obliteration of the stalk of the processus vaginalis. Note that the extended fascial layers of the abdominal wall now form the coverings of the spermatic cord.

both testes in the scrotum. During the first 3 months after birth, most undescended testes descend into the scrotum. Spontaneous testicular descent does not occur after the age of 1 year (Behrman et al., 1996).

The mode of descent of the testis explains why the ductus deferens crosses anterior to the ureter (Fig. 13-33*A*); it also explains the course of the testicular vessels. These vessels form when the testis is high on the posterior abdominal wall. When the testis descends it carries its ductus deferens and vessels with it. As the testis and ductus deferens descend, they are ensheathed by the fascial extensions of the abdominal wall (Fig. 13-46*F*).

- The extension of the transversalis fascia becomes the **internal spermatic fascia.**
- The extensions of the internal oblique muscle and fascia become the **cremasteric muscle** and **fascia.**
- The extension of the external oblique aponeurosis becomes the **external spermatic fascia** (Moore, 1992).

Within the scrotum the testis projects into the distal end of the processus vaginalis. During the perinatal period, the connecting stalk of the process normally obliterates, isolating the **tunica vaginalis** as a peritoneal sac related to the testis (Fig. 13-46*F*).

Descent of the Ovaries

The ovaries also descend from the posterior abdominal wall to the pelvis, just inferior to the pelvic brim. The gubernaculum is attached to the uterus near the attachment of the uterine tube. The cranial part of the gubernaculum becomes the **ovarian ligament** and the caudal part forms the round ligament of the uterus (Fig. 13-32*C*). The **round ligaments** pass through the inguinal canals and terminate in the labia majora. The relatively small processus vaginalis in the female usually obliterates and disappears long before birth; a persistent process is called the **canal of Nuck**.

Cryptorchidism or Undescended Testes

Cryptorchidism (Gr. *kryptos*, hidden) occurs in up to 30% of premature males and in about 3 to 4% of full-term males. This reflects the fact that the testes begin to descend into the scrotum at the end of the third trimester. Cryptorchidism may be unilateral or bilateral. In most cases the testes descend into the scrotum by the end of the first year. If both testes remain within or just outside the abdominal cavity, they fail to mature and sterility is common. Undescended testes are often histologically normal at birth, but failure of development and atrophy are detectable by the end of the first year (Behrman et al., 1996). **Cryptorchid testes** may be in the abdominal cavity or anywhere along the usual path of descent of the testis, but they are usually in the inguinal canal (Fig. 13-47*A*). The cause of most cases of cryptorchidism is unknown, but a deficiency of androgen production by the fetal testes is an important factor. Men with a history of cryptorchidism have a 20 to 44% increase in risk of developing testicular cancer (Palmer, 1991; Behrman et al., 1996).

Ectopic Testes

After traversing the inguinal canal, the testis may deviate from its usual path of descent and lodge in various abnormal locations (Fig. 13-47*B*):

- interstitial (external to aponeurosis of external oblique muscle)
- in the proximal part of the medial thigh
- dorsal to the penis
- on the opposite side (crossed ectopia)

All types of ectopic testis are rare, but **interstitial ectopia** occurs most frequently. Ectopic testis occurs when a part of the gubernaculum passes to an abnormal location and the testis follows it (Wensing, 1988).

Congenital Inguinal Hernia

If the communication between the tunica vaginalis and the peritoneal cavity fails to close (Fig. 13-48*A* and *B*), a **persistent processus vaginalis** exists. A loop of intestine may herniate through it into the scrotum or labium majus (Fig. 13-48*B*). Embryonic remnants resembling the ductus deferens or epididymis are often found in inguinal hernial sacs (Popek, 1990). Congenital inguinal hernia is much more common in males, especially when there are undescended testes. Congenital inguinal hernias are also common with ectopic testes and in females with the androgen insensitivity syndrome (Behrman et al., 1996).

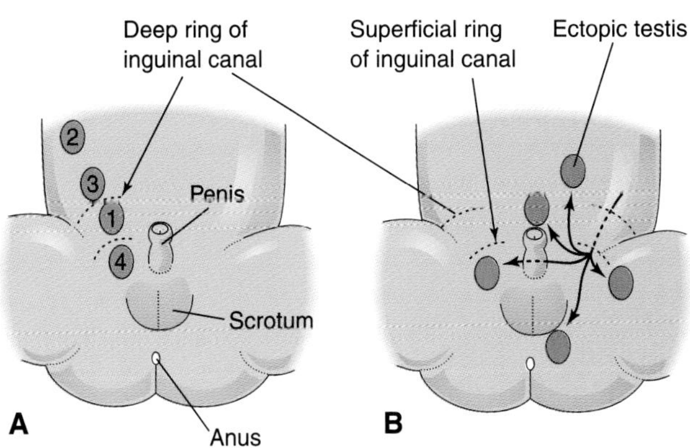

■ **Figure 13-47.** Diagrams showing the possible sites of cryptorchid and ectopic testes. *A*, Positions of cryptorchid testes, numbered in order of frequency. *B*, Usual locations of ectopic testes.

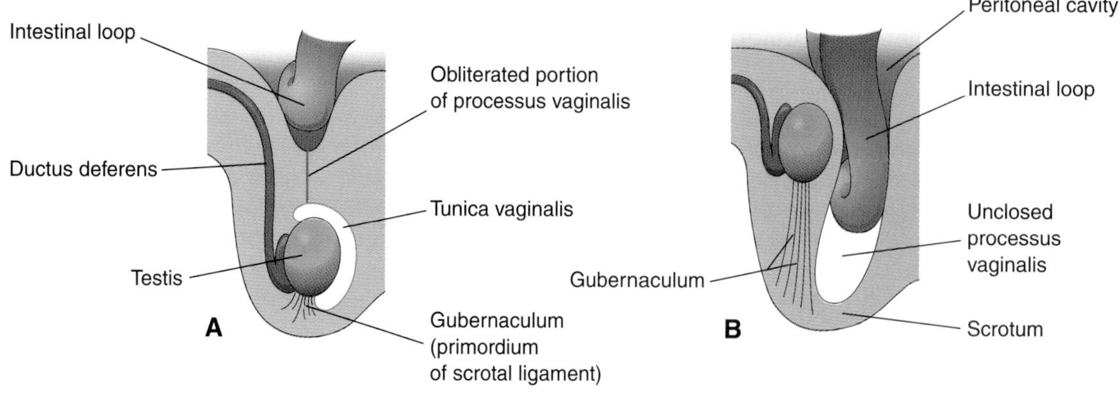

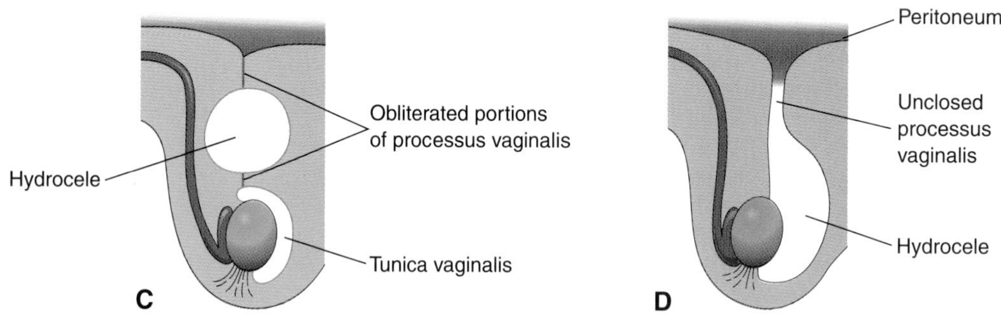

■ **Figure 13–48.** Diagrams of sagittal sections illustrating conditions resulting from failure of closure of the processus vaginalis. *A,* Incomplete congenital inguinal hernia resulting from persistence of the proximal part of the processus vaginalis. *B,* Complete congenital inguinal hernia into the scrotum resulting from persistence of the processus vaginalis. Cryptorchidism, a commonly associated anomaly, is also illustrated. *C,* Large cyst or hydrocele that arose from an unobliterated portion of the processus vaginalis. *D,* Hydrocele of the testis and spermatic cord resulting from peritoneal fluid passing into an unclosed processus vaginalis.

Hydrocele

Occasionally the abdominal end of the processus vaginalis remains open but is too small to permit herniation of intestine (Fig. 13-48*D*). Peritoneal fluid passes into the patent processus vaginalis and forms a **hydrocele of the testis.** If the middle part of the processus vaginalis canal remains open, fluid may accumulate and give rise to a **hydrocele of the spermatic cord** (Fig. 13-48*C*).

SUMMARY OF THE UROGENITAL SYSTEM

The urogenital system develops from the:

- intermediate mesoderm
- mesothelium lining the abdominal cavity
- endoderm of the urogenital sinus

The urinary system begins to develop about 3 weeks before the genital system is evident. Three successive kidney systems develop:

- the *pronephroi*, which are nonfunctional
- the *mesonephroi*, which serve as temporary excretory organs
- the *metanephroi*, which become the permanent kidneys

The **metanephroi** or **permanent kidneys** develop from two sources:

- the *metanephric diverticulum,* or ureteric bud, which gives rise to the ureter, renal pelvis, calices, and collecting tubules
- the *metanephric mass of mesoderm*, which gives rise to the nephrons

At first the kidneys are located in the pelvis but they gradually "ascend" to the abdomen. This apparent migration results from disproportionate growth of the fetal lumbar and sacral regions. Developmental abnormalities of the kidneys and ureters are common. Incomplete division of the metanephric diverticulum results in a double ureter and supernumerary kidney. Failure of the kidney to "ascend" from its embryonic position in the pelvis results in an ectopic kidney that is abnormally rotated.

The **urinary bladder** develops from the urogenital sinus and the surrounding splanchnic mesenchyme. The female urethra and almost all of the male urethra have a similar origin. **Exstrophy of the bladder** results from a rare ventral body wall defect through which the posterior wall of the urinary bladder protrudes onto the abdominal wall. In males, **epispadias** is a common associated anomaly.

The **genital** or **reproductive system** develops in close association with the urinary or excretory system. Genetic sex is established at fertilization, but the gonads do not begin to attain sexual characteristics until the seventh week. **Primordial germ cells** form in the wall of the yolk sac during the fourth week and migrate into the developing gonads, where they differentiate into germ cells (oogonia/spermatogonia). The external genitalia do not acquire distinct masculine or feminine characteristics until the twelfth week. The reproductive organs develop from primordia that are identical in both sexes. During this *indifferent stage* an embryo has the potential to develop into either a male or a female.

Gonadal sex is determined by the testis-determining factor (TDF) on the Y chromosome. TDF is located on the sex-determining region (SRY) of the short arm of the Y chromosome. TDF directs testicular differentiation. The Leydig cells produce testosterone, which stimulates development of the mesonephric ducts into male genital ducts. These androgens also stimulate development of the indifferent external genitalia into the penis and scrotum. A **müllerian inhibiting substance** (MIS), produced by the Sertoli cells of the testes, inhibits development of the paramesonephric ducts (primordia of female genital ducts).

In the absence of a Y chromosome and the presence of two X chromosomes, ovaries develop, the mesonephric ducts regress, the paramesonephric ducts develop into the uterus and uterine tubes, the vagina develops from the vaginal plate derived from the urogenital sinus, and the indifferent external genitalia develop into the clitoris and labia (majora and minora).

Persons with **true hermaphroditism**, an extremely rare intersexual condition, have both ovarian and testicular tissue and variable internal and external genitalia. Errors in sexual differentiation cause pseudohermaphroditism. **Male pseudohermaphroditism** results from failure of the fetal testes to produce adequate amounts of masculinizing hormones, or from the tissue insensitivity of the sexual structures. **Female pseudohermaphroditism** usually results from congenital adrenal hyperplasia (CAH), a disorder of the fetal suprarenal (adrenal) glands that causes excessive production of androgens and masculinization of the external genitalia.

Most anomalies of the female genital tract, such as **double uterus**, result from incomplete fusion of the paramesonephric ducts. **Cryptorchidism** and **ectopic testes** result from abnormalities of testicular descent. **Congenital inguinal hernia** and hydrocele result from persistence of the processus vaginalis. Failure of the urogenital folds to fuse in males results in various types of **hypospadias**.

Clinically Oriented Problems

Case 13–1

A 3-year-old girl was still in diapers because she was continually wet. The pediatrician saw urine coming from the infant's vagina. An *intravenous urogram* showed two renal pelves and two ureters on the right side. One ureter was clearly observed to enter the bladder, but the termination of the other one was not clearly seen. A pediatric urologist examined the child under general anesthesia and observed a small opening in the posterior wall of the vagina. He passed a tiny catheter into it, and injected a radiopaque solution. This procedure showed that the opening in the vagina was the orifice of the second ureter.

- What is the embryological basis for the two renal pelves and ureters?
- Describe the embryological basis of the ectopic ureteric orifice.
- What is the anatomical basis of the continual dribbling of urine into the vagina?

Case 13–2

A seriously injured young man suffered a cardiac arrest. After cardiopulmonary resuscitation (CPR), his heart began to beat again, but spontaneous respirations did not occur. Artificial respiration was instituted but there was no electroencephalographic (EEG) evidence of brain activity. After 2 days the man's family agreed that there was no hope of his recovery and they asked that his kidneys be donated for transplantation. The radiologist carried out femoral artery catheterization and aortography (radiographic visualization of the aorta and its branches). This technique showed a single large renal artery on the right, but two renal arteries on the left, one medium in size and the other small. Only the right kidney was used for transplantation because it is more difficult to implant small arteries than large ones. Grafting of the small accessory renal artery into the aorta would be difficult because of its size, and part of the kidney would die if one of the arteries was not successfully grafted.

- Are accessory renal arteries common?
- What is the embryological basis of the two left renal arteries?
- In what other circumstance might an accessory renal artery be of clinical significance?

Case 13–3

A 32-year-old woman with a short history of cramping lower abdominal pain and tenderness underwent a laparotomy because of a suspected ectopic pregnancy. The operation revealed a pregnancy in a *rudimentary right uterine horn*. The gravid uterine horn was totally removed.

- Is this type of uterine anomaly common?
- What is the embryological basis of the rudimentary uterine horn?

Case 13–4

During the physical examination of a newborn male infant, it was observed that the urethra opened on the ventral surface of the penis at the junction of its glans and body (shaft). The glans was curved toward the undersurface of the penis.

- Give the medical terms for the anomalies described.
- What is the embryological basis of the abnormal urethral orifice?
- Is this anomaly common? Discuss its etiology.

Case 13–5

A 20-year-old woman was prevented from competing in the Olympics because her buccal smear test was chromatin negative, indicating that she had a male sex chromosome complement.

- Is she a male or a female?
- What is the probable basis for her failing to pass the sex chromatin test?
- Is there an anatomical basis for not allowing her to compete in the Olympics?

Case 13–6

A 10-year-old boy suffered pain in his left groin while attempting to lift a heavy box. Later he noticed a lump in his groin. When he told his mother about the lump, she arranged an appointment with the family physician. After a physical examination, a diagnosis of indirect inguinal hernia was made.

- Explain the embryological basis of this type of inguinal hernia.
- On the basis of your embryological knowledge, list the layers of the spermatic cord that would cover the hernial sac.

Discussion of problems appears at the back of the book.

REFERENCES AND SUGGESTED READING

Arant BS Jr: Postnatal development of renal function during the first year of life. *Pediatr Nephrol 1:*308, 1987.

Badawy SA, Kasello DJ, Powers C, et al: Supernumerary ovary with an endometrioma and osseous metaplasia: a case report. *Am J Obstet Gynecol 173:*1623, 1995.

Bard J: A new role for the stromal cells in kidney development. *BioEssays 18:*705, 1996.

Barr ML: Correlations between sex chromatin patterns and sex chromosome complexes in man. *In* Moore KL (ed): *The Sex Chromatin*. Philadelphia, WB Saunders, 1966.

Behrman RE, Kliegman RM, Arvin AM (eds): *Nelson Textbook of Pediatrics,* 15th ed. Philadelphia, WB Saunders, 1996.

Belman AB: Hypospadias update. *Urology 49:*166, 1997.

Berta P, Hawkins JR, Sinclair AH, et al: Genetic evidence equating SRY and the testis-determining factor. *Nature 348:*448, 1990.

Bruch SW, Adzick NS, Goldstein RB, Harrison MR: Challenging the embryogenesis of cloacal exstrophy. *J Pediatr Surg 31:*768, 1996.

Brun JL, Lemoine P: Les malformations utérines. Diagnostic, pronostic et traitement. *Presse Med 24:*1658, 1995.

Carr DH, Haggar RA, Hart AG: Germ cells in the ovaries of XO female infants. *Am J Clin Pathol 49:*521, 1968.

Crelin ES: Normal and abnormal development of ureter. *Urology 12:* 2, 1978.

Cunha GR: The dual origin of vaginal epithelium. *Am J Anat 143:* 387, 1975.

Daneman A, Alton DJ. Radiographic manifestations of renal anomalies. *Radiol Clin North Am 29:*351, 1991.

Davies JA: Mesenchyme to epithelium transition during development of the mammalian kidney tubule. *In* Newgreen D (ed): *Epithelial-Mesenchymal Transitions,* Part 2. Basel, Karger, 1997.

DeKretser DM, Burger HG: The Y chromosome and spermatogenesis. *N Engl J Med 336:*576, 1997.

DiGeorge AM: Hermaphroditism. *In* Behrman RE, Kliegman RM, Arvin AM (eds): *Nelson Textbook of Pediatrics,* 15th ed. Philadelphia, WB Saunders, 1996.

Dische F: *Renal Pathology,* 2nd ed. Oxford, Oxford University Press, 1995.

Eppig JJ: The ovary: oogenesis. *In* Hillier SG, Kitchener HC, Neilson JP (eds): *Scientific Essentials of Reproductive Medicine*. Philadelphia, WB Saunders, 1996.

Fine RN: Diagnosis and treatment of fetal urinary tract abnormalities. *J Pediatr 121:*333, 1992.

Fleming S: N-linked oligosaccharides during human renal organogenesis. *J Anat 170:*151, 1990.

Fouda-Neel K, Ahmed S, Borghol M: Complete bladder duplication with exstrophy of 1 moiety in a male infant. *J Urol 156:*1468, 1996.

Fukuda T: Ultrastructure of primordial germ cells in human embryos. *Virchows Arch B Cell Pathol 20:*85, 1975.

Gardner LI: Development of the normal fetal and neonatal adrenal. *In* Gardner LI (ed): *Endocrine and Genetic Diseases of Childhood and Adolescence,* 2nd ed. Philadelphia, WB Saunders, 1975.

Gasser B, Mauss Y, Ghnassia JP, et al: A quantitative study of normal nephrogenesis in the human fetus: its implication in the natural history of kidney changes due to low obstructive uropathies. *Fetal Diagn Ther 8:*371, 1993.

Goldberg JM, Friedman CI. Noncanalization of the fallopian tube. *J Reprod Med 40:*317, 1995.

Gray SW, Skandalakis JE: *Embryology for Surgeons,* 2nd ed. Baltimore, Williams & Wilkins, 1993.

Grobstein C: Some transmission characteristics of the tubule inducing influence on mouse metanephrogenic mesenchyme. *Exp Cell Res 13:*575, 1957.

Grootegoed JA: The testis: spermatogenesis. *In* Hillier SG, Kitchener HC, Neilson JP (eds): *Scientific Essentials of Reproductive Medicine*. Philadelphia, WB Saunders, 1996.

Hammerman MR, Rodgers SA, Ryan G: Growth factors and metanephrogenesis. *Am J Physiol 262(4 Pt 2):*F523, 1992.

Hawkins EP, Perlman EJ (eds): Germ cell tumors. *In* Parham DM (ed): *Pediatric Neoplasia: Morphology and Biology*. Philadelphia, Lippincott-Raven Publishers, 1996.

Hay ED: Epithelial-mesenchymal transitions. *Seminars in Devel Biol 1:*347, 1990.

Herzlinger D, Oiao J, Cohen D, et al: Wnt-1 and Wnt-2 are potent inducers of nephrogenesis. *FASEB J 8:*A822, 1994.

Houston IB, Oetliker O: The growth and development of the kidneys. *In* Davis JA, Dobbing J (eds): *Scientific Foundations of Paediatrics*. Philadelphia, WB Saunders, 1974.

Jones HH, Scott WW: *Hermaphroditism, Genital Anomalies and Related Endocrine Disorders*. Baltimore, Williams & Wilkins, 1958.

Jost A: Development of sexual characteristics. *Sci J 6:*67, 1970.

Kim HH, Laufer MR: Developmental abnormalities of the female reproductive tract. *Curr Opin Obstet Gynecol 6:*518, 1994.

Lennox B: The sex chromatin in hermaphroditism. *In* Moore KL (ed): *The Sex Chromatin*. Philadelphia, WB Saunders, 1966.

Mack WS: Testicular maldescent. *In* Rashad MN, Morton WRM (eds): *Selected Topics on Genital Anomalies and Related Subjects*. Springfield, Charles C Thomas, 1969.

Mahony BS: Ultrasound evaluation of the genitourinary system. *In* Callen PW (ed): *Ultrasonography in Obstetrics and Gynecology,* 3rd ed. Philadelphia, WB Saunders, 1994.

McDonough PG: Gonadal dysgenesis. *In* Quilligan EJ, Zuspan FP (eds): *Current Therapy in Obstetrics and Gynecology,* Vol 3. Philadelphia, WB Saunders, 1990.

McElreavey K, Vilain E, Cotinot C, et al: Control of sex determination in animals. *Eur J Biochem 218:*769, 1993.

Meacham LR, Winn KJ, Culler FL, Parks JS: Double vagina, cardiac, pulmonary, and other genital malformations with 46,XY karyotype. *Am J Med Genet 41:*478, 1991.

Mesrobian HG, Rushton HG, Bulas D: Unilateral renal agenesis may result from in utero regression of multicystic renal dysplasia. *J Urol 150:*793, 1993.

Minh HN, Hervé de Sigalony JP, Smadja A, Orcel L: Nouvelles acquisitions sur l'embryogénèe du vagin. *J Gynecol Obstet Biol Reprod 18:*589, 1989.

Mittwoch U: Sex determination and sex reversal: genotype, phenotype, dogma and semantics. *Hum Genet 89:*467, 1992.

Möbus VJ, Kortenhorn K, Kreienberg R, Friedberg V: Long-term results after operative correction of vaginal aplasia. *Am J Obstet Gynecol 175:*617, 1996.

Moffatt DB: Developmental abnormalities of the urogenital system. *In* Chisholm GD, Williams DI (eds): *Scientific Foundations of Urology,* 2nd ed. London, Heinemann Medical, 1982.

Moore KL: *Clinically Oriented Anatomy,* 3rd ed. Baltimore, Williams & Wilkins, 1992.

Moore KL: The development of clinical sex chromatin tests. *In* Moore KL (ed): *The Sex Chromatin*. Philadelphia, WB Saunders, 1966.

Morton WRM: Development of the urogenital systems. *In* Rashad MN, Morton WRM (eds): *Selected Topics on Genital Anomalies and Related Subjects*. Springfield, Charles C Thomas, 1969.

Muram D: Developmental anomalies. *In* Copeland LJ, Jarrell J, McGregor J (eds): *Textbook of Gynecology*. Philadelphia, WB Saunders, 1993.

Nader S: Polycystic ovary syndrome and the androgen-insulin connection. *Obstet Gynecol 165:*346, 1991.

New MI, White PC, Pang S, et al: The adrenal hyperplasias. *In* Scriver CR, Beaudet AL, Sly WS, Valle D (eds): *The Metabolic Basis of Inherited Diseases,* 6th ed. New York, McGraw-Hill, 1989.

Nishi T: Prenatal diagnosis of urinary tract abnormalities. *Acta Obstet Gynecol Scand 76:*409, 1997.

O'Rahilly R: The development of the vagina in the human. *In* Blandau RJ, Bergsma D (eds): *Morphogenesis and Malformations of the Genital Systems*. Original Article Series. New York, Alan R Liss, 1977.

Palmer JM: The undescended testicle. *Endocrinol Metab Clin North Am 20:*231, 1991.

Peña A: Total urogenital mobilization—An easier way to repair cloacas. *J Pediatr Surg 32:*263, 1997.

Peipert JF, Donnenfeld AE: Oligohydramnios: a review. *Obstet Gynecol Surv 46:*325, 1991.

Pepe GJ, Albrecht ED: Regulation of the primate fetal adrenal cortex. *Endocr Rev 11:*151, 1990.

Persaud TVN: Embryology of the female genital tract and gonads. *In* Copeland LJ, Jarrell J, McGregor J (eds): *Textbook of Gynecology*. Philadelphia, WB Saunders, 1993.

Polani P: Hormonal and clinical aspects of hermaphroditism and the testicular feminizing syndrome in man. *Philos Trans R Soc Lond [Biol Sci] 259:*187, 1970.

Popek EJ: Embryonal remnants in inguinal sac hernias. *Human Pathol 21:*339, 1990.

Powell DM, Newman KD, Randolph J: A proposed classification of vaginal anomalies and their surgical correction. *J Pediatr Surg 30:* 271, 1995.

Pryor JL, Kent-First M, Muallem A, et al: Microdeletions in the Y chromosome of infertile men. *New Engl J Med 336:*534, 1997.

Reid RL: Amenorrhea. *In* Copeland LJ, Jarrell J, McGregor J (eds): *Textbook of Gynecology*. Philadelphia, WB Saunders, 1993.

Rutgers JL: Advances in the pathology of intersex conditions. *Human Pathol 22:*884, 1991.

Sariola H, Saarma M, Sainio K, et al: Dependence of kidney morphogenesis on the expression of nerve growth factor receptor. *Science 254:*571, 1991.

Schlegel RJ, Gardner LI: Ambiguous and abnormal genitalia in infants: differential diagnosis and clinical management. *In* Gardner LI (ed): *Endocrine and Genetic Diseases of Childhood and Adolescence,* 2nd ed. Philadelphia, WB Saunders, 1975.

Sivan E, Koch S, Recce EA: Sonographic prenatal diagnosis of ambiguous genitalia. *Fetal Diagn Ther 10:*311, 1995.

Soules MR, Pagon RA, Burns MW, Matsumoto AM: Normal and abnormal sexual development. *In* Carr BR, Blackwell RE (eds): *Textbook of Reproductive Medicine*. Norwalk, Appleton & Lange, 1993.

Speiser PW, New MI: Prenatal diagnosis and management of congenital adrenal hyperplasia. *Clin Perinatol 21:*631, 1994.

Stempfel RS Jr: Abnormalities of sexual differentiation. *In* Gardner LI (ed): *Endocrine and Genetic Diseases of Childhood and Adolescence,* 2nd ed. Philadelphia, WB Saunders, 1975.

Thompson MW, McInnes RR, Willard HF: *Thompson & Thompson Genetics in Medicine,* 5th ed. Philadelphia, WB Saunders, 1991.

Vaughan ED Jr, Middleton GW: Pertinent genitourinary embryology. Review for the practicing urologist. *Urology 6:*139, 1975.

Verga G, Avolio L: Agenesis of the scrotum: an extremely rare anomaly. *J Urol 156:*1467, 1996.

Welling LW, Grantham JJ: Cystic and developmental diseases of the kidney. *In* Brenner BM, Rector FC Jr (eds): *The Kidney,* 5th ed. Philadelphia, WB Saunders, 1997.

Wensing CJG: The embryology of testicular descent. *Hormone Res 30:*144, 1988.

Wernert N, Kern L, Heitz P, et al: Morphological and immunohistochemical investigations of the utriculus prostaticus from the fetal period up to adulthood. *Prostate 17:*19, 1990.

Witschi E: Migration of the germ cells of human embryos from the yolk sac to the primitive gonadal folds. *Contr Embryol Carneg Instn 32:*67, 1948.

Woolf AS (ed): Nephrogenesis. *Exp Nephrology 4:*1, 1996.

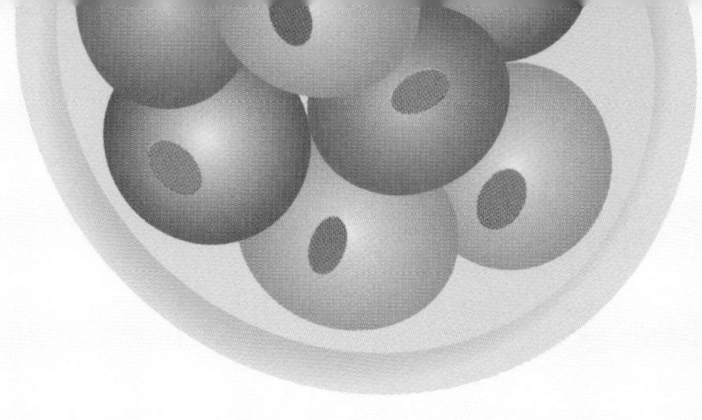

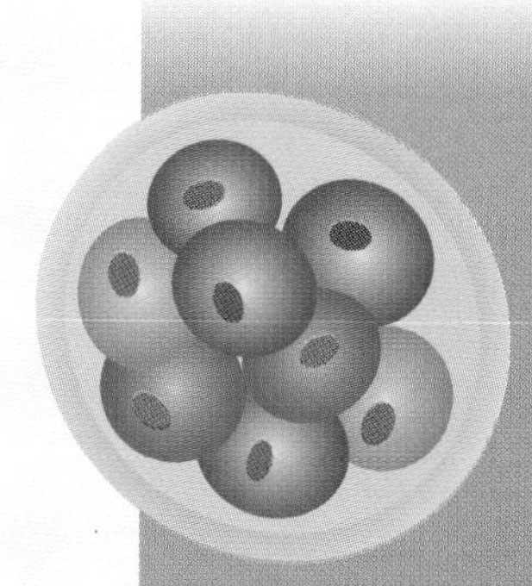

The Cardiovascular System

14

■ *The cardiovascular system is the first major system to function in the embryo.* The primordial heart and vascular system appear in the middle of the third week of embryonic development. *The heart starts to function at the beginning of the fourth week.* This precocious cardiac development is necessary because the rapidly growing embryo can no longer satisfy its nutritional and oxygen requirements by diffusion alone. Consequently, there is a need for an efficient method of acquiring oxygen and nutrients from the maternal blood and disposing of carbon dioxide and waste products. The cardiovascular system is derived mainly from:

- *splanchnic mesoderm,* which forms the primordium of the heart (Fig. 14-1*A* and *B*)
- *paraxial and lateral mesoderm* near the otic placodes (thickened ectodermal areas located midway along the hindbrain), from which the internal (inner) ears develop
- neural crest cells originating from the region between the otic vesicles (primordia of membranous labyrinths of internal ears) and the caudal limits of the third pair of somites

Blood vessel development—**angiogenesis** (Hanahan, 1997)—is described in Chapter 4. Primordial blood vessels cannot be distinguished structurally as arteries or veins, but are named according to their future fates and relationship to the heart.

EARLY DEVELOPMENT OF THE HEART AND VESSELS

The earliest sign of the heart is the appearance of paired endothelial strands—**angioblastic cords**—during the third week (Fig. 14-1*B* and *C*). These cords canalize to form **endocardial heart tubes**, which fuse to form the tubular heart late in the third week (see Fig. 14-7). The heart begins to beat at 22 to 23 days (Fig. 14-2). An inductive influence from the embryonic endoderm appears to stimulate early formation of the heart (Carlson, 1994). Blood flow begins during the fourth week and can be visualized by Doppler ultrasonography (Fig. 14-3). For recent molecular, genetic, and biochemical studies of early cardiac development, see Harvey (1996), Olson and Srivastava (1996), and Lin et al. (1997).

Development of Veins Associated With the Heart

Three paired veins drain into the tubular heart of a 4-week-old embryo (Fig. 14-2):

- *Vitelline veins* return poorly oxygenated blood from the yolk sac.
- *Umbilical veins* carry well-oxygenated blood from the chorionic villi of the embryonic placenta; only the left umbilical vein persists.
- *Common cardinal veins* return poorly oxygenated blood from the body of the embryo.

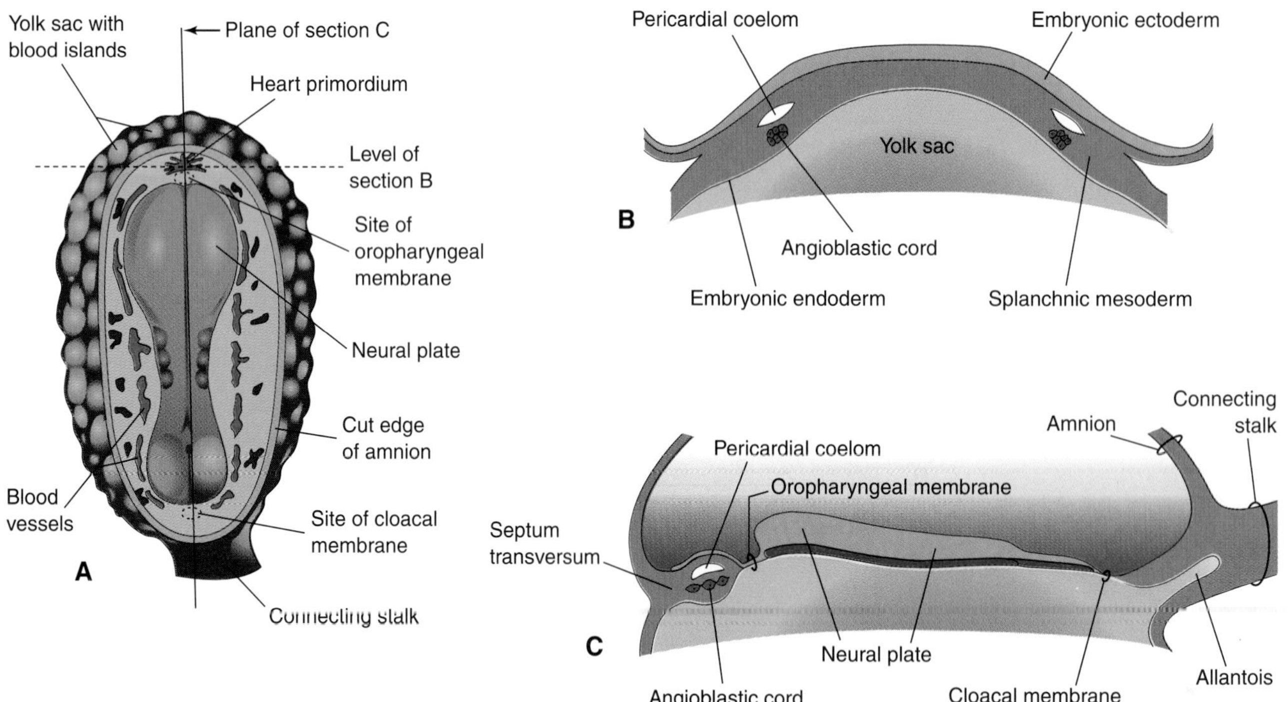

■ **Figure 14-1.** *A,* Drawing of a dorsal view of an embryo (about 18 days). *B,* Transverse section of the embryo demonstrating the angioblastic cords and their relationship to the pericardial coelom. *C,* Longitudinal section through the embryo illustrating the relationship of the angioblastic cords to the oropharyngeal membrane, pericardial coelom, and septum transversum.

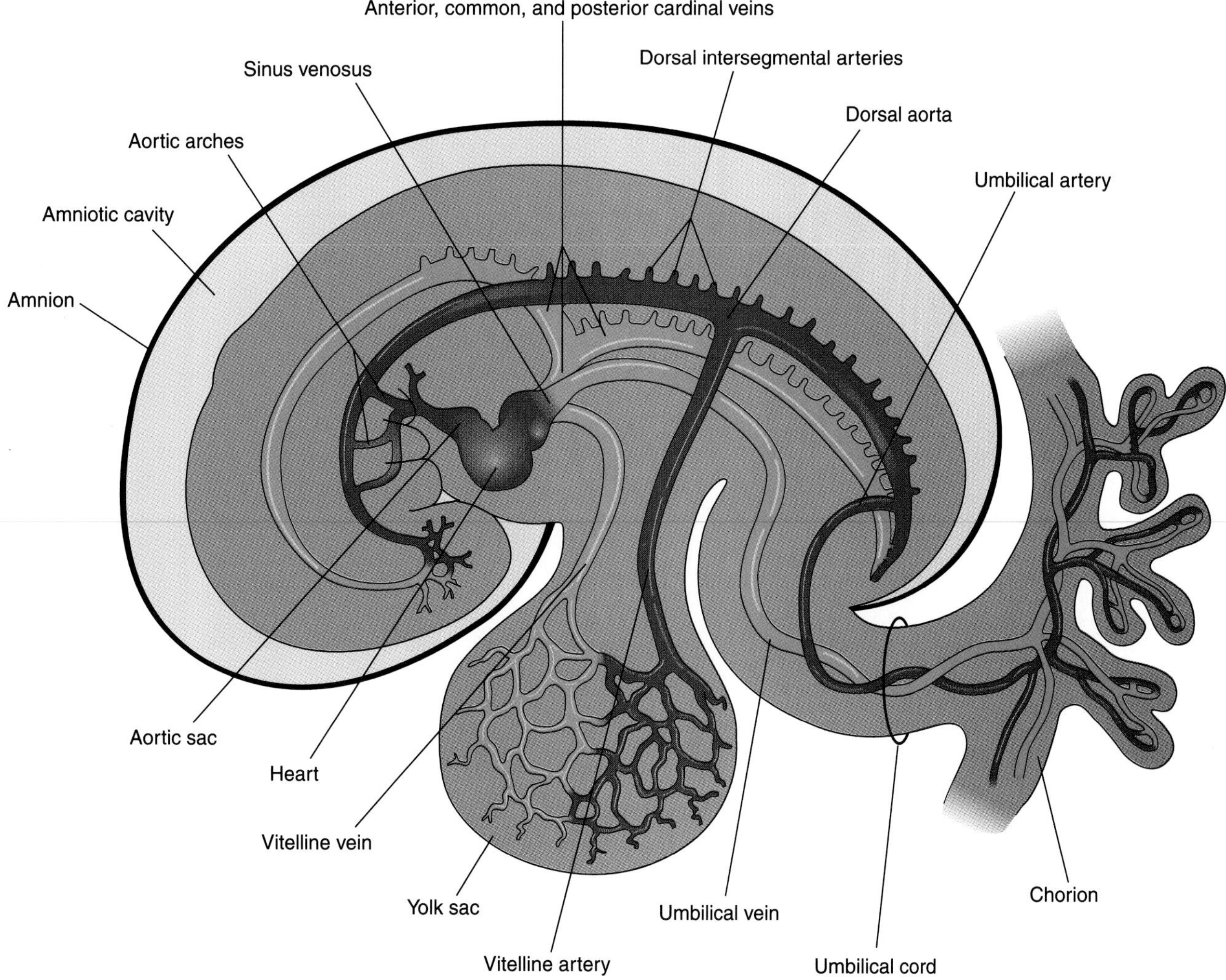

■ **Figure 14–2.** Sketch of the embryonic cardiovascular system (about 26 days) showing vessels on the left side only. The umbilical vein carries well-oxygenated blood and nutrients from the chorion (embryonic part of placenta) to the embryo. The umbilical arteries carry poorly oxygenated blood and waste products to the chorion.

The **vitelline veins** follow the yolk stalk into the embryo. The *yolk stalk* is the narrow tube connecting the yolk sac with the midgut (see Fig. 12-1). After passing through the septum transversum, the vitelline veins enter the venous end of the heart—the **sinus venosus** (Figs. 14-2 and 14-4*A*). As the liver primordium grows into the septum transversum (see Chapter 12), the *hepatic cords* anastomose around preexisting endothelium-lined spaces. These spaces, the primordia of the **hepatic sinusoids** of the liver, later become linked to the vitelline veins. The **hepatic veins** form from the remains of the right vitelline vein in the region of the developing liver. The **portal vein** develops from an anastomotic network formed by the vitelline veins around the duodenum (Fig. 14-5*B*).

The **umbilical veins** run on each side of the liver and carry well-oxygenated blood from the placenta to the sinus venosus. As the liver develops, the umbilical veins lose their connection with the heart and empty into the liver. The right umbilical vein disappears at the end of the embryonic period, leaving the left umbilical vein as the only vessel carrying well-oxygenated blood from the placenta to the embryo. Transformation of the umbilical veins may be summarized as follows (Fig. 14-5):

- The right umbilical vein and the caudal part of the left umbilical vein between the liver and the sinus venosus degenerate.
- The persistent caudal part of the left umbilical vein becomes the **umbilical vein,** which carries all the blood from the placenta to the embryo.
- A large venous shunt—the **ductus venosus**—develops within the liver (Fig. 14-5*B*) and connects the umbilical vein with the inferior vena cava (IVC). The ductus venosus forms a bypass through the liver, enabling most of the blood from the placenta to pass directly to the heart without passing through the capillary networks of the liver.

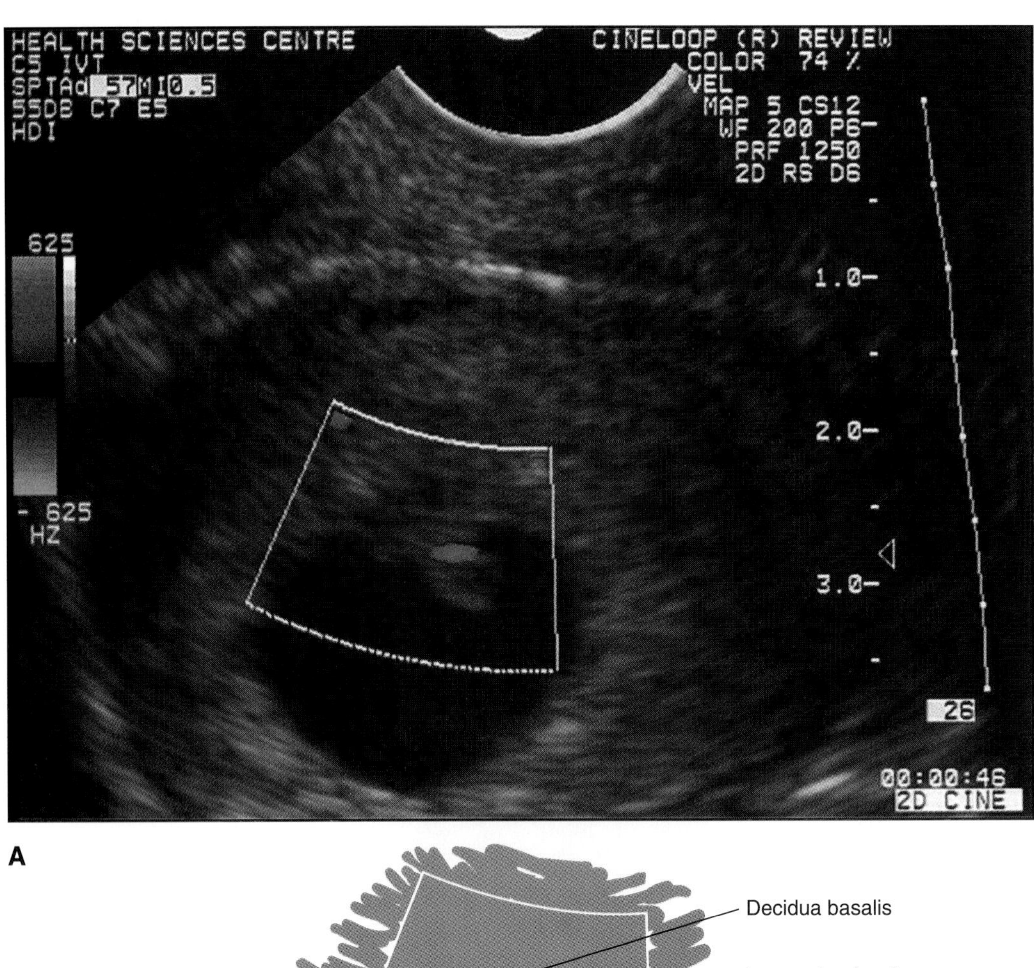

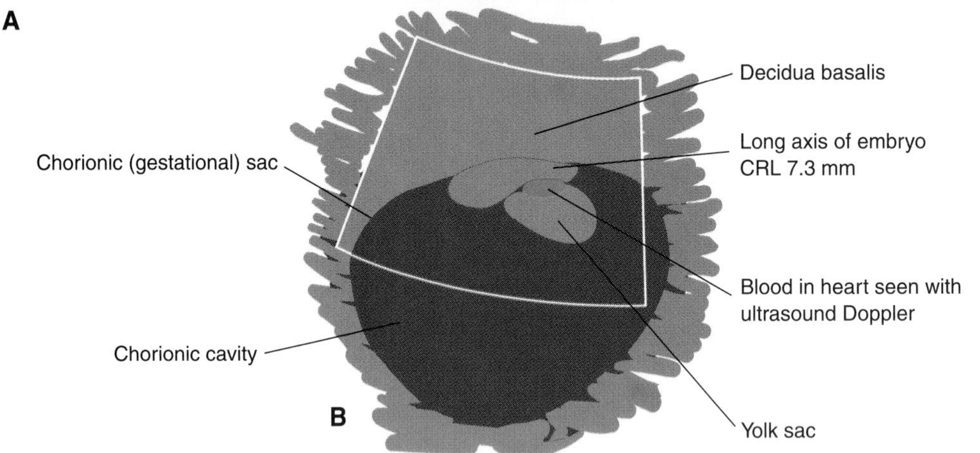

■ **Figure 14–3.** *A,* Sonogram of a 5-week embryo (crown rump length: 7.3 mm) and its yolk sac within its chorionic (gestational) sac. The red pulsating heart of the embryo was visualized using Doppler ultrasound. *B,* Sketch of the sonogram for orientation and identification of structures. (Courtesy of E. A. Lyons, MD, Professor of Radiology and Obstetrics and Gynecology, University of Manitoba, Winnipeg, Manitoba, Canada.)

The **cardinal veins** (Figs. 14-2 and 14-4*A*) constitute the main venous drainage system of the embryo. The anterior and posterior cardinal veins drain cranial and caudal parts of the embryo, respectively. The anterior and posterior cardinal veins join the **common cardinal veins**, which enter the *sinus venosus* (Fig. 14-2). During the eighth week of embryonic development, the **anterior cardinal veins** become connected by an oblique anastomosis (Fig. 14-5*A* and *B*), which shunts blood from the left to the right anterior cardinal vein. This anastomotic shunt becomes the **left brachiocephalic vein** when the caudal part of the left anterior cardinal vein degenerates (Figs. 14-4*D* and 14-5*C*). The **superior vena cava** (SVC) forms from the right anterior cardinal vein and the right common cardinal vein.

The **posterior cardinal veins** develop primarily as the vessels of the mesonephroi and largely disappear with these transitory kidneys (see Chapter 13). The only adult derivatives of the posterior cardinal veins

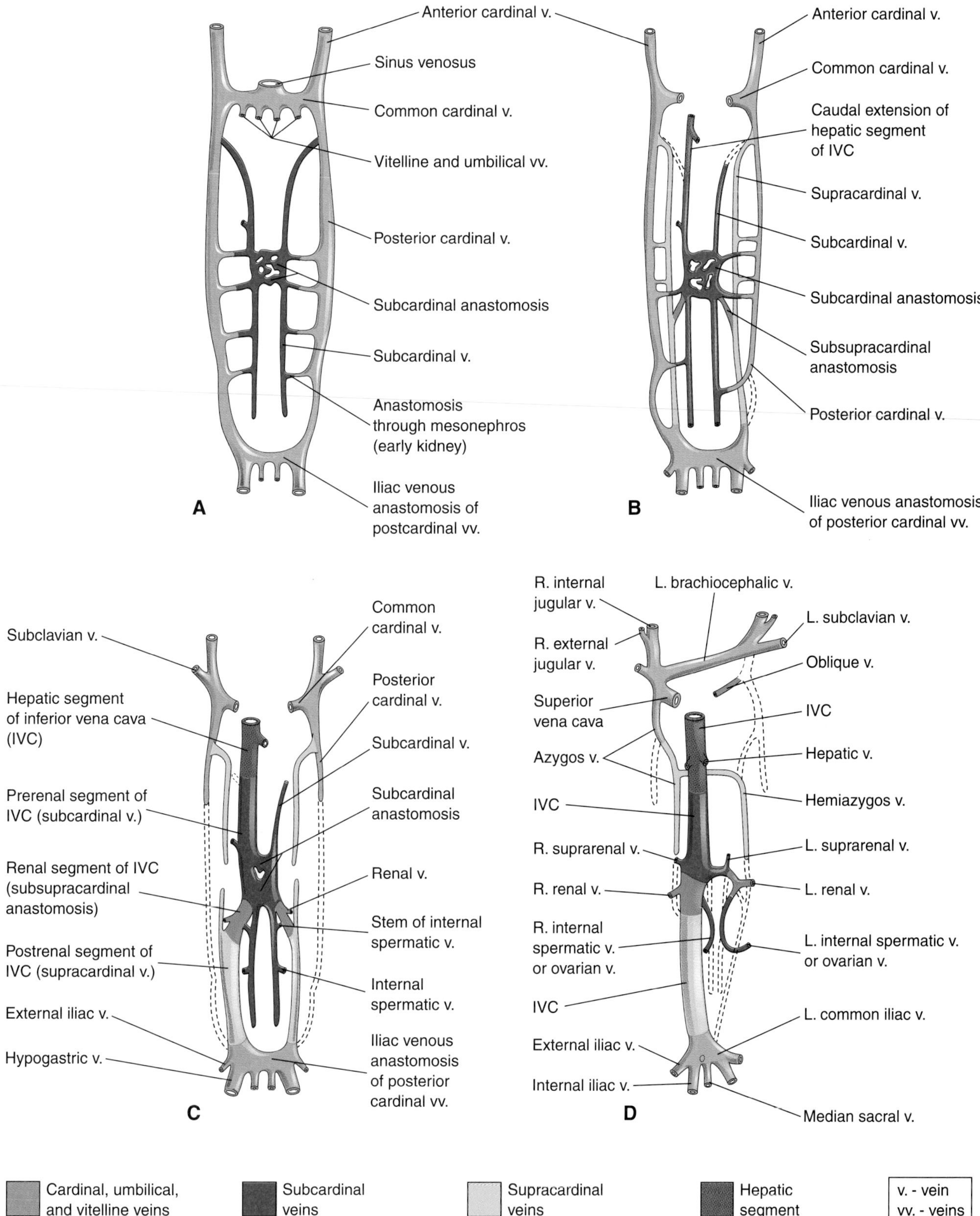

■ **Figure 14–4.** Drawings illustrating the primordial veins of the trunk in the human embryo (ventral views). Initially, three systems of veins are present: the umbilical veins from the chorion, the vitelline veins from the yolk sac, and the cardinal veins from the body of the embryo. Next the subcardinal veins appear, and finally the supracardinal veins develop. *A,* 6 weeks. *B,* 7 weeks. *C,* 8 weeks. *D,* Adult. This drawing illustrates the transformations that produce the adult venous pattern. (Modified from Arey LB: *Developmental Anatomy,* revised 7th ed. Philadelphia, WB Saunders, 1974.)

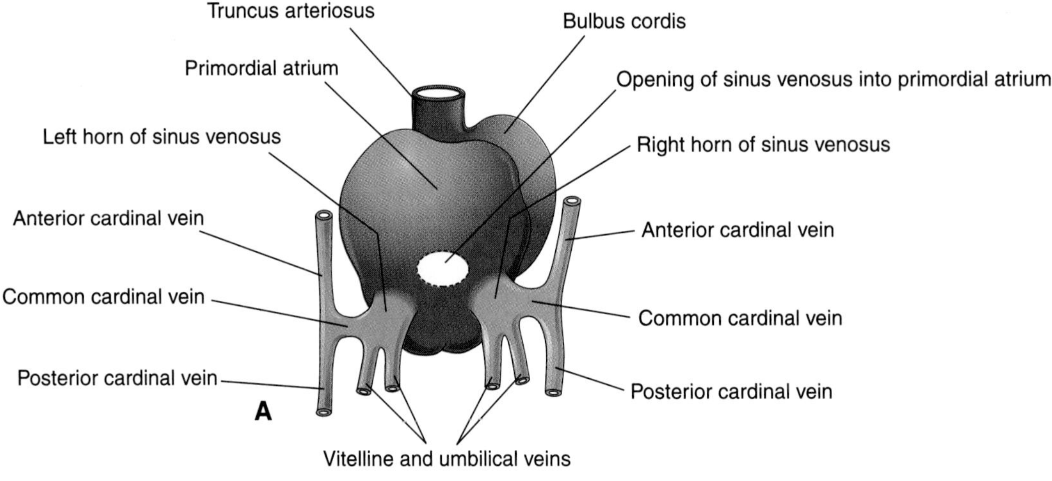

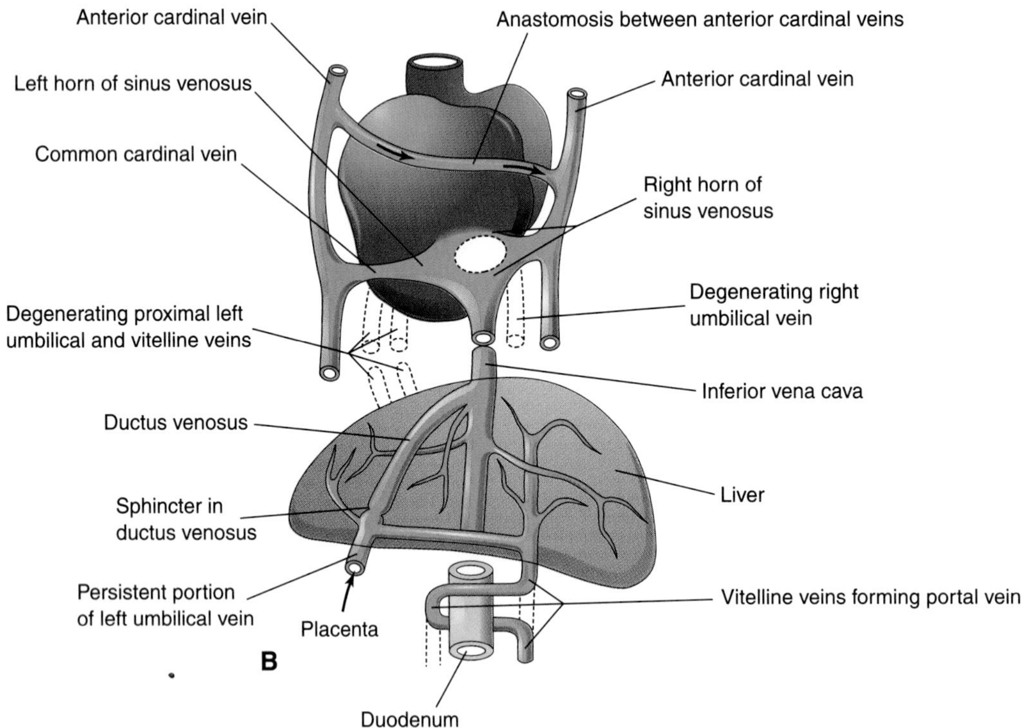

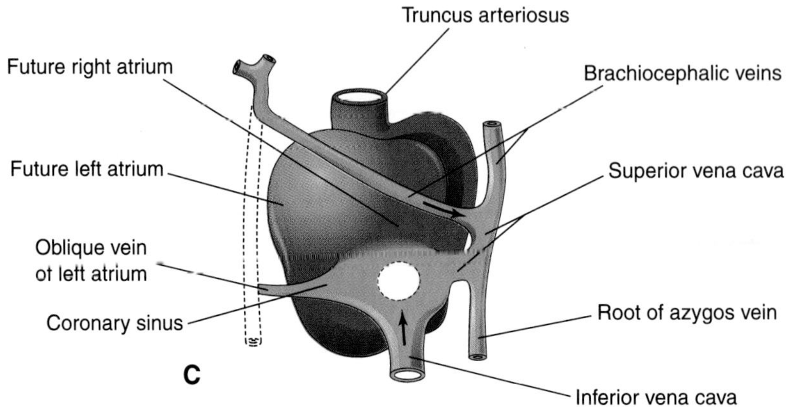

■ **Figure 14–5.** Dorsal views of the developing heart. *A,* During the fourth week (about 24 days), showing the primordial atrium and sinus venosus and veins draining into them. *B,* 7 weeks, showing the enlarged right horn of the sinus venosus and venous circulation through the liver. The organs are not drawn to scale. *C,* 8 weeks, indicating the adult derivatives of the cardinal veins.

are the *root of the azygos vein* and the *common iliac veins* (Fig. 14-4*D*). The subcardinal and supracardinal veins gradually replace and supplement the posterior cardinal veins. The **subcardinal veins** appear first (Fig. 14-4*A*). They are connected with each other through the subcardinal anastomosis and with the posterior cardinal veins through the mesonephric sinusoids. The subcardinal veins form the stem of the left renal vein, the suprarenal (adrenal) veins, the gonadal veins (testicular and ovarian), and a segment of the IVC (Fig. 14-4*D*). The **supracardinal veins** are the last pair of vessels to develop. They become disrupted in the region of the kidneys (Fig. 14-4*C*). Cranial to this they become united by an anastomosis that is represented in the adult by the **azygos** and **hemiazygos veins** (Figs. 14-4*D* and 14-5*C*). Caudal to the kidneys, the left supracardinal vein degenerates, but the right supracardinal vein becomes the inferior part of the IVC (Fig. 14-4*D*).

DEVELOPMENT OF THE INFERIOR VENA CAVA (IVC)

The IVC forms during a series of changes in the primordial veins of the trunk that occur as blood, returning from the caudal part of the embryo, is shifted from the left to the right side of the body. The IVC is composed of four main segments (Fig. 14-4*C*):

- a *hepatic segment* derived from the hepatic vein (proximal part of right vitelline vein) and hepatic sinusoids
- a *prerenal segment* derived from the right subcardinal vein
- a *renal segment* derived from the subcardinal-supracardinal anastomosis
- a *postrenal segment* derived from the right supracardinal vein

Anomalies of the Venae Cavae

Because of the many transformations that occur during the formation of the SVC and IVC, variations in their adult form occur, but they are not common. The most common anomaly is a persistent left SVC, which drains into the right atrium through the enlarged orifice of the *coronary sinus* (Fig. 14-6), a short trunk receiving most of the cardiac veins. The most common anomaly of the IVC is for its abdominal course to be interrupted; as a result, blood drains from the lower limbs, abdomen, and pelvis to the heart through the azygos system of veins.

Double Superior Venae Cavae

Persistence of the left anterior cardinal vein results in a left SVC; hence there are two superior venae cavae (Fig. 14-6). The anastomosis that usually forms the left brachiocephalic vein is small or absent. The abnormal left SVC, derived from the left anterior cardinal and common cardinal veins, opens into the right atrium through the coronary sinus.

Left Superior Vena Cava

The left anterior cardinal vein and common cardinal vein may form a left SVC, and the right anterior cardinal vein and common cardinal vein, which usually form the SVC, degenerate. As a result, blood from the right side is carried by the brachiocephalic vein to the unusual left SVC, which empties into the coronary sinus.

Absence of Hepatic Segment of IVC

Occasionally the hepatic segment of the IVC fails to form. As a result, blood from inferior parts of the body drains into the right atrium through the azygos and hemiazygos veins. The hepatic veins open separately into the right atrium.

Double Inferior Venae Cavae

In unusual cases, the IVC inferior to the renal veins is represented by two vessels. Usually the left one is much smaller (Moore, 1992). This condition probably results from failure of an anastomosis to develop between the primitive veins of the trunk (Fig. 14-4*B*). As a result, the inferior part of the left supracardinal vein persists as a second IVC.

Aortic Arches and Other Branches of the Dorsal Aorta

As the *pharyngeal arches* form during the fourth and fifth weeks, they are supplied by arteries—the **aortic**

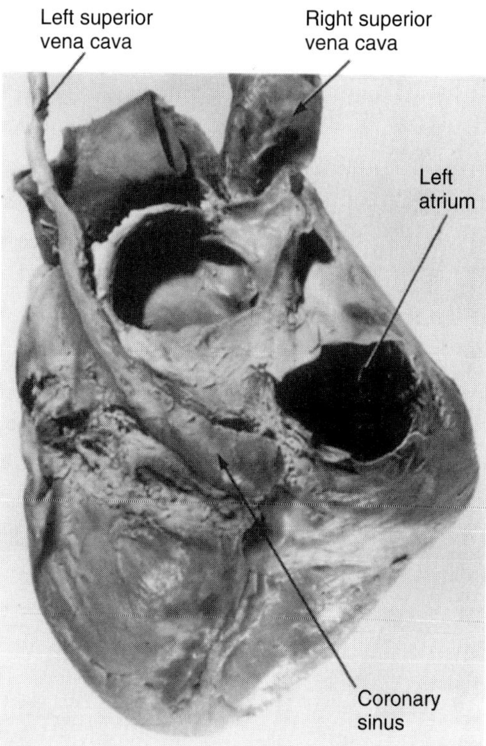

■ **Figure 14-6.** Photograph of the posterior aspect of an adult heart with double superior venae cavae. Parts of the walls of the atria have been removed. The small anomalous left superior vena cava opens into the coronary sinus.

arches—that arise from the **aortic sac** and terminate in the dorsal aortae (Fig. 14-2). Initially, the paired dorsal aortae run through the entire length of the embryo, but they soon fuse to form a single **dorsal aorta**, just caudal to the pharyngeal arches.

INTERSEGMENTAL ARTERIES

Thirty or so branches of the dorsal aorta, the *intersegmental arteries*, pass between and carry blood to the somites and their derivatives (Fig. 14-2). The dorsal intersegmental arteries in the neck join to form a longitudinal artery on each side, the **vertebral artery**. Most of the original connections of the intersegmental arteries to the dorsal aorta disappear. In the thorax, the dorsal intersegmental arteries persist as **intercostal arteries**. Most of the dorsal intersegmental arteries in the abdomen become **lumbar arteries**, but the fifth pair of lumbar intersegmental arteries remains as the **common iliac arteries** (Fig. 14-4*D*). In the sacral region, the intersegmental arteries form the **lateral sacral arteries**. The caudal end of the dor-

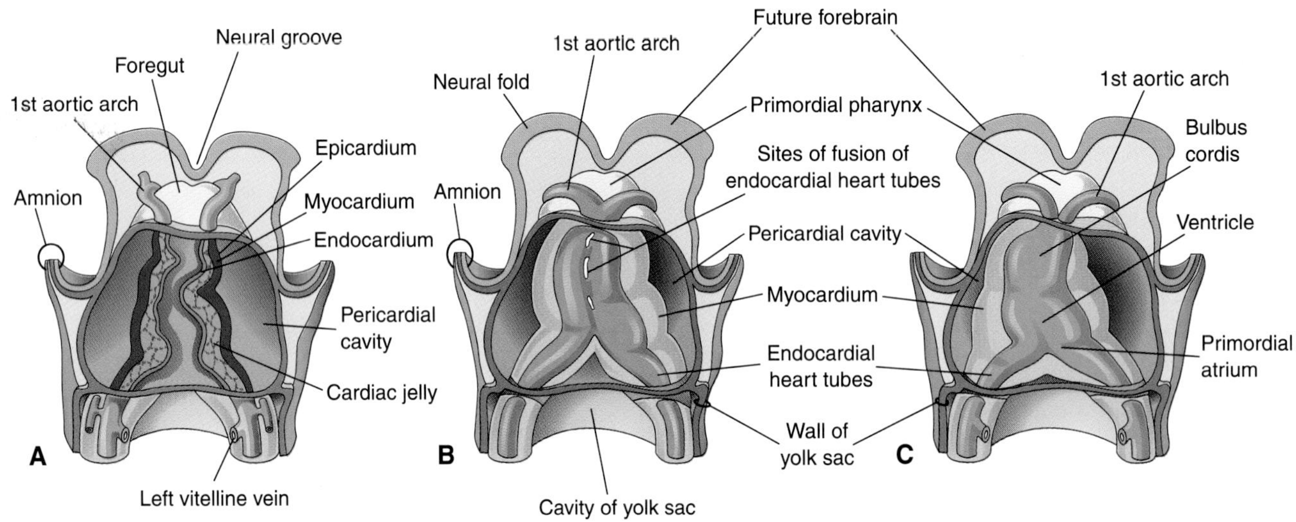

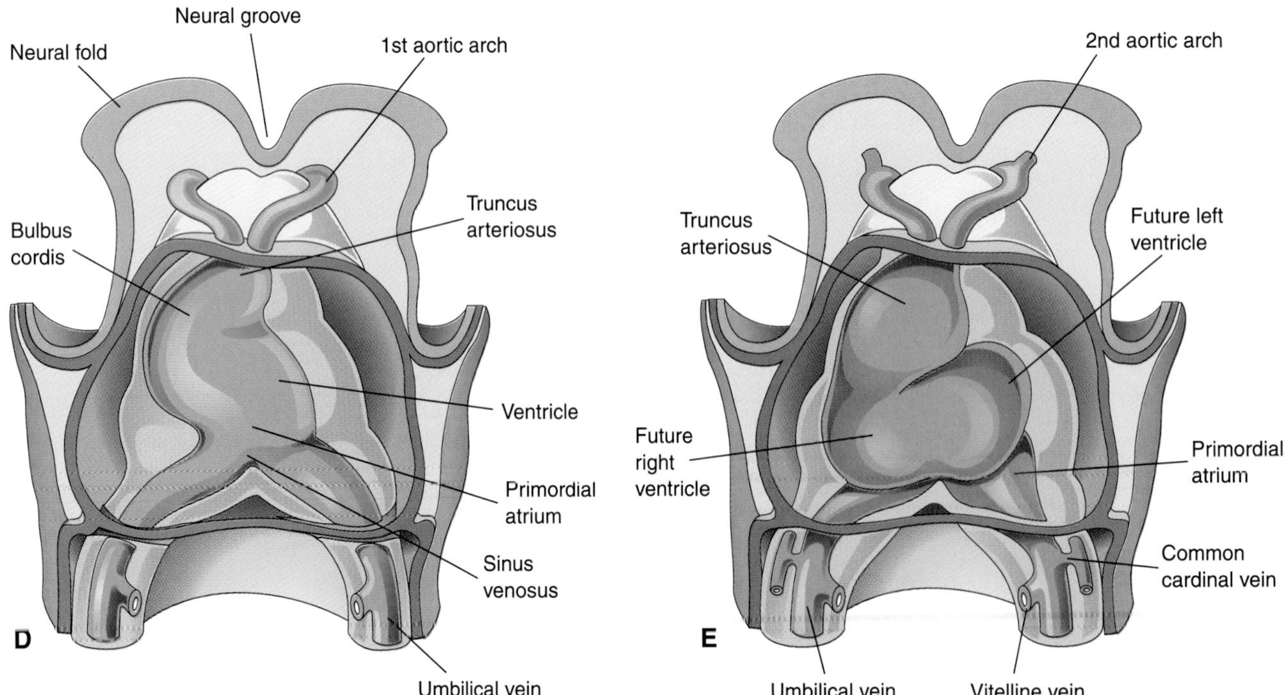

■ **Figure 14-7.** *A* to *C*, Sketches of ventral views of the developing heart and pericardial region (22 to 35 days). The ventral pericardial wall has been removed to show the developing myocardium and fusion of the endothelial tubes to form a single endocardial tube. The fusion begins at the cranial ends of the tubes and extends caudally until a single tubular heart is formed. The endothelium of the heart tube forms the endocardium of the heart. As the heart elongates, it bends upon itself, forming an S-shaped heart (*D* and *E*).

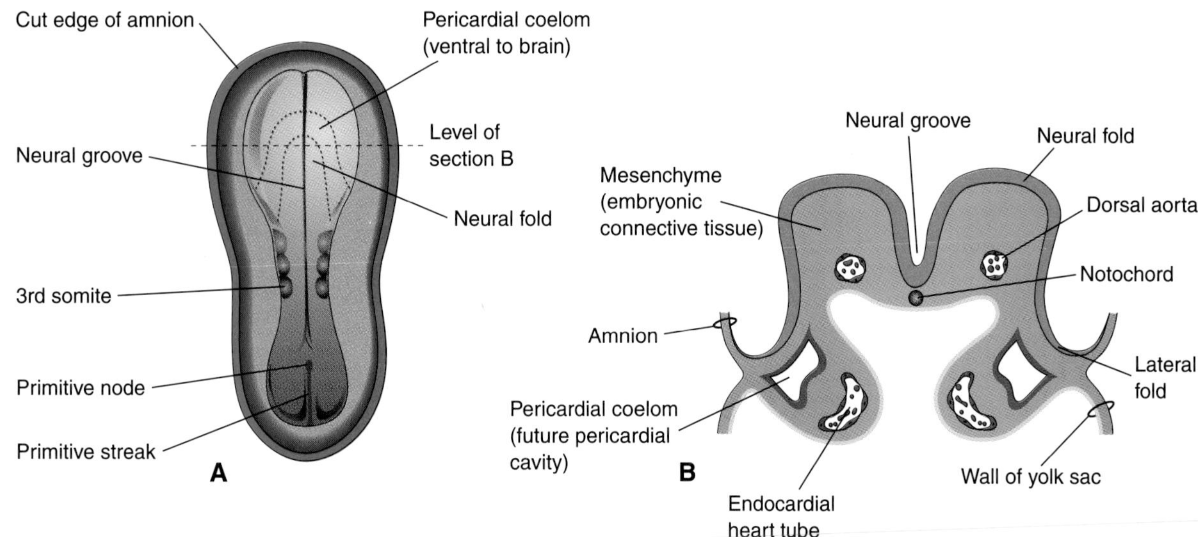

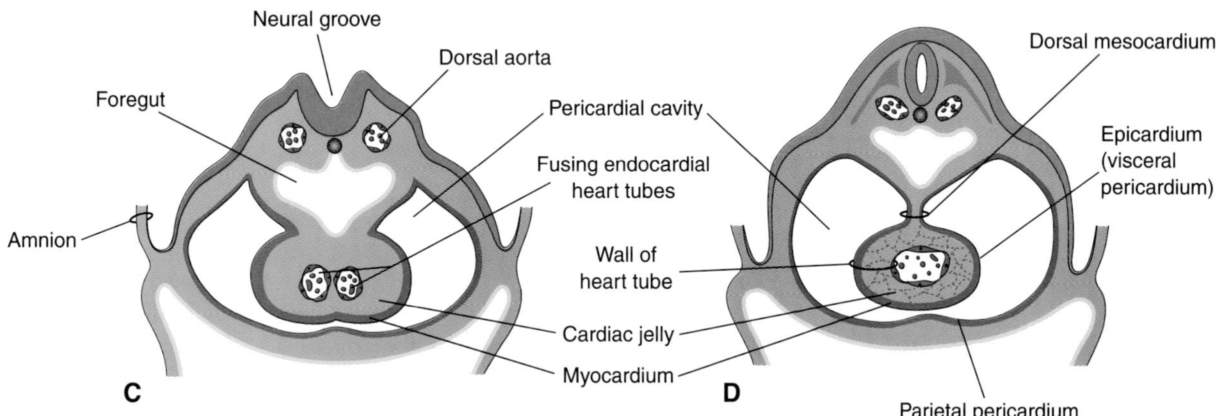

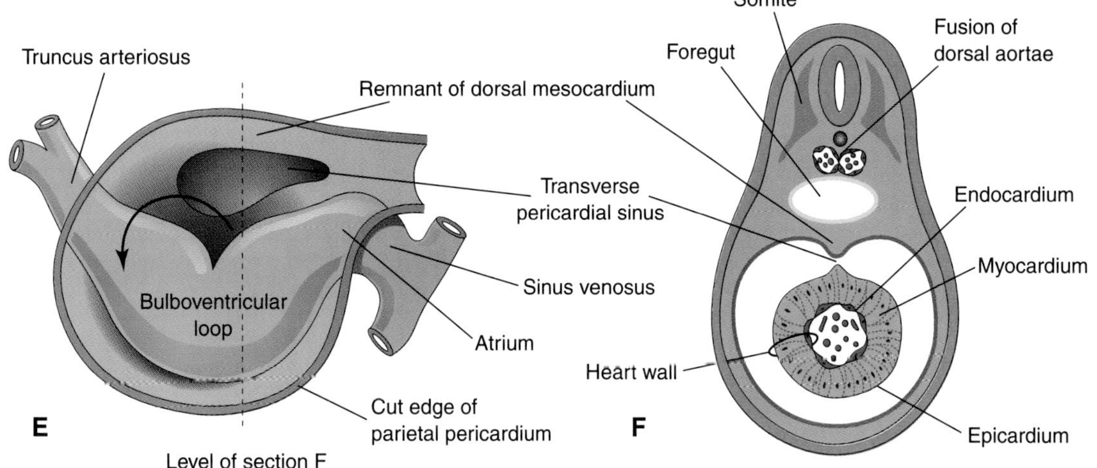

■ **Figure 14–8.** *A,* Drawing of a dorsal view of an embryo (about 20 days). *B,* Schematic transverse section of the heart region of the embryo illustrated in *A,* showing the two endocardial heart tubes and the lateral folds of the body. *C,* Transverse section of a slightly older embryo, showing the formation of the pericardial cavity and the fusing heart tubes. *D,* Similar section (about 22 days), showing the single heart tube suspended by the dorsal mesocardium. *E,* Schematic drawing of the heart (about 28 days) showing degeneration of the central part of the dorsal mesocardium and formation of the transverse sinus of the pericardium. *F,* Transverse section of the embryo at the level shown in *E,* showing the layers of the heart wall.

sal aorta becomes the median sacral artery (Moore, 1992).

FATE OF VITELLINE AND UMBILICAL ARTERIES

The unpaired ventral branches of the dorsal aorta supply the yolk sac, allantois, and chorion (Fig. 14-2). The **vitelline arteries** pass to the yolk sac and later the primordial gut, which forms from the incorporated part of the yolk sac. Three vitelline arteries remain as the

- *celiac artery* to the foregut
- *superior mesenteric artery* to the midgut
- *inferior mesenteric artery* to the hindgut

The paired **umbilical arteries** pass through the connecting stalk (later the *umbilical cord*) and become continuous with vessels in the chorion, the embryonic part of the placenta (see Chapter 7). The umbilical arteries carry poorly oxygenated blood to the placenta (Fig. 14-2). Proximal parts of the umbilical arteries become the *internal iliac arteries* and *superior vesical arteries*, whereas distal parts obliterate after birth and become the *medial umbilical ligaments*. The major changes leading to the definitive arterial system, especially the *transformation of the aortic arches*, are described later.

FINAL PRENATAL DEVELOPMENT OF THE HEART

The primordium of the heart is first evident at 18 days (Fig. 14-1) and begins to beat at 22 to 23 days (Fig. 14-3). In the **cardiogenic area**, splanchnic mesenchymal cells ventral to the pericardial coelom aggregate and arrange themselves side-by-side to form two longitudinal, cellular cardiac primordia—**angioblastic cords**. These cords become canalized to form two thin-walled **endocardial heart tubes** (Figs. 14-7 and 14-8*B*). As lateral embryonic folding occurs, the endocardial tubes approach each other and fuse to form a single endocardial tube (Figs. 14-7*C* and 14-8*D*). Fusion of the endocardial tubes begins at the cranial end of the developing heart and extends caudally. Molecular studies in mouse and chick embryos have demonstrated the presence of two 6HLH (basic helix-loop-helix) genes, dHAND and eHAND, in the paired primordial endocardial tubes and in later stages of cardiac morphogenesis (Srivastava et al., 1995). The murine MEF2C gene, which is expressed in cardiogenic precursor cells before formation of the heart tubes, appears to be an essential regulator in early cardiac development (Lin et al., 1997). Their role remains to be elucidated.

As the heart tubes fuse, an external layer of the embryonic heart—the **primordial myocardium**—is formed from splanchnic mesoderm surrounding the pericardial coelom (Fig. 14-8*B* and *C*). At this stage the developing heart is composed of a thin endothelial tube, separated from a thick muscular tube, the primordial myocardium, by gelatinous connective tissue—**cardiac jelly** (Fig. 14-8*D*). The endothelial tube becomes the internal endothelial lining of the heart or **endocardium**, and the primordial myocardium becomes the muscular wall of the heart or **myocardium**. The visceral pericardium or **epicardium** is derived from mesothelial cells that arise from the external surface of the sinus venosus and spread over the myocardium.

As folding of the head region occurs, the heart and pericardial cavity come to lie ventral to the foregut and caudal to the oropharyngeal membrane (Fig. 14-9). Concurrently, the tubular heart elongates and develops alternate dilations and constrictions (Fig. 14-7*C* to *E*):

- truncus arteriosus
- bulbus cordis
- ventricle
- atrium
- sinus venosus

The tubular **truncus arteriosus** is continuous cranially with the **aortic sac** (Fig. 14-10*A*), from which the *aortic arches* arise. The **sinus venosus** receives the umbilical, vitelline, and common cardinal veins from the chorion, yolk sac, and embryo, respectively (Fig. 14-10*B*).

The arterial and venous ends of the heart are fixed by the pharyngeal arches and septum transversum, respectively. Because the bulbus cordis and ventricle grow faster than other regions, the heart bends upon itself, forming a U-shaped *bulboventricular loop* (Fig. 14-8*E*). The signaling molecule(s) and cellular mechanisms responsible for cardiac looping are largely unknown (for details, see Olson and Srivastava, 1996; Lin et al., 1997). As the primordial heart bends, the atrium and sinus venosus come to lie dorsal to the truncus arteriosus, bulbus cordis, and ventricle (Fig. 14-10*A* and *B*). By this stage the sinus venosus has developed lateral expansions, the right and left **horns of the sinus venosus**.

As the heart elongates and bends, it gradually invaginates into the **pericardial cavity** (Figs. 14-8*C* and *D* and 14-9C). The heart is initially suspended from the dorsal wall by a mesentery, the **dorsal mesocardium**, but the central part of this mesentery soon degenerates, forming a communication, the **transverse pericardial sinus**, between the right and left sides of the pericardial cavity (Fig. 14-8*E* and *F*). The heart is now attached only at its cranial and caudal ends.

Circulation Through the Primordial Heart

The initial contractions of the heart originate in muscle, i.e., they are of myogenic origin (Anderson, 1996). The muscle layers of the atrium and ventricle are continuous, and contractions occur in peristalsis-like waves that begin in the sinus venosus. At first circulation through the primordial heart is of an ebb-and-flow type; however, by the end of the fourth week coordinated contractions of the heart result in unidirectional

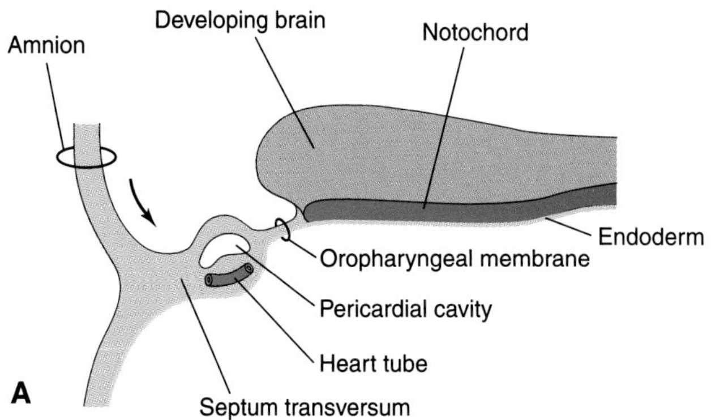

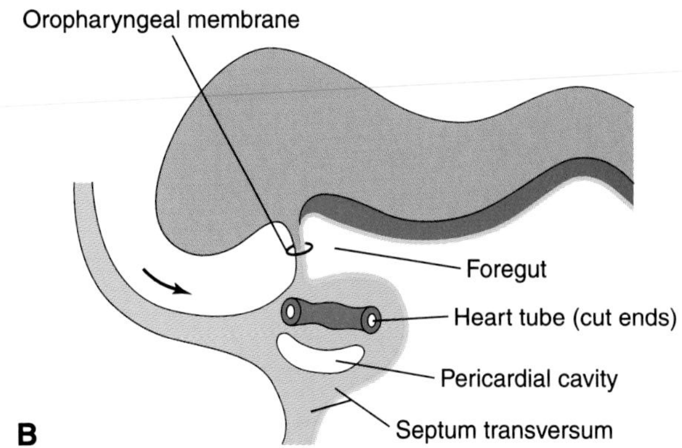

■ **Figure 14–9.** Schematic drawings of longitudinal sections through the cranial half of human embryos during the fourth week, showing the effect of the head fold *(arrow)* on the position of the heart and other structures. *A* and *B*, As the head fold develops, the heart tube and pericardial cavity come to lie ventral to the foregut and caudal to the oropharyngeal membrane. *C*, Note that the positions of the pericardial cavity and septum transversum have reversed with respect to each other. The septum transversum now lies posterior to the pericardial cavity, where it will form the central tendon of the diaphragm.

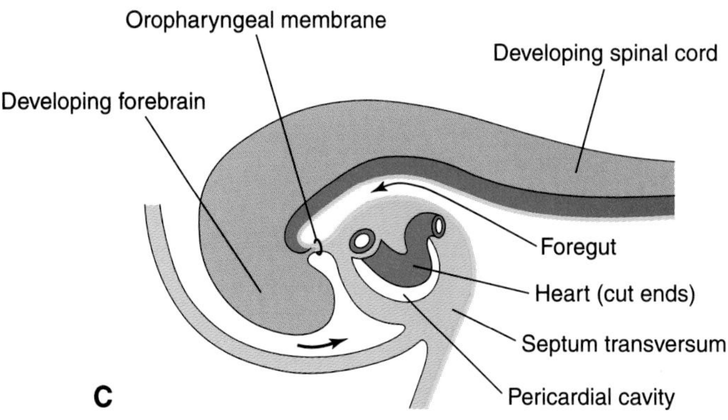

flow. Blood enters the sinus venosus (Fig. 14-10*A* and *B*) from:

- the embryo through the common cardinal veins
- the developing placenta through the umbilical veins
- the yolk sac through the vitelline veins

Blood from the sinus venosus enters the primordial atrium; flow from it is controlled by **sinoatrial valves** (Figs. 14-10*A* and 14-11*A*). The blood then passes through the **atrioventricular canal** into the primordial ventricle. When the ventricle contracts, blood is pumped through the **bulbus cordis** and **truncus arteriosus** into the aortic sac, from which it is distributed to the **aortic arches** in the pharyngeal arches (Fig. 14-10*C*). The blood then passes into the dorsal aortae for distribution to the embryo, yolk sac, and placenta.

Text continued on page 365

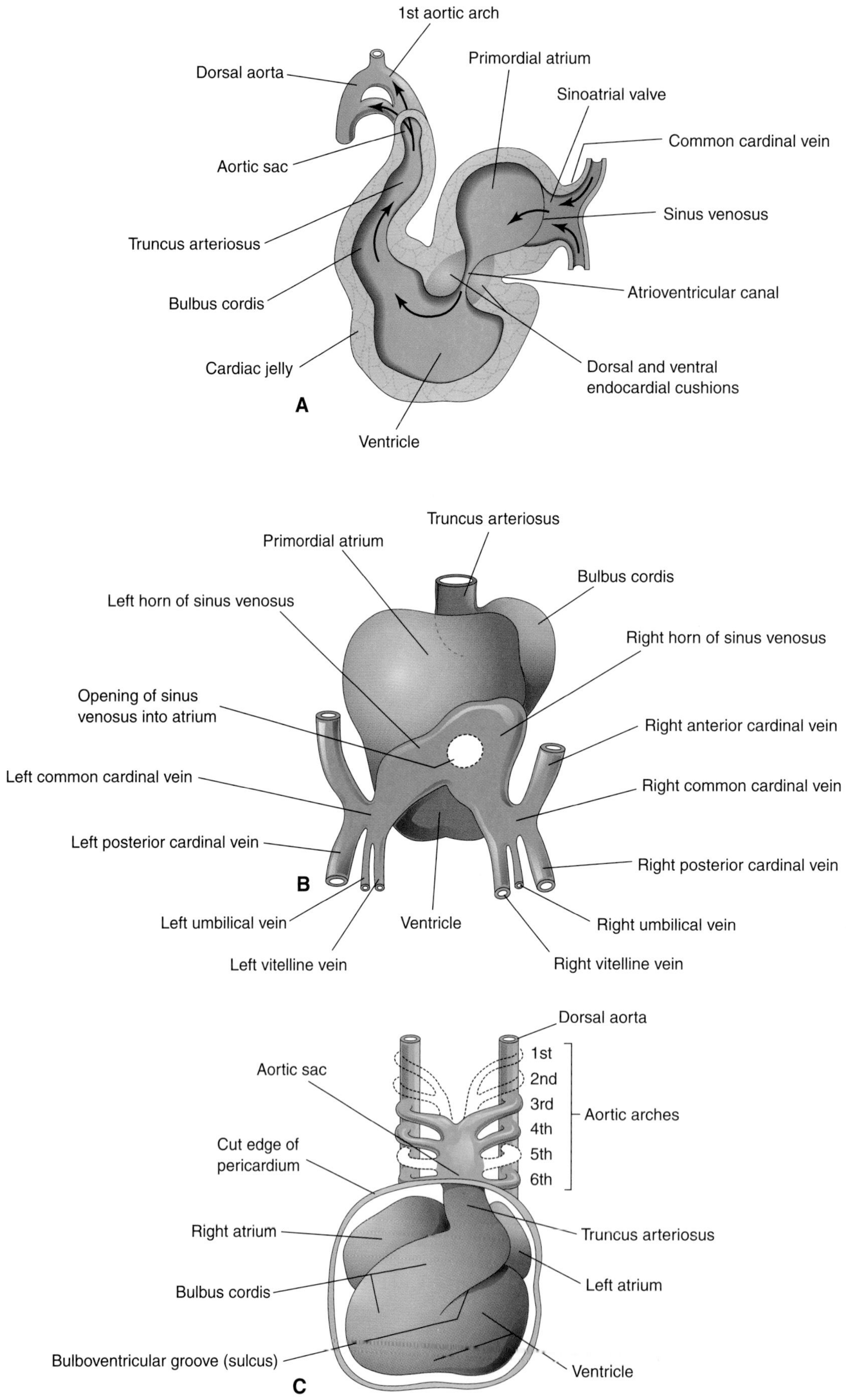

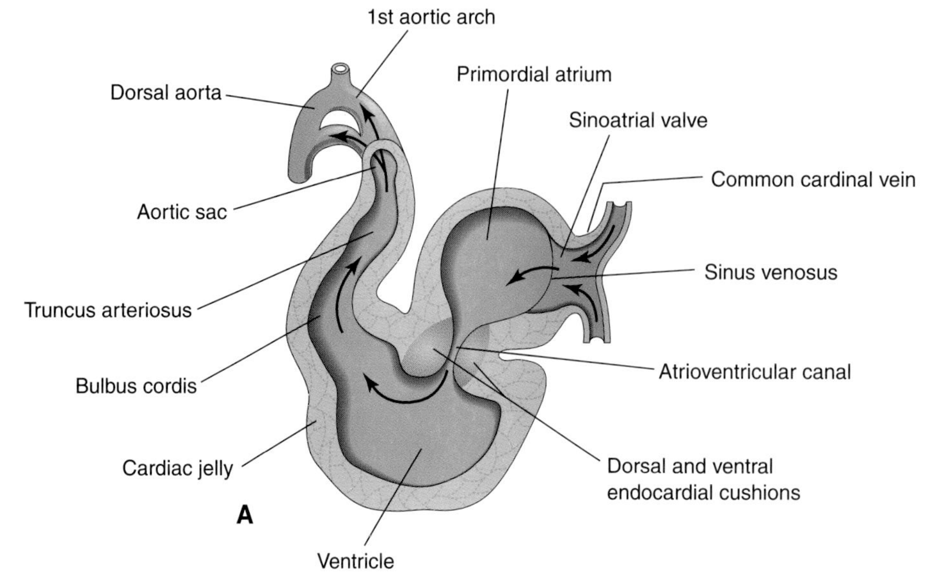

■ **Figure 14–10.** *A,* Schematic sagittal section of the primordial heart (about 24 days), showing blood flow through it *(arrows). B,* Dorsal view of the heart (about 26 days), illustrating the horns of the sinus venosus and the dorsal location of the primordial atrium. *C,* Ventral view of the heart and aortic arches (about 35 days). The ventral wall of the pericardial sac has been removed to show the heart in the pericardial cavity.

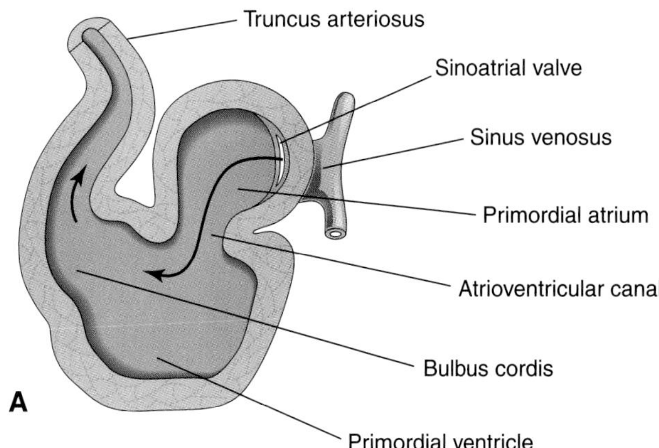

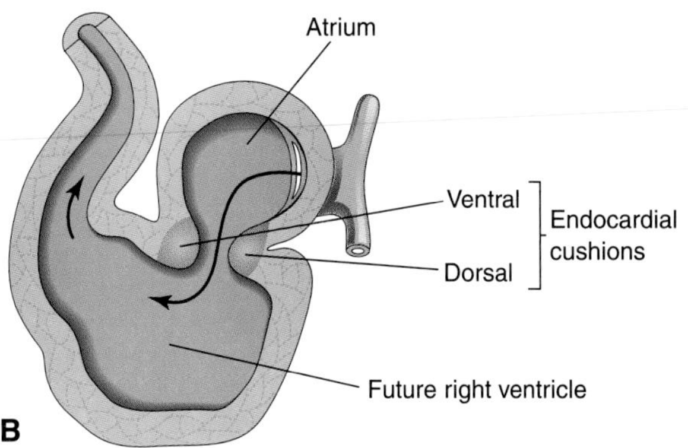

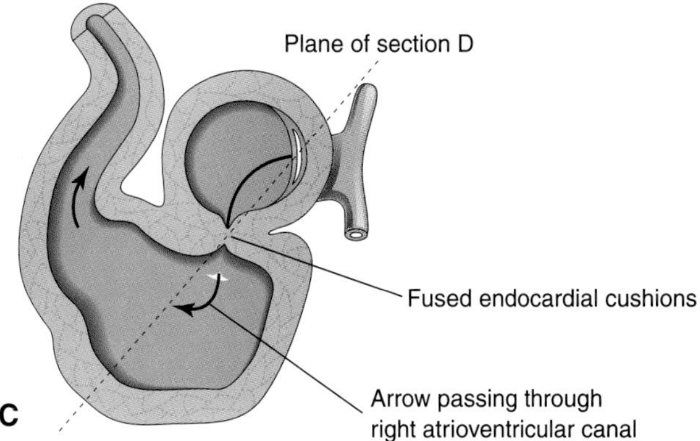

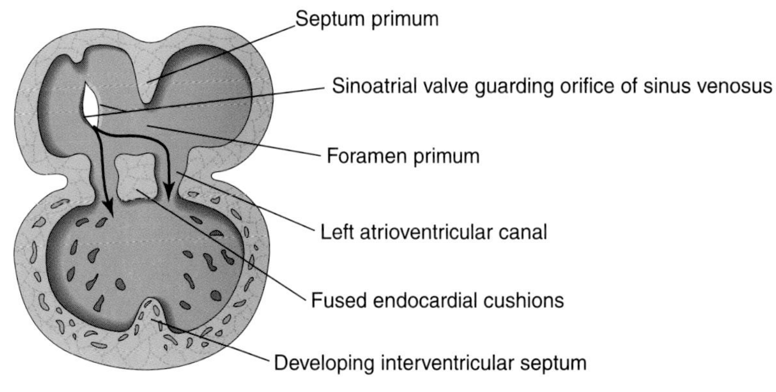

■ **Figure 14–11.** *A* to *C,* Schematic sketches of sagittal sections of the heart during the fourth and fifth weeks, illustrating blood flow through the heart and division of the atrioventricular canal. *D,* Coronal section of the heart at the plane shown in *C.* Note that the interatrial and interventricular septa have also started to develop.

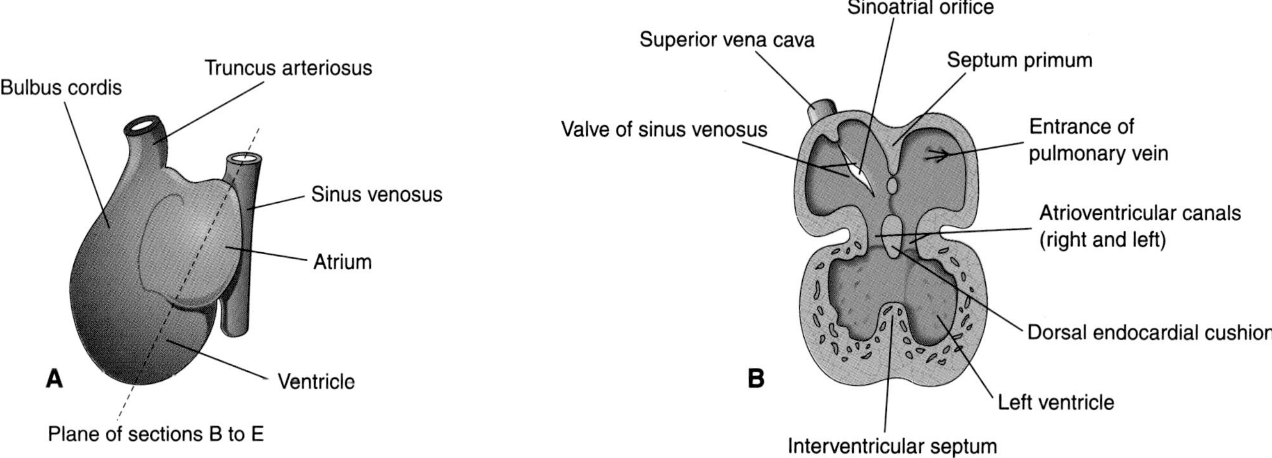

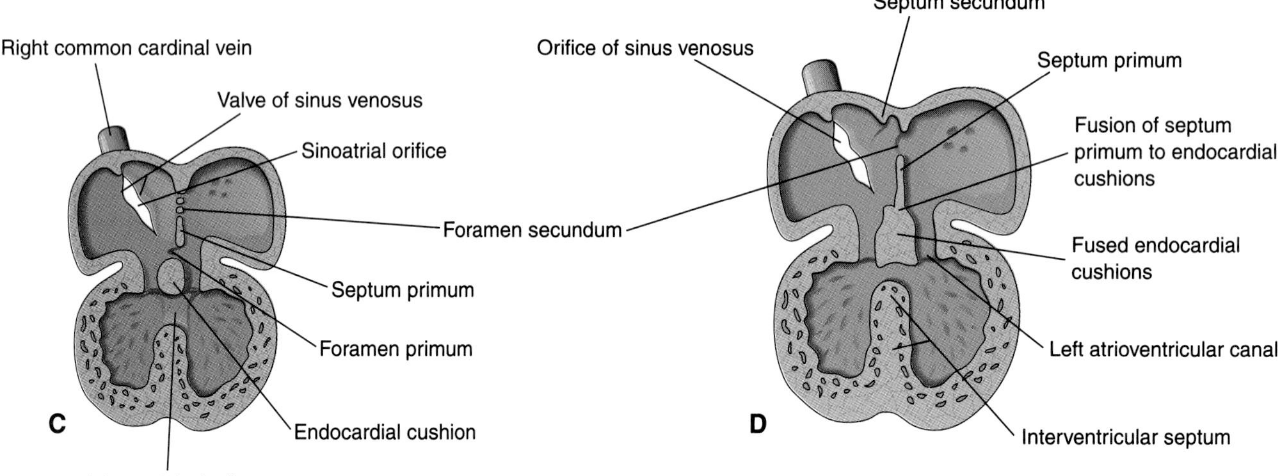

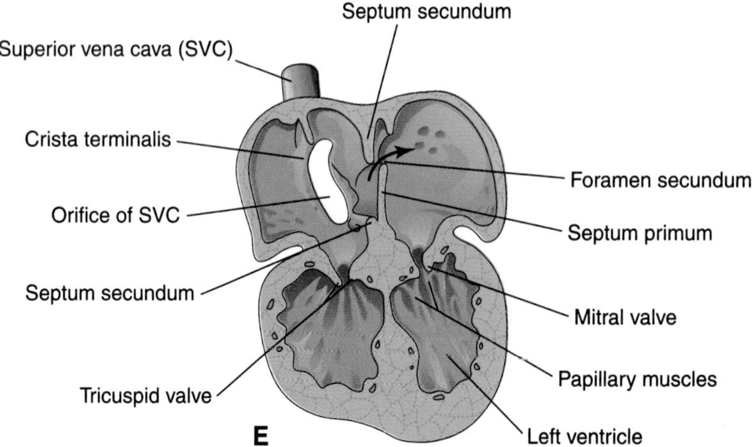

■ **Figure 14–12.** Schematic drawings of the developing heart showing partitioning of the atrioventricular canal, primordial atrium, and ventricle. *A,* Sketch showing the plane of the sections. *B,* During the fourth week (about 28 days), showing the early appearance of the septum primum, interventricular septum, and dorsal endocardial cushion. *C,* Section of the heart (about 32 days), showing perforations in the dorsal part of the septum primum. *D,* Section of the heart (about 35 days) showing the foramen secundum. *E,* About 8 weeks, showing the heart after it is partitioned into four chambers. The arrow indicates the flow of well-oxygenated blood from the right to the left atrium.

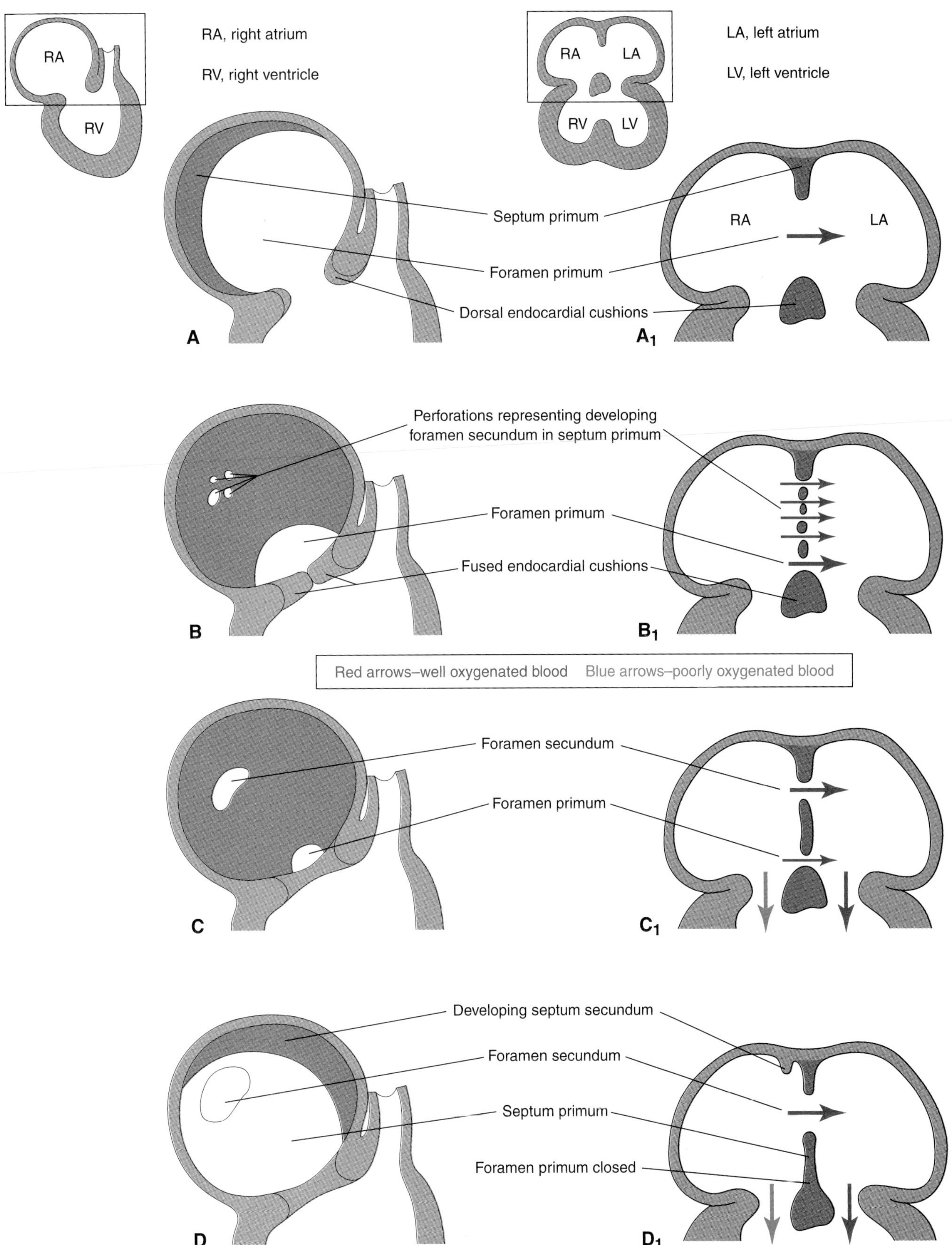

■ **Figure 14–13.** Diagrammatic sketches illustrating progressive stages in partitioning of the primitive atrium. *A* to *H* are views of the developing interatrial septum as viewed from the right side. A_1 to H_1 are coronal sections of the developing interatrial septum. As the septum secundum grows, note that it overlaps the opening in the septum primum (foramen secundum).

Illustration continued on following page

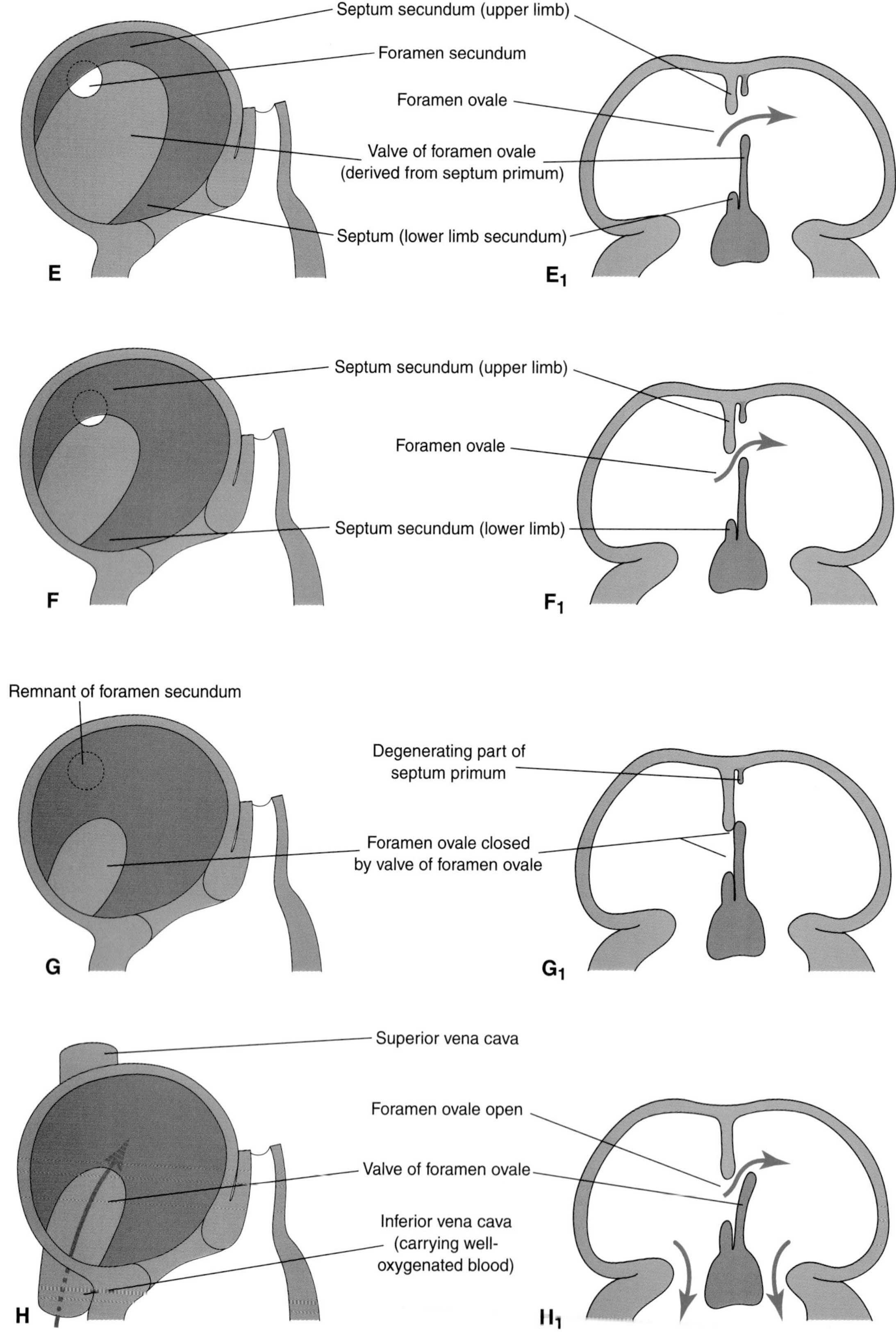

■ **Figure 14–13.** *Continued.* Observe the valve of the foramen ovale in G_1 and H_1. When pressure in the right atrium exceeds that in the left atrium, blood passes from the right to the left side of the heart. When the pressures are equal or higher in the left atrium, the valve formed by the septum primum closes the foramen ovale.

Partitioning of the Primordial Heart

Partitioning of the atrioventricular canal, primordial atrium, and ventricle begins around the middle of the fourth week and is essentially completed by the end of the fifth week. Although described separately, these processes occur concurrently. For details of the molecular processes that have been implicated in cardiac development, refer to Olson and Srivastava (1996) and Lin et al. (1997).

PARTITIONING OF ATRIOVENTRICULAR CANAL

Toward the end of the fourth week, **endocardial cushions** form on the dorsal and ventral walls of the atrioventricular (AV) canal. As these masses of tissue are invaded by mesenchymal cells during the fifth week (Fig. 14-11*B*), the AV endocardial cushions approach each other and fuse, dividing the AV canal into right and left *AV canals* (Fig. 14-11*C*). These canals partially separate the primordial atrium from the ventricle, and the endocardial cushions function as AV valves.

PARTITIONING OF PRIMORDIAL ATRIUM

Beginning at the end of the fourth week, the primordial atrium is divided into right and left atria by the formation and subsequent modification and fusion of two septa, the septum primum and septum secundum (Figs. 14-12 and 14-13).

The **septum primum,** a thin crescent-shaped membrane, grows toward the fusing endocardial cushions from the roof of the primordial atrium, partially dividing the common atrium into right and left halves. As this curtainlike septum grows, a large opening—the **foramen primum** (ostium primum), forms between its crescentic free edge and the endocardial cushions (Figs. 14-12*C* and 14-13*A* to *C*). The foramen primum serves as a shunt, enabling oxygenated blood to pass from the right to the left atrium. The foramen primum becomes progressively smaller and disappears as the septum primum fuses with the fused endocardial cushions to form a **primordial AV septum** (Fig. 14-13*D* and D_1. Before the foramen primum disappears, perforations—produced by programmed cell death—appear in the central part of the septum primum. As the septum fuses with the fused endocardial cushions, the perforations coalesce to form another opening, the **foramen secundum** (ostium secundum). Concurrently, the free edge of the septum primum fuses with the left side of the fused endocardial cushions, obliterating the foramen primum (Figs. 14-12*D* and 14-13*D*). The foramen secundum ensures a continuous flow of oxygenated blood from the right to the left atrium.

The **septum secundum,** a crescentic muscular membrane, grows from the ventrocranial wall of the atrium, immediately to the right of the septum primum (Fig. 14-13D_1). As this thick septum grows during the fifth and sixth weeks, it gradually overlaps the foramen secundum in the septum primum (Fig. 14-13*E*). The septum secundum forms an incomplete partition between the atria; consequently, an oval foramen—the **foramen ovale**—forms. The cranial part of the septum primum, initially attached to the roof of the left atrium, gradually disappears (Fig. 14-13G_1 and H_1). The remaining part of the septum primum, attached to the fused endocardial cushions, forms the flaplike **valve of the foramen ovale**.

Before birth the foramen ovale allows most of the oxygenated blood entering the right atrium from the IVC to pass into the left atrium (Fig. 14-14*A*), and

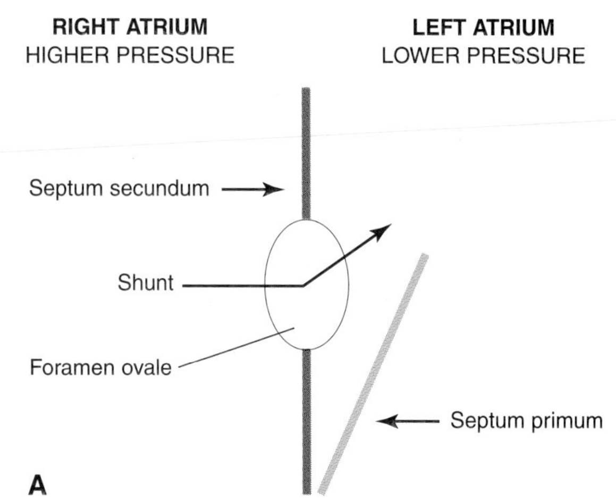

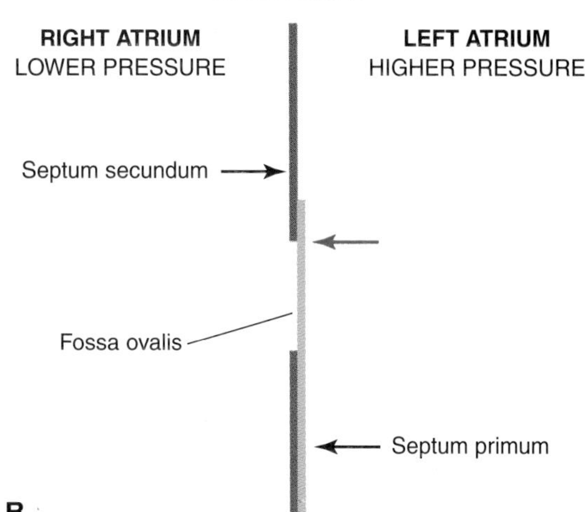

■ **Figure 14-14.** Diagrams illustrating the relationship of the septum primum to the foramen ovale and septum secundum. *A,* Before birth well-oxygenated blood is shunted from the right atrium through the foramen ovale into the left atrium when the pressure rises. When the pressure falls in the right atrium, the flaplike valve of the foramen ovale is pressed against the relatively rigid septum secundum. This closes the foramen ovale. *B,* After birth the pressure in the left atrium rises as the blood returns from the lungs, which are now functioning. Eventually the septum primum is pressed against the septum secundum and adheres to it, permanently closing the foramen ovale and forming the fossa ovalis.

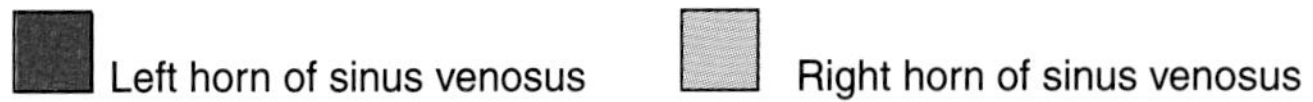

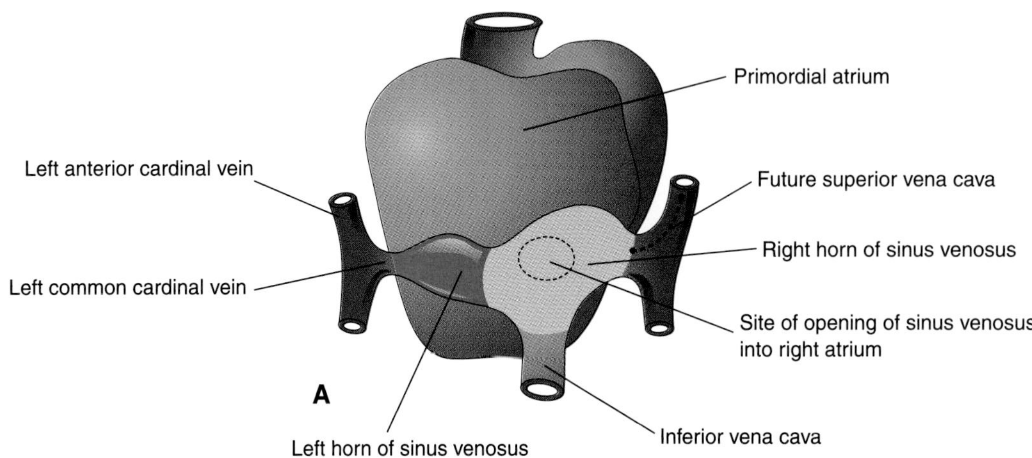

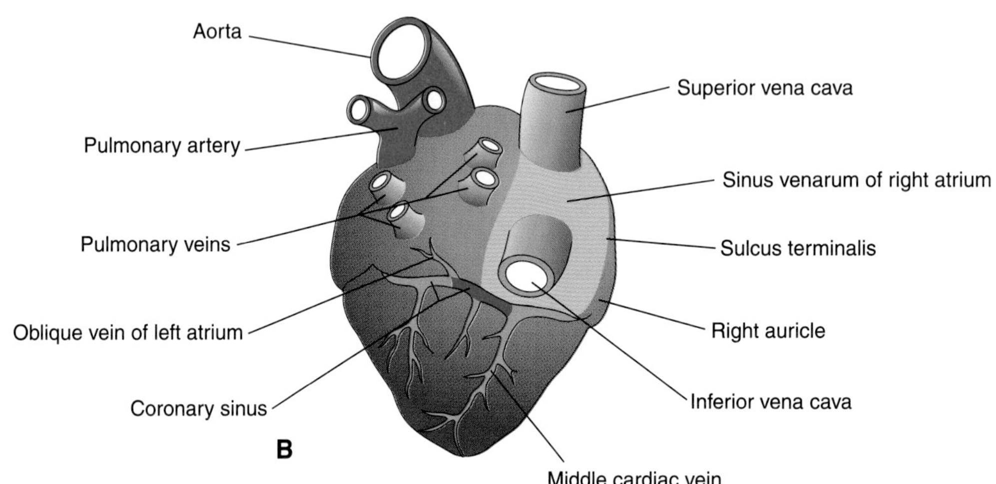

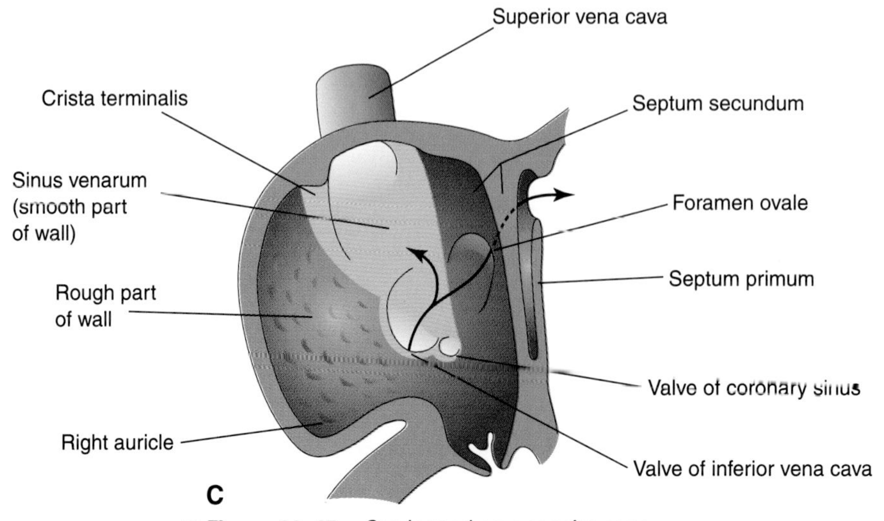

■ **Figure 14–15.** *See legend on opposite page*

prevents the passage of blood in the opposite direction because the septum primum closes against the relatively rigid septum secundum (Fig. 14-14*B*). *After birth* the foramen ovale normally closes and the valve of the foramen ovale fuses with the septum primum. As a result, the interatrial septum becomes a complete partition between the atria.

Changes in the Sinus Venosus

Initially the sinus venosus opens into the center of the dorsal wall of the primitive atrium and its right and left horns are about the same size (Fig. 14-5*A*). Progressive enlargement of the right horn of the sinus venosus results from *two left-to-right shunts of blood*:

- The first shunt of blood results from transformation of the vitelline and umbilical veins, discussed previously.
- The second shunt of blood occurs when the anterior cardinal veins become connected by an oblique anastomosis (Fig. 14-5*B* and *C*). This communication shunts blood from the left to the right anterior cardinal vein. The shunt eventually becomes the left *brachiocephalic vein*. The right anterior cardinal vein and the right common cardinal vein become the SVC.

By the end of the fourth week, the right horn is noticeably larger than the left (Fig. 14-15*B*). As this occurs the sinoatrial orifice moves to the right and opens in the part of the primordial atrium that will become the adult right atrium (Figs. 14-11*D* and 14-15*C*). The results of the two left-to-right venous shunts (Fig. 14-15) are:

- The left horn of the sinus venosus decreases in size and importance.
- The right horn enlarges and receives all the blood from the head and neck through the SVC, and from the placenta and caudal regions of the body through the IVC.

Initially the sinus venosus is a separate chamber of the heart and opens into the dorsal wall of the right atrium (Fig. 14-10*A* and *B*). As heart development proceeds, the left horn of the sinus venosus becomes the **coronary sinus**, and the right horn becomes incorporated into the wall of the right atrium (Fig. 14-15*B* and *C*).

Because it is derived from the sinus venosus, the smooth part of the wall of the right atrium is called the **sinus venarum** (Fig. 14-15*B* and *C*). The remainder of the internal surface of the wall of the right atrium and the conical muscular pouch, the **auricle** (auricular appendage), have a rough trabeculated appearance. These two parts are derived from the primordial atrium. The smooth part (sinus venarum) and the rough part (primordial atrium) are demarcated internally in the right atrium by a vertical ridge, the **crista terminalis** (Fig. 14-15*C*), and externally by a shallow inconspicuous groove, the **sulcus terminalis** (Fig. 14-15*B*). The crista terminalis represents the cranial part of the right sinoatrial valve (Fig. 14-15*C*); the caudal part of this valve forms the valves of the IVC and coronary sinus. The left sinoatrial valve fuses with the septum secundum and is incorporated with it into the interatrial septum.

PRIMORDIAL PULMONARY VEIN AND FORMATION OF THE LEFT ATRIUM

Most of the wall of the left atrium is smooth because it is formed by incorporation of the primordial pulmonary vein (Fig. 14-16). This vein develops as an outgrowth of the dorsal atrial wall, just to the left of the septum primum. As the atrium expands, the primordial pulmonary vein and its main branches are gradually incorporated into the wall of the left atrium; as a result, four pulmonary veins are formed (Fig. 14-16*C* and *D*). Molecular studies have confirmed that atrial myoblasts migrate into the walls of the pulmonary veins. The functional significance of this pulmonary cardiac muscle (pulmonary myocardium) is uncertain (Jones et al., 1994). The small left auricle (auricular appendage) is derived from the primordial atrium; its internal surface has a rough trabeculated appearance.

Anomalous Pulmonary Venous Connections

In total anomalous pulmonary venous connections, none of the pulmonary veins connects with the left atrium. They open into the right atrium or into one of the systemic veins or into both. In partial anomalous pulmonary venous connections, one or more pulmonary veins have similar anomalous connections; the others have normal connections.

PARTITIONING OF THE PRIMORDIAL VENTRICLE

Division of the primordial ventricle into two ventricles is first indicated by a median muscular ridge—the **primordial interventricular (IV) septum**—in the floor

■ **Figure 14–15.** Diagrams illustrating the fate of the sinus venosus. *A,* Dorsal view of the heart (about 26 days) showing the primitive atrium and sinus venosus. *B,* Dorsal view at 8 weeks after incorporation of the right horn of the sinus venosus into the right atrium. The left horn of the sinus venosus has become the coronary sinus. *C,* Internal view of the fetal right atrium showing (1) the smooth part of the wall of the right atrium (sinus venarum) derived from the right horn of the sinus venosus, and (2) the crista terminalis and the valves of the inferior vena cava and coronary sinus derived from the right sinuatrial valve. The primitive right atrium becomes the right auricle, a conical muscular pouch.

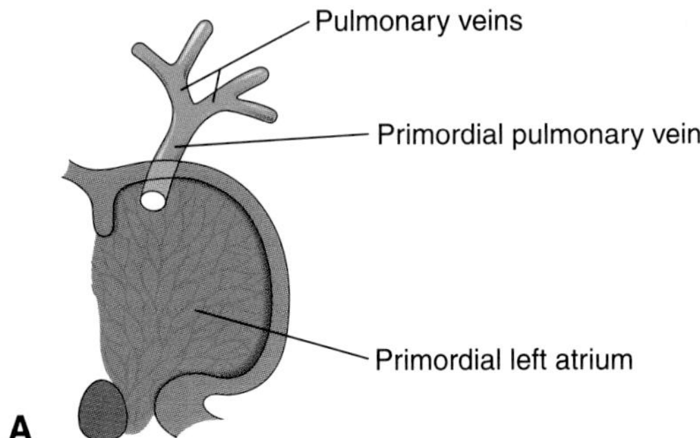

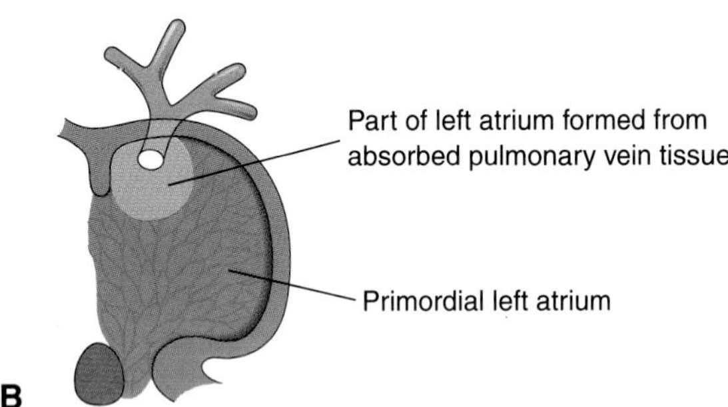

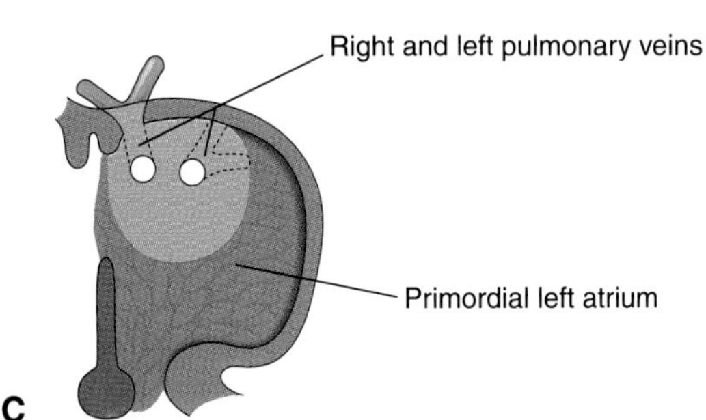

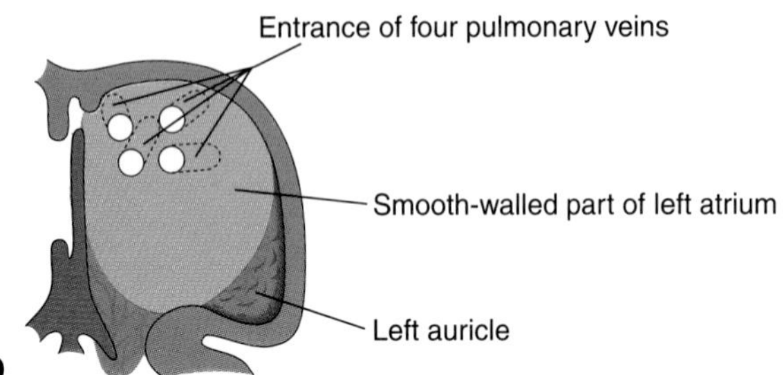

■ **Figure 14–16.** Diagrammatic sketches illustrating absorption of the pulmonary vein into the left atrium. *A*, 5 weeks, showing the common pulmonary vein opening into the primordial left atrium. *B*, Later stage, showing partial absorption of the common pulmonary vein. *C*, 6 weeks, showing the openings of two pulmonary veins into the left atrium resulting from absorption of the common pulmonary vein. *D*, 8 weeks, showing four pulmonary veins with separate atrial orifices. The primordial left atrium becomes the left auricle, a tubular appendage of the atrium. Most of the left atrium is formed by absorption of the primordial pulmonary vein and its branches.

of the ventricle near its apex (Fig. 14-12*B*). This thick crescentic fold has a concave free edge (Fig. 14-17*A*). Initially, most of its increase in height results from dilation of the ventricles on each side of the IV septum (Fig. 14-17*B*). The medial walls of the enlarging ventricles approach each other and fuse to form the primordium of the **muscular part of the IV septum**. Later, there is active proliferation of myoblasts in the septum, which increase its size. Until the seventh week there is a crescent-shaped **interventricular (IV) foramen** between the free edge of the IV septum and the fused endocardial cushions. The IV foramen permits communication between the right and left ventricles (Figs. 14-17 and 14-18*B*). The IV foramen usually closes by the end of the seventh week as the bulbar ridges fuse with the endocardial cushion (Fig. 14-18*C* to *E*).

Closure of the IV foramen and formation of the membranous part of the IV septum result from fusion of tissues from three sources:

- the right bulbar ridge
- the left bulbar ridge
- the endocardial cushion

The **membranous part of the IV septum** is derived from an extension of tissue from the right side of the endocardial cushion to the muscular part of the IV septum. This tissue merges with the aorticopulmonary septum and the thick muscular part of the IV septum (Fig. 14-19*C*). After closure of the IV foramen and formation of the membranous part of the IV septum, the pulmonary trunk is in communication with the right ventricle and the aorta communicates with the left ventricle (Fig. 14-18*E*).

Cavitation of the ventricular walls forms a spongework of muscular bundles. Some of these bundles remain as the **trabeculae carneae** (muscular bundles on the lining of the ventricular walls) and others become the **papillary muscles** and tendinous cords (*chordae tendineae*). The tendinous cords run from the papillary muscles to the atrioventricular valves (Fig. 14-19*C* and *D*).

Fetal Cardiac Ultrasonography

Technological advances in ultrasonography have made it possible for sonographers to recognize normal and abnormal fetal anatomy (Fig. 14-20). In the presence of a very slow heart beat (less than 80 beats per minute), the fetus is at risk of associated heart disease (Silverman and Schmidt, 1994). Most studies are performed between 18 and 22 weeks of gestation because the heart is large enough to examine easily; however, fetal cardiac anatomy can be studied as early as 18 weeks if necessary. For details concerning the ultrasound evaluation of the heart, including color flow studies, see Silverman and Schmidt (1994) and Lee et al. (1995).

PARTITIONING OF BULBUS CORDIS AND TRUNCUS ARTERIOSUS

During the fifth week of development, active proliferation of mesenchymal cells in the walls of the bulbus cordis results in the formation of **bulbar ridges** (Figs. 14-18*C* and *D* and 14-21*B* and *C*). Similar ridges form in the truncus arteriosus that are continuous with the bulbar ridges. The bulbar and **truncal ridges** are derived largely from neural crest mesenchyme (Kirby et al., 1983; Clark, 1986). **Neural crest cells** migrate through the primordial pharynx and pharyngeal arches to reach the ridges. As this occurs, the bulbar and truncal ridges undergo an 180 degree spiraling. The spiral orientation of the bulbar and truncal ridges, possibly caused by the streaming of blood from the ventricles, results in the formation of a spiral **aorticopulmonary septum** when the ridges fuse (Fig. 14-21*D* to *G*). This septum divides the bulbus cordis and truncus arteriosus into two arterial channels, the **aorta** and **pulmonary trunk** (Yu and Hutchins, 1996). Because of the spiraling of the aorticopulmonary septum, the pulmonary trunk twists around the ascending aorta (Fig. 14-21*H*).

The **bulbus cordis** is incorporated into the walls of the definitive ventricles (Fig. 14-18*A* and *B*):

- In the right ventricle, the bulbus cordis is represented by the **conus arteriosus** (infundibulum), which gives origin to the pulmonary trunk.
- In the left ventricle, the bulbus cordis forms the walls of the **aortic vestibule**, the part of the ventricular cavity just inferior to the aortic valve.

DEVELOPMENT OF CARDIAC VALVES

When partitioning of the truncus arteriosus is nearly completed (Fig. 14-21*A* to *C*), the **semilunar valves** begin to develop from three swellings of subendocardial tissue around the orifices of the aorta and pulmonary trunk. These swellings are hollowed out and reshaped to form three thin-walled cusps (Figs. 14-19*C* and *D* and 14-22). The **atrioventricular (AV) valves** (tricuspid and mitral valves) develop similarly from localized proliferations of tissue around the AV canals.

Conducting System of the Heart

Initially the muscle layers of the atrium and ventricle are continuous. The primordial atrium acts as the interim pacemaker of the heart, but the sinus venosus soon takes over this function. The **sinuatrial node** (sinoatrial node) develops during the fifth week. It is originally in the right wall of the sinus venosus, but it is incorporated into the wall of the right atrium with the sinus venosus (Fig. 14-19*D*). The sinuatrial node (SA node) is located high in the right atrium, near the entrance of the SVC. After incorporation of the sinus venosus, cells from its left wall are found in the base of the interatrial septum just anterior to the opening of the coronary sinus. Together with cells from the AV region, they form the **AV node and bundle**, which are located just superior to the endocardial cushions. The fibers arising from the **AV bundle** pass from the atrium into the ventricle and split into right and left **bundle branches**, which are distributed throughout the ventricular myocardium (Fig. 14-19*D*). The SA

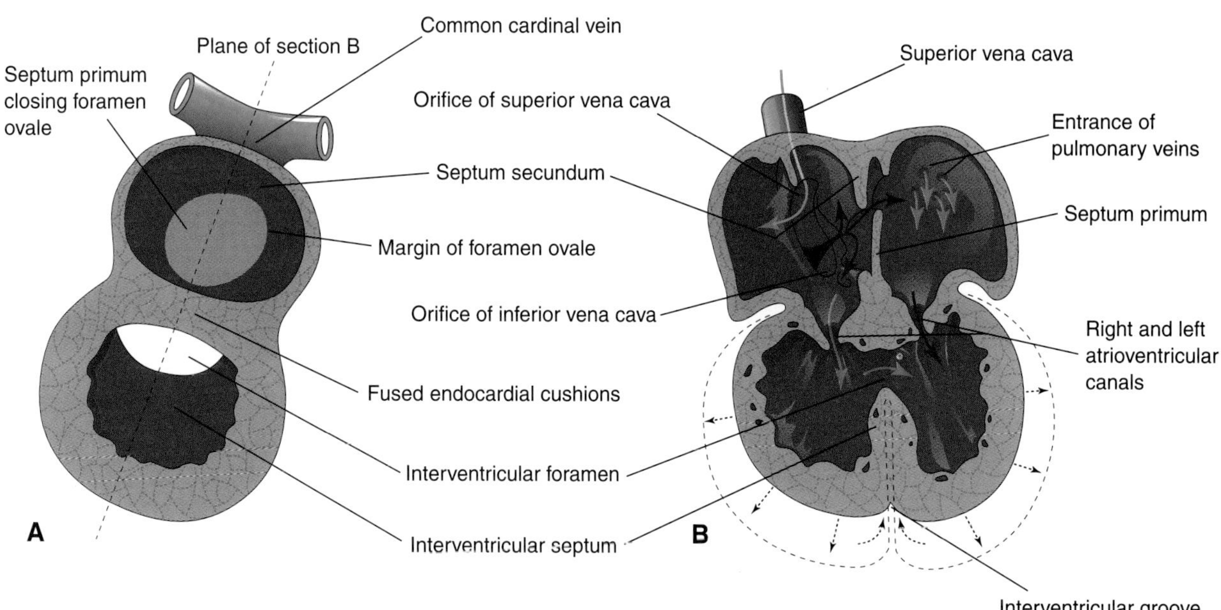

■ **Figure 14-17.** Schematic diagrams illustrating partitioning of the primordial heart. *A,* Sagittal section late in the fifth week showing the cardiac septa and foramina. *B,* Coronal section at a slightly later stage illustrating the directions of blood flow through the heart and expansion of the ventricles.

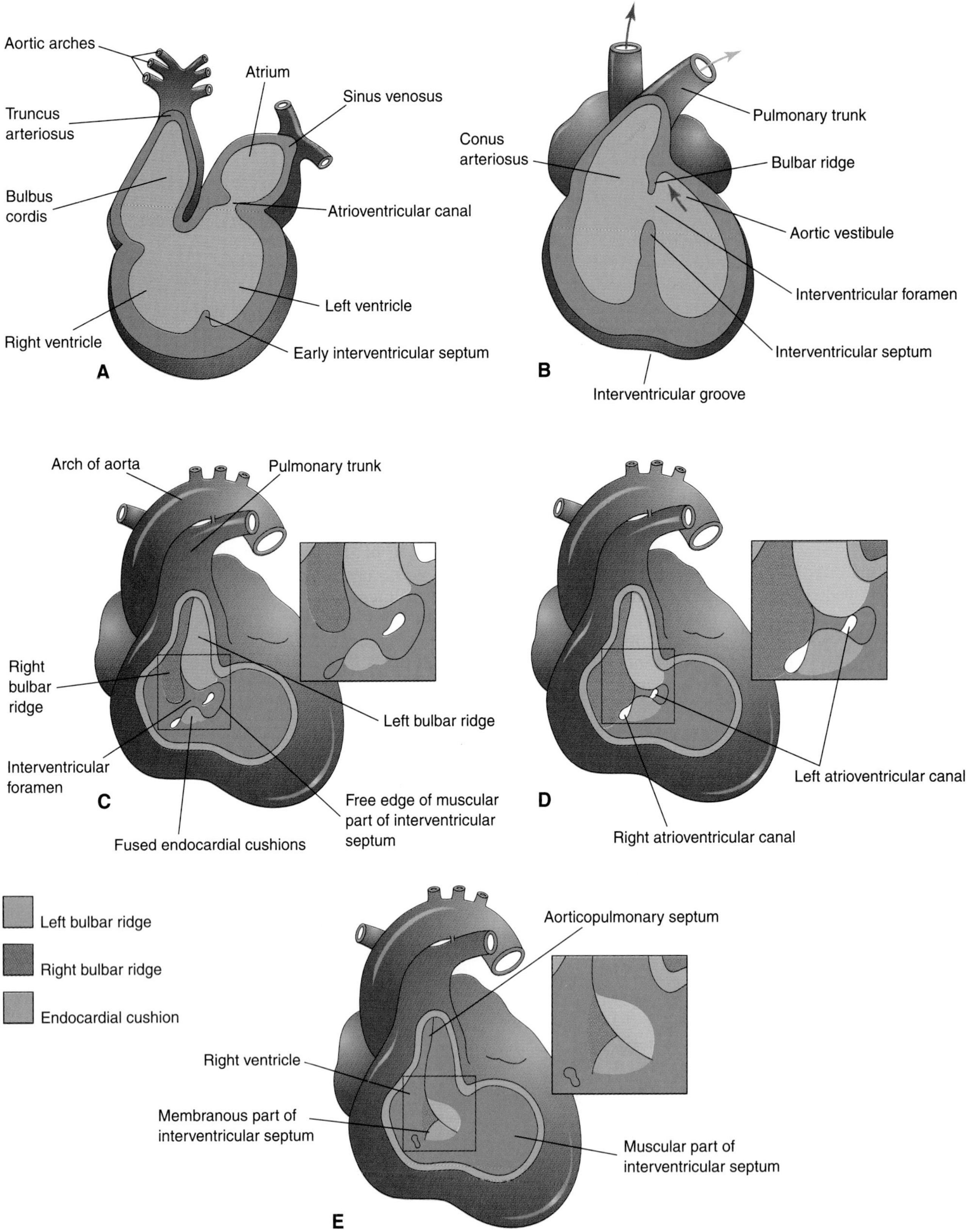

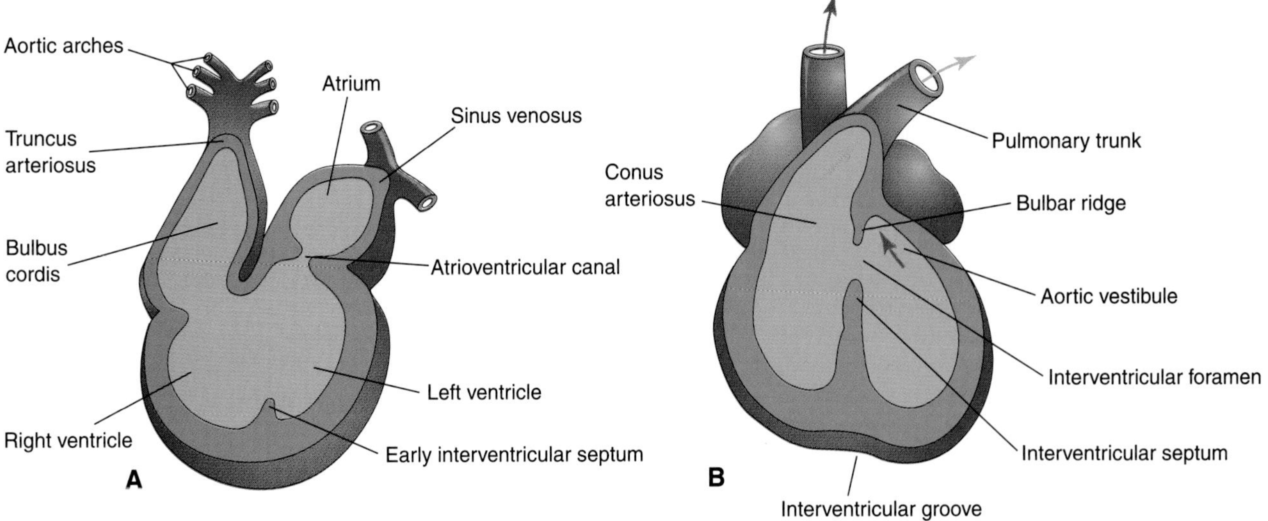

■ **Figure 14–18.** Sketches illustrating incorporation of the bulbus cordis into the ventricles and partitioning of the bulbus cordis and truncus arteriosus into the aorta and pulmonary trunk. *A,* Sagittal section at 5 weeks, showing the bulbus cordis as one of the chambers of the primordial heart. *B,* Schematic coronal section at 6 weeks, after the bulbus cordis has been incorporated into the ventricles to become the conus arteriosus (infundibulum) of the right ventricle and the aortic vestibule of the left ventricle. *C* to *E,* Schematic drawings illustrating closure of the interventricular foramen and formation of the membranous part of the interventricular septum. The walls of the truncus arteriosus, bulbus cordis, and right ventricle have been removed. *C,* 5 weeks, showing the bulbar ridges and fused endocardial cushions. *D,* 6 weeks, showing how proliferation of subendocardial tissue diminishes the interventricular foramen. *E,* 7 weeks, showing the fused bulbar ridges, the membranous part of the interventricular septum formed by extensions of tissue from the right side of the endocardial cushions, and closure of the interventricular foramen.

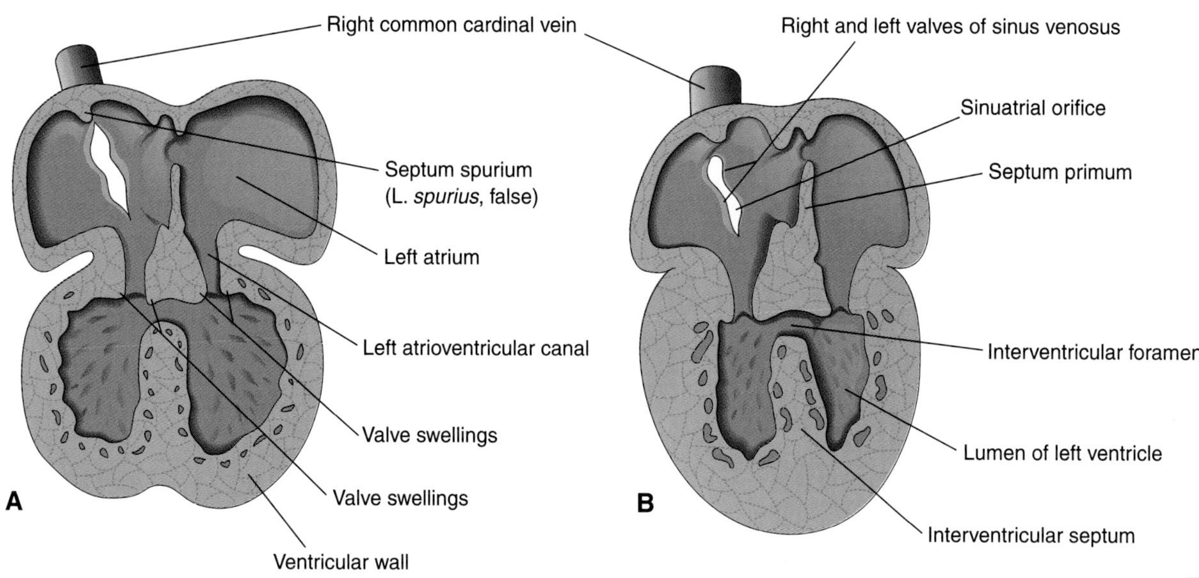

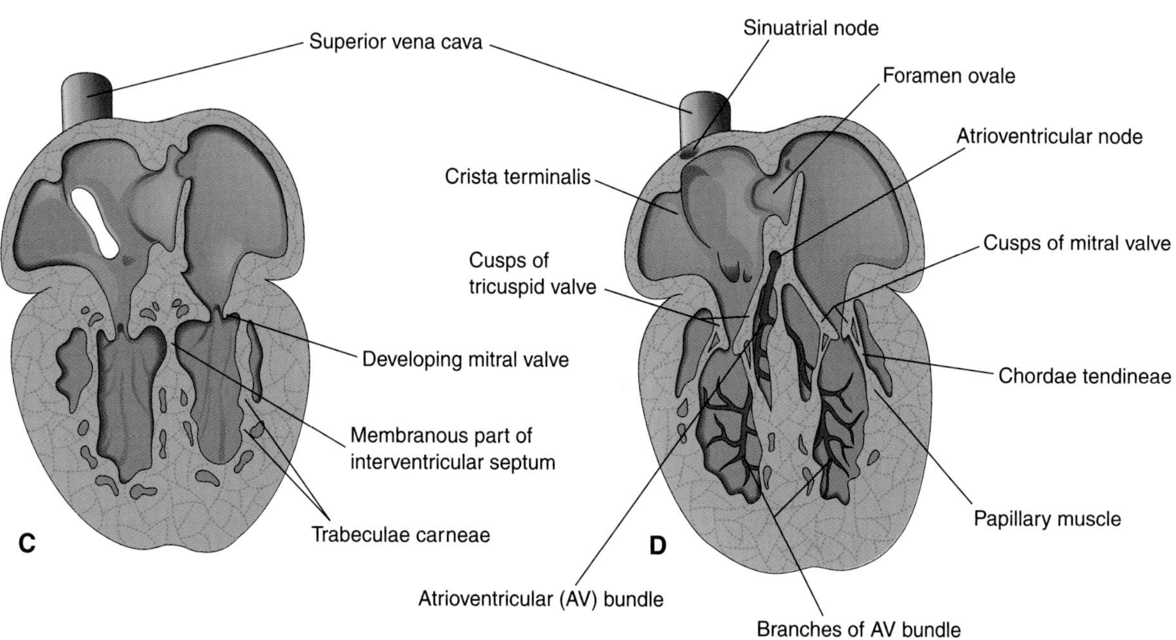

■ **Figure 14–19.** Schematic sections of the heart illustrating successive stages in the development of the atrioventricular valves, chordae tendineae, and papillary muscles. *A,* 5 weeks. *B,* 6 weeks. *C,* 7 weeks. *D,* 20 weeks, showing the conducting system of the heart.

node, AV node, and AV bundle are richly supplied by nerves; however, the conducting system is well developed before these nerves enter the heart. This specialized tissue is normally the only pathway from the atria to the ventricles because, as the four chambers of the heart develop, a band of connective tissue grows in from the epicardium. This tissue subsequently separates the muscle of the atria from that of the ventricles and forms part of the **cardiac skeleton**.

Abnormalities of the Conducting System

Abnormalities of the conducting tissue may cause unexpected death during infancy. Anderson and Ashley (1974) observed conducting tissue abnormalities in the hearts of several infants who died unexpectedly from a

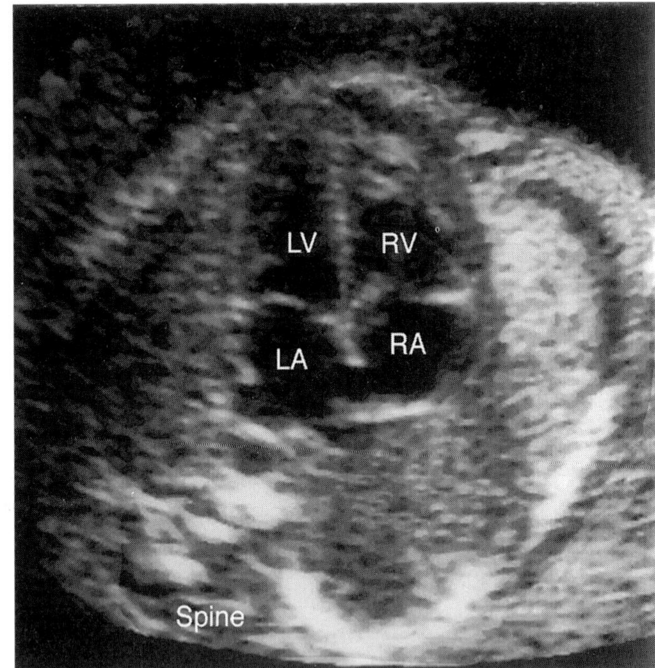

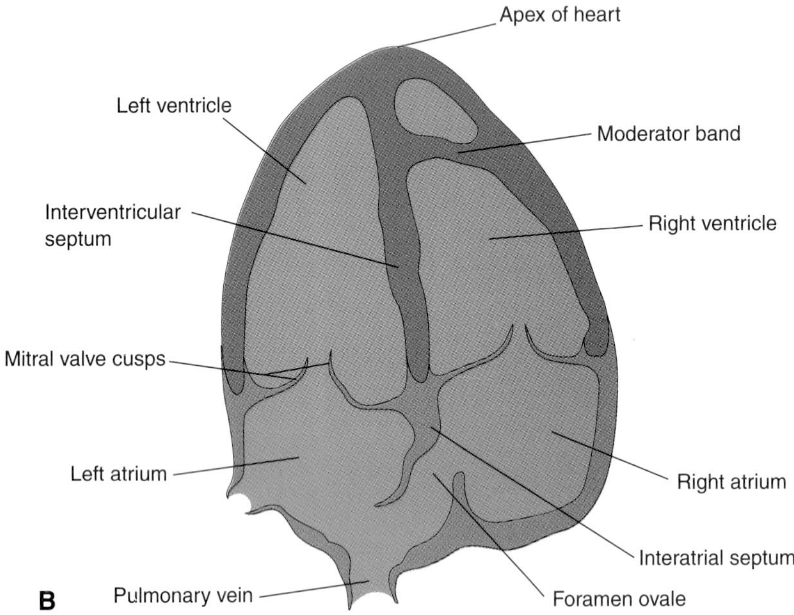

■ **Figure 14–20.** *A,* Ultrasound image showing the normal four-chamber view of the heart in a fetus of about 20 weeks' gestation. *B,* Orientation sketch (modified from the AIUM Technical Bulletin—Performance of the Basic Fetal Cardiac Ultrasound Examination). The scan was obtained across the fetal thorax. The ventricles and atria are well formed and two atrioventricular (AV) valves are present. The moderator band is one of the trabeculae carneae that carries part of the right branch of the AV bundle. (LA, left atrium; LV, left ventricle; RA, right atrium; RV, right ventricle.) (Courtesy of Wesley Lee, MD, Division of Fetal Imaging, William Beaumont Hospital, Royal Oak, Michigan.)

disorder classified as "crib death" or **sudden infant death syndrome (SIDS)**. There remains a lack of consensus that a single mechanism is responsible for the sudden and unexpected deaths of apparently healthy infants. Some findings in infants who later died of SIDS suggest that they have an abnormality in the autonomic nervous system. **SIDS** is the most common cause of postnatal death in developed countries, generally accounting for 40 to 50% of infant deaths during the first year. A **brain stem developmental abnormality** or maturational delay related to neuroregulation of cardiorespiratory control appears to be the most compelling hypothesis (Hunt, 1996).

ANOMALIES OF THE HEART AND GREAT VESSELS

Congenital heart defects (CHDs) are common, with a frequency of 6 to 8 cases per 1000 births (Bernstein, 1996). Some cases of CHD are caused by single-gene or chromosomal mechanisms (Thompson et al., 1991) and others result from exposure to teratogens such as the *rubella virus* (see Chapter 8); however, in most cases the cause is unknown. Most CHDs are thought to be caused by multiple factors, genetic and environmental (Clark, 1996), each of which has a minor effect (i.e., **multifactorial inheritance**). The molecular aspects of abnormal cardiac development are poorly un-

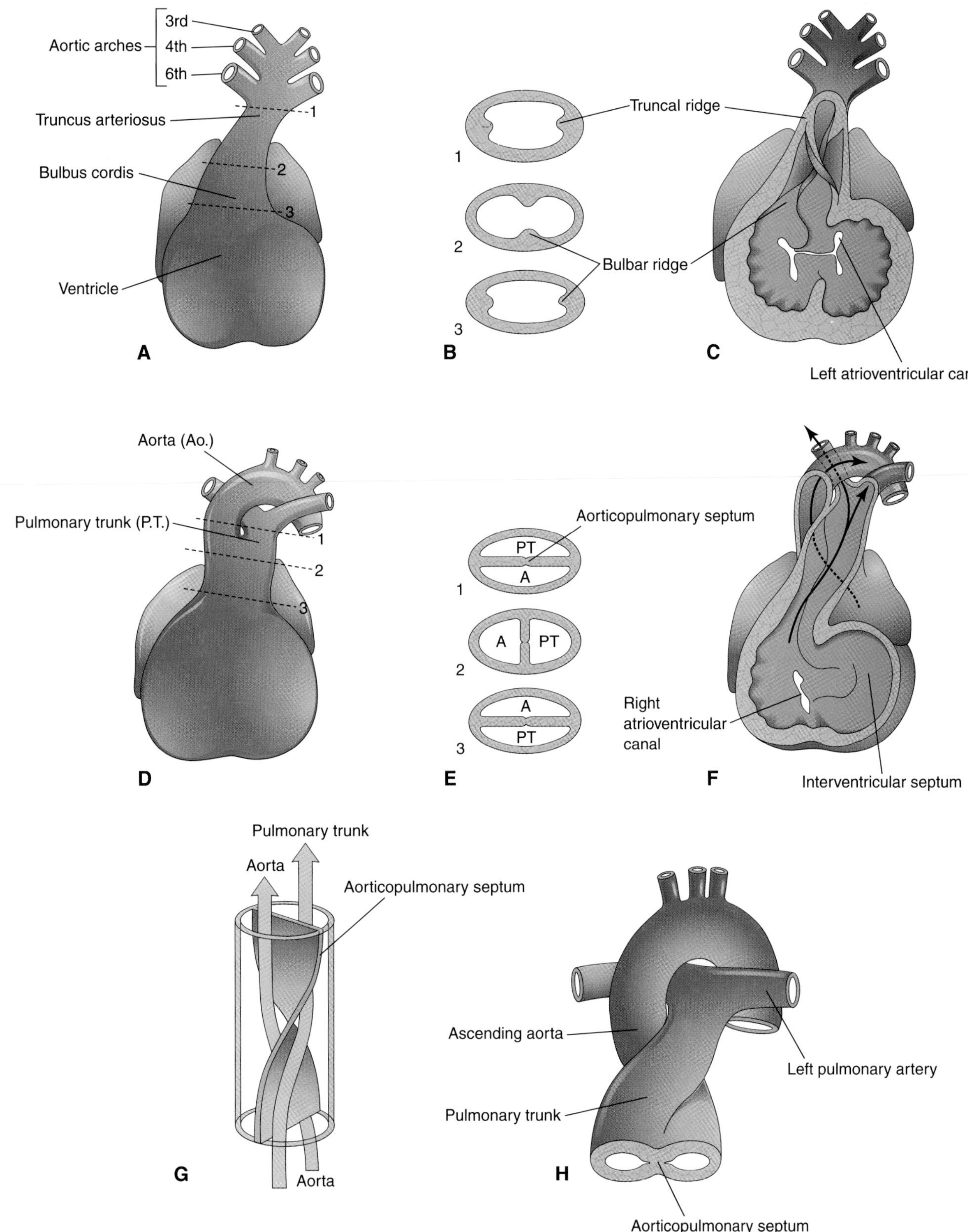

■ **Figure 14–21.** Schematic drawings illustrating partitioning of the bulbus cordis and truncus arteriosus. *A,* Ventral aspect of heart at 5 weeks. *B,* Transverse sections of the truncus arteriosus and bulbus cordis, illustrating the truncal and bulbar ridges. *C,* The ventral wall of the heart and truncus arteriosus has been removed to demonstrate these ridges. *D,* Ventral aspect of heart after partitioning of the truncus arteriosus. *E,* Sections through the newly formed aorta **(A)** and pulmonary trunk **(PT),** showing the aorticopulmonary septum. *F,* 6 weeks. The ventral wall of the heart and pulmonary trunk have been removed to show the aorticopulmonary septum. *G,* Diagram illustrating the spiral form of the aorticopulmonary septum. *H,* Drawing showing the great arteries twisting around each other as they leave the heart.

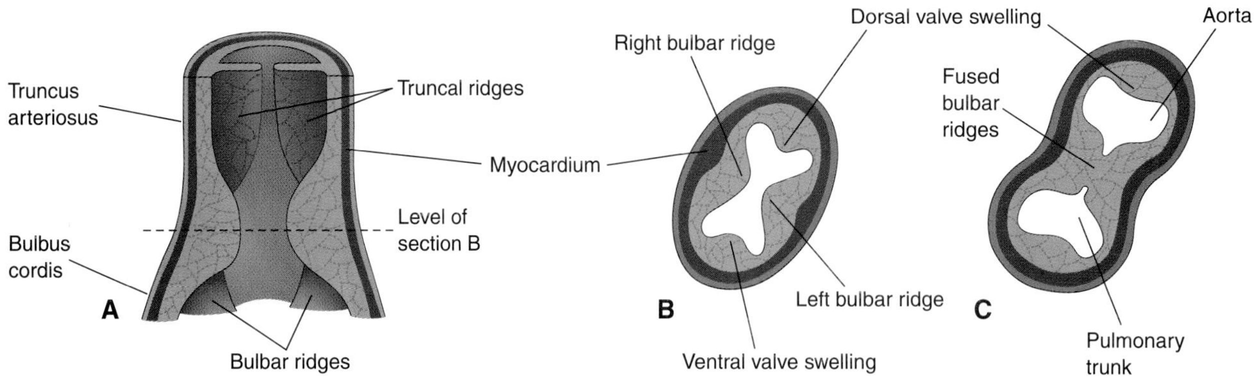

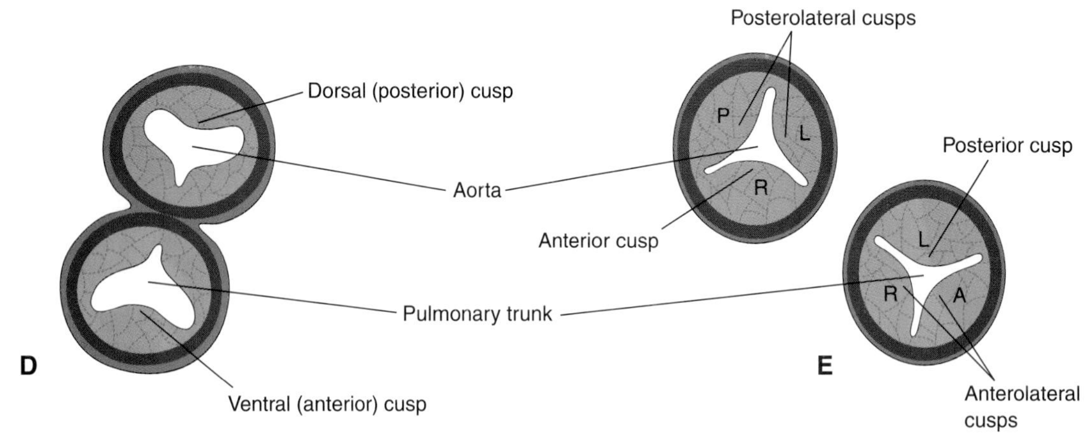

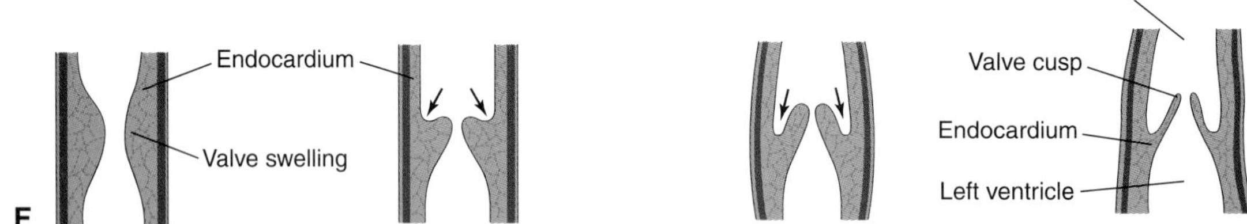

■ **Figure 14–22.** Schematic drawings illustrating development of the semilunar valves of the aorta and pulmonary trunk. *A*, Sketch of a section of the truncus arteriosus and bulbus cordis, showing the valve swellings. *B*, Transverse section of the bulbus cordis. *C*, Similar section after fusion of the bulbar ridges. *D*, Formation of the walls and valves of the aorta and pulmonary trunk. *E*, Rotation of the vessels has established the adult relations of the valves. *F*, Longitudinal sections of the aorticoventricular junction, illustrating successive stages in the hollowing *(arrows)* and thinning of the valve swellings to form the valve cusps.

derstood, and gene therapy for infants with CHDs is at present a remote prospect (Olson and Srivastava, 1996). Recent technology, such as real-time two-dimensional echocardiography, permits detection of fetal CHDs as early as the seventeenth or eighteenth week of gestation (Veille et al., 1989; Silverman and Schmidt, 1994; Lee et al., 1995).

Most CHDs are well tolerated during fetal life; however, at birth when the fetus loses its contact with the maternal circulation, the impact of CHDs become apparent. Some types of CHD cause very little disability; others are incompatible with extrauterine life. Because of recent advances in cardiovascular surgery, many types of CHD can be corrected surgically, and fetal cardiac surgery may soon be possible for complex CHDs (Verrier et al., 1991). Not all CHDs are described in this book. Emphasis is on those that are compatible with life or are currently amenable to surgery. The subsequent discussion of cardiac anomalies is understandably brief. Readers interested in more comprehensive discussions should consult Bernstein (1996).

Dextrocardia

If the heart tube bends to the left instead of to the right (Fig. 14-23), the heart is displaced to the right

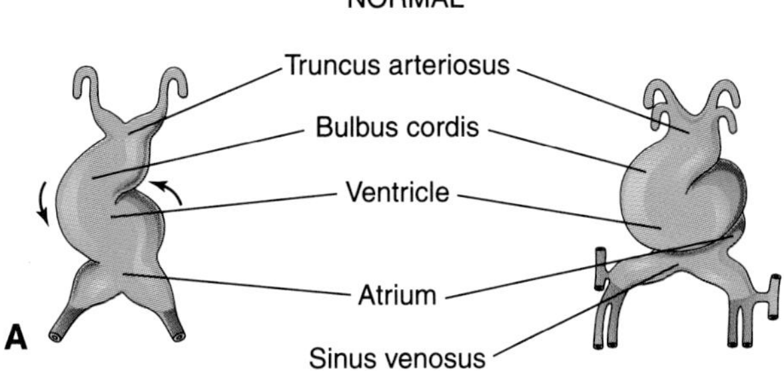

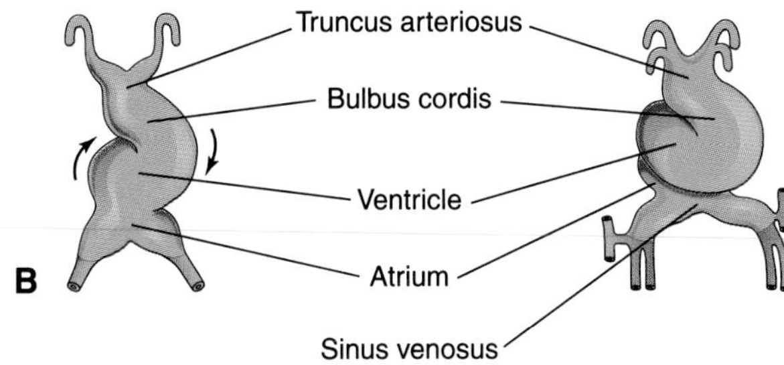

■ **Figure 14–23.** Sketches of the primordial heart tube during the fourth week. *A,* Normal bending to the right. *B,* Abnormal bending to the left.

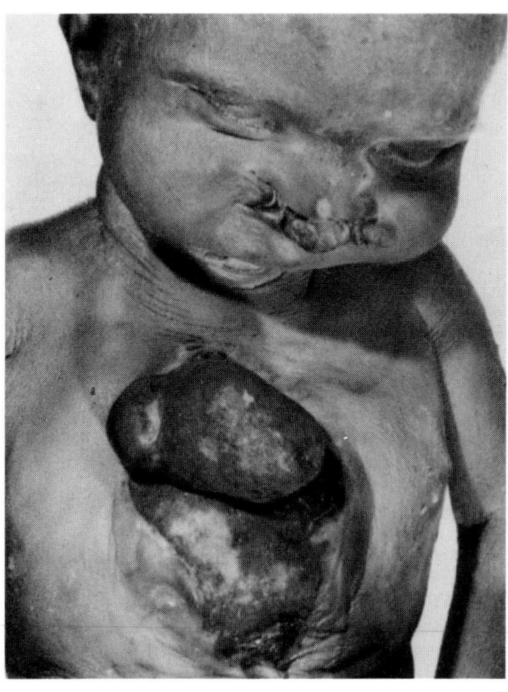

■ **Figure 14–24.** Photograph of a newborn infant with ectopic cordis, cleft sternum, and bilateral cleft lip. Death occurred in the first days of life from infection, cardiac failure, and hypoxemia.

and there is transposition in which the heart and its vessels are reversed left to right as in a mirror image. **Dextrocardia** is the most frequent positional abnormality of the heart. In **dextrocardia with situs inversus** (transposition of viscera such as the liver), the incidence of accompanying cardiac defects is low. If there are no other associated vascular abnormalities, these hearts function normally. In **isolated dextrocardia**, the abnormal position of the heart is not accompanied by displacement of other viscera. This anomaly is usually complicated by severe cardiac anomalies (e.g., single ventricle and arterial transposition). For a discussion of the prognosis and treatment of dextrocardia, see Bernstein (1996).

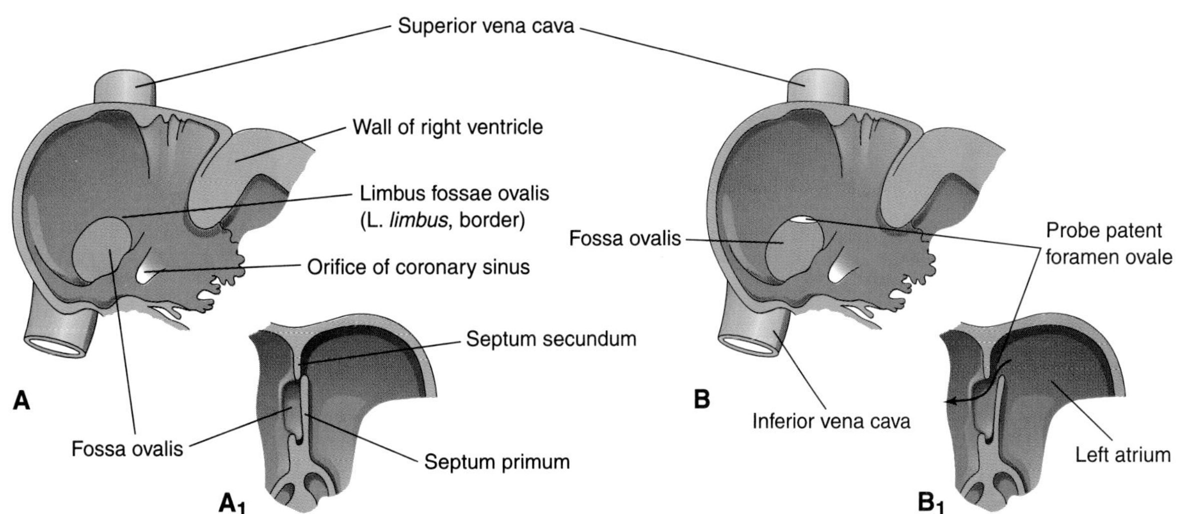

■ **Figure 14–25.** *A,* Drawing illustrating the normal postnatal appearance of the right side of the interatrial septum after adhesion of the septum primum to the septum secundum. A_1, Sketch of a section of the interatrial septum illustrating formation of the fossa ovalis in the right atrium. Note that the floor of this fossa is formed by the septum primum. *B* and B_1, Similar views of a probe patent foramen ovale resulting from incomplete adhesion of the septum primum to the septum secundum.

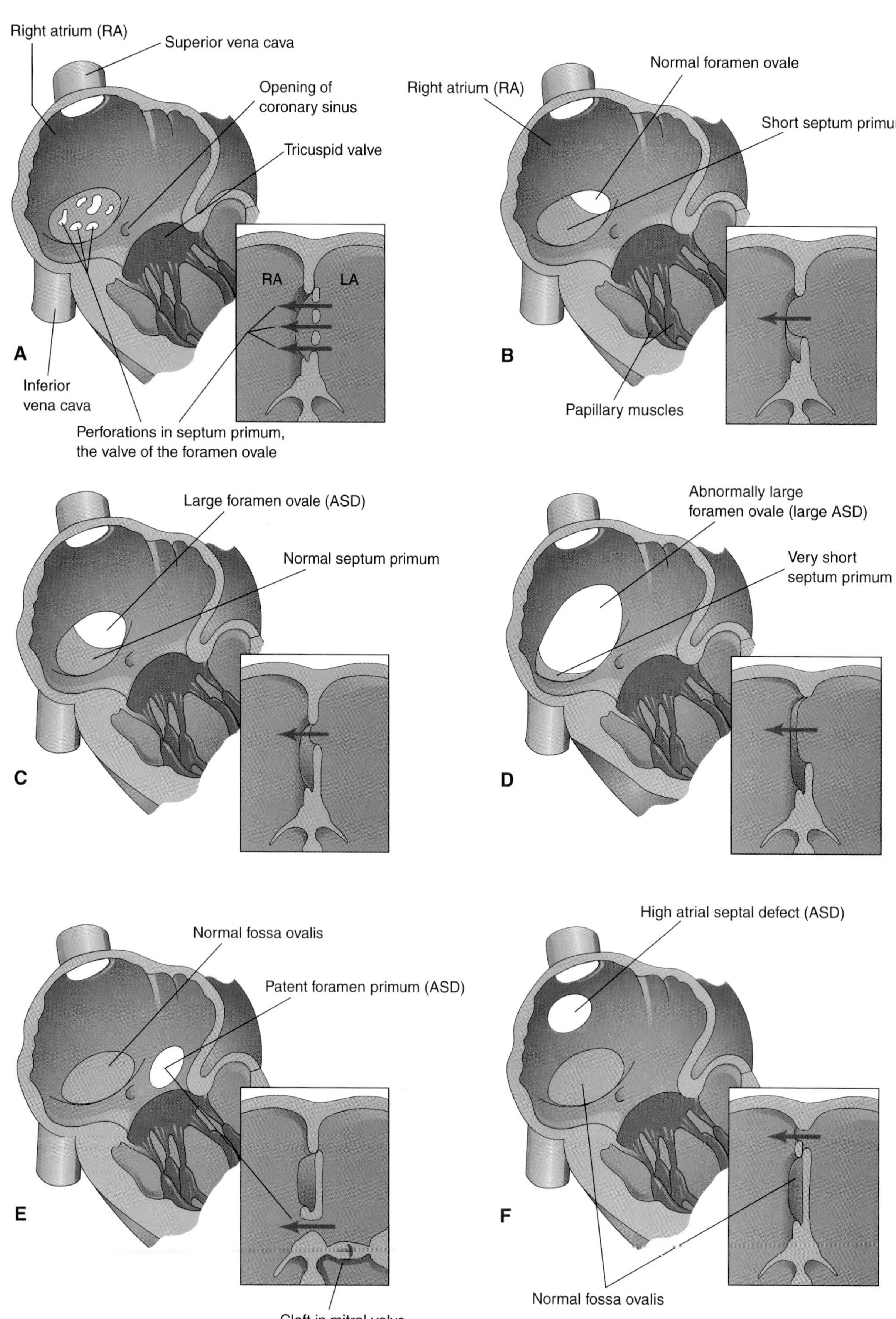

■ **Figure 14–26.** *Legend on opposite page*

Ectopia Cordis

In ectopia cordis, an extremely rare condition, the heart is in an abnormal location (Fig. 14-24). In the thoracic form of ectopia cordis, the heart is partly or completely exposed on the surface of the thorax. It is usually associated with widely separated halves of the sternum and an open pericardial sac. Death occurs in most cases during the first few days after birth, usually from infection, cardiac failure, or hypoxemia (Bernstein, 1996). If there are not severe cardiac defects, surgical therapy usually consists of covering the heart with skin. In some cases of ectopia cordis, the heart protrudes through the diaphragm into the abdomen. The clinical outcome for patients with ectopia cordis has improved and many have survived to adulthood (Hornberger et al., 1996). The most common thoracic form of ectopia cordis results from faulty development of the sternum and pericardium because of failure of complete fusion of the lateral folds in the formation of the thoracic wall during the fourth week.

Atrial Septal Defects

Atrial septal defect (ASD) is a common congenital heart anomaly and occurs more frequently in females than in males. The most common form of ASD is **patent foramen ovale** (Fig. 14-25*B*). A small isolated patent foramen ovale is of no hemodynamic significance; however, if there are other defects (e.g., pulmonary stenosis or atresia), blood is shunted through the foramen ovale into the left atrium and produces **cyanosis**, a dark bluish or purplish coloration of the skin and mucous membranes resulting from deficient oxygenation of the blood.

A **probe patent foramen ovale** is present in up to 25% of people (Fig. 14-25*B*). A probe can be passed from one atrium to the other through the superior part of the floor of the fossa ovalis. This defect, usually small, is not clinically significant, but a probe patent foramen ovale may be forced open because of other cardiac defects and contribute to the functional pathology of the heart. Probe patent foramen ovale results from incomplete adhesion between the original flap of the valve of the foramen ovale and the septum secundum after birth.

There are four clinically significant types of ASD (Figs. 14-26 and 14-27):

- ostium secundum defect
- endocardial cushion defect with ostium primum defect
- sinus venosus defect
- common atrium

The first two types of ASD are relatively common.

Ostium secundum ASDs (Figs. 14-26*A* to *D* and 14-27) are in the area of the fossa ovalis and include both defects of the septum primum and septum secundum. The defects may be multiple and, in symptomatic older children, defects of 2 cm or more in diameter are not unusual (Bernstein, 1996). Females with these defects outnumber males 3:1. Ostium secundum ASDs are one of the most common types of CHD. The patent foramen ovale usually results from abnormal resorption of the septum primum during the formation of the foramen secundum. If resorption occurs in abnormal locations, the septum primum is fenestrated or netlike (Fig. 14-26*A*). If excessive resorption of the septum primum occurs, the resulting short septum primum will not close the foramen ovale (Fig. 14-26*B*). If an abnormally large foramen ovale occurs because of defective development of the septum secundum, a normal septum primum will not close the abnormal foramen ovale at birth (Fig. 14-26*C*). Large ostium secundum ASDs may occur because of a combination of excessive resorption of the septum primum and a large foramen ovale (Figs. 14-26*D* and 14-27). Ostium secundum ASDs are well tolerated during childhood; symptoms such as pulmonary hypertension usually appear in the 30s or later. Closure of the ASD is carried out at open heart surgery and the mortality rate is less than 1% (Bernstein, 1996).

Endocardial cushion and AV septal defects with ostium primum ASDs (Fig. 14-26*E*) are less common forms of ASD. Several cardiac abnormalities are grouped together under this heading because they result from the same developmental defect, a deficiency of the endocardial cushions and the AV septum. The septum primum does not fuse with the endocardial cushions; as a result, there is a **patent foramen primum**. Usually there is also a cleft in the anterior cusp of the mitral valve. In the less common complete type of endocardial cushion and AV septal defects, fusion of the endocardial cushions fails to occur. As a result, there is a large defect in the center of the heart known as an **AV canal** or **AV septal defect** (Fig. 14-28). This type of ASD occurs in about 20% of persons with Down syndrome; otherwise it is a relatively uncommon cardiac defect. It consists of a continuous interatrial and interventricular defect with markedly abnormal AV valves (Bernstein, 1996). This severe cardiac defect can be detected during an ultrasound evaluation of the fetal heart.

All **sinus venosus defects** are located in the superior part of the interatrial septum close to the entry of the SVC (Fig. 14-26*F*). A sinus venosus defect is one of the rarest types of ASD. It results from incomplete absorption of the sinus venosus into the right atrium and/or abnormal development of the septum secundum. This type of ASD is commonly associated with partial anomalous pulmonary venous connections.

■ **Figure 14-26.** Drawings of the right aspect of the interatrial septum (*A* to *F*). The adjacent sketches of sections of the septa illustrate various types of atrial septal defect (ASD). *A,* Patent foramen ovale resulting from resorption of the septum primum in abnormal locations. *B,* Patent foramen ovale caused by excessive resorption of the septum primum ("short flap defect"). *C,* Patent foramen ovale resulting from an abnormally large foramen ovale. *D,* Patent foramen ovale resulting from an abnormally large foramen ovale and excessive resorption of the septum primum. *E,* Endocardial cushion defect with primum-type ASD. The adjacent section shows the cleft in the anterior cusp of the mitral valve. *F,* Sinus venosus ASD. The high septal defect resulted from abnormal absorption of the sinus venosus into the right atrium. In *E* and *F,* note that the fossa ovalis has formed normally.

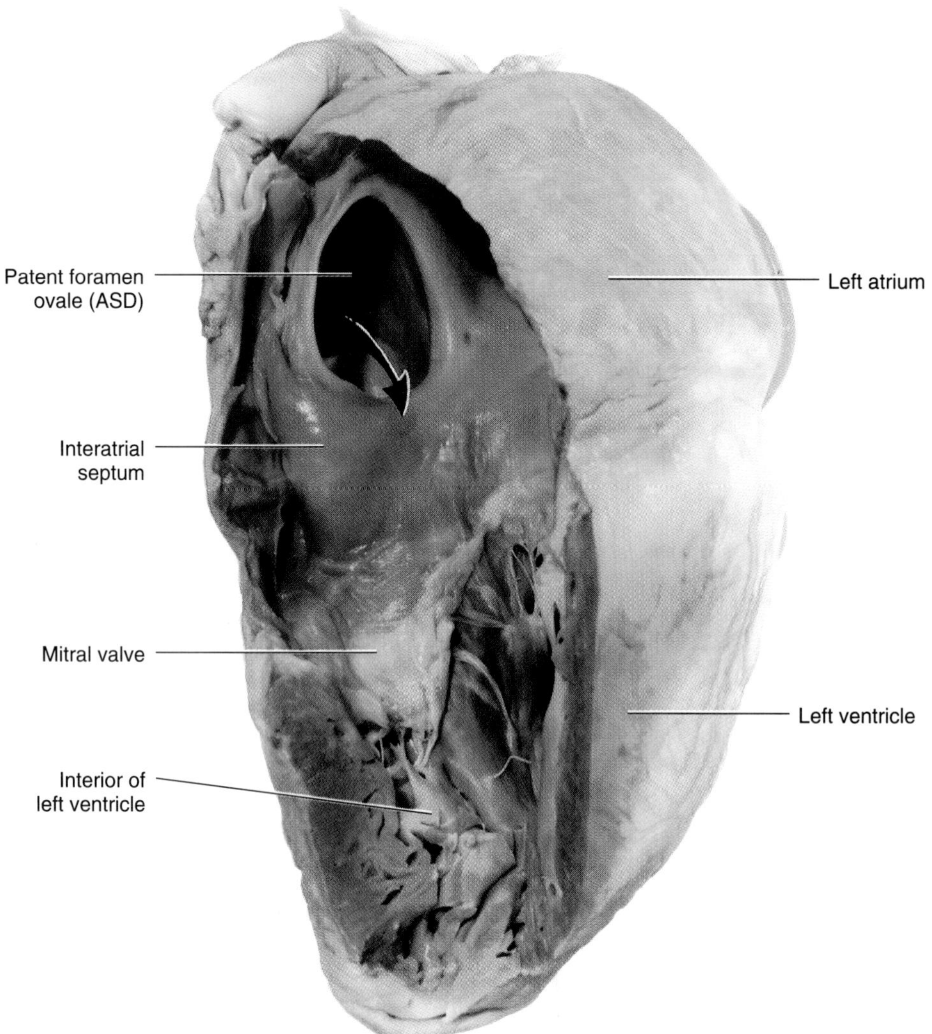

■ **Figure 14–27.** Photograph of a dissection of an adult male heart with a large patent foramen ovale. The arrow passes through a large ASD, which resulted from an abnormally large foramen ovale and excessive resorption of the septum primum. This is referred to as a secundum type ASD and is one of the most common types of CHD. The right ventricle and atrium are enlarged.

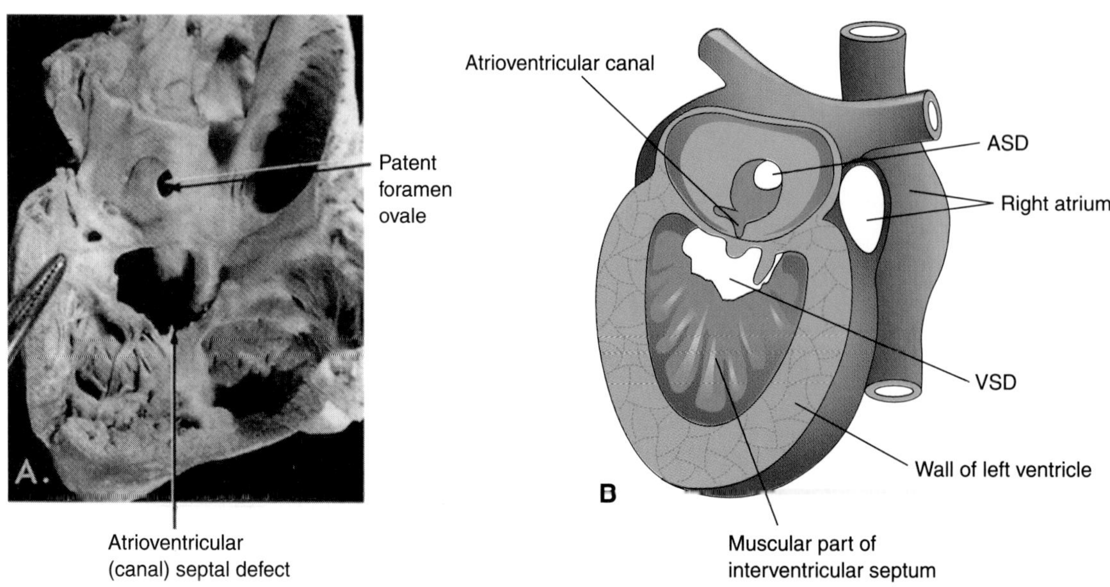

■ **Figure 14–28.** *A,* Photograph of an infant's heart, sectioned and viewed from the right side, showing a patent foramen ovale and an atrioventricular (canal) septal defect. (From Lev M: *Autopsy Diagnosis of Congenitally Malformed Hearts.* Springfield, IL: Charles C Thomas, 1953.) *B,* Schematic drawing of a heart illustrating various septal defects.

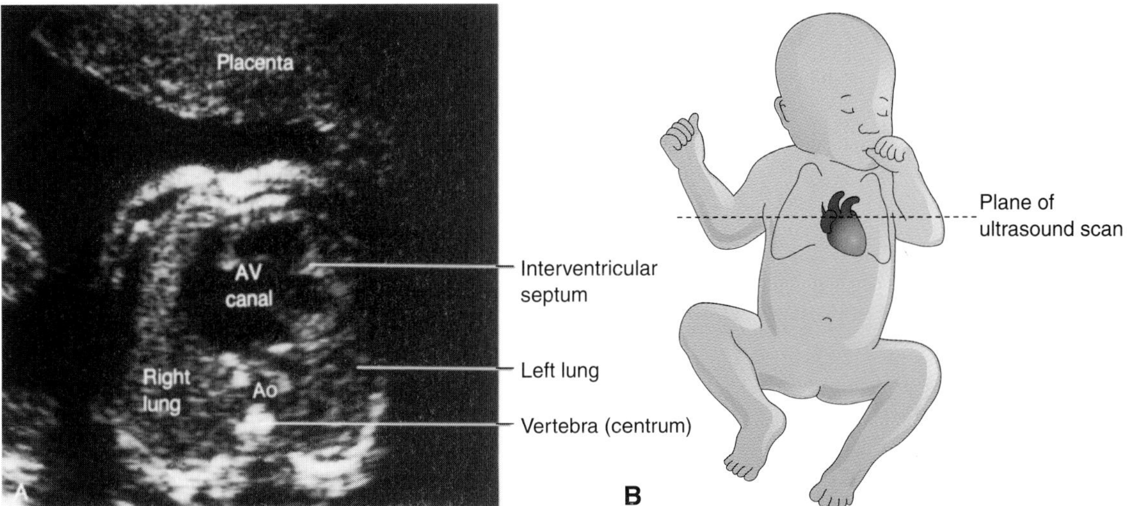

■ **Figure 14–29.** *A,* Ultrasound image of the heart of a second-trimester fetus with an atrioventricular (AV) canal (atrioventricular septal) defect. An ASD and VSD are also present (Ao, aorta.) (Courtesy of B. Benacerraf, MD, Diagnostic Ultrasound Associates, P.C., Boston, MA.) *B,* Orientation drawing.

Common Atrium

Common atrium is a rare cardiac defect in which the interatrial septum is absent. This situation is the result of failure of the septum primum and septum secundum to develop.

Ventricular Septal Defects

Ventricular septal defect (VSD) is the most common type of CHD, accounting for about 25% of defects. VSD occurs more frequently in males than in females. Most VSDs occur in the membranous part of the IV septum (Fig. 14-28); however, they may occur in any part of the IV septum (Bernstein, 1996). Many small VSDs close spontaneously (30-50%), most frequently during the first year. Isolated VSDs are detected at a rate of 10 to 12 per 10,000 between birth and 5 years (Fink, 1985). Most patients with a large VSD have a massive left-to-right shunt of blood. For a full discussion of the complications of VSDs, see Bernstein (1996).

Membranous VSD is the most common type of VSD (Figs. 14-28*B* and 14-29*A* and *B*). Incomplete closure of the IV foramen results from failure of the membranous part of the IV septum to develop. It also arises from failure of an extension of subendocardial tissue to grow from the right side of the endocardial cushion and fuse with the aorticopulmonary septum and the muscular part of the IV septum (Fig. 14-18*C* to *E*). Large VSDs with excessive pulmonary blood flow (Fig. 14-30) and pulmonary hypertension result in dyspnea (difficult breathing) and cardiac failure early in infancy (Bernstein, 1996).

Muscular VSD is a less common type of defect and may appear anywhere in the muscular part of the interventricular septum. Sometimes there are multiple small defects, producing the **Swiss cheese VSD**. Mus-

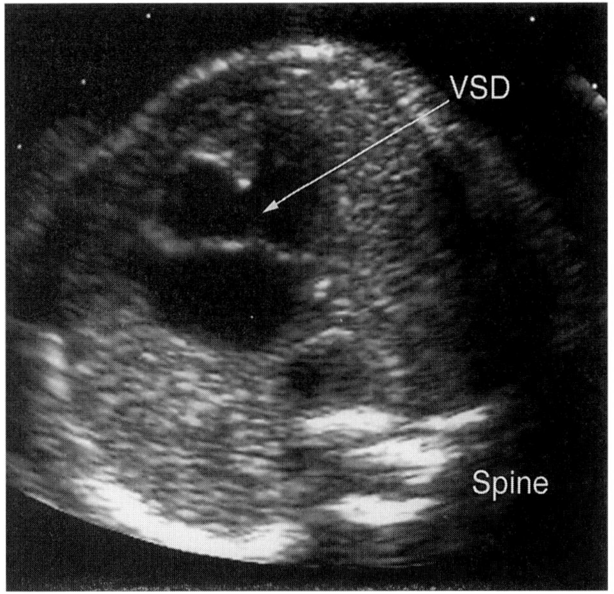

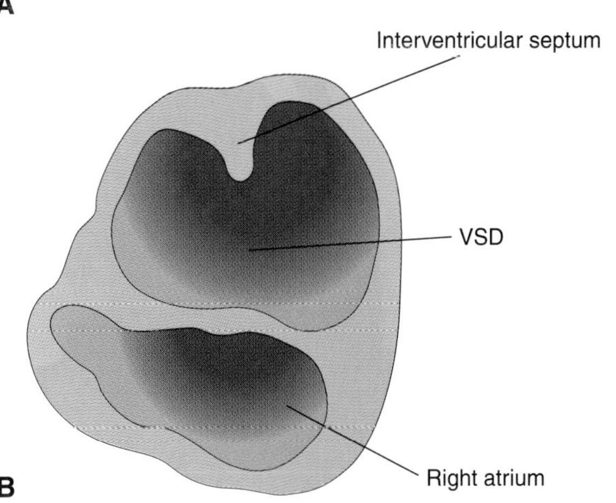

■ **Figure 14–30.** Ultrasound scan of a fetal heart at 23.4 weeks' gestation with an atrioventricular septal defect and a large VSD. (Courtesy of Wesley Lee, MD, Division of Fetal Imaging, William Beaumont Hospital, Royal Oak, Michigan.)

cular VSDs probably occur because of excessive cavitation of myocardial tissue during formation of the ventricular walls and the muscular part of the interventricular septum.

Absence of the IV septum—**single ventricle or common ventricle**—resulting from failure of the IV septum to form, is extremely rare and results in a three-chambered heart (cor triloculare biatriatum). When there is a single ventricle, both atria empty through a common valve or two separate AV valves into a single ventricular chamber. The aorta and pulmonary trunk arise from the single ventricle. **Transposition of the great arteries** (see Fig. 14-32) and a rudimentary outlet chamber are present in most infants with this severe CHD. Some patients die during infancy from congestive heart failure, but others survive until early adult life. For discussion of the treatment of this defect, see Bernstein (1996).

Truncus Arteriosus

Truncus arteriosus (TA) or **persistent TA** results from failure of the truncal ridges and aorticopulmonary septum to develop normally and divide the truncus arteriosus into the aorta and pulmonary trunk (Fig. 14-31). In this anomaly a single arterial trunk, the TA, arises from the heart and supplies the systemic, pulmonary, and coronary circulations (Bernstein, 1996). A VSD is always present with the TA anomaly and the TA overrides the VSD (Fig 14-31*B*). Recent studies indicate that developmental arrest of the outflow tract, semilunar valves, and aortic sac in the early embryo (Carnegie stage 14, days 31-32) is involved in the pathogenesis of TA anomalies. The etiology of this condition is largely unknown (Yu and Hutchins, 1996). The most common type of TA is a single arterial vessel that

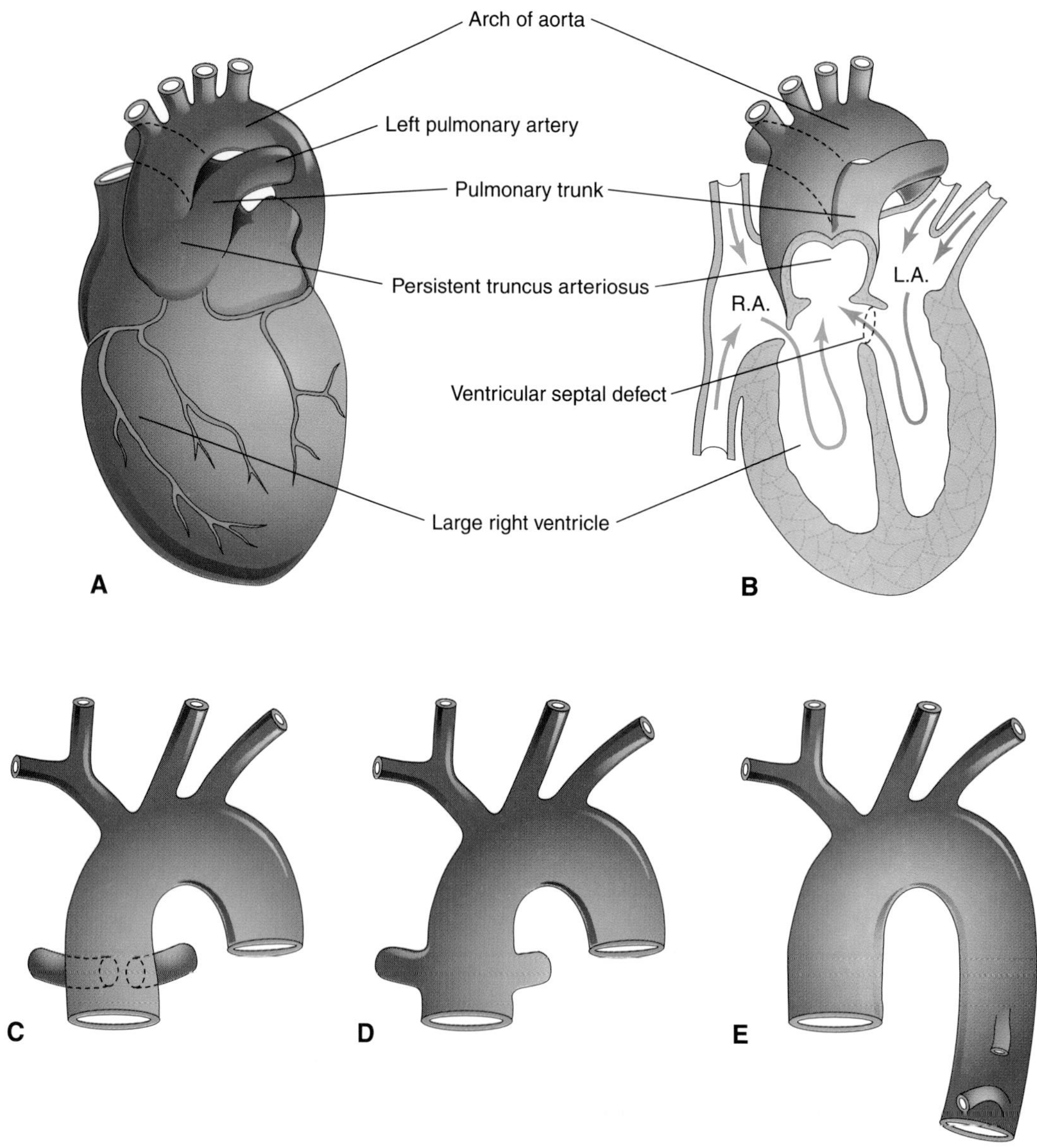

■ **Figure 14-31.** Drawings illustrating the main types of persistent truncus arteriosus. *A,* The common trunk divides into the aorta and a short pulmonary trunk. *B,* Coronal section of the heart shown in *A.* Observe the circulation in this heart *(arrows)* and the VSD. *C,* The right and left pulmonary arteries arise close together from the truncus arteriosus. *D,* The pulmonary arteries arise independently from the sides of the truncus arteriosus. *E,* No pulmonary arteries are present; the lungs are supplied by the bronchial arteries.

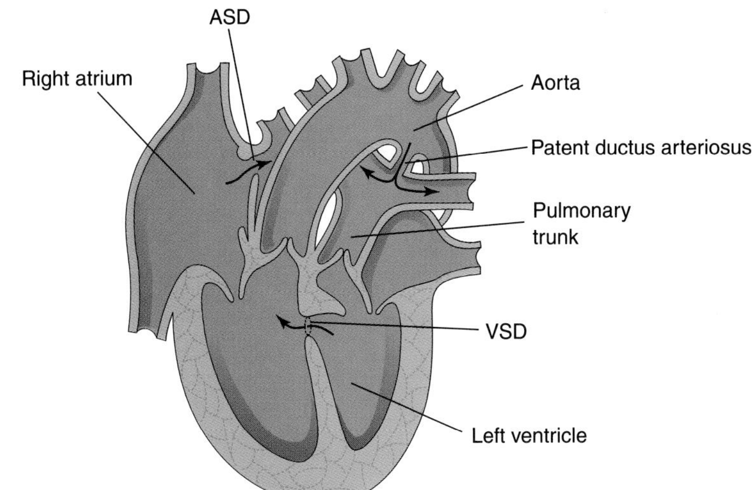

■ **Figure 14–32.** Diagram of a malformed heart illustrating transposition of the great arteries (TGA). The ventricular and atrial septal defects allow mixing of the arterial and venous blood. TGA is the most common single cause of cyanotic heart disease in newborn infants. As here, it is often associated with other cardiac anomalies (VSD and ASD).

branches to form the pulmonary trunk and ascending aorta (Fig. 14–31*A* and *B*). In the next most common type, the right and left pulmonary arteries arise close together from the dorsal wall of the TA (Fig. 14–31*C*). Less common types are illustrated in Figure 14–31*D* and *E*.

Aorticopulmonary Septal Defect

Aorticopulmonary septal defect is a rare condition in which there is an opening (*aortic window*) between the aorta and pulmonary trunk near the aortic valve (**aorticopulmonary window defect**). This defect is a result of a localized defect in the formation of the aorticopulmonary septum. The presence of pulmonary and aortic valves and an intact IV septum distinguishes this anomaly from the TA defect (Bernstein, 1996).

Transposition of the Great Arteries

Transposition of the great arteries (TGA) is the most common cause of **cyanotic heart disease** in newborn infants (Fig. 14–32). TGA is often associated with other cardiac anomalies. In typical cases the aorta lies anterior and to the right of the pulmonary trunk and arises anteriorly from the morphological right ventricle, and the pulmonary trunk arises from the morphological left ventricle. There is also an *ASD* with or without an associated *patent ductus arteriosus* (PDA) (see Fig. 14–33*A* and *B*) and VSD. These associated defects permit some interchange between the pulmonary and systemic circulations. Because of these anatomical abnormalities, deoxygenated systemic venous blood returning to the right atrium enters the right ventricle and then passes to the body through the aorta. Oxygenated pulmonary venous blood passes through the left ventricle back into the pulmonary

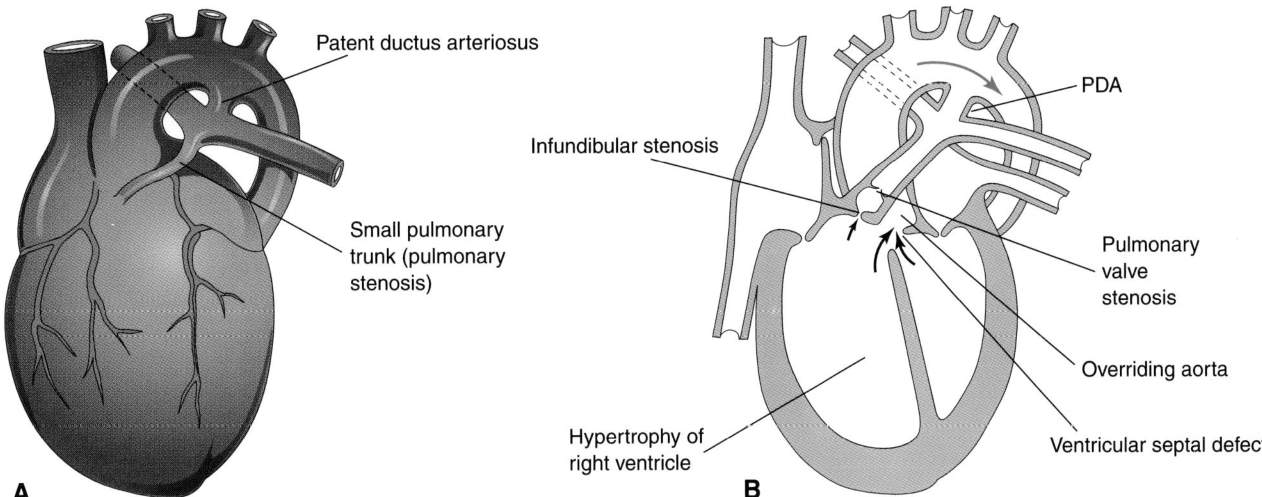

■ **Figure 14–33.** *A,* Drawing of an infant's heart, showing a small pulmonary trunk (pulmonary stenosis) and a large aorta resulting from unequal partitioning of the truncus arteriosus. There is also hypertrophy of the right ventricle and a PDA. *B,* Frontal section of a heart illustrating tetralogy of Fallot. Observe the four cardiac deformities: pulmonary valve stenosis, VSD, overriding aorta, and hypertrophy of the right ventricle. In this case, there is also infundibular stenosis.

circulation. Because of the patent foramen ovale, there is some mixing of the blood; without surgical correction of the transposition, these infants usually die within a few months.

Many attempts have been made to explain the embryological basis of TGA, but the **conal growth hypothesis** is favored by many investigators. According to this explanation, the aorticopulmonary septum fails to pursue a spiral course during partitioning of the bulbus cordis and TA. This defect is thought to result from failure of the conus arteriosus to develop normally during incorporation of the bulbus cordis into the ventricles.

Unequal Division of the Truncus Arteriosus

Unequal division of the truncus arteriosus (Figs. 14-33*A* and 14-34*B* and *C*) results when partitioning of the TA superior to the valves is unequal; one great artery is large and the other small. As a result, the aorticopulmonary septum is not aligned with the IV septum and a VSD results. The larger vessel (aorta or pulmonary trunk) usually straddles (overrides) the VSD (Fig. 14-33*B*). In **pulmonary valve stenosis**, the

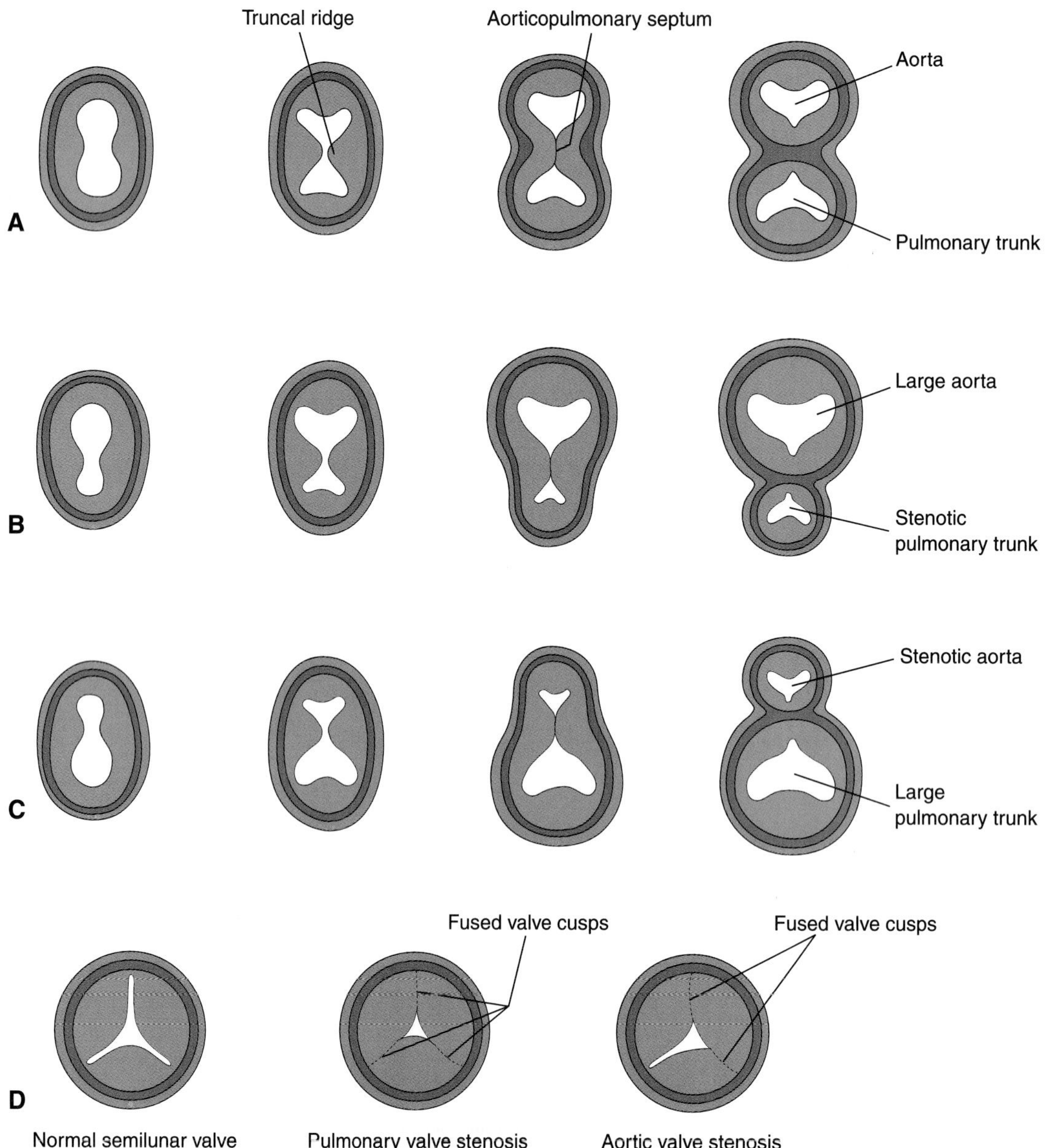

■ **Figure 14–34.** Abnormal division of the truncus arteriosus (TA). *A* to *C*, Sketches of transverse sections of the TA illustrating normal and abnormal partitioning of the TA. *A*, Normal. *B*, Unequal partitioning of the TA resulting in a small pulmonary trunk. *C*, Unequal partitioning resulting in a small aorta. *D*, Sketches illustrating a normal semilunar valve and stenotic pulmonary and aortic valves.

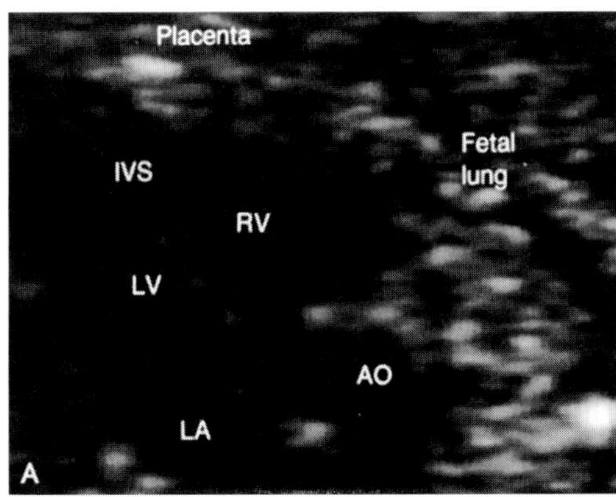

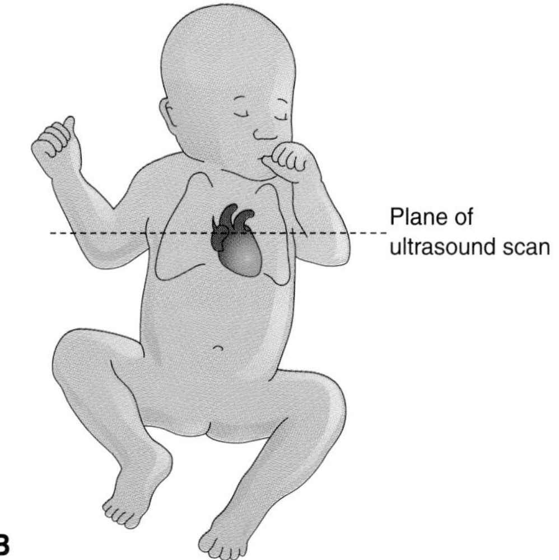

■ **Figure 14–35.** *A,* Ultrasound image of the heart of a 20-week fetus with tetralogy of Fallot. Note that the large overriding aorta **(AO)** straddles the interventricular septum. As a result it receives blood from the left **(LV)** and right **(RV)** ventricles. (IVS, interventricular septum; LA, left atrium.) (Courtesy of B. Benacerraf, MD, Diagnostic Ultrasound Associates, P.C., Boston, MA.) *B,* Orientation drawing.

cusps of the pulmonary valve are fused to form a dome with a narrow central opening (Fig. 14-34*D*). In **infundibular stenosis**, the conus arteriosus (infundibulum) of the right ventricle is underdeveloped. The two types of pulmonary stenosis may occur together. Depending upon the degree of obstruction to blood flow, there is a variable degree of hypertrophy of the right ventricle (Fig. 14-33*A* and *B*).

Tetralogy of Fallot

This classic group of four cardiac defects (Figs. 14-33*B*, 14-35, and 14-36) consists of :

- pulmonary stenosis (obstruction to right ventricular outflow)
- ventricular septal defect (VSD)
- dextroposition of aorta (overriding aorta)
- right ventricular hypertrophy

The pulmonary trunk is usually small (Fig. 14-33*A*), and there may be various degrees of pulmonary artery stenoses as well (Bernstein, 1996). **Cyanosis** is one of the obvious signs of tetralogy, but it is not often present at birth.

Pulmonary Atresia

This anomaly results when division of the truncus arteriosus is so unequal that the pulmonary trunk has no lumen, or there is no orifice at the level of the pulmonary valve. Pulmonary atresia may or may not be associated with a VSD. Pulmonary atresia with VSD is an extreme form of tetralogy of Fallot. The entire right ventricular output is through the aorta. Pulmonary blood flow is dependent on a PDA or on bronchial collateral vessels. If the pulmonary arteries are severely hypoplastic, **heart-lung transplantation** may be the only therapy (Bernstein, 1996).

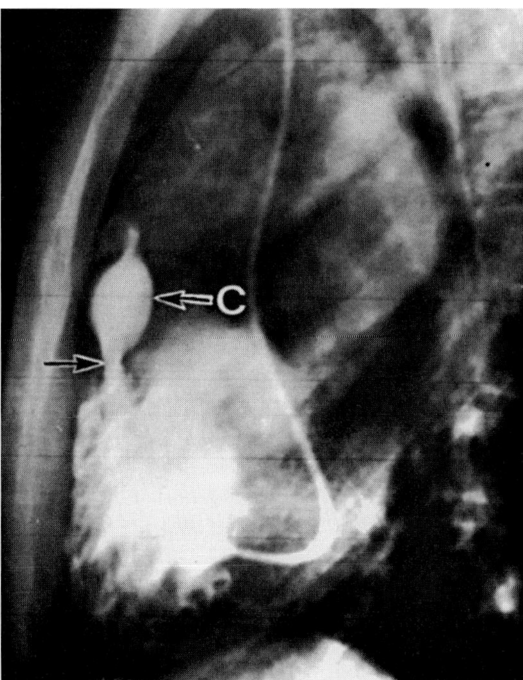

■ **Figure 14–36.** Lateral view of a selective right ventriculogram in a patient with tetralogy of Fallot. The arrows point to an infundibular stenosis that is below the infundibular chamber **(C)**. (From Bernstein D: Cyanotic congenital heart disease. *In* Behrman RE, Kliegman RM, Arvin AM [eds]: *Nelson Textbook of Pediatrics,* 15th ed. Philadelphia, WB Saunders, 1996.)

Aortic Stenosis and Atresia

In **aortic valve stenosis**, the edges of the valve are usually fused to form a dome with a narrow opening (Fig. 14-34*D*). This anomaly may be present at birth (congenital) or it may develop after birth (acquired). The valvular stenosis causes extra work for the heart and results in hypertrophy of the left ventricle and abnormal heart sounds (**heart murmurs**). In *subaortic stenosis*, there is often a band of fibrous tissue just inferior to the aortic valve. The narrowing of the aorta results from persistence of tissue that normally degenerates as the valve forms. Aortic atresia is present when obstruction of the aorta or its valve is complete.

Hypoplastic Left Heart Syndrome

The left ventricle is small and nonfunctional (Fig. 14-37); the right ventricle maintains both pulmonary and systemic circulations (Bernstein, 1996). The blood passes through an ASD or a dilated foramen ovale from the left to the right side of the heart, where it mixes with the systemic venous blood. In addition to the underdevelopment of the left side of the heart, there is atresia of the aortic or mitral orifice and hypoplasia of the ascending aorta. Infants with this severe anomaly usually die during the first few weeks after birth. *Disturbances in the migration of neural crest cells* (Leatherbury and Kirby, 1996), in hemodynamic function, in cell death, and in the proliferation of the extracellular matrix are likely responsible for the pathogenesis of many CHDs (Clarke, 1986).

AORTIC ARCH DERIVATIVES

As the pharyngeal arches develop during the fourth week, they are supplied by arteries—the **aortic arches**—from the *aortic sac*, the homolog of the ventral aorta in other mammals (Fig. 14-38*B*). The aortic arches terminate in the dorsal aorta of the ipsilateral side. Although six pairs of aortic arches usually develop, they are not all present at the same time. By the time the sixth pair of aortic arches has formed, the first two pairs have disappeared (Fig. 14-38*C*). During the sixth to eighth weeks, the primordial aortic arch pattern is transformed into the adult arterial arrangement.

Derivatives of the First Pair of Aortic Arches

These arteries largely disappear but the remaining parts form the **maxillary arteries**, which supply the ears, teeth, and muscles of the eye and face. These aortic arches may also contribute to the formation of the **external carotid arteries**.

Derivatives of the Second Pair of Aortic Arches

Dorsal parts of these vessels persist and form the stems of the **stapedial arteries**, which are small vessels that run through the ring of the stapes, a small ear bone, in the embryo.

Derivatives of the Third Pair of Aortic Arches

Proximal parts of these arteries form the **common carotid arteries**, which supply structures in the head.

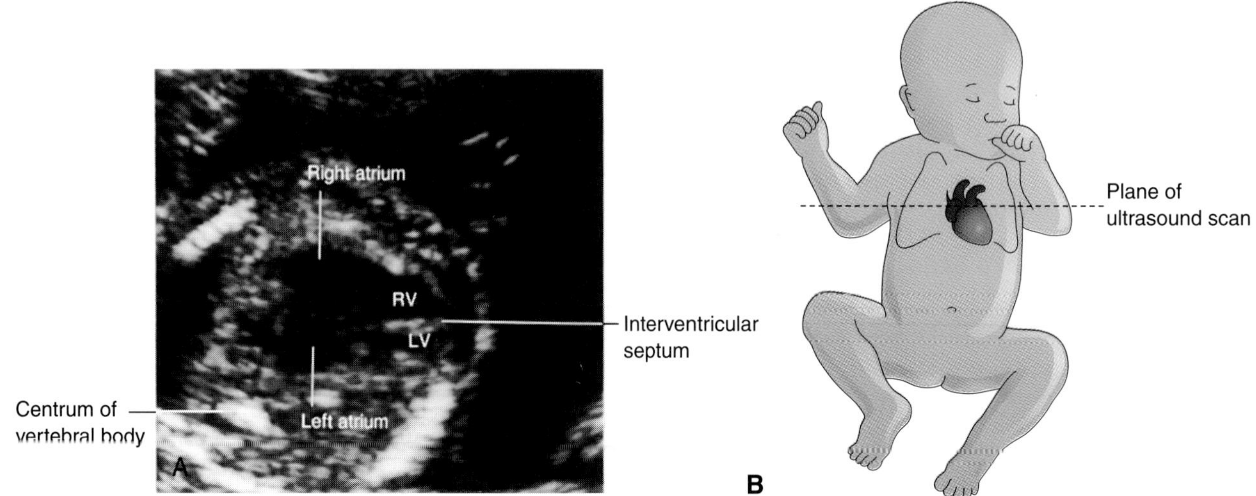

■ **Figure 14-37.** *A,* Ultrasound image of the heart of a second-trimester fetus with a hypoplastic left heart. Note that the left ventricle **(LV)** is much smaller than the right ventricle **(RV)**. This is an oblique scan of the fetal thorax through the long axis of the ventricles. (Courtesy of B. Benacerraf, MD, Diagnostic Ultrasound Associates, P.C., Boston, MA.) *B,* Orientation drawing.

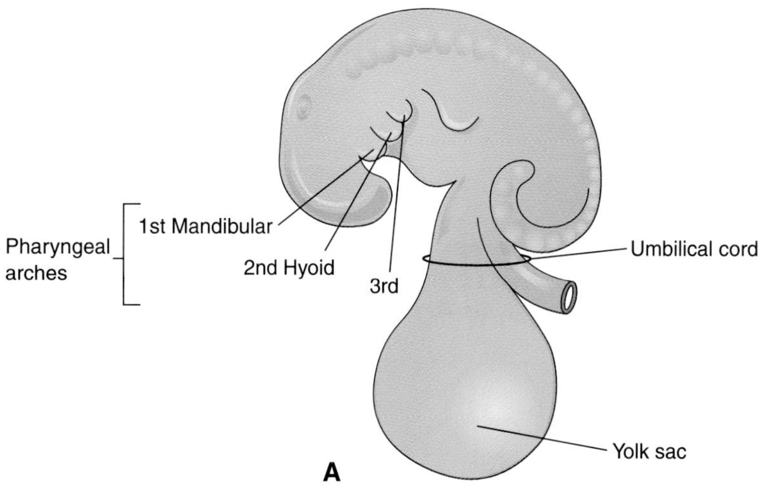

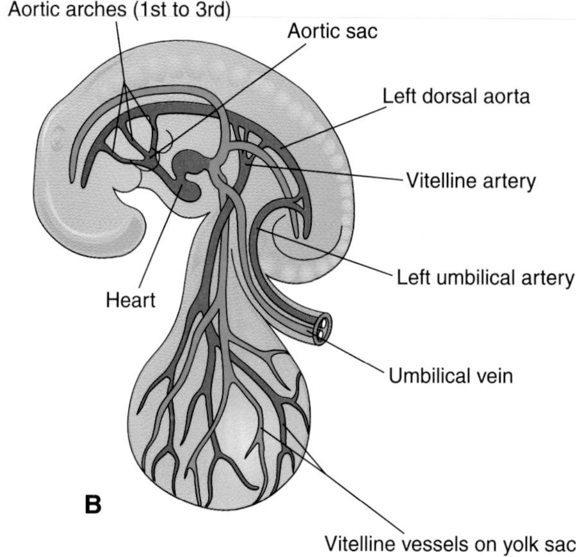

■ **Figure 14–38.** Drawings illustrating the pharyngeal arches and aortic arches. *A,* Left side of an embryo (about 26 days). *B,* Schematic drawing of this embryo, showing the left aortic arches arising from the aortic sac, running through the pharyngeal arches, and terminating in the left dorsal aorta. *C,* An embryo (about 37 days), showing the single dorsal aorta and that most of the first two pairs of aortic arches have degenerated.

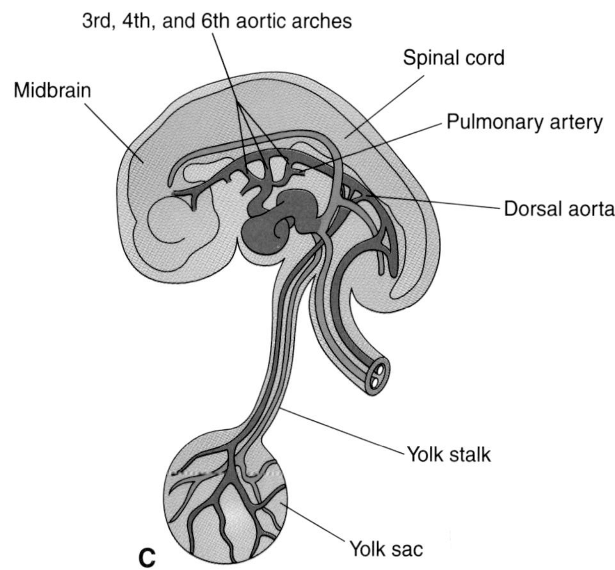

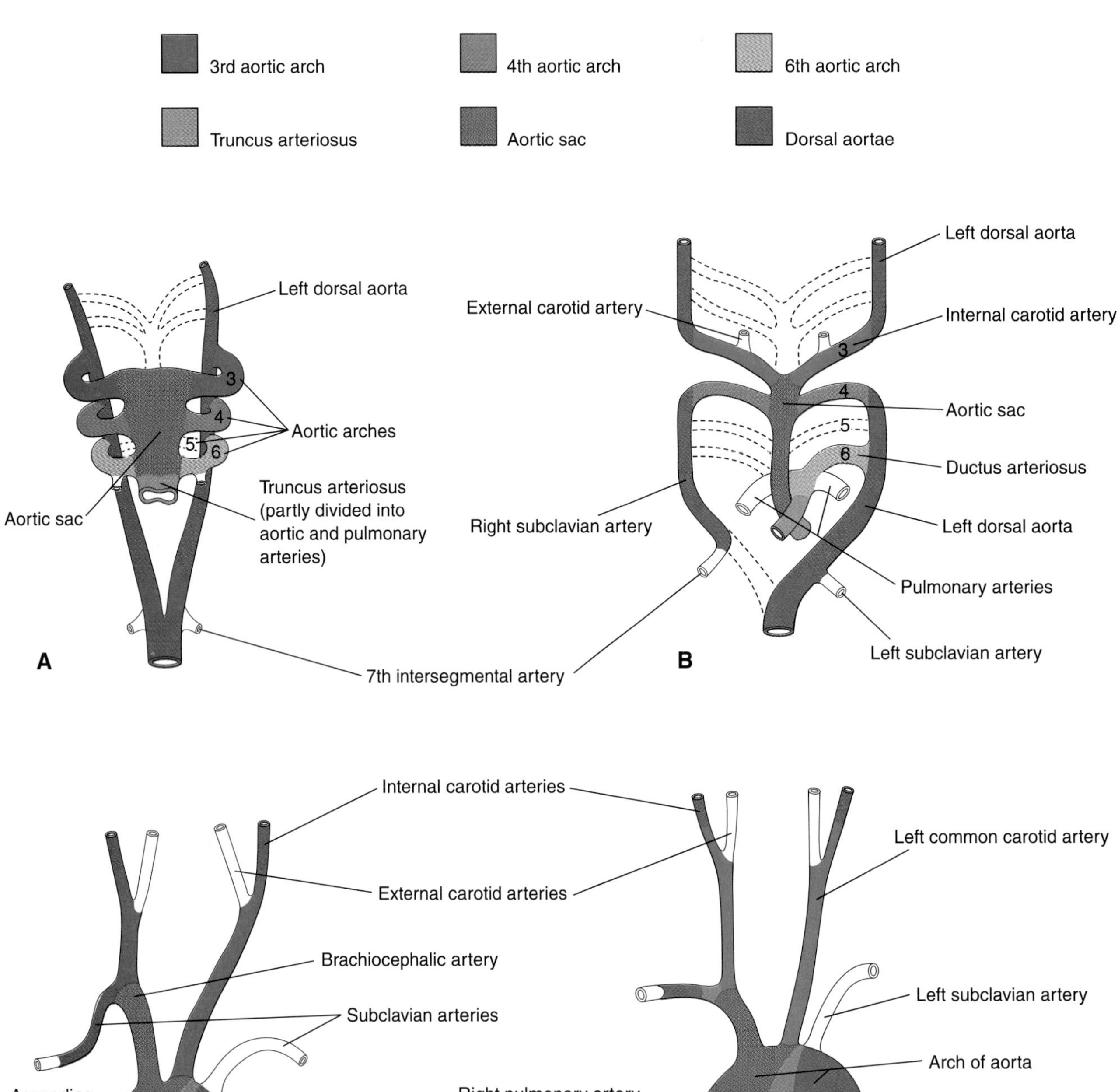

■ **Figure 14–39.** Schematic drawings illustrating the arterial changes that result during transformation of the truncus arteriosus, aortic sac, aortic arches, and dorsal aortae into the adult arterial pattern. The vessels that are not colored are not derived from these structures. *A,* Aortic arches at 6 weeks; by this stage the first two pairs of aortic arches have largely disappeared. *B,* Aortic arches at 7 weeks; the parts of the dorsal aortae and aortic arches that normally disappear are indicated with broken lines. *C,* Arterial arrangement at 8 weeks. *D,* Sketch of the arterial vessels of a 6-month-old infant. Note that the ascending aorta and pulmonary arteries are considerably smaller in *C* than in *D.* This represents the relative flow through these vessels at the different stages of development. Observe the large size of the ductus arteriosus (DA) in *C,* and that it is essentially a direct continuation of the pulmonary trunk. The DA normally becomes functionally closed within the first few days after birth. Eventually the DA becomes the ligamentum arteriosum, as shown in *D.*

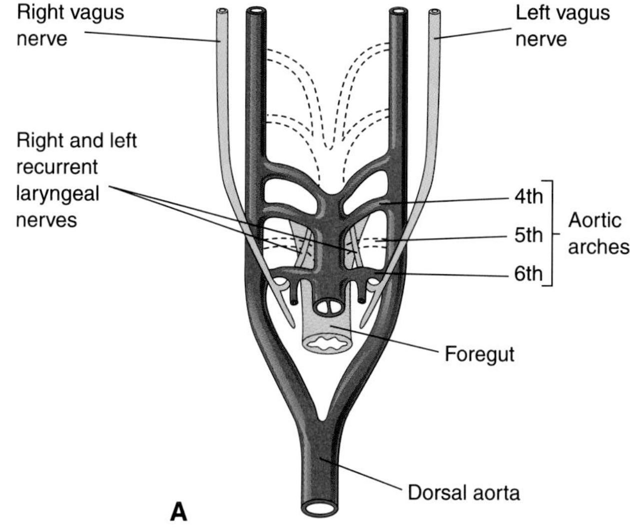

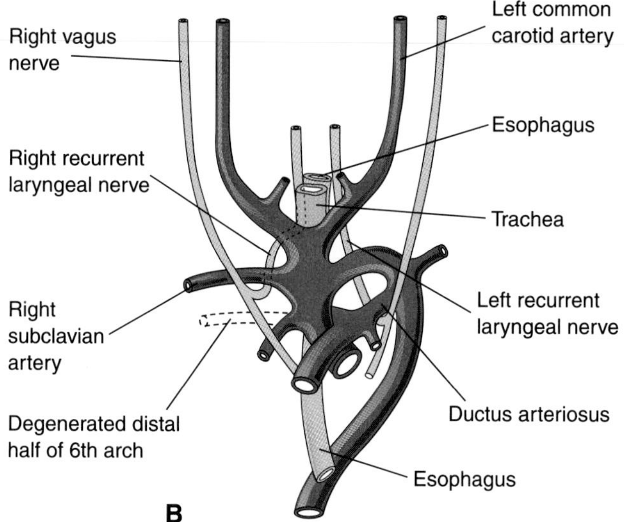

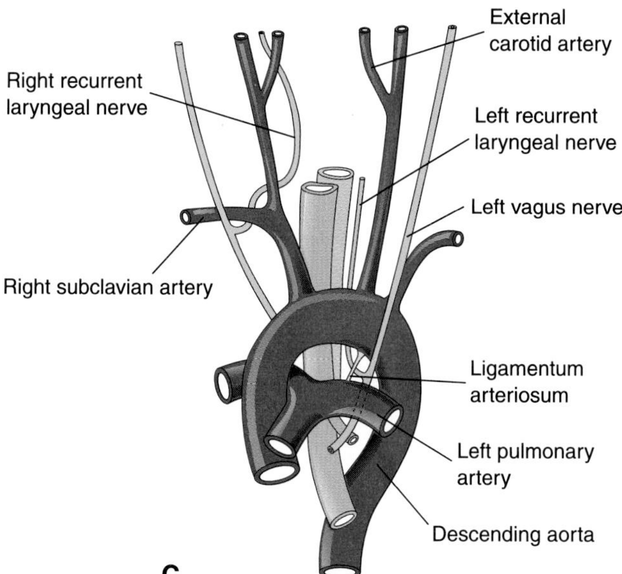

Distal parts of the third pair of aortic arches join with the dorsal aortae to form the **internal carotid arteries**, which supply the ears, orbits, brain and its meninges (protective membranes for the brain).

Derivatives of the Fourth Pair of Aortic Arches

The **left fourth aortic arch** forms part of the arch of the aorta (Fig. 14-39*C*). The proximal part of the arch develops from the aortic sac and the distal part is derived from the left dorsal aorta.

The **right fourth aortic arch** becomes the proximal part of the **right subclavian artery**. The distal part of the subclavian artery forms from the right dorsal aorta and right seventh intersegmental artery. The left subclavian artery is not derived from an aortic arch; it forms from the left seventh intersegmental artery (Fig. 14-39*A*). As development proceeds, differential growth shifts the origin of the left subclavian artery cranially; consequently, it comes to lie close to the origin of the left common carotid artery (Fig. 14-39*D*).

Derivatives of the Fifth Pair of Aortic Arches

In about 50% of embryos the fifth pair of aortic arches are rudimentary vessels that soon degenerate, leaving no vascular derivatives. In other embryos, these arteries do not develop.

Derivatives of the Sixth Pair of Aortic Arches

The **left sixth aortic arch** develops as follows (Fig. 14-39*B* and *C*):

- The proximal part of the arch persists as the proximal part of the **left pulmonary artery**.
- The distal part of the arch passes from the left pulmonary artery to the dorsal aorta to form a prenatal shunt, the **ductus arteriosus**.

The **right sixth aortic arch** develops as follows:

- The proximal part of the arch persists as the proximal part of the **right pulmonary artery**.
- The distal part of the arch degenerates.

The transformation of the sixth pair of aortic arches explains why the course of the **recurrent laryngeal nerves** differs on the two sides. These nerves supply the sixth pair of pharyngeal arches and hook around the sixth pair of aortic arches on their way to the developing larynx (Fig. 14-40*A*). **On the right**, be-

■ **Figure 14–40.** Diagrams showing the relation of the recurrent laryngeal nerves to the aortic arches. *A,* 6 weeks, showing the recurrent laryngeal nerves hooked around the sixth pair of aortic arches. *B,* 8 weeks showing the right recurrent laryngeal nerve hooked around the right subclavian artery, and the left recurrent laryngeal nerve hooked around the ductus arteriosus and arch of the aorta. *C,* Child, showing the left recurrent laryngeal nerve hooked around the ligamentum arteriosum and arch of the aorta.

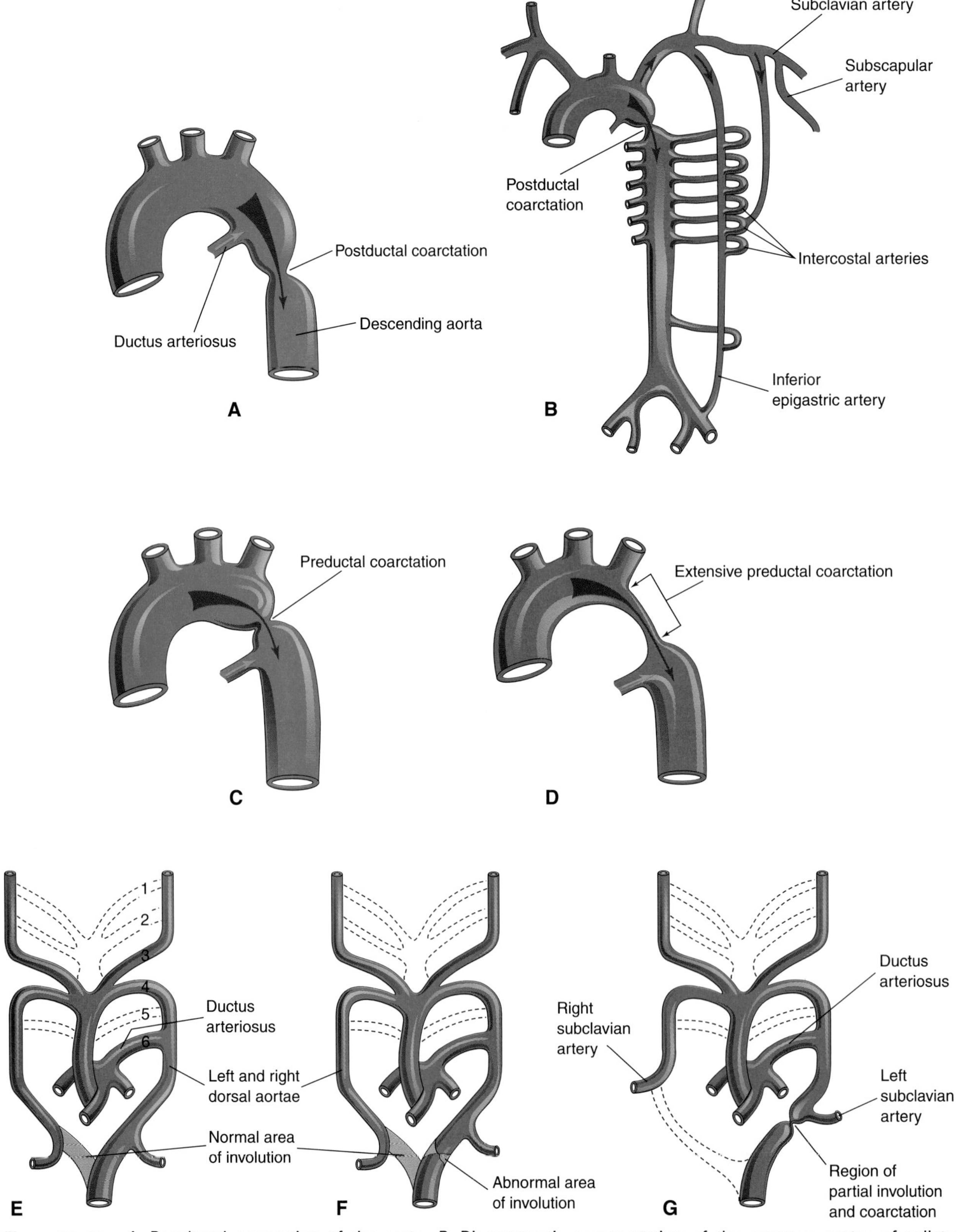

■ **Figure 14–41.** *A,* Postductal coarctation of the aorta. *B,* Diagrammatic representation of the common routes of collateral circulation that develop in association with postductal coarctation of the aorta. *C* and *D,* Preductal coarctation. *E,* Sketch of the aortic arch pattern in a 7-week embryo, showing the areas that normally involute. Note that the distal segment of the right dorsal aorta normally involutes as the right subclavian artery develops. *F,* Abnormal involution of a small distal segment of the left dorsal aorta. *G,* Later stage, showing the abnormally involuted segment appearing as a coarctation of the aorta. This moves to the region of the ductus arteriosus with the left subclavian artery. These drawings (*E* to *G*) illustrate one hypothesis about the embryological basis of coarctation of the aorta.

cause the distal part of the right sixth aortic arch degenerates, the right recurrent laryngeal nerve moves superiorly and hooks around the proximal part of the right subclavian artery, the derivative of the fourth aortic arch (Fig. 14-40*B*). **On the left**, the left recurrent laryngeal nerve hooks around the ductus arteriosus (DA) formed by the distal part of the sixth aortic arch. When this vessel involutes after birth, the nerve hooks around the *ligamentum arteriosum* (remnant of DA), and the arch of the aorta (Fig. 14-40*C*).

AORTIC ARCH ANOMALIES

Because of the many changes involved in transformation of the embryonic pharyngeal arch system of arteries into the adult arterial pattern, it is understandable why anomalies may occur. Most irregularities result from the persistence of parts of aortic arches that usually disappear, or from disappearance of parts that normally persist.

Coarctation of the Aorta

Aortic coarctation (constriction) occurs in about 10% of children and adults with congenital heart diseases (Tikkanen and Heinonen, 1993). Coarctation is characterized by a constriction of varying length of the aorta (Fig. 14-41). Most constrictions of the aorta occur distal to the origin of the left subclavian artery at the entrance of the ductus arteriosus (**juxtaductal coarctation**). The classification into preductal and postductal coarctations is commonly used; however, in 90% of instances, the coarctation is directly opposite the ductus arteriosus (Bernstein, 1996). Coarctation of the aorta occurs twice as often in males as in females, and is associated with a bicuspid aortic valve in 70% of cases.

In **postductal coarctation** (Fig. 14-41*A* and *B*), the constriction is just distal to the ductus arteriosus (DA). This permits development of a collateral circulation during the fetal period (Fig. 14-41*B*), thereby assisting with passage of blood to inferior parts of the body. In **preductal coarctation** (Fig. 14-41*C*), the fetal prototype, the constriction is proximal to the DA. The narrowed segment may be extensive (Fig. 14-41*D*); before birth, blood flows through the DA to the descending aorta for distribution to the lower body.

In an infant with severe aortic coarctation, closure of the DA results in hypoprofusion and rapid deterioration. These patients are usually infused with prostaglandin E_2, in an attempt to reopen the DA and establish an adequate blood flow to the lower limbs (Bernstein, 1996). The causes of coarctation of the aorta are not clearly understood (Tikkanen and Heinonen, 1993), a statement that is denied by Hutchins (1993). Aortic coarctation may be a feature of Turner syndrome (see Chapter 8). This and other observations suggest that genetic and/or environmental factors cause coarctation. There are three main views about the embryological basis of coarctation of the aorta:

- During formation of the arch of the aorta, muscle tissue of the ductus arteriosus may be incorporated into the wall of the aorta; then, when the DA contracts at birth, the ductal muscle in the aorta also contracts, forming a coarctation.
- There may be abnormal involution of a small seg-

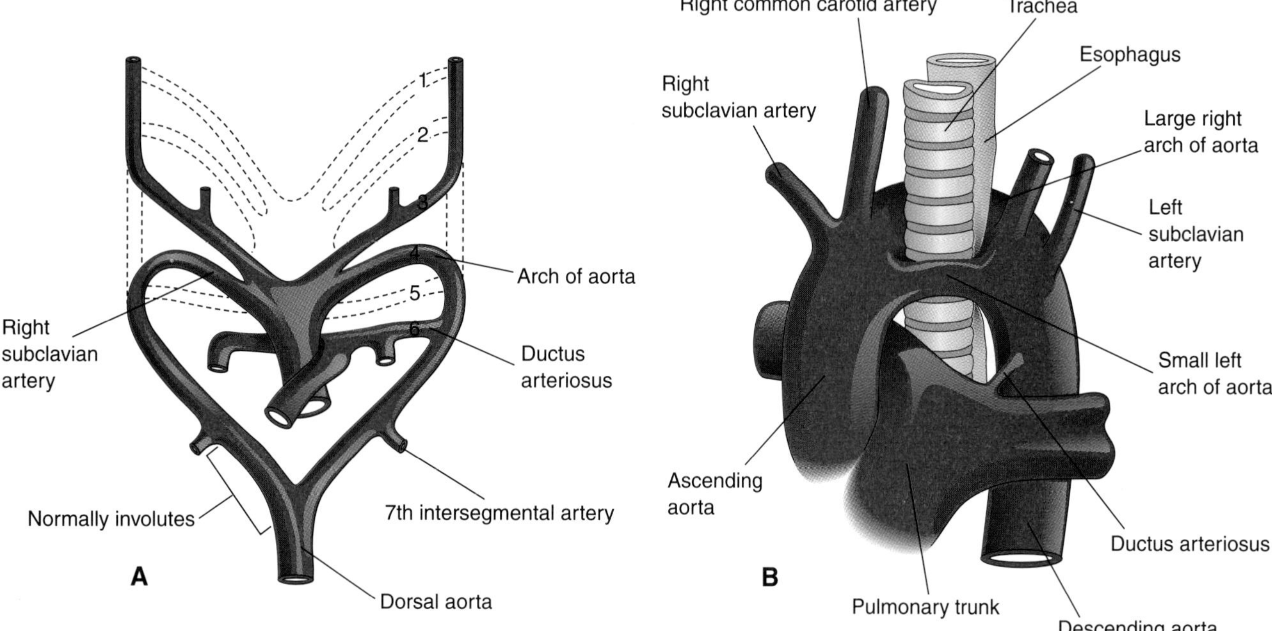

■ **Figure 14-42.** *A,* Drawing of the embryonic aortic arches illustrating the embryological basis of double aortic arch. The distal portion of the right dorsal aorta persists and forms a right aortic arch. *B,* A large right aortic arch and a small left aortic arch arise from the ascending aorta and form a vascular ring around the trachea and esophagus. Note that there is compression of the esophagus and trachea. The right common carotid and subclavian arteries arise separately from the large right arch of the aorta.

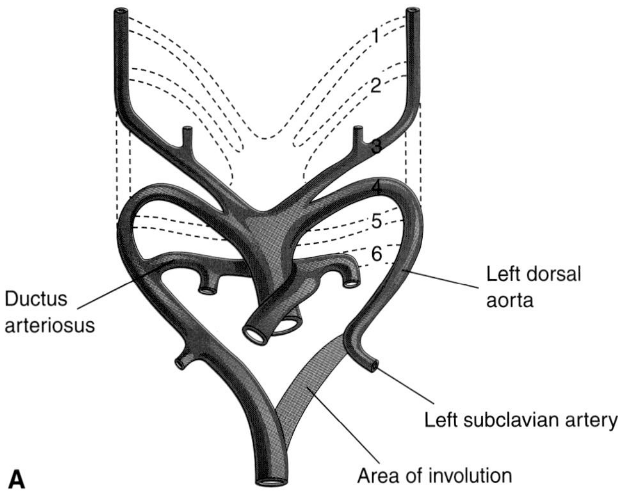

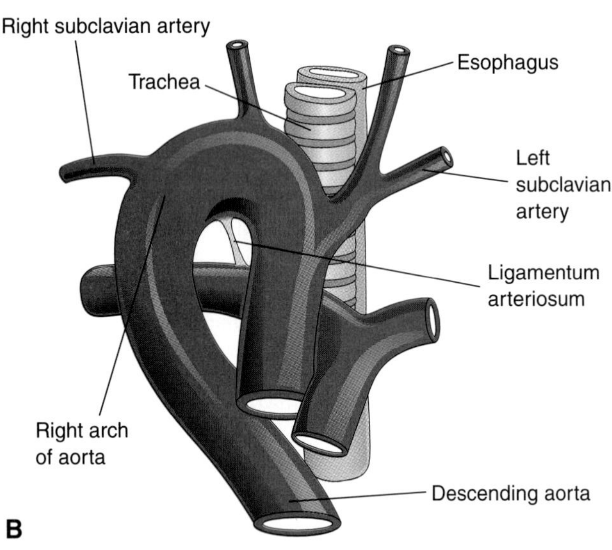

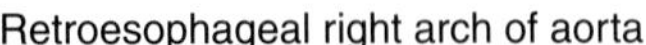

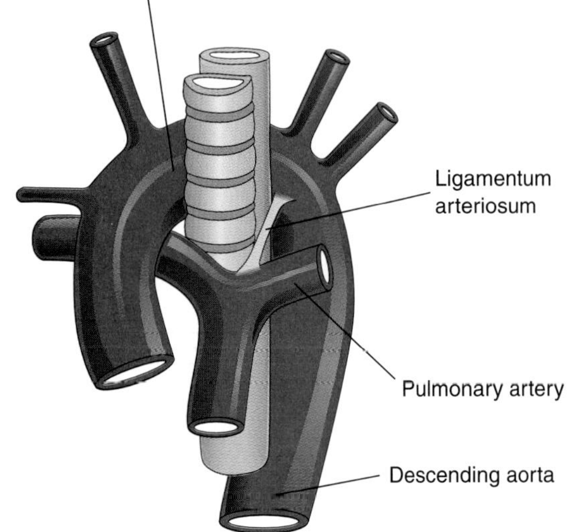

ment of the left dorsal aorta (Fig. 14–41*F*). Later this stenotic segment (area of coarctation) moves cranially with the left subclavian artery (Fig. 14–41*G*).

- During fetal life the segment of the arch of the aorta between the left subclavian artery and the DA is normally narrow because it carries very little blood. Following closure of the DA, this *isthmus* normally enlarges until it is the same diameter as the aorta. If the isthmus persists, a coarctation forms.

Double Aortic Arch

This rare anomaly is characterized by a **vascular ring** around the trachea and esophagus (Fig. 14–42). Varying degrees of compression of these structures may occur. If the compression is significant, it causes wheezing respirations that are aggravated by crying, feeding, and flexion of the neck (Bernstein, 1996). The vascular ring results from failure of the distal part of the right dorsal aorta to disappear (Fig. 14–42*A*); as a result, right and left arches form. Usually the right arch of the aorta is larger and passes posterior to the trachea and esophagus (Fig. 14–42*B*).

Right Arch of Aorta

When the entire right dorsal aorta persists (Fig. 14–43*A* and *B*) and the distal part of the left dorsal aorta involutes, a right aortic arch results. There are two main types:

- *Right arch of the aorta without a retroesophageal component* (Fig. 14–43*B*). The DA (or ligamentum arteriosum) passes from the right pulmonary artery to the right arch of the aorta. Because no vascular ring is formed, this condition is usually asymptomatic.
- *Right arch of the aorta with a retroesophageal component* (Fig. 14–43*C*). Originally there was probably a small left arch of the aorta that involuted, leaving the right arch of the aorta posterior to the esophagus. The DA (or ligamentum arteriosum) attaches to the distal part of the arch of the aorta and forms a ring, which may constrict the esophagus and trachea.

■ **Figure 14–43.** *A,* Sketch of the aortic arches, showing abnormal involution of the distal portion of the left dorsal aorta. There is also persistence of the entire right dorsal aorta and the distal part of the right sixth aortic arch artery. *B,* Right aortic arch without a retroesophageal component. *C,* Right aortic arch with a retroesophageal component. The abnormal right aortic arch and the ligamentum arteriosum (postnatal remnant of DA) form a vascular ring that compresses the esophagus and trachea.

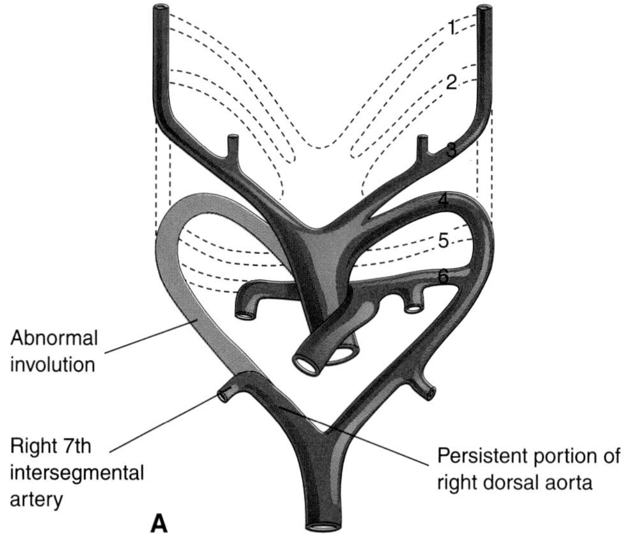

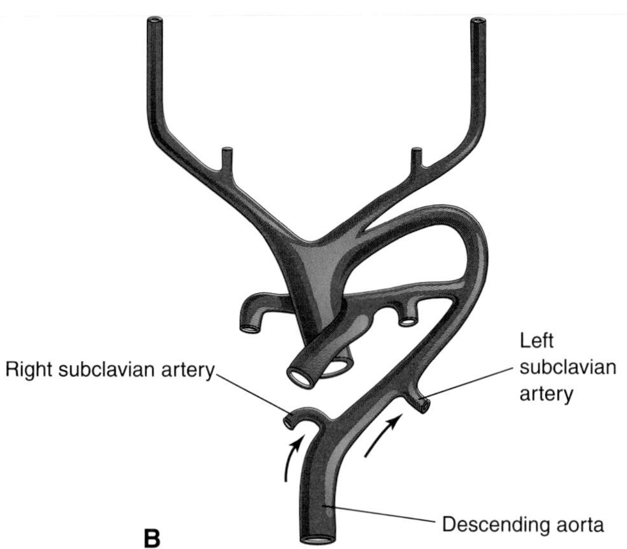

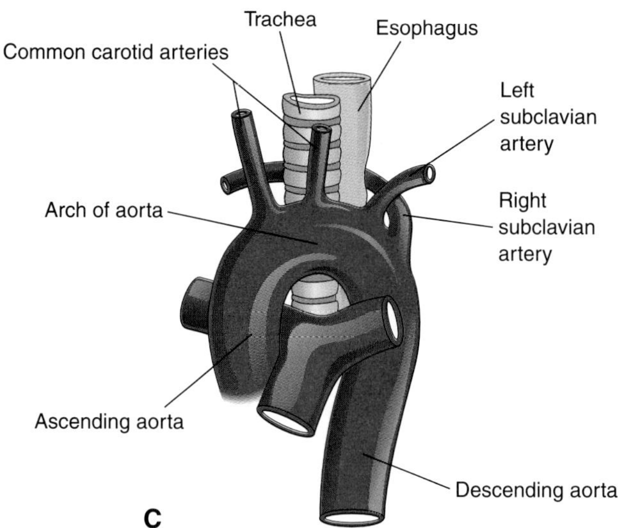

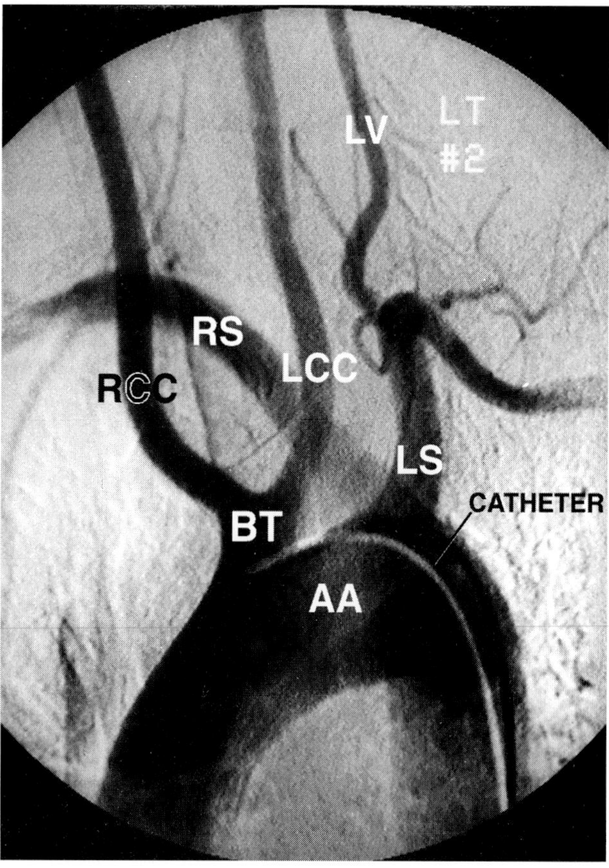

■ **Figure 14–45.** Abnormal origin of right subclavian artery. This left anterior oblique view of aortic arch arteriogram shows both common carotid arteries arising from a common stem of the arch of the aorta. The origin of the right subclavian artery **(RS)** is distal to the separate origin of the left subclavian artery **(LS),** but is superimposed in this view. The right subclavian artery then courses cranially and to the right, posterior to the esophagus and trachea. **AA,** arch of aorta; **BT,** brachiocephalic trunk; **RCC,** right and **LCC,** left common carotid arteries; **LV,** left vertebral artery. (Courtesy of Gerald S. Smyser, MD, Altru Health System, Grand Forks, ND.)

Anomalous Right Subclavian Artery

The right subclavian artery arises from the distal part of the arch of the aorta and passes posterior to the trachea and esophagus to supply the right upper limb (Figs. 14-44 and 14-45).

■ **Figure 14–44.** Sketches illustrating the possible embryological basis of abnormal origin of the right subclavian artery. *A,* The right fourth aortic arch and cranial part of the right dorsal aorta have involuted. As a result, the right subclavian artery forms from the right seventh intersegmental artery and the distal segment of the right dorsal aorta. *B,* As the arch of the aorta forms, the right subclavian artery is carried cranially (*arrows*) with the left subclavian artery. *C,* The abnormal right subclavian artery arises from the aorta and passes posterior to the trachea and esophagus.

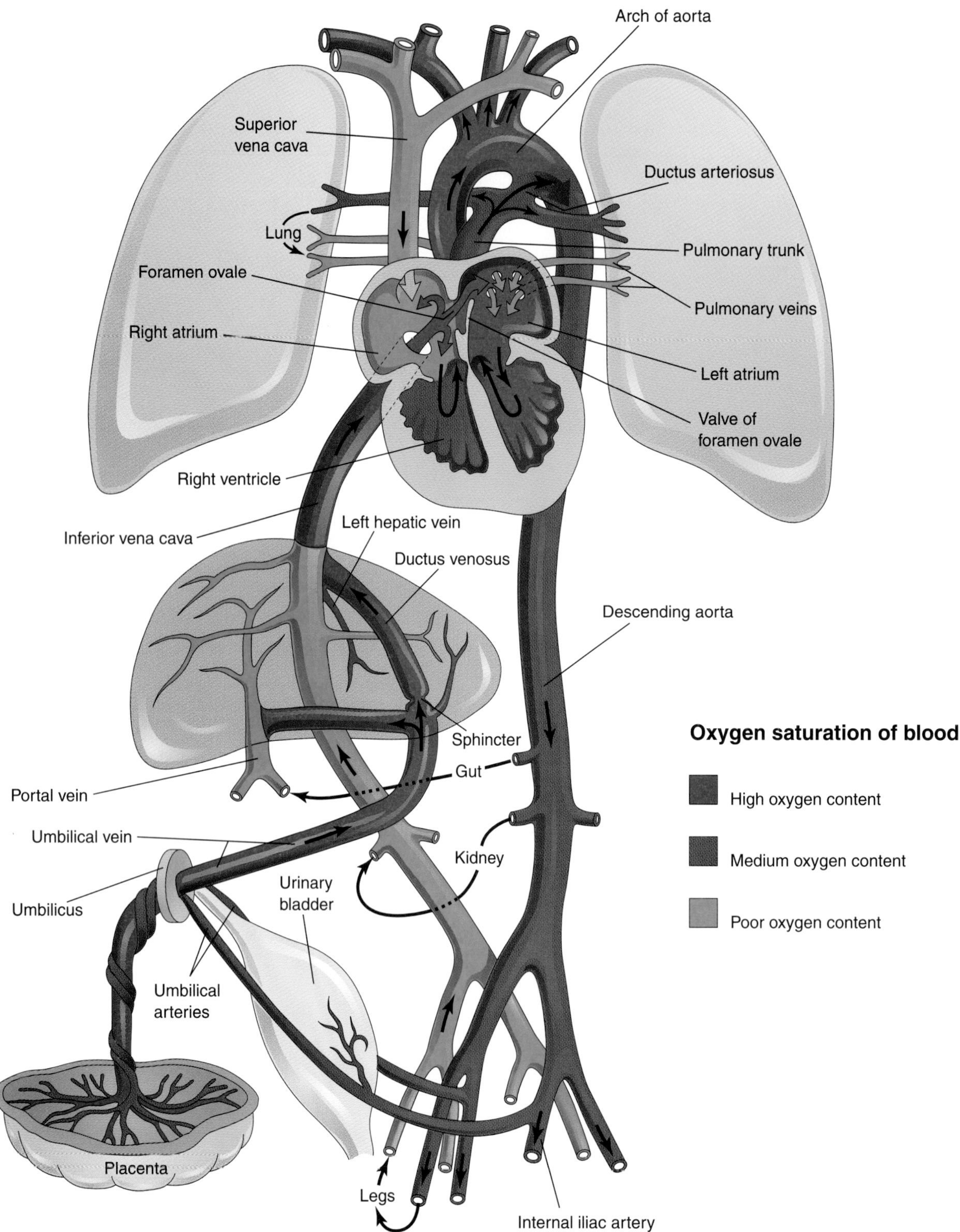

■ **Figure 14–46.** Schematic illustration of the fetal circulation. The colors indicate the oxygen saturation of the blood, and the arrows show the course of the blood from the placenta to the heart. The organs are not drawn to scale. Observe that three shunts permit most of the blood to bypass the liver and lungs: (1) ductus venosus; (2) foramen ovale; and (3) ductus arteriosus. The poorly oxygenated blood returns to the placenta for oxygen and nutrients through the umbilical arteries.

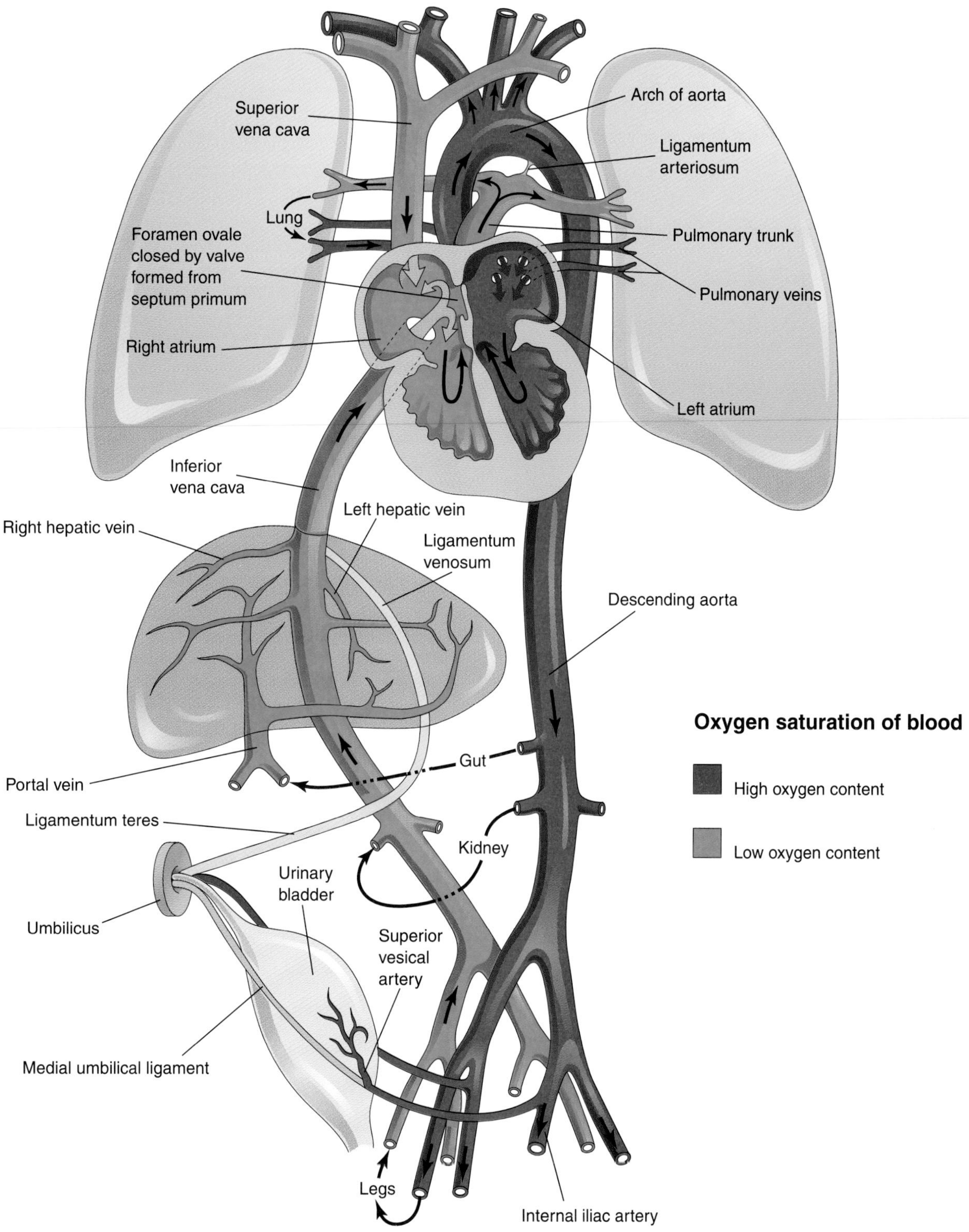

■ **Figure 14–47.** Schematic illustration of the neonatal circulation. The adult derivatives of the fetal vessels and structures that become nonfunctional at birth are also shown. The arrows indicate the course of the blood in the infant. The organs are not drawn to scale. After birth the three shunts that short-circuited the blood during fetal life cease to function, and the pulmonary and systemic circulations become separated.

A **retroesophageal right subclavian artery** occurs when the right fourth aortic arch and the right dorsal aorta disappear cranial to the seventh intersegmental artery. As a result, the right subclavian artery forms from the right seventh intersegmental artery and the distal part of the right dorsal aorta. As development proceeds, differential growth shifts the origin of the right subclavian artery cranially until it comes to lie close to the origin of the left subclavian artery. Although an anomalous right subclavian artery is fairly common and always forms a vascular ring, it is rarely significant clinically because the ring is usually not tight enough to constrict the esophagus and trachea.

FETAL AND NEONATAL CIRCULATION

The fetal cardiovascular system (Fig. 14-46) is designed to serve prenatal needs and permit modifications at birth that establish the neonatal circulatory pattern (Fig. 14-47). Good respiration in the newborn infant is dependent upon normal circulatory changes at birth, which result in oxygenation of the blood occurring in the lungs when fetal blood flow through the placenta ceases (Sansoucie and Cavaliere, 1997). Prenatally the lungs do not provide gas exchange and the pulmonary vessels are vasoconstricted. The three vascular structures most important in the transitional circulation are:

- ductus venosus
- foramen ovale
- ductus arteriosus

Fetal Circulation

Highly oxygenated, nutrient rich blood returns from the placenta in the **umbilical vein** (Fig. 14-46). On approaching the liver, about half of the blood under high pressure passes directly into the **ductus venosus**, a fetal vessel connecting the umbilical vein to the IVC (Figs. 14-48 and 14-49); consequently, this blood bypasses the liver. The other half of the blood in the umbilical vein flows into the *sinusoids of the liver* and enters the IVC through the **hepatic veins**. Blood flow through the ductus venosus is regulated by a *sphincter mechanism* close to the umbilical vein. When the sphincter relaxes, more blood passes through the ductus venosus. When the sphincter contracts, more blood is diverted to the portal vein and hepatic sinusoids (Fig. 14-49). Although an *anatomical sphincter* in the ductus venosus has been described (Dickson, 1957), its presence is not universally accepted. However, it is generally agreed that there is a *physiological sphincter* that prevents overloading of the heart when venous flow in the umbilical vein is high, e.g., during uterine contractions.

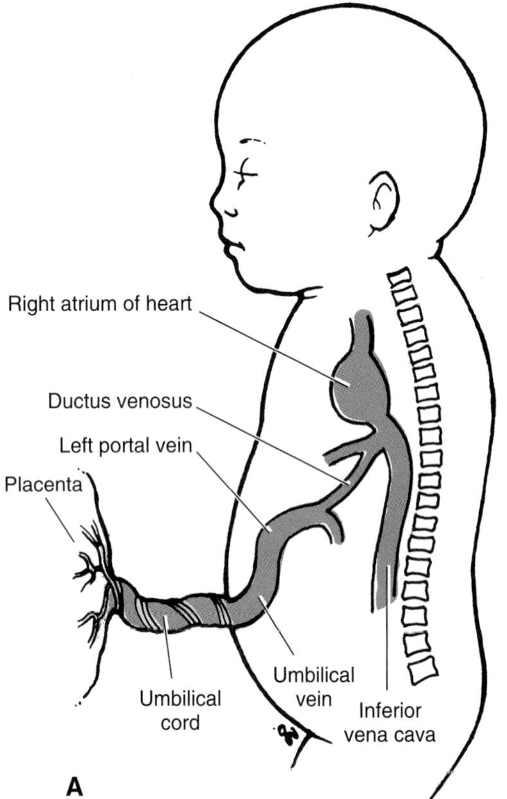

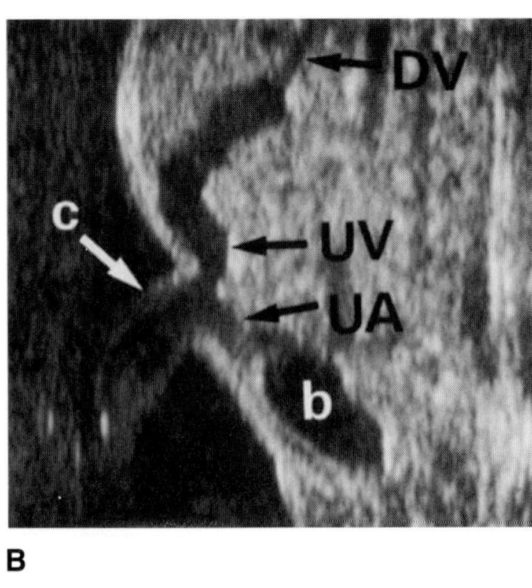

■ **Figure 14-48.** *A,* Schematic illustration of the course of the umbilical vein from the umbilical cord to the liver. *B,* Ultrasound scan showing the umbilical cord and the course of its vessels in the embryo. **c,** umbilical cord; **b,** bladder; **UV,** umbilical vein; **UA,** umbilical artery; **DV,** ductus venosus. (From Goldstein RB: Ultrasound evaluation of the fetal abdomen. *In* Callen PW [ed]: *Ultrasonography in Obstetrics and Gynecology,* 3rd ed. Philadelphia, WB Saunders, 1996.)

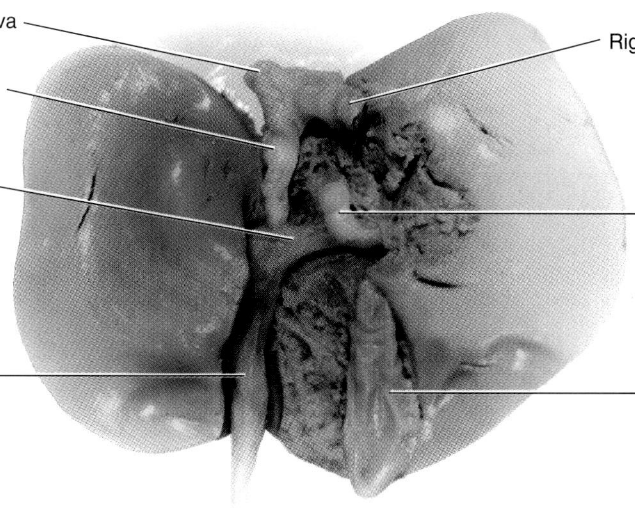

■ **Figure 14–49.** Photograph of a dissection of the visceral surface of the fetal liver. About 50% of umbilical venous blood bypasses the liver and joins the IVC through the ductus venosus.

After a short course in the IVC, the blood enters the right atrium of the heart. Because the IVC contains poorly oxygenated blood from the lower limbs, abdomen, and pelvis, the blood entering the right atrium is not as well oxygenated as that in the umbilical vein, but it still has a high oxygen content (Fig. 14-46). Most blood from the IVC is directed by the inferior border of the septum secundum, the **crista dividens**, through the **foramen ovale** into the left atrium (Fig. 14-50). Here it mixes with the relatively small amount of poorly oxygenated blood returning from the lungs through the pulmonary veins. The fetal lungs extract oxygen from the blood instead of providing it. From the left atrium, the blood passes to the left ventricle and leaves through the ascending aorta.

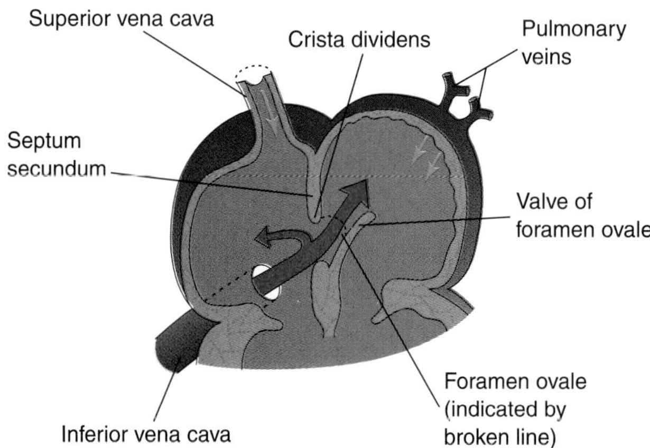

■ **Figure 14–50.** Schematic diagram of blood flow through the fetal atria, illustrating how the crista dividens (lower edge of the septum secundum) separates the blood from the inferior vena cava into two streams. The larger stream passes through the foramen ovale into the left atrium, where it mixes with the small amount of deoxygenated blood coming from the lungs through the pulmonary veins. The smaller stream of blood from the IVC remains in the right atrium and mixes with poorly oxygenated blood from the SVC and coronary sinus.

The arteries to the heart, head, neck, and upper limbs receive well-oxygenated blood. The liver also receives well-oxygenated blood from the umbilical vein (Figs. 14-48 and 14-49). The small amount of well-oxygenated blood from the IVC that remains in the right atrium mixes with poorly oxygenated blood from the SVC and coronary sinus and passes into the right ventricle. This blood, with a medium oxygen content, leaves through the pulmonary trunk. About 10% of the blood goes to the lungs, but most of it passes through the **ductus arteriosus** (DA) into the descending aorta to perfuse the caudal part of the fetal body and return to the placenta through the umbilical arteries (Fig. 14-46). The DA protects the lungs from circulatory overloading and allows the right ventricle to strengthen in preparation for functioning at full capacity at birth (Carlson, 1994). Because of the high pulmonary vascular resistance in fetal life, pulmonary blood flow is low. Only a small volume of blood from the ascending aorta (about 10% of the cardiac output) enters the descending aorta. About 65% of the blood in the descending aorta passes into the umbilical arteries and is returned to the placenta for reoxygenation. The remaining 35% of the blood supplies the viscera and the inferior half of the body (Bernstein, 1996).

Transitional Neonatal Circulation

Important circulatory adjustments occur at birth when the circulation of fetal blood through the placenta ceases and the infant's lungs expand and begin to function (Fig. 14-47). The three shunts that permitted much of the blood to bypass the liver and lungs close and cease to function (Sansoucie and Cavaliere, 1997).

As soon as the baby is born, the foramen ovale, ductus arteriosus, ductus venosus, and umbilical vessels are no longer needed. The sphincter in the ductus venosus constricts, so that all blood entering the liver passes through the hepatic sinusoids. Occlusion of the placental circulation causes an immediate fall of blood pressure in the IVC and right atrium.

Aeration of the lungs at birth is associated with:

- a dramatic fall in pulmonary vascular resistance
- a marked increase in pulmonary blood flow
- a progressive thinning of the walls of the pulmonary arteries; the thinning of the walls of these arteries results mainly from stretching as the lungs increase in size with the first few breaths

The foramen closes at birth. Because of increased pulmonary blood flow, the pressure in the left atrium is higher than in the right atrium. The increased left atrial pressure closes the foramen ovale by pressing the valve of the foramen ovale against the septum secundum (Fig. 14-47). The output from the right ventricle now flows entirely into the pulmonary circulation. Because pulmonary vascular resistance is lower than the systemic vascular resistance, blood flow in the DA reverses, passing from the aorta to the pulmonary trunk.

The right ventricular wall is thicker than the left ventricular wall in fetuses and newborn infants because the right ventricle has been working harder. By the end of the first month, the left ventricular wall is thicker than the right ventricular wall because the left ventricle is now working harder than the right one. The right ventricular wall becomes thinner, because of the atrophy associated with its lighter workload.

The ductus arteriosus constricts at birth, but there is often a small shunt of blood from the aorta to the left pulmonary artery for 24 to 48 hours in a normal healthy, full-term infant. At the end of 24 hours, 20% of ducts are functionally closed, 82% by 48 hours, and 100% at 96 hours (see Sansoucie and Cavaliere, 1997). In premature infants and in those with persistent hypoxia, the ductus arteriosus (DA) may remain open much longer. Oxygen is the most important factor in controlling closure of the ductus arteriosus in full-term infants (Bernstein, 1996). Closure of the DA appears to be mediated by **bradykinin**, a substance released from the lungs during their initial inflation. Bradykinin has potent contractile effects on smooth muscle. The action of this substance appears to be dependent on the high oxygen content of the aortic blood resulting from aeration of the lungs at birth. When the PO_2 of the blood passing through the DA reaches about 50 mm Hg, the wall of the ductus constricts. The mechanisms by which oxygen causes ductal restrictions are not well understood. The effects of oxygen on the ductal smooth muscle may be direct or may be mediated by its effects on prostaglandin E_2 (PGE_2) secretion. Transforming growth factor-β (TGF-β) is probably involved in the anatomical closure of the DA after birth (Tannenbaum et al., 1996). The DA of a premature infant is less responsive to oxygen.

During fetal life the patency of the DA before birth is controlled by the low content of oxygen in the blood passing through it and by endogenously produced **prostaglandins** that act on the smooth muscle in the wall of the DA, causing them to relax (Hammerman, 1995). *Hypoxia* and other ill-defined influences cause the local production of PGE_2 and prostacyclin (PGI_2), which keep the DA open. Inhibitors of prostaglandin synthesis, such as **indomethacin**, can cause constriction of a patent ductus arteriosus in premature infants (Kliegman, 1996).

The umbilical arteries constrict at birth, preventing loss of the infant's blood. The umbilical cord is not tied for a minute or so; consequently, blood flow through the umbilical vein continues, transferring fetal blood from the placenta to the infant.

The change from the fetal to the adult pattern of blood circulation is not a sudden occurrence. Some changes occur with the first breath; others are effected over hours and days (Bernstein, 1996). During the transitional stage, there may be a right-to-left flow through the foramen ovale. The closure of fetal vessels and the foramen ovale is initially a functional change. Later anatomical closure results from proliferation of endothelial and fibrous tissues (Sansoucie and Cavaliere, 1997).

Adult Derivatives of Fetal Vascular Structures

Because of the changes in the cardiovascular system at birth, certain vessels and structures are no longer required. Over a period of months, these fetal vessels form nonfunctional ligaments, and fetal structures such as the foramen ovale persist as anatomical vestiges of the prenatal circulatory system.

UMBILICAL VEIN AND LIGAMENTUM TERES

The intra-abdominal part of the *umbilical vein* eventually becomes the *ligamentum teres* (Fig. 14-47), which passes from the umbilicus to the porta hepatis (Moore, 1992); here it is attached to the left branch of the portal vein (Fig. 14-51). The umbilical vein remains patent for a considerable period and may be used for *exchange transfusions of blood* during early infancy. These transfusions are done to prevent brain damage and death of anemic erythroblastotic infants. Most of the infant's blood is replaced with donor blood. The lumen of the umbilical vein usually does not disappear completely; hence, the ligamentum teres can usually be cannulated even in adults, if necessary, for the injection of contrast media or chemotherapeutic drugs. The potential patency of this vein may also be of functional significance in hepatic cirrhosis (Moore, 1992).

DUCTUS VENOSUS AND LIGAMENTUM VENOSUM

The *ductus venosus* becomes the *ligamentum venosum*; however, its closure is more prolonged than the DA (Carlson, 1994). The ligamentum venosum passes through the liver from the left branch of the portal vein to the IVC, to which it is attached (Fig. 14-51).

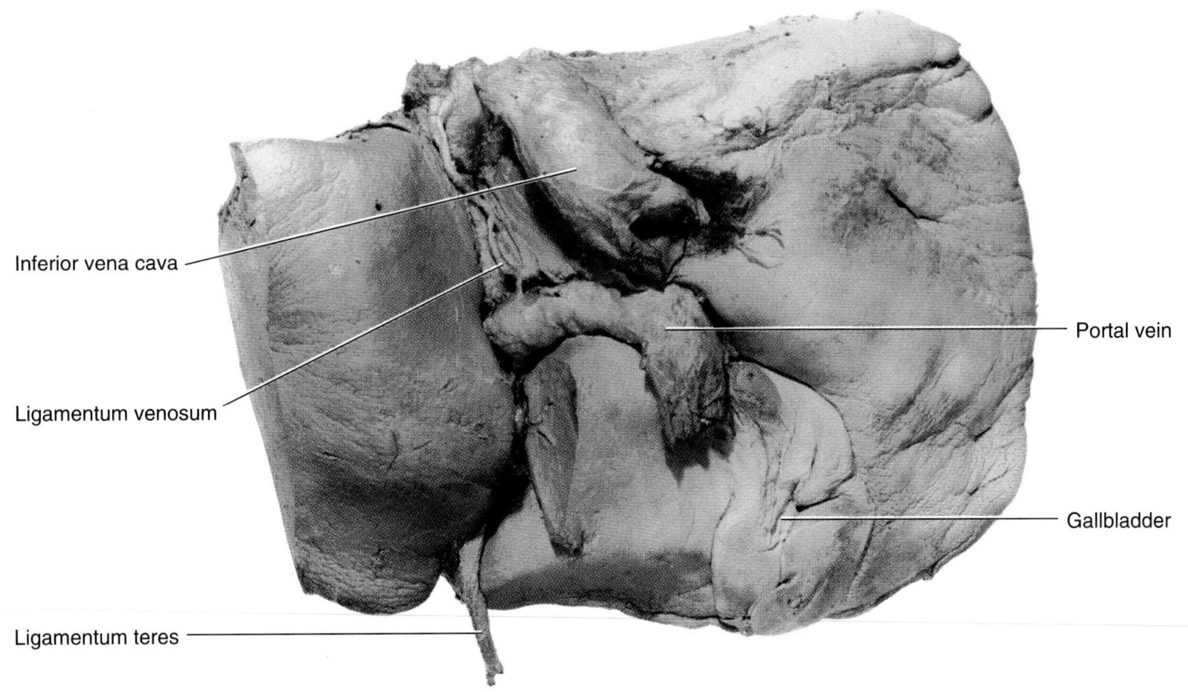

■ **Figure 14–51.** Photographs of a dissection of the visceral surface of an adult liver. Note that in the adult the umbilical vein is represented by the ligamentum teres and the ductus venosus by the ligamentum venosum.

UMBILICAL ARTERIES AND ABDOMINAL LIGAMENTS

Most of the intra-abdominal parts of the umbilical arteries become the *medial umbilical ligaments* (Fig. 14-47); the proximal parts of these vessels persist as the *superior vesical arteries*, which supply the urinary bladder (Moore, 1992).

FORAMEN OVALE AND FOSSA OVALIS

The foramen ovale normally closes functionally at birth. Anatomical closure occurs by the third month and results from tissue proliferation and adhesion of the septum primum (valve of foramen ovale) to the left margin of the septum secundum. The septum primum forms the floor of the fossa ovalis (Fig. 14-52). The inferior edge of the septum secundum forms a rounded fold, the *limbus fossae ovalis* (anulus ovalis), which marks the former boundary of the foramen ovale. There is often a lunate impression on the left side of the interatrial septum, which indicates the former site of the foramen ovale.

DUCTUS ARTERIOSUS AND LIGAMENTUM ARTERIOSUM

Functional closure of the DA is usually completed within the first few days after birth (Fig. 14-53*A*). It passes from the left pulmonary artery to the arch of the aorta. Anatomical closure of the ductus and formation of the ligamentum arteriosum normally occurs by the twelfth week (Fig. 14-53*C*).

Patent Ductus Arteriosus (PDA)

This common anomaly is two to three times more frequent in females than in males (Fig. 14-53*B*). The reason for this preponderance is not known. A dominant form of PDA has been reported in the medical literature. Functional closure of the DA usually occurs soon after birth; however, if it remains patent, aortic blood is shunted into the pulmonary artery. It has been suggested that persistent patency of the DA may result from failure of TGF-β induction after birth (Tannenbaum et al., 1996). PDA is the most common congenital anomaly associated with maternal rubella infection during early pregnancy (see Chapter 8), but the mode of action of the rubella virus is unclear. *Premature infants usually have a PDA*; the patency is the result of hypoxia and immaturity. Virtually all infants whose birth weight is less than 1750 gm have a PDA in the first 24 hours of postnatal life. A PDA that persists in a full-term infant is a pathological entity. Surgical closure of a PDA is the usual treatment. Closure is achieved by ligation and division of the DA.

The embryological basis of PDA is failure of the ductus arteriosus to involute after birth and form the ligamentum arteriosum. Failure of contraction of the muscular wall of the ductus arteriosus after birth is the primary cause of patency. There is some evidence that the low oxygen content of the blood in newborn infants with the *respiratory distress syndrome* can adversely affect closure of the ductus arteriosus; for example, PDA commonly occurs in small premature infants with respiratory difficulties associated with a deficiency of surfactant. Isolated PDA is more common in infants born at high altitude. PDA may occur as an isolated anomaly or in association with cardiac defects. Large differences between aortic and pulmonary blood pressures can cause a heavy flow of blood through the DA, thereby preventing normal constriction. Such pressure differences may be caused by coarctation of the aorta (Fig. 14-41*C*), transposition of the great arteries (Fig. 14-32), or pulmonary stenosis and atresia (Fig. 14-34).

DEVELOPMENT OF THE LYMPHATIC SYSTEM

The lymphatic system begins to develop at the end of the sixth week, about 2 weeks after the primordia of the cardiovascular system are recognizable. Lymphatic vessels develop in a manner similar to that previously described for blood vessels (see Chapter 4) and make connections with the venous system. The early lymphatic capillaries join each other to form a network of lymphatics (Fig. 14-54*A*).

Development of Lymph Sacs and Lymphatic Ducts

There are **six primary lymph sacs** at the end of the embryonic period (Fig. 14-54*A*):

- two *jugular lymph sacs* near the junction of the subclavian veins with the anterior cardinal veins (the future internal jugular veins)

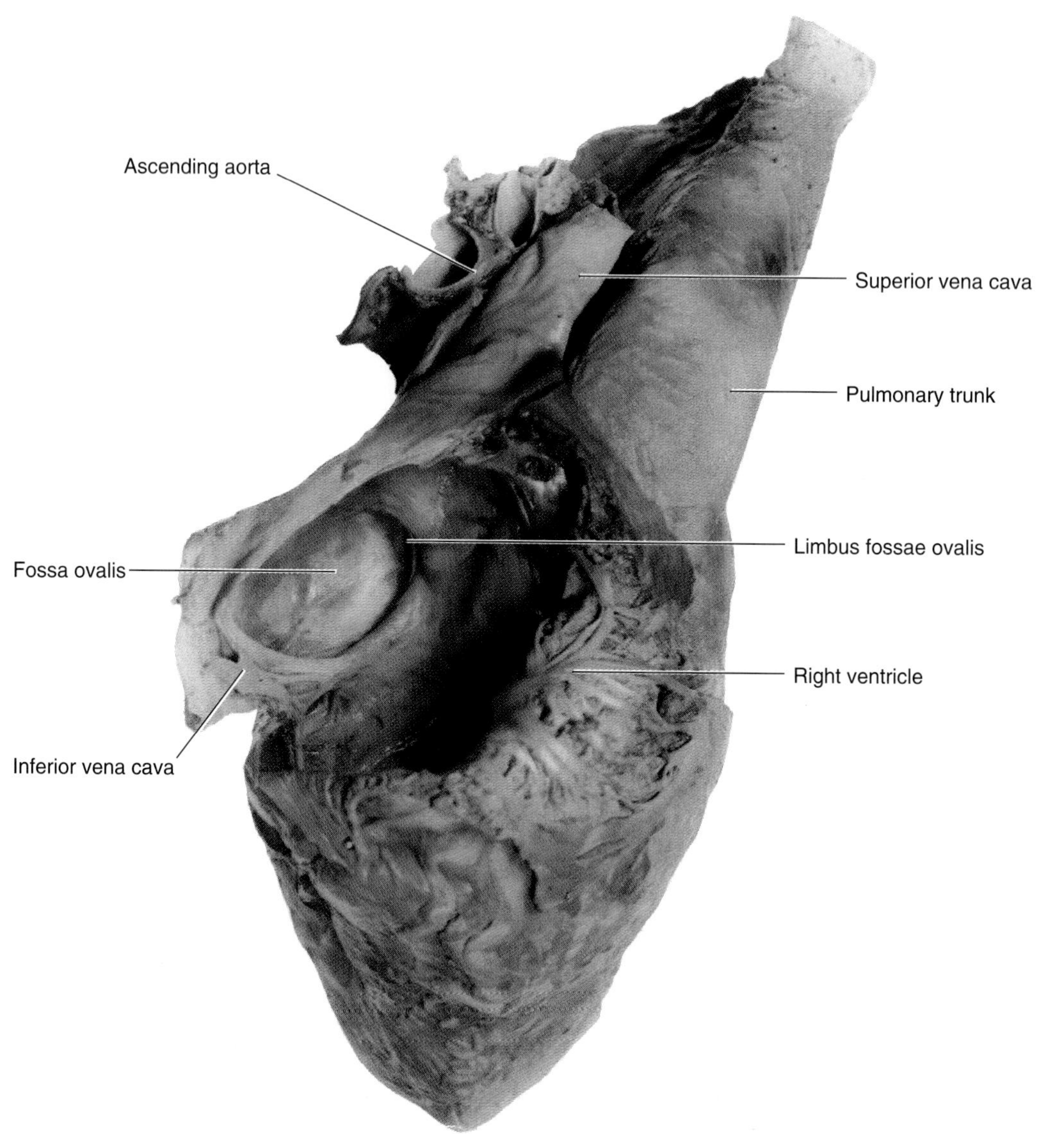

■ **Figure 14-52.** Photograph of a dissection of the right atrial aspect of the interatrial septum of an adult heart. Observe the fossa ovalis and the limbus fossae ovalis. The floor of this oval fossa is formed by the septum primum, whereas the limbus fossae ovalis is formed by the free edge of the septum secundum. Aeration of lungs at birth is associated with a dramatic fall in pulmonary vascular resistance and a marked increase in pulmonary flow. Because of the increased pulmonary blood flow, the pressure in the left atrium is raised above that in the right atrium. This increased left atrial pressure closes the foramen ovale by pressing the valve of the foramen ovale against the septum secundum. This forms the fossa ovalis, a landmark of the interatrial septum.

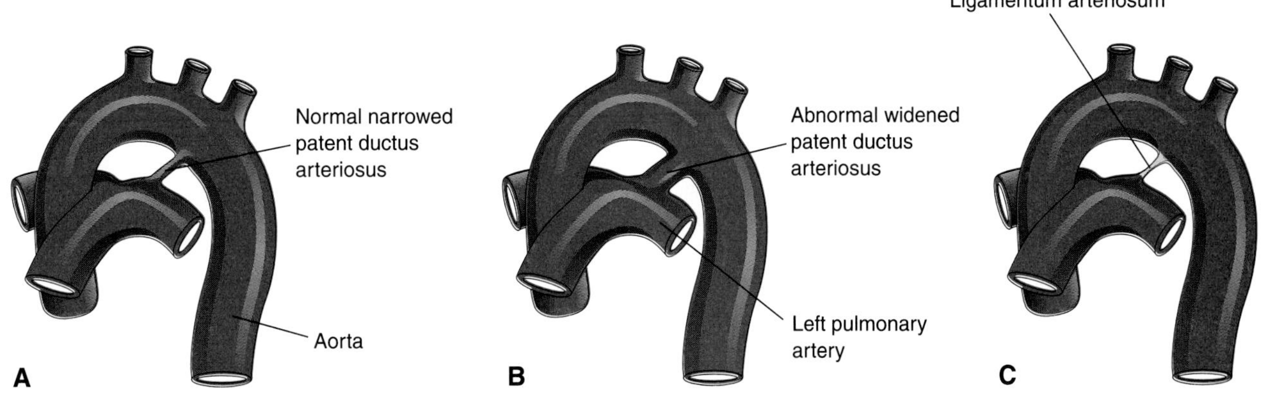

■ **Figure 14–53.** Closure of the ductus arteriosus. *A,* The ductus arteriosus (DA) of a newborn infant. *B,* Abnormal patent DA in a 6-month-old infant. The large ductus is nearly the same size as the left pulmonary artery. *C,* The ligamentum arteriosum in a 6-month-old infant.

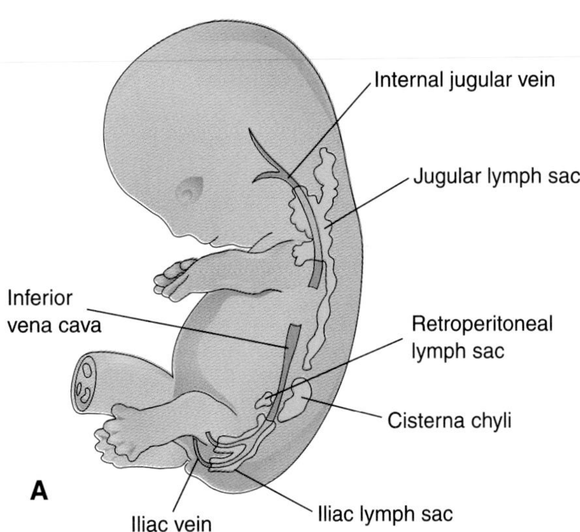

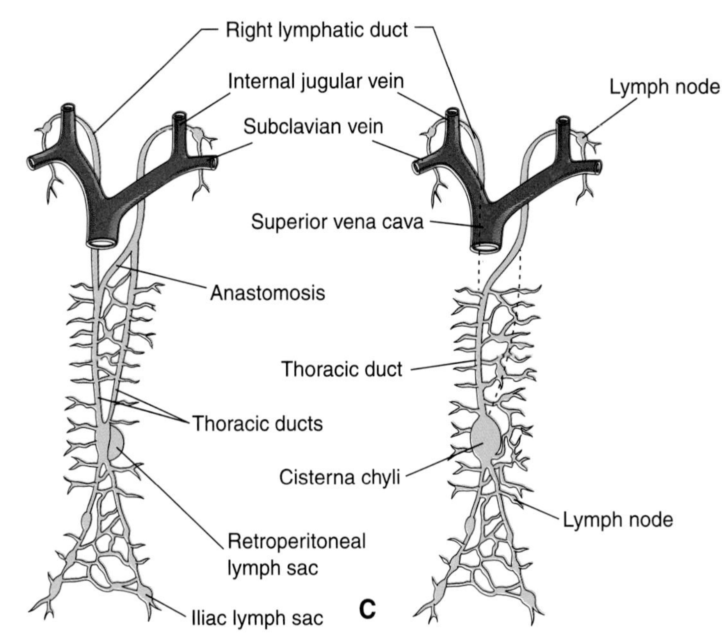

■ **Figure 14–54.** Drawings illustrating development of the lymphatic system. *A,* Left side of an 8-week embryo, showing the primary lymph sacs. *B,* Ventral view of the lymphatic system at 9 weeks, showing the paired thoracic ducts. *C,* Later in the fetal period, illustrating formation of the definitive thoracic duct and right lymphatic duct.

- two *iliac lymph sacs* near the junction of the iliac veins with the posterior cardinal veins
- one *retroperitoneal lymph sac* in the root of the mesentery on the posterior abdominal wall
- one *cisterna chyli* located dorsal to the retroperitoneal lymph sac

Lymphatic vessels soon join the lymph sacs and pass along main veins to the head, neck, and upper limbs from the jugular lymph sacs; to the lower trunk and lower limbs from the iliac lymph sacs; and to the primitive gut from the retroperitoneal lymph sac and the cisterna chyli. Two large channels (right and left thoracic ducts) connect the jugular lymph sacs with the cisterna chyli. Soon a large anastomosis forms between these channels (Fig. 14-54*B*).

THORACIC DUCT

The thoracic duct develops from

- the caudal part of the right thoracic duct
- the anastomosis between the thoracic ducts and the cranial part of the left thoracic duct

Because there are initially right and left thoracic ducts, there are many variations in the origin, course, and termination of the adult thoracic duct.

The *right lymphatic duct* is derived from the cranial part of the right thoracic duct (Fig. 14-54*C*). The thoracic duct and right lymphatic duct connect with the venous system at the angle between the internal jugular and subclavian veins. The superior part of the embryonic **cisterna chyli** persists. In the adult the cisterna chyli is about 5 cm long and 6 mm wide (Moore, 1992).

DEVELOPMENT OF LYMPH NODES

Except for the superior part of the cisterna chyli, the lymph sacs are transformed into groups of lymph nodes during the early fetal period. Mesenchymal cells invade each lymph sac and break up its cavity into a network of lymphatic channels—the primordia of the *lymph sinuses*. Other mesenchymal cells give rise to the capsule and connective tissue framework of the lymph node.

DEVELOPMENT OF LYMPHOCYTES

The lymphocytes are derived originally from primitive stem cells in the yolk sac mesenchyme and later from the liver and spleen. The lymphocytes eventually enter the bone marrow, where they divide to form *lymphoblasts*. The lymphocytes that appear in lymph nodes before birth are derived from the *thymus gland*, a derivative of the third pair of pharyngeal pouches (see Chapter 10). Small lymphocytes leave the thymus and circulate to other lymphoid organs. Later some mesenchymal cells in the lymph nodes differentiate into lymphocytes. Lymph nodules do not appear in the lymph nodes until just before and/or after birth.

DEVELOPMENT OF THE SPLEEN AND TONSILS

The spleen develops from an aggregation of mesenchymal cells in the dorsal mesentery of the stomach (see Chapter 12). The **palatine tonsils** develop from the second pair of pharyngeal pouches. The **tubal tonsils** develop from aggregations of lymph nodules around

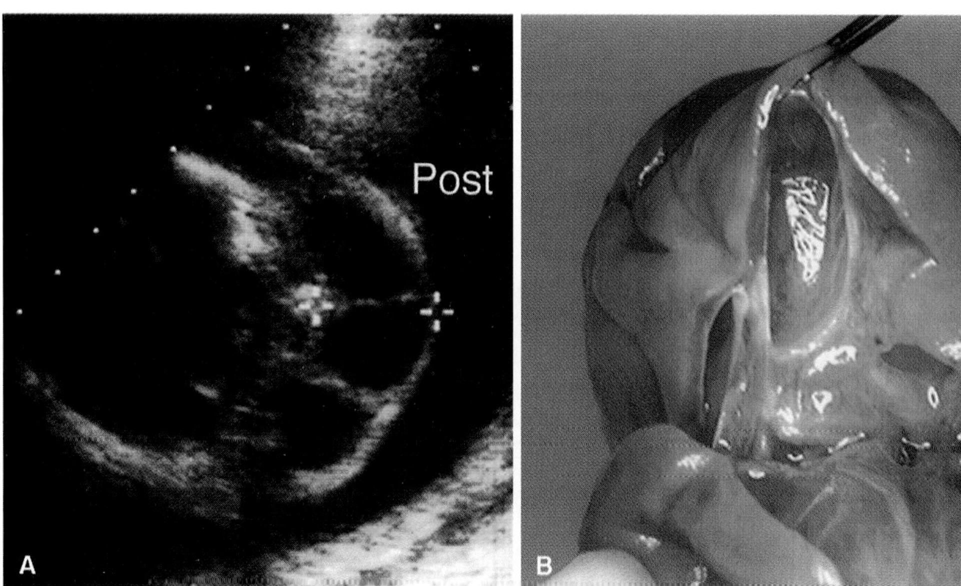

■ **Figure 14-55.** Cystic hygroma. *A,* Transverse axial sonogram of the neck in a fetus with a large nuchal cystic hygroma. *B,* Photograph of a neck dissection. **Post,** posterior. Cystic hygroma was demonstrated from this cross-sectional view of the posterior fetal neck at 18.5 weeks' gestation. The lesion was characterized by multiple, septated cystic areas within the mass itself as shown in the pathology specimen *(B).* (Courtesy of Wesley Lee, MD, Division of Fetal Imaging, William Beaumont Hospital, Royal Oak, Michigan.)

the pharyngeal openings of the pharyngotympanic (auditory, eustachian) tubes. The **pharyngeal tonsils** (adenoids) develop from an aggregation of lymph nodules in the wall of the nasopharynx. The **lingual tonsil** develops from an aggregation of lymph nodules in the root of the tongue. Lymph nodules also develop in the mucosa of the respiratory and digestive systems.

Anomalies of the Lymphatic System

Congenital anomalies of the lymphatic system are uncommon. There may be diffuse swelling of a part of the body—**congenital lymphedema**. This condition may result from dilation of primitive lymphatic channels or from congenital hypoplasia of lymphatic vessels. More rarely, diffuse cystic dilation of lymphatic channels involves widespread portions of the body. In **cystic hygroma,** large swellings usually appear in the inferolateral part of the neck and consist of large single or multilocular, fluid-filled cavities (Fig. 14-55). Hygromas may be present at birth, but they often enlarge and become evident during infancy. Most hygromas appear to be derived from abnormal transformation of the jugular lymph sacs. Hygromas are believed to arise from parts of a jugular lymph sac that are pinched off, or from lymphatic spaces that fail to establish connections with the main lymphatic channels.

SUMMARY OF THE CARDIOVASCULAR SYSTEM

The cardiovascular system begins to develop toward the end of the third week and the heart starts to beat at the beginning of the fourth week. Mesenchymal cells derived from the splanchnic mesoderm proliferate and form isolated cell clusters, which soon develop into endothelial tubes that join to form the primordial vascular system. The heart develops from splanchnic mesenchyme in the *cardiogenic area*. Paired endothelial tubes form and fuse into a single endocardial heart tube. Splanchnic mesoderm surrounding the heart tube forms the *primordial myocardium*.

The primordium of the heart consists of four chambers:

- bulbus cordis
- ventricle
- atrium
- sinus venosus

The **truncus arteriosus** (primordium of ascending aorta and pulmonary trunk) is continuous caudally with the **bulbus cordis**, which becomes part of the ventricles. As the heart grows, it bends to the right and soon acquires the general external appearance of the adult heart. The heart becomes partitioned into four chambers between the fourth and seventh weeks. Three systems of paired veins drain into the primordial heart:

- the *vitelline system*, which becomes the *portal system*
- the *cardinal veins*, which form the *caval system*
- the *umbilical system*, which involutes after birth

As the pharyngeal arches form during the fourth and fifth weeks, they are penetrated by arteries—the **aortic arches**—that arise from the **aortic sac**. During the sixth to eighth weeks, the aortic arches are transformed into the adult arterial arrangement of the carotid, subclavian, and pulmonary arteries.

The critical period of heart development is from day 20 to day 50 after fertilization. Numerous critical events occur during cardiac development, and deviation from the normal pattern at any time may produce one or more congenital heart defects. Because partitioning of the primordial heart results from complex processes, defects of the cardiac septa are relatively common, particularly VSDs. Some congenital anomalies result from abnormal transformation of the aortic arches into the adult arterial pattern (e.g., right aortic arch).

Because the lungs are nonfunctional during prenatal life, the **fetal cardiovascular system** is structurally designed so that the blood is oxygenated in the placenta and largely bypasses the lungs. The modifications that establish the postnatal circulatory pattern at birth are not abrupt, but extend into infancy. Failure of these changes in the circulatory system to occur at birth results in two of the most common congenital anomalies of the heart and great vessels:

- patent foramen ovale
- patent ductus arteriosus

The **lymphatic system** begins to develop late in the sixth week in close association with the venous system. Six primary **lymph sacs** develop, which later become interconnected by lymphatic vessels. Lymph nodes develop along the network of lymphatic vessels; lymph nodules do not appear until just before or after birth. Sometimes a part of a jugular lymph sac becomes pinched off and may give rise to a mass of dilated lymphatic spaces, a **cystic hygroma**.

Clinically Oriented Problems

Case 14–1

A pediatrician detected a cardiac defect in an infant, and he explained to the baby's mother that this is a common birth defect.

- What is the most common type of congenital cardiac defect?
- What percentage of congenital heart disease results from this defect?
- Discuss blood flow in infants with this defect.
- What problems would the infant likely encounter if the cardiac defect were large?

Case 14–2

A female infant was born normally after a pregnancy complicated by a *rubella infection* during the first trimester of pregnancy. She had *congenital cataracts* and *congenital heart disease*. A radiograph of the infant's chest at 3 weeks showed generalized *cardiac enlargement* with some increase in pulmonary vascularity.

- What congenital cardiovascular anomaly is commonly associated with maternal rubella during early pregnancy?
- What probably caused the cardiac enlargement?

Case 14–3

A newborn infant was referred to a pediatrician because of the blue color of his skin (cyanosis). An ultrasound examination was ordered to confirm the preliminary diagnosis.

- In the *tetralogy of Fallot* there are four cardiac abnormalities. What are they?
- What is one of the most obvious signs of the tetralogy of Fallot?
- What radiographic technique might be used to confirm a tentative diagnosis of this type of congenital heart disease?
- What do you think would be the main aim of therapy in these cases?

Case 14–4

A male infant was born after a full-term normal pregnancy. Severe generalized cyanosis was observed on the first day. A chest film revealed a *slightly enlarged heart* with a narrow base and increased pulmonary vascularity. A clinical diagnosis of *transposition of the great arteries* (TGA) was made.

- What radiographic technique would likely be used to verify the diagnosis?
- What would this technique reveal in the present case?
- How was the infant able to survive after birth with this severe congenital anomaly of the great arteries?

Case 14–5

During an autopsy on a 72-year-old man who had died following *chronic heart failure*, it was observed that his heart was very large and that the pulmonary artery and its main branches were dilated. Opening the heart revealed a very large *atrial septal defect*.

- What type of ASD was probably present?
- Where would the defect likely be located?
- Explain why the pulmonary artery and its main branches were dilated.

Discussion of these problems appears at the back of the book.

REFERENCES AND SUGGESTED READING

Anderson PAW: The heart and development. *Semin Perinatol 20:*482, 1996.

Anderson RH, Ashley GT: Growth and development of the cardiovascular system. *In* Davis JA, Dobbing J (eds): *Scientific Foundation of Paediatrics*. Philadelphia, WB Saunders, 1974.

Behrman RE, Kliegman RM, Arvin AM (eds): *Nelson Textbook of Pediatrics,* 15th ed. Philadelphia, WB Saunders, 1996.

Bernstein E: The cardiovascular system. *In* Behrman RE, Kliegman RM, Arvin AM (eds): *Nelson Textbook of Pediatrics,* 15th ed. Philadelphia, WB Saunders, 1996.

Blausen BE, Johannes RS, Hutchins GM: Computer-based reconstructions of the cardiac ventricles of human embryos. *Am J Cardiovasc Pathol 3:*37, 1989.

Bowman JM: Hemolytic disease (erythroblastosis fetalis). *In* Creasy RK, Resnik R (eds): *Maternal-Fetal Medicine: Principles and Practice,* 3rd ed. Philadelphia, WB Saunders, 1994.

Bruyer Jr HJ, Kargas SA, Levy JM: The causes and underlying developmental mechanisms of congenital cardiovascular malformation: A critical review. *Am J Med Genet (Suppl) 3:*411, 1987.

Butler J, Vincent RN, Reed M, Collins GF: Cardiac embryogenesis: a three-dimensional approach. *Can J Cardiol 3:*111, 1987.

Carlson BM: *Human Embryology and Developmental Biology*. St Louis, Mosby, 1994.

Chinn A, Fitzsimmons J, Shepard TH, Fantel AG: Congenital heart disease among spontaneous abortuses and stillborn fetuses: prevalence and associations. *Teratology 40:*475, 1989.

Clark EB: Cardiac embryology. Its relevance to congenital heart disease. *Am J Dis Child 140:*41, 1986.

Clark EB: Pathogenetic mechanisms of congenital cardiovascular malformations revisited. *Semin Perinatol 20:*465, 1996.

Collet RW, Edwards JE: Persistent truncus arteriosus: a classification according to anatomic types. *Surg Clin North Am 29:*1245, 1949.

Conte G, Grieco M: Closure of the interventricular foramen and morphogenesis of the membranous septum and ventricular septal defects in the human heart. *Anat Anz 155:*39, 1984.

Conte G, Pellegrini A: On the development of the coronary arteries in human embryos, stages 14–19. *Anat Embryol 169:*209, 1984.

Creazzo TL, Burch J, Redmond S, Kumiski D: Myocardial enlargement in defective heart development. *Anat Rec 239:*170, 1994.

Deanfield JE: Transposition of the great arteries: to switch or not to switch? *Curr Opin Pediatr 1:*85, 1989.

Dickson AD: The development of the ductus venosus in man and the goat. *J Anat 91:*358, 1957.

Fananapazir K, Kaufman MH: Observations on the development of the aortico-pulmonary spiral septum in the mouse. *J Anat 158:*157, 1988.

Feinberg RN (ed): *The Development of the Vascular System*. Farmington, CT, S Karger Publishers, 1990.

Feinberg RN, Sherer GK, Auerbach R (eds): *The Development of the Vascular System*. Basel, Karger, 1991.

Ferencz C: The etiology of congenital cardiovascular malformations: observations on genetic risks with implications for further birth defects research. *J Med 16:*497, 1985.

Ferencz C, Rubin JD, McCarter RB, et al: Cardiac and noncardiac malformations: observations in a population-based study. *Teratology 35:*367, 1987.

Fink BW: *Congenital Heart Disease,* 2nd ed. Chicago, Year Book Medical Publishers, 1985.

Freed MD: Congenital cardiac malformations. *In* Avery ME, Taeusch Jr HW (eds): *Schaffer's Diseases of the Newborn,* 5th ed. Philadelphia, WB Saunders, 1994.

Gilbert-Barness E (ed): *Potter's Pathology of the Fetus and Infant*. St Louis, Mosby, 1997.

Goldstein RB: Ultrasound evaluation of the fetal abdomen. *In* Callen PW (ed): *Ultrasonography in Obstetrics and Gynecology,* 3rd ed. Philadelphia, WB Saunders, 1996.

Gootman N, Gootman PM (eds): *Perinatal Cardiovascular Function*. New York, Marcel Dekker, 1983.

Hammerman C: Patent ductus arteriosus: Clinical relevance of prostaglandins and prostaglandin inhibitors in PDA pathophysiology and treatment. *Clin Perinatol 22(2):*457, 1995.

Hanahan D: Signaling vascular morphogenesis and maintenance. *Science 277:*48, 1997.

Harvey RP: NK-2 homeobox genes and heart development. *Dev Biol 178:*203, 1996.

Hirakow R: Development of the vertebrate heart and the extracellular matrix. *Congen Anom 26:*205, 1986.

Hornberger LK, Colan SD, Lock JE, et al: Outcome of patients with ectopia cordis and significant intracardiac defects. *Circulation 94(Suppl II)*:32, 1996.

Hunt CE: Sudden infant death syndrome. *In* Behrman RE, Kliegman RM, Arvin AM (eds): *Nelson Textbook of Pediatrics,* 15th ed. Philadelphia, WB Saunders, 1996.

Jones WK, Sanchez A, Robbins J: Murine pulmonary myocardium: developmental analysis of cardiac gene analysis. *Dev Dyn 200*:117, 1994.

Kirby ML, Gale TF, Stewart DE: Neural crest cells contribute to normal aorticopulmonary septation. *Science 220*:1059, 1983.

Kirklin JW, Colvin EV, McConnell ME, et al: Complete transposition of the great arteries: treatment in the current era. *Pediatr Clin North Am 37*:171, 1990.

Kliegman RM: Respiratory tract disorders. *In* Behrman RE, Kliegman RM, Arvin AM (eds): *Nelson Textbook of Pediatrics,* 15th ed. Philadelphia, WB Saunders, 1996.

Leatherbury L, Kirby ML: Cardiac development and perinatal care of infants with neural crest-associated conotruncal defects. *Semin Perinatol 20*:473, 1996.

Lee W, Smith RS, Comstock CH, et al: Tetralogy of fallot: prenatal diagnosis and postnatal survival. *Obstet Gynecol 86*:583, 1995.

Lilja M: Infants with single umbilical artery studied in a national registry. 3: A case control study of risk factors. *Paediatr Perinat Epidemiol 8*:325, 1994.

Lin Q, Schwarz J, Bucana C, Olson EN: Control of mouse cardiac morphogenesis and myogenesis by transcription factor MEF2C. *Science 276*:1404, 1997.

Long WA: *Fetal and Neonatal Cardiology*. Philadelphia, WB Saunders, 1990.

Merrill WH, Bender HW: The surgical approach to congenital heart disease. *Curr Probl Surg 22*:4, 1985.

Moller JF, Neal WA: *Fetal, Neonatal and Infant Cardiac Disease*. Norwalk, Appleton & Lange, 1989.

Moore KL: *Clinically Oriented Anatomy,* 3rd ed. Baltimore, Williams & Wilkins, 1992.

Morris GK, Hampton J: Congenital heart lesions—an introduction. *Med Internat 18*:745, 1985.

Nathanielsz PW: *Life Before Birth. The Challenges of Fetal Development*. New York, WH Freeman and Company, 1996.

Olson EN, Srivastava D: Molecular pathways controlling heart development. *Science 272*:671, 1996.

O'Malley CD, Shaw GM, Wasserman CR, Lammer EJ: Epidemiological characteristics of conotruncal heart defects in California, 1987–1988. *Teratology 53*:374, 1996.

O'Rahilly R: The timing and sequence of events in human cardiogenesis. *Acta Anat 79*:70, 1971.

Page EW, Villee CA, Villee DB: *Human Reproduction. Essentials of Reproductive and Perinatal Medicine,* 3rd ed. Philadelphia, WB Saunders, 1981.

Papp JG: Autonomic responses and neurohumoral control in the human early antenatal heart. *Basic Res Cardiol 83*:2, 1988.

Persaud TVN: Historical development of the concept of a pulmonary circulation. *Can J Cardiol 5*:12, 1989.

Pexieder T: Genetic aspects of congenital heart disease. *In* Pexieder T (ed): *Perspectives in Cardiovascular Research,* vol 5. *Mechanisms of Cardiac Morphogenesis and Teratogenesis*. New York, Raven Press, 1981.

Pezzati M, Cianciulli D, Danesi G: Acardiac twins. Two case reports. *J Perinat Med 25*:119, 1997.

Riva E, Hearse DK: *The Developing Myocardium*. New York, Futura Publishing, 1991.

Sansoucie DA, Cavaliere TA: Transition from fetal to extrauterine circulation. *Neonat Network 16*:5, 1997.

Schats R, Jansen CAM, Wladimiroff JW: Embryonic heart activity: appearance and development in early pregnancy. *Brit J Obstet Gynaecol 97*:989, 1990.

Schmidt KG, Silverman NH: The fetus with a cardiac malformation. *In* Harrison MR, Golbus MS, Filly RA (eds): *The Unborn Patient. Prenatal Diagnosis and Treatment,* 2nd ed. Philadelphia, WB Saunders, 1991.

Schoenwolf GC, Garcia-Martinez V: Primitive-streak origin and state of commitment of cells of the cardiovascular system in avian and mammalian embryos. *Cell Mol Biol Res 41*:233, 1995.

Schultheiss TM, Burch JBE, Lassar AB: A role for bone morphogenetic proteins in the induction of cardiac myogenesis. *Genes Dev 11*:451, 1997.

Schwartz SM, Heimark RL, Majesky MW: Developmental mechanisms underlying pathology of arteries. *Physiol Rev 70*:1177, 1990.

Seeds JW, Azizkhan RG: *Congenital Malformations. Antenatal Diagnosis, Perinatal Management, and Counseling*. Rockville, MD, Aspen Publishers, 1990.

Sherer DM, Divon MY: Prenatal ultrasonographic assessment of the ductus arteriosus: a review. *Obstet Gynecol 87*:630, 1996.

Silverman NH, Schmidt KG: Ultrasound evaluation of the fetal heart. *In* Callen PW (ed): *Ultrasonography in Obstetrics and Gynecology,* 3rd ed. Philadelphia, WB Saunders, 1994.

Skandalakis JE, Gray SW: *Embryology for Surgeons. The Embryological Basis for the Treatment of Congenital Anomalies,* 3rd ed. Baltimore, Williams & Wilkins, 1994.

Skovránek J: Prenatal development of the heart and the blood circulatory system. *Physiol Res 40*:25, 1991.

Srivastava D, Cserjesi P, Olson EN: A subclass of 6HLH proteins required for cardiac morphogenesis. *Science 270*:1995, 1995.

Tannenbaum JE, Waleh NS, Mauray F, et al: Transforming growth factor—protein and messenger RNA expression is increased in the closing ductus arteriosus. *Pediatr Res 39*:427, 1996.

Thompson MW, McInnes RR, Willard HF: *Thompson & Thompson Genetics in Medicine,* 5th ed. Philadelphia, WB Saunders, 1991.

Tikkanen J, Heinonen OP: Risk factors for coarctation of the aorta. *Teratology 47*:565, 1993.

Ueland K: Cardiac diseases. *In* Creasy RK, Resnik R (eds): *Maternal-Fetal Medicine: Principles and Practice,* 3rd ed. Philadelphia, WB Saunders, 1994.

Veille JC, Mahowald MB, Sivakoff M: Ethical dilemmas in fetal echocardiography. *Obstet Gynecol 73*:710, 1989.

Verrier ED, Vlahakes GJ, Hanley FL, Bradley SM: Experimental Fetal Cardiac Surgery. *In* Harrison MR, Golbus MS, Filly RA (eds): *The Unborn Patient. Prenatal Diagnosis and Treatment,* 2nd ed. Philadelphia, WB Saunders, 1991.

Virmani R, Atkinson JD, Fenoglio JJ: *Cardiovascular Pathology*. Philadelphia, WB Saunders, 1991.

Yoffey JM, Courtice, FC: *Lymphatics, Lymph and Lymphomyeloid Complex*. London, Academic Press, 1970.

Yu IT, Hutchins GM; Truncus arteriosus malformation: a developmental arrest at Carnegie stage 14. *Teratology 53*:31, 1996.

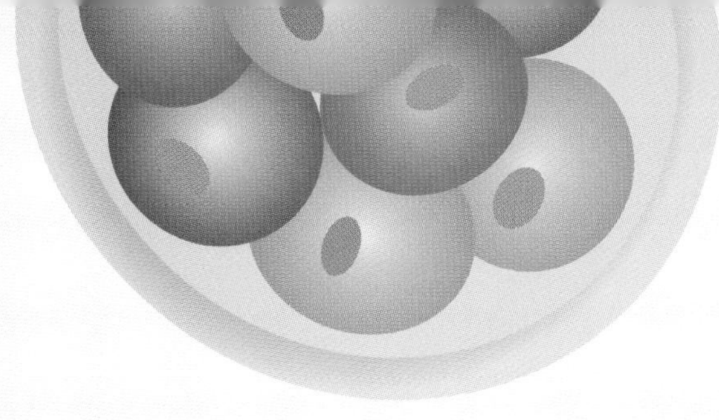

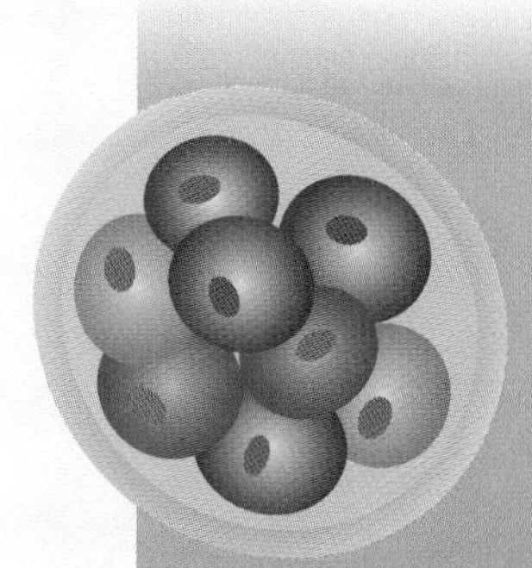

The Skeletal System

15

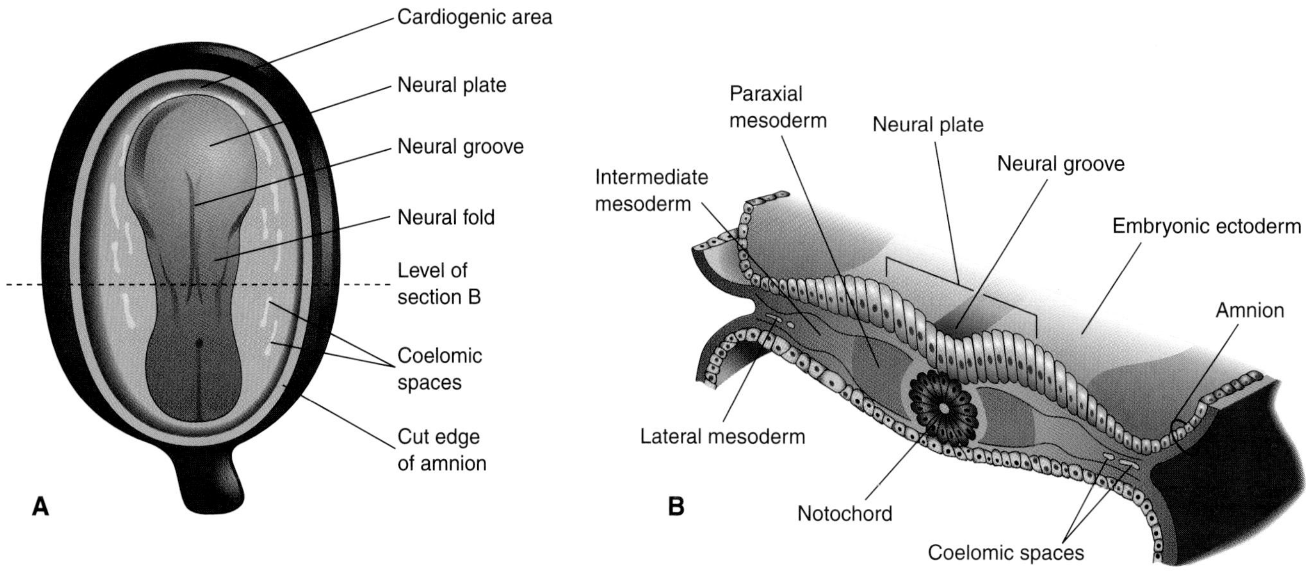

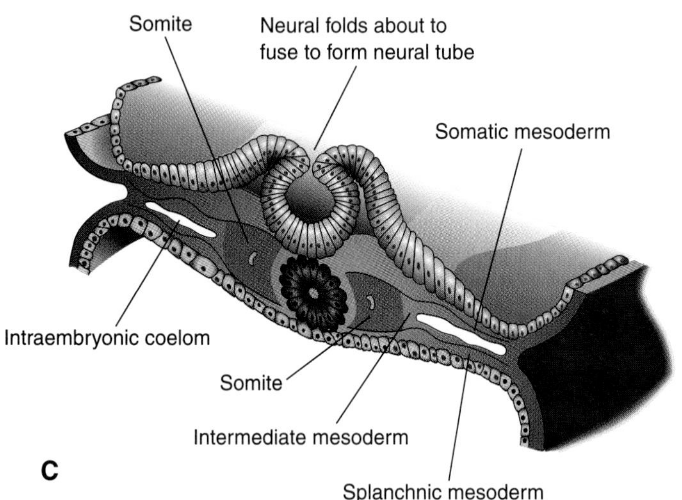

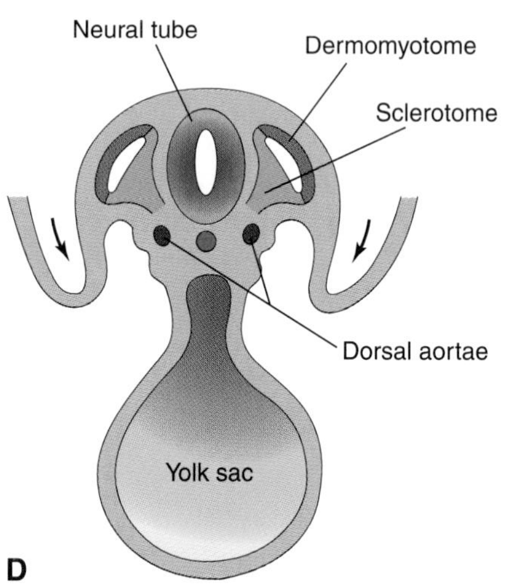

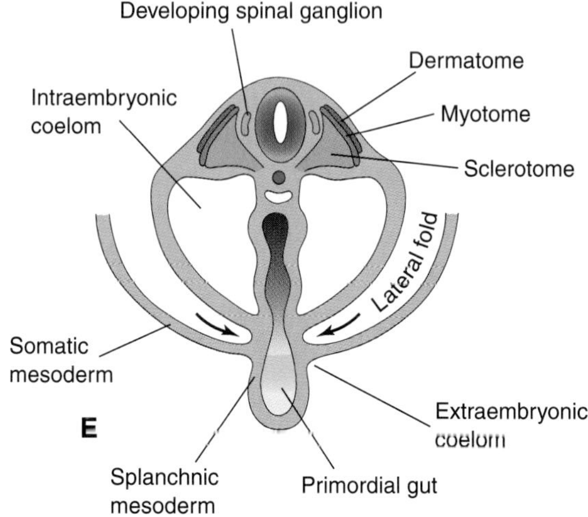

■ **Figure 15–1.** Drawings illustrating formation and early differentiation of somites. *A,* Dorsal view of a presomite embryo (about 18 days). *B,* Transverse section of the embryo shown in *A,* illustrating the paraxial mesoderm from which the somites are derived. *C,* Transverse section of an embryo of about 22 days, showing the appearance of the early somites. Note that the neural folds are about to fuse to form the neural tube. *D,* Transverse section of an embryo of about 24 days, showing folding of the embryo in the horizontal plane *(arrows).* The dermomyotome region of the somite gives rise to the dermatome and myotome. *E,* Transverse section of an embryo of about 26 days, showing the dermatome, myotome, and sclerotome regions of the somite.

■ The skeletal system develops from mesodermal and neural crest cells. As the notochord and neural tube form, the *intraembryonic mesoderm* lateral to these structures thickens to form two longitudinal columns of *paraxial mesoderm* (Fig. 15-1*A* and *B*). Toward the end of the third week, these columns become segmented into blocks of mesodermal tissue, the **somites** (Fig. 15-1*C*). Externally the somites appear as beadlike elevations along the dorsolateral surface of the embryo (see Chapter 5). Each somite differentiates into two parts (Fig. 15-1*D* and *E*):

- The ventromedial part is the **sclerotome**; its cells form the vertebrae and ribs.
- The dorsolateral part is the **dermomyotome**; cells from its *myotome* region form myoblasts (primordial muscle cells), and those from its *dermatome* region form the dermis of the skin.

Mesodermal cells give rise to a *mesenchyme*—loosely organized embryonic connective tissue. Considerable mesenchyme in the head region is also derived from the neural crest. **Neural crest cells** migrate into the pharyngeal arches and form the bones and connective tissue of craniofacial structures. Regardless of their origin, mesenchymal cells have the ability to differentiate in many different ways (e.g., into fibroblasts, chondroblasts, or osteoblasts).

DEVELOPMENT OF BONE AND CARTILAGE

Bones first appear as condensations of mesenchymal cells that form models of the bones. Condensation marks the beginning of selective gene activity, which precedes cell differentiation (Figs. 15-2 and 15-3).

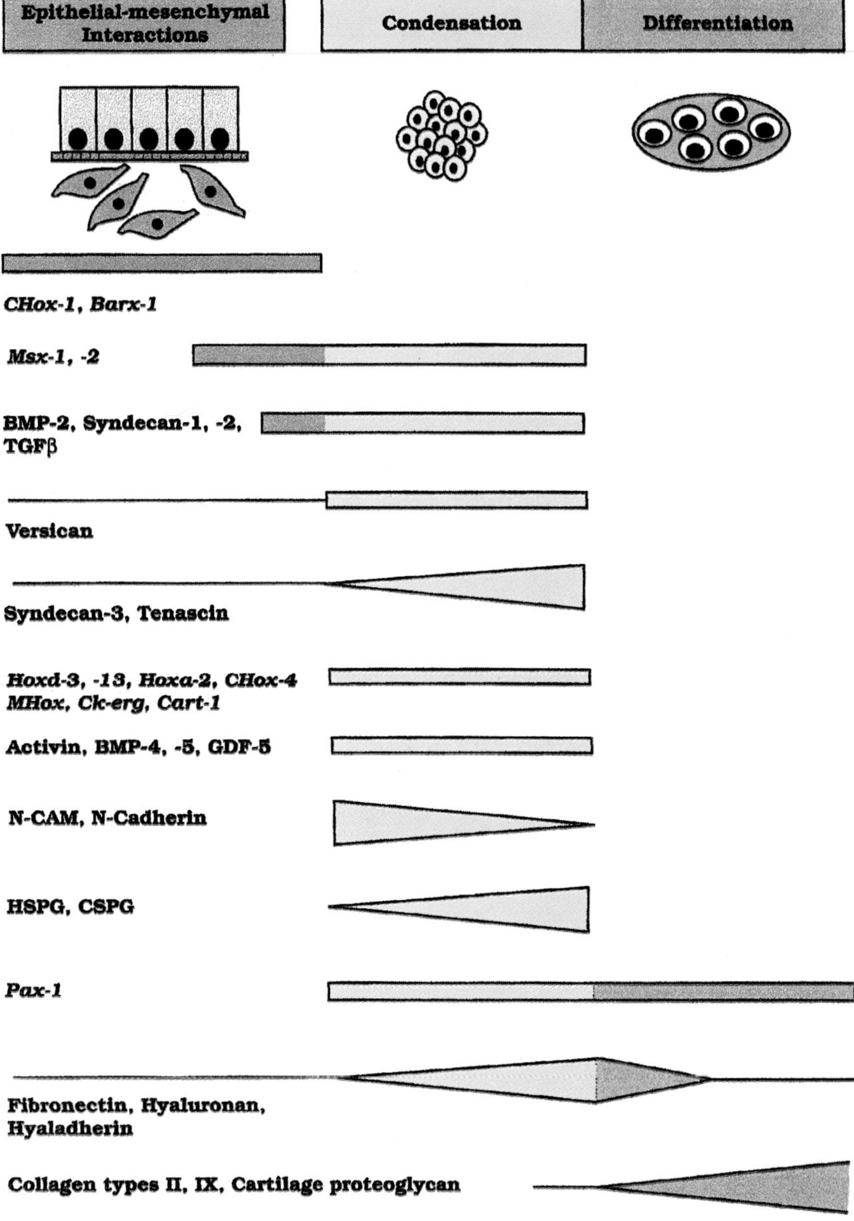

■ **Figure 15-2.** A summary of the molecules known to be associated with the three major phases of chondrogenesis in the craniofacial skeleton. The three phases are: precondensation, characterized by epithelial-mesenchymal interactions (brown); condensation (yellow); and differentiation (blue). The precondensation phase is characterized by expression of Hox genes (CHox-1 [Hoxa4], Barx-1), Msx-1, -2, the growth factors BMP-2 and TGFβ, and syndecan-1. Versican, syndecan-3, and tenascin, which are present in low concentrations precondensation, are up-regulated at condensation. Other Hox genes and transcription factors (Hoxd-3, -13, Hoxa-2, Cdxa [Chox-4], Mhox, Ck-erg and Cart-1) and other growth factors (activin, BMP-4, -5 and GDF-5) are expressed at condensation. The cell adhesion molecules N-CAM and N-cadherin also appear with condensation but are down-regulated during condensation. Heparan sulfate and chondroitin sulfate proteoglycans appear at condensation and are up-regulated during condensation. The transcriptional factor Pax-1 is present during and following condensation. Extracellular matrix molecules such as fibronectin, hyaluronan, and hyaladherin increase during condensation (yellow) but are down-regulated thereafter (blue). Collagen types II and IX and cartilage proteoglycan appear postcondensation, although mRNAs for the collagens and for the core protein of the proteoglycan are up-regulated during condensation. (From Hall BK, Miyake T: Divide, accumulate, differentiate: cell condensation in skeletal development revisited. *Int J Dev Biol* 39:881, 1995. See this publication for more details.)

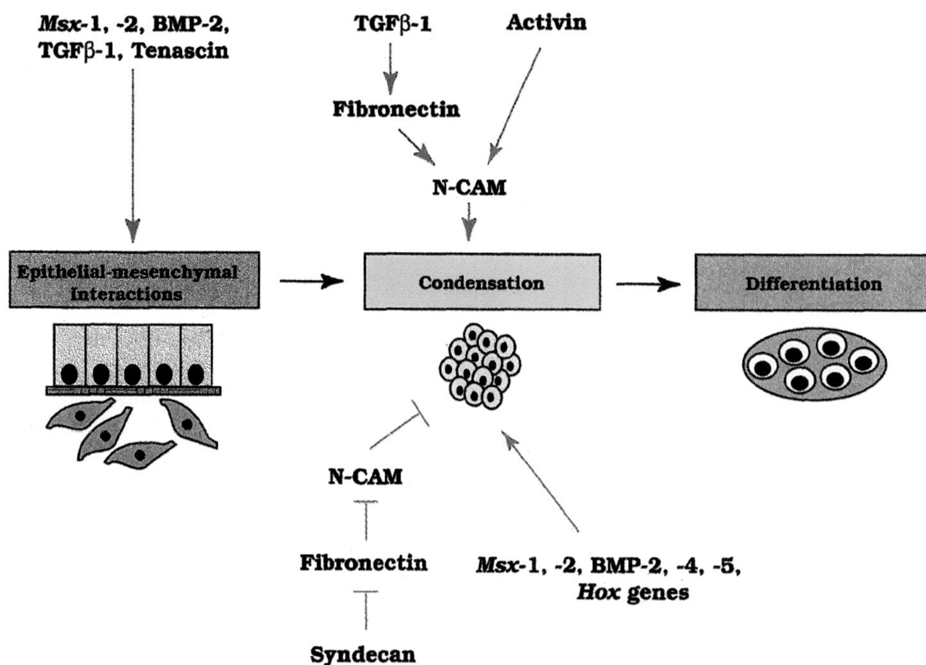

■ **Figure 15–3.** A summary of the molecular pathways leading to condensation formation and to differentiation of prechondrogenic cells in the three major phases of chondrogenesis shown in Figure 15–2. Condensation is initiated by Msx-1, -2, growth factors, and tenascin regulating epithelial-mesenchymal interactions that in turn control condensation. TGFβ-1, by up-regulating fibronectin, and activin, by direct action, stimulate accumulation of N-CAM and so promote condensation. Transition from condensation to overt cell differentiation is mediated negatively by suppression of further condensation and positively by direct enhancement of differentiation. Syndecan, by inhibiting fibronectin, breaks the link to N-CAM and so terminates condensation formation. Cessation of activin synthesis has the same effect. A number of Hox and Msx tenes and BMP-2, -4, and -5 enhance differentiation directly by acting on condensed cells. (From Hall BK, Miyake T: Divide, accumulate, differentiate: cell condensation in skeletal development revisited. *Int J Dev Biol 39*:881, 1995. See this publication for more details.)

See Hall and Miyake (1995) for details on the molecular characteristics of condensations. Members of the transforming growth factor-β (TGF-β) family of genes are involved in various stages of bone formation (Centrella et al., 1994). Most flat bones develop in mesenchyme within preexisting membranous sheaths (Gartner and Hiatt, 1997); this type of osteogenesis is **intramembranous bone formation**. Mesenchymal models of most limb bones are transformed into cartilage bone models, which later become ossified by **endochondral bone formation**. The protooncogenes C-fos and C-myc probably play an essential role in bone and cartilage development (Sakano et al., 1997). There are significant differences in the kinetics of the mineralization process in endochondral and intramembranous bone formation (Dziedzic-Goclawska et al., 1988).

Histogenesis of Cartilage

Cartilage develops from mesenchyme and first appears in embryos during the fifth week. In areas where cartilage is to develop, the mesenchyme condenses to form **chondrification centers**. The mesenchymal cells proliferate and become rounded. Cartilage-forming cells—**chondroblasts**—secrete collagenous fibrils and the ground substance of the matrix. Subsequently, collagenous and/or elastic fibers are deposited in the intercellular substance or matrix. *Three types of cartilage* are distinguished according to the type of matrix that is formed:

- hyaline cartilage, the most widely distributed type (e.g., in joints)
- fibrocartilage (e.g., in the intervertebral discs)
- elastic cartilage (e.g., in the auricle of the ear)

For more details about the histogenesis and growth of cartilage, see Gartner and Hiatt (1997).

Histogenesis of Bone

Bone develops in two types of connective tissue, mesenchyme and cartilage. Like cartilage, bone consists of cells and an organic intercellular substance—the **bone matrix**—that comprises collagen fibrils embedded in an amorphous component. For an account of bone cells with respect to the regulation of development, structure, matrix formation, and mineralization, see Marks and Popoff (1988), Dziedzic-Goclawska et al. (1988), and Gartner and Hiatt (1997).

INTRAMEMBRANOUS OSSIFICATION

This type of bone formation occurs in mesenchyme that has formed a membranous sheath (Fig. 15-4); hence, the name *intramembranous ossification*. The mesenchyme condenses and becomes highly vascular; some cells differentiate into **osteoblasts** (bone-forming cells) and begin to deposit matrix or intercellular substances—**osteoid tissue**—or prebone. The osteoblasts are almost completely separated from one another, contact being maintained by a few tiny processes. Calcium phosphate is then deposited in the osteoid tissue as it is organized into bone. Bone osteoblasts are trapped in the matrix and become **osteocytes**. At first, new bone has no organized pattern. Spicules of bone soon become organized and coalesce into lamellae or layers. Concentric lamellae develop around blood vessels, forming **haversian systems**. Some osteoblasts remain at the periphery of the developing bone and continue to lay down layers, forming plates of compact bone on the surfaces. Between the surface plates, the intervening bone remains spiculated or spongy. This spongy environment is somewhat accentuated by the action of cells with a different origin—**osteoclasts**—which absorb bone (Hughes and Boyce, 1997). In the interstices of spongy bone, the mesenchyme differentiates into **bone marrow**.

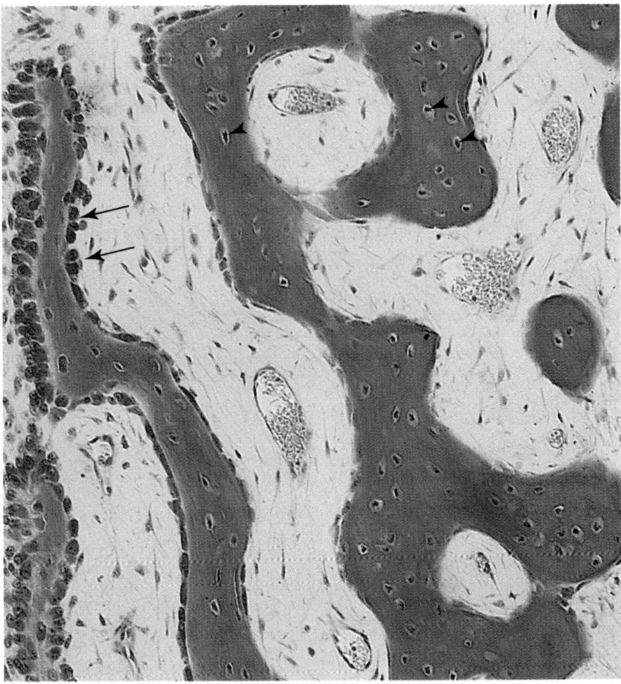

■ **Figure 15-4.** Light micrograph of intramembranous ossification (×132). Trabeculae of bone are being formed by osteoblasts lining their surface (*arrows*). Observe osteocytes trapped in lacunae (*arrowheads*) and that primitive osteons are beginning to form. The primitive osteons (canals) contain blood capillaries. (From Gartner LP, Hiatt JL: *Color Textbook of Histology.* Philadelphia, WB Saunders, 1997.)

During fetal and postnatal life, there is continuous remodeling of bone by the simultaneous action of osteoclasts and osteoblasts. Studies on the cellular and molecular events during embryonic bone formation suggest that osteogenesis and chondrogenesis are programmed early in development (Sakano et al., 1997) and are independent events under the influence of vascular factors.

INTRACARTILAGINOUS OSSIFICATION

This type of bone formation occurs in preexisting cartilaginous models (Fig. 15-5*A* to *E*). In a long bone, for example, the **primary center of ossification** appears in the *diaphysis*—the part of a long bone between its ends—which forms the **body** or **shaft** of the bone. Here the cartilage cells increase in size (hypertrophy), the matrix becomes calcified, and the cells die. Concurrently a thin layer of bone is deposited under the **perichondrium** surrounding the diaphysis; thus the perichondrium becomes the **periosteum**. Invasion of vascular connective tissue from the periosteum breaks up the cartilage. Some invading cells differentiate into **hemopoietic cells**—responsible for the formation of blood cells—of the bone marrow. Other invading cells differentiate into osteoblasts that deposit bone matrix on the spicules of calcified cartilage. This process continues toward the **epiphyses** or ends of the bone. The spicules of bone are remodeled by the action of osteoclasts and osteoblasts.

Lengthening of long bones occurs at the diaphyseal-epiphyseal junction. The lengthening of bone depends on the **epiphyseal cartilage plates** (growth plates), whose chondrocytes proliferate and participate in endochondral bone formation. Cartilage cells in the diaphyseal-epiphyseal region proliferate by mitosis. Toward the diaphysis, the cartilage cells hypertrophy and the matrix becomes calcified and broken up into spicules by vascular tissue from the marrow or medullary cavity. Bone is deposited on these spicules; absorption of this bone keeps the spongy bone masses relatively constant in length and enlarges the marrow cavity.

Ossification of limb bones begins at the end of the embryonic period and thereafter makes demands on the maternal supply of calcium and phosphorus. Pregnant women are therefore advised to maintain an adequate intake of these elements in order to preserve healthy bones and teeth. The region of bone formation at the center of the body or shaft of a long bone is the **primary ossification center** (Fig. 15-5*B*). At birth the bodies or diaphyses are largely ossified, but most of the ends or *epiphyses* are still cartilaginous. Most **secondary ossification centers** appear in the epiphyses during the first few years after birth. The epiphyseal cartilage cells hypertrophy, and there is invasion by vascular connective tissue. Ossification spreads in all directions, and only the articular cartilage and a transverse plate of cartilage, the **epiphyseal cartilage plate**, remain cartilaginous (Fig. 15-5*E*).

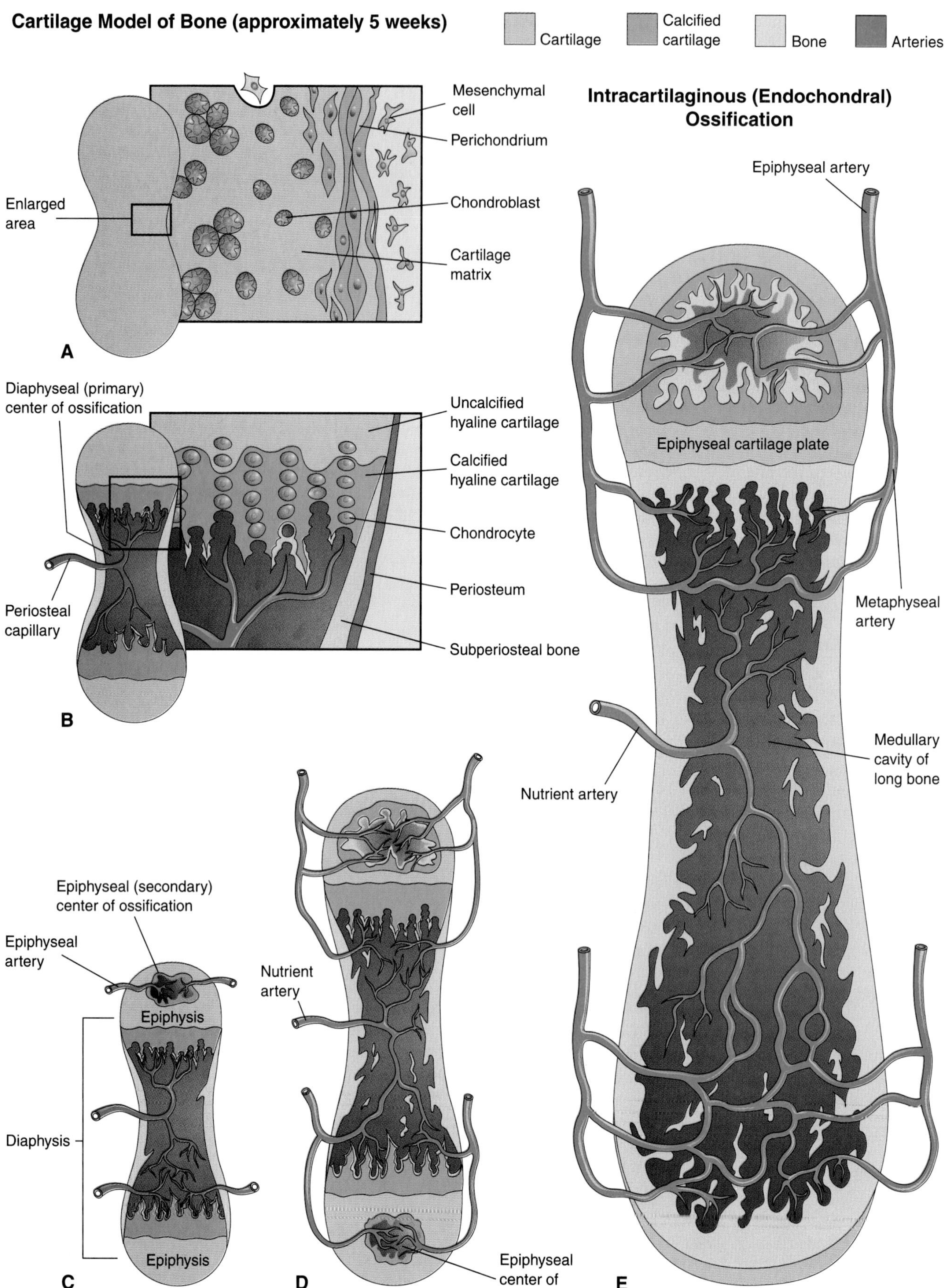

■ **Figure 15–5.** *A* to *E,* Schematic longitudinal sections illustrating intracartilaginous or endochondral ossification in a developing long bone.

Upon completion of growth, this plate is replaced by spongy bone; the epiphyses and diaphysis are united, and further elongation of the bone does not occur.

In most bones the epiphyses have fused with the diaphysis by about the age of 20 years. Growth in the diameter of a bone results from deposition of bone at the periosteum and from absorption on the medullary surface. The rate of deposition and absorption is balanced to regulate the thickness of the compact bone and the size of the medullary (marrow) cavity. The internal reorganization of bone continues throughout life. The development of irregular bones is similar to that of the epiphyses of long bones. Ossification begins centrally and spreads in all directions. In addition to membranous and endochondral ossification, **chondroid tissue**, which also differentiates from mesenchyme, is now recognized as an important factor for skeletal growth (Dhem et al., 1989). For a comprehensive description of bone formation, see Gartner and Hiatt (1997).

Rickets

Rickets is a disease that occurs in children who have a vitamin D deficiency. Calcium absorption by the intestine is impaired, which causes disturbances of ossification of the epiphyseal cartilage plates (e.g., they are not adequately mineralized), and there is disorientation of cells at the metaphysis (Gartner and Hiatt, 1997). The limbs are shortened and deformed, with severe bowing of the limb bones (Moore, 1992). For more information about the clinical manifestations of and the radiological and pathological findings in rickets, see Behrman et al. (1996).

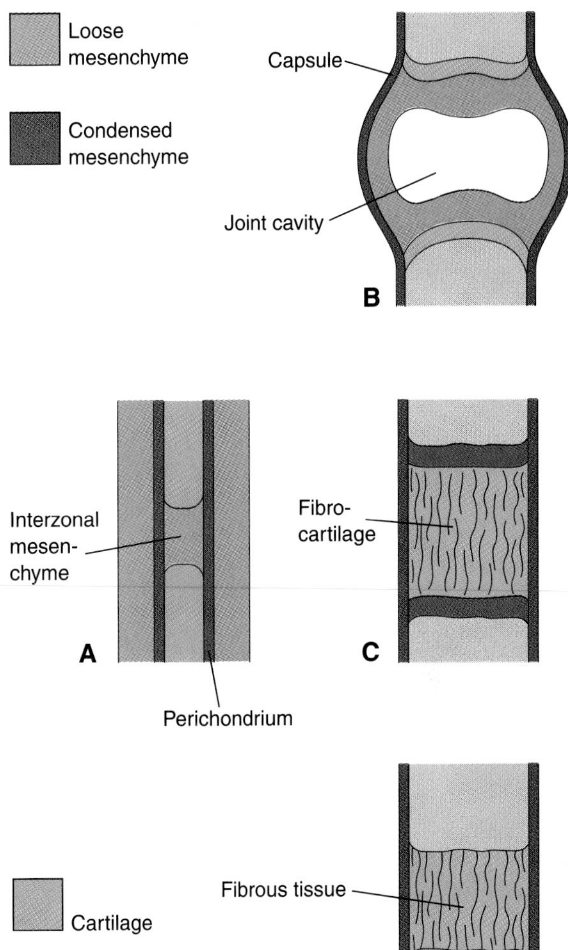

■ **Figure 15–6.** Schematic drawings illustrating the development of joints during the sixth and seventh weeks. *A,* Condensed mesenchyme continues across the gap, or interzone, between the developing bones, enclosing some mesenchyme (the interzonal mesenchyme) between them. This primitive joint may differentiate into *B,* a synovial joint, *C,* a cartilaginous joint, or *D,* a fibrous joint.

DEVELOPMENT OF JOINTS

Joints begin to develop during the sixth week, and by the end of the eighth week they resemble adult joints (Fig. 15-6). The terms *articulation* and *joint* are used synonymously to refer to the structural arrangements that join two or more bones together at their place of meeting. Joints are classified as:

- fibrous joints
- cartilaginous joints
- synovial joints

Joints with little or no movement are classified according to the type of material holding the bones together; e.g., the bones involved in fibrous joints are joined by fibrous tissue (Fig. 15-6*D*).

Fibrous Joints

During the development of the fibrous joint, the interzonal mesenchyme between the developing bones differentiates into dense fibrous tissue (Fig. 15-6*D*); e.g., the sutures of the skull are fibrous joints.

Cartilaginous Joints

During the development of cartilaginous joints, the interzonal mesenchyme between the developing bones differentiates into hyaline cartilage (e.g., the costochondral joints) or fibrocartilage (Fig. 15-6*C*), for example, the pubic symphysis between the bodies of the pubic bones (Moore, 1992).

Synovial Joints

During the development of this common type of joint (e.g., the knee joint), the interzonal mesenchyme between the developing bones differentiates as follows (Fig. 15-6*B*):

- Peripherally it forms the capsular and other ligaments.
- Centrally it disappears and the resulting space becomes the joint or synovial cavity.

- Where it lines the fibrous capsule and articular surfaces, it forms the synovial membrane, a part of the articular capsule.

Probably as a result of joint movements, the mesenchymal cells subsequently disappear from the surfaces of the articular cartilages. An abnormal intrauterine environment restricting embryonic and fetal movements may interfere with limb development and cause joint fixation (Davis and Kalousek, 1988).

DEVELOPMENT OF AXIAL SKELETON

The axial skeleton is composed of the:

- skull
- vertebral column
- ribs
- sternum

During formation of this part of the skeleton, the cells in the sclerotomes of the somites change their position (Fig. 15-1). During the fourth week, they surround the neural tube (primordium of spinal cord) and the notochord, the structure about which the primordia of the vertebrae develop. This positional change of the sclerotomal cells is effected by differential growth of the surrounding structures and not by active migration of sclerotomal cells (Gasser, 1979). The *Pax-1* gene, which is expressed in all prospective sclerotomal cells of epithelial somites in chick and mouse embryos, seems to play an essential role in the development of the vertebral column (Wilting et al., 1996).

Development of Vertebral Column

During the precartilaginous or mesenchymal stage, mesenchymal cells from the sclerotomes are found in three main areas (Fig. 15-7*A*):

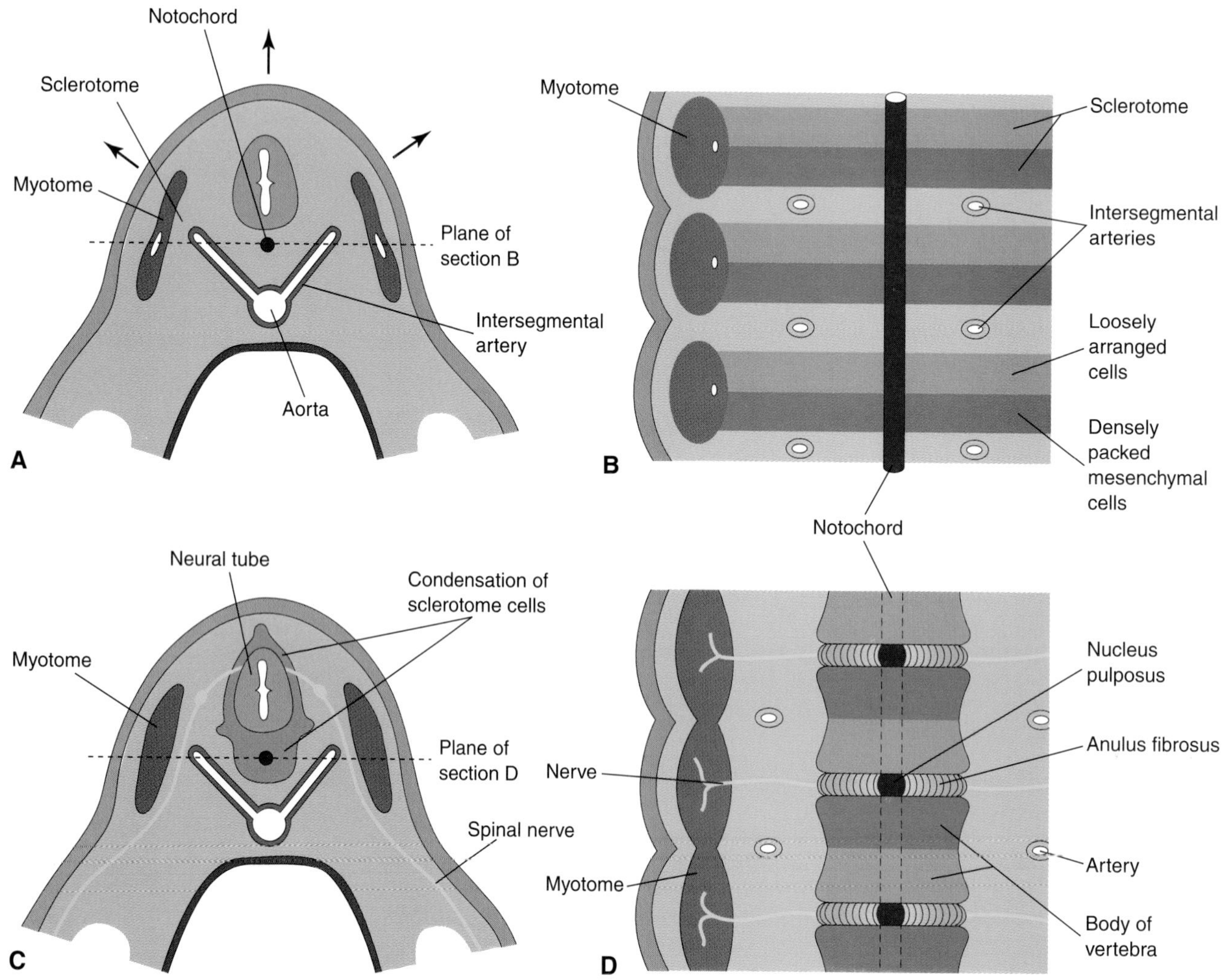

■ **Figure 15-7.** *A,* Transverse section through a 4-week embryo. The arrows indicate the dorsal growth of the neural tube and the simultaneous dorsolateral movement of the somite remnant, leaving behind a trail of sclerotomal cells. *B,* Diagrammatic frontal section of this embryo, showing that the condensation of sclerotomal cells around the notochord consists of a cranial area of loosely packed cells and a caudal area of densely packed cells. *C,* Transverse section through a 5-week embryo, showing the condensation of sclerotomal cells around the notochord and neural tube, which forms a mesenchymal vertebra. *D,* Diagrammatic frontal section, illustrating that the vertebral body forms from the cranial and caudal halves of two successive sclerotomal masses. The intersegmental arteries now cross the bodies of the vertebrae, and the spinal nerves lie between the vertebrae. The notochord is degenerating except in the region of the intervertebral disc, where it forms the nucleus pulposus.

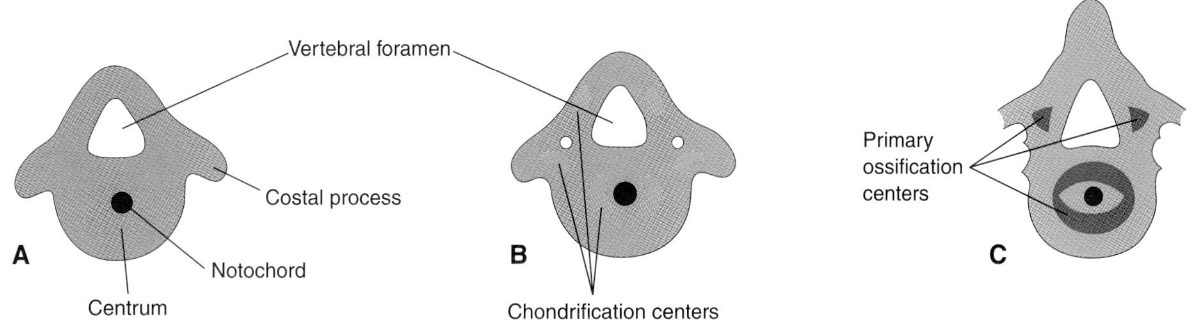

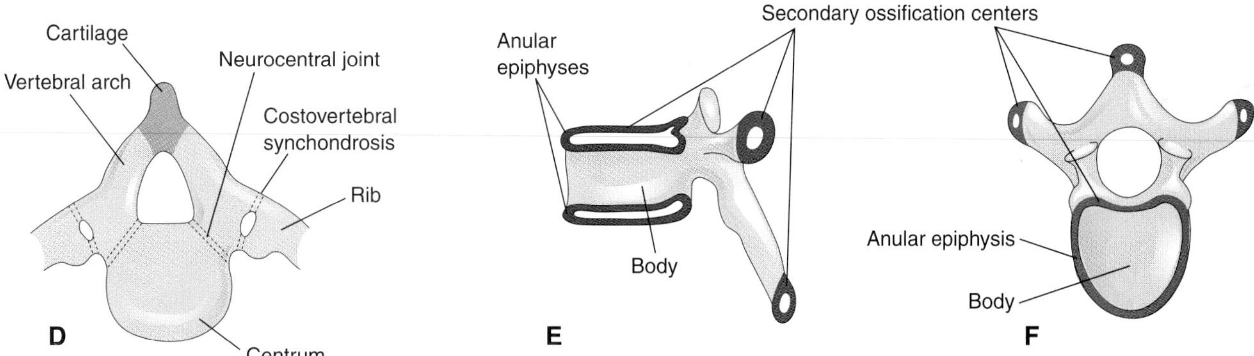

■ **Figure 15–8.** Drawings illustrating the stages of vertebral development. *A,* Mesenchymal vertebra at 5 weeks. *B,* Chondrification centers in a mesenchymal vertebra at 6 weeks. *C,* Primary ossification centers in a cartilaginous vertebra at 7 weeks. *D,* Thoracic vertebra at birth consisting of three bony parts. Note the cartilage between the halves of the vertebral arch and between the arch and the centrum (neurocentral joint). *E* and *F,* Two views of a typical thoracic vertebra at puberty showing the location of the secondary centers of ossification.

- around the notochord
- surrounding the neural tube
- in the body wall

In a frontal section of a 4-week embryo, the sclerotomes appear as paired condensations of mesenchymal cells around the notochord (Fig. 15-7*B*). Each sclerotome consists of loosely arranged cells cranially and densely packed cells caudally. Some densely packed cells move cranially opposite the center of the myotome, where they form the **intervertebral disc** (Fig. 15-7*C* and *D*). The remaining densely packed cells fuse with the loosely arranged cells of the immediately caudal sclerotome to form the mesenchymal **centrum**, the primordium of the body of a vertebra. Thus each centrum develops from two adjacent sclerotomes and becomes an intersegmental structure. The nerves now lie in close relationship to the intervertebral discs, and the *intersegmental arteries* lie on each side of the vertebral bodies. In the thorax the dorsal intersegmental arteries become the *intercostal arteries*.

The **notochord** degenerates and disappears where it is surrounded by the developing vertebral bodies. Between the vertebrae the notochord expands to form the gelatinous center of the intervertebral disc, the **nucleus pulposus** (Fig. 15-7*D*). This nucleus is later surrounded by the circularly arranged fibers that form the **anulus fibrosus**. The nucleus pulposus and anulus fibrosus together constitute the **intervertebral disc**. The mesenchymal cells, surrounding the neural tube, form the vertebral (neural) arch. The mesenchymal cells in the body wall form the costal processes that form ribs in the thoracic region.

Chordoma

Remnants of the notochord may persist and give rise to a **chordoma**. About a third of these slow-growing malignant tumors occur at the base of the skull and extend to the nasopharynx. They infiltrate bone and are difficult to remove. Few patients survive longer than 5 years (Rubin and Farber, 1988). Chordomas also develop in the lumbosacral region.

CARTILAGINOUS STAGE OF VERTEBRAL DEVELOPMENT

During the sixth week chondrification centers appear in each mesenchymal vertebra (Fig. 15-8*A* and *B*). The two centers in each centrum fuse at the end of the embryonic period to form a cartilaginous centrum. Concomitantly the centers in the vertebral arches fuse with each other and the centrum. The spinous and transverse processes develop from extensions of chondrification centers in the vertebral arch. Chondrification spreads until a cartilaginous vertebral column is formed.

BONY STAGE OF VERTEBRAL DEVELOPMENT

Ossification of typical vertebrae begins during the embryonic period and usually ends by the twenty-fifth year. There are two primary ossification centers, ventral and dorsal, for the centrum (Fig. 15-8*C*). These **primary ossification centers** soon fuse to form one center. Three primary centers are present by the end of the embryonic period:

- one in the centrum
- one in each half of the vertebral arch

Ossification becomes evident in the vertebral arches during the eighth week. At birth each vertebra consists of three bony parts connected by cartilage (Fig. 15-8*D*). The bony halves of the vertebral arch usually fuse during the first 3 to 5 years. The arches first unite in the lumbar region, and union progresses cranially. The vertebral arch articulates with the centrum at cartilaginous **neurocentral joints**. These articulations permit the vertebral arches to grow as the spinal cord enlarges. These joints disappear when the vertebral arch fuses with the centrum during the third to sixth years. See Wilting et al. (1996) for more details on the development of the vertebral column. Five **secondary ossification centers** appear in the vertebrae after puberty:

- one for the tip of the spinous process
- one for the tip of each transverse process
- two *anular epiphyses*, one on the superior and one on the inferior rim of the vertebral body (Fig. 15-8*E* and *F*).

The **vertebral body** is a composite of the anular epiphyses and the mass of bone between them. The vertebral body includes the centrum, parts of the vertebral arch, and the facets for the heads of the ribs. All secondary centers unite with the rest of the vertebra around 25 years of age.

Exceptions to the typical ossification of vertebrae occur in the atlas (C1), axis (C2), C7, lumbar vertebrae, sacrum, and coccyx. For details of their ossification, consult Bannister et al. (1995) and Moore (1992).

Variation in the Number of Vertebrae

About 95% of people have 7 cervical, 12 thoracic, 5 lumbar, and 5 sacral vertebrae. About 3% of people have one or two additional vertebrae and about 2% have one fewer. To determine the number of vertebrae, it is necessary to examine the entire vertebral column because an apparent extra (or absent) vertebra in one segment of the column may be compensated for by an absent (or extra) vertebra in an adjacent segment, for example, 11 thoracic-type vertebrae with 6 lumbar-type vertebrae.

Development of Ribs

The ribs develop from the mesenchymal costal processes of the thoracic vertebrae (Fig. 15-8*A*). They become cartilaginous during the embryonic period and ossify during the fetal period. The original site of union of the costal processes with the vertebra is replaced by *costovertebral joints*. These are the plane type of synovial joint (Fig. 15-8*D*). Seven pairs of ribs (1 to 7)—**true ribs**—attach through their own cartilages to the sternum. Five pairs of ribs (8 to 12)—**false ribs**—attach to the sternum through the cartilage of another rib or ribs. The last two pairs of ribs (11 and 12) do not attach to the sternum; they are **floating ribs**.

Development of Sternum

A pair of mesenchymal vertical bands, **sternal bars**, develop ventrolaterally in the body wall. *Chondrification* occurs in these bars as they move medially. They fuse craniocaudally in the median plane to form cartilaginous models of the manubrium, sternebrae (segments of the sternal body), and xiphoid process. Fusion at the inferior end of the sternum is sometimes incomplete; as a result, the xiphoid process in these infants is bifid or perforated. Centers of ossification appear craniocaudally in the sternum before birth, except that for the xiphoid process, which appears during childhood.

Development of Skull

The skull develops from mesenchyme around the developing brain. The skull consists of:

- the **neurocranium**, a protective case for the brain
- the **viscerocranium**, the skeleton of the face

See Hall and Miyake (1995) for details of molecular events related to chondrogenesis in the craniofacial skeleton.

CARTILAGINOUS NEUROCRANIUM

Initially the cartilaginous neurocranium or **chondrocranium** consists of the cartilaginous base of the developing skull, which forms by fusion of several cartilages (Fig. 15-9*A* to *D*). Later endochondral ossification of the chondrocranium forms the bones of the base of the skull. The ossification pattern of these bones has a definite sequence, beginning with the occipital bone, basisphenoid bone (body of sphenoid), and ethmoid bone (Kjaer, 1990).

The **parachordal cartilage**, or **basal plate**, forms

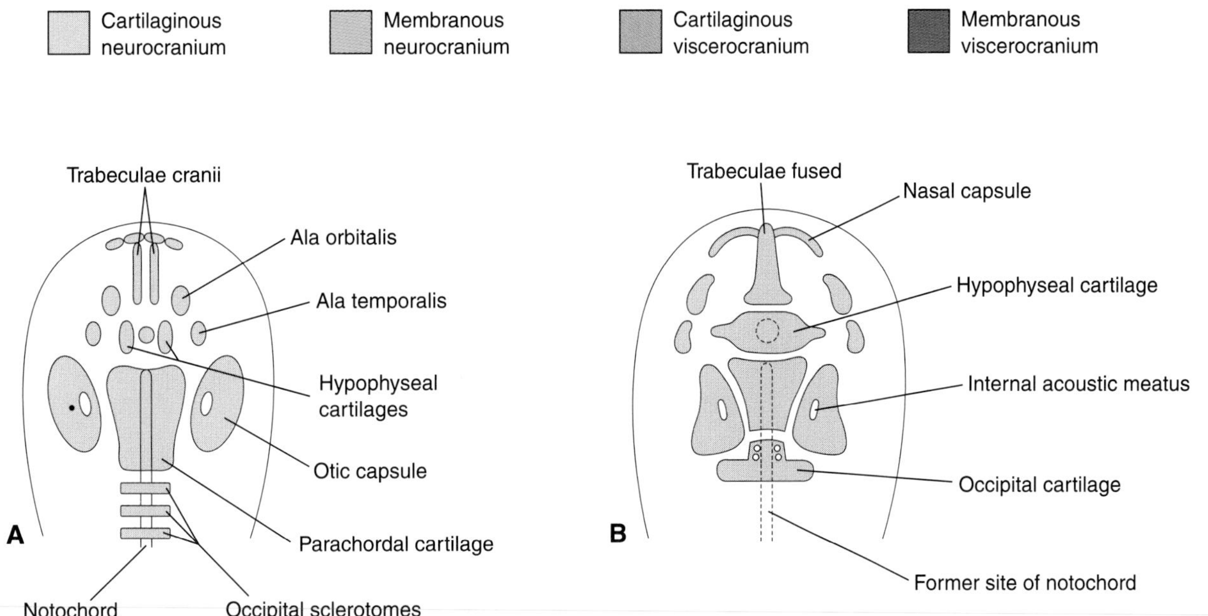

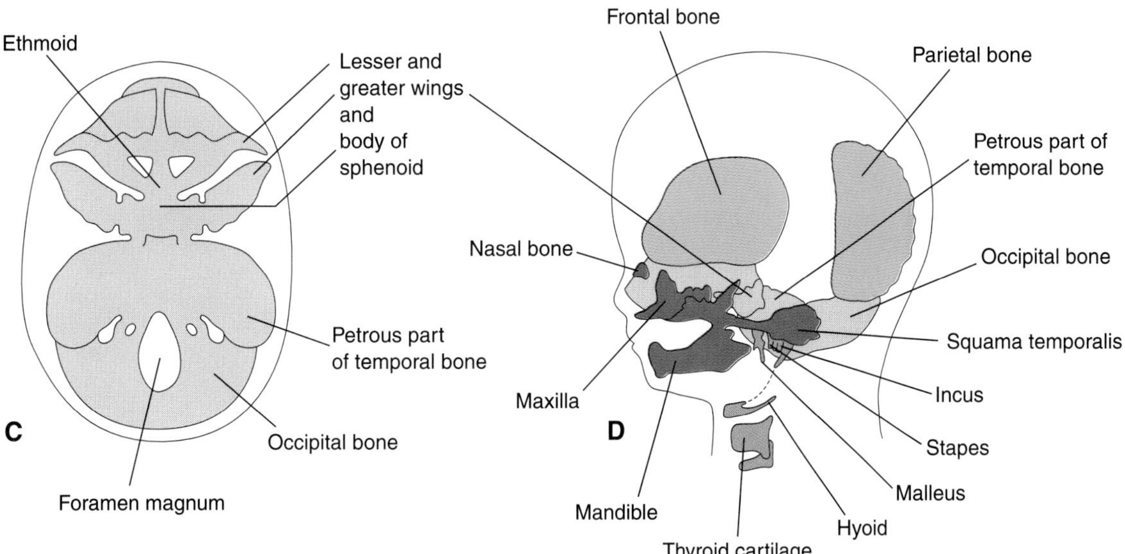

■ **Figure 15–9.** Diagrams illustrating stages in the development of the skull. *A* to *C* are views of the base of the developing skull (viewed superiorly). *D* is a lateral view. *A,* 6 weeks, showing the various cartilages that will fuse to form the chondrocranium. *B,* 7 weeks, after fusion of some of the paired cartilages. *C,* 12 weeks, showing the cartilaginous base of the skull or chondrocranium formed by the fusion of various cartilages. *D,* 20 weeks, indicating the derivation of the bones of the fetal skull.

around the cranial end of the notochord (Fig. 15-9*A*) and fuses with the cartilages derived from the sclerotome regions of the occipital somites. This cartilaginous mass contributes to the base of the occipital bone; later, extensions grow around the cranial end of the spinal cord and form the boundaries of the foramen magnum (Fig. 15-9*C*).

The **hypophyseal cartilage** forms around the developing pituitary gland (hypophysis cerebri) and fuses to form the body of the sphenoid bone. The *trabeculae cranii* fuse to form the body of the ethmoid bone, and the *ala orbitalis* forms the lesser wing of the sphenoid bone. *Otic capsules* develop around the otic vesicles, the primordia of the internal ears (see Chapter 19), and form the petrous and mastoid parts of the temporal bone. *Nasal capsules* develop around the nasal sacs (see Chapter 10) and contribute to the formation of the ethmoid bone.

MEMBRANOUS NEUROCRANIUM

Intramembranous ossification occurs in the mesenchyme at the sides and top of the brain, forming the **calvaria** (cranial vault). During fetal life the flat bones of the calvaria are separated by dense connective tissue membranes that form fibrous joints, the **sutures**

(Fig. 15-10). Six large fibrous areas—**fontanelles**—are present where several sutures meet (Sundaresan et al., 1990; Moore and Agur, 1995). The softness of the bones and their loose connections at the sutures enable the calvaria to undergo changes of shape during birth, called molding. During **molding of the fetal skull** (adaptation of the fetal head to the pelvic cavity during birth), the frontal bone becomes flat, the occipital bone is drawn out, and one parietal bone slightly overrides the other one. Within a few days after birth, the shape of the calvaria usually returns to normal.

CARTILAGINOUS VISCEROCRANIUM

These parts of the fetal skull are derived from the cartilaginous skeleton of the first two pairs of pharyngeal arches (see Chapter 10).

- The dorsal end of the *first arch cartilage* (Meckel cartilage) forms two middle ear bones, the malleus and incus.
- The dorsal end of the *second arch cartilage* (Reichert cartilage) forms the stapes of the middle

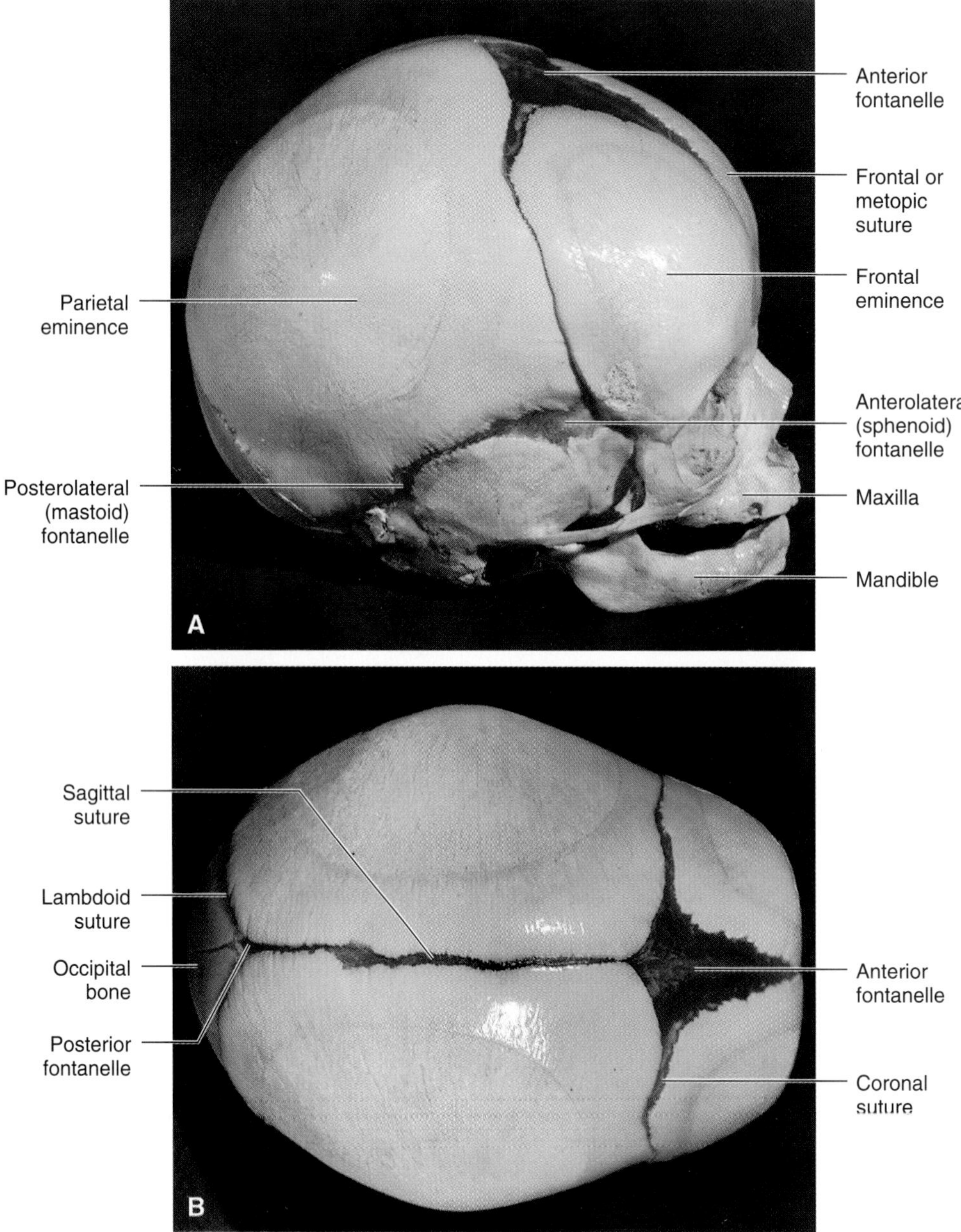

■ **Figure 15–10.** Photographs of a fetal skull showing the bones, fontanelles, and connecting sutures. *A,* Lateral view. *B,* Superior view. The posterior and anterolateral fontanelles disappear because of growth of surrounding bones, within 2 or 3 months after birth, but they remain as sutures for several years. The posterolateral fontanelles disappear in a similar manner by the end of the first year and the anterior fontanelle by the end of the second year. The halves of the frontal bone normally begin to fuse during the second year, and the frontal or metopic suture is usually obliterated by the eighth year. The other sutures disappear during adult life, but the times when the sutures close are subject to wide variations.

ear and the styloid process of the temporal bone. Its ventral end ossifies to form the lesser cornu (L., horn) and superior part of the body of the hyoid bone.
- The third, fourth, and sixth arch cartilages form only in the ventral parts of the arches. The *third arch cartilages* give rise to the greater cornua and inferior part of the body of the hyoid bone.
- The *fourth and sixth arch cartilages* fuse to form the laryngeal cartilages, except for the epiglottis (see Chapter 10).

MEMBRANOUS VISCEROCRANIUM

Intramembranous ossification occurs in the maxillary prominence of the first pharyngeal arch (see Chapter 10) and subsequently forms the squamous temporal, maxillary, and zygomatic bones. The squamous temporal bones become part of the neurocranium. The mesenchyme in the mandibular prominence of the first arch condenses around its cartilage (Meckel cartilage) and undergoes intramembranous ossification to form the mandible. Some endochondral ossification occurs in the median plane of the chin and in the mandibular condyle.

NEWBORN SKULL

After recovering from molding, the newborn skull is rather round and its bones are thin. Like the fetal skull (Fig. 15-10), it is large in proportion to the rest of the skeleton and the face is relatively small compared with the calvaria. The small facial region of the skull results from:

- the small size of the jaws
- the virtual absence of paranasal (air) sinuses
- the underdevelopment of the facial bones at birth

POSTNATAL GROWTH OF SKULL

The fibrous sutures of the newborn calvaria permit the brain to enlarge during infancy and childhood. The increase in the size of the calvaria is greatest during the first 2 years, the period of most rapid postnatal growth of the brain. The calvaria normally increases in capacity until about 16 years of age. After this, it usually increases slightly in size for 3 to 4 years because of thickening of its bones. There is also rapid growth of the face and jaws, coinciding with eruption of the primary or deciduous teeth. These facial changes are more marked after the secondary or permanent teeth erupt (see Chapter 20). There is concurrent enlargement of the frontal and facial regions, associated with the increase in the size of the paranasal sinuses. Most paranasal sinuses are rudimentary or absent at birth. Growth of these sinuses is important in altering the shape of the face and in adding resonance to the voice.

Klippel-Feil Syndrome (Brevicollis)

The main features of this syndrome are short neck, low hairline, and restricted neck movements. In most cases the number of cervical vertebral bodies is less than normal. In some cases there is a lack of segmentation of several elements of the cervical region of the vertebral column. The number of cervical nerve roots may be normal but they are small, as are the intervertebral foramina. Patients with this syndrome are often otherwise normal, but the association of this anomaly with other congenital anomalies is not uncommon.

Spina Bifida

Failure of fusion of the halves of the vertebral arch results in a major defect—spina bifida. The incidence of this vertebral defect ranges from 0.04 to 0.15%, and it occurs more frequently in girls than boys (Sarwark, 1996). Most cases of spina bifida (80%) are "open" and covered by a thin membrane. A "closed" spina bifida or spina bifida occulta is covered by a thick membrane or skin. This defect of the vertebral arch is a consequence of failure of fusion of the halves of the vertebral arch.

Spina bifida occulta is commonly observed in radiographs of the cervical, lumbar, and sacral regions. Frequently only one vertebra is affected. Spina bifida occulta is a relatively minor, insignificant anomaly of the vertebral column that usually causes no clinical symptoms. It can be diagnosed in utero by sonography (Filly, 1991a). Spina bifida occulta of the first sacral vertebra occurs in about 20% of vertebral columns that are examined radiographically (Behrman et al., 1996). The spinal cord and spinal nerves are usually normal and neurological symptoms are commonly absent. The skin over the bifid vertebral arch is intact and there may be no external evidence of the vertebral defect. Sometimes the anomaly is indicated by a dimple or a tuft of hair. In about 3% of normal adults, there is spina bifida occulta of the atlas. At other cervical levels this condition is rare and when present, it is sometimes accompanied by other abnormalities of the cervical region of the vertebral column.

Spina bifida cystica, a severe type of spina bifida involving the spinal cord and meninges, is discussed in Chapter 18. Neurological symptoms are present in these cases. See Chapter 18 for illustrations and photographs of infants with spina bifida.

Accessory Ribs

Accessory ribs, usually rudimentary, result from the development of the costal processes of cervical or

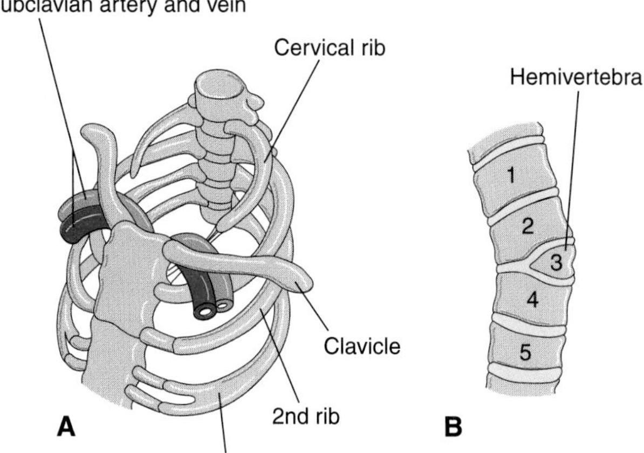

■ **Figure 15–11.** Drawings of vertebral and rib abnormalities. *A,* Cervical and forked ribs. Observe that the left cervical rib has a fibrous band that passes posterior to the subclavian vessels and attaches to the sternum. This condition very likely produced neurovascular changes in the left upper limb. *B,* Anterior view of the vertebral column showing a hemivertebra. The right half of the third thoracic vertebra is absent. Note the associated lateral curvature (scoliosis) of the vertebral column.

lumbar vertebrae (Fig. 15–11*A*). These processes form ribs in the thoracic region. The most common type of accessory rib is a **lumbar rib**, but it usually causes no problems (Moore, 1992). **Cervical ribs** occur in 0.5 to 1% of people. A cervical rib is attached to the seventh cervical vertebra and may be unilateral or bilateral (McNally et al., 1990). Pressure of a cervical rib on the brachial plexus or the subclavian artery often produces symptoms (Moore and Agur, 1995).

Fused Ribs

Fusion of ribs occasionally occurs posteriorly when two or more ribs arise from a single vertebra. Fused ribs are often associated with a hemivertebra.

Hemivertebra

The developing vertebral bodies have two chondrification centers that soon unite. A hemivertebra results from failure of one of the chondrification centers to appear and subsequent failure of half of the vertebra to form (Fig. 15–11*B*). These defective vertebrae produce **scoliosis** (lateral curvature) of the vertebral column (Moore, 1992). There are other causes of scoliosis (e.g., myopathic scoliosis resulting from weakness of the spinal muscles).

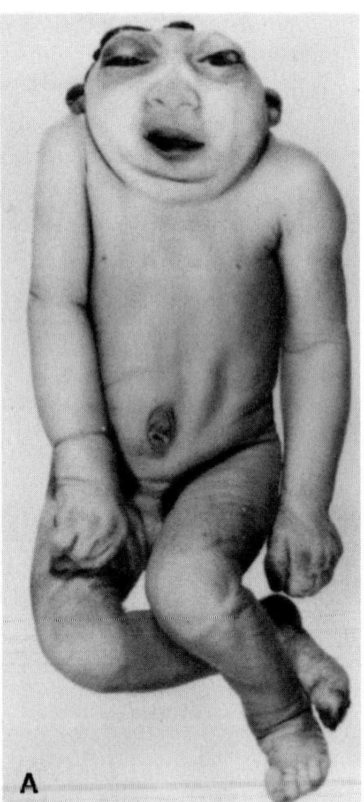

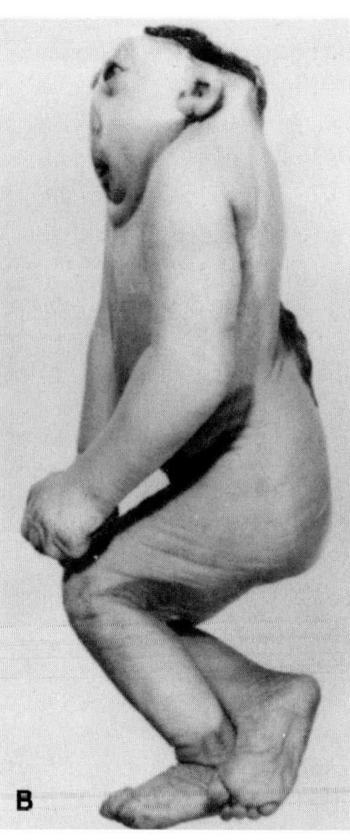

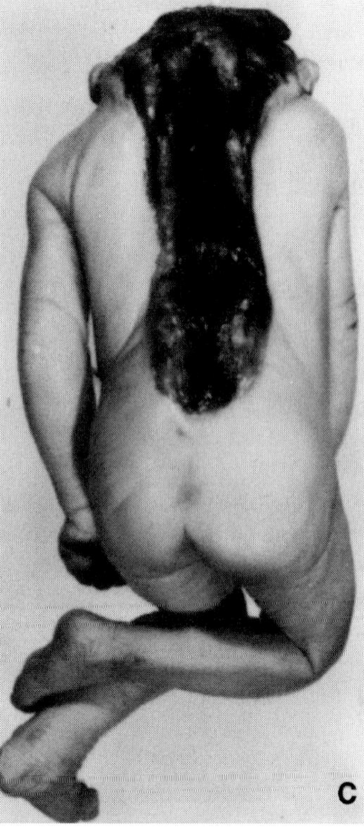

■ **Figure 15–12.** Photographs of anterior (*A*), lateral (*B*), and posterior (*C*) views of a newborn infant with acrania (absence of calvaria), meroanencephaly (partial absence of brain), rachischisis (extensive cleft in vertebral arches of the vertebral column), and myeloschisis (severe anomaly of spinal cord). Infants with these severe craniovertebral anomalies involving the brain and spinal cord usually die within a few days after birth. For more information about meroanencephaly and spina bifida with myeloschisis, see Chapter 18.

Rachischisis

The term *rachischisis* (cleft vertebral column) refers to the vertebral abnormalities in a complex group of anomalies (*axial dysraphic disorders*) that primarily affect axial structures (Fig. 15-12*C*). In these infants, the neural folds fail to fuse, either because of faulty induction by the underlying notochord or from the action of teratogenic agents on the neuroepithelial cells in the neural folds. The neural and vertebral defects may be extensive or be restricted to a small area.

Cleft Sternum

Minor sternal clefts (e.g., a notch or foramen in the xiphoid process) are common and are of no clinical concern. A *sternal foramen* of varying size and form occurs occasionally at the junction of the third and fourth sternebrae. This insignificant foramen is the result of incomplete fusion of the cartilaginous sternal bars during the embryonic period.

Skull Anomalies

These abnormalities range from major defects that are incompatible with life to those that are minor and insignificant. With large defects, there is often herniation of the meninges and/or brain (see Chapter 18).

Acrania

In this condition the calvaria is absent and extensive defects of the vertebral column are often present (Fig. 15-12). Acrania associated with **meroanencephaly** or **anencephaly** (partial absence of the brain) occurs about once in 1000 births and is incompatible with life. Meroanencephaly results from failure of the cranial end of the neural tube to close during the fourth week. This anomaly causes subsequent failure of the calvaria to form (Fig. 15-12*A* and *B*).

Craniosynostosis

Several skull deformities result from premature closure of the skull sutures. Prenatal closure results in the most severe abnormalities. The cause of craniosynostosis is unknown, but genetic factors appear to be important. These abnormalities are much more common in males than in females and they are often associated with other skeletal anomalies. The type of deformed skull produced depends upon which sutures close prematurely. If the sagittal suture closes early, the skull becomes long, narrow, and wedge-shaped—**scaphocephaly** (Fig. 15-13). This type of skull deformity constitutes about half the cases of craniosynostosis. Another 30% of cases involve premature closure of the coronal sutures, which results in a high, towerlike skull—**oxycephaly** or turricephaly (Fig. 15-14*A*). If the coronal or lambdoid suture closes prematurely on one side only, the skull is twisted and asymmetrical—**plagiocephaly** (Fig. 15-14*B*).

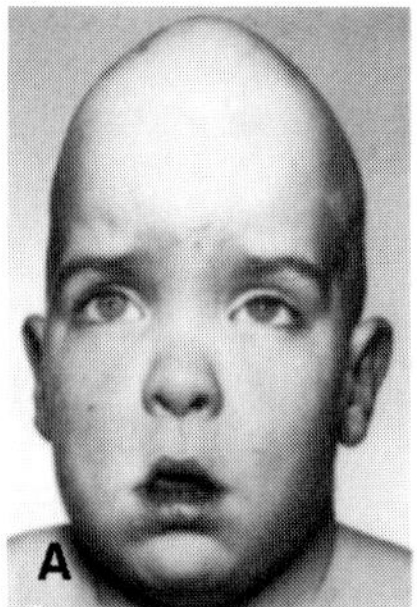

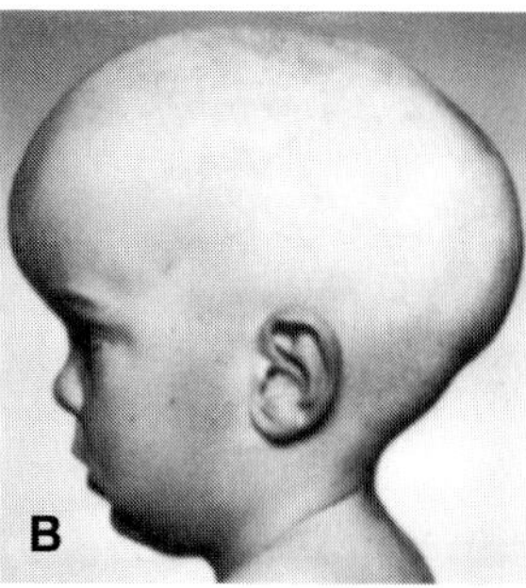

■ **Figure 15-13.** *A* and *B*, Photographs of a boy with a long, wedge-shaped skull (scaphocephaly) resulting from craniosynostosis—premature closure of the sagittal suture. (From Laurence KM, Weeks R: Abnormalities of the central nervous system. *In* Norman AP [ed]: *Congenital Abnormalities of Infancy,* 2nd ed. Oxford, Blackwell Scientific Publications, 1971.)

Microcephaly

Infants with this condition are born with a normal-sized or slightly small calvaria. The fontanelles close during early infancy, and the sutures close during the first year. This anomaly is not caused by premature closure of sutures. Microcephaly is the result of abnormal development of the central nervous system (CNS) in which the brain and, consequently, the skull fail to grow. Generally, microcephalics are severely mentally retarded. This anomaly is also discussed in Chapter 18.

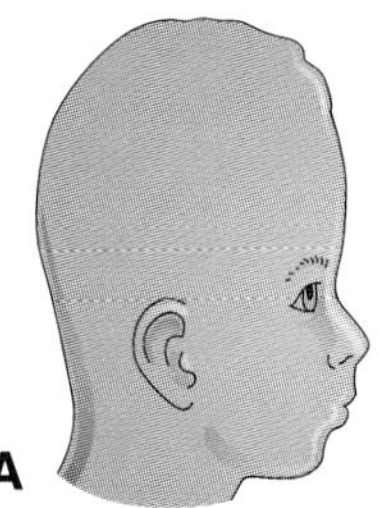

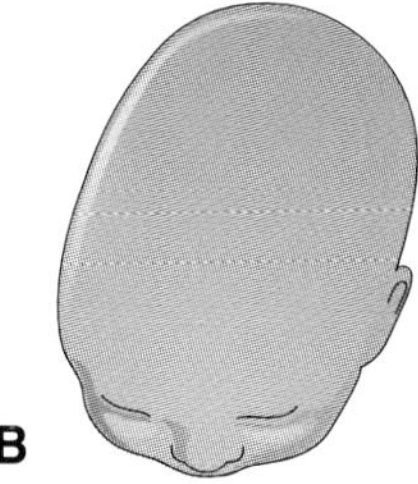

■ **Figure 15-14.** Drawings illustrating skull anomalies. *A*, Oxycephaly (turricephaly), showing the towerlike skull resulting from premature closure of the coronal suture. *B*, Plagiocephaly, illustrating an asymmetrical skull resulting from premature closure of the coronal and lambdoid sutures on the left side.

Anomalies at the Craniovertebral Junction

Congenital abnormalities at the craniovertebral junction are present in about 1% of newborn infants, but they may not produce symptoms until adult life. The following are examples of these anomalies: *basilar invagination* (superior displacement of the bone around the foramen magnum); *assimilation of the atlas* (nonsegmentation at the junction of the atlas and occipital bone); *atlantoaxial dislocation*; Arnold-Chiari malformation (see Chapter 18); and *separate dens* or odontoid process (failure of the centers in the dens to fuse with the centrum of the axis).

DEVELOPMENT OF APPENDICULAR SKELETON

The appendicular skeleton consists of the pectoral and pelvic girdles and the limb bones. Mesenchymal bones form during the fifth week as condensations of mesenchyme appear in the limb buds (Fig. 15-15*A* to *C*). *During the sixth week the mesenchymal bone models in the limbs undergo chondrification to form hyaline cartilage bone models* (Fig. 15-15*D* and *E*). The clavicle initially develops by intramembranous ossification, and it later forms growth cartilages at both ends. The models of the pectoral girdle (shoulder girdle) and upper limb bones appear slightly before those of the pelvic girdle and lower limbs; the bone models appear in a proximodistal sequence. Patterning in the developing limbs is regulated by **homeobox-containing genes**. The molecular mechanisms of these *HOX* genes in limb morphogenesis remain uncertain (Muragaki et al., 1996).

Ossification begins in the long bones by the eighth week of embryonic development and initially occurs in the diaphyses of the bones from **primary centers of ossification** (Fig. 15-5). By 12 weeks primary ossification centers have appeared in nearly all bones of the limbs (Fig. 15-16). The clavicles begin to ossify before any other bones in the body. The femora are the next bones to show traces of ossification. The first

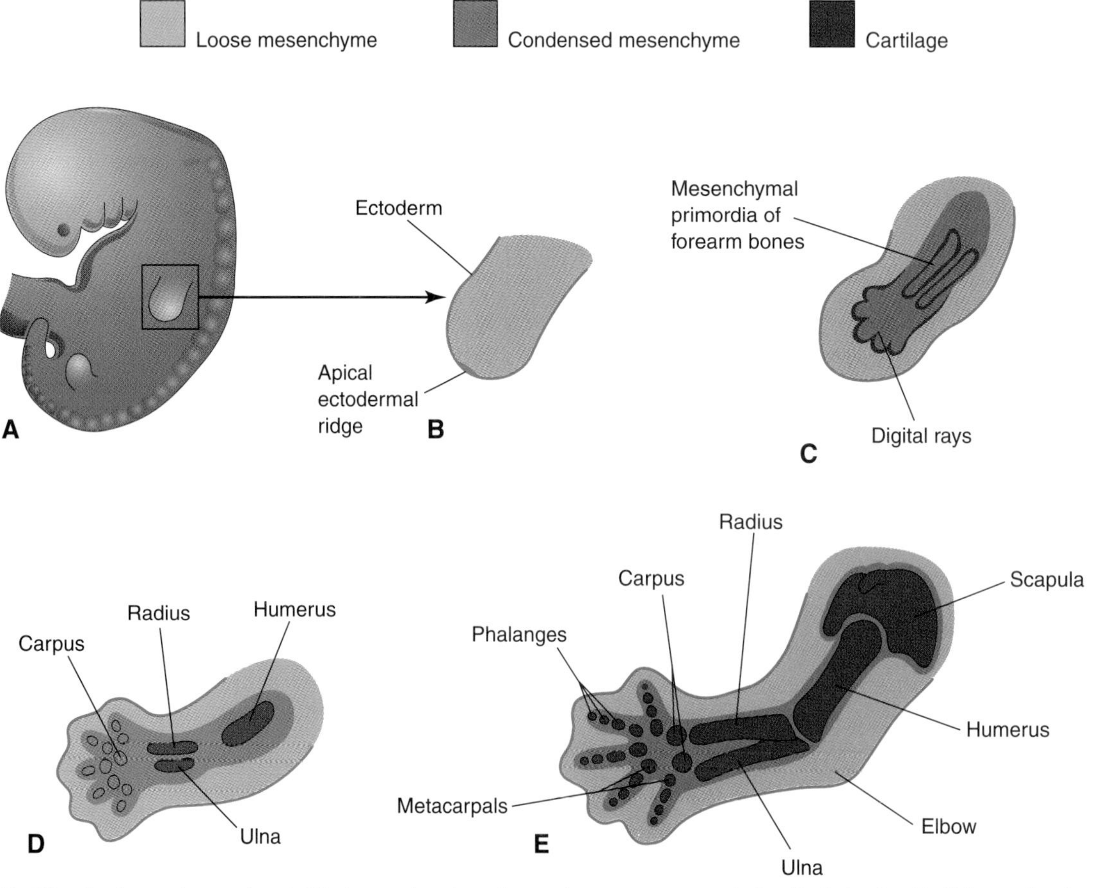

■ **Figure 15-15.** *A,* An embryo about 28 days, showing the early appearance of the limb buds. *B,* Schematic drawing of a longitudinal section through an upper limb bud. The apical ectodermal ridge has an inductive influence on the mesenchyme in the limb bud; it promotes growth of the mesenchyme and appears to give it the ability to form specific cartilaginous elements. *C,* Similar sketch of an upper limb bud at about 33 days, showing the mesenchymal primordia of the limb bones. The digital rays are mesenchymal condensations that undergo chondrification and ossification to form the bones of the hand. *D,* Upper limb at 6 weeks, showing the cartilage models of the bones. *E,* Later in the sixth week, showing the completed cartilaginous models of the bones of the upper limb.

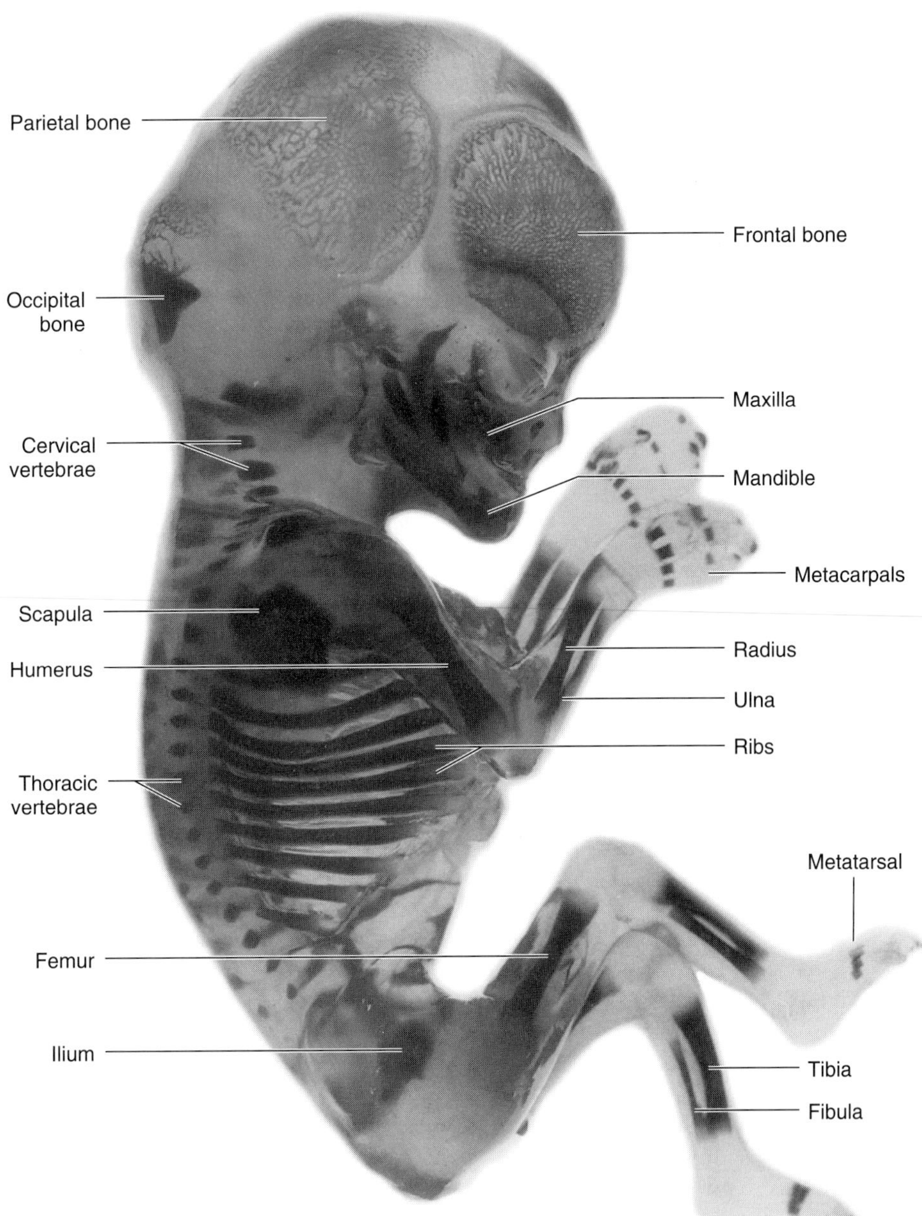

■ **Figure 15–16.** Alizarin-stained and cleared 12-week human fetus. Observe the degree of progression of ossification from the primary centers of ossification, which is endochondral in the appendicular and axial parts of the skeleton except for most of the cranial bones (i.e., those that form the calvaria). Observe that the carpus and tarsus are wholly cartilaginous at this stage, as are the epiphyses of all long bones. (Courtesy of Gary Geddes, MD, Lake Oswego, Oregon.)

indication of ossification in the cartilaginous model of a long bone is visible near the center of the future body (shaft); this is the primary center of ossification. Primary centers appear at different times in different bones, but most of them appear between the seventh and twelfth weeks of development. Virtually all primary centers of ossification are present at birth. The part of a bone ossified from a primary center is the **diaphysis.**

The secondary ossification centers of the bones at the knee are the first to appear. The centers for the distal end of the femur and the proximal end of the tibia usually appear during the last month of intrauterine life (34 to 38 weeks after fertilization). Consequently they are usually present at birth; however, most secondary centers of ossification appear after birth. The part of a bone ossified from a secondary center is the **epiphysis.**

The bone formed from the primary center in the diaphysis does not fuse with that formed from the secondary centers in the epiphyses until the bone grows to its adult length. This delay enables lengthening of the bone to continue until the final size is reached. During bone growth, a plate of cartilage known as the **epiphyseal cartilage plate** intervenes between the diaphysis and the epiphysis (Fig. 15-5). The epiphyseal plate is eventually replaced by bone development on each of its two sides, diaphyseal and epiphyseal. When this occurs, growth of the bone ceases.

Bone Age

Bone age is a good index of general maturation. Determination of the number, size, and fusion of epiphyseal centers from radiographs is a commonly used method. A radiologist determines the bone age of a person by assessing the ossification centers using two criteria:

- The appearance of calcified material in the diaphysis and/or the epiphysis is specific for each diaphysis and epiphysis and for each bone and sex.
- The disappearance of the dark line representing the epiphyseal cartilage plate indicates that the epiphysis has fused with the diaphysis.

Fusion of the epiphyseal centers, which occurs at specific times for each epiphysis, happens 1 to 2 years earlier in females than in males. Real-time ultrasonography is now increasingly used for the evaluation and measurement of fetal bones, as well as for the determination of gestational age (van der Harten et al., 1990; Filly, 1991b).

Generalized Skeletal Malformations

Achondroplasia is the most common cause of **dwarfism**—shortness of stature (see Chapter 8). It occurs about once in 15,000 births. The limbs are bowed and short because of disturbance of endochondral ossification at the epiphyseal cartilage plates, particularly of long bones, during fetal life. The trunk is usually short, and the head is enlarged with a bulging forehead and "scooped-out" nose (flat nasal bridge). Achondroplasia is an *autosomal dominant disorder*, and about 80% of cases arise from new mutations; the rate increases with paternal age (Behrman et al., 1996). For details of its inheritance, see Thompson et al. (1991).

Hyperpituitarism

Congenital infantile hyperpituitarism, which causes an infant to grow at an abnormally rapid rate, is rare. This may result in **gigantism** (excessive height and body proportions), or *acromegaly* (enlargement of the soft tissues, visceral organs, and bones of the face, hands, and feet). In acromegaly, the epiphyseal and diaphyseal centers of the long bones fuse, thereby preventing elongation of these bones. Both gigantism and acromegaly result from an excessive secretion of growth hormone (McCann, 1988).

Hypothyroidism and Cretinism

A severe deficiency of fetal thyroid hormone production results in cretinism, a condition characterized by growth retardation, mental deficiency, skeletal abnormalities, and auditory and neurological disorders. Bone age appears as less than chronological age because epiphyseal development is delayed (Griffin, 1988). Cretinism is very rare except in areas where there is a lack of iodine in the soil and water. Agenesis of the thyroid gland also results in cretinism.

SUMMARY OF THE SKELETAL SYSTEM

The skeletal system develops from mesenchyme, derived from mesoderm and the neural crest. In most bones, such as the long bones in the limbs, the condensed mesenchyme undergoes chondrification to form cartilage bone models. Ossification centers appear in these models by the end of the embryonic period, and the bones ossify later by **endochondral ossification**. Some bones, the flat bones of the skull for example, develop by **intramembranous ossification**. The vertebral column and ribs develop from mesenchymal cells from the sclerotomes of the somites. Each vertebra is formed by fusion of a condensation of the caudal half of one pair of **sclerotomes** with the cranial half of the subjacent pair of sclerotomes.

The developing skull consists of a neurocranium and a viscerocranium, each of which has membranous and cartilaginous components. The neurocranium forms the **calvaria**, a protective case for the brain. The viscerocranium forms the skeleton of the face. The **appendicular skeleton** develops from endochondral ossification of the cartilaginous bone models, which form from mesenchyme in the developing limbs. Joints are classified as:

- fibrous joints
- cartilaginous joints
- synovial joints

They develop from interzonal mesenchyme between the primordia of bones. In a fibrous joint the intervening mesenchyme differentiates into dense fibrous connective tissue. In a cartilaginous joint the mesenchyme between the bones differentiates into cartilage. In a synovial joint, a *synovial cavity* is formed within the intervening mesenchyme by breakdown of the cells. The mesenchyme also gives rise to the synovial membrane and the capsular and other ligaments of the joint.

Although there are numerous types of skeletal anomaly, most of them, except for spina bifida occulta and accessory ribs, are uncommon.

Clinically Oriented Problems

Case 15–1

A newborn infant presented with a lesion in his lower back, which was thought to be a vertebral arch defect.

- What is the most common congenital anomaly of the vertebral column?
- Where is the defect usually located?
- Does this congenital anomaly usually cause symptoms (e.g., back problems)?

Case 15–2

A young girl presented with pain in her upper limb, which worsened when she lifted heavy objects. After a radiographical examination, the physician told her parents that she had a rudimentary rib in her neck.

- Occasionally rudimentary ribs are associated with the seventh cervical vertebra and the first lumbar vertebra. Are these accessory ribs of clinical importance?
- What is the embryological basis of accessory ribs?

Case 15–3

The mother of a girl with a "crooked spine" was told that her daughter had scoliosis.

- What vertebral defect can produce scoliosis?
- Define this condition.
- What is the embryological basis of the vertebral defect?

Case 15–4

A boy presented with a long, thin, head. His mother was concerned that her son might become mentally retarded.

- What is meant by the term craniosynostosis?
- What results from this developmental abnormality?
- Give a common example and describe it.

Case 15–5

A child presented with characteristics of the Klippel-Feil syndrome.

- What are the main features of this condition?
- What vertebral anomalies are usually present?

Discussion of these problems appears at the back of the book.

REFERENCES AND SUGGESTED READING

Bannister LH, Berry MM, Collins P, et al (eds): *Gray's Anatomy,* 38th ed. New York, Churchill Livingstone, 1995.

Behrman RE, Kliegman RM, Arvin AM (eds): *Nelson Textbook of Pediatrics,* 15th ed. Philadelphia, WB Saunders, 1996.

Bruder SP, Caplan AL: Cellular and molecular events during embryonic bone development. *Connect Tissue Res 20:*65, 1989.

Budorick NE, Pretorius DH, Grafe MR, Lou KV: Ossification of the fetal spine. *Radiology 181:*561, 1991.

Caplan AL: Mesenchymal stem cells. *J Orthop Res 9:*641, 1991.

Centrella M, Horowitz MC, Wozney JM, McCarthy TL: Transforming growth factor-β gene family members and bone. *Endocr Rev 15:* 27, 1994.

Cohen Jr MM: Syndrome delineation and its implications for the study of pathogenetic mechanisms. *In* Persaud TVN (ed): Advances in the Study of Birth Defects, vol 5. *Genetic Disorders.* New York, Alan R. Liss, 1982.

Cole DEC, Cohen Jr MM: Osteogenesis imperfecta. An update. *J Pediatr 119:*73, 1991.

Craig FM, Bayliss MT, Bentley G, Archer CW: A role for hyaluronan in joint development. *J Anat 171:*17, 1990.

Daniels K, Solursh M: Modulation of chondrogenesis by the cytoskeleton and extracellular matrix. *J Cell Sci 100(Pt. 2):*249, 1991.

Davis JE, Kalousek DK: Fetal akinesia deformation sequence in previable fetuses. *Am J Med Genet 29:*77, 1988.

Dhem A, Goret-Nicaise M, Dambrain R, Nyssen-Behets C, et al: Skeletal growth and chondroid tissue. *Arch Ital Anat Embriol 94:*237, 1989.

Dunlop L-LT, Hall BK: Relationships between cellular condensation, preosteoblast formation and epithelial-mesenchymal interactions in initiation of osteogenesis. *Int J Dev Biol 39:*357, 1995.

Dziedzic-Goclawska A, Emerich J, Grzesik W, et al: Differences in the kinetics of the mineralization process in endochondral and intramembranous osteogenesis in human fetal development. *J Bone Miner Res 3:*533, 1988.

Filly RA: The fetus with a CNS malformation: ultrasound evaluation. *In* Harrison MR, Golbus MS, Filly RA (eds): *The Unborn Patient. Prenatal Diagnosis and Treatment,* 2nd ed. Philadelphia, WB Saunders, 1991a.

Filly RA: Sonographic anatomy of the normal fetus. *In* Harrison MR, Golbus MS, Filly RA (eds): *The Unborn Patient. Prenatal Diagnosis and Treatment,* 2nd ed. Philadelphia, WB Saunders, 1991b.

Filly RA, Golbus MS: Ultrasonography of the normal and pathologic fetal skeleton. *Radiol Clin North Am 20:*311, 1982.

Gartner LP, Hiatt JL: *Color Textbook of Histology*. Philadelphia, WB Saunders, 1997.

Gasser RF: Evidence that sclerotomal cells do not migrate medially during normal embryonic development of the rat. *Am J Anat 154:* 509, 1979.

Griffin JE: The thyroid. *In* Griffin JE, Ojeda SR (eds): *Textbook of Endocrine Physiology*. New York, Oxford Press, 1988.

Hall BK, Miyake T: Divide, accumulate, differentiate: cell condensation in skeletal development revisited. *Int J Dev Biol 39:*881, 1995.

Hughes DE, Boyce BF: Apoptosis in bone physiology and disease. *J Clin Pathol Mol Pathol 50:*132, 1997.

Hunter AGW: Craniofacial anthropometric analysis in several types of chondrodysplasia. *Am J Med Genet 65:*5, 1996.

Kjaer I: Ossification of the human fetal basicranium. *J Craniofac Genet Dev Biol* 10:29, 1990.

Mahony BS: Ultrasound evaluation of the fetal musculoskeletal system. *In* Callen PW (ed): *Ultrasonography in Obstetrics and Gynecology,* 3rd ed. Philadelphia, WB Saunders, 1994.

Marin-Padilla M: Cephalic axial skeletal-neural dysraphic disorders: embryology and pathology. *Can J Neurol Sci 18:*153, 1991.

Marks Jr SC, Popoff SN: Bone cell biology: the regulation of development, structure, and function in the skeleton. *Am J Anat 183:*1, 1988.

McCann SM: The anterior pituitary and hypothalamus. *In* Griffin JE, Ojeda SR (eds): *Textbook of Endrocine Physiology*. New York, Oxford Press, 1988.

McNally E, Sandin B, Wilkins RA: The ossification of the costal element of the seventh cervical vertebra with particular reference to cervical ribs. *J Anat 170:*125, 1990.

Meizner I, Barnhard Y: Achondrogenesis type 1 diagnosed by transvaginal ultrasonography at 13 weeks' gestation. *Am J Obstet Gynecol 173:*1620, 1995.

Moore KL: *Clinically Oriented Anatomy,* 3rd ed. Baltimore, Williams & Wilkins, 1992.

Moore KL, Agur AMR: *Essential Clinical Anatomy*. Baltimore, Williams & Wilkins, 1995.

Muragaki Y, Mundlos S, Upton J, Olsen BR: Altered growth and branching patterns in synpolydactyly caused by mutations in HOXD 13. *Science 272:*548, 1996.

Ohta Y, Suwa F, Yang L, et al: Development and histology of fibrous architecture of the fetal temporomandibular joint. *Okajimas Folia Anat Jpn 70:*1, 1993.

O'Rahilly R, Müller F, Meyer DB: The human vertebral column at the end of the embryonic period proper. 3. The thoracolumbar region. *J Anat 168:*81, 1990a.

O'Rahilly R, Müller F, Meyer DB: The human vertebral column at the end of the embryonic period proper. 4. The sacrococcygeal region. *J Anat 168:*95, 1990b.

Romero R, Athanassiadis AP, Sirtori M, Inati M: Fetal skeletal anomalies. *In* Fleischer AC, Romero R, Manning FA, et al (eds): *The Principles and Practice of Ultrasonography in Obstetrics and Gynecology,* 4th ed. Norwalk, Appleton & Lange, 1991.

Rubin E, Farber JL (eds): *Pathology*. Philadelphia, JB Lippincott, 1988.

Sabbagha RE: Ultrasound diagnosis of fetal structural anomalies. In Simpson JL, Elias S (eds): *Essentials of Prenatal Diagnosis*. New York, Churchill Livingstone, 1993.

Sakano S, Murata Y, Iwata H, et al: Protooncogene expression in osteogenesis induced by bone morphogenetic protein. *Clin Orthop 33:*240, 1997.

Sarwark JF: Spina bifida. *Pediatr Clin North Am 43:*1151, 1996.

Smith MM, Hall BK: Development and evolutionary origins of vertebrate skeletogenic and odontogenic tissue. *Biol Rev Camb Philos Soc 65:*277, 1990.

Sperber GH: *Craniofacial Embryology,* 4th ed (revised reprint). London, Butterworths, 1993.

Sundaresan M, Wright M, Price AB: Anatomy and development of the fontanelle. *Arch Dis Child 65:*386, 1990.

Thompson MW, McInnes RR, Willard HF: *Thompson & Thompson Genetics in Medicine,* 5th ed. Philadelphia, WB Saunders, 1991.

Uhthoff HK: *The Embryology of the Human Locomotor System*. New York, Springer Verlag, 1990.

van der Harten HJ, Brons JT, Schipper NW, et al: The prenatal development of the normal human skeleton: a combined ultrasonographic and post-mortem radiographic study. *Pediatr Radiol 21:* 52, 1990.

Wilting J, Müller TS, Ebensperger C, et al: Development of the vertebral column: morphogenesis and genes. *In* Vogel R, Fanghänel J, Giebel J (eds): *Aspects of Terminology,* vol 1. Marburg, Tectum Verlag, 1996.

Wolpert L: Positional information and pattern formation in development. *Develop Genet 15:*485, 1994.

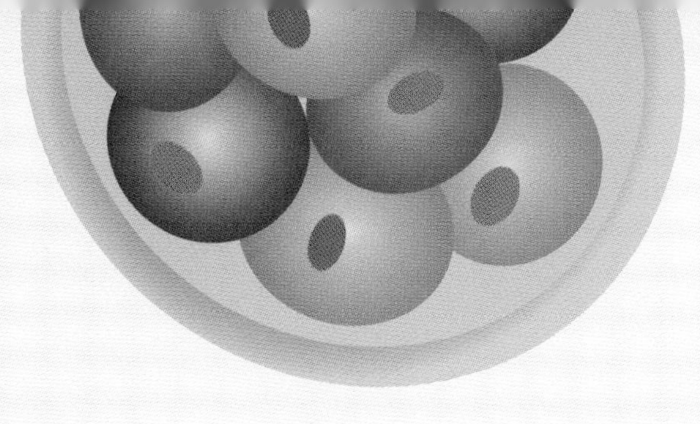

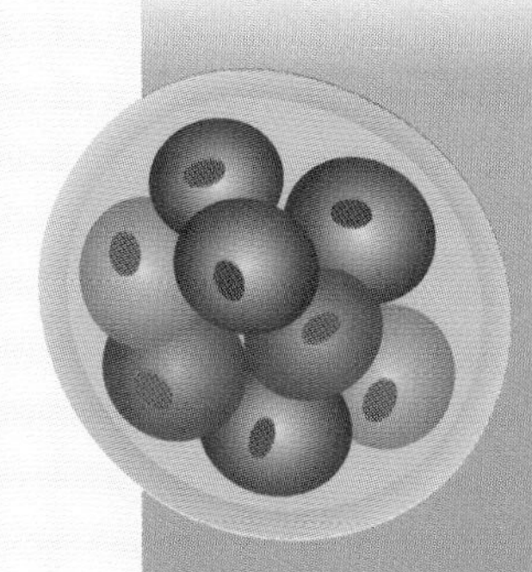

The Muscular System

16

■ The muscular system develops from **mesoderm**, except for the muscles of the iris, which develop from **neuroectoderm** (Uusitalo and Kivela, 1995). Muscle tissue develops **myoblasts**, embryonic muscle cells that are derived from mesenchyme (embryonic connective tissue). MyoD, a member of the family of myogenic regulatory factors (MRFs), activates transcription of muscle-specific genes and is considered to be an important regulatory gene for the induction of myogenic differentiation (Pin et al., 1997). The induction of myogenesis in mesenchymal cells by MyoD is dependent on their degree of differentiation (Filvaroff and Derynck, 1996). Much of the mesenchyme in the head is derived from the **neural crest** (see Chapters 4 and 5), particularly the tissues derived from the pharyngeal arches (see Chapter 10); however, the original mesenchyme in the arches gives rise to the musculature of the face and neck (see Table 10-1).

DEVELOPMENT OF SKELETAL MUSCLE

The myoblasts that form the skeletal muscles of the trunk are derived from mesoderm in the myotome regions of the somites (Fig. 16-1; see Fig. 15-1). The

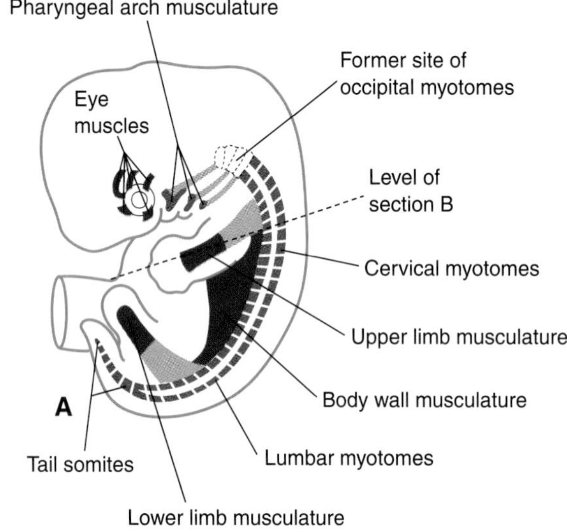

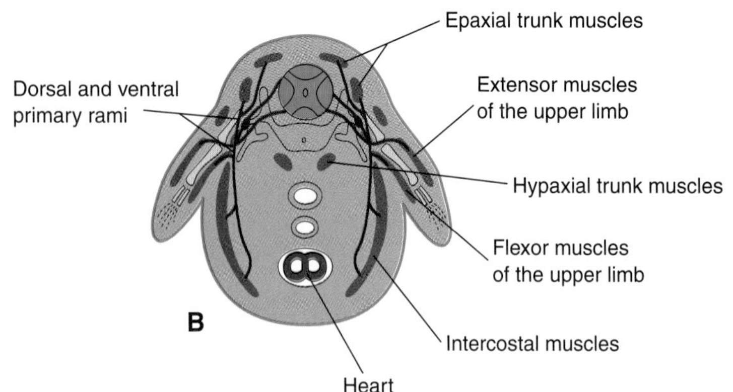

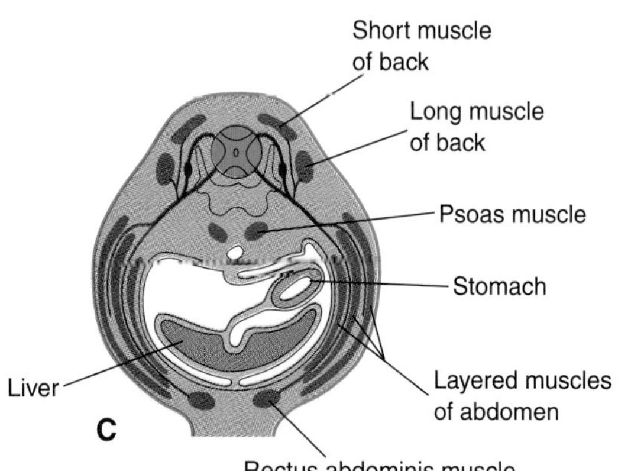

■ **Figure 16-1.** *A,* Sketch of an embryo (about 41 days), showing the myotomes and developing muscular system. *B,* Transverse section of the embryo, illustrating the epaxial and hypaxial derivatives of a myotome. *C,* Similar section of a 7-week embryo, showing the muscle layers formed from the myotomes.

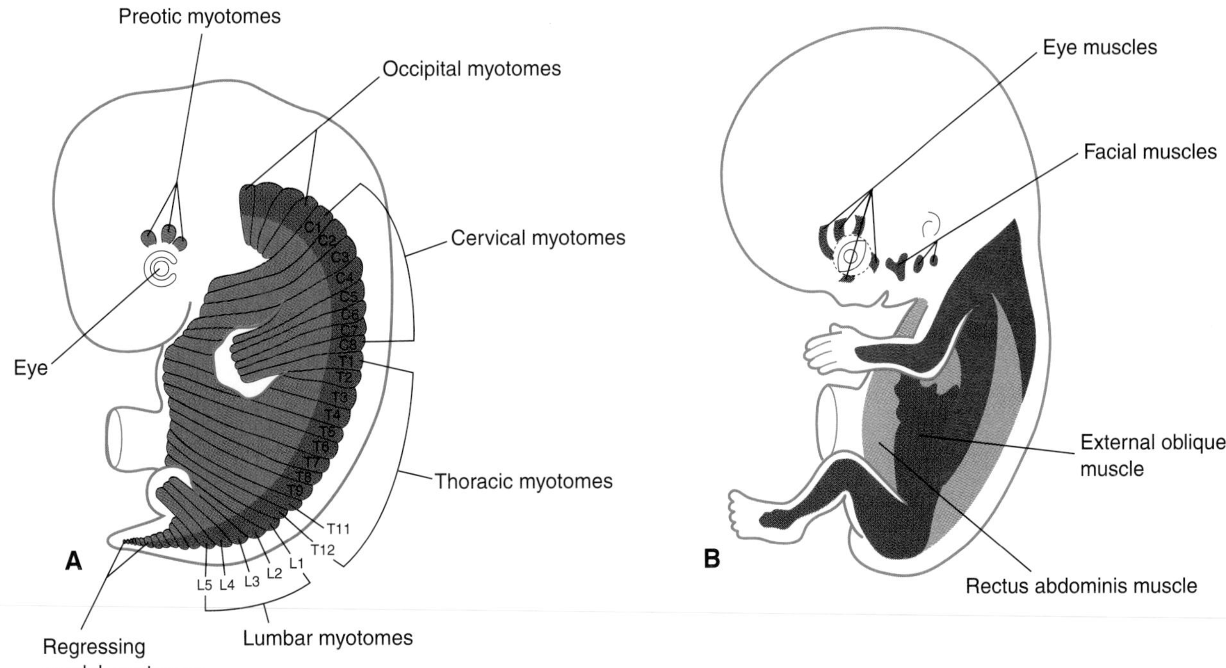

■ **Figure 16–2.** Drawings illustrating the developing muscular system. *A,* 6-week embryo, showing the myotome regions of the somites that give rise to most skeletal muscles. *B,* 8-week embryo, showing the developing trunk and limb musculature.

limb muscles develop from myogenic precursor cells in the limb buds. In mammals, at least two separate populations of muscle precursor cells have been identified within the limb bud. Recent experimental studies showed that these cells originate from the somites in response to signals from nearby tissues (Brand-Saberi et al., 1996). The first indication of **myogenesis** is the elongation of the nuclei and cell bodies of mesenchymal cells as they differentiate into **myoblasts**. Soon these primordial muscle cells fuse to form elongated, multinucleated, cylindrical structures —**myotubes**. At the molecular level, these events are preceded by the activation of genes and expression of the MyoD family of muscle-specific basic helix-loop-helix (bHLH) transcription factors or MRFs in the precursor myogenic cells. For a review of recent work on the genetic control and regulation of muscle differentiation, see Buonanno and Rosenthal (1996), Pin and Merrifield (1997), and Pin et al. (1997).

Muscle growth during development results from the ongoing fusion of myoblasts and myotubes. **Myofilaments** develop in the cytoplasm of the myotubes during or after fusion of the myoblasts. Soon myofibrils and other organelles characteristic of striated muscle cells develop. Because muscle cells are long and narrow, they are usually called **muscle fibers**. As the myotubes differentiate, they become invested with external laminae, which segregate them from the surrounding connective tissue. Fibroblasts produce the perimysium and epimysium layers of the fibrous sheath; the endomysium is formed by the external lamina, which is derived from the muscle fiber, and reticular fibers. Most skeletal muscle develops before birth, and almost all remaining ones are formed by the end of the first year. The increase in the size of a muscle after the first year results from an increase in the diameter of the fibers because of the formation of more myofilaments. Muscles increase in length and width in order to grow with the skeleton. Their ultimate size depends on the amount of exercise that is performed. Not all embryonic muscle fibers persist; many of them fail to establish themselves as necessary units of the muscle and soon degenerate.

Myotomes

Each typical myotome part of a somite divides into a dorsal *epaxial division* and a ventral *hypaxial division* (Fig. 16-1*B*). Each developing **spinal nerve** also divides and sends a branch to each division, the *dorsal primary ramus* supplying the epaxial division and the *ventral primary ramus*, the hypaxial division. Some muscles, the intercostal muscles for example, remain segmentally arranged like the somites, but most myoblasts migrate away from the myotome and form nonsegmented muscles.

DERIVATIVES OF THE EPAXIAL DIVISIONS OF MYOTOMES

Myoblasts from these divisions of the myotomes form the extensor muscles of the neck and vertebral column (Fig. 16-2). The embryonic extensor muscles derived from the sacral and coccygeal myotomes degenerate; their adult derivatives are the dorsal sacrococcygeal ligaments (Moore, 1992).

DERIVATIVES OF THE HYPAXIAL DIVISIONS OF MYOTOMES

Myoblasts from these divisions of the cervical myotomes form the scalene, prevertebral, geniohyoid, and infrahyoid muscles (Fig. 16-2). The thoracic myotomes form the lateral and ventral flexor muscles of the vertebral column, and the lumbar myotomes form the quadratus lumborum muscle. The sacrococcygeal myotomes form the muscles of the pelvic diaphragm (Moore and Agur, 1995) and probably the striated muscles of the anus and sex organs.

Pharyngeal Arch Muscles

The migration of myoblasts from the pharyngeal arches to form the muscles of mastication, facial expression, pharynx, and larynx is described in Chapter 10. These muscles are innervated by pharyngeal arch nerves.

Ocular Muscles

The origin of the extrinsic eye muscles is unclear, but it is thought that they may be derived from mesenchymal cells near the prechordal plate (Figs. 16-1 and 16-2). The mesoderm in this area is thought to give rise to three *preotic myotomes*. Myoblasts differentiate from mesenchymal cells derived from these myotomes. Groups of myoblasts, each supplied by its own nerve (CN III, CN IV, or CN VI), form the extrinsic muscles of the eye.

Tongue Muscles

Initially there are four *occipital (postotic) myotomes*; the first pair disappears. Myoblasts from the remaining myotomes form the tongue muscles, which are innervated by the hypoglossal nerve (CN XII).

Limb Muscles

The musculature of the limbs develops from the myogenic cells (**myoblasts**) surrounding the developing bones (Fig. 16-1). Grafting and gene targeting studies in birds and mammals have demonstrated that at least some of the precursor myogenic cells in the limb buds originate from the somites. These cells are first located in the ventral part of the dermomyotome and are epithelial in nature (see Fig. 15-1*D*). Following mesenchymal-epithelial transformation, the cells then migrate into the primordium of the limb. The molecular mechanisms that initiate and control the migration of myogenic precursor cells from the somites to the limb buds and subsequent muscle formation are largely unknown (Brand-Saberi et al., 1996; Pin and Merrifield, 1997).

DEVELOPMENT OF SMOOTH MUSCLE

Smooth muscle fibers differentiate from splanchnic mesenchyme surrounding the endoderm of the primordial gut and its derivatives (see Fig. 15-1). The smooth muscle in the walls of many blood and lymphatic vessels arises from somatic mesoderm. The muscles of the iris (sphincter and dilator pupillae) and the myoepithelial cells in mammary and sweat glands are thought to be derived from mesenchymal cells that originate from ectoderm. The first sign of differentiation of smooth muscle is the development of elongated nuclei in spindle-shaped myoblasts. During early development new myoblasts continue to differentiate from mesenchymal cells but do not fuse; they remain mononucleated. During later development, division of existing myoblasts gradually replaces the differentiation of new myoblasts in the production of new smooth muscle tissue. As smooth muscle cells differentiate, filamentous but non-sarcomeric contractile elements develop in their cytoplasm and the external surface of each cell acquires a surrounding external lamina. As smooth muscle fibers develop into sheets or bundles, they receive autonomic innervation; fibroblasts and muscle cells synthesize and lay down collagenous, elastic, and reticular fibers.

DEVELOPMENT OF CARDIAC MUSCLE

Cardiac muscle develops from splanchnic mesenchyme surrounding the developing heart tube (see Chapter 14). **Cardiac myoblasts** differentiate from the primordial myocardium. Heart muscle is recognizable in the fourth week and likely develops through expression of cardiac-specific genes. Immunohistochemical studies have revealed a spatial distribution of "tissue-specific" antigens (myosin heavy chain isoforms) in the embryonic heart between the fourth and eighth weeks of development (Wessels et al., 1991). **Cardiac muscle fibers** arise by differentiation and growth of single cells, unlike striated skeletal muscle fibers, which develop by fusion of cells. Growth of cardiac muscle fibers results from the formation of new **myofilaments**. The myoblasts adhere to each other as in developing skeletal muscle, but the intervening cell membranes do not disintegrate; these areas of adhesion give rise to **intercalated discs** (Cormack, 1993). Late in the embryonic period, special bundles of muscle cells develop with relatively few myofibrils and relatively larger diameters than typical cardiac muscle fibers. These atypical cardiac muscle cells—**Purkinje fibers**—form the conducting system of the heart (see Chapter 14).

Anomalies of Muscles

Absence of one or more skeletal muscles is more common than is generally recognized. Usually only a single muscle is absent on one side of the body, or only part of the muscle fails to develop. Occasionally the same muscle or muscles may be absent on both sides of the body. Any muscle in the body may occasionally be absent; common examples are the sternocostal head of the pectoralis major (Fig. 16-3), the palmaris longus, trapezius, serratus anterior, and quadratus femoris (Moore, 1992). Absence of the pectoralis major, often its sternal part, is usually associated with syndactyly

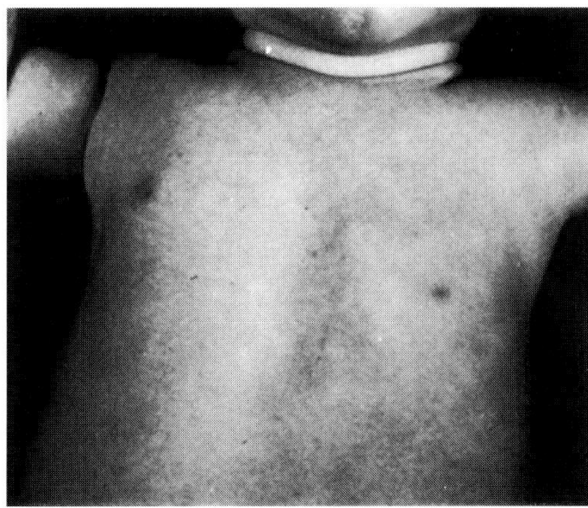

■ **Figure 16–3.** Photograph of the thorax of an infant with congenital absence of the left pectoralis major muscle. Note the absence of the anterior axillary fold on the left and low location of the left nipple. (From Behrman RE, Kliegman RM, Arvin AM [eds]: *Nelson Textbook of Pediatrics,* 15th ed. Philadelphia, WB Saunders, 1996.)

(fusion of digits). These anomalies are part of the *Poland syndrome*. Absence of the pectoralis major is occasionally associated with absence of the mammary gland and/or hypoplasia of the nipple.

In rare instances, failure of normal muscle development may be widespread, leading to immobility of multiple joints—**arthrogryposis multiplex congenita** (Fig. 16–4). Persons with this disorder have congenital stiffness of one or more joints associated with hypoplasia of the associated muscles (Behrman et al., 1996). The causes encompass both neurogenic and primary myopathic diseases. The involved muscles are replaced partially or completely by fat and fibrous tissue.

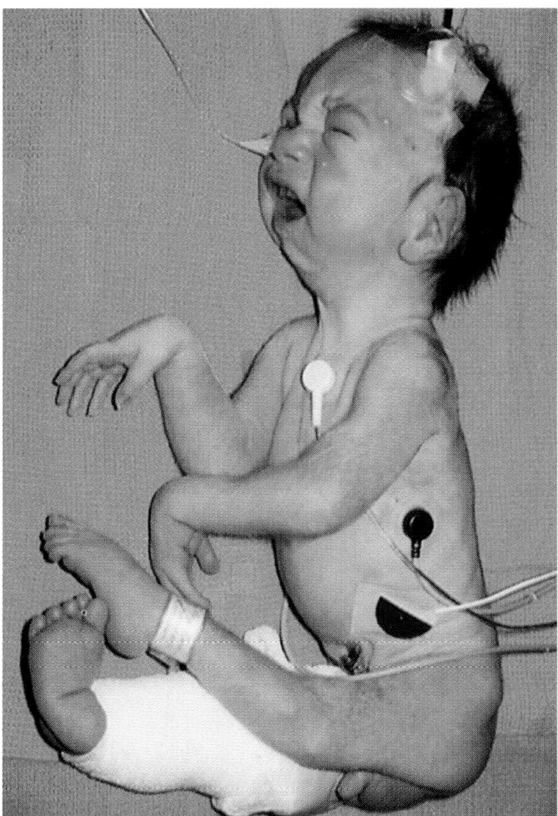

■ **Figure 16–4.** Neonate with multiple joint contractures—arthrogryposis. (Courtesy of Dr. A. E. Chudley, Section of Genetics and Metabolism, Department of Pediatrics and Child Health, Children's Hospital and University of Manitoba, Winnipeg, Manitoba, Canada.)

Some muscular anomalies cause difficulty in breathing, such as **congenital absence of the diaphragm**, which is usually associated with incomplete expansion of the lungs or part of a lung (**pulmonary atelectasis**) and pneumonitis (pneumonia). Absence of muscles of the anterior abdominal wall may be associated with severe gastrointestinal and genitourinary anomalies, exstrophy of the bladder for example (see Chapter 13). Occasionally individuals with congenital absence of a muscle develop **muscular dystrophy** in later life. The most common association is between congenital absence of the pectoralis major muscle and the Landouzy-Dejerine facioscapulohumeral form of muscular dystrophy (Mastaglia, 1974). Both muscle development and muscle repair have distinctive dependence upon expression of muscle regulatory genes (Anderson et al., 1996; Megeney et al., 1996).

Variations in Muscles

All muscles are subject to a certain amount of variation, but some are affected more often than others. Certain muscles are functionally vestigial, such as those of the external ear and scalp. Some muscles present in other primates appear in only some humans (e.g., the sternalis muscle). Variations in the form, position, and attachments of muscles are common and are usually functionally insignificant.

The sternocleidomastoid muscle is sometimes injured at birth, resulting in **congenital torticollis** (Moore, 1992). There is fixed rotation and tilting of the head because of fibrosis and shortening of the sternocleidomastoid muscle on one side (Fig. 16–5). Some cases of torticollis (wryneck) result from tearing of fibers of the sternocleidomastoid muscle during childbirth. Bleeding into the muscle occurs in a localized area, forming a small swelling called a *hematoma*. Later a mass develops because of necrosis (death) of muscle fibers and fibrosis (formation of fibrous tissue). Shortening of the muscle usually follows; this causes lateral bending of the head to the affected side and a slight turning away of the head from the side of the short muscle. Although birth trauma is commonly considered as a cause of congenital torticollis, the fact that the condition has been observed in infants delivered by cesarean section suggests that there are other causes in some cases (Davids et al., 1993; Behrman et al., 1996).

Accessory Muscles

Accessory muscles occasionally develop and some are clinically significant. For example, an *accessory soleus muscle* is present in about 6% of the population (Agur, 1998). It has been suggested that the primordium of the soleus muscle undergoes early splitting to form an accessory soleus (Romanus et al., 1986).

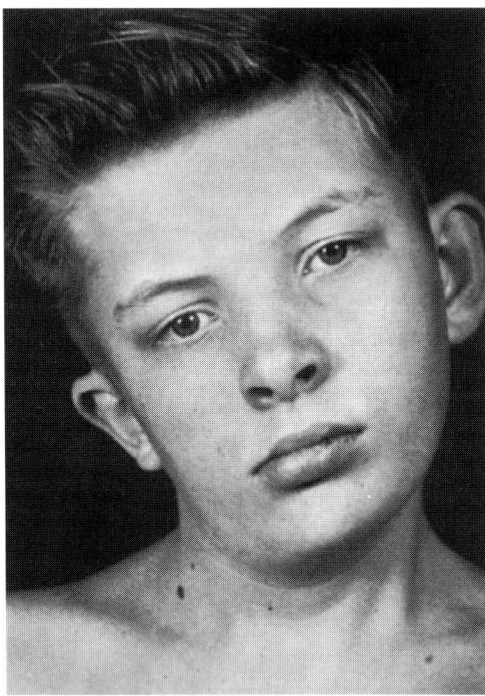

■ **Figure 16–5.** Photograph of the head and neck of a 12-year-old boy with congenital torticollis (wryneck). Shortening of the right sternocleidomastoid muscle has caused tilting of the head to the right and turning of the chin to the left. There is also asymmetrical development of the face and skull. (From Behrman RE, Vaughan III VC: *Nelson Textbook of Pediatrics,* 13th ed. Philadelphia, WB Saunders, 1987.)

SUMMARY OF THE MUSCULAR SYSTEM

Most skeletal muscle is derived from the myotome regions of somites. Some head and neck muscles are derived from pharyngeal arch mesoderm. The limb muscles develop from myogenic precursor cells, which are derived from somites. Cardiac muscle and most smooth muscle are derived from splanchnic mesoderm. Absence or variation of some muscles is common and is usually of little consequence.

Clinically Oriented Problems

Case 16–1

An infant presented with absence of the left anterior axillary fold. In addition, the left nipple was much lower than usual.

- Absence of which muscle probably caused these unusual observations?
- What syndrome would you suspect may be present?
- For what features would you look?
- Would the infant be likely to suffer any disability if absence of this muscle was the only anomaly present?

Case 16–2

A medical student was concerned when she learned that she had only one palmaris longus muscle.

- Is this a common occurrence?
- What is its incidence?
- Does the absence of this muscle cause a disability?

Case 16–3

The parents of a 4-year-old girl observed that she always held her head slightly tilted to the right side and that one of her neck muscles was more prominent than the others. The clinical history revealed that hers had been a breech birth, one in which the buttocks presented.

- Name the muscle that was likely prominent.
- Did it pull the child's head to the right side?
- What is this deformity called?
- What probably caused the muscle shortening that resulted in this condition?

Case 16–4

A newborn infant presented with an abdominal wall defect. Failure of striated muscle to develop in the median plane of the anterior abdominal wall is associated with the formation of a severe congenital anomaly of the urinary system.

- What is this anomaly called?
- What is the probable embryological basis of the failure of muscle to form in these persons?

Discussion of these problems appears at the back of the book.

REFERENCES AND SUGGESTED READING

Agur AMR: Personal communication, 1998.

Anderson JE, McIntosh L, Garrett K, et al: The absence of MyoD increases MDX mouse dystrophy and reduces muscle repair. *Molec Biol Cell Supp 7:*468a, 1996.

Behrman RE Kliegman RM, Arvin AM (eds): *Nelson Textbook of Pediatrics,* 15th ed. Philadelphia, WB Saunders, 1996.

Brand-Saberi B, Müller TS, Wilting J, et al: Scatter factor/hepatocyte growth factor (SF/HGF) induces emigration of myogenic cells at interlimb level in vivo. *Dev Biol 179:*303, 1996.

Buonanno A, Rosenthal N: Molecular control of muscle diversity and plasticity. *Dev Genet 19:*95, 1996.

Caplan AL: Mesenchymal stem cells. *J Orthop Res 9:*641, 1991.

Chen T-C, Wallace MC, Merlie JP, Olson EN: Separable regulatory elements governing *myogenin* transcription in mouse embryogenesis. *Science 261:*215, 1993.

Cormack DH: *Essential Histology.* Philadelphia, JB Lippincott, 1993.

Davids JR, Wenger DR, Mubarak SJ: Congenital muscular torticollis: sequela of intrauterine or perinatal compartment syndrome. *J Pediatr Orthop 13:*141, 1993.

Dubowitz V: *Muscle Disorders in Childhood,* 2nd ed. Philadelphia, WB Saunders, 1995.

Filvaroff EH, Derynck R: Induction of myogenesis in mesenchymal cells by MyoD depends on their degree of differentiation. *Dev Biol 178:*459, 1996.

Gasser RF: The development of the facial muscles in man. *Am J Anat 120:*357, 1967.

Jones KJ, North KN: Recent advances in diagnosis of the childhood muscular dystrophies. *J Paediatr Child Health 33:*195, 1997.

Levi AC, Borghi F, Garavoglia M: Development of the anal canal muscles. *Dis Colon Rectum 34:*262, 1991.

Mahony BS: Ultrasound evaluation of the fetal musculoskeletal system. *In* Callen PW (ed): *Ultrasonography in Obstetrics and Gynecology,* 2nd ed. Philadelphia, WB Saunders, 1994.

Mastaglia FL: The growth and development of skeletal muscles. *In* Davis JA, Dobbing J (eds): *Scientific Foundations of Paediatrics*. Philadelphia, WB Saunders, 1974.

Megeney A, Kablar B, Garrett K, et al: MyoD is required for myogenic stem cell function in adult skeletal muscle. *Genes Dev 10:* 1173, 1996.

Moore KL: *Clinically Oriented Anatomy,* 3rd ed. Baltimore, Williams & Wilkins, 1992.

Moore KL, Agur, AMR: *Essential Clinical Anatomy*. Baltimore, Williams & Wilkins, 1995.

Murakami G, Nakamura H: Somites and pattern formation of trunk muscles—a study in quail-chick chimera. *Arch Histol Cytol 54:* 249, 1991.

Noden DM: Vertebrate craniofacial development—the relation between ontogenetic process and morphological outcome. *Brain Behav Evol 38:*190, 1991.

Olson EN: MyoD family: a paradigm for development? *Genes Dev 4:* 1454, 1990.

O'Rahilly R, Gardner E: The timing and sequence of events in the development of the limbs of the human embryo. *Anat Embryol 148:*1, 1975.

Pin CL, Ludolph DC, Cooper ST, et al: Distal regulatory elements control MRF4 gene expression in early and late myogenic cell populations. *Dev Dyn 208:*299, 1997.

Pin CL, Merrifield PA: Regionalized expression of myosin isoforms in heterotypic myotubes formed from embryonic and fetal rat myoblasts in vitro. *Dev Dyn 208:*420, 1997.

Romanus B, Lindahl S, Stener B: Accessory soleus muscle. A clinical and radiographic presentation of eleven cases. *J Bone Joint Surg 68A:*731, 1986.

Rudnicki MA, Jaenisch R: The MyoD family of transcriptional factors and skeletal myogenesis. *Bio Essays 17:*2584, 1995.

Sutherland CJ, Elsom VL, Gordon ML, et al: Coordination of skeletal muscle gene expression occurs late in mammalian development. *Dev Biol 146:*167, 1991.

Uusitalo M, Kivela T: Development of cytoskeleton in neuroectodermally derived epithelial and muscle cells of human eye. *Invest Ophthalmol Vis Sci 36:*2584, 1995.

Wessels A, Vermeulen JL, Viragh S, et al: Spatial distribution of "tissue-specific" antigens in the developing heart and skeletal muscle. II. An immunohistochemical analysis of myosin heavy chain isoform expression patterns in the embryonic heart. *Anat Rec 229:*355, 1991.

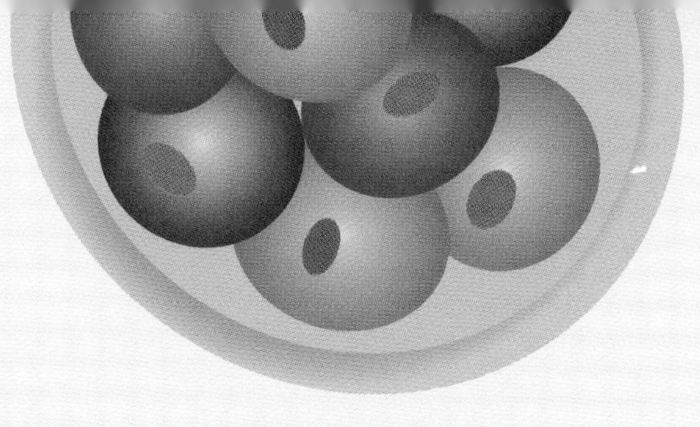

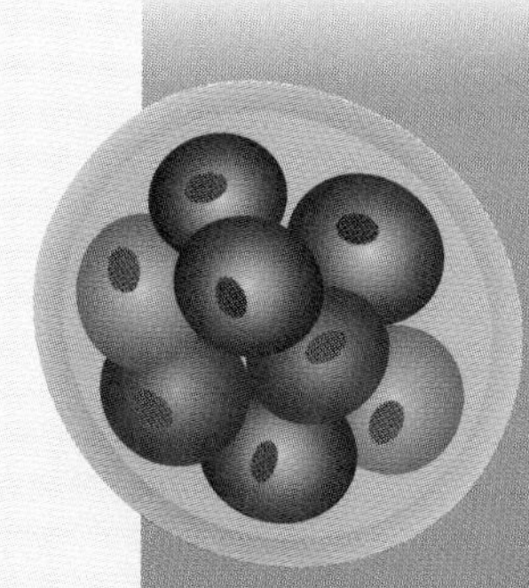

The Limbs

17

■ The general features of limb development are described and illustrated in Chapter 5. Development of limb bones is described in Chapter 15, and formation of limb musculature is outlined in Chapter 16. The purpose of this chapter is to consolidate this material and provide more information about limb development.

EARLY STAGES OF LIMB DEVELOPMENT

The **limb buds** first appear as small elevations of the ventrolateral body wall during the fourth week (Fig. 17-1*A*). Limb development begins with the activation of a group of mesenchymal cells in the lateral meso-

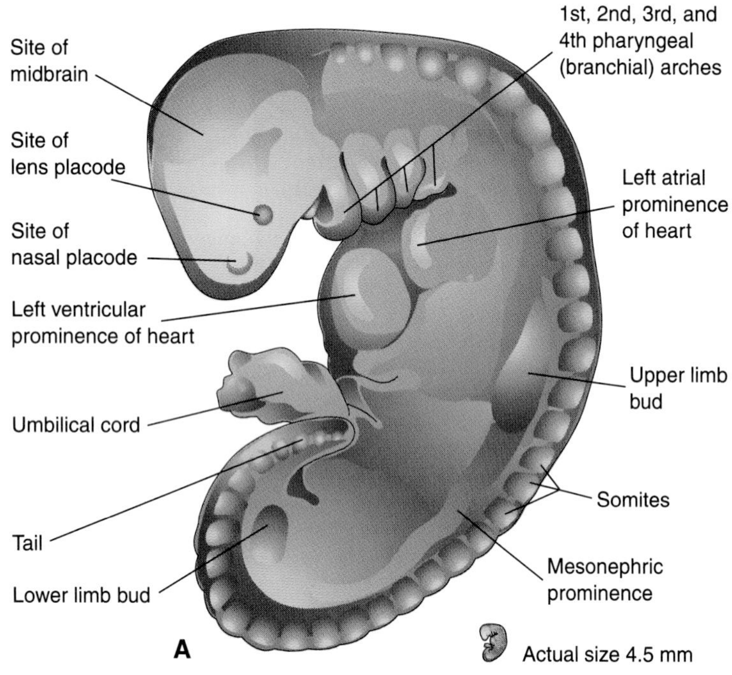

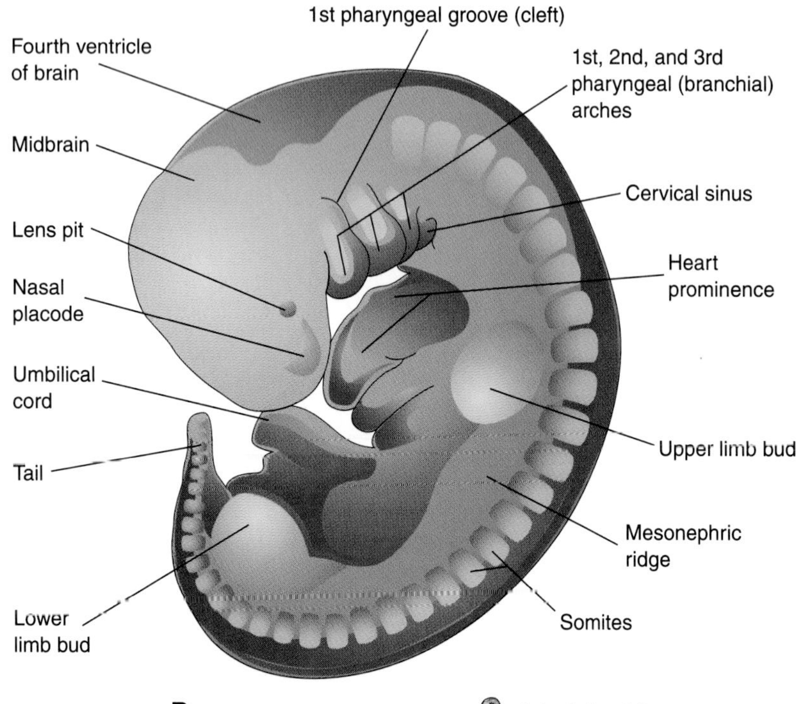

■ **Figure 17-1.** *A,* Lateral view of a human embryo at Carnegie stage 13, about 28 days. The upper limb buds appear as swellings on the ventrolateral body wall. The lower limbs are not as well developed. *B,* Lateral view of an embryo at Carnegie stage 14, about 32 days. The upper limb buds are paddle-shaped and the lower limb buds are flipperlike. (Modified from Nishimura H, Semba R, Tanimura T, Tanaka O: *Prenatal Development of the Human with Special Reference to Craniofacial Structures: An Atlas.* Washington, DC, National Institutes of Health, 1977.)

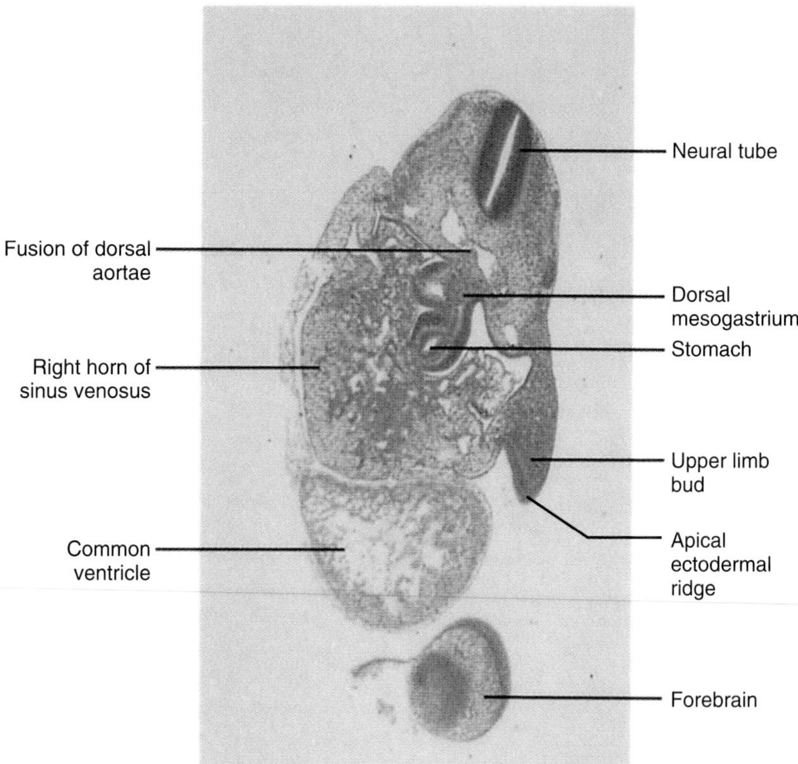

■ **Figure 17–2.** Oblique section of an embryo at Carnegie stage 13, about 28 days. Observe the flipperlike upper limb bud lateral to the embryonic heart. (From Moore KL, Persaud, TVN, Shiota K: *Color Atlas of Clinical Embryology.* Philadelphia, WB Saunders, 1994.)

derm (Carlson, 1994). Homeobox-containing (*Hox*) genes regulate patterning in vertebrate limb development (Muragaki et al., 1996; Cohn et al., 1997). The limb buds form deep to a thick band of ectoderm. The upper limb buds are visible by day 26 or 27, and the lower limb buds appear a day or two later. Each limb bud consists of a mass of mesenchyme covered by ectoderm. The mesenchyme is derived from the somatic layer of lateral mesoderm. The limb buds elongate by the proliferation of the mesenchyme within them. The upper limb buds appear disproportionately low on the embryo's trunk because of the early development of the cranial half of the embryo.

The early stages of limb development are alike for the upper and lower limbs; however, development of the upper limb buds precedes that of the lower limb buds by about 2 days (Figs. 17-1*B* and 17-4). In addition, there are distinct differences between the development of the hand and foot because of their form and function. The upper limb buds develop opposite the caudal cervical segments, and the lower limb buds form opposite the lumbar and upper sacral segments.

At the apex of each limb bud the ectoderm thickens to form an **apical ectodermal ridge** (AER). Interaction between the AER and mesenchymal cells in the limb is essential to limb development (Hinrichsen et al., 1994). The AER, a multilayered epithelial structure (Fig. 17-2), interacts with mesenchyme in the limb bud, promoting outgrowth of the bud (Carlson, 1994). *The AER exerts an inductive influence on the limb mesenchyme that initiates growth and development of the limbs.* The mesenchyme adjacent to the AER consists of undifferentiated, rapidly proliferating cells, whereas mesenchymal cells proximal to it differentiate into blood vessels and cartilage bone models. Members of the transforming growth factor-β gene family, activin-A and bone morphogenetic proteins (BMPs), play an important role in bone development and remodeling (Centrella et al., 1994; Russell, 1996). The distal ends of the flipperlike limb buds flatten into paddlelike hand and foot plates (Fig. 17-3). Experimental studies have shown that endogenous *retinoic acid* is involved in limb development and pattern formation (see Tabin [1991] for a review of the role of retinoids in limb morphogenesis).

By the end of the sixth week, mesenchymal tissue in the **hand plates** has condensed to form **digital rays** (Figs. 17-3 and 17-4*A* to *C*). These mesenchymal condensations outline the pattern of the digits (fingers). During the seventh week, similar condensations of mesenchyme form digital rays in the **foot plates** (Fig. 17-4*G* to *I*). At the tip of each digital ray, a part of the AER induces development of the mesenchyme into the mesenchymal primordia of the bones (phalanges) in the digits. The intervals between the digital rays are occupied by loose mesenchyme. Soon, the intervening regions of mesenchyme break down, forming *notches between the digital rays* (Figs. 17-3, 17-4*D* and *J*, and 17-5*A* to *D*). As the tissue break-

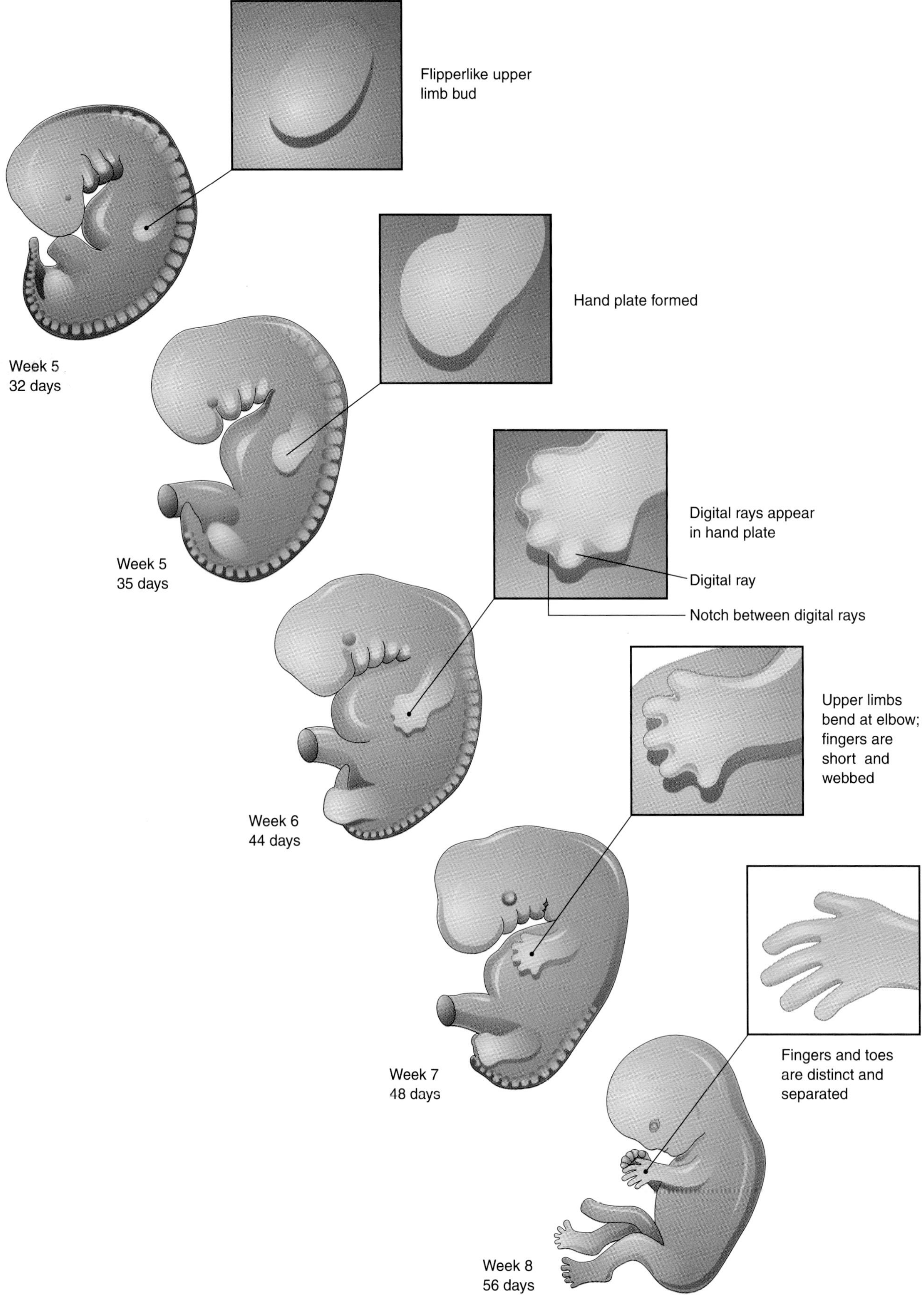

■ **Figure 17–3.** Drawings illustrating development of the limbs (32–56 days).

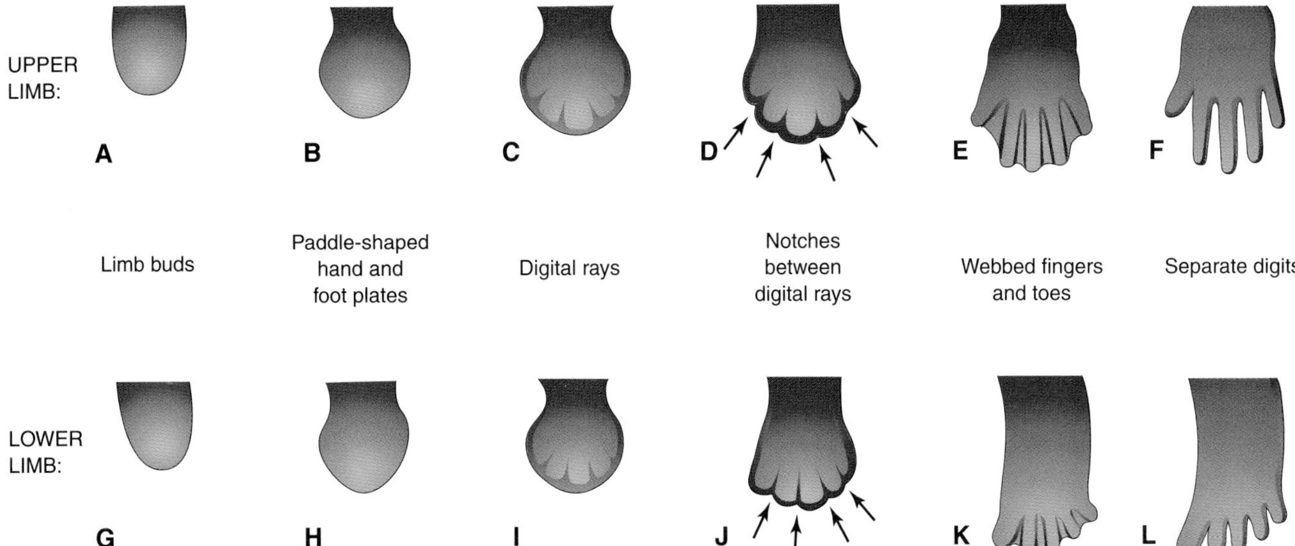

■ **Figure 17–4.** Drawings illustrating development of the hands and feet between the fourth and eighth weeks. The early stages of limb development are alike, except that development of the hands precedes that of the feet by a day or so. *A,* 27 days. *B,* 32 days. *C,* 41 days. *D,* 46 days. *E,* 50 days. *F,* 52 days. *G,* 28 days. *H,* 36 days. *I,* 46 days. *J,* 49 days. *K,* 52 days. *L,* 56 days.

down progresses, separate digits are produced by the end of the eighth week (Fig. 17-4*E, F, K,* and *L*). **Programmed cell death** (apoptosis) is responsible for the tissue breakdown in the interdigital regions, and it is probably mediated by signaling molecules known as **bone morphogenetic proteins** (BMP). Blocking these cellular and molecular events could account for **syndactyly**, webbing or fusion of fingers or toes (Zou and Niswander, 1996).

FINAL STAGES OF LIMB DEVELOPMENT

As the limbs elongate during the fifth week, mesenchymal models of the bones are formed by cellular aggregations (Fig. 17-7*B*). **Chondrification centers** appear later in the fifth week. By the end of the sixth week, the entire limb skeleton is cartilaginous (Figs. 17-6*A* to *D* and 17-7*C* and *D*). **Osteogenesis of long bones** begins in the seventh week from primary ossification centers in the middle of the cartilaginous models of the long bones. **Primary ossification centers** are present in all long bones by the twelfth week (see Chapter 15). Ossification of the carpal (wrist) bones begins during the first year after birth.

As the long bones form, myoblasts aggregate and form a large muscle mass in each limb bud (see Fig. 16-1). In general this muscle mass separates into dorsal (extensor) and ventral (flexor) components. The mesenchyme in the limb bud gives rise to bones, ligaments, and blood vessels (Fig. 17-6). From the dermomyotome regions of the somites, myogenic precursor cells also migrate into the limb bud and later differentiate into **myoblasts**—precursors of muscle cells (see Hinrichsen et al. [1994] for more information). The cervical and lumbosacral myotomes contribute to the muscles of the pectoral and pelvic girdles.

Early in the seventh week the limbs extend ventrally. The developing upper and lower limbs rotate in opposite directions and to different degrees (Figs. 17-8 and 17-9):

- *The upper limbs rotate laterally through 90 degrees* on their longitudinal axes; thus the future elbows point dorsally and the extensor muscles lie on the lateral and posterior aspects of the limb.
- *The lower limbs rotate medially* through almost 90 degrees; thus the future knees face ventrally and the extensor muscles lie on the anterior aspect of the lower limb.

It should now be clear that the radius and the tibia are homologous bones, as are the ulna and fibula, just as the thumb and great toe are homologous digits. Originally the flexor aspect of the limbs is ventral and the extensor aspect dorsal, and the preaxial and postaxial borders are cranial and caudal, respectively (Fig. 17-10*A* and *D*). **Synovial joints** appear at the beginning of the fetal period, coinciding with functional differentiation of the limb muscles and their innervation (Kabak and Boizow, 1990).

DERMATOMES AND CUTANEOUS INNERVATION OF LIMBS

Because of its relationship to the growth and rotation of the limbs, the cutaneous segmental nerve supply of the limbs is considered in this chapter rather than in Chapter 18 on the nervous system. See Lamb (1988) for details on the embryology of the peripheral nerves in relation to the innervation of the muscle fibers in

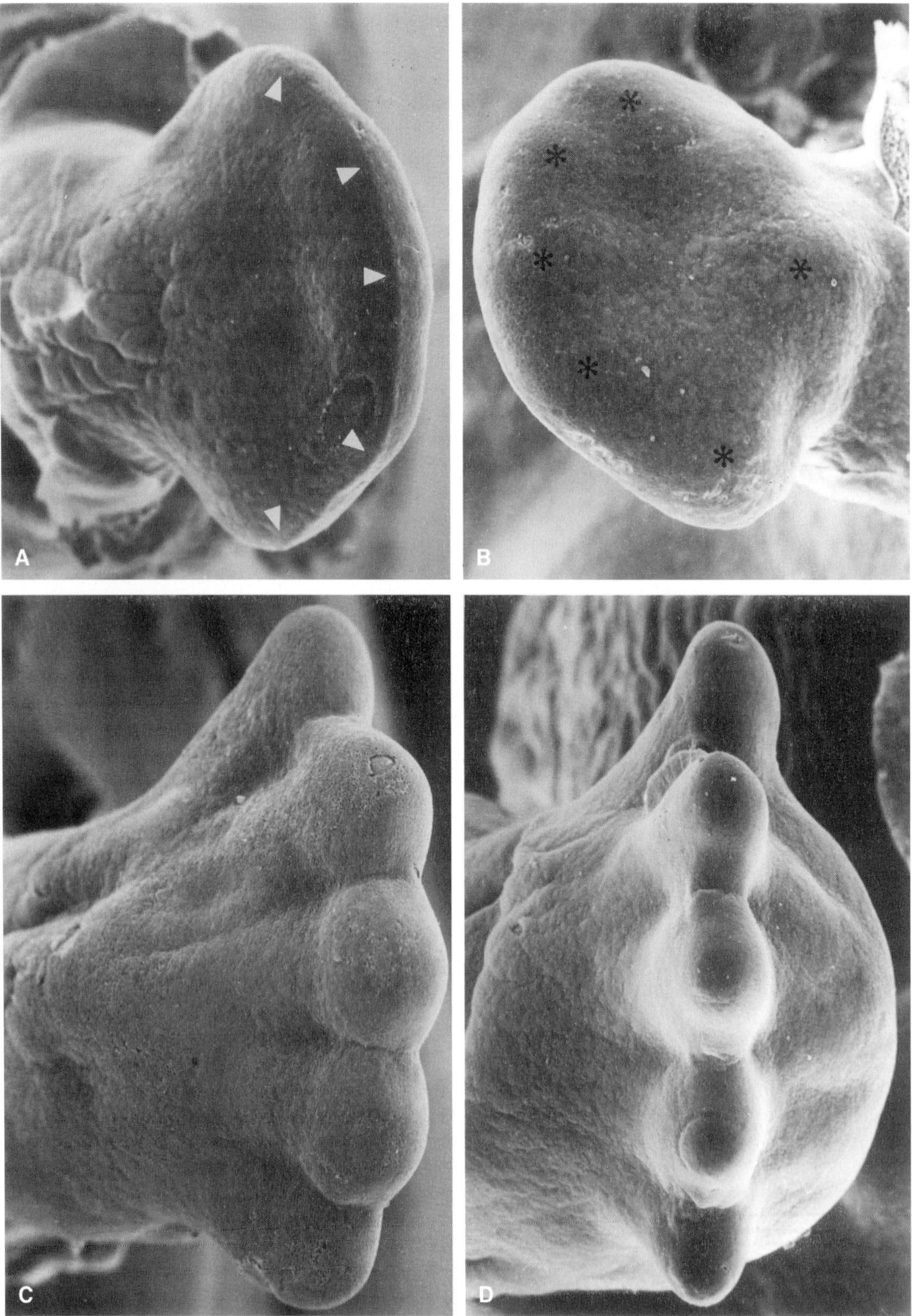

■ **Figure 17–5.** Scanning electron micrographs. Dorsal *(A)* and plantar *(B)* views of the right foot of human embryo, Carnegie stage 19 (about 48 days). The toe buds (*arrowheads* in *A*) and the heel cushion and metatarsal tactile elevation (*asterisks* in *B*) have just appeared. Dorsal *(C)* and distal *(D)* views of the right foot of human embryos, Carnegie stage 22 (about 55 days). The tips of the toes are separated and interdigital degeneration has begun. Note the dorsiflexion of the metatarsus and toes *(C)*, as well as the thickened heel cushion *(D)*. (From Hinrichsen KV, Jacob HJ, Jacob M, et al.: Principles of ontogenesis of leg and foot in man. *Ann Anat 176*:121, 1994.)

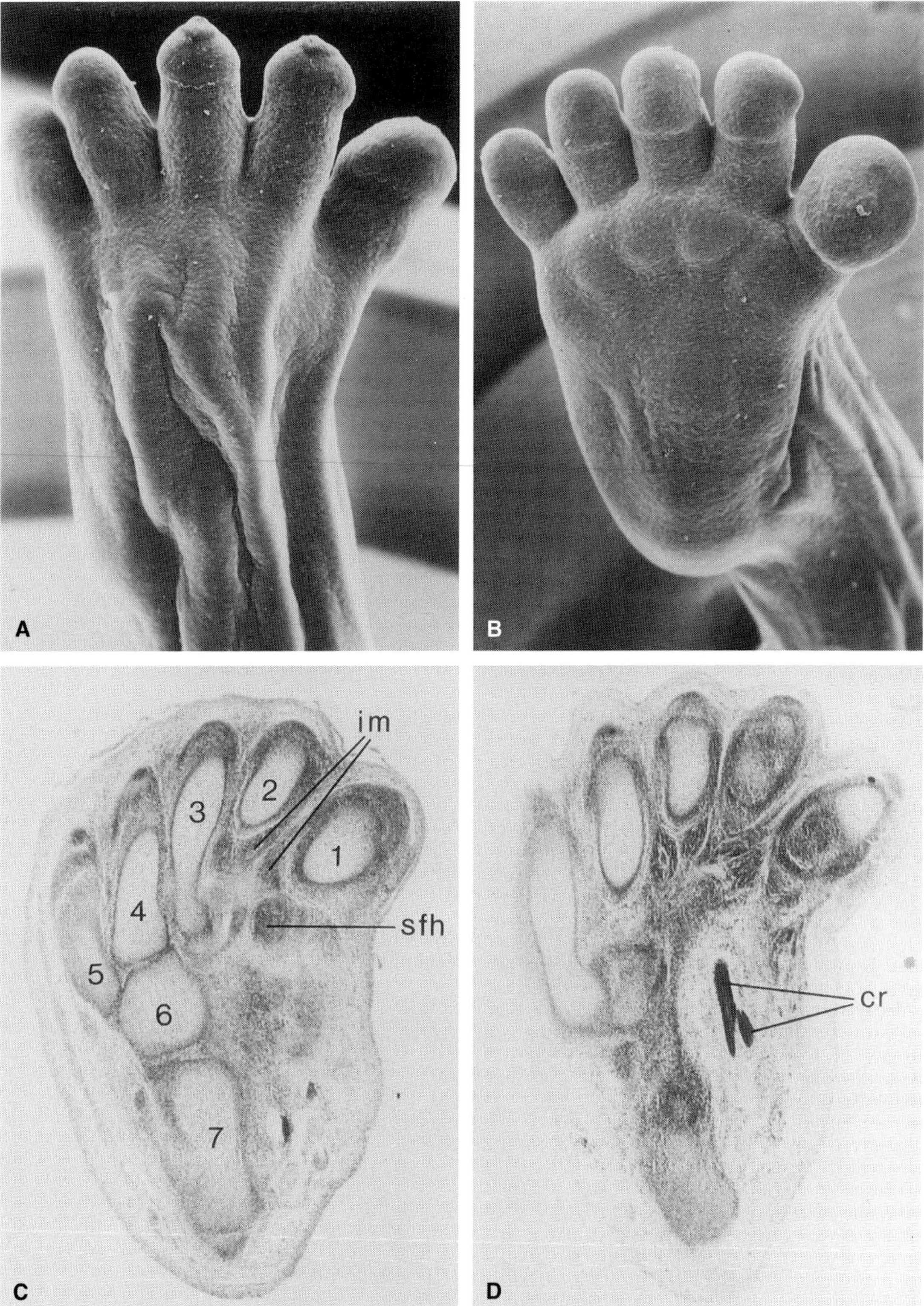

■ **Figure 17–6.** *A* and *B,* Scanning electron micrographs. *A,* Dorsal view of right leg and foot. *B,* Plantar view of the left foot of a human embryo at 8 weeks. Although supinated, dorsiflexion of the foot is distinct. Note the elongation of the foot. *C* and *D,* Paraffin sections of the tarsus and metatarsus of a young human fetus, stained with hematoxylin and eosin. **1–5**: metatarsal cartilages; **6**: cubital cartilage; **7**: calcaneus. The separation of the interosseous muscles **(im)** and short flexor muscles of the big toe **(sfh)** is clearly seen. The plantar crossing **(cr)** of the tendons of the long flexors of the digits and hallux is shown in *D.* (From Hinrichsen KV, Jacob HJ, Jacob M, et al.: Principles of ontogenesis of leg and foot in man. *Ann Anat 176:*121, 1994.)

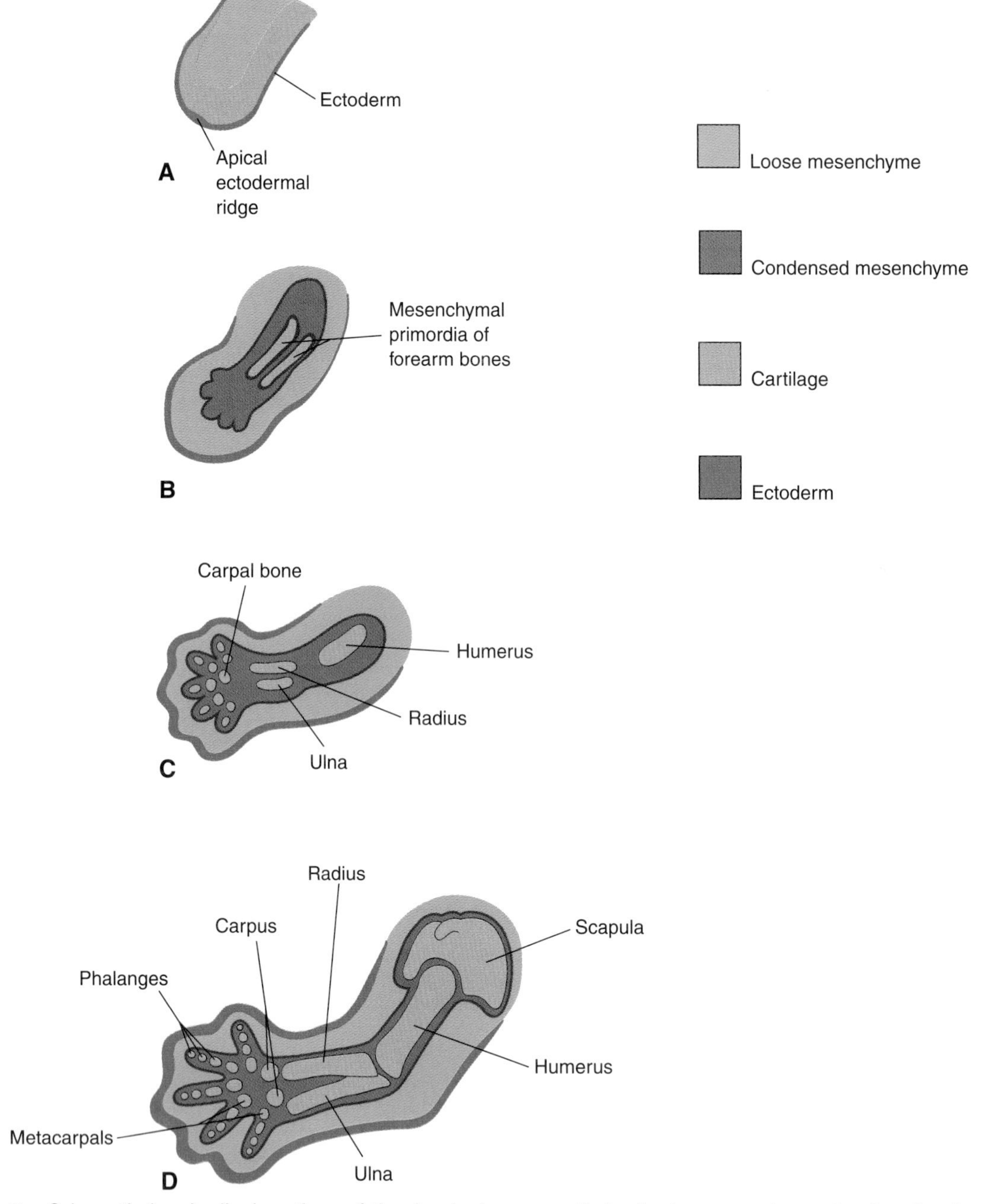

■ **Figure 17–7.** Schematic longitudinal sections of the developing upper limb of a human embryo, showing development of the cartilaginous bones.

the limbs. **Motor axons** arising from the spinal cord enter the limb buds during the fifth week and grow into the dorsal and ventral muscle masses. **Sensory axons** enter the limb buds after the motor axons and use them for guidance (Carlson, 1994). **Neural crest cells**, the precursors of Schwann cells, surround the motor and sensory nerve fibers in the limbs and form the *neurolemmal* (Schwann cell) and *myelin sheaths* (see Chapter 18).

A **dermatome** is the area of skin supplied by a single spinal nerve and its spinal ganglion. During the fifth week, the peripheral nerves grow from the developing limb plexuses (brachial and lumbosacral) into the mesenchyme of the limb buds (Fig. 17-10*B* and *E*). The spinal nerves are distributed in segmental bands, supplying both dorsal and ventral surfaces of the limb buds. As the limbs elongate, the cutaneous distribution of the spinal nerves migrates along the limbs and no longer reaches the surface in the distal part of the limbs. Although the original dermatomal pattern changes during growth of the limbs, an orderly sequence of distribution can still be recognized in the adult (Fig. 17-10*C* and *F*). In the upper limb, observe that the areas supplied by C5 and C6 adjoin the areas supplied by T2, T1, and C8, but the overlap between them is minimal at the *ventral axial line*.

A **cutaneous nerve area** is the area of skin supplied by a peripheral nerve. Cutaneous nerve areas and dermatomes show considerable overlapping. If the dorsal root supplying the area is cut, the dermatomal patterns indicate that there may be a slight deficit in the area indicated. Because there is overlapping of dermatomes, a particular area of skin is not exclusively innervated by a single segmental nerve. The limb dermatomes may be traced progressively down the lateral aspect of the upper limb and back up its medial aspect. A comparable distribution of dermatomes occurs in the lower limbs, which may be traced down the ventral aspect and then up the dorsal aspect of the lower limb. When the limbs descend they carry their nerves with them; this explains the oblique course of the nerves arising from the brachial and lumbosacral plexuses.

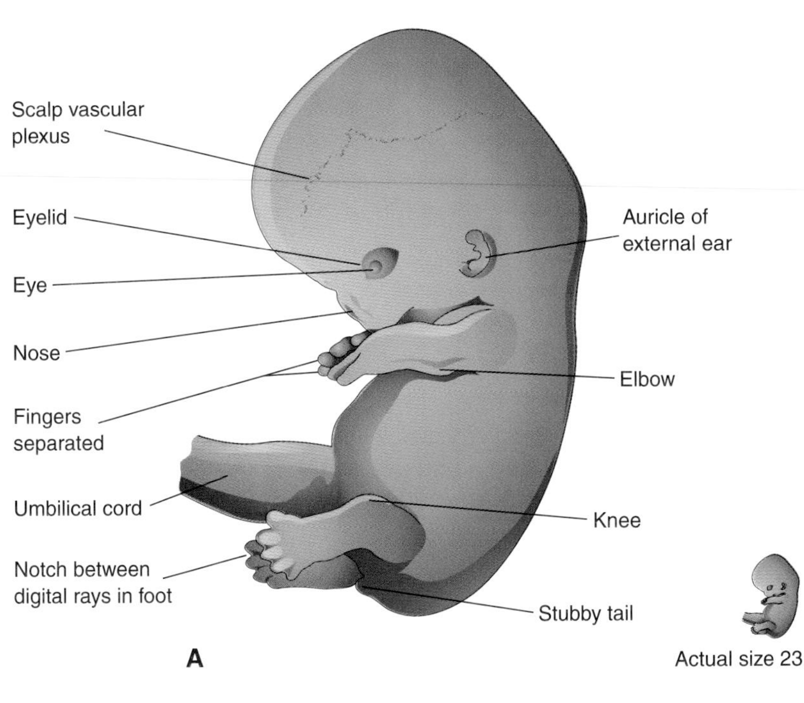

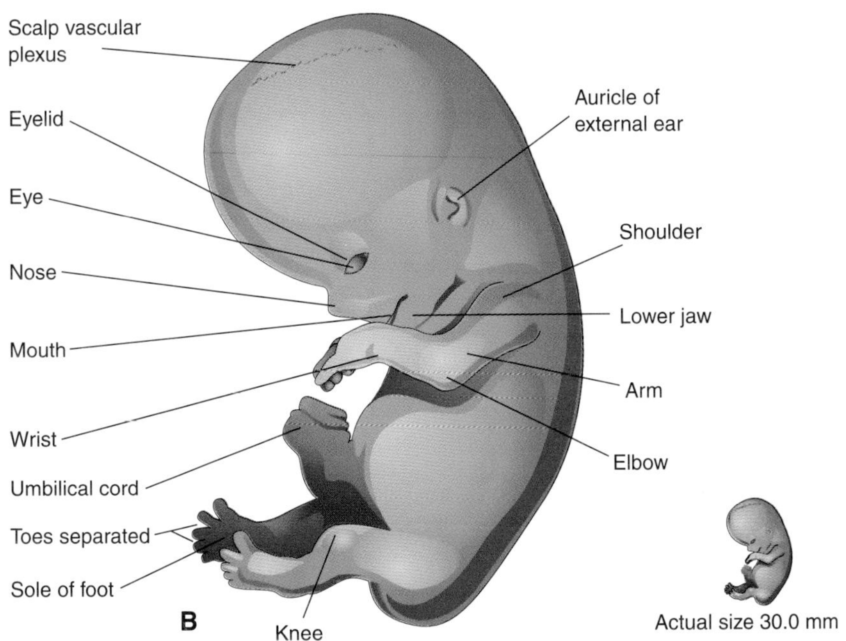

■ **Figure 17–8.** *A,* Lateral view of an embryo at Carnegie stage 21, about 52 days. The fingers are separated and the toes are beginning to separate. Note that the feet are fan-shaped. *B,* Lateral view of an embryo at Carnegie stage 23, about 56 days. All regions of the limbs are apparent and the digits in the hands and feet are separated. (Modified from Nishimura H, Semba R, Tanimura T, Tanaka O: *Prenatal Development of the Human with Special Reference to Craniofacial Structures: An Atlas.* Washington, DC, National Institutes of Health, 1977.)

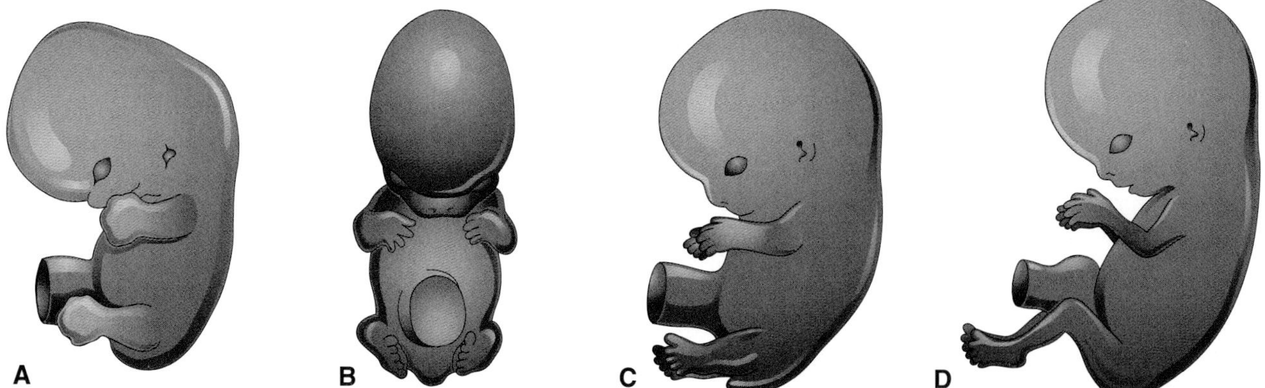

■ **Figure 17–9.** Drawings illustrating positional changes of the developing limbs of human embryos. *A,* About 48 days, showing the limbs extending ventrally and the hand and foot plates facing each other. *B,* About 51 days, showing the upper limbs bent at the elbows and the hands curved over the thorax. *C,* About 54 days, showing the soles of the feet facing medially. *D,* About 56 days. Note that the elbows now point caudally and the knees cranially.

BLOOD SUPPLY TO THE LIMBS

The limb buds are supplied by branches of the *intersegmental arteries* (Fig. 17-11*A*), which arise from the aorta and form a fine capillary network throughout the mesenchyme. The primitive vascular pattern consists of a **primary axial artery** and its branches (Fig. 17-11*B*), which drain into a peripheral marginal sinus. Blood in the **marginal sinus** drains into a peripheral vein. The vascular pattern changes as the limbs develop, chiefly by vessels sprouting from existing vessels. The new vessels coalesce with other sprouts to form new vessels. The primary axial artery becomes the **brachial artery** in the arm and the **common interosseous artery** in the forearm, which has anterior and posterior interosseous branches. The ulnar and radial arteries are terminal branches of the brachial artery. As the digits form, the marginal sinus breaks up and the final venous pattern, represented by the basilic and cephalic veins and their tributaries, develops. In the thigh the primary axial artery is represented by the **deep artery of the thigh** (profunda

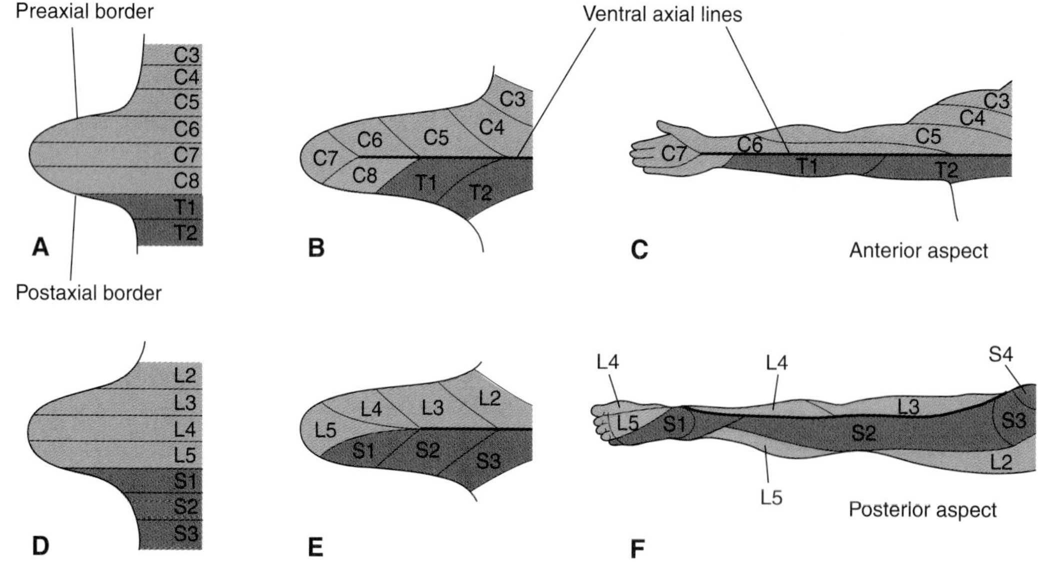

■ **Figure 17–10.** Diagrams illustrating development of the dermatomal patterns of the limbs. The axial lines indicate where there is no sensory overlap. *A* and *D,* Ventral aspect of the limb buds early in the fifth week. At this stage the dermatomal patterns show the primitive segmental arrangement. *B* and *E,* Similar views later in the fifth week showing the modified arrangement of dermatomes. *C* and *F,* The dermatomal patterns in the adult upper and lower limbs. The primitive dermatomal pattern has disappeared but an orderly sequence of dermatomes can still be recognized. In *F,* note that most of the original ventral surface of the lower limb lies on the back of the adult limb. This results from the medial rotation of the lower limb that occurs toward the end of the embryonic period. In the upper limb the ventral axial line extends along the anterior surface of the arm and forearm. In the lower limb, the ventral axial line extends along the medial side of the thigh and knee to the posteromedial aspect of the leg to the heel.

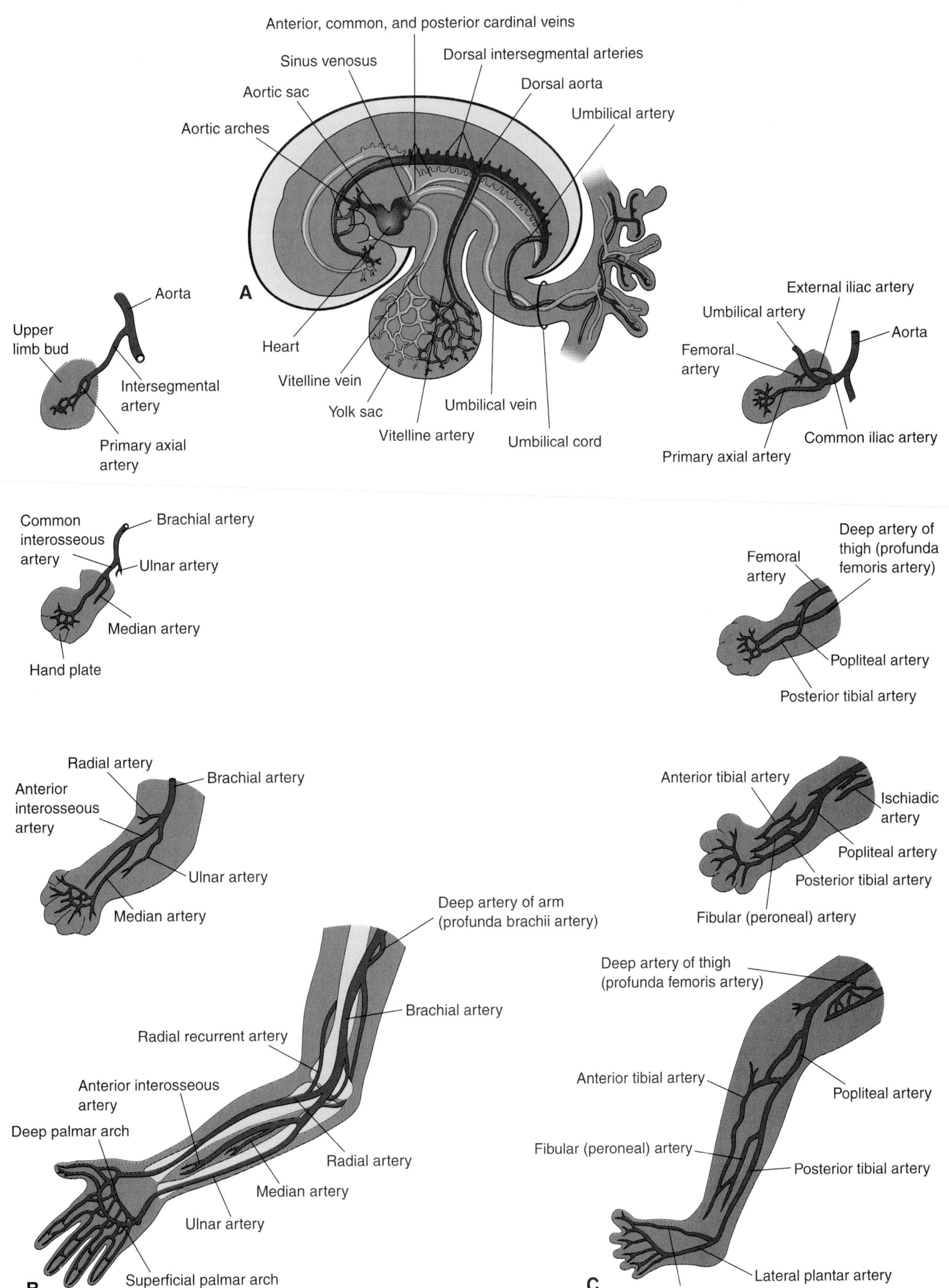

■ **Figure 17–11.** Development of limb arteries. *A,* Sketch of the primitive cardiovascular system in a 4-week embryo, about 26 days. *B,* Development of arteries in the upper limb. *C,* Development of arteries in the lower limb.

femoris artery). In the leg, the primary axial artery is represented by the anterior and posterior tibial arteries (Moore, 1992).

ANOMALIES OF LIMBS

Minor limb anomalies are relatively common but they can usually be corrected surgically (Hoffinger, 1996; van Heest, 1996). Although minor anomalies are usually of no serious medical consequence, they may serve as indicators of more serious anomalies and they may be part of a recognizable pattern of defects (Jones, 1997).

The most critical period of limb development is from 24 to 36 days after fertilization. The statement is based on clinical studies of infants exposed to thalidomide, a potent human teratogen that produced limb defects and other anomalies (Newman, 1986). Exposure to a potent teratogen before day 33 may cause severe anomalies, such as absence of the limbs and hands (Figs. 17-12*A* and 17-13*C*). Exposure to a teratogen from days 34 to 36 produces absence or hypoplasia of the thumbs (Fig. 17-14*B*). Consequently, a teratogen that could cause absence of the limbs or parts of them must act before the end of the critical period of limb development. Many severe limb anomalies occurred from 1957 to 1962 as a result of maternal ingestion of **thalidomide** (Fig. 17-12). This drug, widely used as a sedative and antinauseant, was withdrawn from the market in December 1961. Since that time similar limb anomalies have rarely been observed. Because thalidomide is still available as an investigational agent, it must be emphasized that *thalidomide is absolutely contraindicated in women of childbearing age* (Behrman et al., 1996).

Major limb anomalies appear about twice in 1000 newborns (Connor and Ferguson-Smith, 1988). Most of these defects are caused by genetic factors (Fig. 17-

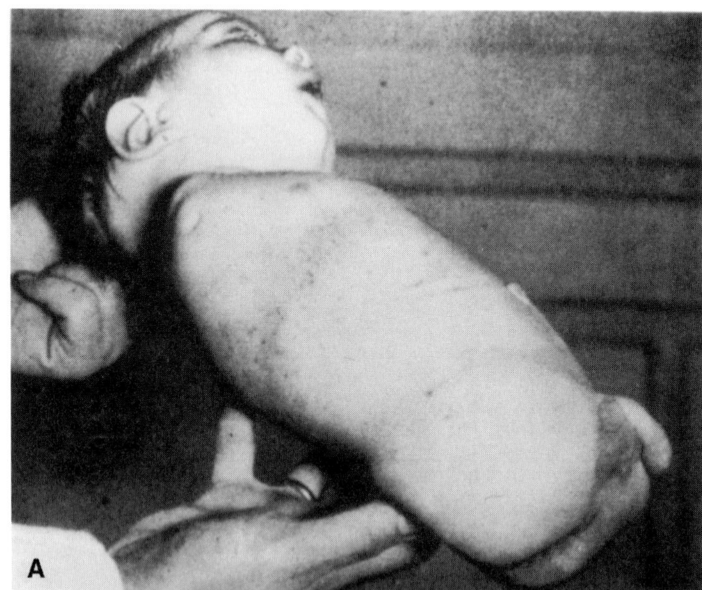

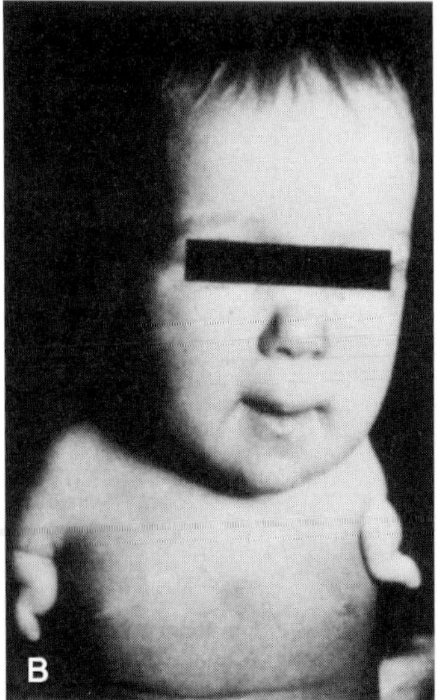

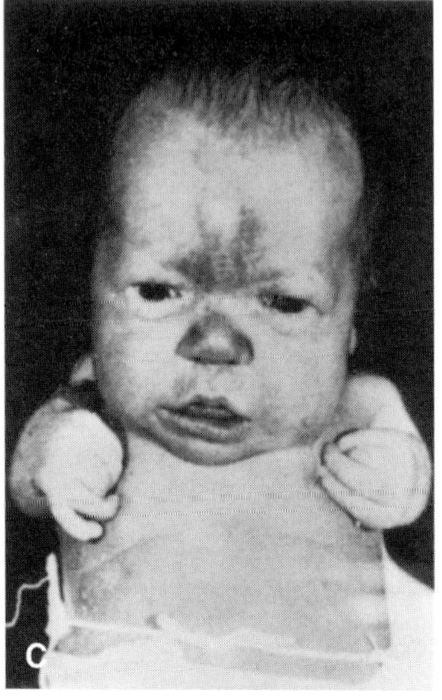

■ **Figure 17-12.** Limb anomalies caused by thalidomide. *A,* Quadruple amelia: absence of the upper and lower limbs. *B,* Meromelia of the upper limbs: the limbs are represented by rudimentary stumps. *C,* Meromelia with the rudimentary upper limbs attached directly to the trunk. (From Lenz W, Knapp K: Foetal malformation due to thalidomide. *Ger Med Mon* 7:253, 1962.)

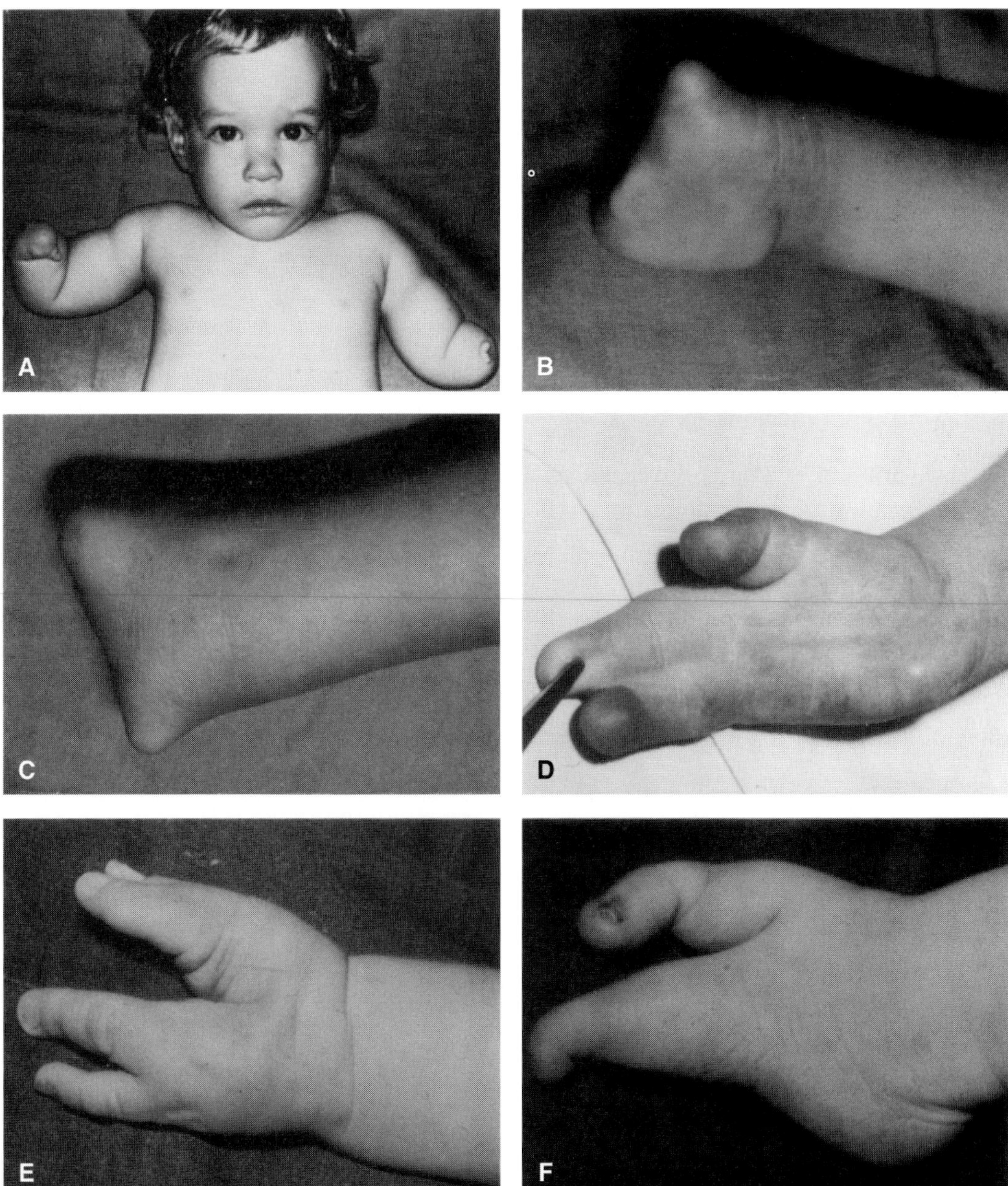

■ **Figure 17–13.** Various types of meromelia (partial absence of limbs). *A,* Absence of the hands and most of the forearms. *B,* Absence of the digits. *C,* Absence of the hand. *D,* Absence of the fourth and fifth digits and syndactyly of the second and third digits. *E,* Absence of the third digit, resulting in a cleft hand. *F,* Absence of the second and third toes and syndactyly of the fourth and fifth toes, resulting in a cleft foot. (*D* is from Swenson O: *Pediatric Surgery.* 1958. Courtesy of Appleton-Century-Crofts.)

14*C* to *F*). Several unrelated congenital anomalies of the lower limb were found to be associated with a similar aberrant arterial pattern, which might be of some importance in the pathogenesis of these defects (Levinsohn et al., 1991).

Limb Defects

The terminology used to describe limb defects in this book follows the international nomenclature, in which only two basic descriptive terms are used:

- *amelia*, complete absence of a limb or limbs
- *meromelia* (Gr. *meros*, part, and *melos*, extremity), partial absence of a limb or limbs (Fig. 17-13).

Descriptive terms such as hemimelia, peromelia, ectromelia, and phocomelia are not used in current nomenclature because of their imprecision.

Cleft Hand and Cleft Foot

In these rare anomalies (lobster-claw deformities), there is absence of one or more central digits, resulting from failure of development of one or more digital rays (Fig. 17-13*E* and *F*). The hand or foot is divided into two parts that oppose each other like lobster claws. The remaining digits are partially or completely fused (syndactyly).

Congenital Absence of Radius

The radius is partially or completely absent. The hand deviates laterally (radially) and the ulna bows with the concavity on the lateral side of the forearm. This anomaly results from failure of the mesenchymal primordium of the radius to form during the fifth week of development. Absence of the radius is usually caused by genetic factors.

Brachydactyly

Shortness of the digits (fingers or toes) is uncommon and is the result of reduction in the length of the phalanges (Fig. 17-14*A*). This anomaly is usually inherited as a dominant trait and is often associated with shortness of stature.

Polydactyly

Supernumerary digits are common (Figs. 17-14*C* and *D* and 17-15). Often the extra digit is incompletely formed and lacks proper muscular development; it is thus useless. If the hand is affected, the extra digit is most commonly medial or lateral rather than central. In the foot the extra toe is usually on the lateral side. Polydactyly is inherited as a dominant trait.

Syndactyly

Syndactyly occurs in 1:2200 births (Behrman et al., 1996). Cutaneous syndactyly (simple webbing of digits) is the most common limb anomaly. It is more frequent in the foot than in the hand (Fig. 17-16). **Cutaneous syndactyly** results from failure of the webs to degenerate between two or more digits (Fig. 17-17A and *D*). In severe cases there is fusion of several digits (Fig. 17-17*B*, *E*, and *F*). In some cases there is fusion of the bones (synostosis). **Osseous syndactyly** occurs when the notches between the digital rays fail to develop during the seventh week; as a result, separation of the digits does not occur. Syndactyly is most frequently observed between the third and fourth fingers and between the second and third toes. It is inherited as a simple dominant or simple recessive trait (Thompson et al., 1991). A case of synpolydactyly (syndactyly and polydactyly), caused by mutations in the NH_2-terminal, non-DNA binding part of HOXD13, has been reported (Muragaki et al., 1996).

Congenital Clubfoot

Any deformity of the foot involving the talus (ankle bone) is called clubfoot or talipes (L. *talus*, heel, ankle + *pes*, foot). Clubfoot is a common anomaly, occurring about once in 1000 births. It is characterized by an abnormal position of the foot that prevents normal

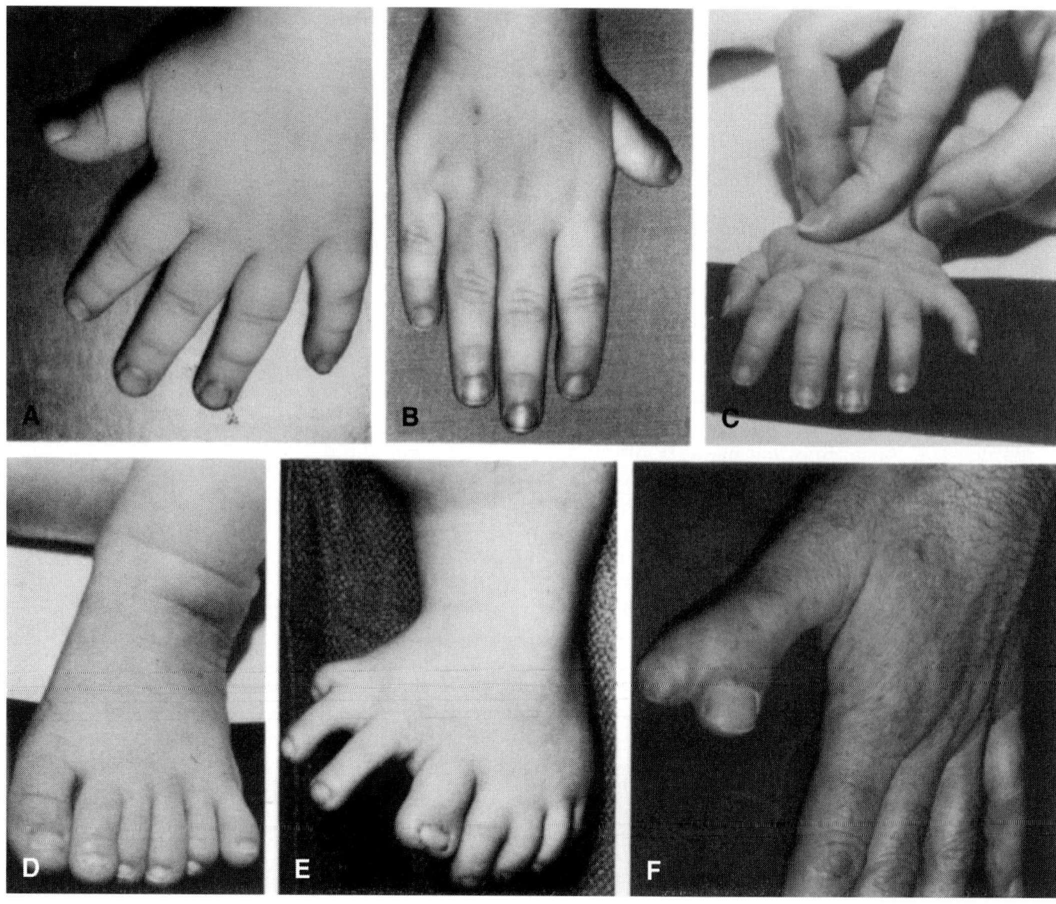

■ **Figure 17-14.** Various types of limb anomaly. *A,* Brachydactyly. *B,* Hypoplasia of the thumb. *C,* Polydactyly showing a supernumerary fifth finger. *D,* Polydactyly showing a supernumerary fifth toe. *E,* Partial duplication of the foot. *F,* Partial duplication of the thumb. (*C* and *D* are from Swenson O: *Pediatric Surgery.* 1958. Courtesy of Appleton-Century-Crofts.)

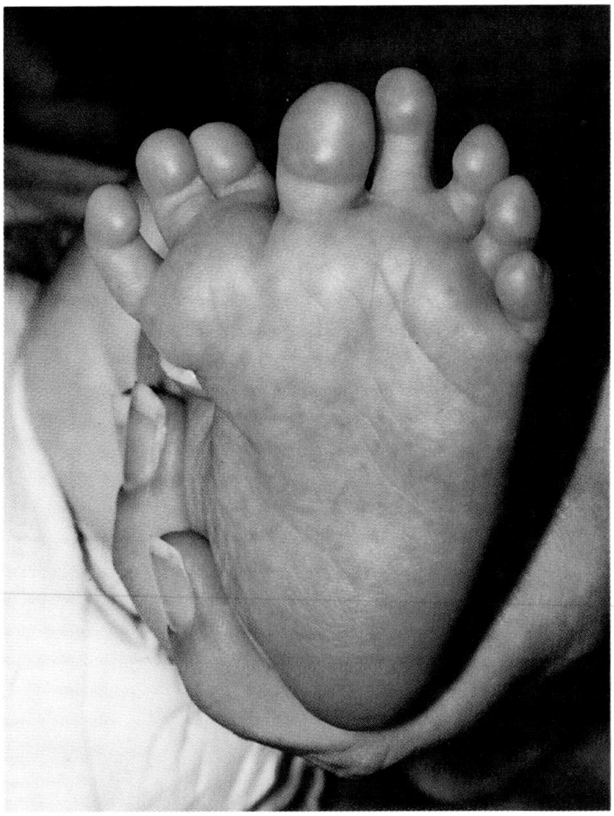

■ **Figure 17–15.** Polydactyly showing partial duplication of the right foot and toes. (Courtesy of Dr. A. E. Chudley, Section of Genetics and Metabolism, Department of Pediatrics and Child Health, Children's Hospital and University of Manitoba, Winnipeg, Manitoba, Canada.)

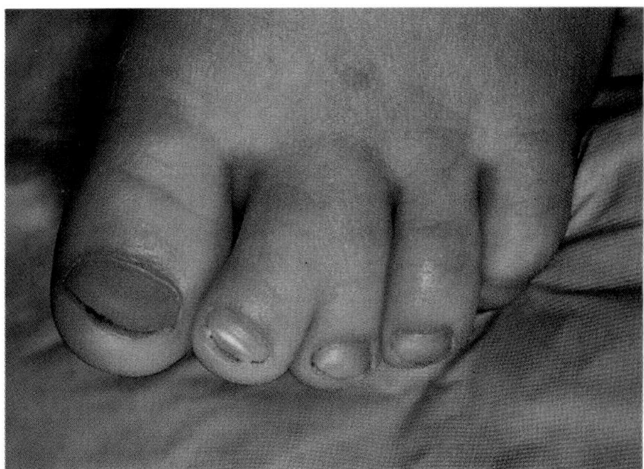

■ **Figure 17–16.** Syndactyly of the second and third toes. (Courtesy of Dr. A. E. Chudley, Section of Genetics and Metabolism, Department of Pediatrics and Child Health, Children's Hospital and University of Manitoba, Winnipeg, Manitoba, Canada.)

weight bearing. As the child develops, he or she tends to walk on the ankle rather than on the sole of the foot. **Talipes equinovarus**, the most common type of clubfoot (Figs. 17-17*C* and 17-18), occurs about twice as frequently in males. The sole of the foot is turned medially and the foot is inverted. There is much uncertainty about the cause of clubfoot (Robertson and Corbett, 1997). Although it is commonly stated that clubfoot results from abnormal positioning or restricted movement of the fetus's lower limbs in utero, the evidence for this is inconclusive. When the

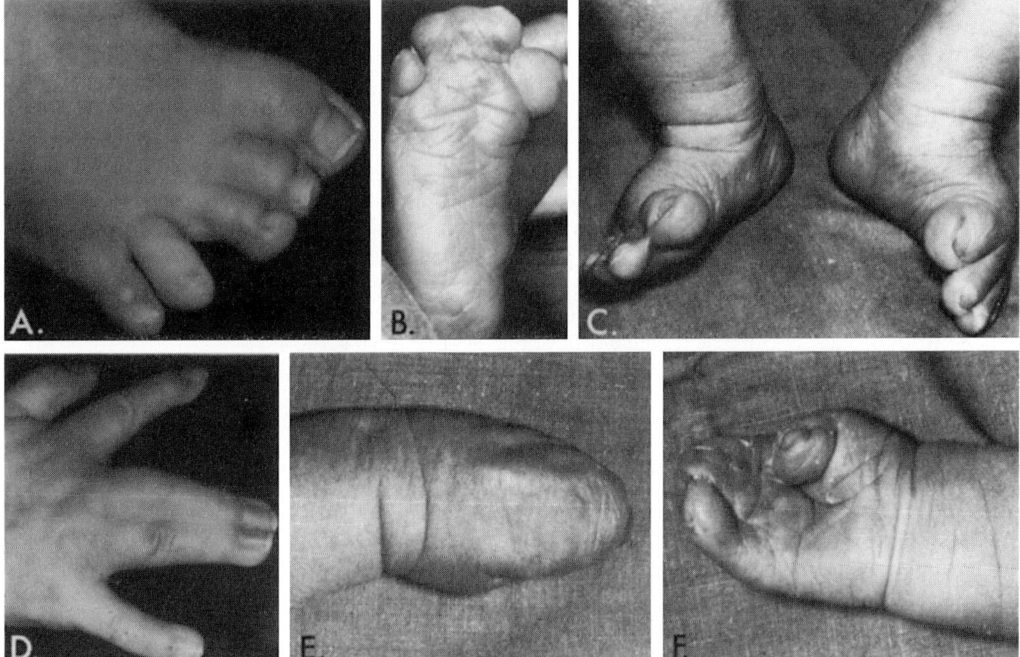

■ **Figure 17–17.** Various types of limb anomaly. *A,* Cutaneous syndactyly showing skin webs between the first and second and second and third toes. *B,* Severe cutaneous syndactyly involving fusion of all the toes except the fifth. *C,* Cutaneous syndactyly associated with clubfoot (talipes equinovarus). *D,* Cutaneous syndactyly involving webbing of the third and fourth fingers. *E* and *F,* Dorsal and palmar views of a child's right hand, showing osseous syndactyly (fusion) of the second to fifth fingers. (*A* and *D* are from Swenson O: *Pediatric Surgery.* 1958. Courtesy of Appleton-Century-Crofts).

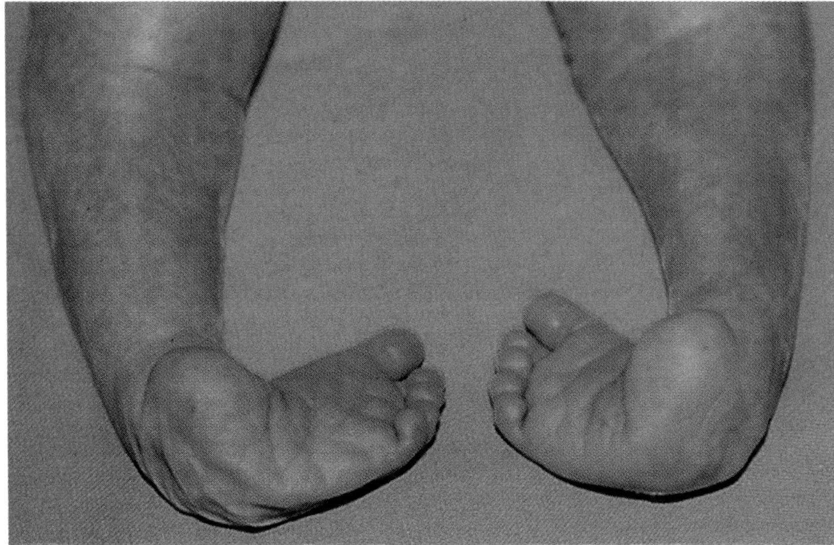

■ **Figure 17–18.** Neonate with bilateral talipes equinovarus deformities (clubfeet). This is the classic type with sharp and tight hyperextension and incurving of the feet. (Courtesy of Dr. A. E. Chudley, Section of Genetics and Metabolism, Department of Pediatrics and Child Health, Children's Hospital and University of Manitoba, Winnipeg, Manitoba, Canada.)

abnormal position of the foot results from the position of the fetus in utero, the foot can easily be positioned normally (Nichols and Zwelling, 1997). Hereditary factors are involved in some cases, and it appears that environmental factors are involved in most cases. Clubfoot appears to follow a **multifactorial pattern of inheritance**; hence, any intrauterine position that results in abnormal positioning of the feet may cause clubfeet if the fetus is genetically predispositioned to this deformity.

Congenital Dislocation of the Hip

This deformity occurs in about one of every 1500 newborn infants and is more common in females than in males. The capsule of the hip joint is very relaxed at birth, and there is underdevelopment of the acetabulum of the hip bone and the head of the femur. The actual dislocation almost always occurs after birth. Two causative factors are commonly given:

- **Abnormal development of the acetabulum** occurs in about 15% of infants with congenital dislocation of the hip, which is common after breech deliveries, suggesting that breech posture during the terminal months of pregnancy may result in abnormal development of the acetabulum and head of the femur.
- **Generalized joint laxity** is often a dominantly inherited condition, which appears to be associated with congenital dislocation of the hip. Congenital dislocation of the hip follows a multifactorial pattern of inheritance (Thompson et al., 1991).

Causes of Limb Anomalies

Anomalies of the limbs originate at different stages of development. Suppression of limb bud development during the early part of the fourth week results in *absence of the limbs*—**amelia** (Fig. 17-12*A*). Arrest or disturbance of differentiation or growth of the limbs during the fifth week results in various types of **meromelia** (Figs. 17-12*B* and *C* and 17-13*A* to *C*). *Meromelia denotes partial absence of a limb.*

Like other congenital anomalies, some limb defects are caused by:

- genetic factors, e.g., chromosomal abnormalities associated with trisomy 18 (see Chapter 8)
- mutant genes as in brachydactyly or osteogenesis imperfecta (Marini and Gerber, 1997)
- environmental factors, e.g., teratogens such as thalidomide
- a combination of genetic and environmental factors (*multifactorial inheritance*), e.g., congenital dislocation of the hip (Thompson et al., 1991)
- vascular disruption and ischemia, e.g., limb reduction defects (Van Allen, 1992).

Experimental studies support the suggestion that mechanical influences during intrauterine development may cause some limb defects (Kennedy and Persaud, 1977, 1979). A reduced quantity of amniotic fluid (**oligohydramnios**) is commonly associated with limb deformations (Dunn, 1976); however, the significance of in utero mechanical influences on congenital postural deformation is still open to question (Light and Ogden, 1993). For more information on congenital limb defects, see Van Heest (1966) and Hoffinger (1996).

SUMMARY OF LIMB DEVELOPMENT

The limbs begin to appear toward the end of the fourth week as slight elevations of the ventrolateral body wall. The upper limb buds develop about 2 days before the lower limb buds. The tissues of the limb buds are derived from two main sources: mesoderm and ectoderm. The **apical ectodermal ridge** (AER) exerts an inductive influence on the limb mesenchyme, promoting growth and development of the limbs. The limb buds elongate by proliferation of the mesenchyme within them. **Programmed cell death** is an important mechanism in limb development; e.g., in the formation of the digits. Limb muscles are derived from mesenchyme (myogenic precursor cells) originating in the somites. The muscle-forming cells (myoblasts) form dorsal and ventral muscle masses. Nerves grow into the limb buds after the muscle masses have formed. Most blood vessels of the limb buds arise as buds from the aorta and cardinal veins.

Initially, the developing limbs are directed caudally; later, they project ventrally, and finally, they rotate on their longitudinal axes. The upper and lower limbs rotate in opposite directions and to different degrees. The majority of limb anomalies are caused by genetic factors; however many limb abnormalities probably result from an interaction of genetic and environmental factors (multifactorial inheritance). Relatively few congenital anomalies of the limbs can be attributed to specific environmental teratogens, except those resulting from thalidomide.

Clinically Oriented Problems

Case 17–1

A mother consulted her pediatrician after noticing that when her 11-month-old daughter began to stand independently, her legs seemed to be of different lengths.

- Do more female infants have congenital dislocation of the hip than male infants?
- Are the hip joints of these infants usually dislocated at birth?
- What are the probable causes of congenital dislocation of the hip?

Case 17–2

A male infant was born with limb defects. His mother said that one of her relatives had a similar defect.

- Are limb anomalies similar to those caused by the drug thalidomide common?
- What was the characteristic *malformation syndrome* produced by thalidomide?
- Name the limb and other defects commonly associated with the thalidomide syndrome.

Case 17–3

A newborn infant was born with an obvious clubfoot. The physician explained that this was a common type of anomaly.

- What is the most common type of clubfoot?
- How common is it?
- Describe the feet of infants born with this anomaly.

Case 17–4

A baby was born with webbing between his fingers. The doctor stated this minor defect could be easily corrected surgically.

- Is syndactyly common?
- Does it occur more often in the hands than in the feet?
- What is the embryological basis of syndactyly?

Discussion of these problems appears at the back of the book.

REFERENCES AND SUGGESTED READING

Behrman RE, Kliegman RM, Arvin AM (eds): *Nelson Textbook of Pediatrics,* 15th ed. Philadelphia, WB Saunders, 1996.

Bernhardt DB: Prenatal and postnatal growth and development of the foot and ankle. *Phys Ther 68:*1831, 1988.

Brook WJ, Diaz-Benjumea FJ, Cohen SM: Organizing spatial pattern in limb development. *Ann Rev Cell Develop Biol 12:*161, 1996.

Carlson BM: *Human Embryology and Developmental Biology*. St Louis, Mosby, 1994.

Centrella M, Horowitz MC, Wozney JM, McCarthy TL: Transforming growth factor-β gene family members and bone. *Endocr Rev 15:* 27, 1994.

Cohn MJ, Patel K, Krumlauf R, et al: *HOX* 9 genes and vertebrate limb specification. *Nature 387:*97, 1997.

Connor JM, Ferguson-Smith MA: *Essential Medical Genetics,* 2nd ed. Oxford, Blackwell Scientific Publications, 1988.

Dunn PM: Congenital postural deformities. *Br Med Bull 32:*65, 1976.

Filly RA: Sonographic anatomy of the normal fetus. *In* Harrison MR, Golbus MS, Filly RA (eds): *The Unborn Patient. Prenatal Diagnosis and Treatment,* 2nd ed. Philadelphia, WB Saunders, 1991.

Frantz CH, O'Rahilly R: Congenital skeletal limb deficiencies. *J Bone Joint Surg 43A:*1202, 1961.

Guidera KJ, Ganey TM, Keneally CR, Ogden JA: The embrology of lower-extremity torsion. *Clin Orthop 259:*17, 1994.

Hartwig NG, Vermeij-Keers C, DeVries HE, et al: Limb body wall malformation complex: an embryologic etiology? *Hum Pathol 20:* 1071, 1989.

Hinrichsen KV, Jacob HJ, Jacob M, et al: Principles of ontogenesis of leg and foot in man. *Ann Anat 176:*121, 1994.

Hoffinger SA: Evaluation and management of pediatric foot deformities. *Pediatr Clin North Am 43:*1091, 1996.

Jones KL: *Smith's Recognizable Patterns of Human Malformation,* 5th ed. Philadelphia, WB Saunders, 1997.

Kabak S, Boizow L: Organogenese des Extremitätenskeletts und der Extremitätengelenke beim Menschenembryo. *Anat Anz 170:*349, 1990.

Keegan JJ, Garrett FD: The segmental distribution of the cutaneous nerves in the limbs of man. *Anat Rec 102:*409, 1948.

Kennedy LA, Persaud TVN: Pathogenesis of developmental defects induced in the rat by amniotic sac puncture. *Acta Anat 97:*23, 1977.

Kennedy LA, Persaud TVN: Experimental amniocentesis and teratogenesis: clinical implications. *In* Persaud TVN (ed): *Advances in the Study of Birth Defects, Vol 1. Teratogenic Mechanisms*. New York, Alan R Liss, 1979.

Lamb AH: Aspects of peripheral motor system development. *Aust Paediatr J 24(Suppl 1):*37, 1988.

Lenz W: How can the teratogenic action of a factor be established in man? *South Med J Supp 64:*41, 1971.

Lenz W, Knapp K: Foetal malformations due to thalidomide. *Ger Med Mon 7:*253, 1962.

Levinsohn EM, Hootnick DR, Packard DS Jr: Consistent arterial abnormalities associated with a variety of congenital malformations of the lower limb. *Invest Radiol 26:*364, 1991.

Light TR, Ogden JA: Congenital constriction band syndrome: pathophysiology and treatment. *Yale J Biol Med 66:*143, 1993.

Lubinsky MS: Explaining certain limb anomalies and the limb-hematopoiesis community of syndromes using a model of determination. *Teratology 43:*295, 1991.

Mahony BS: Ultrasound evaluation of the fetal musculoskeletal system. *In* Callen PW (ed): *Ultrasonography in Obstetrics and Gynecology,* 3rd ed. Philadelphia, WB Saunders, 1994.

Mahony BS, Filly RA: High-resolution sonographic assessment of the fetal extremities. *J Ultrasound Med 3:*489, 1984.

Maini PK, Solursh M: Cellular mechanisms of pattern formation in the developing limb. *Int Rev Cytol 129:*91, 1991.

Marini JC, Gerber NL: Osteogenesis imperfecta. *JAMA 277:*746, 1997.

Martin JH: Anatomical substrates for somatic sensation. *In* Kandel ER, Schwartz JH (eds): *Principles of Neural Science*. New York, Elsevier, 1985.

McCarthy D: The developmental anatomy of pes valgo planus. *Clin Podiatr Med Surg 6:*491, 1989.

Moore KL: *Clinically Oriented Anatomy,* 3rd ed. Baltimore, Williams & Wilkins, 1992.

Mundy GR: *Bone Remodelling and Its Disorders*. London, Martin Dunitz, 1995.

Muragaki Y, Mundlos S, Upton J, Olsen BR: Altered growth and branching patterns in synpolydactyly caused by mutations in HOXD13. *Science 272:*548, 1996.

Newman CGH: Clinical aspects of thalidomide embryopathy—a continuing preoccupation. *Teratogen Update. Environmentally Induced Birth Risks*. New York, Alan R Liss, 1986.

Nichols FH, Zwelling E (eds): *Maternal-Newborn Nursing. Theory and Practice*. Philadelphia, WB Saunders, 1997.

O'Rahilly R, Gardner E: The timing and sequence of events in the development of the limbs in the human embryo. *Anat Embryol 148:*1, 1975.

O'Rahilly R, Müller F: *Developmental Stages in Human Embryos*. Washington, Carnegie Institution of Washington, 1987.

Oransky M, Canero G, Maiotti M: Embryonic development of the posterolateral structures of the knee. *Anat Rec 225:*347, 1989.

Robertson WW Jr, Corbett D: Congenital clubfoot. *Clin Orthop 338:* 14, 1997.

Russell RGG: Cytokines and growth factors involved in bone metabolism and disease. *Bull Royal College of Pathologists 95:*ii, 1996.

Seyfer AE, Wind G, Martin RR: Study of upper extremity growth and development using human embryos and computer-reconstructed models. *J Hand Surg 14:*927, 1989.

Tabin CJ: Retinoids, homeoboxes, and growth factors: toward molecular models for limb development. *Cell 66:*199, 1991.

Thompson MW, McInnes RR, Willard HF: *Thompson & Thompson Genetics in Medicine,* 5th ed. Philadelphia, WB Saunders, 1991.

Uhthoff HK: *The Embryology of the Human Locomotor System*. New York, Springer-Verlag, 1990.

Van Allen MI: Structural anomalies resulting from vascular disruption. *Pediatr Clin North Am 39:*255, 1992.

Van Heest AE: Congenital disorders of the hand and upper extremity. *Pediatr Clin North Am 43:*1113, 1996.

Wolpert L: Mechanisms of limb development and malformation. *Br Med Bull 32:*65, 1976.

Wolpert L: Positional information and pattern formation in development. *Dev Genet 15:*485, 1994.

Zou H, Niswander L: Requirement for BMP signaling in interdigital apoptosis and scale formation. *Science 272:*738, 1996.

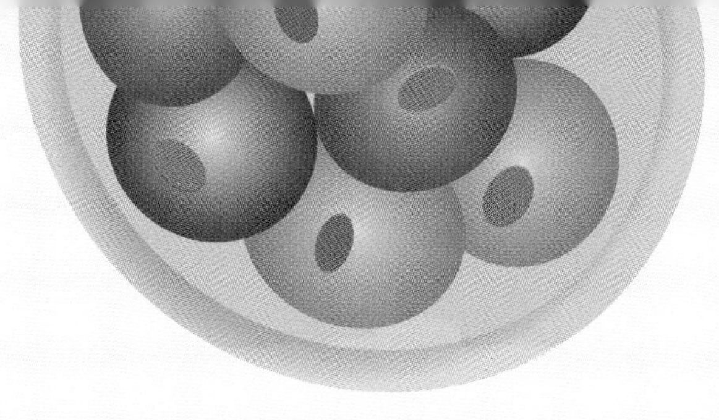

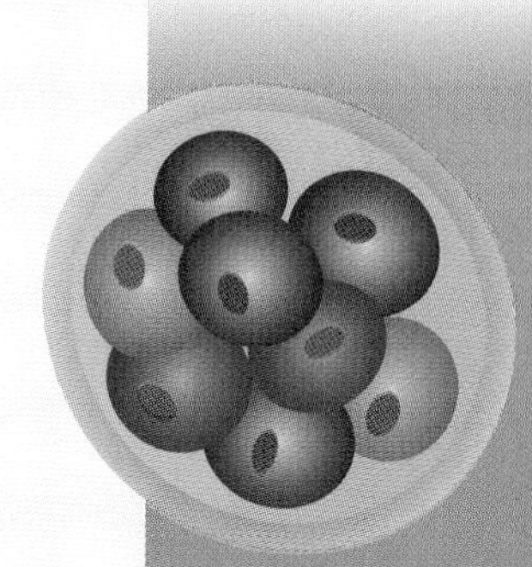

The Nervous System

18

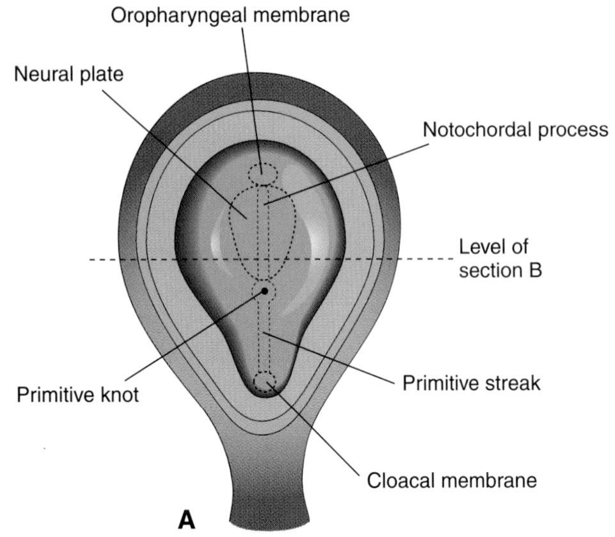

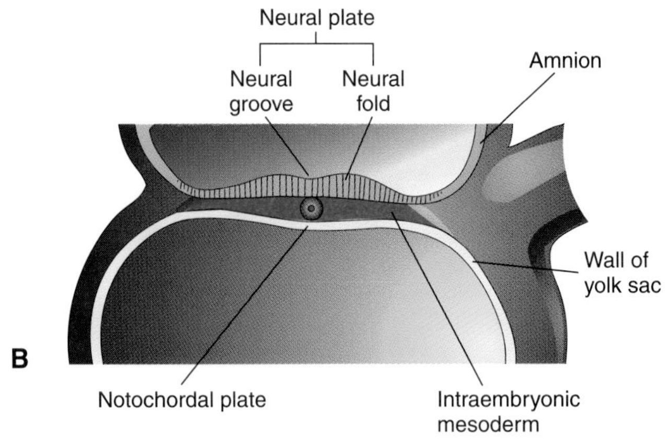

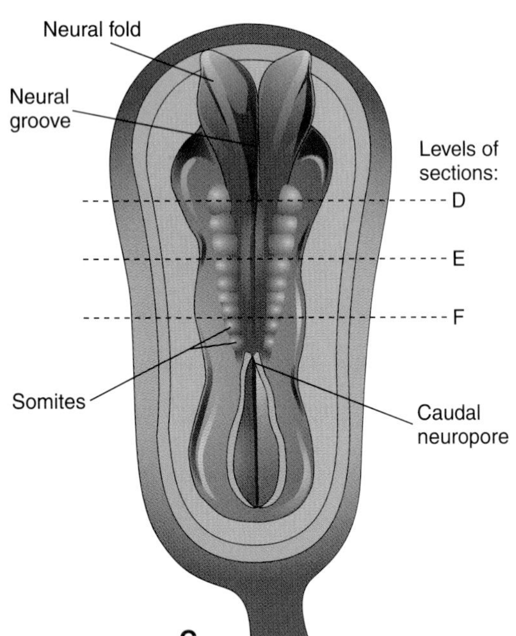

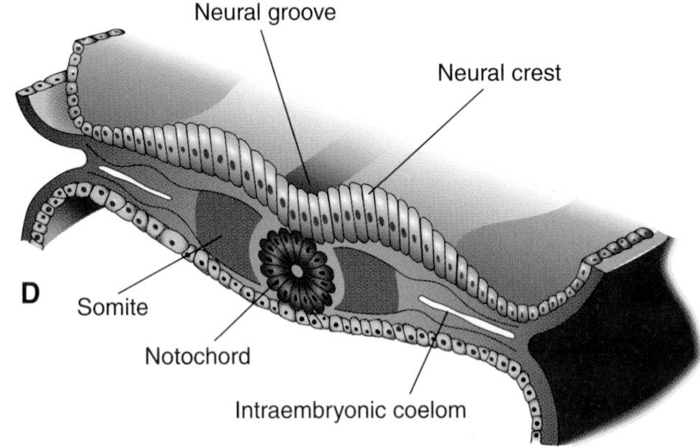

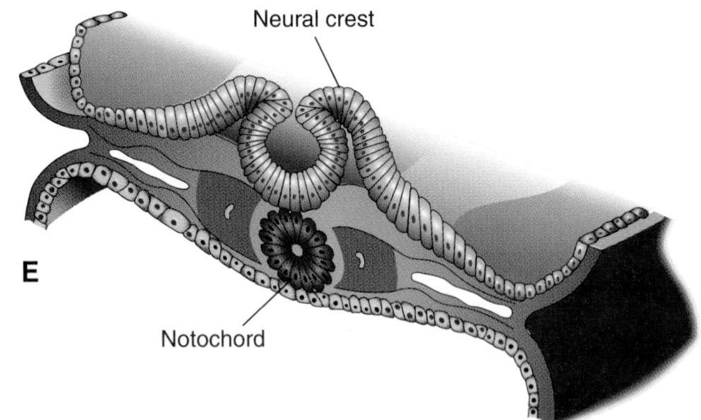

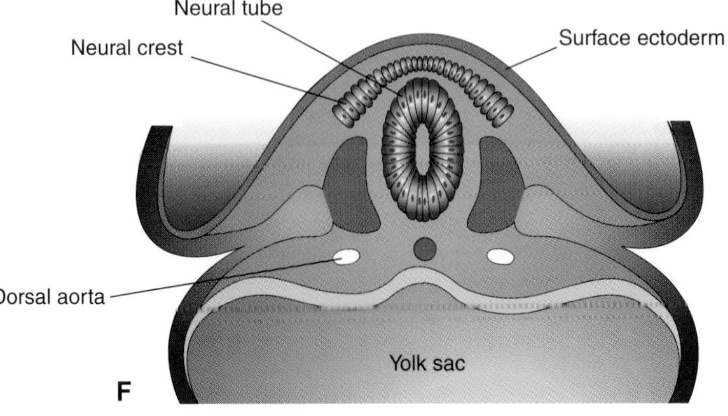

■ **Figure 18–1.** Diagrams illustrating the neural plate and folding of it into the neural tube. *A,* Dorsal view of an embryo of about 18 days, exposed by removing the amnion. *B,* Transverse section of the embryo showing the neural plate and early development of the neural groove. The developing notochord is also shown. *C,* Dorsal view of an embryo of about 22 days. The neural folds have fused opposite the fourth to sixth somites but are widely spread apart at both ends. *D* to *F,* Transverse sections of this embryo at the levels shown in *C,* illustrating formation of the neural tube and its detachment from the surface ectoderm. Note that some neuroectodermal cells are not included in the neural tube but remain between it and the surface ectoderm as the neural crest.

■ The nervous system consists of three parts:

- *Central nervous system* (CNS), which includes the brain and spinal cord
- *Peripheral nervous system* (PNS), which includes neurons (nerve cells) outside the CNS and cranial and spinal nerves that connect the brain and spinal cord with peripheral structures
- *Autonomic nervous system* (ANS), which has parts in both the CNS and PNS and consists of neurons that innervate smooth muscle, cardiac muscle, or glandular epithelium, or combinations of these tissues (Haines, 1997)

ORIGIN OF THE NERVOUS SYSTEM

The nervous system develops from the **neural plate** (Fig. 18-1*A*), a thickened, slipper-shaped area of embryonic ectoderm. It is the notochord and paraxial mesoderm that induce the overlying ectoderm to differentiate into the neural plate. Signaling molecules appear to involve members of the *transforming growth factor-β* (TGF-β) family, which includes activin and *fibroblast growth factors* (FGFs). Formation of the neural folds, neural tube, and neural crest from the neural plate is illustrated in Figure 18-1*B* to *F*. For detailed descriptions of the mechanisms involved in

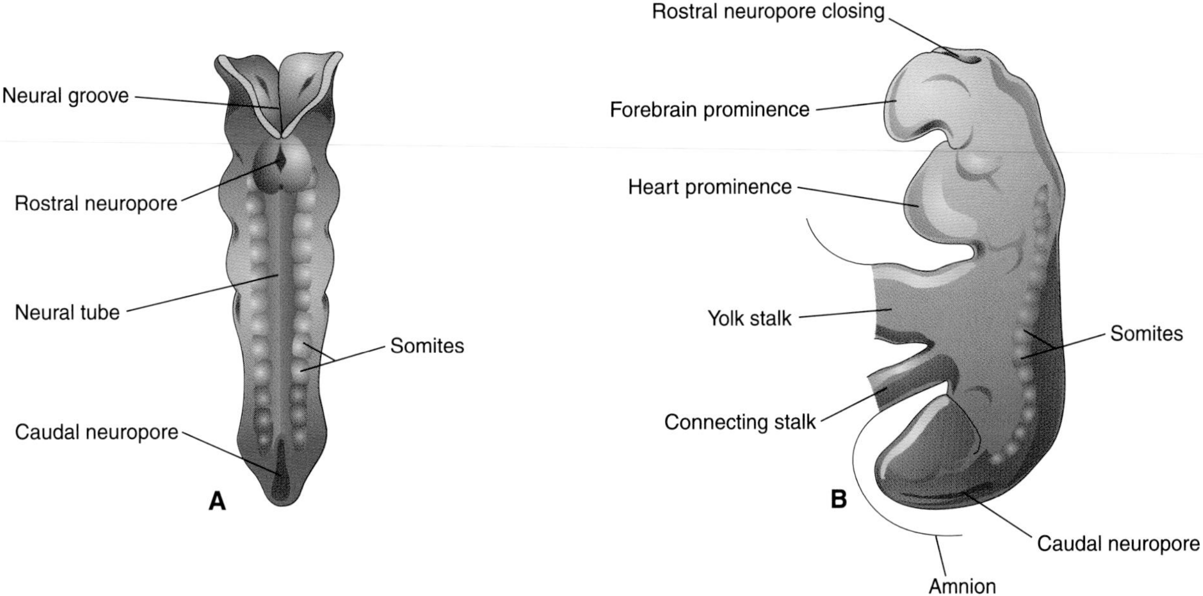

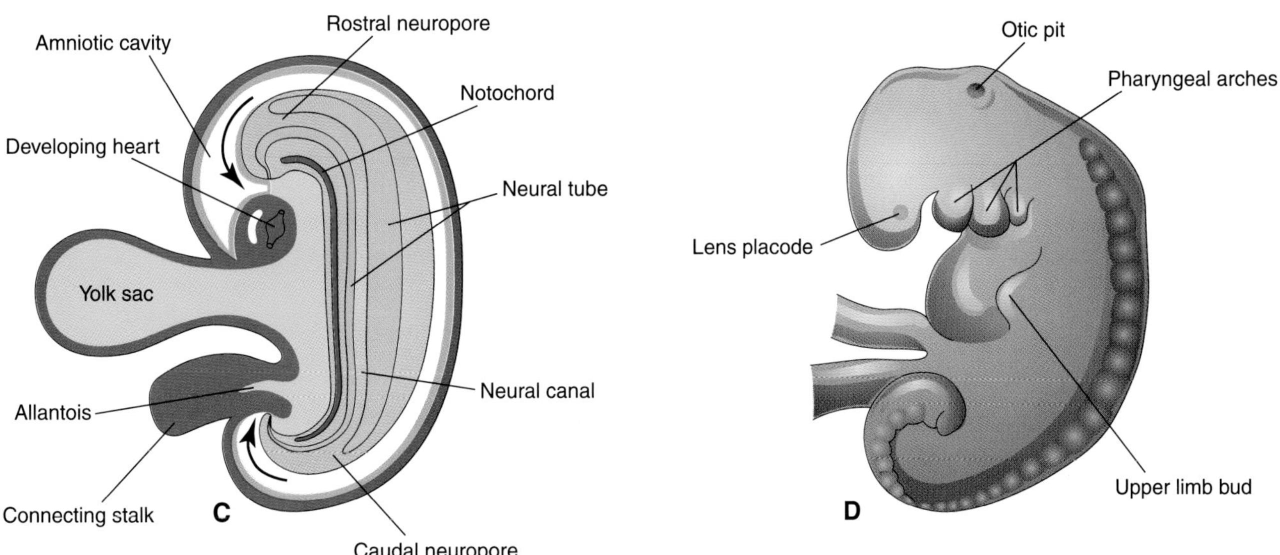

■ **Figure 18-2.** *A,* Dorsal view of an embryo of about 23 days, showing advanced fusion of the neural folds, forming the neural tube. *B,* Lateral view of an embryo of about 24 days, showing the forebrain prominence and closing of the rostral neuropore. *C,* Diagrammatic sagittal section of this embryo, showing the transitory communication of the neural canal with the amniotic cavity *(arrows)*. *D,* Lateral view of an embryo of about 27 days. Note that the neuropores shown in *B* are closed.

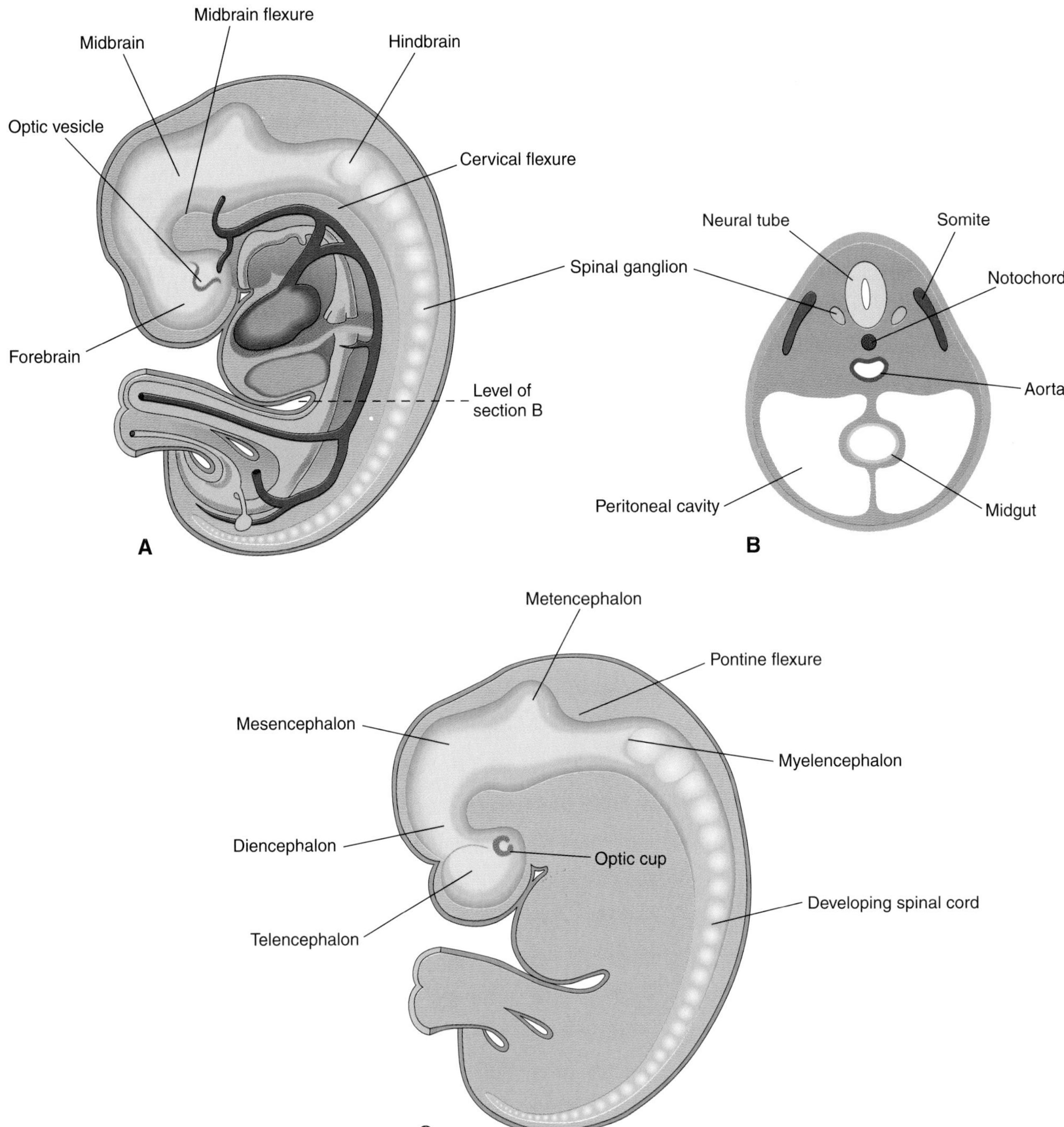

■ **Figure 18–3.** *A*, Schematic lateral view of an embryo of about 28 days, showing the three primary brain vesicles: forebrain, midbrain, and hindbrain. Two flexures demarcate the primary divisions of the brain. *B*, Transverse section of this embryo, showing the neural tube that will develop into the spinal cord in this region. The spinal (dorsal root) ganglia derived from the neural crest are also shown. *C*, Schematic lateral view of the central nervous system of a 6-week embryo, showing the secondary brain vesicles and pontine flexure. The flexure (bend) occurs as the brain grows rapidly.

neural tube formation, see Jacobson (1992), Carlson (1994), Darnell and Schoenwolf (1997), Evans and Hutchins (1997), and Sausedo et al. (1997).

- The **neural tube** differentiates into the CNS, consisting of the brain and spinal cord.
- The **neural crest** gives rise to cells that form most of the PNS and ANS, consisting of cranial, spinal, and autonomic ganglia.

Formation of the neural tube—**neurulation**—begins during the early part of the fourth week (22 to 23 days) in the region of the fourth to sixth pairs of somites. At this stage the cranial two-thirds of the neural plate and tube, as far caudal as the fourth pair of somites, represent the future brain, and the caudal one-third of the neural plate and tube represents the future spinal cord. Fusion of the neural folds proceeds in cranial and caudal directions until only small areas remain open at both ends (Fig. 18-2*A* and *B*). Here the lumen of the neural tube—**neural canal**—commu-

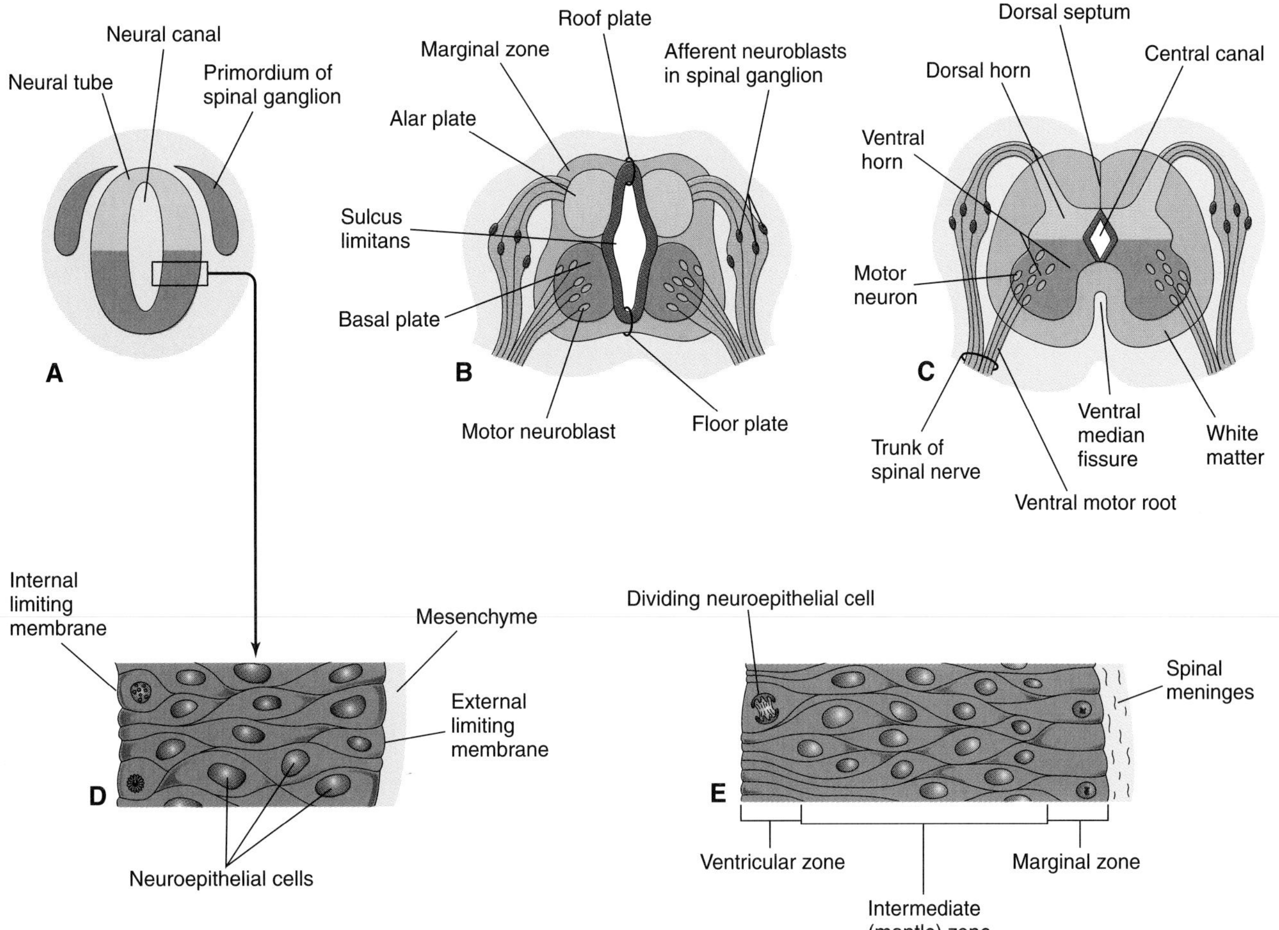

■ **Figure 18–4.** Diagrams illustrating development of the spinal cord. *A*, Transverse section of the neural tube of an embryo of about 23 days. *B* and *C*, Similar sections at 6 and 9 weeks, respectively. *D*, Section of the wall of the neural tube shown in *A*. *E*, Section of the wall of the developing spinal cord, showing its three zones. In *A* to *C*, note that the neural canal of the neural tube is converted into the central canal of the spinal cord.

nicates freely with the amniotic cavity (Fig. 18–2*C*). The cranial opening, the **rostral (anterior) neuropore,** closes on about the twenty-fifth day, and the **caudal (posterior) neuropore** 2 days later (Fig. 18–2*D*). Closure of the neuropores coincides with the establishment of a blood vascular circulation for the neural tube. The walls of the neural tube thicken to form the brain and the spinal cord (Fig. 18–3). The neural canal of the neural tube is converted into the *ventricular system* of the brain and the *central canal* of the spinal cord.

Nonfusion of the Neural Tube

Observations from studies carried out in laboratory animals, including mice, led to the formulation of a hypothesis that there are multiple, possibly five, closure sites involved in the formation of the neural tube in humans. Failure of closure of site 1 results in spina bifida cystica; meroanencephaly or anencephaly from failure of closure of site 2; craniorachischisis results from failure of sites 2, 4, and 1 to close; and site 3 nonfusion is rare. Descriptions of these severe CNS anomalies will be given later. It has been suggested that the most caudal region may have a fifth closure site from the second lumbar vertebra to the second sacral vertebra, and that closure inferior to the second sacral vertebra is by secondary neurulation (Van Allen et al., 1993). Epidemiological analysis of infants born with neural tube defects (NTDs) supports the concept that there is multisite closure of the neural tube in humans (Martinez-Frias et al., 1996).

DEVELOPMENT OF THE SPINAL CORD

The neural tube caudal to the fourth pair of somites develops into the spinal cord (Figs. 18–3 and 18–4). The lateral walls of the neural tube thicken, gradually reducing the size of the neural canal until only a minute **central canal** of the spinal cord is present at 9 to 10 weeks (Fig. 18–4*C*). Initially the wall of the neural tube is composed of a thick, pseudostratified, columnar neuroepithelium (Fig. 18–4*D*). These neuroepithelial cells constitute the **ventricular zone** (ependymal layer), which gives rise to all neurons and macroglial cells (macroglia) in the spinal cord (Fig. 18–5).

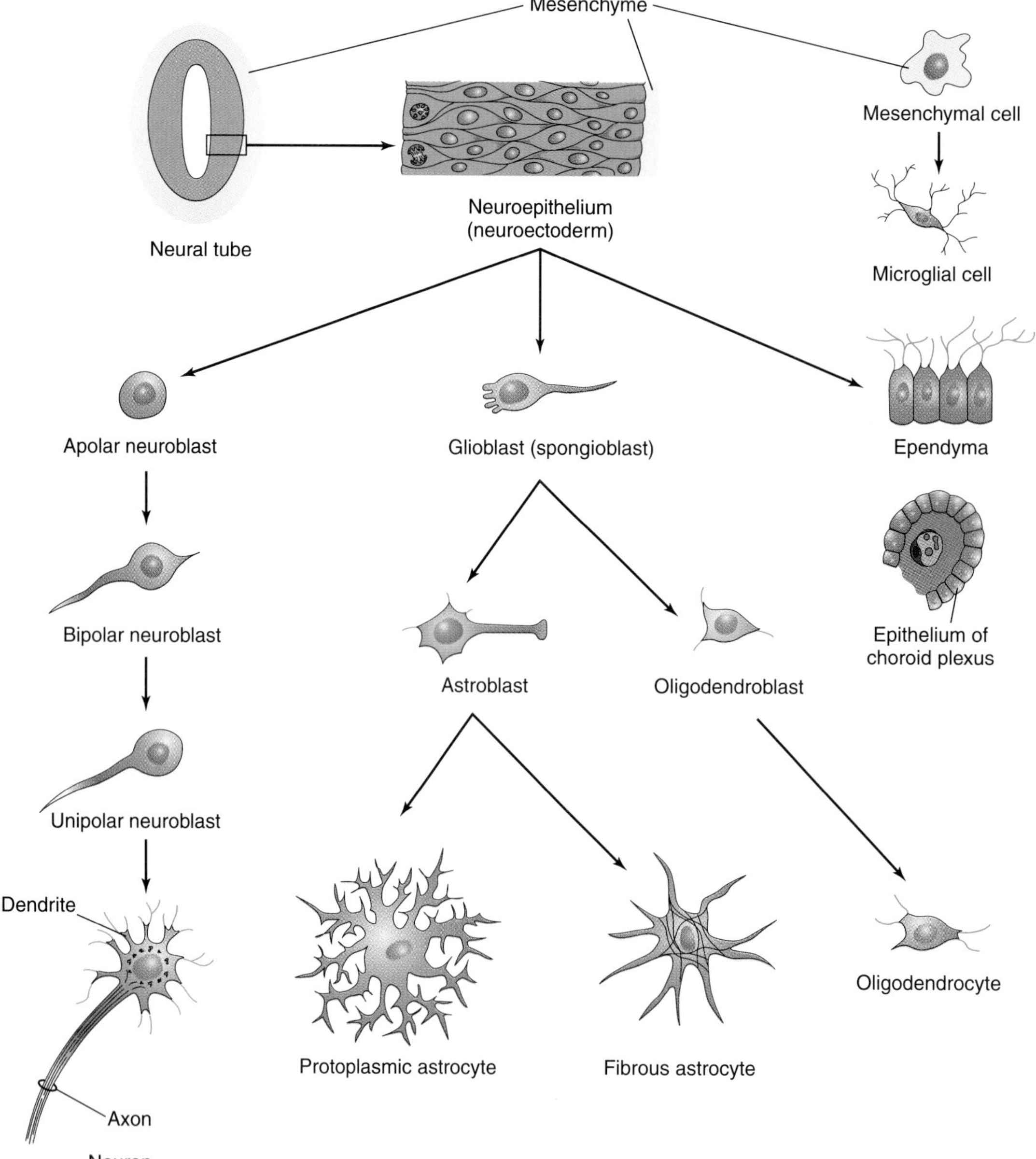

■ **Figure 18–5.** Schematic diagrams illustrating histogenesis of cells in the central nervous system. After further development the multipolar neuroblast *(lower left)* becomes a nerve cell or neuron. Neuroepithelial cells give rise to all neurons and macroglial cells. Microglial cells are derived from mesenchymal cells that invade the developing nervous system with the blood vessels.

Macroglial cells are the larger types of neuroglial cells (e.g., astrocytes and oligodendrocytes). Soon a **marginal zone** composed of the outer parts of the neuroepithelial cells becomes recognizable (Fig. 18-4*E*). This zone gradually becomes the *white matter of the spinal cord* as axons grow into it from nerve cell bodies in the spinal cord, spinal ganglia, and brain. Some dividing neuroepithelial cells in the ventricular zone differentiate into primordial neurons—**neuroblasts.** These embryonic cells form an **intermediate zone** (mantle layer) between the ventricular and marginal zones. Neuroblasts become neurons as they develop cytoplasmic processes (Fig. 18-5).

The primordial supporting cells of the central nervous system—**glioblasts** (spongioblasts)—differentiate from neuroepithelial cells, mainly after neuroblast formation has ceased. The glioblasts migrate from the ventricular zone into the intermediate and marginal zones. Some glioblasts become **astroblasts** and later *astrocytes,* whereas others become **oligodendroblasts** and eventually *oligodendrocytes* (Fig. 18-5). When the neuroepithelial cells cease producing neuroblasts and glioblasts, they differentiate into ependymal cells, which form the **ependyma** (ependymal epithelium) lining the central canal of the spinal cord.

Microglial cells (microglia), which are scattered throughout the gray and white matter, are small cells that are derived from *mesenchymal cells* (Fig. 18-5); however, the origin of microglia is controversial. Microglial cells invade the central nervous system rather late in the fetal period after it has been penetrated by blood vessels. The current view is that microglia develop from blood cells of the monocyte-macrophage lineage, which enter the CNS with the blood vessels (Hutchins et al., 1997).

Proliferation and differentiation of neuroepithelial cells in the developing spinal cord produce thick walls and thin roof and floor plates (Fig. 18-4*B*). Differential thickening of the lateral walls of the spinal cord soon produces a shallow longitudinal groove on each side—the **sulcus limitans** (Figs. 18-4*B* and 18-6). This groove separates the dorsal part, the **alar plate** (lamina) from the ventral part, the **basal plate** (lamina). The alar and basal plates produce longitudinal bulges extending through most of the length of the developing spinal cord. This regional separation is of fundamental importance because the alar and basal plates are later associated with afferent and efferent functions, respectively.

Cell bodies in the alar plates form the dorsal gray columns that extend the length of the spinal cord. In transverse sections of the cord, these columns are the **dorsal (gray) horns** (Fig. 18-7). Neurons in these columns constitute afferent nuclei, and groups of these nuclei form the **dorsal gray columns.** As the alar plates enlarge, the *dorsal septum* or raphe forms (Parkinson and Del Bigio, 1996). Cell bodies in the basal plates form the ventral and lateral gray columns. In transverse sections of the spinal cord these columns are the **ventral (gray) horns** and **lateral (gray) horns,** respectively. Axons of ventral horn cells grow out of the spinal cord and form the **ventral roots of the spinal nerves** (Fig. 18-7). As the basal plates enlarge, they bulge ventrally on each side of the median plane. As this occurs, the *ventral median septum* forms, and a deep longitudinal groove—the **ventral median fissure**—develops on the ventral surface of the spinal cord.

Development of Spinal Ganglia

The unipolar neurons in the spinal ganglia (dorsal root ganglia) are derived from **neural crest cells** (Figs. 18-8 and 18-9). The axons of cells in the spinal ganglia are at first bipolar but the two processes soon unite in a T-shaped fashion. Both processes of spinal ganglion cells have the structural characteristics of axons, but the peripheral process is a dendrite in that

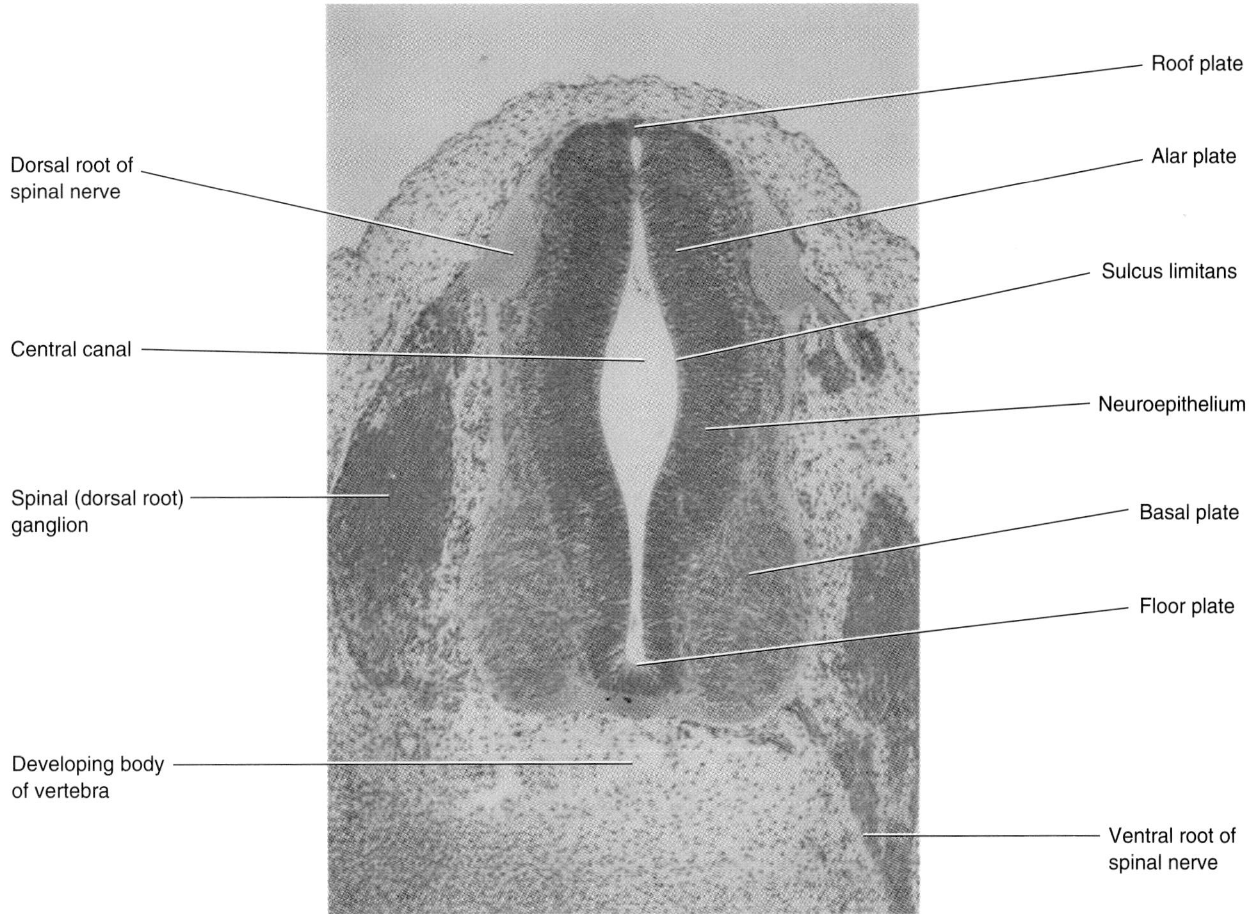

■ **Figure 18-6.** Transverse section of an embryo (×100) at Carnegie stage 16, about 40 days. The ventral root of the spinal nerve is composed of nerve fibers arising from neuroblasts in the basal plate (developing ventral horn of spinal cord), whereas the dorsal root is formed by nerve processes arising from neuroblasts in the spinal (dorsal root) ganglion. (From Moore KL, Persaud TVN, Shiota K: *Color Atlas of Clinical Embryology.* Philadelphia, WB Saunders, 1994.)

Dorsal septum
Central canal
Dorsal nerve root
Ventricular zone
Ventral median septum
Ventral median fissure
Dorsal (gray) horn
Intermediate zone
Marginal zone
Ventral (gray) horn
Spinal ganglion
Developing centrum

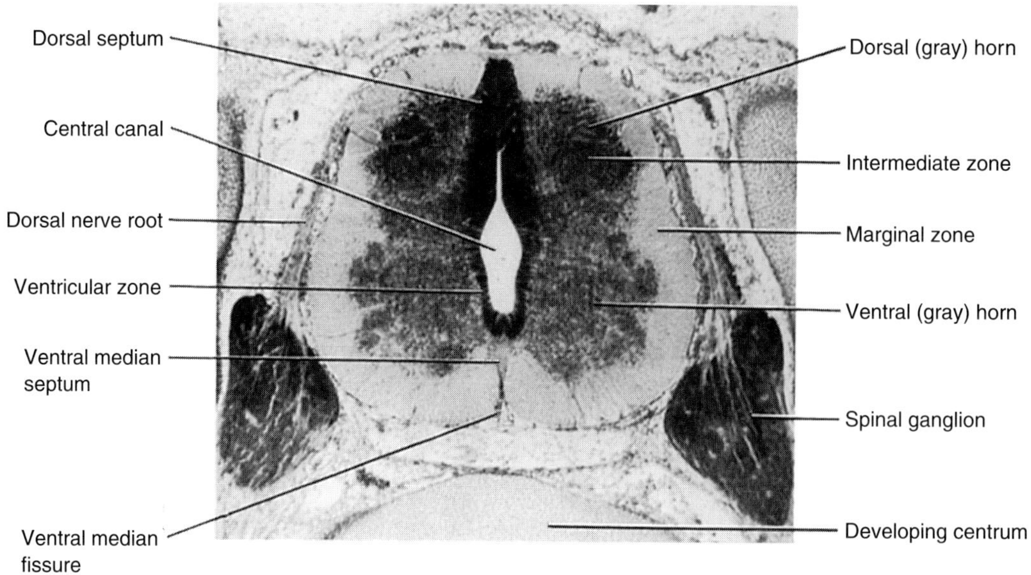

■ **Figure 18–7.** Photomicrograph of a transverse section of the developing spinal cord in a 20-mm human embryo of about 50 days (× 60). (Courtesy of Professor Jean Hay [retired], Department of Anatomy, University of Manitoba, Winnipeg, Canada.)

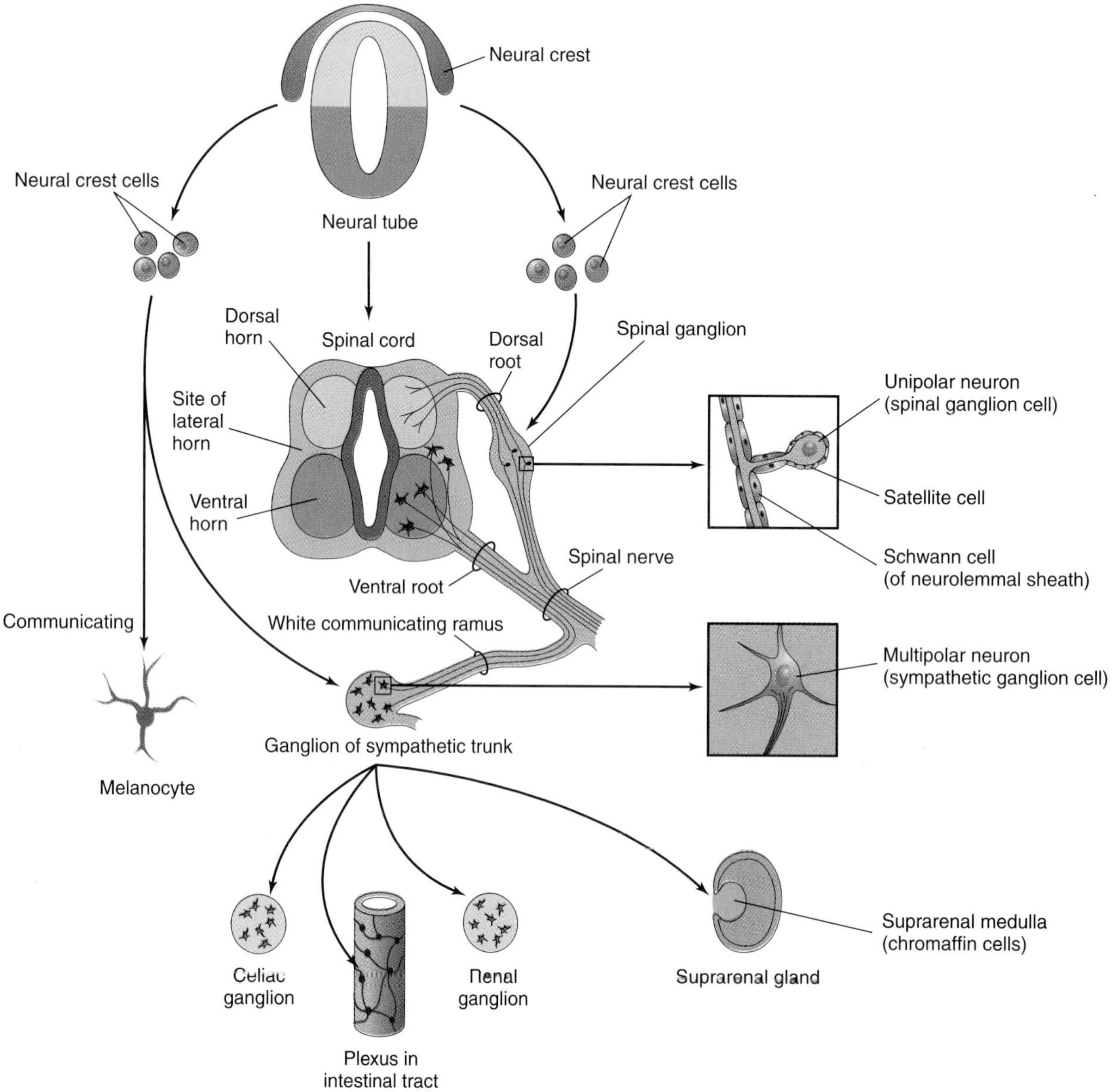

Neural crest
Neural crest cells
Neural tube
Neural crest cells
Dorsal horn
Spinal cord
Dorsal root
Spinal ganglion
Site of lateral horn
Ventral horn
Unipolar neuron (spinal ganglion cell)
Satellite cell
Schwann cell (of neurolemmal sheath)
Spinal nerve
Ventral root
Communicating
White communicating ramus
Multipolar neuron (sympathetic ganglion cell)
Ganglion of sympathetic trunk
Melanocyte
Suprarenal medulla (chromaffin cells)
Celiac ganglion
Renal ganglion
Suprarenal gland
Plexus in intestinal tract

■ **Figure 18–8.** Diagrams showing some derivatives of the neural crest. Neural crest cells also differentiate into the cells in the afferent ganglia of cranial nerves and many other structures (see Chapter 5). The formation of a spinal nerve is also illustrated.

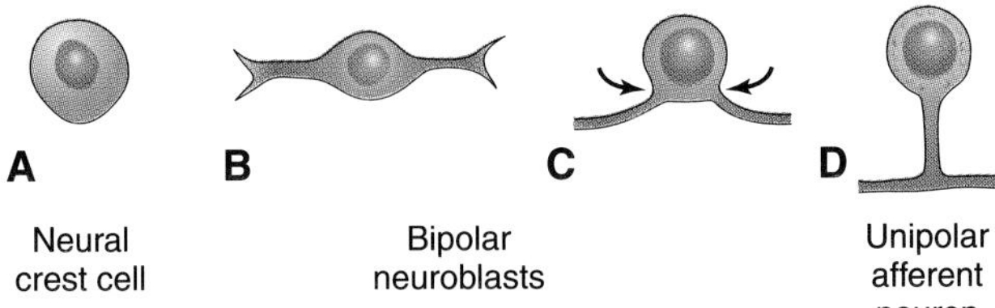

■ **Figure 18-9.** *A-D,* Diagrams illustrating successive stages in the differentiation of a neural crest cell into a unipolar afferent neuron in a spinal ganglion.

there is conduction toward the cell body. The peripheral processes of spinal ganglion cells pass in the spinal nerves to sensory endings in somatic or visceral structures (Fig. 18-8). The central processes enter the spinal cord and constitute the *dorsal roots of the spinal nerves.*

Development of Spinal Meninges

The mesenchyme surrounding the neural tube condenses to form a membrane called the *primordial meninx* (membrane). The external layer of this membrane thickens to form the **dura mater** (Fig. 18-10). The internal layer remains thin and forms the pia-arachnoid, composed of **pia mater** and **arachnoid mater;** together these layers form the leptomeninges. **Neural crest cells** mingle with the mesenchyme, forming the **leptomeninges,** and appear to be involved in the function of the pia mater. Fluid-filled spaces appear within the leptomeninges that soon coalesce to form the **subarachnoid space.** The origin of the pia mater and arachnoid from a single layer is indicated in the adult by the **arachnoid trabeculae**—numerous delicate strands of connective tissue that pass between the pia and arachnoid (Moore, 1992). Embryonic **cerebrospinal fluid** (CSF) begins to form during the fifth week.

Positional Changes of Spinal Cord

The spinal cord in the embryo extends the entire length of the vertebral canal (Fig. 18-10*A*). The spinal nerves pass through the intervertebral foramina near their levels of origin. Because the vertebral column and dura mater grow more rapidly than the spinal cord, this relationship does not persist. The caudal end of the spinal cord gradually comes to lie at relatively higher levels. At 6 months it lies at the level of the first sacral vertebra (Fig. 18-10*B*). The spinal cord in the newborn terminates at the level of the second or third lumbar vertebra (Fig. 18-10*C*). The spinal cord in the adult usually terminates at the inferior border of the first lumbar vertebra (Fig. 18-10*D*). This is an average level because the caudal end of the spinal cord may be as superior as the twelfth thoracic vertebra or as inferior as the third lumbar vertebra (Moore, 1992). As a result the spinal nerve roots, especially those of the lumbar and sacral segments, run obliquely from the spinal cord to the corresponding level of the vertebral column. The nerve roots inferior to the end

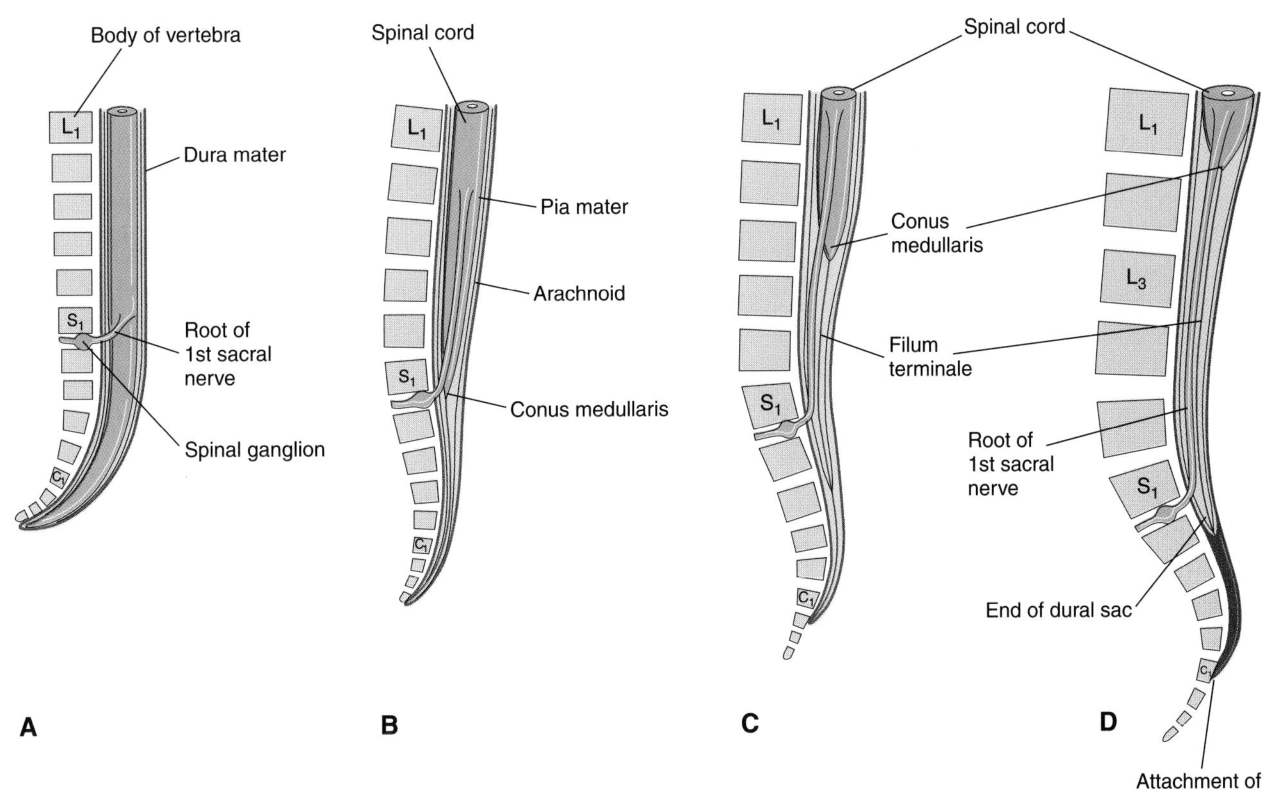

■ **Figure 18-10.** Diagrams showing the position of the caudal end of the spinal cord in relation to the vertebral column and meninges at various stages of development. The increasing inclination of the root of the first sacral nerve is also illustrated. *A,* 8 weeks. *B,* 24 weeks. *C,* Newborn. *D,* Adult.

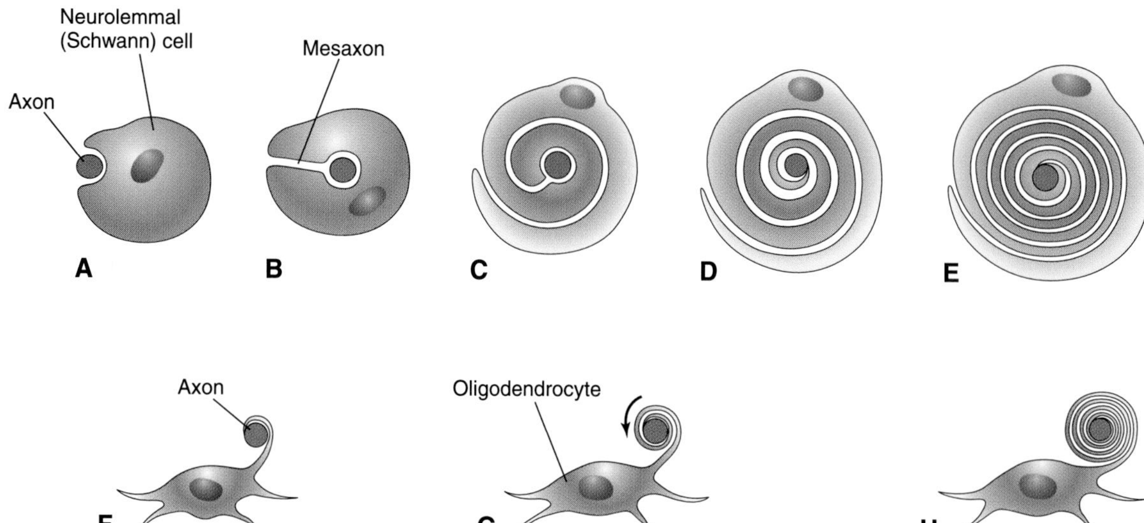

■ **Figure 18–11.** Diagrammatic sketches illustrating myelination of nerve fibers. *A* to *E*, Successive stages in the myelination of an axon of a peripheral nerve fiber by a neurolemmal or Schwann cell. The axon first indents the cell; the Schwann cell then rotates around the axon as the mesaxon (site of invagination) elongates. The cytoplasm between the layers of cell membrane gradually condenses. Cytoplasm remains on the inside of the sheath between the myelin and axon. *F* to *H*, Successive stages in the myelination of a nerve fiber in the CNS by an oligodendrocyte. A process of the neuroglial cell wraps itself around an axon, and the intervening layers of cytoplasm move to the body of the cell.

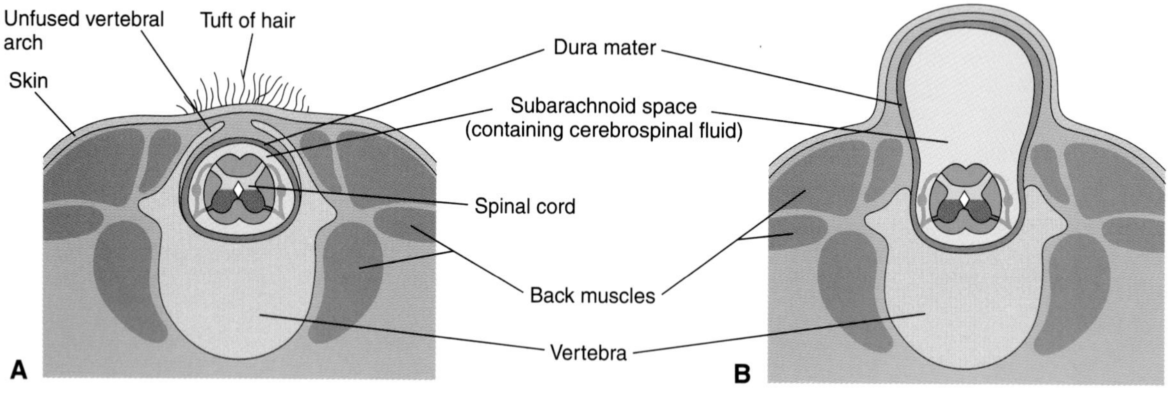

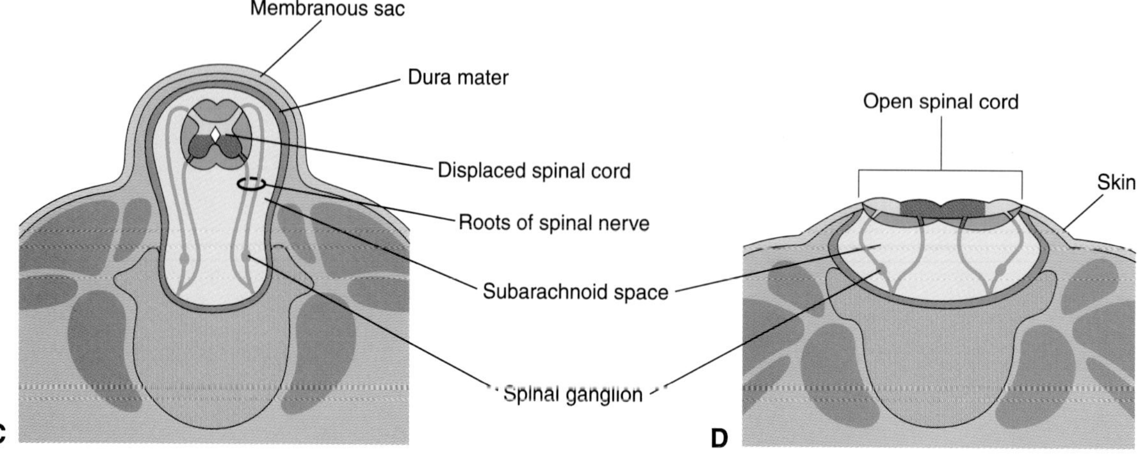

■ **Figure 18–12.** Diagrammatic sketches illustrating various types of spina bifida and the commonly associated anomalies of the vertebral arch, spinal cord, and meninges. *A*, Spina bifida occulta. Observe the unfused vertebral arch. *B*, Spina bifida with meningocele. *C*, Spina bifida with meningomyelocele. *D*, Spina bifida with myeloschisis. The types illustrated in *B* to *D* are referred to collectively as spina bifida cystica because of the cystlike sac that is associated with them.

of the cord—the **conus medullaris**—form a sheaf of nerve roots, the **cauda equina** (L., horse's tail). Although the dura mater and arachnoid mater usually end at S2 vertebra in adults, the pia mater does not. Distal to the caudal end of the spinal cord, the pia mater forms a long fibrous thread, the **filum terminale** (Fig. 18-10*C* and *D*), which indicates the line of regression of the caudal end of the embryonic spinal cord. This thread extends from the conus medullaris and attaches to the periosteum of the first coccygeal vertebra.

Myelination of Nerve Fibers

Myelin sheaths in the spinal cord begin to form during the late fetal period and continue to form during the first postnatal year. Myelin basic proteins, a family of related polypeptide isoforms, are essential in myelination (Staugaitis et al., 1996). In general, fiber tracts become myelinated at about the time they become functional. The **myelin sheaths** surrounding nerve fibers within the spinal cord are formed by **oligodendrocytes.** The plasma membranes of these cells wrap around the axon, forming a number of layers (Fig. 18-11*F* to *H*). The myelin sheaths around the axons of peripheral nerve fibers are formed by the plasma membranes of **neurolemmal (Schwann) cells,** which are analogous to oligodendrocytes (Hutchins et al., 1997). These neuroglial cells are derived from **neural crest cells** that migrate peripherally and wrap themselves around the axons of somatic motor neurons and preganglionic autonomic motor neurons as they pass out of the central nervous system (Figs. 18-8 and 18-11*A* to *E*). These cells also wrap themselves around both the central and peripheral processes of somatic and visceral sensory neurons, as well as around the axons of postganglionic autonomic motor neurons. For more details of this process, see Barr and Kiernan (1993) and Hutchins et al. (1997). Beginning at about 20 weeks, peripheral nerve fibers have a whitish appearance, resulting from the deposition of myelin. Motor roots are myelinated before sensory roots.

CONGENITAL ANOMALIES OF THE SPINAL CORD

Most congenital anomalies of the spinal cord result from defective closure of the neural tube during the fourth week of development. These **neural tube defects** (NTDs) affect the tissues overlying the spinal cord: meninges, vertebral arches, muscles, and skin (Fig. 18-12*B* to *D*). Anomalies involving the vertebral arches are referred to as **spina bifida.** This term denotes *nonfusion of the embryonic halves of the vertebral arches,* which is common to all types of spina bifida. (For information on the level of the lesion and other associated congenital defects, see Hunter et al. [1996].) Severe anomalies also involve the spinal cord and meninges. Spina bifida ranges from clinically significant types to minor anomalies that are unimportant.

Spina Bifida Occulta

This *defect in the vertebral arch* (neural arch) is the result of failure of the embryonic halves of the arch to grow normally and fuse in the median plane (Fig. 18-12*A*). Spina bifida occulta occurs in L5 or S1 vertebrae in about 10% of otherwise normal people (Moore, 1992). In its most minor form, the only evidence of its presence may be a small dimple with a tuft of hair arising from it (Fig. 18-13). Spina bifida occulta usually produces no clinical symptoms. A small percentage of affected infants have functionally significant defects of the underlying spinal cord and dorsal roots (Behrman et al., 1996).

Spinal Dermal Sinus

A posterior skin dimple in the median plane of the sacral region of the back may be associated with a spinal dermal sinus (Fig. 18-14*A*). The dimple indi-

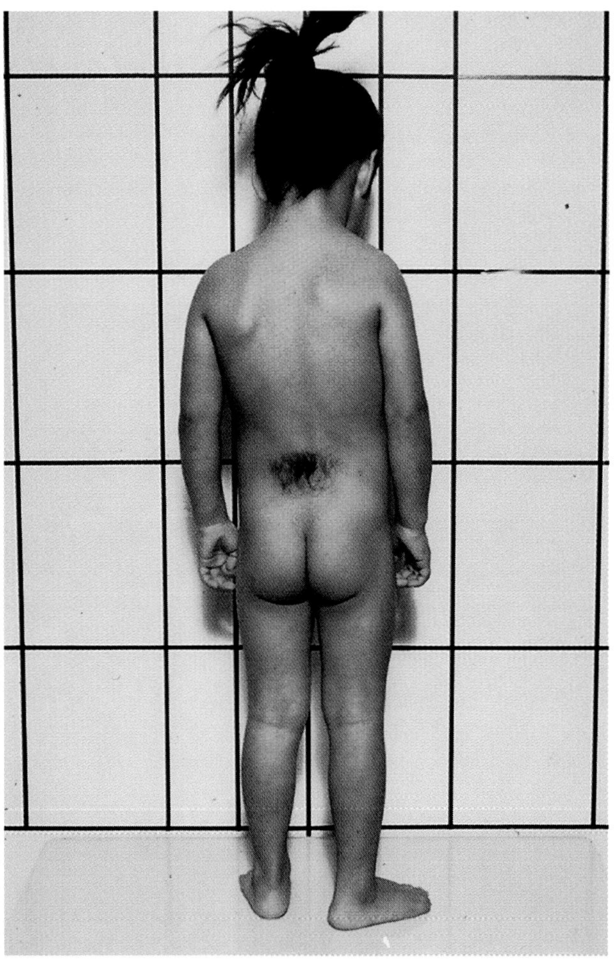

■ **Figure 18-13.** Photograph of a female child with a hairy patch in the lumbosacral region, indicating the site of a spina bifida occulta. (Courtesy of Dr. A. E. Chudley, Section of Genetics and Metabolism, Department of Pediatrics and Child Health, Children's Hospital and University of Manitoba, Winnipeg, Manitoba, Canada.)

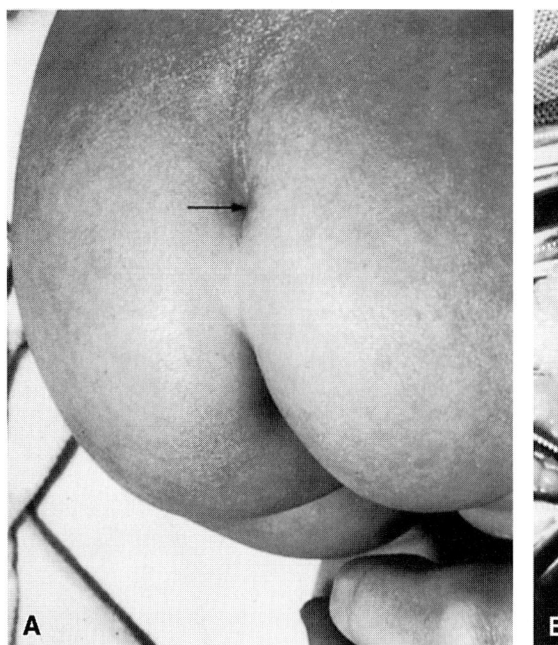

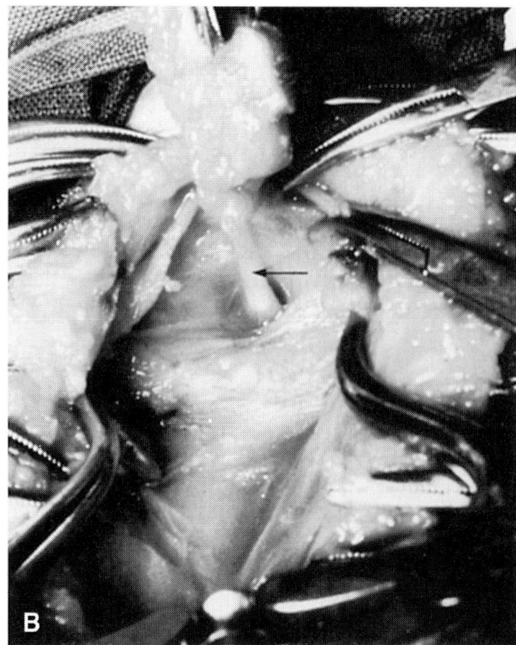

■ **Figure 18–14.** *A*, Photograph of a skin dimple in the sacral region. The opening of a spinal dermal sinus in the dimple is indicated by an arrow. *B*, Photograph taken during removal of this sinus showing a cord *(arrow)* connecting the dimple to the spinal dura mater. (Courtesy of Dr. Dwight Parkinson, Department of Surgery and Department of Human Anatomy and Cell Science, University of Manitoba, Winnipeg, Canada.)

cates the region of closure of the caudal neuropore at the end of the fourth week; therefore, the dimple represents the last place of separation between the surface ectoderm and the neural tube. In some cases the dimple is connected with the dura mater by a fibrous cord (Fig. 18-14*B*).

Spina Bifida Cystica

Severe types of spina bifida, involving protrusion of the spinal cord and/or meninges through the defect in the vertebral arches, are referred to collectively as *spina bifida cystica* because of the cystlike sac that is associated with these anomalies (Figs. 18-12*B* to *D*, 18-15, and 18-16). Spina bifida cystica occurs about once in every 1000 births. When the sac contains meninges and cerebrospinal fluid, the anomaly is called **spina bifida with meningocele** (Fig. 18-12*B*). The spinal cord and spinal roots are in their normal position, but there may be spinal cord abnormalities. If the spinal cord and/or nerve roots are included in the sac, the anomaly is called **spina bifida with meningomyelocele** (Figs. 18-12*C* and 18-17). Myelo refers to the spinal cord, which used to be called the spinal medulla (Gr. *myelos*, medulla). Meningoceles are rare compared with meningomyeloceles (Filly, 1994).

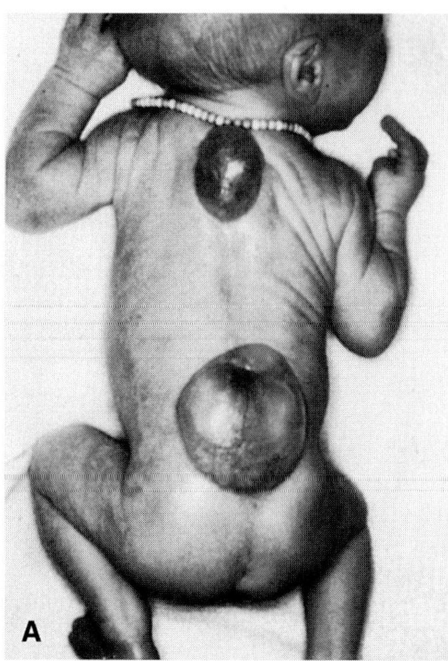

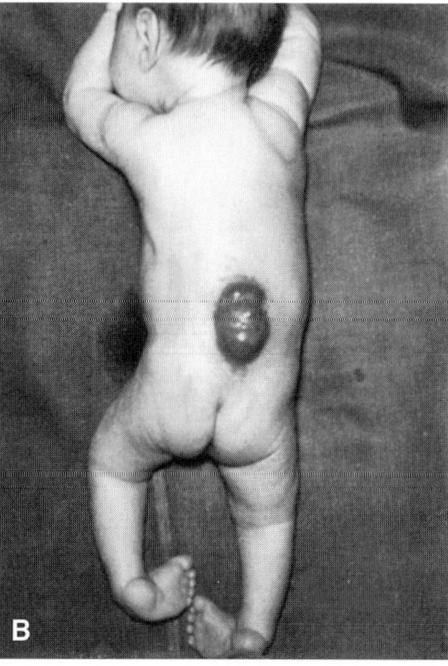

■ **Figure 18–15.** Photographs of infants with spina bifida cystica. *A*, Spina bifida with meningomyelocele in the thoracic and lumbar regions. *B*, Spina bifida with myeloschisis in the lumbar region. Note that nerve involvement has affected the lower limbs. (Courtesy of Dr. Dwight Parkinson, Department of Surgery and Department of Human Anatomy and Cell Science, University of Manitoba, Winnipeg, Canada.)

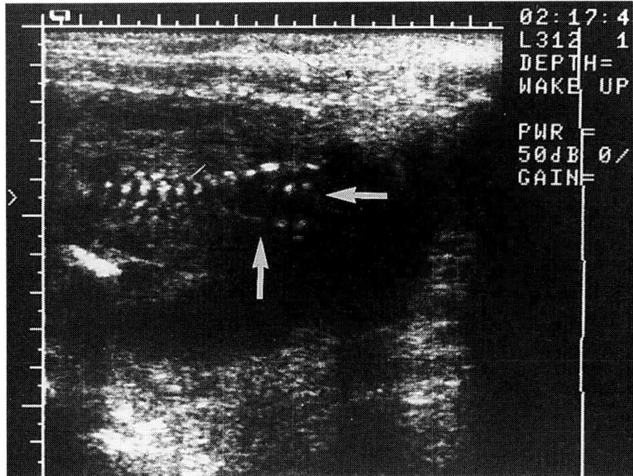

■ **Figure 18–16.** Sonogram of the back of a fetus of 18 weeks' gestation. The mother had a grossly elevated serum alpha-fetoprotein (AFP) (see Chapter 6). Observe the large spina bifida comprising the lower thoracic and entire lumbosacral region of the vertebral column (arrows). (Courtesy of Dr. C. R. Harman, Department of Obstetrics, Gynecology and Reproductive Sciences, Women's Hospital and University of Manitoba, Winnipeg, Manitoba, Canada.)

Spina bifida cystica shows considerable geographical variation in incidence. In the British Isles, for example, the incidence varies from 4.2 per 1000 newborn infants in South Wales to 1.5 per 1000 in southeastern England (Laurence and Weeks, 1971). Severe cases of spina bifida with the meningomyelocele involving several vertebrae are often associated with partial absence of the brain—**meroanencephaly** or **anencephaly** (Fig. 18–18). Spina bifida cystica shows varying degrees of neurological deficit, depending on the position and extent of the lesion. There is usually a corresponding dermatome loss of sensation, along with complete or partial skeletal muscle paralysis. The level of the lesion determines the area of anesthesia (area of skin without sensation) and the muscles affected.

Sphincter paralysis (bladder and/or anal sphincters) is common with lumbosacral meningomyeloceles (Figs. 18–15 and 18–17). There is almost invariably a *saddle anesthesia* when the sphincters are involved, that is, loss of sensation in the region that impinges on the saddle during riding.

Spina bifida cystica and/or meroanencephaly is strongly suspected in utero when there is a high level of alpha-fetoprotein (AFP) in the amniotic fluid (see Chapter 7). AFP may also be elevated in the maternal blood serum. *Amniocentesis* is usually performed on pregnant women with high levels of serum AFP for the determination of the AFP level in the amniotic fluid. An ultrasound scan reveals the presence of an NTD that has resulted in spina bifida cystica. The fetal vertebral column can be detected by ultrasound at 2 to 12 weeks' gestation (8 to 10 weeks after conception), and if present, *spina bifida cystica* is sometimes visible as a cystic mass adjacent to the affected area of the vertebral column (Fig. 18–19).

Meningomyelocele

This severe type of spinal bifida cystica is often associated with a marked *neurological deficit* inferior to the level of the protruding sac. This deficit occurs because nervous tissue is incorporated in the wall of the sac, impairing development of nerve fibers. Meningomyeloceles may be covered by skin or a thin, easily ruptured membrane (Figs. 18–15*B* and 18–17). Spina bifida with meningomyelocele is a more common and a much more severe anomaly than spina bifida with meningocele. Meningoceles and meningomyeloceles may occur anywhere along the vertebral column, but they are most common in the lumbar and sacral region (Fig. 18–19). Some cases of meningomyelocele are associated with *craniolacunia* (defective development of the calvaria). This results in depressed nonossified areas on the inner surfaces of the flat bones of the calvaria.

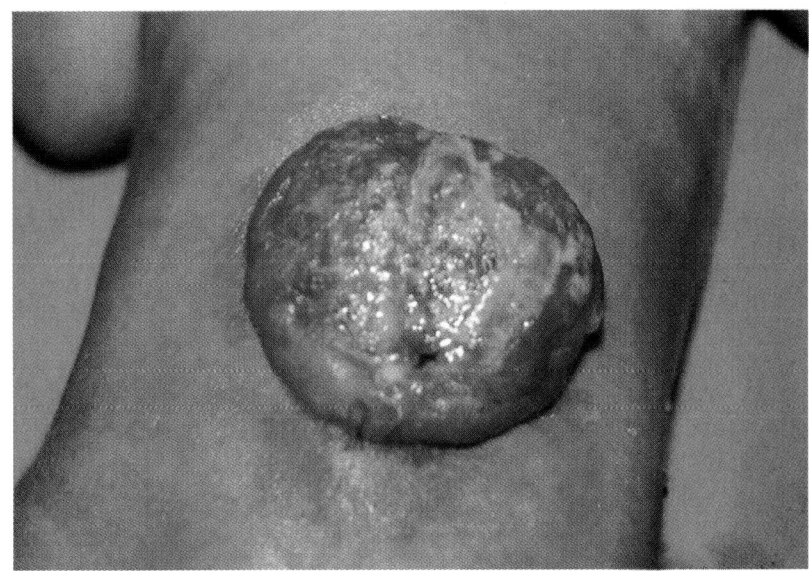

■ **Figure 18–17.** Photograph of the back of a newborn with a large lumbar meningomyelocele. The neural tube defect (NTD) is covered with a thin membrane. (Courtesy of Dr. A. E. Chudley, Section of Genetics and Metabolism, Department of Pediatrics and Child Health, Children's Hospital and University of Manitoba, Winnipeg, Manitoba, Canada.)

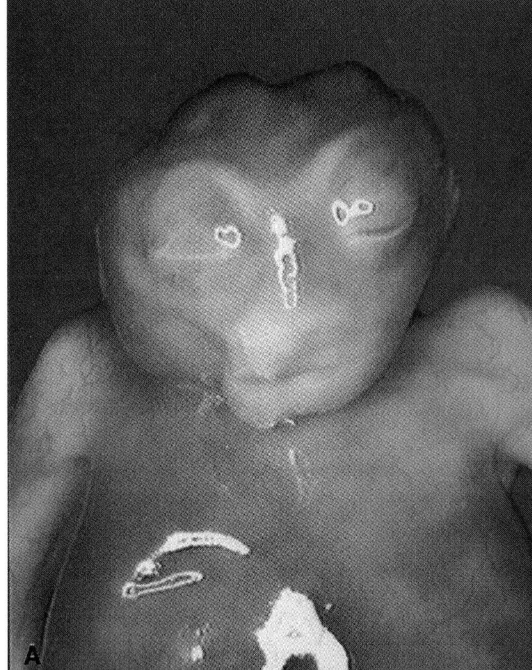

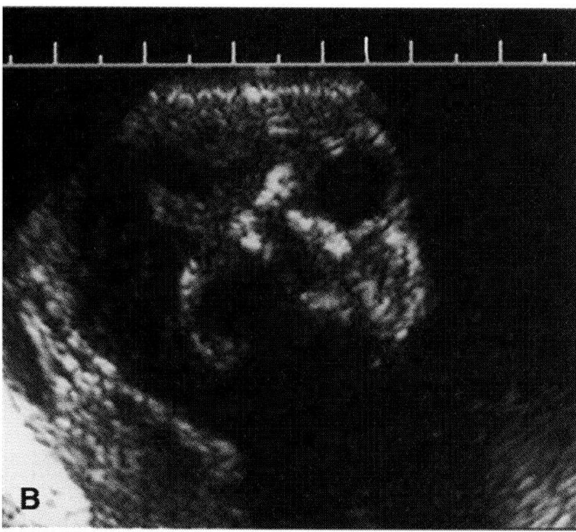

■ **Figure 18–18.** *A*, Photograph of a fetus with meroanencephaly or anencephaly. The NTD was detected by ultrasound at 18 weeks' gestation *(B)*. Note the absence of the calvaria and the large orbits. (Courtesy of Dr. Wesley Lee, Division of Fetal Imaging, Department of Obstetrics and Gynecology, William Beaumont Hospital, Royal Oak, Michigan.)

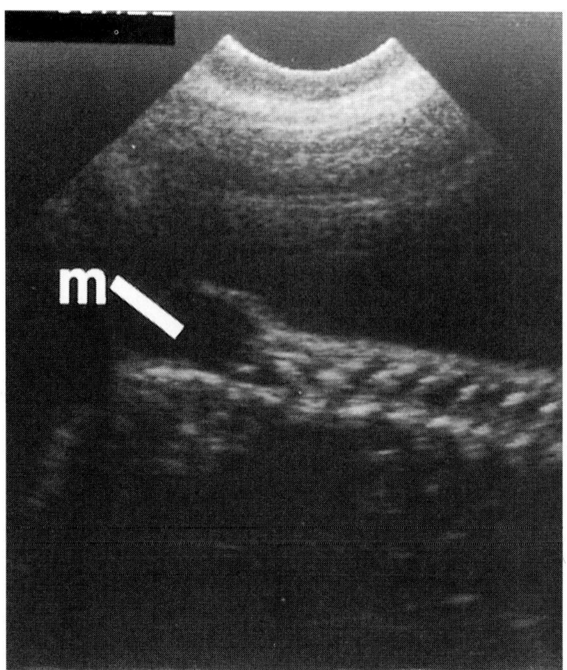

■ **Figure 18–19.** Ultrasound scan of a 14-week-old fetus showing a cystlike protrusion representing a meningomyelocele **(m)** in the sacral region of the vertebral column. The well-formed vertebral arches of the vertebrae superior to the neural tube defect are clearly visible. (Courtesy of Dr. Lyndon M. Hill, Magee-Women's Hospital, Pittsburgh, PA.)

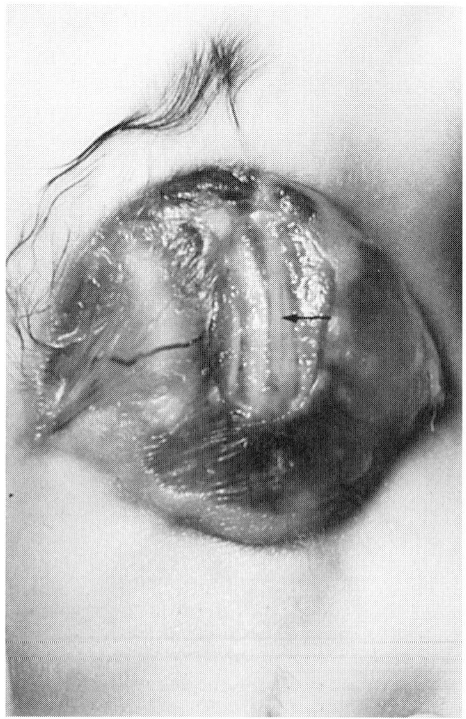

■ **Figure 18–20.** Photograph of an infant's back, exhibiting spina bifida with myeloschisis in the lumbar region. The open spinal cord *(arrow)* is covered by a delicate, semitransparent membrane. This anomaly is the result of a defect in closure of the neural tube during the fourth week (Fig. 18–12*D*). Note the tufts of hair on the surrounding skin. (From Laurence KM, Weeks R: Abnormalities of the central nervous system. *In* Norman AP [ed]: *Congenital Abnormalities in Infancy,* 2nd ed. 1971. Courtesy of Blackwell Scientific Publications.)

Myeloschisis

The most severe type of spina bifida is **spina bifida with myeloschisis** (Figs. 18-12*D* and 18-20). In these cases the spinal cord in the affected area is open because the neural folds failed to fuse (Gr. *schisis,* a cleaving). As a result the spinal cord is represented by a flattened mass of nervous tissue. Spina bifida with myeloschisis may result from an NTD that is caused by a local overgrowth of the neural plate (Fig. 18-21). As a result the caudal neuropore fails to close at the end of the fourth week.

Etiology of Neural Tube Defects

Nutritional and environmental factors undoubtedly play a role in the production of NTDs. Studies have shown that vitamins and folic acid supplements taken prior to conception reduce the incidence of NTDs (Van Allen et al., 1993; Forman et al., 1995; Murphy et al., 1996). Certain drugs increase the risk of meningomyelocele (e.g., valproic acid). This anticonvulsant causes NTDs in 1 to 2% of pregnancies if given during early pregnancy (fourth week of development) when the neural folds are fusing (Fig. 18-22). Pregnant animals exposed to hypothermia or high levels of vitamin A produce offspring with NTDs (Behrman et al., 1996). Studies have also suggested that NTDs might result from specific biochemical abnormalities of the basement membrane, particularly hyaluronate, which plays a role in cell division and the shape of the primordial neuroepithelium (Copp and Bernfield, 1988).

DEVELOPMENT OF THE BRAIN

The neural tube cranial to the fourth pair of somites develops into the brain. Fusion of the neural folds in the cranial region and closure of the rostral neuropore form **three primary brain vesicles** from which the brain develops (Fig. 18-23). The three primary brain vesicles form the:

- *forebrain* (prosencephalon)
- *midbrain* (mesencephalon)
- *hindbrain* (rhombencephalon)

During the fifth week the forebrain partly divides into two secondary vesicles, the *telencephalon* and *diencephalon;* the midbrain does not divide; the hindbrain partly divides into the *metencephalon* and *myelencephalon;* consequently, there are **five secondary brain vesicles.**

Brain Flexures

During the fourth week the embryonic brain grows rapidly and bends ventrally with the head fold. This produces the **midbrain flexure** in the midbrain region and the **cervical flexure** at the junction of the hindbrain and spinal cord (Fig. 18-24). Later, unequal growth of the brain between these flexures produces the **pontine flexure** in the opposite direction. This flexure results in thinning of the roof of the hindbrain. Initially the primordial brain has the same basic structure as the developing spinal cord; however, the brain flexures produce considerable variation in the outline of transverse sections at different levels of the brain, and in the position of the gray and white matter. The **sulcus limitans** extends cranially to the junction of the midbrain and forebrain, and the alar and basal plates are recognizable only in the midbrain and hindbrain.

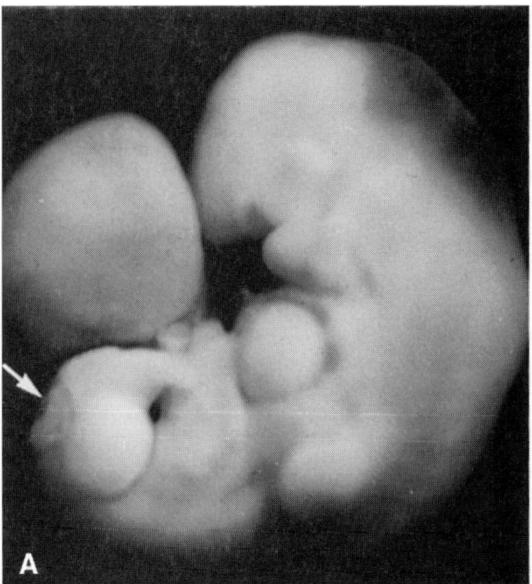

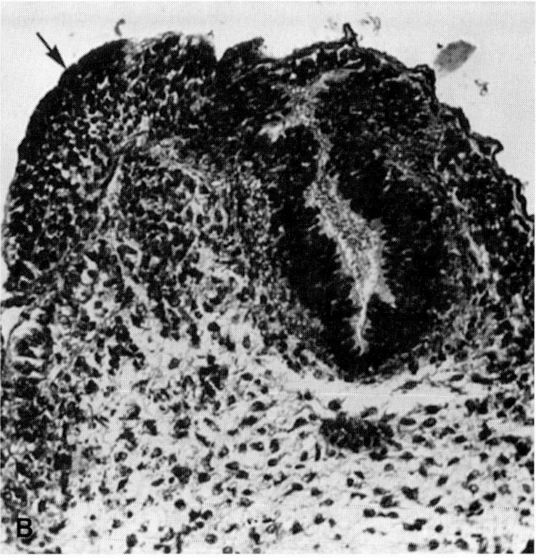

■ **Figure 18-21.** *A,* Photograph of a human embryo of about 30 days. The white arrow indicates the site of the NTD resulting from failure of closure of the caudal neuropore. Normally this neuropore is closed by day 28. *B,* Photomicrograph of a transverse section through the NTD. The black arrow indicates an abnormal fold of neural tissue extending over the left side of the embryo. It appears that this overgrown neural fold has prevented closure of the neural tube. (From Lemire RJ, Shepard TH, Alvord Jr EJ: *Anat Rec 152:*9, 1965.)

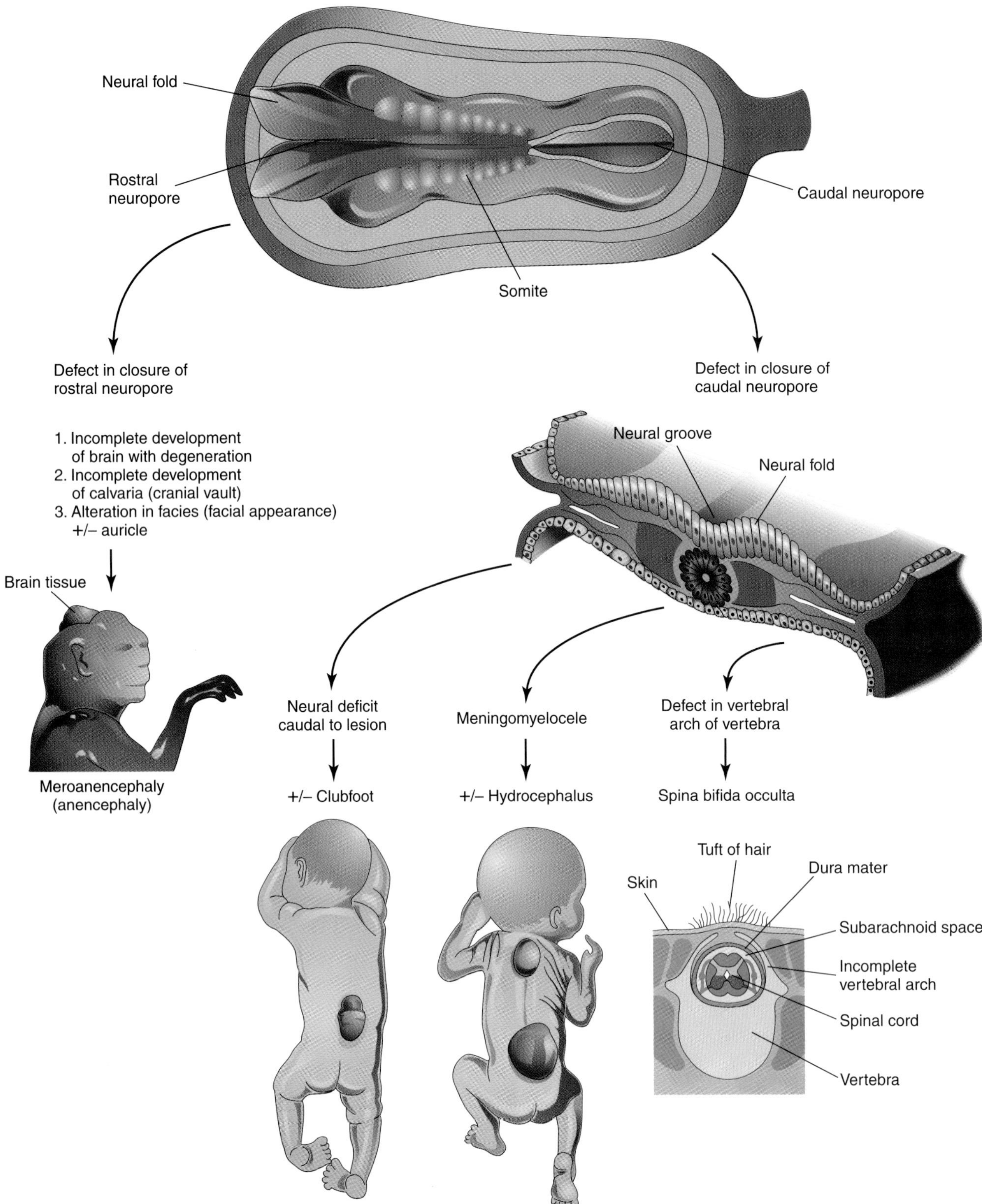

■ **Figure 18–22.** Schematic illustrations explaining the embryological basis of NTDs. Meroanencephaly—partial absence of the brain—results from defective closure of the rostral neuropore, and meningomyelocele results from defective closure of the caudal neuropore. (Modified from Jones KL: *Smith's Recognizable Patterns of Human Malformations,* ed 4. Philadelphia, WB Saunders, 1988.)

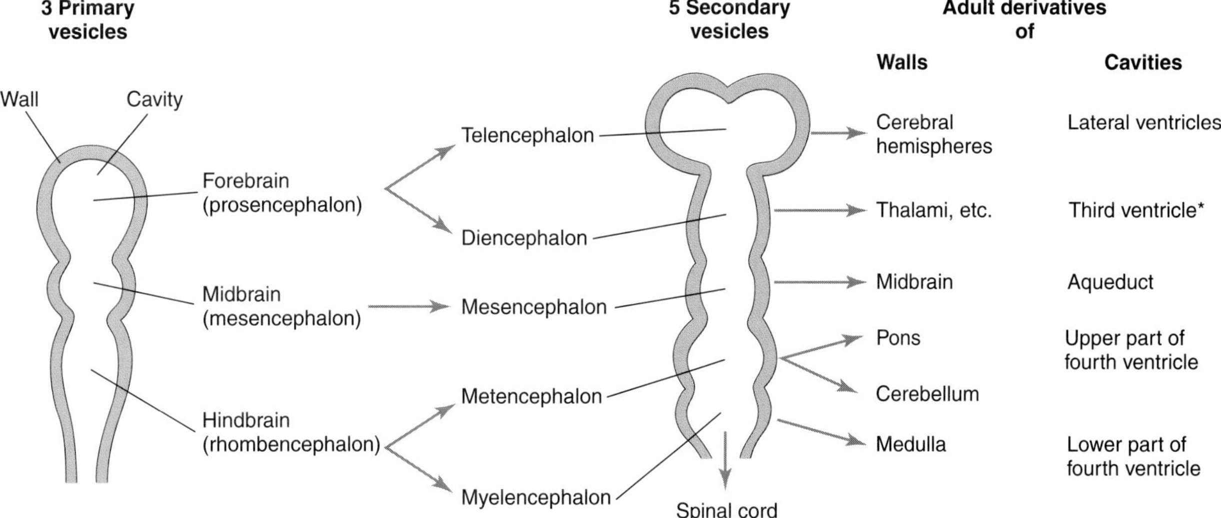

■ **Figure 18–23.** Diagrammatic sketches of the brain vesicles, indicating the adult derivatives of their walls and cavities. *The rostral (anterior) part of the third ventricle forms from the cavity of the telencephalon; most of the third ventricle is derived from the cavity of the diencephalon.

Hindbrain

The **cervical flexure** demarcates the hindbrain from the spinal cord (Fig. 18–24*A*). Later, this junction is arbitrarily defined as the level of the superior rootlet of the first cervical nerve, which is located roughly at the foramen magnum. The **pontine flexure,** located in the future pontine region, divides the hindbrain into

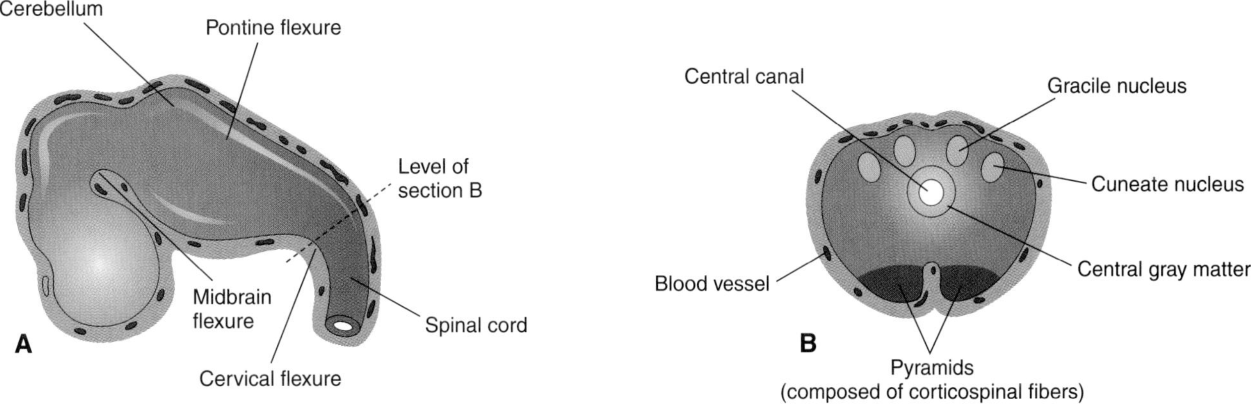

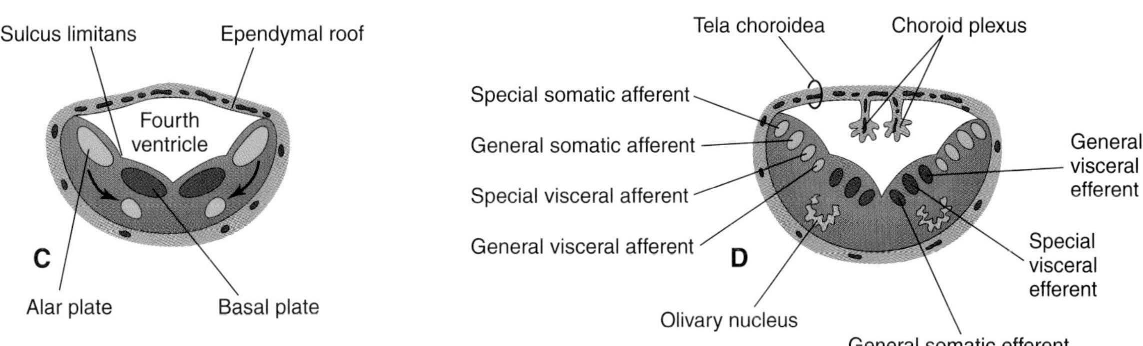

■ **Figure 18–24.** *A,* Sketch of the developing brain at the end of the fifth week, showing the three primary divisions of the brain and the brain flexures. *B,* Transverse section of the caudal part of the myelencephalon (developing closed part of the medulla). *C* and *D,* Similar sections of the rostral part of the myelencephalon (developing "open" part of the medulla), showing the position and successive stages of differentiation of the alar and basal plates. The arrows in *C* show the pathway taken by neuroblasts from the alar plates to form the olivary nuclei.

caudal (myelencephalon) and rostral (metencephalon) parts. The myelencephalon becomes the **medulla oblongata** and the metencephalon the **pons** and **cerebellum.** The cavity of the hindbrain becomes the fourth ventricle and the central canal in the caudal part of the medulla.

MYELENCEPHALON

The caudal part of the myelencephalon (closed part of medulla oblongata) resembles the spinal cord both developmentally and structurally (Fig. 18-24*B*). The neural canal of the neural tube forms a small central canal. Unlike those of the spinal cord, neuroblasts from the alar plates in the myelencephalon migrate into the marginal zone and form isolated areas of gray matter — the **gracile nuclei** medially and the **cuneate nuclei** laterally. These nuclei are associated with correspondingly named tracts that enter the medulla from the spinal cord. The ventral area of the medulla contains a pair of fiber bundles — the **pyramids** — which consist of corticospinal fibers descending from the developing cerebral cortex.

The rostral part of the myelencephalon ("open" part of medulla) is wide and rather flat, especially opposite the pontine flexure (Fig. 18-24*C* and *D*). The pontine flexure causes the lateral walls of the medulla to move laterally like the pages of an open book. It also causes the roof plate to become stretched and greatly thinned. In addition, the cavity of this part of the myelencephalon (part of future fourth ventricle) becomes somewhat rhomboidal (diamond-shaped). As the walls of the medulla move laterally, the alar plates come to lie lateral to the basal plates. As the positions of the plates change, the motor nuclei generally develop medial to the sensory nuclei (Fig. 18-24*C*). Neuroblasts in the basal plates of the medulla, like those in the spinal cord, develop into motor neurons. In the medulla the neuroblasts form nuclei (groups of nerve cells) and organize into three cell columns on each side (Fig. 18-24*D*). From medial to lateral, they are:

- *general somatic efferent,* represented by neurons of the hypoglossal nerve
- *special visceral efferent,* represented by neurons innervating muscles derived from the pharyngeal arches (see Chapter 10)

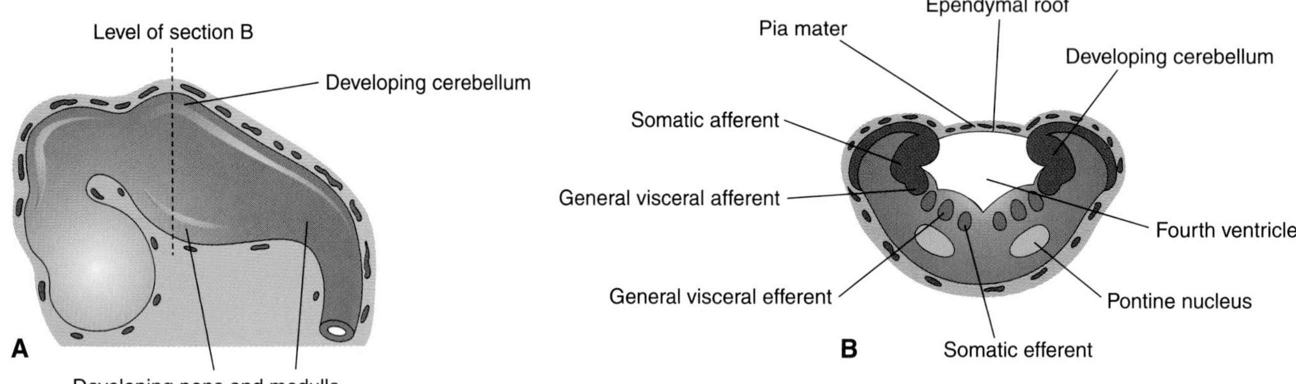

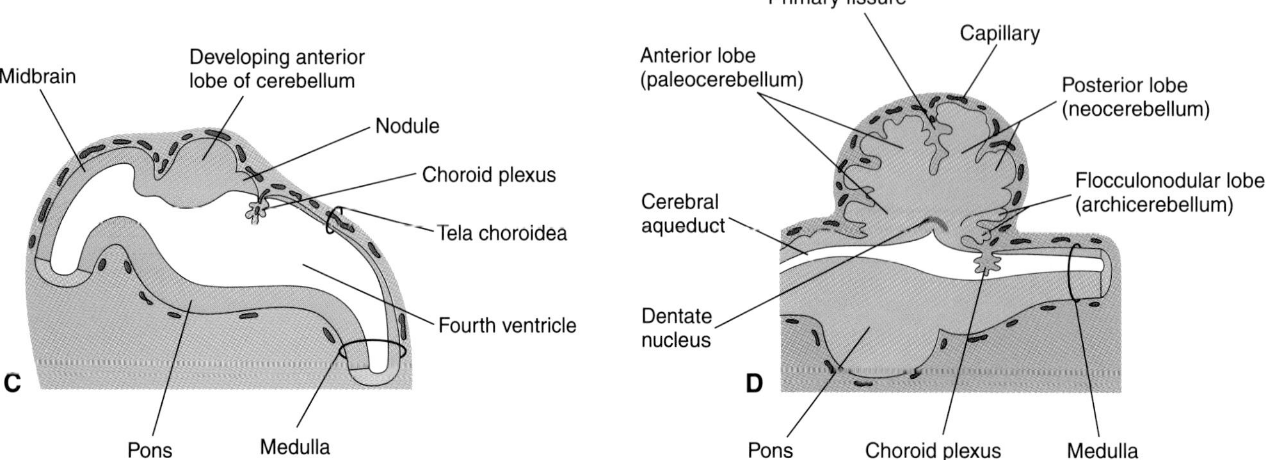

■ **Figure 18-25.** *A,* Sketch of the developing brain at the end of the fifth week. *B,* Transverse section of the metencephalon (developing pons and cerebellum), showing the derivatives of the alar and basal plates. *C* and *D,* Sagittal sections of the hindbrain at 6 and 17 weeks, respectively, showing successive stages in the development of the pons and cerebellum.

- *general visceral efferent,* represented by some neurons of the vagus and glossopharyngeal nerves

Neuroblasts of the alar plates form neurons that are arranged in four columns on each side. From medial to lateral, they are:

- *general visceral afferent* receiving impulses from the viscera
- *special visceral afferent* receiving taste fibers
- *general somatic afferent* receiving impulses from the surface of the head
- *special somatic afferent* receiving impulses from the ear

Some neuroblasts from the alar plates migrate ventrally and form the neurons in the **olivary nuclei** (Fig. 18-24*C* and *D*).

METENCEPHALON

The walls of the metencephalon form the pons and cerebellum, and the cavity of the metencephalon forms the superior part of the fourth ventricle (Fig. 18-25*A*). As in the rostral part of the myelencephalon, the pontine flexure causes divergence of the lateral walls of the pons, which spreads the gray matter in the floor of the fourth ventricle (Fig. 18-25*B*). As in the myelencephalon, neuroblasts in each basal plate develop into motor nuclei and organize into three columns on each side.

The **cerebellum** develops from thickenings of dorsal parts of the alar plates. Initially the cerebellar swellings project into the fourth ventricle (Fig. 18-25*B*). As the swellings enlarge and fuse in the median plane, they overgrow the rostral half of the fourth ventricle and overlap the pons and medulla (Fig. 18-25*D*). Some neuroblasts in the intermediate zone of the alar plates migrate to the marginal zone and differentiate into the neurons of the **cerebellar cortex.** Other neuroblasts from these plates give rise to the central nuclei, the largest of which is the **dentate nucleus** (Fig. 18-25*D*). Cells from the alar plates also give rise to the pontine nuclei, the cochlear and vestibular nuclei, and the sensory nuclei of the trigeminal nerve.

The structure of the cerebellum reflects its phylogenetic development (Fig. 18-25*C* and *D*):

- The *archicerebellum* (flocculonodular lobe), the oldest part phylogenetically, has connections with the vestibular apparatus.
- The *paleocerebellum* (vermis and anterior lobe), of more recent development, is associated with sensory data from the limbs.
- The *neocerebellum* (posterior lobe), the newest part phylogenetically, is concerned with selective control of limb movements.

Nerve fibers connecting the cerebral and cerebellar cortices with the spinal cord pass through the marginal layer of the ventral region of the metencephalon. This region of the brain stem is called the **pons** (L., bridge) because of the robust band of nerve fibers that crosses the median plane and forms a bulky ridge on its anterior and lateral aspects.

Choroid Plexuses and Cerebrospinal Fluid (CSF)

The thin ependymal roof of the fourth ventricle is covered externally by *pia mater,* derived from mesenchyme associated with the hindbrain (Fig. 18-25*C* and *D*). This vascular pia mater, together with the ependymal roof, forms the **tela choroidea.** Because of the active proliferation of the pia mater, the tela choroidea invaginates the fourth ventricle, where it differentiates into the **choroid plexus.** Similar choroid plexuses develop in the roof of the third ventricle and in the medial walls of the lateral ventricles. The choroid plexuses secrete ventricular fluid, which becomes **cerebrospinal fluid** (CSF) when additions are made to it from the surfaces of the brain and spinal cord, and from the pia-arachnoid layer of the meninges. The thin roof of the fourth ventricle evaginates in three locations. These outpouchings rupture to form openings. The **median** and **lateral apertures** (foramen of Magendie and foramina of Luschka, respectively) permit the CSF to enter the **subarachnoid space** from the fourth ventricle. The main site of absorption of CSF into the venous system is through the **arachnoid villi,** which are protrusions of the arachnoid into the dural venous sinuses (Moore, 1992). These villi consist of a thin, cellular layer derived from the epithelium of the arachnoid and the endothelium of the sinus.

Midbrain

The midbrain (mesencephalon) undergoes less change than any other part of the developing brain (Fig. 18-26*A*), except for the most caudal part of the hindbrain. The neural canal narrows and becomes the **cerebral aqueduct** (Fig. 18-25*D*), a canal that connects the third and fourth ventricles. Neuroblasts migrate from the alar plates of the midbrain into the *tectum* (roof) and aggregate to form four large groups of neurons, the paired *superior and inferior colliculi* (Fig. 18-26*A* and *B*), which are concerned with visual and auditory reflexes, respectively. Neuroblasts from the basal plates may give rise to groups of neurons in the **tegmentum** (red nuclei, nuclei of the third and fourth cranial nerves, and the reticular nuclei). The **substantia nigra,** a broad layer of gray matter adjacent to the cerebral peduncle (Fig. 18-26*D* and *E*), may also differentiate from the basal plate, but some authorities believe it is derived from cells in the alar plate that migrate ventrally. Fibers growing from the cerebrum form the cerebral peduncles anteriorly (Fig. 18-26*B*). The **cerebral peduncles** become progressively more prominent as more descending fiber groups (corticopontine, corticobulbar, and corticospinal) pass through the developing midbrain on their way to the brain stem and spinal cord.

Forebrain

As closure of the rostral neuropore occurs, two lateral outgrowths—**optic vesicles**—appear (Fig. 18-3*A*), one on each side of the forebrain. The optic vesicles are the primordia of the *retinae* and *optic nerves* (see Chapter 19). A second pair of diverticula soon arise

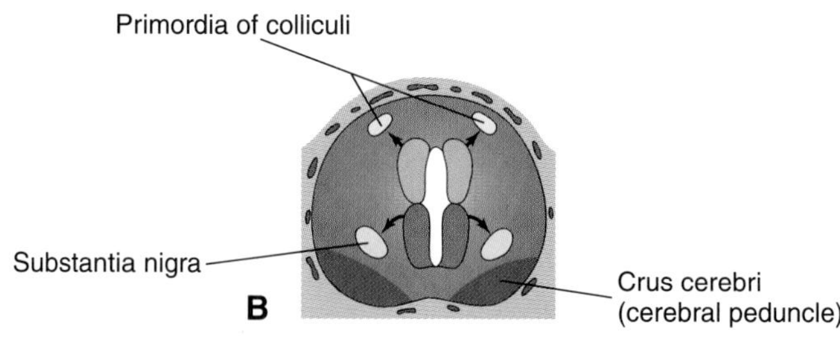

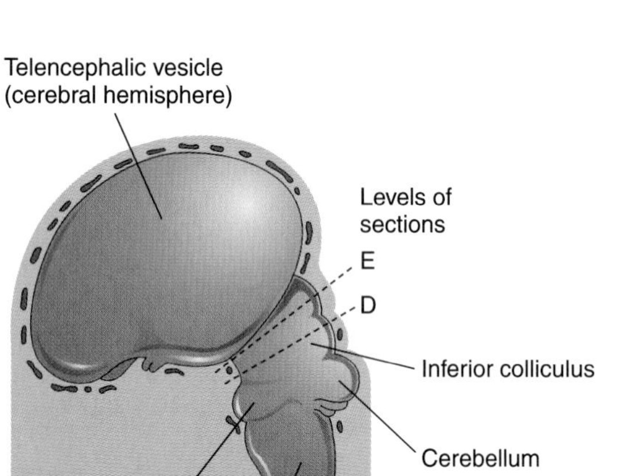

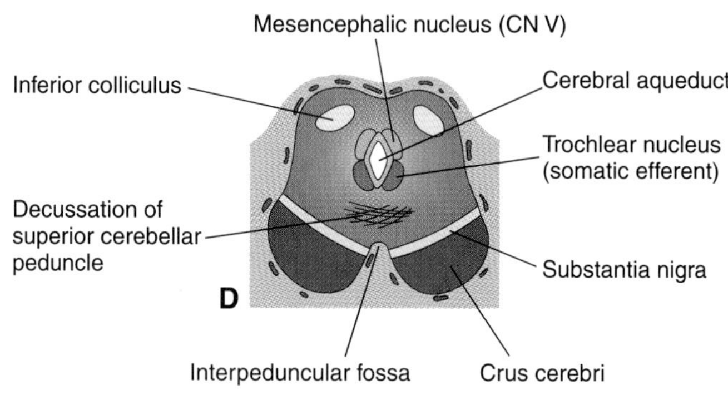

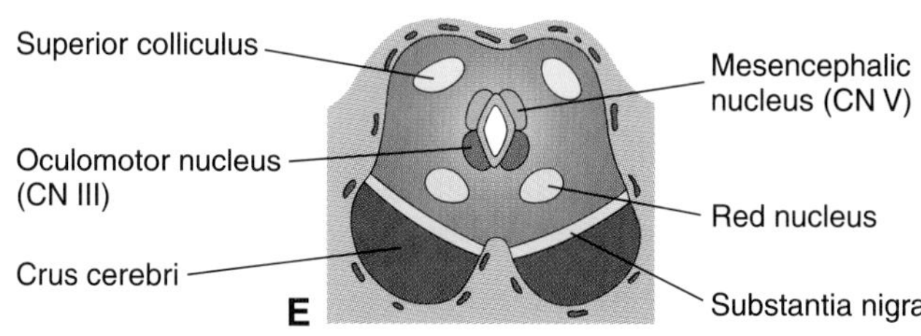

■ **Figure 18–26.** *A*, Sketch of the developing brain at the end of the fifth week. *B*, Transverse section of the developing midbrain, showing the early migration of cells from the basal and alar plates. *C*, Sketch of the developing brain at 11 weeks. *D* and *E*, Transverse sections of the developing midbrain at the level of the inferior and superior colliculi, respectively.

more dorsally and rostrally; these are the **cerebral vesicles** or telencephalic vesicles (Fig. 18-26*C*). They are the primordia of the **cerebral hemispheres,** and their cavities become the *lateral ventricles* (Fig. 18-27*B*). The rostral or anterior part of the forebrain, including the primordia of the cerebral hemispheres, is the **telencephalon** and the caudal or posterior part of the forebrain is the **diencephalon.** The cavities of the telencephalon and diencephalon contribute to the formation of the **third ventricle,** although the cavity of the diencephalon contributes more.

DIENCEPHALON

Three swellings develop in the lateral walls of the third ventricle, which later become the *epithalamus, thalamus,* and *hypothalamus* (Fig. 18-27*C* to *E*). The **thalamus** is separated from the epithalamus by the *epithalamic sulcus* and from the hypothalamus by the *hypothalamic sulcus.* The latter sulcus is not a continuation of the sulcus limitans into the forebrain and does not, like the sulcus limitans, divide sensory and motor areas. The thalamus develops rapidly on each side and bulges into the cavity of the third ventricle, reducing it to a narrow cleft. The thalami meet and fuse in the midline in about 70% of brains, forming a bridge of gray matter across the third ventricle—the *interthalamic adhesion* (massa intermedia).

The **hypothalamus** arises by proliferation of neuroblasts in the intermediate zone of the diencephalic walls, ventral to the hypothalamic sulci. Later a number of nuclei concerned with endocrine activities and homeostasis develop. A pair of nuclei, the **mamillary bodies,** form pea-sized swellings on the ventral surface of the hypothalamus (Fig. 18-27*C*). The **epithalamus** develops from the roof and dorsal portion of the lateral wall of the diencephalon. Initially the epithalamic swellings are large, but later they become relatively small. The **pineal body** develops as a median diverticulum of the caudal part of the roof of the diencephalon (Fig. 18-27*C* and *D*). Proliferation of cells in its walls soon converts it into a solid cone-shaped gland.

Pituitary Gland (Fig. 18-28; Table 18-1). The pituitary gland (hypophysis cerebri) is ectodermal in origin. It develops from two sources:

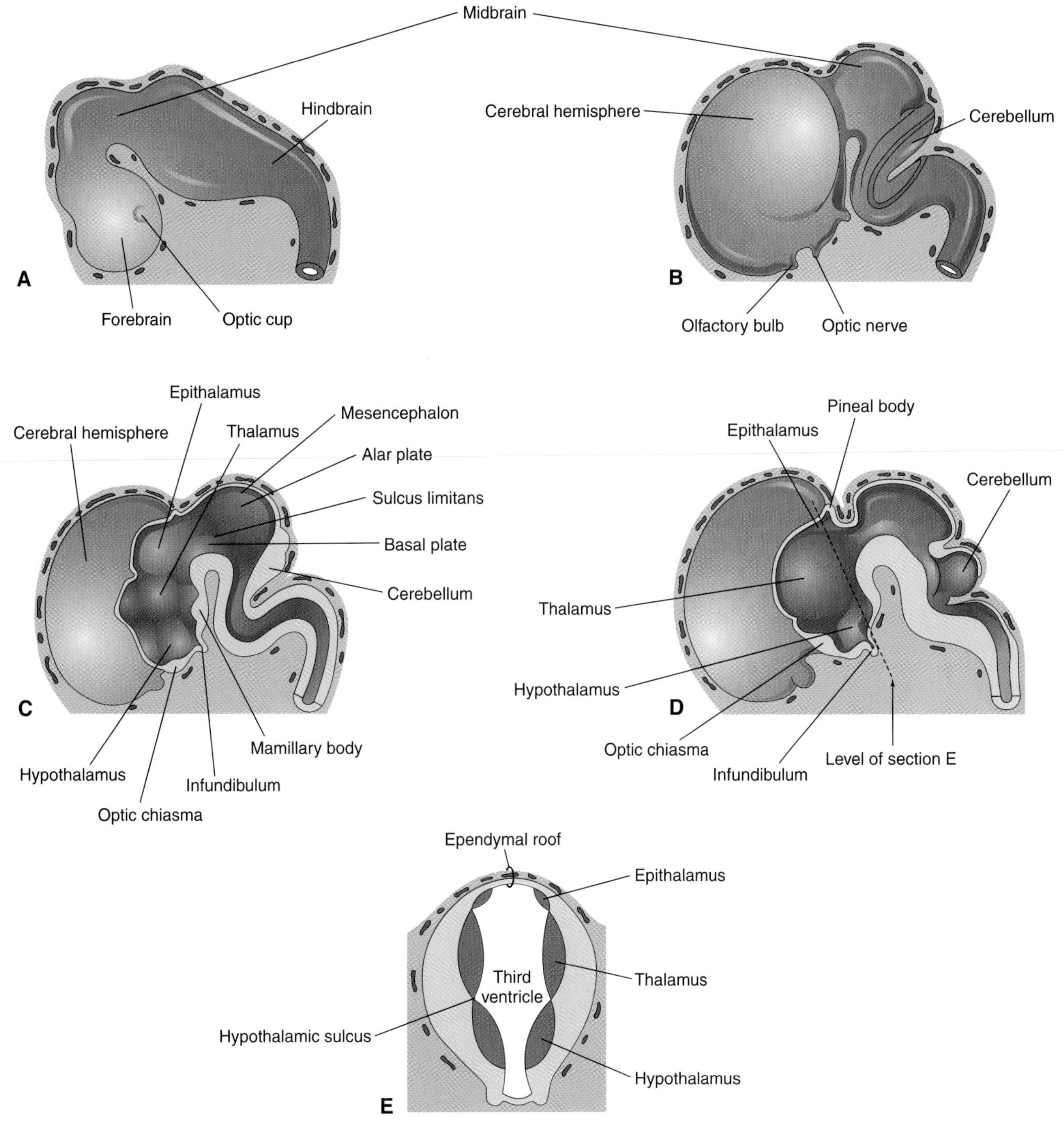

■ **Figure 18–27.** *A*, External view of the brain at the end of the fifth week. *B*, Similar view at 7 weeks. *C*, Median section of this brain, showing the medial surface of the forebrain and midbrain. *D*, Similar section at 8 weeks. *E*, Transverse section of the diencephalon, showing the epithalamus dorsally, the thalamus laterally, and the hypothalamus ventrally.

- an upgrowth from the *ectodermal roof of the stomodeum*
- a downgrowth from the neuroectoderm of the diencephalon, the *neurohypophysial bud*

This double embryonic origin explains why the pituitary gland is composed of two completely different types of tissue.

- The **adenohypophysis** (glandular part) or anterior lobe arises from oral ectoderm.
- The **neurohypophysis** (nervous part) or posterior lobe originates from neuroectoderm.

At the middle of the fourth week, a diverticulum—the **hypophysial pouch** or Rathke pouch—projects from the roof of the stomodeum and lies adjacent to the floor (ventral wall) of the diencephalon (Fig. 18-28*C*). By the fifth week this pouch has elongated and become constricted at its attachment to the oral epithelium, giving it a nipplelike appearance (Fig. 18-28*C*). By this stage it has come into contact with the **infundibulum** (derived from the neurohypophysial bud), a ventral downgrowth (diverticulum) of the diencephalon (Figs. 18-27 and 18-28). The parts of the pituitary gland that develop from the ectoderm of the

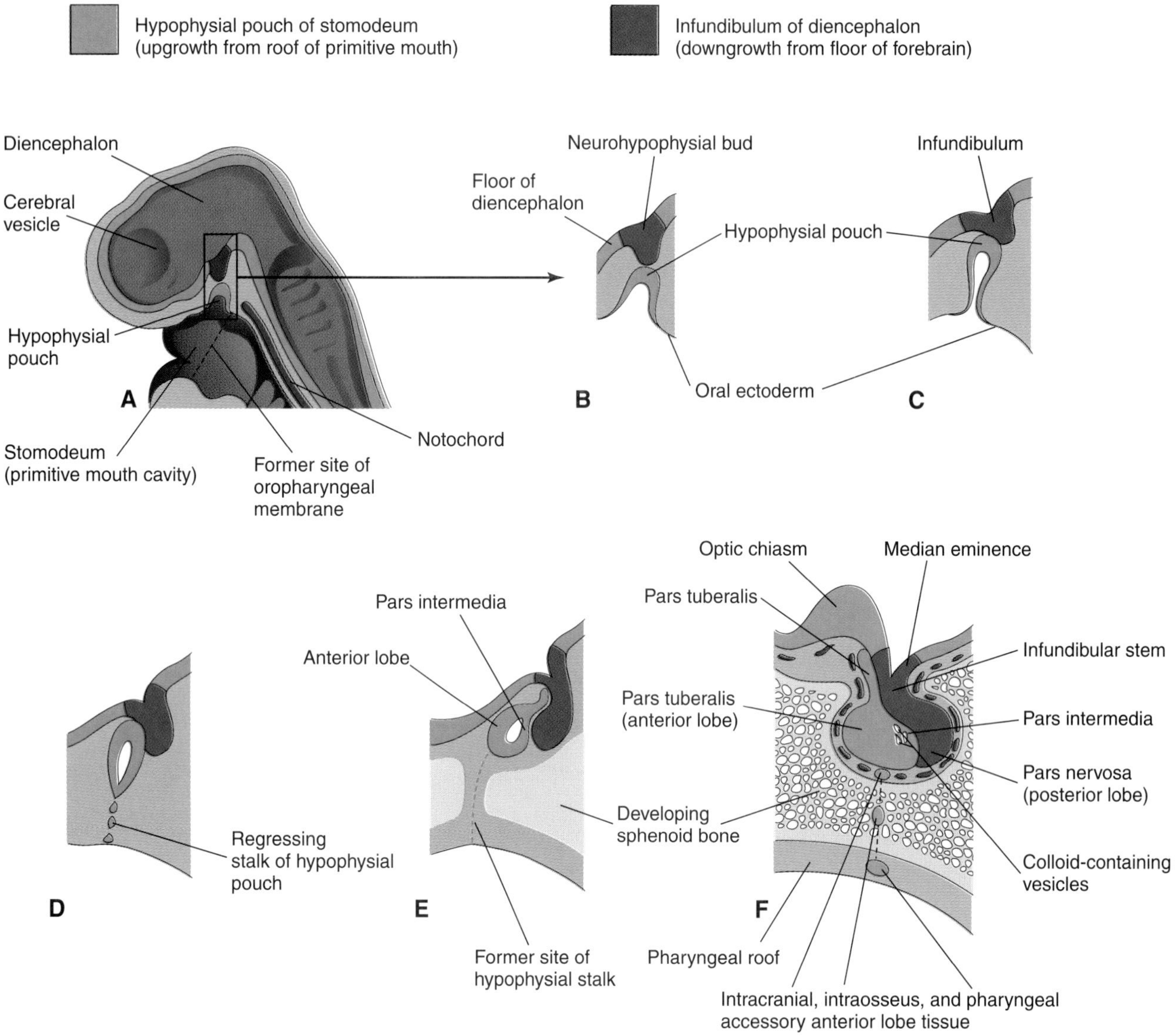

■ **Figure 18–28.** Diagrammatic sketches illustrating development of the pituitary gland. *A*, Sagittal section of the cranial end of an embryo of about 36 days, showing the hypophysial (Rathke) pouch, an upgrowth from the stomodeum, and the neurohypophysial bud, a downgrowth from the forebrain. *B* to *D*, Successive stages of the developing pituitary gland. By 8 weeks, the pouch loses its connection with the oral cavity and is in close contact with the infundibulum and the posterior lobe (neurohypophysis) of the pituitary gland. *E* and *F*, Later stages showing proliferation of the anterior wall of the hypophysial pouch to form the anterior lobe (adenohypophysis) of the pituitary gland.

stomodeum—pars anterior, pars intermedia, and pars tuberalis—form the **adenohypophysis** (Table 18-1). The stalk of the hypophysial pouch passes between the chondrification centers of the developing presphenoid and basisphenoid bones of the skull (Fig. 18-28*E*). During the sixth week the connection of the pouch with the oral cavity degenerates and disappears (Fig. 18-28*D* and *E*).

Table 18–1 ■ Derivation and Terminology of the Pituitary Gland

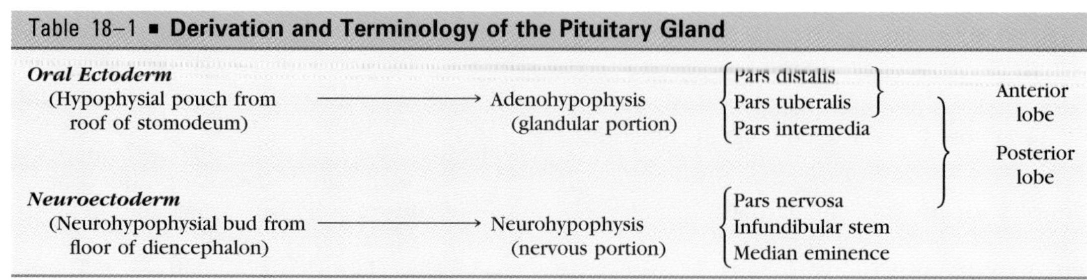

Origin		Division	Parts	Lobe
Oral Ectoderm (Hypophysial pouch from roof of stomodeum)	→	Adenohypophysis (glandular portion)	Pars distalis Pars tuberalis	Anterior lobe
			Pars intermedia	Posterior lobe
Neuroectoderm (Neurohypophysial bud from floor of diencephalon)	→	Neurohypophysis (nervous portion)	Pars nervosa	Posterior lobe
			Infundibular stem Median eminence	

Pharyngeal Hypophysis and Craniopharyngioma

A remnant of the stalk of the hypophysial (Rathke) pouch may persist and form a *pharyngeal hypophysis* in the roof of the oropharynx (Fig. 18-28*F*). Very rarely, accessory masses of anterior lobe tissue develop outside the capsule of the pituitary gland, within the sella turcica of the sphenoid bone. A remnant of the site of the stalk of the hypophysial pouch, the **narrow basipharyngeal canal,** is visible in sections of the newborn sphenoid bone in about 1% of cases. It can also be identified in a small number of radiographs of the skulls of newborn infants (usually those with skull anomalies). Occasionally **craniopharyngiomas** develop in the pharynx or in the basisphenoid (posterior part of sphenoid) from remnants of the stalk of the hypophysial pouch (Fig. 18-29), but most often they form in and/or superior to the sella turcica (Moore, 1992).

Cells of the anterior wall of the hypophysial pouch proliferate actively and give rise to the **pars distalis** of the pituitary gland. Later a small extension, the **pars tuberalis,** grows around the infundibular stem. The extensive proliferation of the anterior wall of the hypophysial pouch reduces its lumen to a narrow cleft (Fig. 18-28*E*). This residual cleft is usually not recognizable in the adult gland, but it may be represented by a zone of cysts. Cells in the posterior wall of the hypophysial pouch do not proliferate; they give rise to the thin, poorly defined **pars intermedia** (Fig. 18-28*F*). The part of the pituitary gland that develops from the neuroectoderm of the brain (infundibulum) is the **neurohypophysis** (Table 18-1). The **infundibulum** gives rise to the *median eminence, infundibular stem,* and *pars nervosa.* Initially the walls of the infundibulum are thin, but the distal end of the infundibulum soon becomes solid as the neuroepithelial cells proliferate. These cells later differentiate into **pituicytes,** the primary cells of the posterior lobe of the pituitary gland, which are closely related to neuroglial cells. Nerve fibers grow into the pars nervosa from the hypothalamic area, to which the infundibular stem is attached.

TELENCEPHALON

The telencephalon consists of a median part and two lateral diverticula, the **cerebral vesicles** (Fig. 18-28*A*). These diverticula are the primordia of the **cerebral hemispheres** (Figs. 18-27*B* and 18-28*A*). The cavity of the median portion of the telencephalon forms the extreme anterior part of the third ventricle (Fig. 18-30). At first, the cerebral vesicles are in wide communication with the cavity of the third ventricle through the **interventricular foramina** (Figs. 18-30 and 18-31*B*). Along a line, the *choroid fissure,* part of the medial wall of the developing cerebral hemisphere, becomes very thin. Initially, this thin ependymal portion lies in the roof of the hemisphere and is continuous with the ependymal roof of the third ventricle (Fig. 18-31*A*). The **choroid plexus** of the lateral ventricle later forms at this site (Figs. 18-30 and 18-32).

As the **cerebral hemispheres** expand, they cover successively the diencephalon, midbrain, and hindbrain. The hemispheres eventually meet each other in the midline, flattening their medial surfaces. The mesenchyme trapped in the longitudinal fissure between them gives rise to the **falx cerebri,** a median fold of

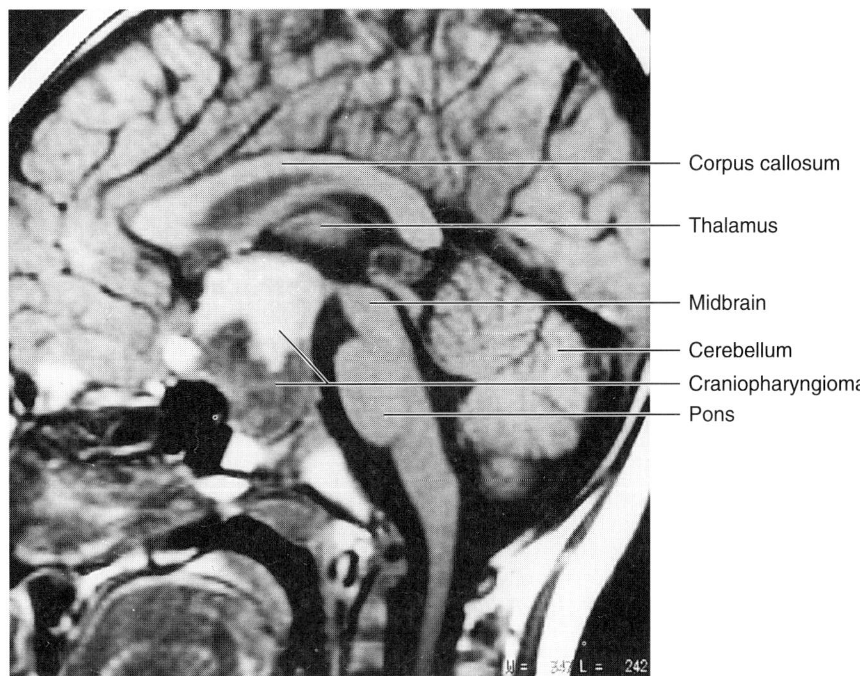

■ **Figure 18–29.** Sagittal magnetic resonance image of a 4-year-old male who presented with a headache and optic atrophy. A large mass (4 cm) occupies an enlarged sella turcica, expanding inferiorly into the sphenoid bone and superiorly into the suprasellar cistern. A craniopharyngioma was confirmed by surgery. There is elevation and compression of the optic chiasm (not discernible in this image). The inferior half of the mass is solid and appears dark, whereas the superior half is cystic and appears brighter. (Courtesy of Dr. Gerald S. Smyser, Altru Health System, Grand Forks, ND.)

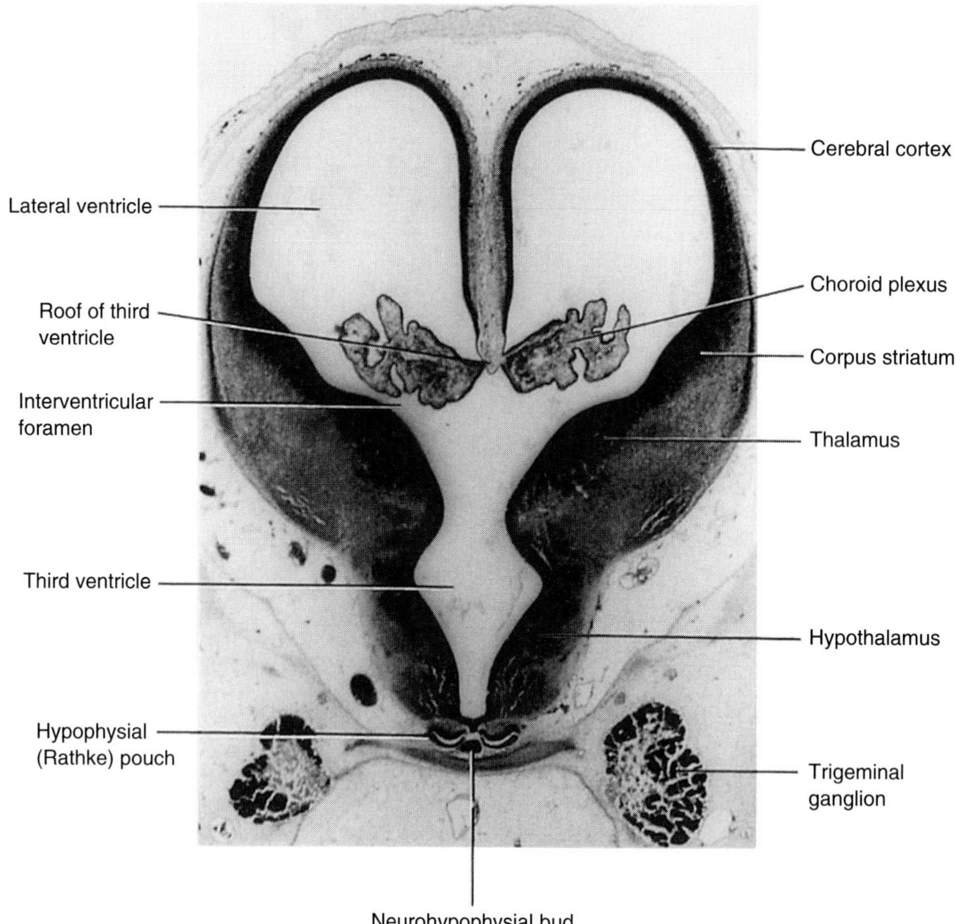

■ **Figure 18–30.** Photomicrograph of a transverse section through the diencephalon and cerebral vesicles of a human embryo (about 50 days) at the level of the interventricular foramina (×20). The choroid fissure is located at the junction of the choroid plexus and the medial wall of the lateral ventricle. (Courtesy of Professor Jean Hay [retired], Department of Anatomy, University of Manitoba, Winnipeg, Canada.)

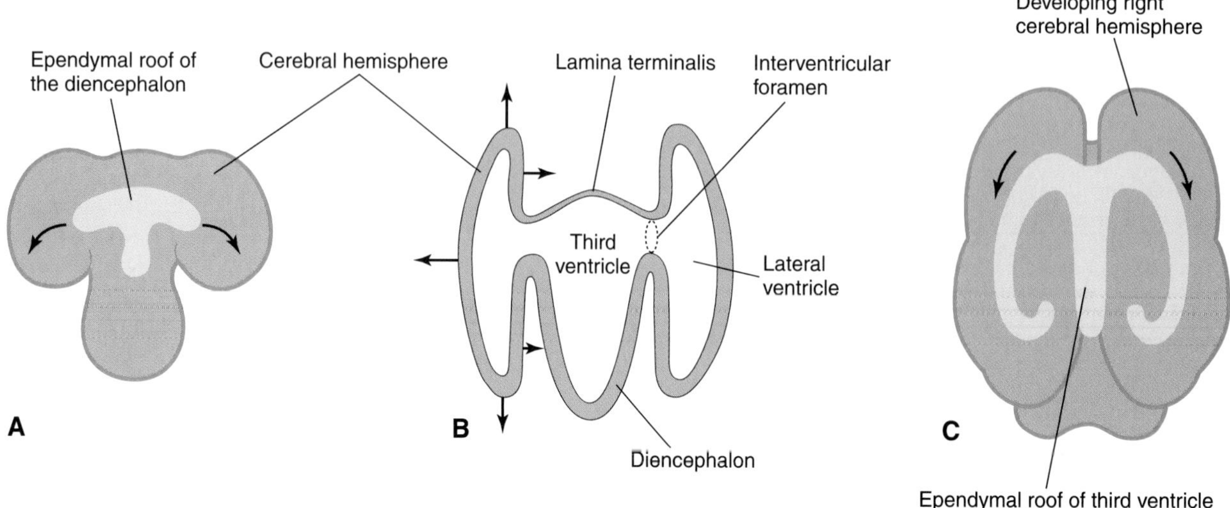

■ **Figure 18–31.** *A,* Sketch of the dorsal surface of the forebrain, indicating how the ependymal roof of the diencephalon is carried out to the dorsomedial surface of the cerebral hemispheres. *B,* Diagrammatic section of the forebrain, showing how the developing cerebral hemispheres grow from the lateral walls of the forebrain and expand in all directions until they cover the diencephalon. The arrows indicate some directions in which the hemispheres expand. The rostral wall of the forebrain, the *lamina terminalis,* is very thin. *C,* Sketch of the forebrain, showing how the ependymal roof is finally carried into the temporal lobes as a result of the C-shaped growth pattern of the cerebral hemispheres.

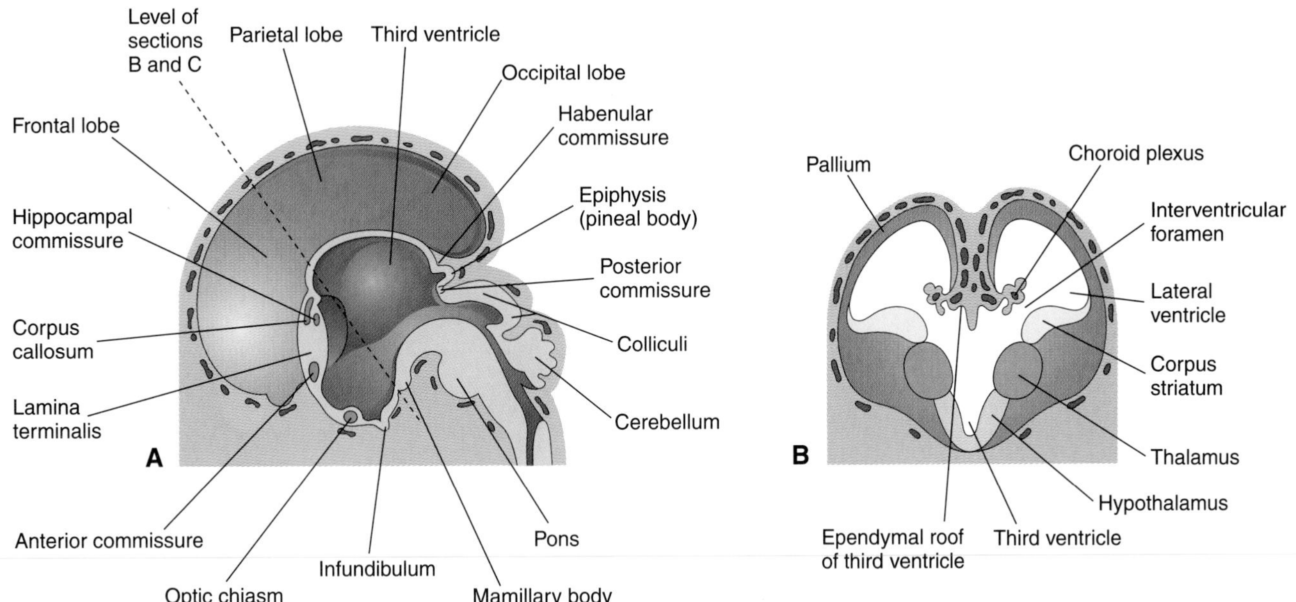

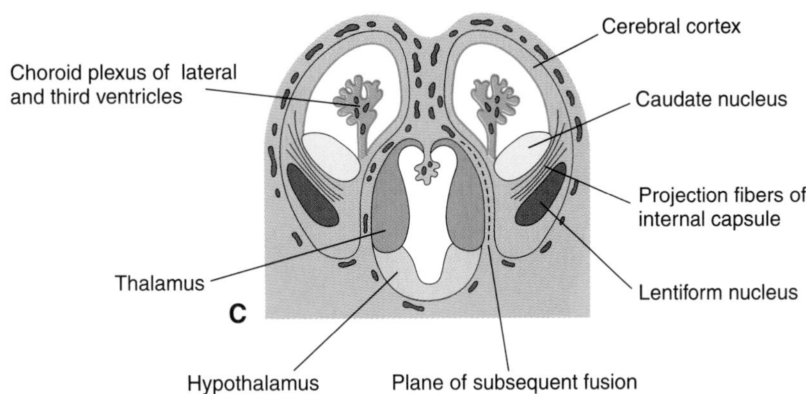

■ **Figure 18–32.** *A*, Drawing of the medial surface of the forebrain of a 10-week embryo showing the diencephalic derivatives, the main commissures, and the expanding cerebral hemispheres. *B*, Transverse section of the forebrain at the level of the interventricular foramina, showing the corpus striatum and choroid plexuses of the lateral ventricles. *C*, Similar section at about 11 weeks, showing division of the corpus striatum into the caudate and lentiform nuclei by the internal capsule. The developing relationship of the cerebral hemispheres to the diencephalon is also illustrated.

dura mater (Moore, 1992). The **corpus striatum** appears during the sixth week as a prominent swelling in the floor of each cerebral hemisphere (Fig. 18-32*B*). The floor of each hemisphere expands more slowly than its thin cortical walls because it contains the rather large corpus striatum; consequently, the cerebral hemispheres become C-shaped (Fig. 18-33).

The growth and curvature of the hemispheres also affect the shape of the lateral ventricles. They become roughly C-shaped cavities filled with CSF. The caudal end of each cerebral hemisphere turns ventrally and then rostrally, forming the temporal lobe; in so doing, it carries the ventricle (forming the temporal horn) and **choroid fissure** with it (Fig. 18-33). Here, the thin medial wall of the hemisphere is invaginated along the choroid fissure by vascular pia mater to form the *choroid plexus of the temporal horn* (Fig. 18-32*B*). As the cerebral cortex differentiates, fibers passing to and from it pass through the **corpus striatum** and divide it into the *caudate* and *lentiform nuclei.* This fiber pathway—the **internal capsule** (Fig. 18-32*C*)—becomes C-shaped as the hemisphere assumes this form. The **caudate nucleus** becomes elongated and C-shaped, conforming to the outline of the lateral ventricle (Fig. 18-33). Its pear-shaped head and elongated body lie in the floor of the frontal horn and body of the lateral ventricle, whereas its tail makes a U-shaped turn to gain the roof of the temporal or inferior horn.

Cerebral Commissures

As the cerebral cortex develops, groups of fibers—**commissures**—connect corresponding areas of the

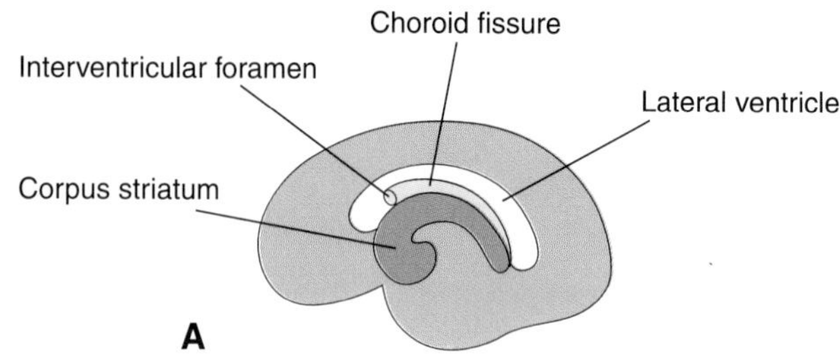

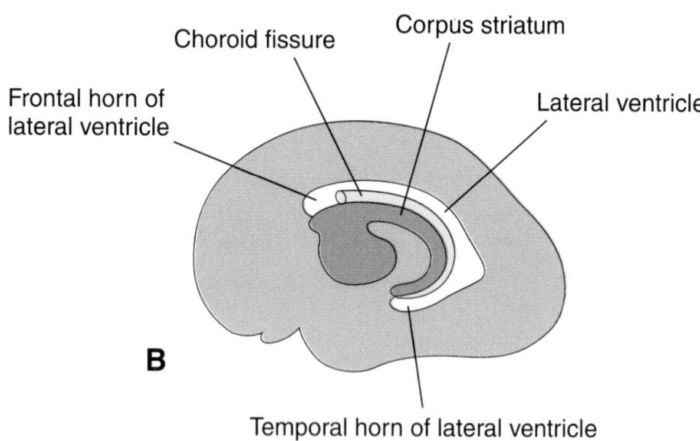

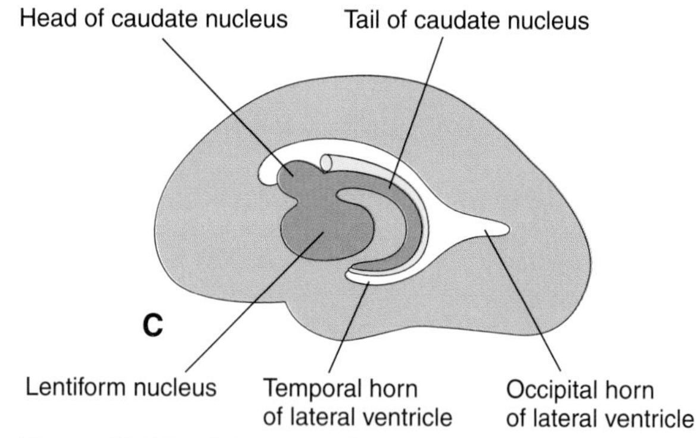

■ **Figure 18–33.** Schematic diagrams of the medial surface of the developing right cerebral hemisphere, showing the development of the lateral ventricle, choroid fissure, and corpus striatum. *A*, 13 weeks. *B*, 21 weeks. *C*, 32 weeks.

cerebral hemispheres with one another (Fig. 18-32). The most important of these commissures cross in the **lamina terminalis,** the rostral end of the forebrain. This lamina extends from the roof plate of the diencephalon to the optic chiasma. It is the natural pathway from one hemisphere to the other. The first commissures to form, the *anterior commissure* and

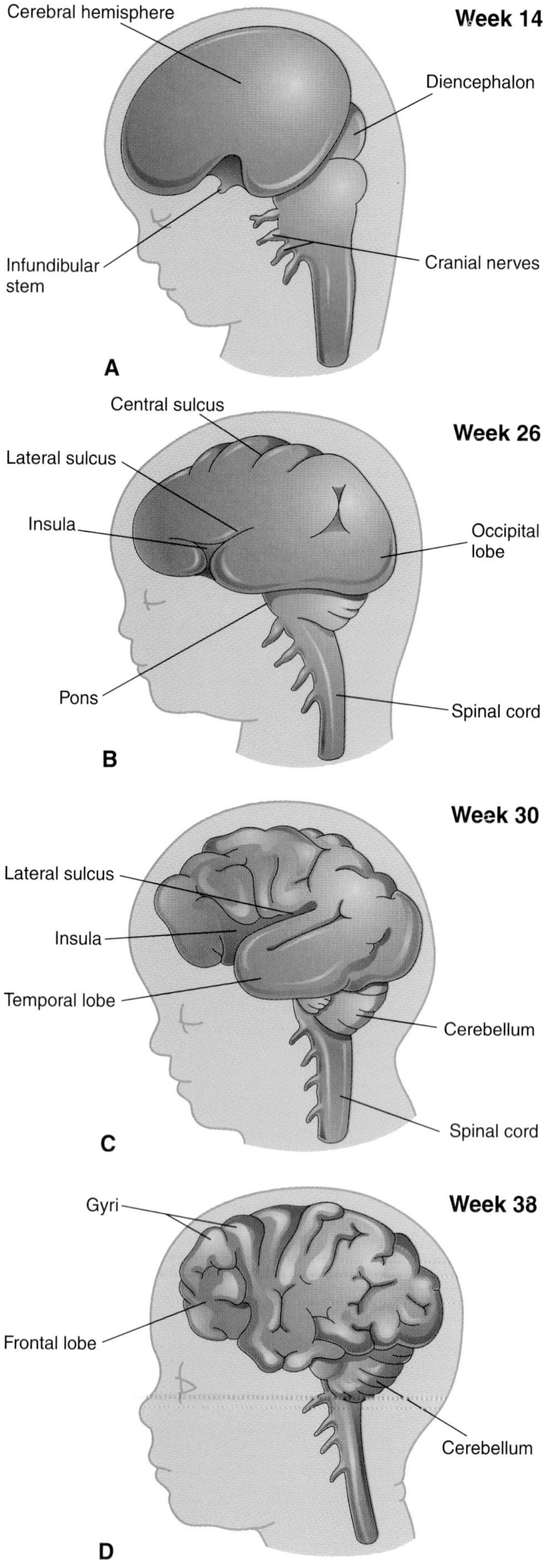

■ **Figure 18–34.** Sketches of lateral views of the left cerebral hemisphere, diencephalon, and brain stem showing successive stages in the development of the sulci and gyri in the cerebral cortex. Note the gradual narrowing of the lateral sulcus and burying of the insula (L., island), an area of cerebral cortex that is concealed from surface view. Note that the surface of the cerebral hemispheres grows rapidly during the fetal period, forming many convolutions (gyri), which are separated by many grooves (sulci). *A*, 14 weeks. *B*, 26 weeks. *C*, 30 weeks. *D*, 38 weeks.

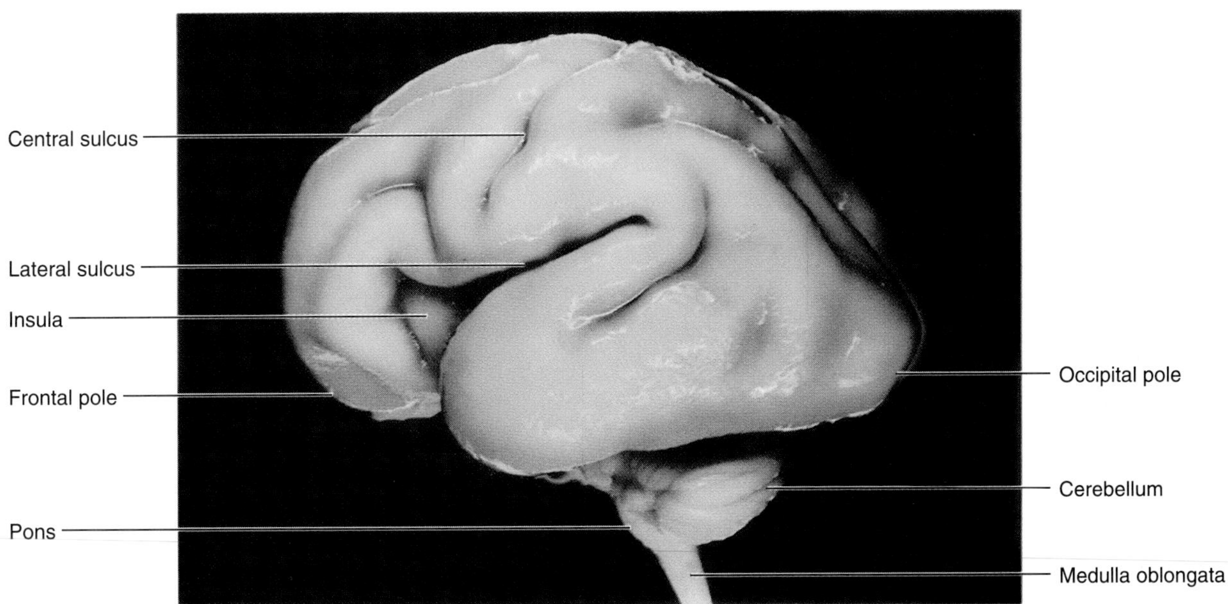

■ **Figure 18–35.** Photograph of a lateral view of the brain of a stillborn fetus (25 weeks). (From Nishimura H, Semba R, Tanimura T, Tanaka O: *Prenatal Development of the Human with Special Reference to Craniofacial Structures: An Atlas.* US Department of Health, Education, and Welfare, National Institutes of Health, Bethesda, 1977.)

hippocampal commissure, are small fiber bundles that connect phylogenetically older parts of the brain. The **anterior commissure** connects the olfactory bulb and related areas of one hemisphere with those of the opposite side. The **hippocampal commissure** connects the hippocampal formations (Haines, 1997).

The largest cerebral commissure is the **corpus callosum** (Fig. 18-32*A*), connecting neocortical areas. The corpus callosum initially lies in the lamina terminalis, but fibers are added to it as the cortex enlarges; as a result, it gradually extends beyond the lamina terminalis. The rest of the **lamina terminalis** lies between the corpus callosum and the fornix. It becomes stretched to form the thin **septum pellucidum,** a thin plate of brain tissue (Koshi et al., 1997). At birth the corpus callosum extends over the roof of the diencephalon. The **optic chiasma,** which develops in the ventral part of the lamina terminalis (Fig. 18-32*A*), consists of fibers from the medial halves of the retinae, which cross to join the optic tract of the opposite side.

The walls of the developing cerebral hemispheres initially show the three typical zones of the neural tube (ventricular, intermediate, and marginal); later a fourth one, the subventricular zone, appears. Cells of the intermediate zone migrate into the marginal zone and give rise to the cortical layers. The gray matter is thus located peripherally, and axons from its cell bodies pass centrally to form the large volume of white matter — the **medullary center.**

Initially the surface of the hemispheres is smooth (Fig. 18-34*A*); however, as growth proceeds, **sulci** (grooves or furrows) and **gyri** (convolutions or elevations) develop (Fig. 18-34*B* and *C*). The sulci and gyri permit a considerable increase in the surface area of the cerebral cortex without requiring an extensive increase in cranial size. As each cerebral hemisphere grows, the cortex covering the external surface of the corpus striatum grows relatively slowly and is soon overgrown (Fig. 18-34*C*). This buried cortex, hidden from view in the depths of the lateral sulcus (fissure) of the cerebral hemisphere (Fig. 18-35), is the **insula** (L., island).

CONGENITAL ANOMALIES OF THE BRAIN

Because of the complexity of its embryological history, abnormal development of the brain is common (about 3 per 1000 births). Most major congenital anomalies of the brain, such as meroanencephaly (anencephaly) and meningoencephalocele, result from defective closure of the rostral neuropore during the fourth week (Fig. 18-36*C*) and involve the overlying tissues (meninges and calvaria). The factors causing the NTDs are genetic, nutritional, and/or environmental in nature (Shaw et al., 1996). Congenital anomalies of the brain may be caused by alterations in the morphogenesis or the histogenesis of the nervous tissue, or they can result from developmental failures occurring in associated structures (notochord, somites, mesenchyme, and skull). Abnormal histogenesis of the cerebral cortex can result in seizures (Fig. 18-37) and various types of **mental retardation.** Subnormal intellectual development may result from exposure of the embryo/fetus during the 8- to 16-week period of development to certain viruses and high levels of radiation (see Chapter 8). Prenatal factors may be involved in the development of **cerebral palsy;** however, this central motor deficit most often results from a normal fetus's brain being damaged at birth. Cerebral palsy is one of the most crippling conditions of childhood (Behrman et al., 1996).

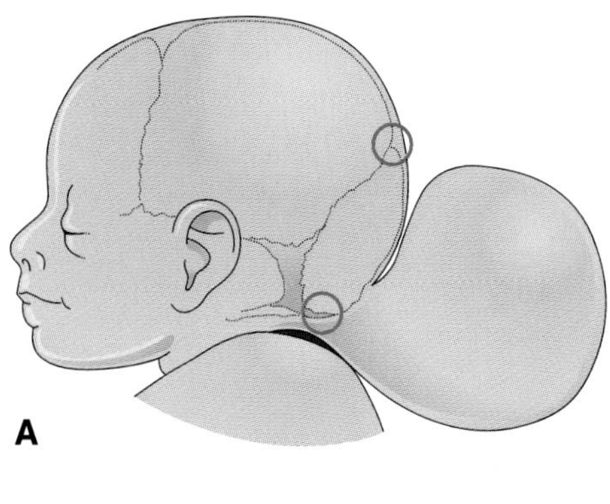

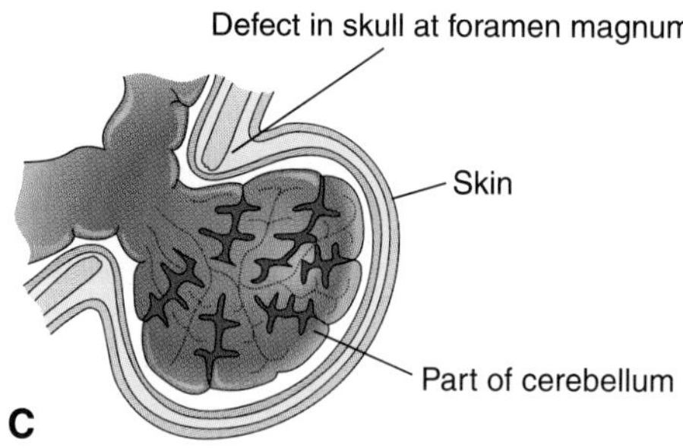

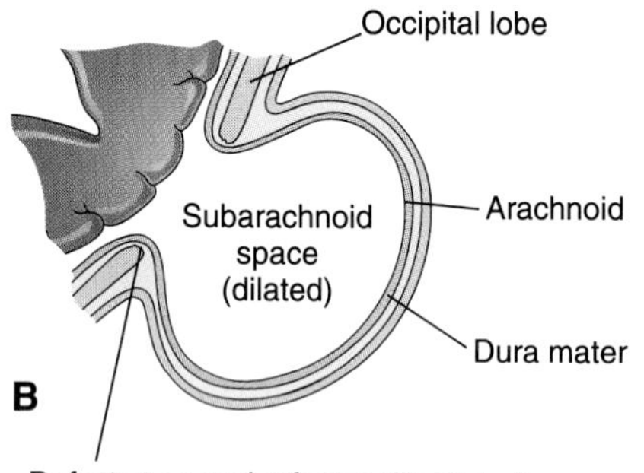

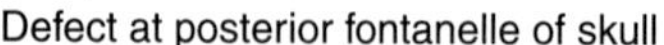

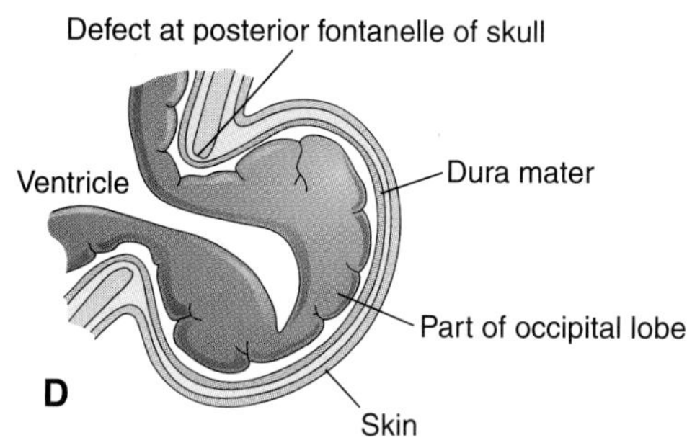

■ **Figure 18-36.** Schematic drawings illustrating cranium bifidum (bony defect in cranium) and various types of herniation of the brain and/or meninges. *A*, Sketch of the head of a newborn infant with a large protrusion from the occipital region of the skull. The upper red circle indicates a cranial defect at the posterior fontanelle. The lower red circle indicates a cranial defect near the foramen magnum. *B*, Meningocele consisting of a protrusion of the cranial meninges that is filled with cerebrospinal fluid (CSF). *C*, Meningoencephalocele consisting of a protrusion of part of the cerebellum that is covered by meninges and skin. *D*, Meningohydroencephalocele consisting of a protrusion of part of the occipital lobe that contains part of the posterior horn of a lateral ventricle.

Cranium Bifidium

Defects in the formation of the cranium *(cranium bifidum)* are often associated with congenital anomalies of the brain and/or meninges. Defects of the cranium are usually in the median plane of the calvaria (Fig. 18-36*A*). The defect is often in the squamous part of the occipital bone and may include the posterior part of the foramen magnum. When the defect is small, usually only the meninges herniate and the anomaly is a **cranial meningocele,** or cranium bifidum with meningocele (Fig. 18-36*B*).

Cranium bifidum associated with herniation of the brain and/or its meninges occurs about once in every 2000 births. When the cranial defect is large, the meninges and part of the brain (Gr. *enkephalos*) herniate, forming a **meningoencephalocele** (Fig. 18-36*C*). If the protruding brain contains part of the ventricular system, the anomaly is a **meningohydroencephalocele** (Figs. 18-36*D* and 18-37).

Exencephaly and Meroanencephaly

These severe anomalies of the brain result from failure of the rostral neuropore to close during the fourth week of development. As a result, the forebrain primordium is abnormal and development of the calvaria is defective (Figs. 18-38 and 18-39). Most of the embryo's brain is exposed or extruding from the skull—**exencephaly.** Because of the abnormal structure and vascularization of the embryonic exencephalic brain, the nervous tissue undergoes degeneration. The remains of the brain appears as a spongy, vascular mass consisting mostly of hindbrain structures. Although this NTD is called *anencephaly* (Gr. *an,* without, + *enkephalos,* brain), a rudimentary brain stem and functioning neural tissue are always present in living infants (Filly, 1994). For this reason, *meroanencephaly* (Gr. *meros,* part) is a better name for this anomaly.

Meroanencephaly is a common lethal anomaly, occurring at least once in every 1000 births. It is two to four times more common in females than in males (Fig. 18-40). It is always associated with acrania (absence of the calvaria) and may be associated with *rachischisis* when defective neural tube closure is extensive (Fig. 18-41). Meroanencephaly accounts for about half of the severe NTDS in Great Britain and it is the most common serious anomaly seen in stillborn fetuses. *Sustained extrauterine life is impossible in infants with meroanencephaly.* Infants with this severe NTD survive for a few hours after birth, at most. Meroanencephaly is suspected in utero when there is an elevated level of alpha-fetoprotein in the amniotic fluid (see Chapter 6). Meroanencephaly can be easily diagnosed by ultrasonography (Fig. 18-40), fetoscopy, and radiography because extensive parts of the brain and calvaria are absent. A therapeutic abortion is usually performed, if the mother requests it, when contin-

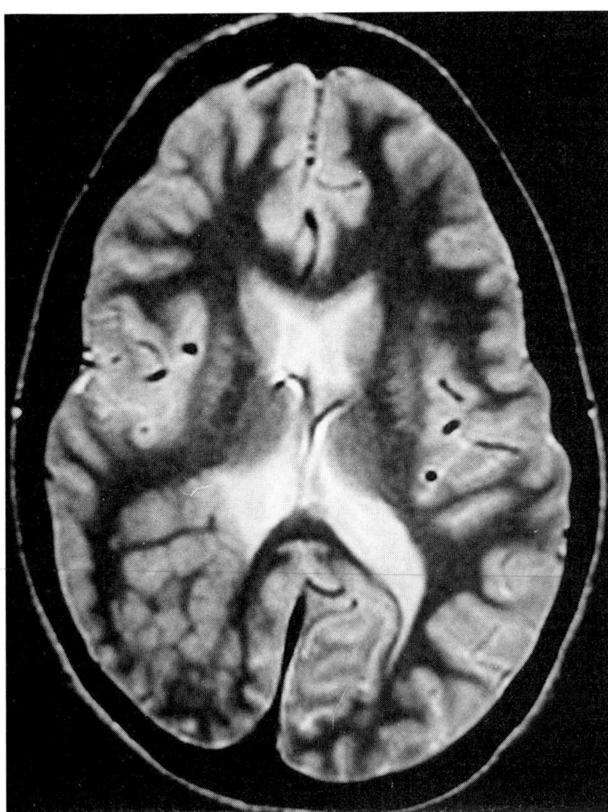

■ **Figure 18–37.** Focal heterotopic cerebral cortex. Magnetic resonance image of a 19-year-old female with seizures showing a focal heterotopic cortex of the right parietal lobe, indenting the right lateral ventricle; note the lack of organized cortex at the overlying surface of the brain. Heterotopic cortex is the result of an arrest of centrifugal migration of neuroblasts along radial processes of glial cells. (Courtesy of Dr. Gerald Smyser, Altru Health System, Grand Forks, ND.)

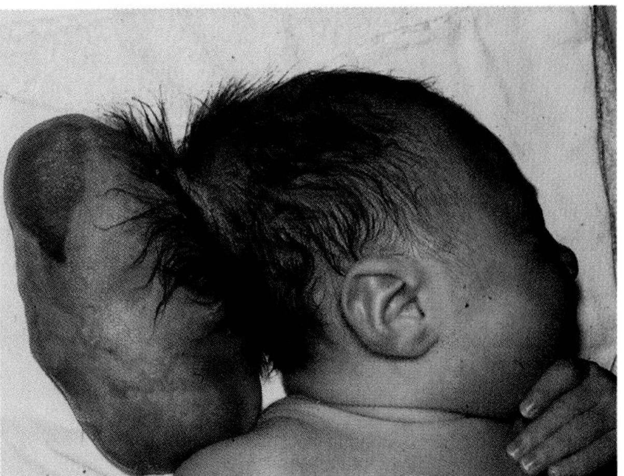

■ **Figure 18–38.** Photograph of an infant with a large meningoencephalocele in the occipital area. (Courtesy of Dr. A. E. Chudley, Section of Genetics and Metabolism, Department of Pediatrics and Child Health, Children's Hospital and University of Manitoba, Winnipeg, Manitoba, Canada.)

uation of the pregnancy will result in the birth of a child with severe anomalies, such as meroanencephaly, that are incompatible with life after birth.

Exencephaly and meroanencephaly can be induced experimentally in rats by using teratogenic agents. Studies of exencephalic human abortuses suggest that the process is similar in humans. Genetic factors are certainly involved because of the well-established familial incidence of these defects. *Meroanencephaly usually has a multifactorial inheritance* (Thompson et al., 1991). An excess of amniotic fluid **(polyhydramnios)** is often associated with meroanencephaly,

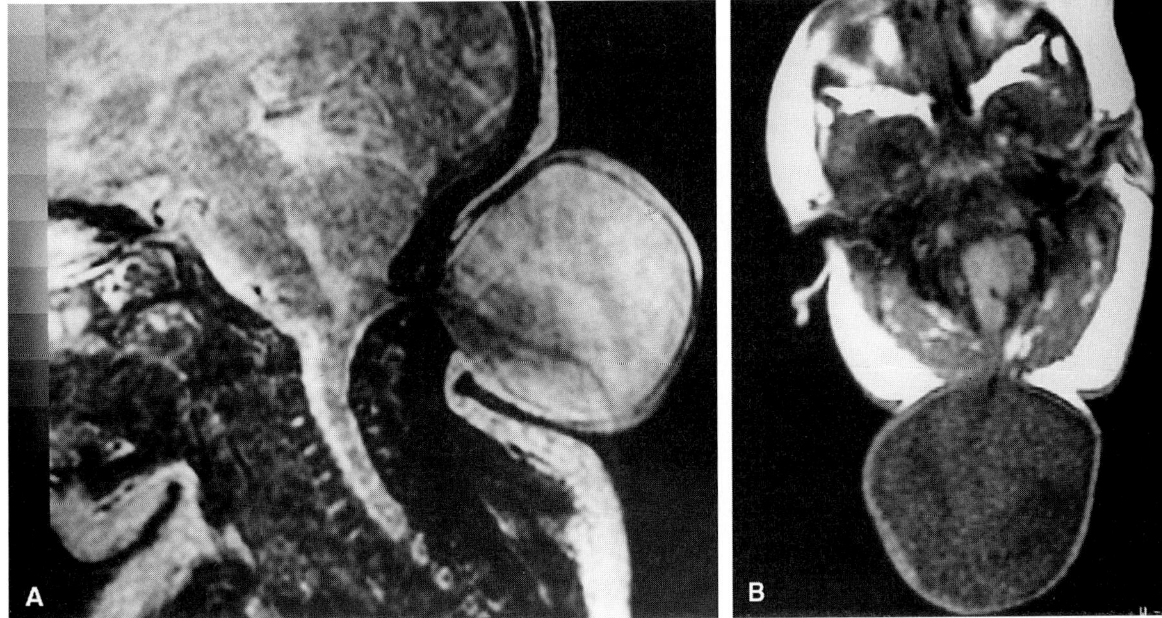

■ **Figure 18–39.** Magnetic resonance images (MRIs) of a 1-day-old infant. *A,* Sagittal MRI taken so that the CSF is bright. The image is blurred because of movement of the infant. *B,* Axial image located at the cranial defect near the foramen magnum and taken so that CSF appears dark. (Compare with Fig. 18–36.) (Courtesy of Dr. Gerald S. Smyser, Altru Health System, Grand Forks, ND.)

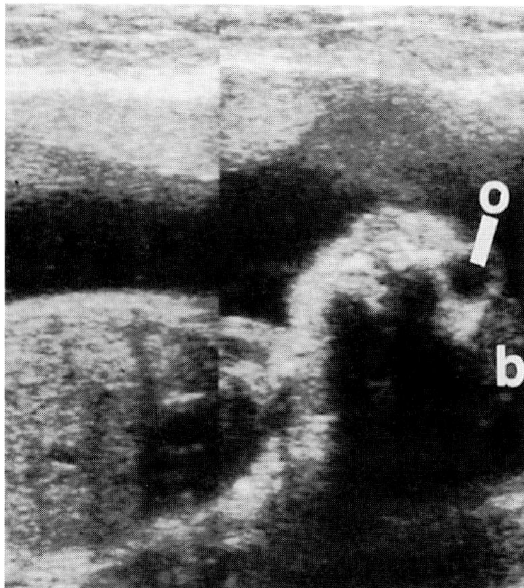

■ **Figure 18–40.** Ultrasound scan of a fetus (about 14 weeks) with meroanencephaly (anencephaly); **o** indicates the orbit and **b** represents the remnant of the brain. (Courtesy of Dr. Lyndon M. Hill, Magee-Women's Hospital, Pittsburgh, PA.)

possibly because the fetus lacks the neural control for swallowing amniotic fluid; thus the fluid does not pass into the intestines for absorption and subsequent transfer to the placenta for disposal.

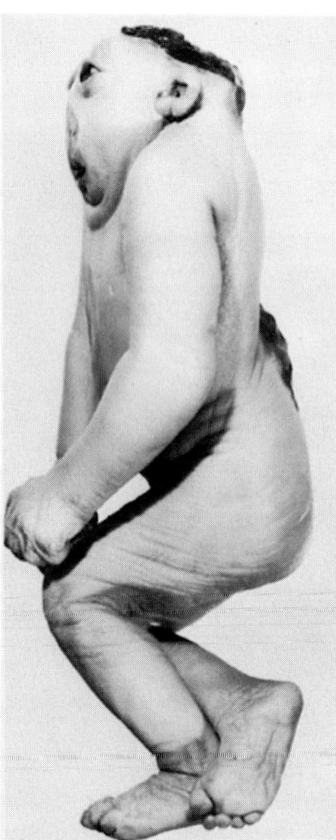

■ **Figure 18–41.** Photograph of an infant with acrania (absence of calvaria), meroanencephaly (absence of most of the brain), rachischisis (failure of fusion of several vertebral arches), and spina bifida with myeloschisis (failure of closure of the neural folds).

Microcephaly

In this uncommon condition, the calvaria and brain are small but the face is normal size (Fig. 18–42). These infants are *grossly mentally retarded* because the brain is underdeveloped—**microencephaly.** Microcephaly (Gr. *mikros,* small, + *kephale,* head) is the result of *microencephaly* (Gr. *mikros,* small, + *enkephalos,* brain), because growth of the *calvaria* is largely the result of pressure from the growing brain. The cause of microcephaly is often uncertain. Some cases appear to be genetic in origin (autosomal recessive), and others are caused by environmental factors (Behrman et al., 1996). Exposure to large amounts of ionizing radiation, infectious agents (e.g., cytomegalovirus, rubella virus, and *Toxoplasma gondii* [see Chapter 8]), and certain drugs (maternal alcohol abuse) during the fetal period are contributing factors in some cases. Microcephaly can be detected in utero by ultrasound scans carried out over the period of gestation. A small head may result from *premature synostosis* (osseous union) of all the cranial sutures (see Chapter 15); however, the calvaria is thin with exaggerated convolutional markings.

Agenesis of the Corpus Callosum

In this condition there is a complete or partial absence of the corpus callosum, the main neocortical commis-

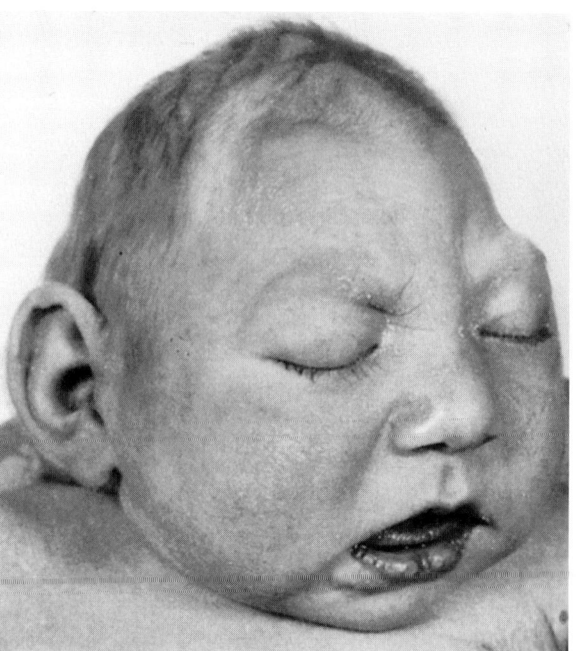

■ **Figure 18–42.** Photograph of an infant with microcephaly, showing the typical normal-sized face and small calvaria, which is covered with loose, wrinkled skin. (From Laurence KM, Weeks R: Abnormalities of the central nervous system. *In* Norman AP [ed]: *Congenital Abnormalities in Infancy,* 2nd ed. 1971. Courtesy of Blackwell Scientific Publications.)

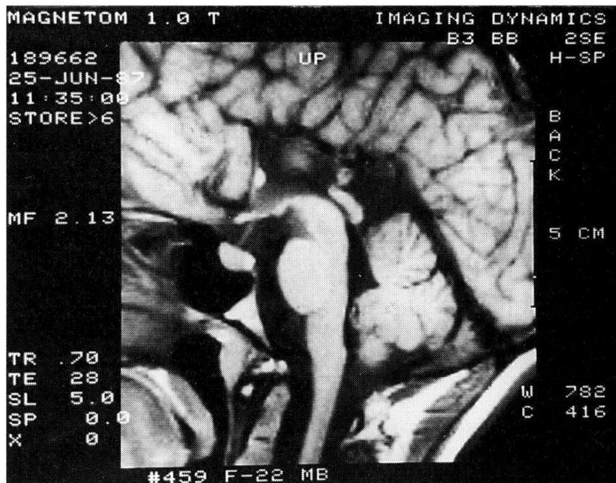

■ **Figure 18–43.** Sagittal magnetic resonance image of the brain of a 22-year-old woman with normal mentation and motor function. There is complete absence of the corpus callosum. (Courtesy of Dr. Gerald S. Smyser, Altru Health System, Grand Forks, ND.)

sure of the cerebral hemispheres (Fig. 18-43). The condition may be asymptomatic, but seizures and mental deficiency are common. In two sisters with agenesis of the corpus callosum, the only symptoms were seizures, recurrent in one but only occasional and minor in the other. Their IQs were average. The cause of this anomaly is unknown; there is no evidence that it is inherited. For more information see Friede (1989) and Lassonde and Jeeves (1994).

Hydrocephalus

Significant enlargement of the head usually results from an imbalance between the production and absorption of cerebrospinal fluid (CSF); as a result, there is **an excess of CSF** in the ventricular system of the brain (Figs. 18-44 and 18-45). *Hydrocephalus results from impaired circulation and absorption of CSF* and, in rare cases, from increased production of CSF by a choroid plexus adenoma (Behrman et al., 1996). Impaired circulation of CSF often results from **congenital aqueductal stenosis** (Fig. 18-46). The cerebral aqueduct is narrow or consists of several minute channels. In a few cases aqueductal stenosis is transmitted by an X-linked recessive trait (Behrman et al., 1996), but most cases appear to result from a *fetal viral infection* (e.g., cytomegalovirus or *Toxoplasma gondii* [see Chapter 8]), or prematurity associated with intraventricular hemorrhage. Blood in the subarachnoid space may cause obliteration of the cisterns or arachnoid villi.

Blockage of CSF circulation results in dilation of the ventricles proximal to the obstruction, internal accumulation of CSF, and pressure on the cerebral hemispheres (Fig. 18-46). This squeezes the brain between the ventricular fluid and the bones of the calvaria. In infants the internal pressure results in an accelerated rate of expansion of the brain and calvaria

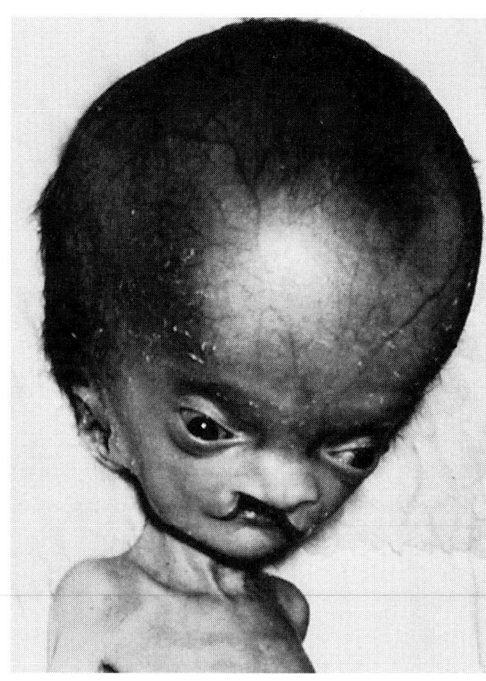

■ **Figure 18–44.** Photograph of an infant with hydrocephalus and bilateral cleft palate.

because the fibrous sutures of the calvaria are not fused. **Hydrocephalus usually refers to obstructive or noncommunicating hydrocephalus,** in which all or part of the ventricular system is enlarged. All ventricles are enlarged if the apertures of the fourth ventri-

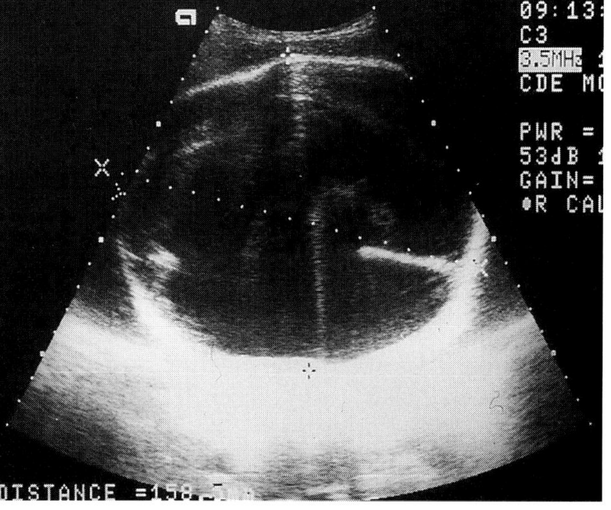

■ **Figure 18–45.** Sonogram showing massive hydrocephalus in a full-term infant. The dimensions of this fetal skull are grossly distorted by the excess of CSF. The large head exceeded maternal pelvic capacity by a wide margin. *Cephalocentesis* (drainage of CSF from the fetal brain by ultrasound-guided percutaneous needle aspiration) was necessary to allow safe delivery. While part of the midline structure of the fetal brain can be seen *(arrow),* this does not exclude some forms of holoprosencephaly (loss of midline structures), as well as all other forms of obstructive hydrocephalus. (Courtesy of Dr. C. R. Harman, Department of Obstetrics, Gynecology and Reproductive Sciences, Women's Hospital and University of Manitoba, Winnipeg, Manitoba, Canada.)

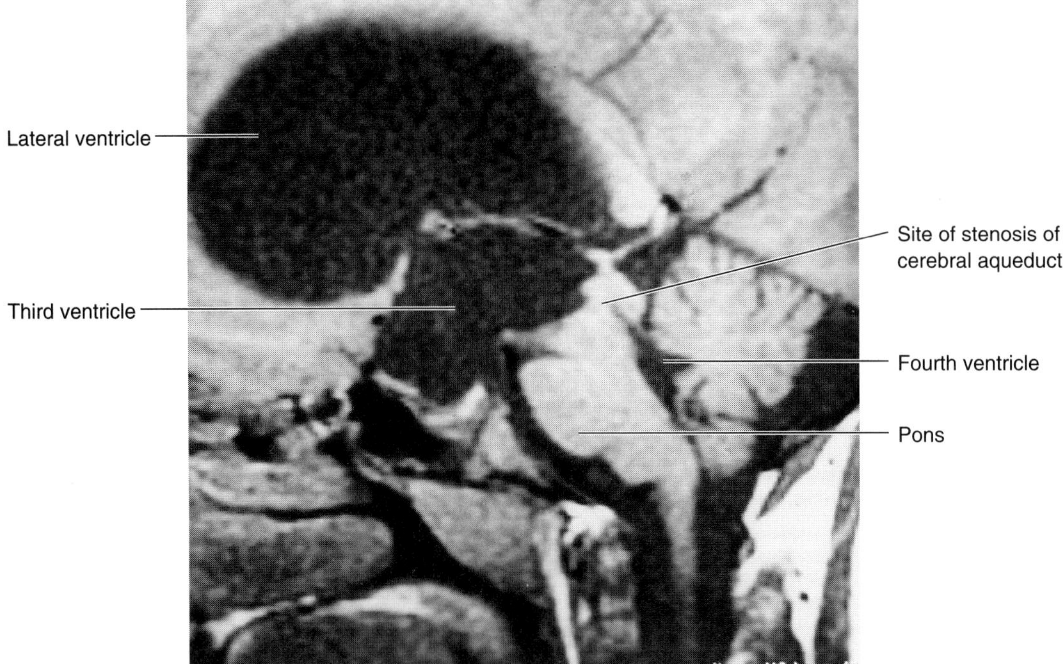

■ **Figure 18–46.** Congenital stenosis of the cerebral aqueduct. This sagittal magnetic resonance image of a 9-month-old infant with a large head shows very large lateral and third ventricles. The CSF appears dark in these images. The cerebral aqueduct appears as a dark line of fluid ventral to the tectum of the midbrain. The cranial end of the aqueduct is stenotic (narrow), which results in the absence of dark CSF. (Courtesy of Dr. Gerald S. Smyser, Altru Health System, Grand Forks, ND.)

cle or the subarachnoid spaces are blocked, whereas the lateral and third ventricles are dilated when only the cerebral aqueduct is obstructed (Fig. 18–46). Although rare, obstruction of one interventricular foramen can produce dilation of one ventricle. Hydrocephalus resulting from obliteration of the subarachnoid cisterns or malfunction of the arachnoid villi is **nonobstructive or communicating hydrocephalus.** Although hydrocephalus may be associated with spina bifida cystica, enlargement of the head may not be obvious at birth. Hydrocephalus often produces thinning of the bones of the calvaria, prominence of the forehead, atrophy of the cerebral cortex and white matter, and compression of the basal ganglia and diencephalon.

Holoprosencephaly

Teratogens, such as high doses of alcohol, can destroy embryonic cells in the median plane of the embryonic disc during the third week, producing a wide range of birth defects resulting from defective formation of the forebrain. The infants have a small forebrain, and the lateral ventricles often merge to form one large ventricle. Defects in forebrain development often cause facial anomalies resulting from a reduction of tissue in the frontonasal prominence (see Chapter 10). Holoprosencephaly is often indicated when the eyes are abnormally close together *(hypotelorism).*

Hydranencephaly

This extremely rare anomaly may be confused with hydrocephalus (Fig. 18–47). *The cerebral hemispheres are absent or represented by membranous sacs* with remnants of the cerebral cortex dispersed over the membranes. The brain stem (midbrain, pons, and medulla) is relatively intact. These infants generally appear normal at birth; however, the head grows excessively after birth because of the accumulation of CSF. A **ventriculoperitoneal shunt** is usually made to prevent further enlargement of the calvaria. Mental development fails to occur and there is little or no cognitive development. The cause of this unusual and severe anomaly is uncertain; however, there is evidence that it may be the result of an early obstruction of blood flow to the areas supplied by the internal carotid arteries (Behrman et al., 1996).

Arnold-Chiari Malformation

This is the most common congenital anomaly involving the cerebellum (Fig. 18–48). A tonguelike projection of the medulla and *inferior displacement of the vermis of the cerebellum herniates through the foramen magnum into the vertebral canal* (Taeusch et al., 1991). The anomaly results in a type of communicating hydrocephalus in which there is interference with

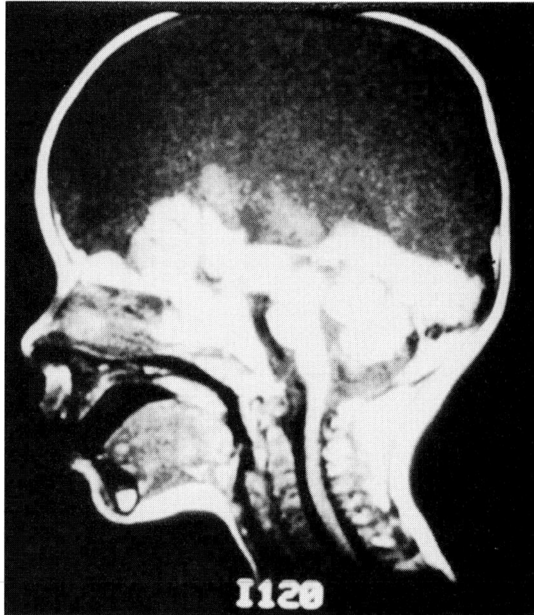

■ **Figure 18–47.** MRI (magnetic resonance image) of the head of an infant with hydranencephaly, showing the brain stem and spinal cord with remnants of the cerebellum and cerebral cortex. The remainder of the cranium is filled with CSF. (From Behrman RE, Kliegman RM, Arvin AM [eds]: *Nelson Textbook of Pediatrics,* 15th ed. Philadelphia, WB Saunders, 1996).

the absorption of CSF; as a result, the entire ventricular system is distended. The **Arnold-Chiari** or **Chiari malformation** occurs once in every 1000 births and is frequently associated with spina bifida with meningomyelocele, spina bifida with myeloschisis, and hydrocephaly. The cause of the Arnold-Chiari malformation is uncertain; however, the posterior cranial fossa is abnormally small in these infants (Friede, 1989; Gilbert-Barnes, 1997).

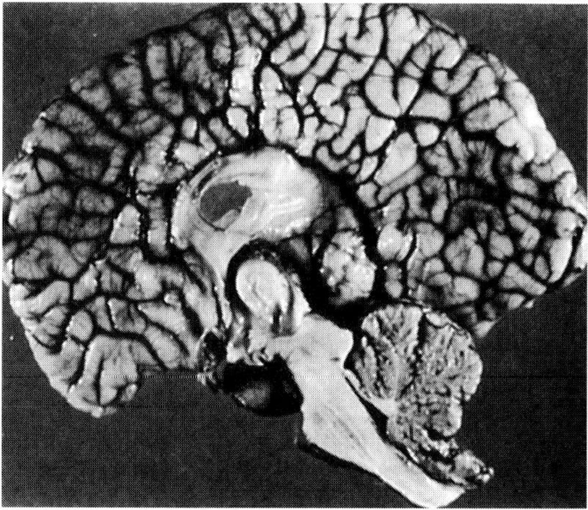

■ **Figure 18–48.** Brain of a child with a thoracolumbar meningomyelocele, showing the Arnold-Chiari malformation. The anomaly consists of elongation of the medulla with inferior displacement of the vermis of the cerebellum through the foramen magnum into the vertebral canal. (From Taeusch HW, Ballard RA, Avery ME [eds]: *Schaffer and Avery's Diseases of the Newborn,* 6th ed. Philadelphia, WB Saunders, 1991.)

Mental Retardation

Congenital impairment of intelligence may result from various genetically determined conditions (e.g., Down syndrome). Mental retardation may result from the action of a mutant gene or from a chromosomal abnormality (e.g., an extra chromosome 13, 18, or 21). Chromosomal abnormalities and mental deficiency are discussed in Chapter 8. **Maternal alcohol abuse is the most common cause of mental retardation.** The 8- to 16-week period of human development is the period of greatest sensitivity for *fetal brain damage resulting from large doses of radiation* (Otake and Schull, 1984; Persaud, 1990). By the end of the sixteenth week, most neuronal proliferation and cell migration to the cerebral cortex are completed. Cell depletion of sufficient degree in the cerebral cortex results in severe mental retardation. Therapeutic abortion is often recommended when exposure exceeds 10,000 mrad (Behrman et al., 1996). Disorders of protein, carbohydrate, or fat metabolism may also cause mental retardation. *Maternal and fetal infections* (e.g., syphilis, rubella virus, toxoplasmosis, and cytomegalovirus) and cretinism are commonly associated with mental retardation (Riley and Vorhees, 1986; Adams, 1989; Persaud, 1990). Retarded mental development throughout the *postnatal growth period* can result from birth injuries, toxins (e.g., lead), cerebral infections (e.g., meningitis), cerebral trauma resulting from head injuries, and poisoning. For a complete discussion of mental retardation and its many causes, see Behrman et al. (1996).

DEVELOPMENT OF THE PERIPHERAL NERVOUS SYSTEM

The peripheral nervous system (PNS) consists of cranial, spinal, and visceral nerves and cranial, spinal, and autonomic ganglia. The PNS develops from various sources, mostly from the *neural crest* (Evans and Hutchins, 1997). All sensory cells (somatic and visceral) of the PNS are derived from **neural crest cells.** The cell bodies of these sensory cells are located outside the CNS. With the exception of the cells in the spiral ganglion of the cochlea and the vestibular ganglion of CN VIII (vestibulocochlear nerve), all peripheral sensory cells are at first bipolar, but the two processes soon unite to form a single process and a unipolar type of neuron (Fig. 18-9*D*). This process has peripheral and central processes. The peripheral process terminates in a sensory ending, whereas the central process enters the spinal cord or brain (Fig. 18-8). The sensory cells in the ganglion of CN VIII remain bipolar. The cell body of each afferent neuron is closely invested by a capsule of modified Schwann cells—**satellite cells** (Fig. 18-8)—which are derived from neural crest cells. This capsule is continuous with the neurolemmal sheath of Schwann cells that surrounds the axons of afferent neurons. External to the satellite cells is a layer of connective tissue that is continuous with the endoneurial sheath of the nerve fibers. This connective tissue and the endoneurial sheath are derived from mesenchyme.

Neural crest cells in the developing brain migrate to form sensory ganglia only in relation to the trigeminal (CN V), facial (CN VII), vestibulocochlear (CN VIII), glossopharyngeal (CN IX), and vagus (CN X) nerves. Neural crest cells also differentiate into multipolar neurons of the *autonomic ganglia* (Fig. 18-8), including ganglia of the sympathetic trunks that lie along the sides of the vertebral bodies; collateral, or prevertebral, ganglia in plexuses of the thorax and abdomen (e.g., the cardiac, celiac, and mesenteric plexuses); and parasympathetic, or terminal, ganglia in or near the viscera (e.g., the submucosal or Meissner plexus). Cells of the paraganglia—**chromaffin cells**—are also derived from the neural crest. The term *paraganglia* includes several widely scattered groups of cells that are similar in many ways to medullary cells of the suprarenal (adrenal) glands. The cell groups largely lie retroperitoneally, often in association with sympathetic ganglia. The carotid and aortic bodies also have small islands of chromaffin cells associated with them. These widely scattered groups of chromaffin cells constitute the **chromaffin system.** Neural crest cells also give rise to melanoblasts (the precursors of the *melanocytes*) and cells of the medulla of the suprarenal gland.

Spinal Nerves

Motor nerve fibers arising from the spinal cord begin to appear at the end of the fourth week (Figs. 18-4 and 18-6 to 18-8). The nerve fibers arise from cells in the *basal plates* of the developing spinal cord and emerge as a continuous series of rootlets along its ventrolateral surface. The fibers destined for a particular developing muscle group become arranged in a bundle, forming a **ventral nerve root.** The nerve fibers of the **dorsal nerve root** are formed by axons derived from neural crest cells that migrate to the dorsolateral aspect of the spinal cord, where they differentiate into the cells of the **spinal ganglion** (Figs. 18-7 to 18-9). The central processes of neurons in the spinal ganglion form a single bundle that grows into the spinal cord, opposite the apex of the dorsal horn of gray matter (Fig. 18-4*B* and *C*). The distal processes of spinal ganglion cells grow toward the ventral nerve root and eventually join it to form a spinal nerve. Immediately after being formed, a **mixed spinal nerve** divides into dorsal and ventral primary rami (L., branches). The **dorsal primary ramus,** the smaller division, innervates the dorsal axial musculature (see Fig. 16-1), vertebrae, posterior intervertebral joints, and part of the skin of the back. The **ventral primary ramus,** the major division of each spinal nerve, contributes to the innervation of the limbs and ventrolateral parts of the body wall. The major **nerve plexuses** (cervical, brachial, and lumbosacral) are formed by ventral primary rami.

As each limb bud develops, the nerves from the spinal cord segments opposite to the bud elongate and grow into the limb. The nerve fibers are distributed to its muscles, which differentiate from myogenic cells that originate from the somites (see Chapter 16). The skin of the developing limbs is also supplied in a segmental manner. Early in development, successive ventral primary rami are joined by connecting loops of nerve fibers, especially those supplying the limbs (e.g., the *brachial plexus* [Moore, 1992]). The dorsal division of the trunks of these plexuses supplies the extensor muscles and the extensor surface of the limbs; the ventral divisions of the trunks supply the flexor muscles and the flexor surface. The dermatomes and cutaneous innervation of the limbs are described in Chapter 17.

Cranial Nerves

Twelve pairs of cranial nerves form during the fifth and sixth weeks of development. They are classified into three groups, according to their embryological origins.

SOMATIC EFFERENT CRANIAL NERVES

The trochlear (CN IV), abducent (CN VI), hypoglossal (CN XII), and the greater part of the oculomotor (CN III) nerves are homologous with the ventral roots of spinal nerves (Fig. 18-49). The cells of origin of these nerves are located in the *somatic efferent column* (derived from the basal plates) of the brain stem. Their axons are distributed to the muscles derived from the head myotomes (preotic and occipital; see Fig. 16-2).

The **hypoglossal nerve** (CN XII) resembles a spinal nerve more than do the other somatic efferent cranial nerves. CN XII develops by the fusion of the ventral root fibers of three or four occipital nerves (Fig. 18-49*A*). Sensory roots, corresponding to the dorsal roots of spinal nerves, are absent. The somatic motor fibers originate from the *hypoglossal nucleus,* consisting of motor cells resembling those of the ventral horn of the spinal cord. These fibers leave the ventrolateral wall of the medulla in several groups, the *hypoglossal nerve roots,* which converge to form the common trunk of CN XII (Fig. 18-49*B*). They grow rostrally and eventually innervate the muscles of the tongue, which are thought to be derived from the occipital myotomes (see Fig. 16-2). With development of the neck, the hypoglossal nerve comes to lie at a progressively higher level.

The **abducent nerve** (CN VI) arises from nerve cells in the basal plates of the metencephalon. It passes from its ventral surface to the posterior of the three preotic myotomes from which the lateral rectus muscle of the eye is thought to originate.

The **trochlear nerve** (CN IV) arises from nerve cells in the somatic efferent column in the posterior part of the midbrain. Although a motor nerve, it emerges from the brain stem dorsally and passes ventrally to supply the superior oblique muscle of the eye.

The **oculomotor nerve** (CN III) supplies most of the muscles of the eye (i.e., the superior, inferior, and medial recti and inferior oblique muscles), which are thought to be derived from the first preotic myotomes.

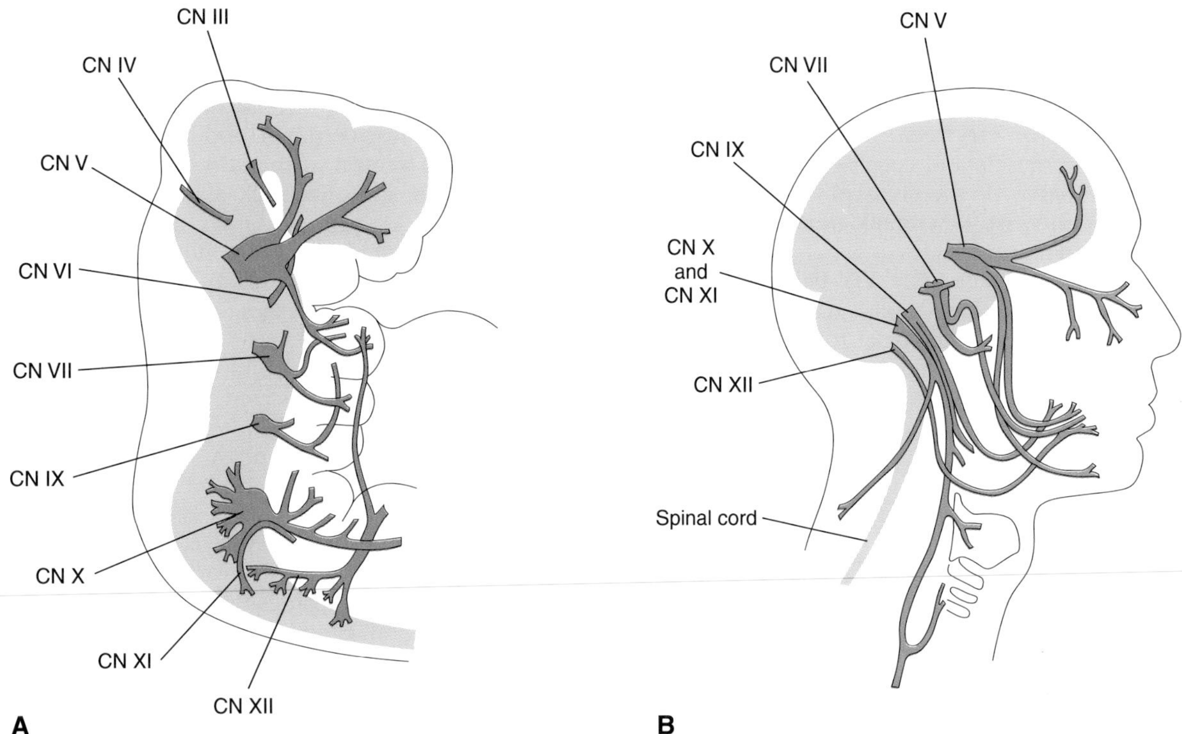

■ **Figure 18–49.** *A*, Schematic drawing of a 5-week-old embryo showing the distribution of most of the cranial nerves, especially those supplying the pharyngeal arches. *B*, Schematic drawing of the head and neck of an adult, showing the general distribution of most of the cranial nerves.

NERVES OF THE PHARYNGEAL ARCHES

Cranial nerves V, VII, IX, and X supply the embryonic pharyngeal arches; thus, the structures that develop from these arches are innervated by these cranial nerves (Fig. 18-49*A*; see Table 10-1).

The **trigeminal nerve** (CN V) is the nerve of the first pharyngeal arch, but it has an ophthalmic division that is not a pharyngeal arch component. *CN V is chiefly sensory and is the principal sensory nerve for the head.* The large **trigeminal ganglion** lies beside the rostral end of the pons, and its cells are derived from the most anterior part of the neural crest. The central processes of cells in this ganglion form the large sensory root of CN V, which enters the lateral portion of the pons. The peripheral processes of cells in this ganglion separate into three large divisions (ophthalmic, maxillary, and mandibular nerves). Their sensory fibers supply the skin of the face as well as the lining of the mouth and nose (see Fig. 10-7). The *motor fibers of CN V* arise from cells in the most anterior part of the *special visceral efferent column* in the metencephalon. The motor nucleus of CN V lies at the midlevel of the pons. The fibers leave the pons at the site of the entering sensory fibers and pass to the muscles of mastication and to other muscles that develop in the mandibular prominence of the first pharyngeal arch (see Table 10-1). The mesencephalic nucleus of CN V differentiates from cells in the midbrain that extend rostrally from the metencephalon.

The **facial nerve** (CN VII) is the nerve of the second pharyngeal arch. It consists mostly of motor fibers that arise principally from a nuclear group in the *special visceral efferent column* in the caudal part of the pons. These fibers are distributed to the *muscles of facial expression* and to other muscles that develop in the mesenchyme of the second pharyngeal arch (see Table 10-1). The small general visceral efferent component of CN VII terminates in the peripheral autonomic ganglia of the head. The sensory fibers of CN VII arise from the cells of the *geniculate ganglion.* The central processes of these cells enter the pons, and the peripheral processes pass to the greater superficial petrosal nerve and, via the chorda tympani nerve, to the taste buds in the anterior two-thirds of the tongue.

The **glossopharyngeal nerve** (CN IX) is the nerve of the third pharyngeal arch. Its motor fibers arise from the special and, to a lesser extent, general visceral efferent columns of the anterior part of the myelencephalon. CN IX forms from several rootlets that arise from the medulla just caudal to the developing internal ear. All the fibers from the special visceral efferent column are distributed to the stylopharyngeus muscle, which is derived from mesenchyme in the third pharyngeal arch (see Table 10-1). The general efferent fibers are distributed to the otic ganglion, from which postganglionic fibers pass to the parotid and posterior lingual glands. The *sensory fibers of CN IX* are distributed as general sensory and special visceral afferent fibers (taste fibers) to the posterior part of the tongue.

The **vagus nerve** (CN X) is formed by fusion of the nerves of the fourth and sixth pharyngeal arches (see

Table 10-1). It has large visceral efferent and visceral afferent components that are distributed to the heart, foregut and its derivatives, and to a large part of the midgut. The nerve of the fourth pharyngeal arch becomes the **superior laryngeal nerve,** which supplies the cricothyroid muscle and constrictor muscles of the pharynx. The nerve of the sixth pharyngeal arch becomes the **recurrent laryngeal nerve,** which supplies various laryngeal muscles.

The **accessory nerve** (CN XI) has two separate origins (Fig. 18-49). The cranial root is a posterior extension of CN X, and the spinal root arises from the cranial five or six cervical segments of the spinal cord. The fibers of the cranial root emerge from the lateral surface of the medulla, where they join the vagus nerve and supply the muscles of the soft palate and intrinsic muscles of the larynx. The fibers of the spinal root supply the sternocleidomastoid and trapezius muscles (Moore, 1992).

SPECIAL SENSORY NERVES

The **olfactory nerve** (CN I) arises from the olfactory bulb. The olfactory cells are bipolar neurons that differentiate from cells in the epithelial lining of the primitive nasal sac. The axons of the olfactory cells are collected into 18 to 20 bundles around which the *cribriform plate* of the ethmoid bone develops. These unmyelinated nerve fibers end in the olfactory bulb.

The **optic nerve** (CN II) is formed by more than a million nerve fibers that grow into the brain from neuroblasts in the primitive retina. Because the optic nerve develops from the evaginated wall of the forebrain, it actually represents a fiber tract of the brain. Development of the optic nerve is described in Chapter 19.

The **vestibulocochlear nerve** (CN VIII) consists of two kinds of sensory fiber in two bundles; these fibers are known as the vestibular and cochlear nerves. The **vestibular nerve** originates in the semicircular ducts and the **cochlear nerve** proceeds from the cochlear duct, in which the **spiral organ** (of Corti) develops. The bipolar neurons of the vestibular nerve have their cell bodies in the vestibular ganglion. The central processes of these cells terminate in the *vestibular nuclei* in the floor of the fourth ventricle. The bipolar neurons of the *cochlear nerve* have their cell bodies in the spiral ganglion. The central processes of these cells end in the ventral and dorsal *cochlear nuclei* in the medulla.

DEVELOPMENT OF THE AUTONOMIC NERVOUS SYSTEM

Functionally, the autonomic system can be divided into sympathetic (thoracolumbar) and parasympathetic (craniosacral) parts.

Sympathetic Nervous System

During the fifth week *neural crest cells* in the thoracic region migrate along each side of the spinal cord, where they form paired cellular masses (ganglia) dorsolateral to the aorta (Fig. 18-8). All these segmentally arranged **sympathetic ganglia** are connected in a bilateral chain by longitudinal nerve fibers. These ganglionated cords—**sympathetic trunks**—are located on each side of the vertebral bodies. Some neural crest cells migrate ventral to the aorta and form neurons in the **preaortic ganglia,** such as the celiac and mesenteric ganglia (Fig. 18-8). Other neural crest cells migrate to the area of the heart, lungs, and gastrointestinal tract, where they form terminal ganglia in sympathetic organ plexuses, located near or within these organs.

After the sympathetic trunks have formed, axons of sympathetic neurons, located in the **intermediolateral cell column** (lateral horn) of the thoracolumbar segments of the spinal cord, pass through the ventral root of a spinal nerve and a **white ramus communicans** (connecting branch) to a paravertebral ganglion (Fig. 18-8). Here they may synapse with neurons or ascend or descend in the sympathetic trunk to synapse at other levels. Other preganglionic fibers pass through the paravertebral ganglia without synapsing, forming splanchnic nerves to the viscera. The postganglionic fibers course through a **gray ramus communicans,** passing from a sympathetic ganglion into a spinal nerve; hence, the sympathetic trunks are composed of ascending and descending fibers.

Parasympathetic Nervous System

The preganglionic parasympathetic fibers arise from neurons in nuclei of the brain stem and in the sacral region of the spinal cord. The fibers from the brain stem leave through the oculomotor (CN III), facial (CN VII), glossopharyngeal (CN IX), and vagus (CN X) nerves. The postganglionic neurons are located in peripheral ganglia or in plexuses near or within the structure being innervated (e.g., the pupil of the eye and salivary glands).

Congenital Aganglionic Megacolon

Congenital aganglionic megacolon or **Hirschsprung disease** results from absence of ganglion cells in the wall of the large intestine, extending proximally and continuously from the anus for a variable distance (Wyllie, 1996). Hirschsprung disease is the most common cause of lower intestinal obstruction in the neonate, with an overall incidence of 1:5000 births (Fig. 18-50). The absence of innervation of the colon results from failure of enteric neuronal precursors to migrate into the wall of the lower bowel (Naftel and Hardy, 1997). The affected segment of colon is paralyzed in a constricted state, which results in distention of the proximal, normally innervated bowel. The aganglionic segment is limited to the rectosigmoid colon in 75% of cases. The clinical symptoms of Hirschsprung disease usually begin within 48 hours of birth with the delayed passage of meconium (fetal feces). Males are affected more often than females (4:1).

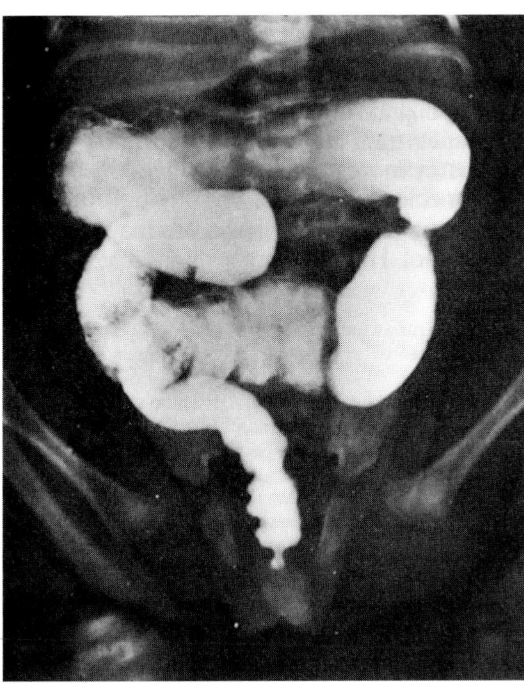

■ **Figure 18–50.** Radiograph of the large bowel showing rectosigmoid narrowing and dilation of the proximal colon, resulting from congenital aganglionic megacolon (Hirschsprung disease). (From Avery ME, Taeusch HW [eds]: *Schaffer's Diseases of the Newborn,* 5th ed. Philadelphia, WB Saunders, 1984.)

SUMMARY OF THE NERVOUS SYSTEM

The central nervous system (CNS) develops from a dorsal thickening of ectoderm—the **neural plate**—which appears around the middle of the third week. The neural plate is induced by the underlying **notochord** and paraxial mesoderm. The neural plate becomes infolded to form a **neural groove** that has neural folds on each side. When the neural folds begin to fuse to form the **neural tube** beginning during the fourth week, some neuroectodermal cells are not included in it, but remain between the neural tube and surface ectoderm as the **neural crest.**

The cranial end of the neural tube forms the brain, the primordia of which are the forebrain, midbrain, and hindbrain. The **forebrain** gives rise to the cerebral hemispheres and diencephalon. The embryonic **midbrain** becomes the adult midbrain, and the **hindbrain** gives rise to the pons, cerebellum, and medulla oblongata. The remainder of the neural tube becomes the spinal cord. The **neural canal,** the lumen of the neural tube, becomes the ventricles of the brain and the central canal of the spinal cord. The walls of the neural tube thicken by proliferation of its neuroepithelial cells. These cells give rise to all nerve and macroglial cells in the central nervous system. The microglia differentiate from mesenchymal cells that enter the central nervous system with the blood vessels. The **pituitary gland** develops from two completely different parts:

- an ectodermal upgrowth from the stomodeum—the *hypophysial pouch*—forms the *adenohypophysis*
- a neuroectodermal downgrowth from the diencephalon—the *neurohypophysial bud*—forms the *neurohypophysis* (Table 18-1).

Cells in the cranial, spinal, and autonomic ganglia are derived from **neural crest cells,** which originate in the neural crest. Schwann cells, which myelinate the axons external to the spinal cord, also arise from neural crest cells. Similarly, most of the autonomic nervous system and all chromaffin tissue, including the suprarenal medulla, develop from neural crest cells.

There are three types of congenital anomaly of the nervous system:

- structural anomalies caused by abnormal organogenesis, such as neural tube defects (NTDs) resulting from defective closure of the neural tube
- disturbances in the organization of the cells of the nervous system (e.g., the effects of high doses of radiation and severe malnutrition) that result in mental retardation
- errors of metabolism, which are often inherited, cause mental retardation because of an accumulation of toxic substances (e.g., phenylketonuria) or a deficiency of essential substances (e.g., congenital hypothyroidism)

Congenital anomalies of the central nervous system are common (about 3 per 1000 births). Defects in the closure of the neural tube (NTDs) account for most severe anomalies (e.g., spinal bifida cystica). The anomalies include the overlying tissues. Some anomalies of the CNS are caused by genetic factors (e.g., numerical chromosomal abnormalities such as trisomy 21); others result from environmental factors such as infectious agents, drugs, and metabolic disease. However, *most CNS anomalies are caused by a combination of genetic and environmental factors.* Gross congenital anomalies (e.g., meroanencephaly) are incompatible with life. Other severe anomalies (e.g., spina bifida with meningomyelocele) cause functional disability (e.g., muscle paralysis in the lower limbs). Severe abnormalities of the CNS also result from congenital anomalies of the ventricular system of the brain. **There are two main types of hydrocephalus:**

- *obstructive or noncommunicating hydrocephalus* (blockage of CSF flow in the ventricular system)
- *nonobstructive or communicating hydrocephalus* (blockage of CSF flow in the subarachnoid space)

In most cases, congenital hydrocephalus is associated with spina bifida with meningomyelocele.

Mental retardation may result from chromosomal abnormalities occurring during gametogenesis, from metabolic disorders, maternal alcohol abuse, or from infections occurring during prenatal life. Various postnatal conditions (e.g., cerebral infection or trauma) may also cause abnormal mental development.

Clinically Oriented Problems

Case 18–1

A pregnant woman developed polyhydramnios over the course of a few days (acute polyhydramnios). After an ultrasonographic examination, a radiologist reported that the fetus had acrania and meroanencephaly.

- How soon can meroanencephaly (anencephaly) be detected by ultrasound scanning?
- Why is polyhydramnios associated with meroanencephaly?
- What other techniques could be used to confirm the diagnosis of meroanencephaly?

Case 18–2

A male infant was born with a large lumbar meningomyelocele that was covered with a thin membranous sac. Within a few days the sac ulcerated and began to leak. A marked neurological deficit was detected inferior to the level of the sac.

- What is the embryological basis of this anomaly?
- What is the basis of the neurological deficit?
- What structures would likely be affected?

Case 18–3

A CT scan of an infant with an enlarged head showed dilation of the lateral and third ventricles.

- What is this condition called?
- Where would the blockage most likely be to produce this abnormal dilation of the ventricles?
- Is this condition usually recognizable before birth?
- How do you think this condition might be treated surgically?

Case 18–4

An infant was born with an abnormally large head.

- Is an enlarged head in an infant synonymous with hydrocephalus?
- What condition is usually associated with an abnormally small head?
- Is growth of the skull dependent on growth of the brain?
- What environmental factors are known to cause microencephaly?

Case 18–5

A radiologist reported that a child's cerebral ventricles were dilated posteriorly, and that the lateral ventricles were widely separated by a dilated third ventricle. Agenesis of the corpus callosum was diagnosed.

- What is the common symptom associated with agenesis of the corpus callosum?
- Are some patients asymptomatic?
- What is the basis of the dilated third ventricle?

Discussion of these problems appears at the back of the book.

REFERENCES AND SUGGESTED READING

Adams J: Prenatal exposure to teratogenic agents and neurodevelopmental outcome. *Res in Infant Assess (BD:OAS) 25:*63, 1989.

Alvarez IS, Schoenwolf GC: Expansion of surface epithelium provides the major extrinsic force for bending of the neural tube. *J Exp Zool 261:*340, 1992.

Barkovich AJ: *Pediatric Neuroimaging.* New York, Raven Press, 1990.

Barr, ML, Kiernan JA: *The Human Nervous System: An Anatomical Viewpoint,* 6th ed. Philadelphia, JB Lippincott, 1993.

Behrman RE, Kliegman RM, Arvin AM (eds): *Nelson Textbook of Pediatrics,* 15th ed. Philadelphia, WB Saunders, 1996.

Bell JE: The pathology of central nervous system defects in human fetuses of different gestational ages. *In* Persaud TVN (ed): *Advances in the Study of Birth Defects, Vol 7. Central Nervous System and Craniofacial Malformations.* New York, Alan R Liss, 1982.

Belzberg AJ, Myles ST, Trevenen CL: The human tail and spinal dysraphism. *J Pediatr Surg 26:*1243, 1991.

Brumfield CG, Aronin PA, Cloud GA, Davis RO: Fetal myelomeningocele. Is antenatal ultrasound useful in predicting neonatal outcome. *J Reprod Med 40:*26, 1995.

Bruni JE, Del Bigio MR: Hydrocephalus. *In Encylopedia of Human Biology,* 2nd ed. New York, Academic Press, 1997.

Bruni JE, Del Bigio MR, Cardoso ER, Persaud TVN: Hereditary hydrocephalus in laboratory animals and humans. *Exp Pathol 35:*239, 1988.

Carlson BM: *Human Embryology and Developmental Biology.* St Louis, Mosby, 1994.

Caviness VS Jr, Takahashi T: Proliferative events in the cerebral ventricular zone. *Brain Dev 17:*159, 1995.

Chuong CM: Adhesion molecules (N-CAM and tenascin) in embryonic development and tissue regeneration. *J Craniofac Genet Dev Biol 10:*147, 1990.

Copp AJ, Bernfield M: Accumulation of basement membrane-associated hyaluronate is reduced in the posterior neuropore region of mutant (curly tail) mouse embryo developing spinal neural tube defects. *Dev Biol 130:*583, 1988.

Cormack DH: *Essential Histology.* Philadelphia, JB Lippincott, 1993.

Darnell DK, Schoenwolf GC: Vertical induction of engrailed-2 and other region-specific markers in the early chick embryo. *Dev Dyn 209:*45, 1997.

DeVellis J, Ciment G, Lauder J (eds): *Neuroembryology. Cellular and Molecular Approaches.* New York, Alan R Liss, 1988.

Dias MS, Pang D: Split cord malformations. *Neurosurg Clin North Am 6:*339, 1995.

Elder GA, Major EO: Early appearance of type II astrocytes in developing human fetal brain. *Brain Res 470:*146, 1988.

Evans OB, Hutchins JB: Development of the nervous system. *In* Haines DE (ed): *Fundamental Neuroscience.* New York, Churchill Livingstone, 1997.

Evrard P: Les troubles du developpement prenatal du cortex cerebral human. *Bull Mem Acad R Med Belg 143:*356, 1988.

Filly RA: Ultrasound evaluation of the fetal neural axis. *In* Callen PW (ed): *Ultrasonography in Obstetrics and Gynecology,* 3rd ed. Philadelphia, WB Saunders, 1994.

Flint G: Embryology of the nervous system. *Br J Neurosurg 3:*131, 1989.

Forman R, Chou S, Koren G: The role of folic acid in preventing neural tube defects. *Contemp Ob/Gyn 4:*16, 1995.

Friede RL: *Developmental Neuropathology,* 2nd ed. Berlin, Springer-Verlag, 1989.

Gabrielli S, Pilu G: Prenatal diagnosis of the head and neck and central nervous system. *In* Reece EA, Hobbins JC, Mahoney MJ, Petrie RH: *Medicine of the Fetus and the Mother.* Philadelphia, JB Lippincott, 1992.

Gilbert-Barnes E (ed): *Potter's Pathology of the Fetus and Infant,* 2 vols. St Louis, Mosby-Year Book, 1997.

Gordon R: A review of the theories of vertebrate neurulation and their relationship to the mechanics of neural tube birth defects. *J Embryol Exp Morph 89(Suppl):*229, 1985.

Graham DI, Lantos PL (eds): *Greenfield's Neuropathology,* 2 vols, 6th ed. New York, Oxford University Press, 1997.

Greenough A, Osborne J, Sutherland S (eds): *Congenital, Perinatal and Neonatal Infections.* Edinburgh, Churchill Livingstone, 1992.

Haines DE (ed): *Fundamental Neuroscience.* New York, Churchill Livingstone, 1997.

Hamburger V: History of the discovery of neuronal death in embryos. *J Neurobiol 23:*116, 1992.

Hanson MA (ed): *The Fetal and Neonatal Brain Stem: Developmental and Clinical Issues.* Cambridge, Cambridge University Press, 1991.

Hunter AGW, Cleveland RH, Blickman JG, Holmes LB: A study of level of lesion, associated malformations and sib occurrence risks in spina bifida. *Teratology 54:*213, 1996.

Hutchins JB, Naftel JP, Ard MD: The cell biology of neurons and glia. *In* Haines DE (ed): *Fundamental Neuroscience.* New York, Churchill Livingstone, 1997.

Jacobson M: *Developmental Neurobiology,* 3rd ed. New York, Plenum Publishing, 1992.

Kollias SS, Ball WS, Prenger EC: Review of the embryologic development of the pituitary gland and report of a case of hypophyseal duplication detected by MRI. *Neuroradiology 37:*3, 1995.

Koshi R, Koshi T, Jeyaseelan L, Vettivel S: Morphology of the corpus callosum in human fetuses. *Clin Anat 10:*22, 1997.

Lassonde M, Jeeves MA (eds): *Callosal Agenesis. A Natural Split Brain?* New York, Plenum Publishing, 1994.

Laurence KM, Weeks R: Abnormalities of the central nervous system. *In* Norman AP (ed): *Congenital Abnormalities in Infancy,* 2nd ed. Oxford, Blackwell Scientific Publications, 1971.

Maden M, Ong DE, Chytil F: Retinoid-binding protein distribution in the developing mammalian nervous system. *Development 109:*75, 1990.

Martinez-Frias M-L, Urioste M, Bermejo E, et al: Epidemiological analysis of multi-site closure failure of neural tube in humans. *Am J Med Genet 66:*64, 1996.

Martinez-Martinez PFA: *Neuroanatomy. Development and Structure of the Central Nervous System.* Philadelphia, WB Saunders, 1982.

Moore KL: *Clinically Oriented Anatomy,* 3rd ed. Baltimore, Williams & Wilkins, 1992.

Müller F, O'Rahilly R: The development of the human brain from a closed neural tube at stage 13. *Anat Embryol (Berl) 177:*203–224, 1988.

Müller F, O'Rahilly R: The development of the human brain, including the longitudinal zoning in the diencephalon at stage 15. *Anat Embryol (Berl) 179:*55, 1988.

Müller F, O'Rahilly R: Development of anencephaly and its variants. *Am J Anat 190:*193, 1991.

Murphy M, Seagroatt V, Hey K, et al: Neural tube defects 1974-1994 — down but not out. *Arch Dis Child 75:*F133, 1996.

Murray RM, Jones P, O'Callaghan E: Fetal brain development and later schizophrenia. *Ciba Found Symp 156:*155, 1991.

Naftel JP, Hardy SGP: Visceral motor pathways. *In* Haines DE (ed): *Fundamental Neuroscience.* New York, Churchill Livingstone, 1997.

Noden DM: Spatial integration among cells forming the cranial peripheral neurons. *J Neurobiol 24:*248, 1993.

Norman MG, McGillivray BC, Kalousek DK, et al: *Congenital Malformations of the Brain.* Oxford, Oxford University Press, 1995.

Okano H: Two major mechanisms regulating cell-fate decisions in the developing nervous system. *Dev Growth Differ 37:*619, 1995.

O'Rahilly R, Gardner E: The timing and sequence of events in the development of the human nervous system during the embryonic period proper. *Z Anat Entwicklungsgesch 134:*1, 1971.

Otake M, Schull WJ: *In utero* exposure to A-bomb radiation and mental retardation: a reassessment. *Br J Radiol 52:*409, 1984.

Parkinson D, Del Bigio MR: Posterior "septum" of human spinal cord: normal developmental variations, composition, and terminology. *Anat Rec 244:*572, 1996.

Persaud TVN: Abnormal development of the central nervous system. *Anat Anz 150:*44, 1981.

Persaud TVN: *Environmental Causes of Human Birth Defects.* Springfield, IL, Charles C Thomas, 1990.

Prechtl HF: Developmental neurology of the fetus. *Baillieres Clin Obstet Gynaecol 2:*21, 1988.

Ralcewicz TA, Persaud TVN: Effects of prenatal exposure to low dose ionizing radiation on the development of the cerebellar cortex in the rat. *Histol Histopathol 10:*371, 1995.

Riley EP, Vorhees CV (eds): *Handbook of Behavioral Teratology.* New York, Plenum Press, 1986.

Rodier PM: Developmental toxicology. *Toxicol Pathol 18:*89, 1990.

Rutishauser U, Jessell TM: Cell adhesion molecules in vertebrate neural development. *Physiol Rev 68:*819, 1988.

Sable DB, Yeh J: Growth factor receptor messenger RNA expression in human fetal brain regions. *Obstet Gynecol 86:*240, 1995.

Sanes JR: Extracellular matrix molecules that influence neural development. *Annu Rev Neurosci 12:*491, 1989.

Sarwark JL: Spina bifida. *Pediatr Clin North Am 43:*1151, 1996.

Sasaki A, Hirato J, Nakazato Y, Ishida Y: Immunohistochemical study of the early human fetal brain. *Acta Neuropathol Berl 76:*128, 1988.

Sausedo RA, Smith JL, Schoenwolf GC: Role of nonrandomly oriented cell division in shaping and bending of the neural plate. *J Comp Neurol 381:*473, 1997.

Schnurch H, Risau W: Differentiating and mature neurons express the acidic fibroblast growth factor gene during chick neural development. *Development 111:*1143, 1991.

Scheoenwolf GG, Smith JL: Mechanisms of neurulation; traditional viewpoint and recent advances. *Development 109:*243, 1990.

Shaw GM, Velie EM, Shaffer D: Risk of neural tube defect-affected pregnancies among obese women. *JAMA 275:*1093, 1996.

Smith AS, Blaser SI, Ross JS, Weinstein MA: Magnetic resonance imaging of disturbances in neuronal migration: illustration of an embryonic process. *Radiographics 9:*509, 1989.

Squier MV: A pathological approach to the diagnosis of hydrocephalus. *Bull Roy Coll of Pathol 95:*iv, 1996.

Stagiannis KD, Sepulveda W, Bower S: Early prenatal diagnosis of holoprosencephaly: the value of transvaginal ultrasonography. *Eur J Obstet Gynecol Reprod Biol 61:*175, 1995.

Staugaitis SM, Colman DR, Pedraza L: Membrane adhesion and other functions for the myelin basic proteins. *BioEssays 18:*13, 1996.

Taeusch HW, Ballard RA, Avery ME (eds): *Schaffer and Avery's Diseases of the Newborn,* 6th ed. Philadelphia, WB Saunders, 1991.

Thompson MW, McInnes RR, Willard HF: *Thompson & Thompson Genetics in Medicine,* 5th ed. Philadelphia, WB Saunders, 1991.

Trojan S, Lodin Z, Mares P, et al: Physiological and pathological aspects of neuroontogenesis. *Physiol Rev 40:*223, 1991.

Van Allen MI, Fraser FC, Dallaire L, et al: Recommendations on the use of folic acid supplementation to prevent the recurrence of neural tube defects. *Can Med Assoc J 149:*1239, 1993.

Van Allen MI, Kalousek DK, Chernoff GF, et al: Evidence for multisite closure of the neural tube in humans. *Am J Genet 47:*723, 1993.

Van Essen DC: A tension-based theory of morphogenesis and compact wiring in the central nervous system. *Nature 385:*313, 1997.

Wald NJ, Cuckle HS: AFP screening in early pregnancy. *In* Spencer JAD (ed): *Fetal Monitoring.* Oxford, Oxford University Press, 1991.

Wyllie R: Congenital aganglionic megacolon (Hirschsprung disease). *In* Behrman RE, Kliegman RM, Arvin AM (eds): *Nelson Textbook of Pediatrics,* 15th ed. Philadelphia, WB Saunders, 1996.

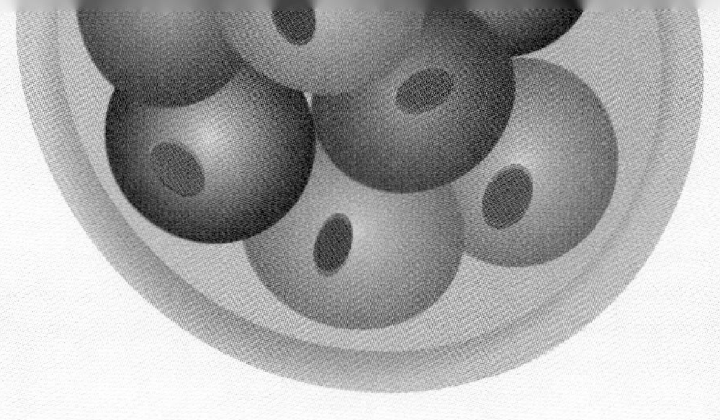

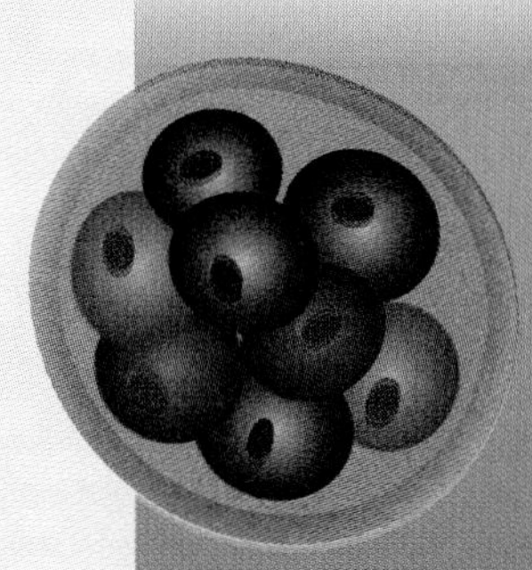

The Eye and Ear

19

DEVELOPMENT OF THE EYE

Early eye development results from a series of inductive signals. For a flow chart of major inductive events and tissue transformations in eye development, see Carlson (1994). The eyes or visual organs are derived from four sources:

- neuroectoderm of the forebrain
- surface ectoderm of the head
- mesoderm between the above layers
- neural crest cells

The neuroectoderm of the forebrain differentiates into the retina, the posterior layers of the iris, and the optic nerve. The surface ectoderm of the head forms the lens of the eye and the corneal epithelium. The mesoderm between the neuroectoderm and surface ectoderm gives rise to the fibrous and vascular coats of the eye. Mesenchymal cells are derived from mesoderm, but neural crest cells migrate into the mesenchyme from the neural crest and differentiate into the choroid, sclera, and corneal endothelium (Wright, 1997). Homeobox-containing genes, including the transcription regulator *Pax6,* play an important role in the development of the vertebrate eye (Mathers et al., 1997).

Eye development is first evident at the beginning of the fourth week. **Optic grooves** (sulci) appear in the neural folds at the cranial end of the embryo (Fig. 19-1*A* and *B*). As the neural folds fuse to form the **forebrain,** the optic grooves evaginate to form hollow diverticula—the **optic vesicles**—which project from the wall of the forebrain into the adjacent mesenchyme (Fig. 19-1*C*). The cavities of the optic vesicles are continuous with the cavity of the forebrain. Formation of optic vesicles is induced by the mesenchyme adjacent to the developing brain, probably through a chemical mediator. As the bulblike optic vesicles grow, their distal ends expand and their connections with the forebrain constrict to form hollow **optic stalks** (Fig. 19-1*D*). The optic vesicles soon come in contact with the surface ectoderm and their lateral surfaces become indented.

Concurrently, the surface ectoderm adjacent to the optic vesicles thickens to form **lens placodes,** the primordia of the lenses (Fig. 19-1*C*). Formation of lens placodes is induced by the optic vesicles after the surface ectoderm has been conditioned by the underlying mesenchyme (Carlson, 1994). An inductive message passes from the optic vesicles, stimulating the surface ectodermal cells to form the lens primordia. The lens placodes invaginate as they sink deep to the surface ectoderm, forming **lens pits** (Figs. 19-1*D* and 19-2). The edges of the lens pits approach each other and fuse to form spherical **lens vesicles** (Fig. 19-1*F* and *H*), which soon lose their connection with the surface ectoderm. Development of the lenses from the lens vesicles is described after formation of the eyeball is discussed.

As the lens vesicles are developing, the optic vesicles invaginate to form double-walled **optic cups** (Figs. 19-1*H* and 19-2). The opening of each cup is large at first but its rim infolds around the lens (Fig. 19-3*A*). By this stage, the lens vesicles have lost their connection with the surface ectoderm and have entered the cavities of the optic cups (see Fig. 19-4). Linear grooves—**optic fissures**—develop on the ventral surface of the optic cups and along the optic stalks (Figs. 19-1*E* to *H* and 19-3*A* to *D*). The optic fissures contain vascular mesenchyme, from which the hyaloid blood vessels develop. The **hyaloid artery,** a branch of the *ophthalmic artery,* supplies the inner layer of the optic cup, the lens vesicle, and the mesenchyme in the optic cup (Figs. 19-1*H* and 19-3). The **hyaloid vein** returns blood from these structures. As the edges of the optic fissure fuse, the hyaloid vessels are enclosed within the optic nerve (Fig. 19-3*C* to *F*). Distal parts of the hyaloid vessels eventually degenerate, but proximal parts persist as the **central artery and vein of the retina** (see Fig. 19-8*D*). For details of the development of blood vessels in the retina, see Penfold et al. (1990). For information on molecular and genetic aspects of eye development, see Graw (1996) and Mathers et al. (1997).

Development of the Retina

The retina develops from the walls of the **optic cup,** an outgrowth of the forebrain (Figs. 19-1 and 19-2). The outer, thinner layer of the optic cup becomes the **retinal pigment epithelium,** and the inner, thicker layer differentiates into the multilayered **neural retina.** During the embryonic and early fetal periods, the two retinal layers are separated by an **intraretinal space,** which is the original cavity of the optic cup. This space gradually disappears as the two layers of the retina fuse (see Fig. 19-8*D*), but this fusion is never firm; hence, when an adult eyeball is dissected, the neural retina is often separated from the retinal pigment epithelium. Because the optic cup is an outgrowth of the forebrain, the layers of the optic cup are continuous with the wall of the brain. Under the influence of the developing lens, the inner layer of the optic cup proliferates to form a thick **neuroepithelium** (Fig. 19-4). Subsequently the cells of this layer differentiate into the **neural retina,** the light-sensitive region of the eye, containing photoreceptors *(rods and cones)* and the cell bodies of neurons (e.g., bipolar and ganglion cells).

Because the optic vesicle invaginates as it forms the optic cup, the neural retina is "inverted"; i.e., light-sensitive parts of the photoreceptor cells are adjacent to the retinal pigment epithelium. As a result, light must pass through most of the retina before reaching the receptors; however, because the retina is thin and transparent, it does not form a barrier to light. The axons of ganglion cells in the superficial layer of the neural retina grow proximally in the wall of the optic stalk to the brain (Figs. 19-3 and 19-4). As a result, the cavity of the optic stalk is gradually obliterated as the axons of the many ganglion cells form the **optic nerve** (Fig. 19-3*F*).

Myelination of optic nerve fibers is incomplete at birth. After the eyes have been exposed to light for about 10 weeks, myelination is complete, but the

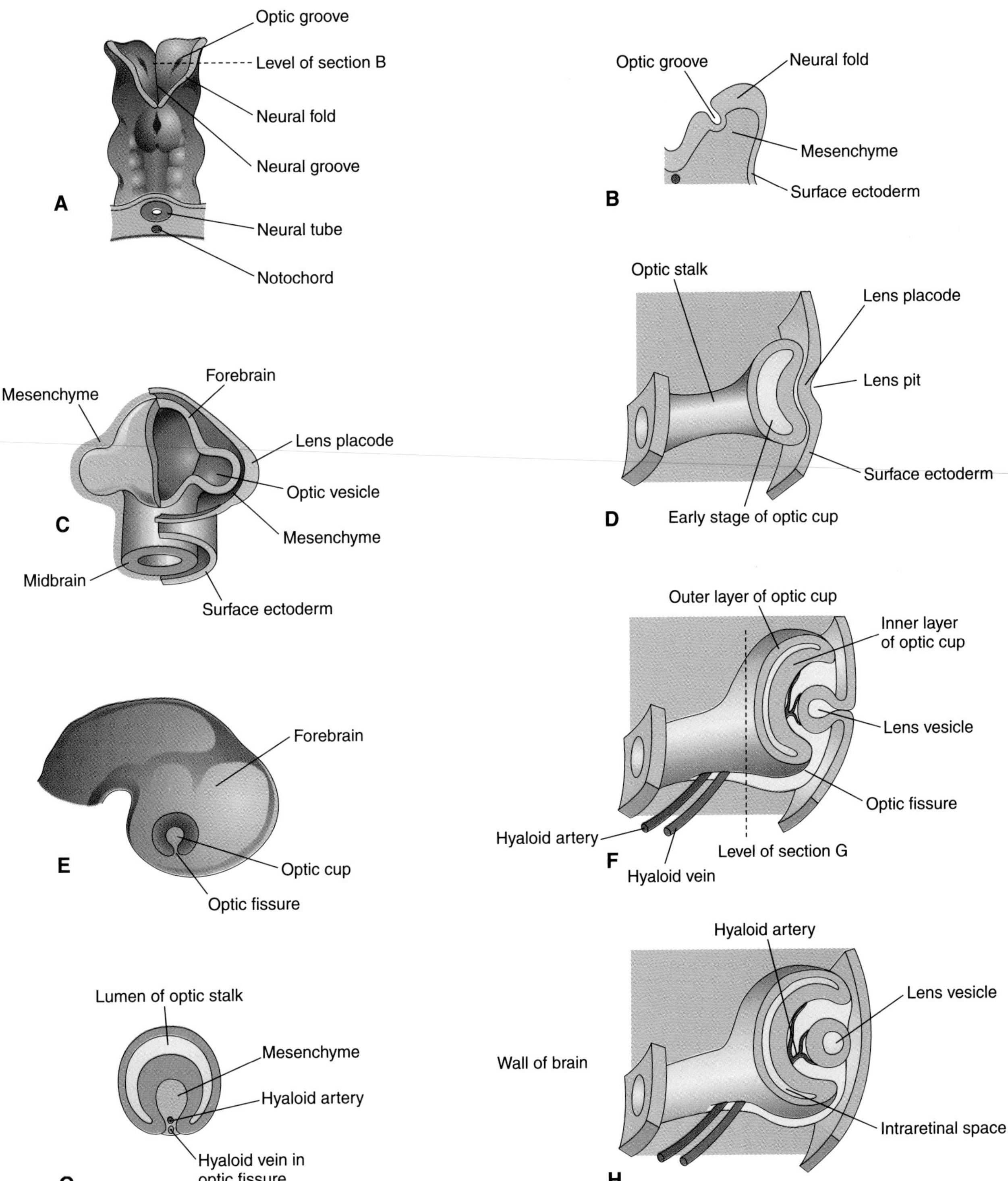

■ **Figure 19–1.** Drawings illustrating early stages of eye development. *A*, Dorsal view of the cranial end of an embryo of about 22 days, showing the optic sulci or grooves, the first indication of eye development. Note that the neural folds have not fused to form the primary forebrain vesicles at this stage. *B*, Transverse section of a neural fold, showing the optic sulcus. *C*, Schematic drawing of the forebrain of an embryo of about 28 days, showing its covering layers of mesenchyme and surface ectoderm. *D*, *F*, and *H*, Schematic sections of the developing eye illustrating successive stages in the development of the optic cup and lens vesicle. *E*, Lateral view of the brain of an embryo of about 32 days, showing the external appearance of the optic cup. *G*, Transverse section of the optic stalk, showing the optic fissure and its contents. Note that the edges of the optic fissure are growing together, thereby completing the optic cup and enclosing the central artery and vein of the retina in the optic stalk and cup.

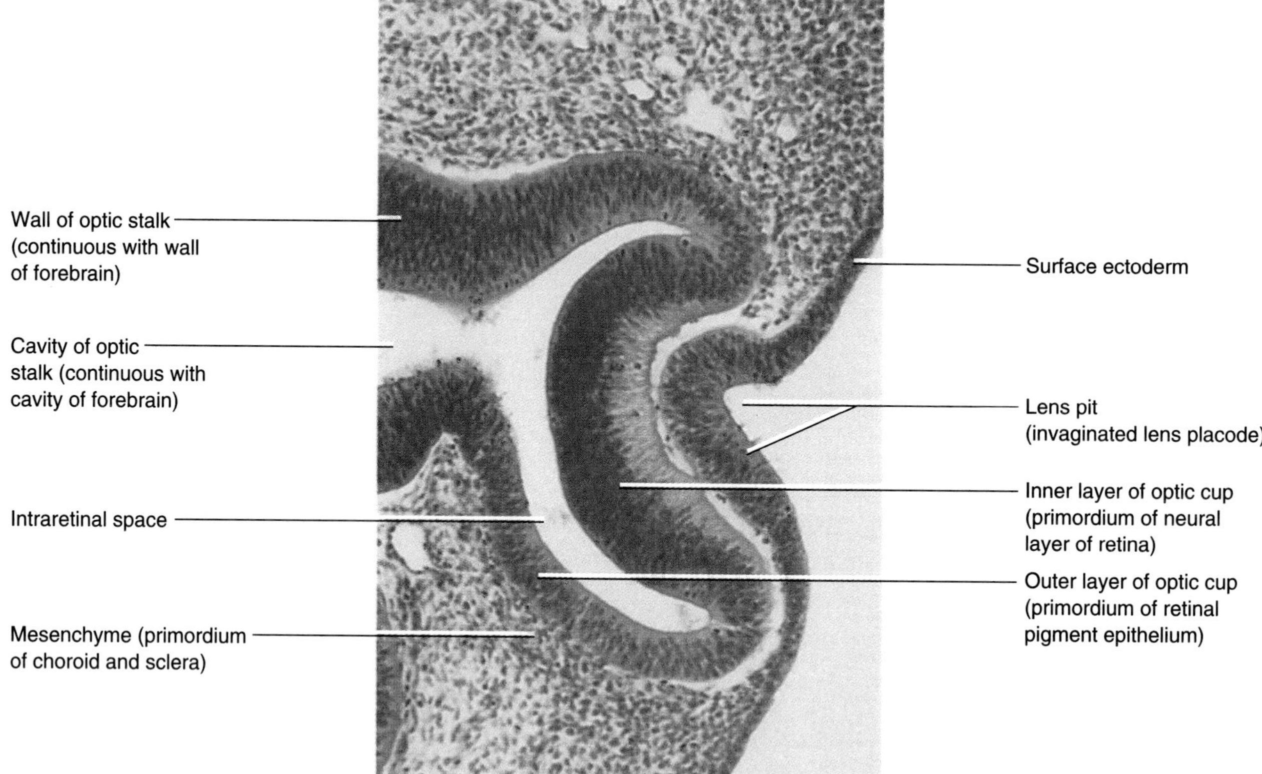

■ **Figure 19–2.** Photomicrograph of a sagittal section of the eye of an embryo (×200) at Carnegie stage 14, about 32 days. Observe the primordium of the lens (invaginated lens placode), the walls of the optic cup (primordium of the retina), and the optic stalk, the primordium of the optic nerve. (From Moore KL, Persaud TVN, Shiota K: *Color Atlas of Clinical Embryology*. Philadelphia, WB Saunders, 1994.)

process normally stops short of the optic disc. The normal newborn infant can see but not too well; it responds to changes in illumination and is able to fixate points of contrast. Visual acuity has been estimated to be in the range of 20/400 (Nelson, 1996). At 2 weeks the infant shows a more sustained interest in large objects.

Congenital Anomalies of the Eye

Because of the complexity of eye development, many anomalies occur but most of them are uncommon. The type and severity of the anomaly depend upon the embryonic stage during which development is disrupted. Several environmental teratogens cause congenital eye defects (Stromland et al., 1991; see Chapter 8). Most common eye anomalies result from *defects in closure of the optic fissure* (Wright, 1997).

Congenital Detachment of the Retina

Congenital detachment of the retina occurs when the inner and outer layers of the optic cup fail to fuse during the fetal period to form the retina and obliterate the intraretinal space (Figs. 19-3 and 19-4). The separation of the neural and pigmented layers of the retina may be partial or complete. Retinal detachment may result from unequal rates of growth of the two retinal layers; as a result, the layers of the optic cup are not in perfect apposition. Sometimes the layers of the optic cup appear to have fused and separated later; such secondary detachments usually occur in association with other anomalies of the eye and head. Knowledge about eye development makes it clear that where there is a detached retina, it is not a detachment of the entire retina, because the retinal pigment epithelium remains firmly attached to the underlying choroid. The detachment is at the site of adherence of the outer and inner layers of the optic cup. Although separated from the retinal pigment epithelium, the neural retina retains its blood supply (central artery of retina), derived from the embryonic hyaloid artery. Normally the retinal pigment epithelium becomes firmly fixed to the choroid, but its attachment to the neural retina is not firm; hence, a **detached retina** may follow a blow to the eyeball, as may occur during a boxing match. As a result, fluid accumulates between the layers and vision is impaired.

Coloboma of the Retina

This defect is characterized by a localized gap in the retina, usually inferior to the optic disc. The defect is bilateral in most cases. *A typical coloboma results from defective closure of the optic fissure.*

Cyclopia

In this very rare anomaly, the eyes are partially or completely fused, forming a single **median eye** enclosed in a single orbit (Fig. 19-5). There is usually a tubular nose (proboscis) superior to the eye. **Cyclopia** (single eye) and **synophthalmia** (fusion of the eyes) represent a spectrum of ocular defects in which the eyes are partially or completely fused. These severe eye anomalies are associated with other craniocerebral defects that are incompatible with life. Cyclopia appears to result from severe suppression of midline cerebral structures—**holoprosencephaly** (see Chapter 18)—that develop from the cranial part of the neural plate (O'Rahilly and Müller, 1989). Cyclopia is transmitted by recessive inheritance.

Microphthalmos

The eye may be very small with other ocular defects or it may be a normal-appearing miniature eye. The affected side of the face is underdeveloped and the orbit is small. Microphthalmos may be associated with other congenital anomalies (e.g., a facial cleft; see Chapter 10), and be part of a syndrome (e.g., trisomy 13; see Chapter 8). Severe microphthalmos results from arrested development of the eye before or

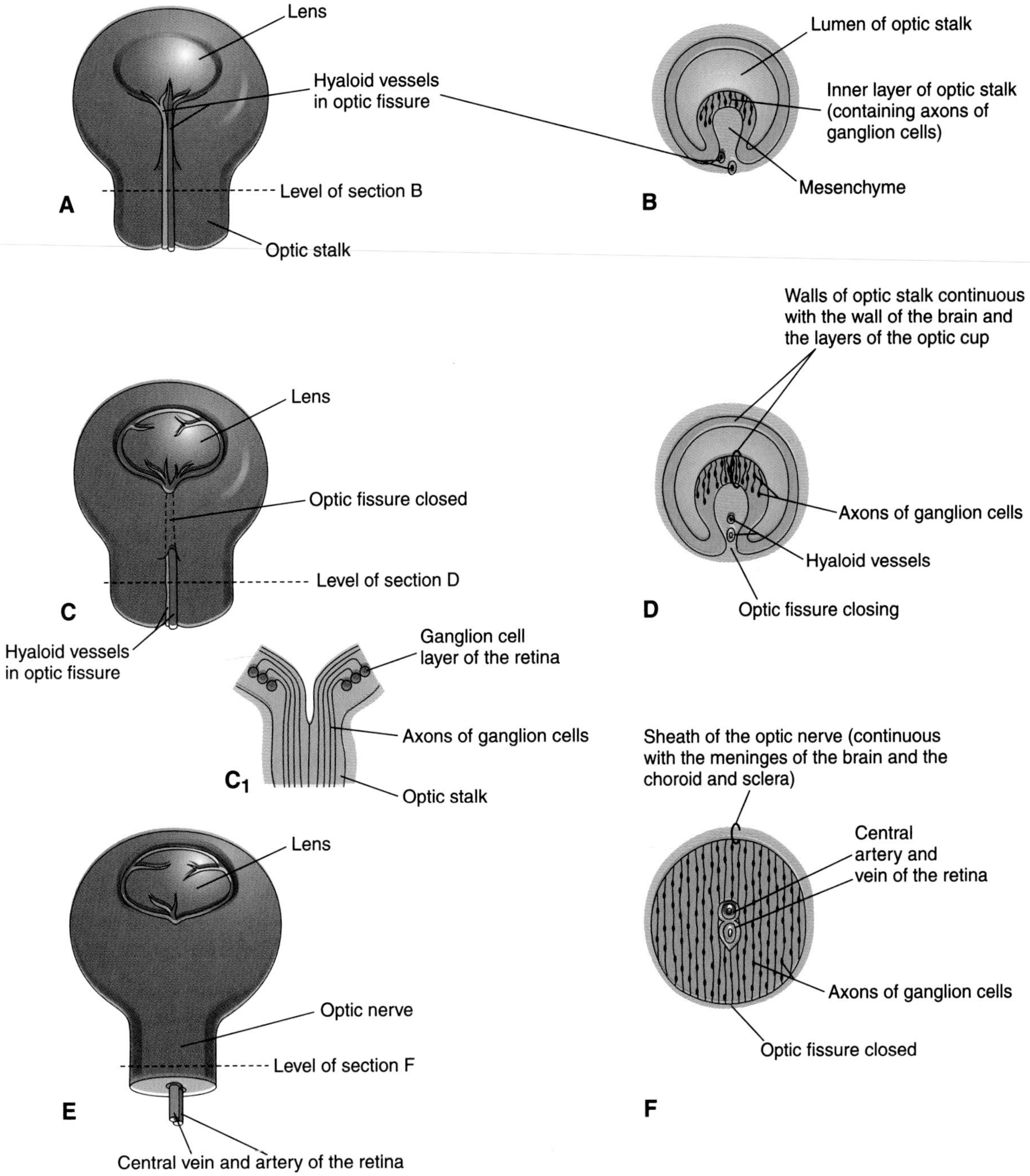

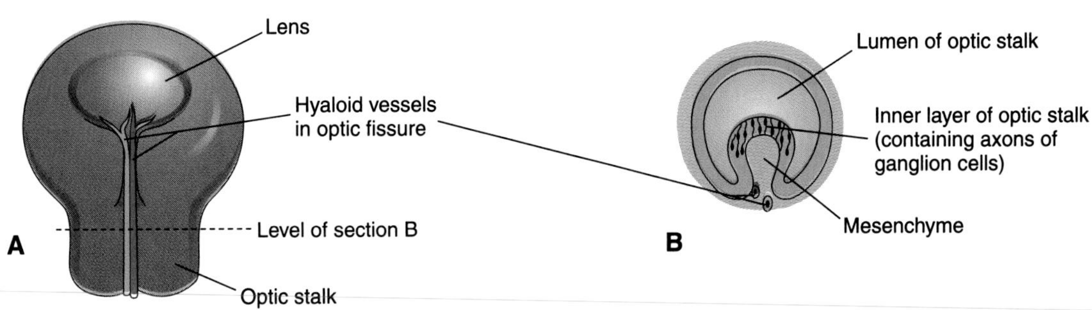

■ **Figure 19–3.** Diagrams illustrating closure of the optic fissure and formation of the optic nerve. *A, C,* and *E,* Views of the inferior surface of the optic cup and stalk, showing progressive stages in the closure of the optic fissure. C_1, Schematic sketch of a longitudinal section of a part of the optic cup and stalk, showing axons of ganglion cells of the retina growing through the optic stalk to the brain. *B, D,* and *F,* Transverse sections of the optic stalk, showing successive stages in closure of the optic fissure and formation of the optic nerve. The optic fissure normally closes during the sixth week. Defects in closure of the fissure result in coloboma of the iris and/or retina. Note that the lumen of the optic stalk is gradually obliterated as axons of ganglion cells accumulate in the inner layer of the optic stalk as the optic nerve forms.

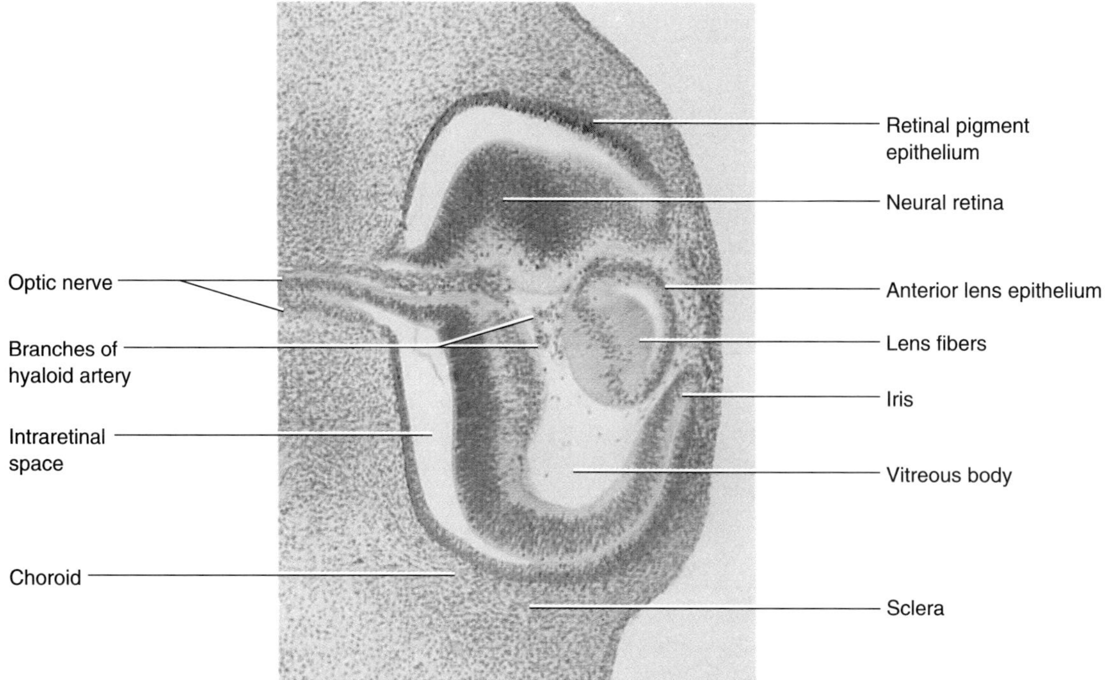

■ **Figure 19–4.** Photomicrograph of a sagittal section of the eye of an embryo (×100) at Carnegie stage 18, about 44 days. Observe that it is the posterior wall of the lens vesicle that forms the lens fibers. The anterior wall does not change appreciably as it becomes the anterior lens epithelium. (From Nishimura H [ed]: *Atlas of Human Prenatal Histology.* Tokyo, Igaku-Shoin, 1983.)

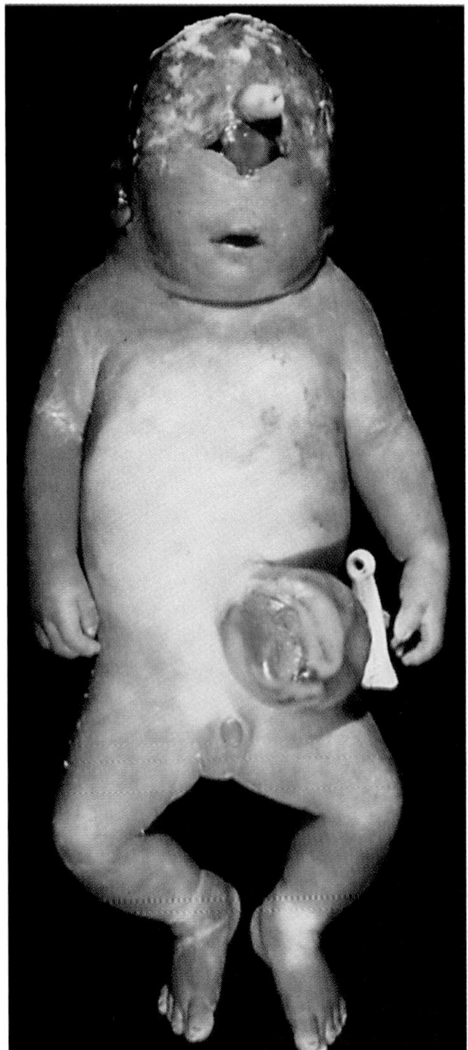

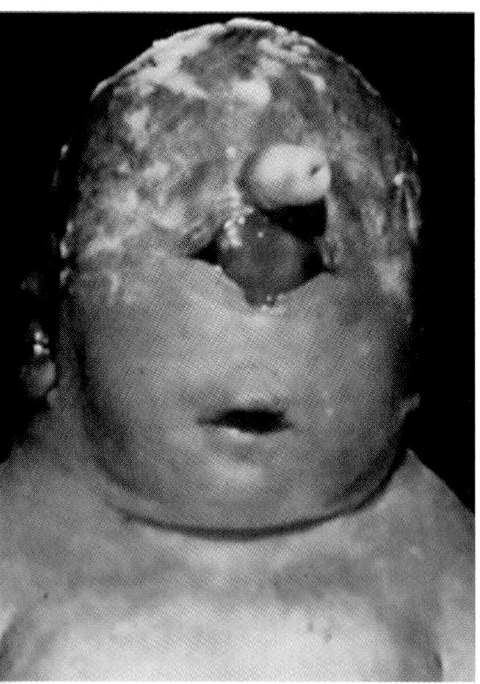

■ **Figure 19–5.** Male neonate with cyclopia (synophthalmia) and omphalocele (herniation of intestines into the proximal part of the umbilical cord). Cyclopia (fusion of the eyes) is a severe, uncommon anomaly of the face and eye associated with a proboscislike appendage superior to the eye. Several facial bones are absent, e.g., nasal bones and ethmoids. (Courtesy of Dr. Susan Phillips, Department of Pathology, Health Sciences Centre, Winnipeg, Manitoba, Canada.)

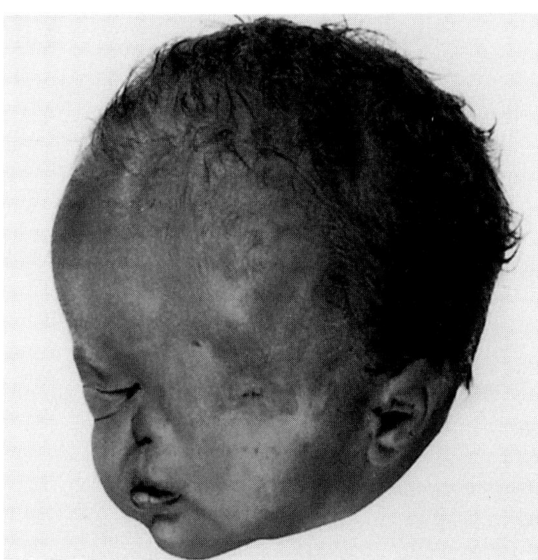

■ **Figure 19-6.** Head of an infant with anophthalmia (congenital absence of all eye tissues) and a single nostril. The eyelids are formed but are mostly fused.

shortly after the optic vesicle has formed in the fourth week. The eye is essentially underdeveloped and the lens does not form. If the interference with development occurs before the optic fissure closes in the sixth week, the eye is larger but the microphthalmos is associated with gross ocular defects. When eye development is arrested in the eighth week or during the early fetal period, simple microphthalmos results (small eye with minor ocular abnormalities). Some cases of microphthalmos are inherited. The hereditary pattern may be recessive or sex-linked with low penetrance. Most cases of simple microphthalmia are caused by infectious agents (e.g., rubella virus, *Toxoplasma gondii,* and herpes simplex virus) that cross the placental membrane during the late embryonic and early fetal periods. See Chapters 7 and 8 for more information.

Anophthalmia

Anophthalmia denotes congenital absence of all tissues of the eye. The eyelids form but no eyeball develops (Fig. 19-6). In some cases eye tissue may be recognizable histologically. Absence of the eye is usually accompanied by other severe craniocerebral anomalies. In **primary anophthalmos,** eye development is arrested early in the fourth week and results from failure of the optic vesicle to form. In **secondary anophthalmos,** development of the forebrain is suppressed and absence of the eye or eyes is one of several associated anomalies.

Development of the Ciliary Body

The ciliary body is the wedge-shaped extension of the choroid (Gartner and Hiatt, 1997). Its medial surface projects toward the lens, forming fingerlike **ciliary processes** (Fig. 19-7). The pigmented portion of the ciliary epithelium is derived from the outer layer of the optic cup and is continuous with the retinal pigment epithelium (Figs. 19-7 and 19-8*D*). The nonpig-

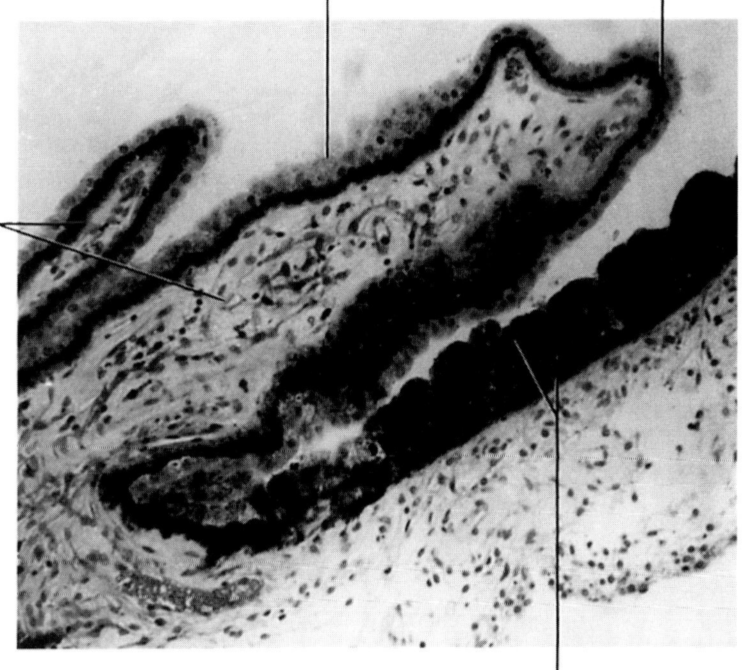

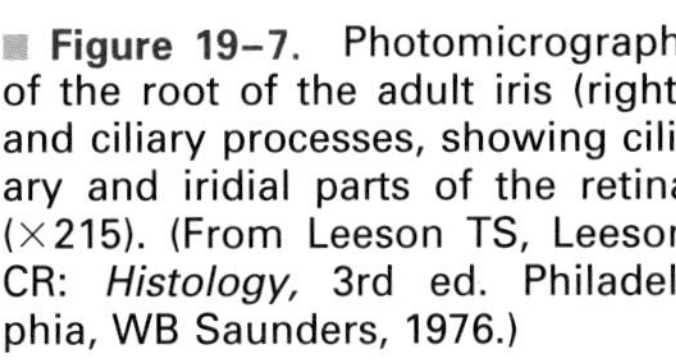

■ **Figure 19-7.** Photomicrograph of the root of the adult iris (right) and ciliary processes, showing ciliary and iridial parts of the retina (×215). (From Leeson TS, Leeson CR: *Histology,* 3rd ed. Philadelphia, WB Saunders, 1976.)

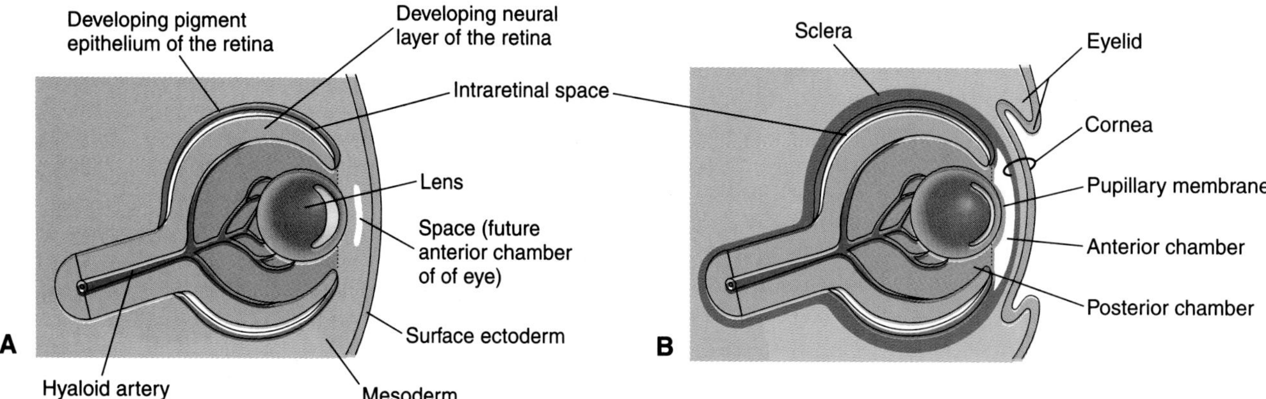

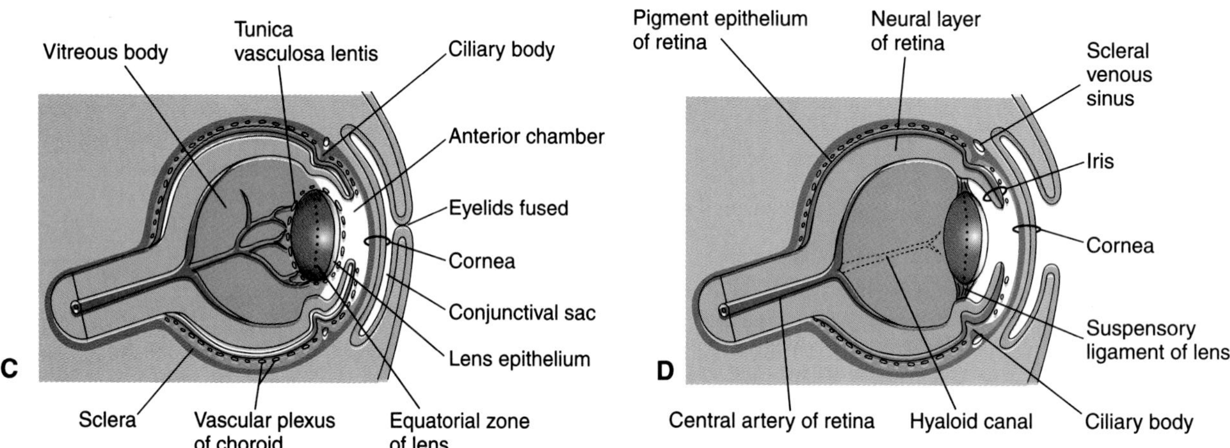

■ **Figure 19–8.** Diagrammatic drawings of sagittal sections of the eye, showing successive developmental stages of the lens, retina, iris, and cornea. *A*, 5 weeks. *B*, 6 weeks. *C*, 20 weeks. *D*, Newborn. Note that the layers of the optic cup fuse to form the retinal pigment epithelium and neural retina and that they extend anteriorly as the double epithelium of the ciliary body and its iris. The retina and optic nerve are formed from the optic cup and optic stalk (outgrowths to the brain). At birth the eye is about three-quarters adult size. Most growth occurs during the first year. After puberty, growth of the eye is negligible.

mented portion of the ciliary epithelium represents the anterior prolongation of the neural retina in which no neural elements differentiate. The **ciliary muscle**—the smooth muscle of the ciliary body—that is responsible for focusing the lens, and the connective tissue in the ciliary body develop from mesenchyme located at the edge of the optic cup in the region between the anterior scleral condensation and the ciliary pigment epithelium.

Development of the Iris

The iris develops from the rim of the optic cup, which grows inward and partially covers the lens (Figs. 19-7 and 19-8). The two layers of the optic cup have remained thin in this area. The epithelium of the iris represents both layers of the optic cup; it is continuous with the double-layered epithelium of the ciliary body and with the retinal pigment epithelium and neural retina. The connective tissue framework (stroma) of the iris is derived from neural crest cells that migrate into the iris (Carlson, 1994). The **dilator pupillae** and **sphincter pupillae muscles** of the iris are *derived from neuroectoderm* of the optic cup. They appear to arise from the anterior epithelial cells of the iris. These smooth muscles result from a transformation of epithelial cells into smooth muscle cells.

Color of the Iris

The iris is typically light blue or gray in most newborn infants. The iris acquires its definitive color as pigmentation occurs during the first 6 to 10 months. The concentration and distribution of pigment-containing cells—**chromatophores**—in the loose vascular connective tissue of the iris determine eye color. If the melanin pigment is confined to the pigmented epithelium on the posterior surface of the iris, the eye appears blue. If melanin is also distributed throughout the stroma of the iris, the eye appears brown.

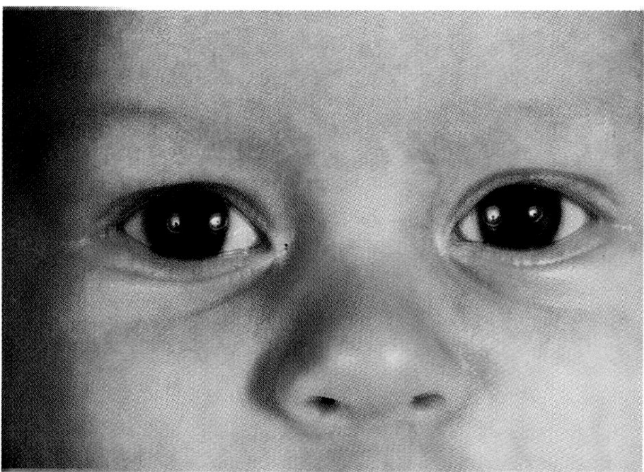

■ **Figure 19–9.** Bilateral coloboma of the iris. Observe the defect in the inferior part of the iris (at the six o'clock position). (Courtesy of A. E. Chudley, Section of Genetics and Metabolism, Department of Pediatrics and Child Health, Children's Hospital, University of Manitoba, Winnipeg, Manitoba, Canada.)

Coloboma of the Iris

In these infants there is a defect in the inferior sector of the iris or a notch in the pupillary margin, giving the pupil a keyhole appearance (Fig. 19-9). The coloboma may be limited to the iris or it may extend deeper and involve the ciliary body and retina. *A typical coloboma results from failure of closure of the optic fissure during the sixth week.* The defect may be genetically determined or caused by environmental factors. A simple coloboma of the iris is frequently hereditary and is transmitted as an autosomal dominant characteristic (Behrman et al., 1996).

Congenital Aniridia

This rare anomaly occurrs in 1 in 64,000 to 96,000 newborns. **There is almost complete absence of the iris.** This anomaly results from an an arrest of development at the rim of the optic cup during the eighth week. The anomaly may be associated with glaucoma and other eye abnormalities. Aniridia may be familial, the transmission being dominant or sporadic. In humans, mutation of the *Pax6* gene results in *aniridia* (Mathers et al., 1997). For a description of the three genetic types of coloboma that occur, see Behrman et al. (1996).

Development of the Lens

The lens develops from the **lens vesicle,** a derivative of the surface ectoderm (Fig. 19-1). The anterior wall of this vesicle, composed of cuboidal epithelium, does not change appreciably as it becomes the **subcapsular lens epithelium** (Fig. 19-8*C*). The nuclei of the tall columnar cells forming the posterior wall of the lens vesicle undergo dissolution. These cells lengthen considerably to form highly transparent epithelial cells, the **primary lens fibers.** As these fibers grow they gradually obliterate the cavity of the lens vesicle (Figs. 19-8*A* to *C* and 19-10). The rim of the lens is known as the equatorial zone or region because it is located midway between the anterior and posterior poles of the lens. The cells in the equatorial zone are cuboidal; as they elongate, they lose their nuclei and become **secondary lens fibers** (Fig. 19-11). These new lens fibers are added to the external sides of the primary lens fibers. Although secondary lens fibers continue to form during adulthood and the lens in-

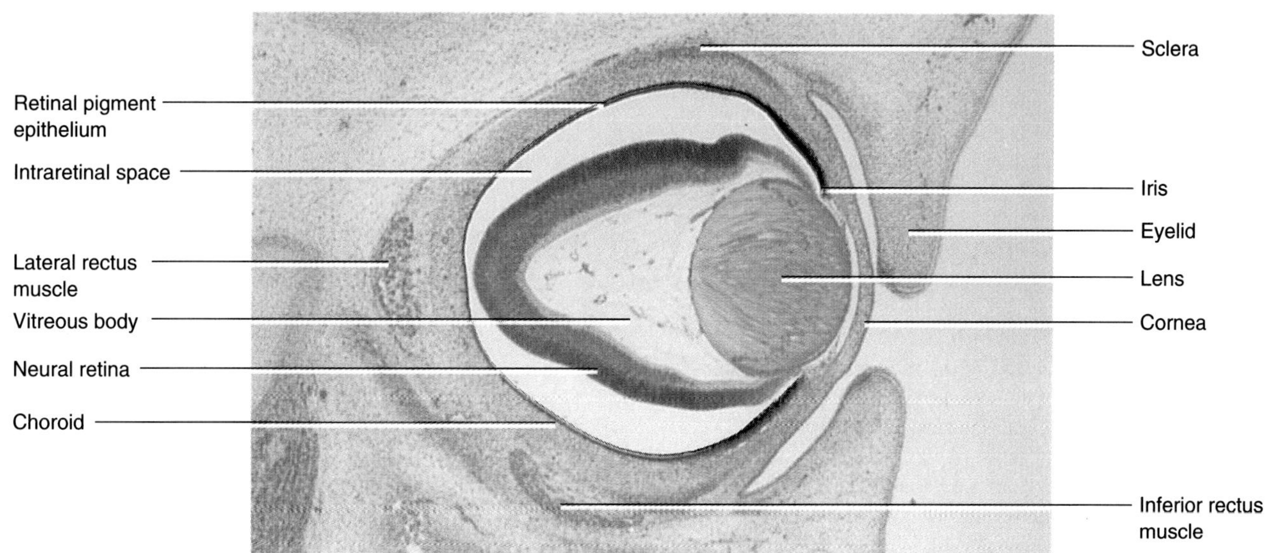

■ **Figure 19–10.** Photomicrograph of a sagittal section of the eye of an embryo (×50) at Carnegie stage 23, about 56 days. Observe the developing neural retina and the retinal pigment epithelium. The intraretinal space normally disappears as these two layers of the retina fuse. (From Moore KL, Persaud TVN, Shiota K: *Color Atlas of Clinical Embryology.* Philadelphia, WB Saunders, 1994.)

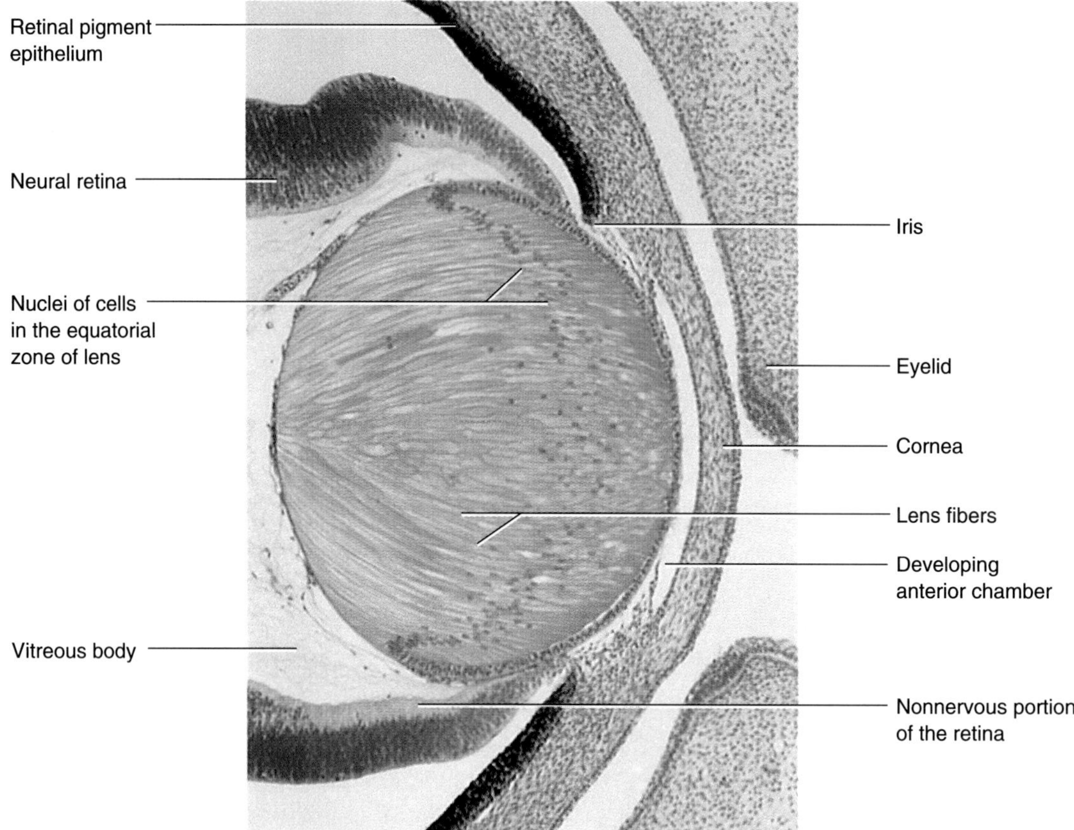

■ **Figure 19–11.** Higher magnification of a portion of the developing eye of the embryo shown in Figure 19–10. Observe that the lens fibers have elongated and obliterated the cavity of the lens vesicle. Note that the inner layer of the optic cup has thickened greatly to form the neural retina and that the outer layer is heavily pigmented (retinal pigment epithelium). (From Moore KL, Persaud TVN, Shiota K: *Color Atlas of Clinical Embryology.* Philadelphia, WB Saunders, 1994.)

creases in diameter, the primary lens fibers must last a lifetime.

The developing lens is supplied by the distal part of the **hyaloid artery** (Figs. 19-4 and 19-8); however, it becomes avascular in the fetal period when this part of the artery degenerates. After this occurs, the lens depends on diffusion from the aqueous humor in the anterior chamber of the eye, which bathes its anterior surface, and from the vitreous humor in other parts. The developing lens is invested by a vascular mesenchymal layer, the **tunica vasculosa lentis.** The anterior part of this capsule is the *pupillary membrane* (Fig. 19-8*B* and *C*). The part of the hyaloid artery that supplies the tunica vasculosa lentis disappears during the late fetal period. As a result, the tunica vasculosa lentis and pupillary membrane degenerate (Fig. 19-8*D*); however, the **lens capsule** produced by the anterior lens epithelium and the lens fibers persists. The lens capsule represents a greatly thickened basement membrane and has a lamellar structure because of its development. The former site of the hyaloid artery is indicated by the **hyaloid canal** in the vitreous body (Fig. 19-8*D*), which is usually inconspicuous in the living eye.

The **vitreous body** forms within the cavity of the optic cup (Fig. 19-8). It is composed of **vitreous humor,** an avascular mass of transparent, gelled, intercellular substance. The **primary vitreous humor** is derived from mesenchymal cells of neural crest origin. The primary vitreous humor does not increase but it is surrounded by a gelatinous **secondary vitreous humor,** the origin of which is uncertain. However, it is generally believed to arise from the inner layer of the optic cup. The secondary vitreous humor consists of primitive hyalocytes, collagenous material, and traces of hyaluronic acid (Wright, 1997).

Persistent Pupillary Membrane

Remnants of the pupillary membrane (iridopupillary membrane), which covers the anterior surface of the lens during the fetal period (Fig. 19-8*B*), may persist as weblike strands of connective tissue or vascular arcades over the pupil in newborns, especially in premature infants. This tissue seldom interferes with vision and tends to atrophy. Very rarely the entire pupillary membrane persists, giving rise to *congenital atresia of the pupil;* surgery is needed in some cases to provide an adequate papillary aperture (Behrman et al., 1996).

Persistence of the Hyaloid Artery

The distal part of the hyaloid artery normally degenerates as its proximal part becomes the central artery of the retina. If a small part of the artery persists distally, it may appear as a freely moving, nonfunctional vessel or as a wormlike structure projecting from the optic disc. Sometimes the hyaloid artery remnant may appear as a fine strand traversing the vitreous body. In other cases a remnant of the hyaloid artery may form a cyst. In unusual cases, the entire distal part of the artery persists and extends from the optic disc through the vitreous body to the lens. In most of these infants, the eye is microphthalmic (very small), but in some cases the eye is otherwise normal.

Congenital Aphakia

Absence of the lens is extremely rare and results from failure of the lens placode to form during the fourth week. Congenital aphakia could also result from failure of lens induction by the optic vesicle (Johnson and Cheng, 1997).

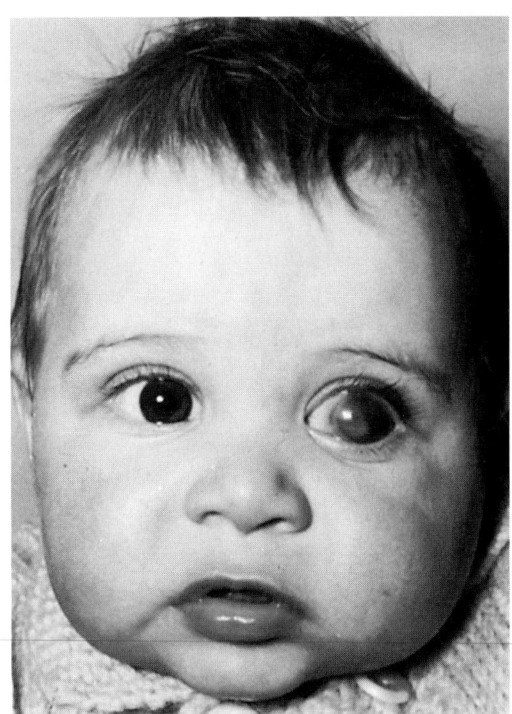

■ **Figure 19–12.** Child with congenital glaucoma of the left eye. (Courtesy of Dr. C. A. Brown, Consultant Ophthalmologist, Bristol Eye Hospital, England.)

Development of Aqueous Chambers

The **anterior chamber of the eye** develops from a cleftlike space that forms in the mesenchyme located between the developing lens and cornea (Figs. 19-4 and 19-11). The mesenchyme superficial to this space forms the substantia propria of the cornea and the mesothelium of the anterior chamber. After the lens is established, it induces the surface ectoderm to develop into the epithelium of the cornea and the conjunctiva. The **posterior chamber of the eye** develops from a space that forms in the mesenchyme posterior to the developing iris and anterior to the developing lens. When the pupillary membrane disappears and the pupil forms (Fig. 19-8*C* and *D*), the anterior and posterior chambers of the eye are able to communicate with each other through a circumferential **scleral venous sinus** (sinus venosus sclerae, canal of Schlemm). This sinus (canal) is the outflow site of aqueous humor from the anterior chamber of the eye to the venous system.

Congenital Glaucoma

Abnormal elevation of intraocular pressure in newborn infants usually results from abnormal development of the drainage mechanism of the aqueous humor during the fetal period (Fig. 19-12). *Intraocular tension* rises because of an imbalance between the production of aqueous humor and its outflow. This imbalance may result from abnormal development of the *scleral venous sinus* in the iridocorneal angle or angle of the anterior chamber (Fig. 19-8*D*). Congenital glaucoma is usually caused by recessive mutant genes, but the condition may result from a rubella infection during early pregnancy (see Chapter 8).

Congenital Cataracts

In this condition the lens is opaque and frequently appears grayish-white. Blindness results. Many lens opacities are inherited, dominant transmission being more common than recessive or sex-linked transmission (Behrman et al., 1996). Some congenital cataracts are caused by teratogenic agents, particularly the *rubella virus* (Fig. 19-13), that affect early development of the lenses. The lenses are vulnerable to rubella virus between the fourth and seventh weeks, when primary lens fibers are forming. Cataract and other ocular abnormalities caused by the **rubella virus** could be completely prevented if immunity to rubella were conferred on all women of reproductive age. Physical agents, such as **radiation,** can also damage the lens and produce cataracts. Another cause of cataract is an enzymatic deficiency—**congenital galactosemia.** These cataracts are not present at birth but they may appear as early as the second week after birth. Because of the enzyme deficiency, large amounts of galactose from milk accumulate in the infant's blood and tissues, causing injury to the lens and resulting in cataract formation (Behrman et al., 1996).

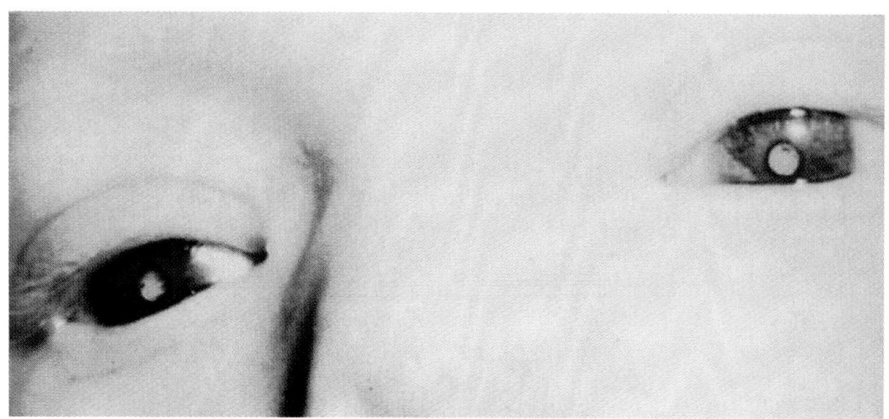

■ **Figure 19–13.** Typical bilateral congenital cataracts resulting from the teratogenic effects of the rubella virus. (Courtesy of Dr. Richard Bargy, Department of Ophthalmology, Cornell–New York Hospital.)

Development of the Cornea

The cornea is formed from three sources:

- The external corneal epithelium is derived from **surface ectoderm.**
- The embryonic connective tissue or **mesenchyme** is derived from **mesoderm,** which is continuous with the developing sclera.
- **Neural crest cells** migrate from the lip of the optic cup through the embryonic connective tissue and differentiate into the corneal endothelium.

Formation of the cornea is induced by the lens vesicle. The inductive influence results in transformation of the surface ectoderm into the transparent, multilayered avascular cornea, the part of the fibrous tunic of the eye that bulges out of the orbit. For more information about induction of the cornea, see Carlson (1994).

Development of the Choroid and Sclera

The mesenchyme surrounding the optic cup (largely of neural crest origin), reacts to the inductive influence of the retinal pigment epithelium by differentiating into an inner vascular layer, the **choroid,** and an outer fibrous layer, the **sclera** (Fig. 19–8*C*). The sclera develops from a condensation of mesenchyme external to the choroid and is continuous with the stroma of the cornea. Toward the rim of the optic cup, the choroid becomes modified to form the cores of the **ciliary processes,** consisting chiefly of capillaries supported by delicate connective tissue. The first choroidal blood vessels appear during the fifteenth week; by the twenty-second week, arteries and veins can be easily distinguished (Sellheyer, 1990).

Edema of the Optic Disc

The optic nerve is surrounded by three sheaths, which evaginated with the optic vesicle and stalk; consequently, they are continuous with the meninges of the brain.

- The outer dural sheath from the dura mater is thick and fibrous and blends with the sclera.
- The intermediate sheath from the arachnoid mater is thin.
- The inner sheath from the pia mater is vascular and closely invests the optic nerve and central vessels of the retina as far as the optic disc.
- Cerebrospinal fluid (CSF) is present in the subarachnoid space between the intermediate and inner sheaths of the optic nerve.

The relationship of the sheaths of the optic nerve to the meninges of the brain and the subarachnoid space is important clinically (Moore and Agur, 1995). An increase in CSF pressure (often resulting from increased intracranial pressure) slows venous return from the retina, causing papilledema (fluid accumulation) of the optic disc. This occurs because the retinal vessels are covered by pia mater and lie in the extension of the subarachnoid space that surrounds the optic nerve.

Development of the Eyelids

The eyelids develop during the sixth week from neural crest cell mesenchyme and from two folds of skin that grow over the cornea (Fig. 19–8*B*). The eyelids adhere to one another by the beginning of the tenth week, and remain adherent until the twenty-sixth to the twenty-eighth week (Fig. 19–8*C*). While the eyelids are adherent, there is a closed **conjunctival sac** anterior to the cornea. When the eyes begin to open, the **bulbar conjunctiva** is reflected over the anterior part of the sclera and the surface epithelium of the cornea. The **palpebral conjunctiva** lines the inner surface of the eyelids. For a detailed account of the development of the eyelids, see Sevel (1988a) and Wright (1997). The eyelashes and glands are derived from the surface ectoderm in a manner similar to that described for other parts of the integument (see Chapter 20). The connective tissue and tarsal plates develop from mesenchyme in the developing eyelids. The *orbicularis oculi muscle* is derived from mesenchyme in the second pharyngeal arch (see Chapter 10) and is supplied by its nerve (CN VII).

Congenital Ptosis of the Eyelid

Drooping of the upper eyelids at birth is relatively common (Fig. 19-14). Ptosis (blepharoptosis) may result from failure of normal development of the **levator palpebrae superioris muscle** (Moore, 1992). Congenital ptosis (Gr., a falling) may also result from prenatal injury or abnormal development of the superior division of the **oculomotor nerve** (CN III), which supplies this muscle. If ptosis is associated with inability to move the eyeball superiorly, there is also failure of the superior rectus muscle of the eye to develop normally. *Congenital ptosis is hereditary* and an isolated defect is usually transmitted as an autosomal dominant trait (Nelson, 1996). Congenital ptosis is associated with several syndromes (for details, see Behrman et al. [1996]).

Coloboma of the Eyelid

Large defects of the eyelid **(palpebral coloboma)** are uncommon (Fig. 19-15). A coloboma is usually characterized by a small notch in the upper eyelid, but the defect may involve almost the entire lid. Coloboma of the lower eyelid is rare. Palpebral colobomas appear to result from local developmental disturbances in the formation and growth of the eyelids.

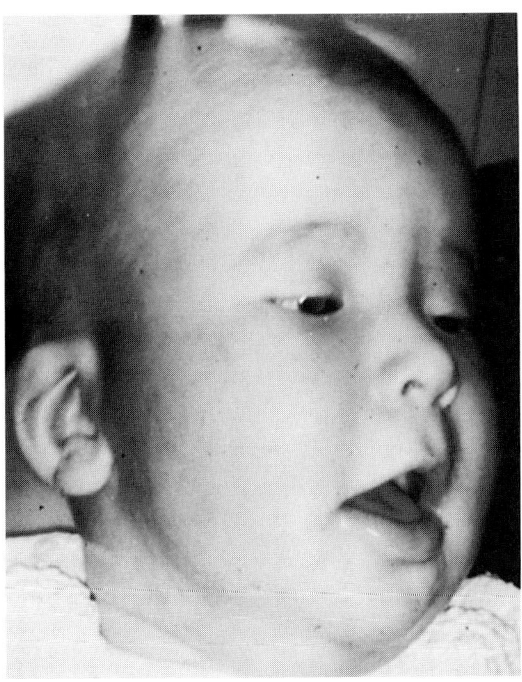

■ **Figure 19-14.** Child with congenital bilateral ptosis. Drooping of the upper eyelid usually results from abnormal development or failure of development of the levator palpebrae superioris, the muscle that elevates the eyelid. In bilateral cases, as here, the infant contracts the frontalis muscle of the forehead in an attempt to raise the eyelids. (From Avery ME, Taeusch Jr HW: *Schaffer's Diseases of the Newborn,* 5th ed. Philadelphia, WB Saunders, 1984.)

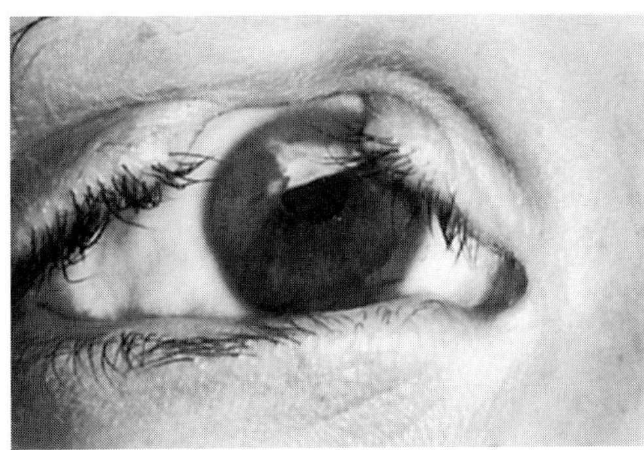

■ **Figure 19-15.** Photograph of the eye of a child with a coloboma of the iris and upper eyelid. (From Brown CA: Abnormalities of the eyes and associated structures. *In* Norman AP [ed]: *Congenital Abnormalities in Infancy,* 2nd ed. 1971. Courtesy of Blackwell Scientific Publications.)

Cryptophthalmos

Cryptophthalmos (L. kryptos, hidden) results from congenital absence of the eyelids—failure of the eyelids to develop; as a result, skin covers the eye. The eyeball is small and defective, and the cornea and conjunctiva usually do not develop. Fundamentally, the defect means *absence of the palpebral fissure (slit);* usually there is varying absence of eyelashes and eyebrows and other eye defects (Jones, 1997). Cryptophthalmos is an autosomal recessive condition that is usually part of the *cryptophthalmos syndrome.*

Development of Lacrimal Glands

At the superolateral angles of the orbits, the lacrimal glands develop from a number of solid invaginations of the surface ectoderm. The buds branch and become canalized to form the ducts and alveoli of the glands. The lacrimal glands are small at birth and do not function fully until about 6 weeks; hence the newborn infant does not produce tears when it cries. Tears are often not present with crying until 1 to 3 months (Nelson, 1996).

DEVELOPMENT OF THE EAR

The ear is composed of three anatomical parts:

- *the external ear,* consisting of the auricle (pinna), the external acoustic (auditory) meatus, and the external layer of the tympanic membrane (eardrum)
- *the middle ear,* consisting of a chain of three auditory ossicles (small ear bones), which connect the internal layer of the tympanic membrane to the oval window of the internal ear
- *the internal ear,* consisting of the vestibulococh-

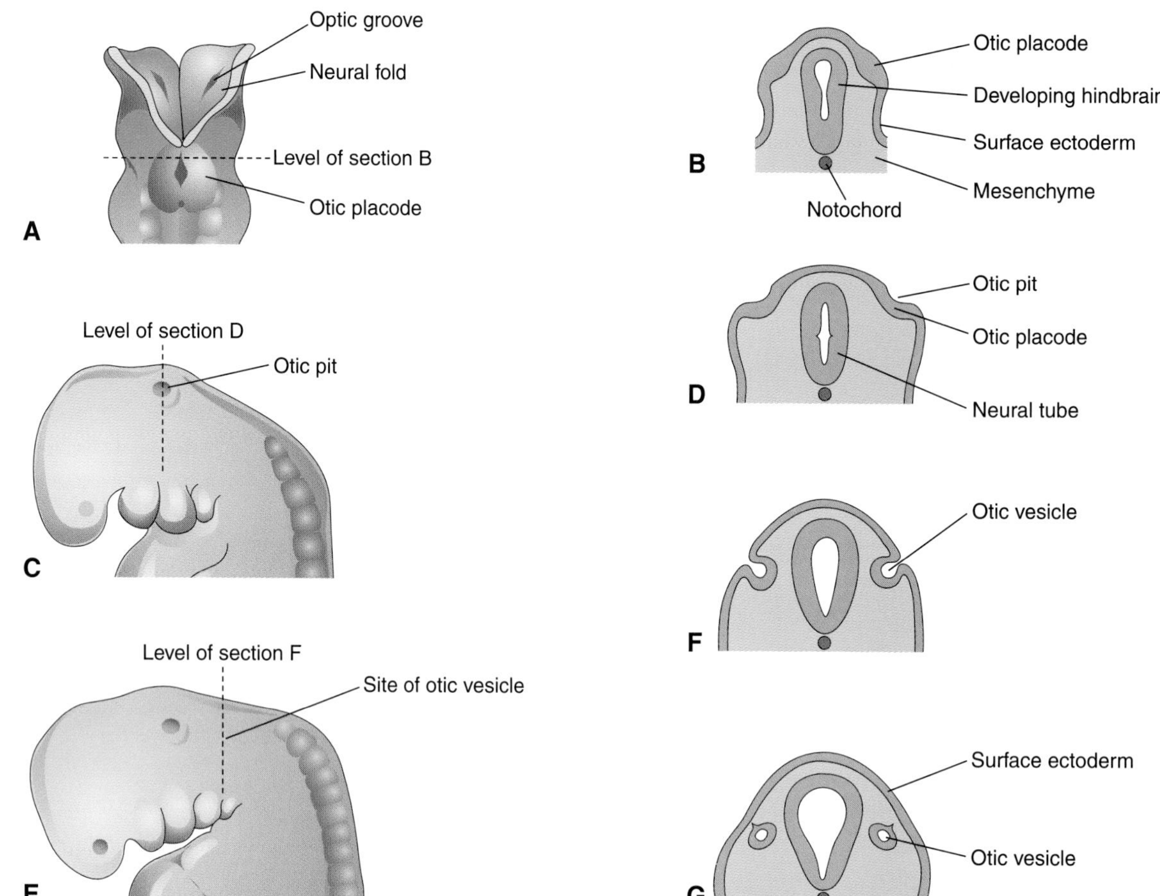

■ **Figure 19–16.** Drawings illustrating early development of the internal ear. *A*, Dorsal view of a 4-week-old embryo (about 22 days), showing the otic placodes. *B, D, F,* and *G*, Schematic coronal sections illustrating successive stages in the development of otic vesicles. *C* and *E*, Lateral views of the cranial region of embryos, about 24 and 28 days, respectively.

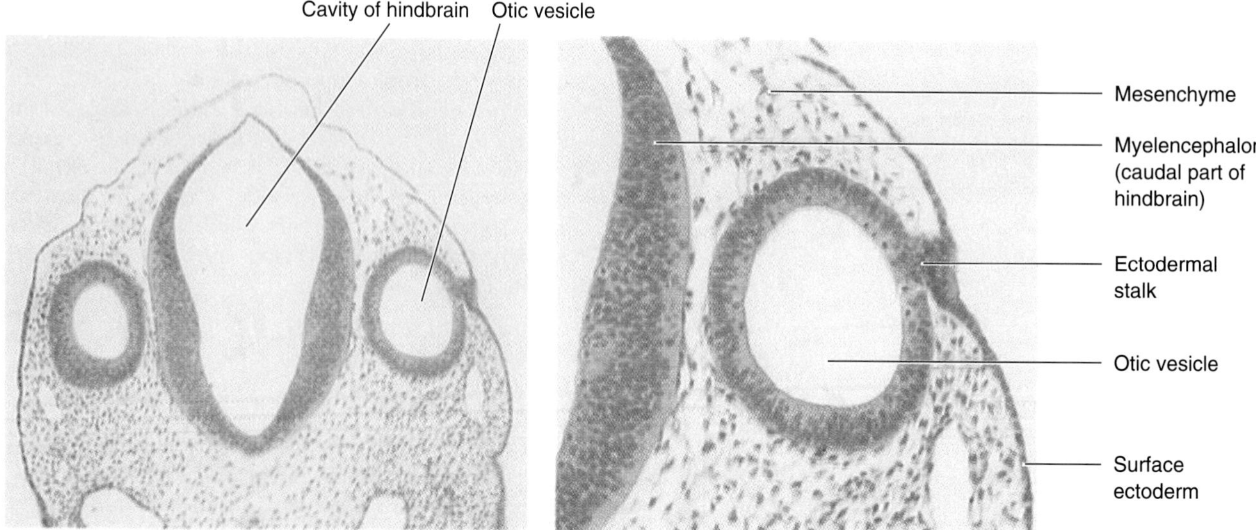

■ **Figure 19–17.** *Left*, Photomicrograph of a transverse section of an embryo (×55) at Carnegie stage 12, about 26 days. Observe the otic vesicles (auditory vesicles), the primordia of the membranous labyrinths, which give rise to the internal ears. *Right*, Higher magnification of the right otic vesicle (×120). Note the ectodermal stalk, which is still attached to the remnant of the otic placode. The otic vesicle will soon lose its connection with the surface ectoderm (primordium of epidermis). (From Nishimura H [ed]: *Atlas of Human Prenatal Histology*. Tokyo, Igaku-Shoin, 1983.)

lear organ, which is concerned with both hearing and balance

The external and middle parts of the ear are concerned with the transference of sound waves to the internal ear, which converts the waves into nerve impulses and registers changes in equilibrium.

Development of the Internal Ear

The internal ear is the first of the three anatomical parts to begin development. Early in the fourth week a thickening of surface ectoderm, the **otic placode,** appears on each side of the myelencephalon, the caudal part of the hindbrain (Fig. 19-16*A* and *B*). Inductive influences from the notochord and paraxial mesoderm stimulate the surface ectoderm to form the otic placodes. Each otic placode soon invaginates and sinks deep to the surface ectoderm into the underlying mesenchyme. In so doing it forms an **otic pit** (Fig. 19-16*C* and *D*). The edges of the otic pit soon come together and fuse to form an **otic vesicle** (otocyst), the primordium of the *membranous labyrinth* (Figs. 19-16*E* to *G* and 19-17). The otic vesicle loses its connection with the surface ectoderm and a diverticulum grows from the otic vesicle and elongates to form the **endolymphatic duct** and **sac** (Fig. 19-18*A* to *E*). Two regions of the otic vesicle are now recognizable:

- a dorsal **utricular part,** from which the endolymphatic duct, utricle, and semicircular ducts arise
- a ventral **saccular part,** which gives rise to the saccule and cochlear duct; this duct contains the **spiral organ** (of Corti)

Three disclike diverticula grow out from the utricular part of the developing **membranous labyrinth.** Soon the central parts of these diverticula fuse and disappear (Fig. 19-18*B* to *E*). The peripheral unfused parts of the diverticula become the **semicircular ducts,** which are attached to the utricle and are later

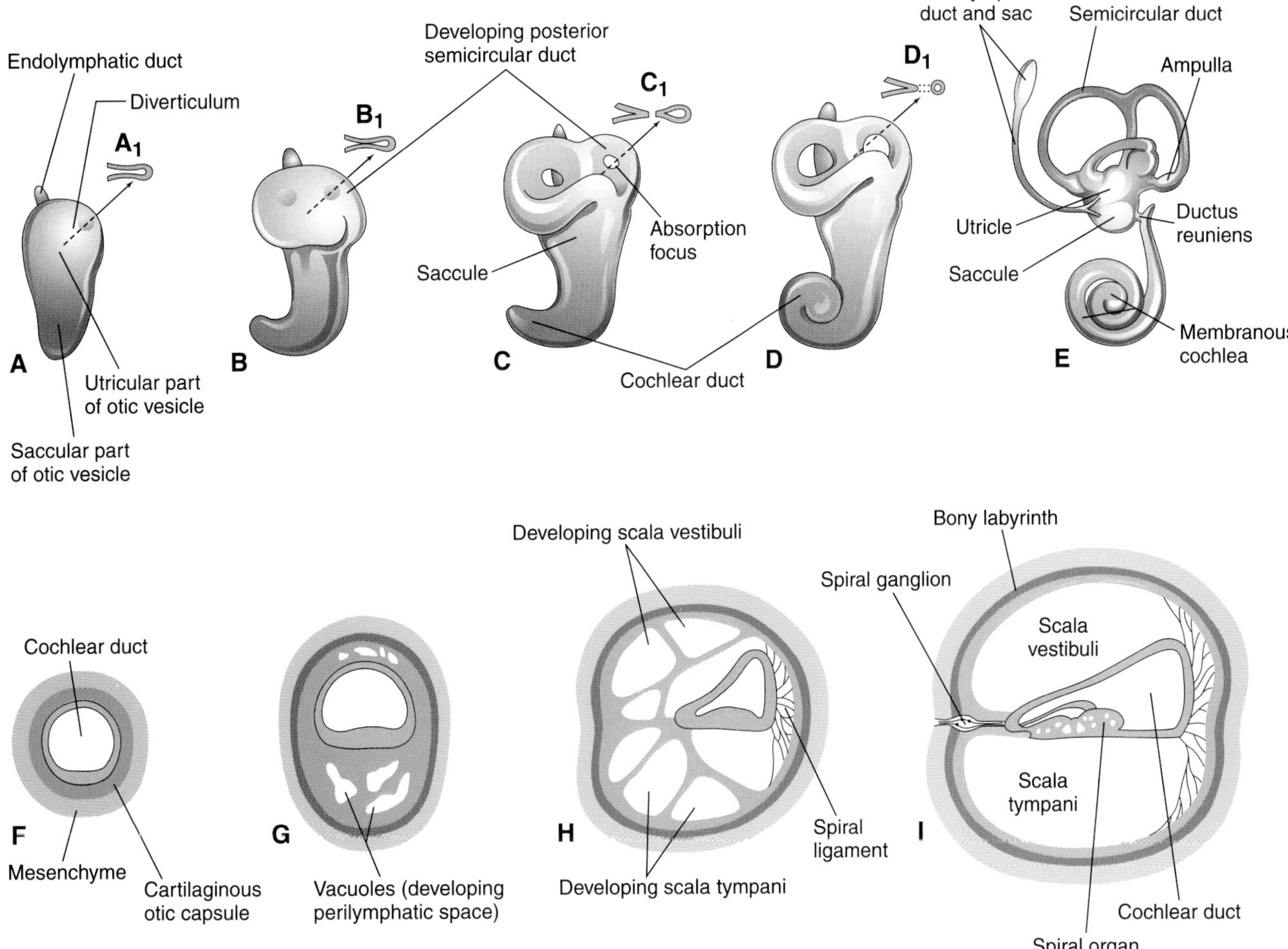

■ **Figure 19-18.** Drawings of the otic vesicle, showing development of the membranous and bony labyrinths of the internal ear. *A* to *E*, Lateral views showing successive stages in the development of the otic vesicle into the membranous labyrinth from the fifth to eighth weeks. A_1 to D_1, Diagrammatic sketches illustrating development of a semicircular duct. *F* to *I*, Sections through the cochlear duct, showing successive stages in the development of the spiral organ (of Corti) and the perilymphatic space from the eighth to the twentieth weeks.

enclosed in the **semicircular canals** of the bony labyrinth. Localized dilatations, the **ampullae,** develop at one end of each semicircular duct. Sensory nerve endings — **cristae ampullares** — differentiate in these ampullae and in the utricle and saccule (maculae utriculi and sacculi).

From the ventral saccular part of the otic vesicle, a tubular diverticulum — the **cochlear duct** — grows and coils to form the *membranous cochlea* (Fig. 19-18*C* to *E*). A connection of the cochlea with the saccule, the **ductus reuniens,** soon forms. The **spiral organ** (of Corti) differentiates from cells in the wall of the cochlear duct (Fig. 19-18*F* to *I*). Ganglion cells of the eighth cranial nerve migrate along the coils of the membranous cochlea and form the **spiral ganglion** (cochlear ganglion). Nerve processes extend from this ganglion to the **spiral organ,** where they terminate on the hair cells. The cells in the spiral ganglion retain their embryonic bipolar condition; that is, they do not become unipolar like spinal ganglion cells.

Inductive influences from the otic vesicle stimulate the mesenchyme around the otic vesicle to condense and differentiate into a cartilaginous **otic capsule** (Fig. 19-18*F*). It was suggested from the results of histochemical and in vitro studies that the transforming growth factor-β_1 (TGF-β_1) may play a role in modulating epithelial-mesenchymal interaction in the internal ear and in directing the formation of the otic capsule (Frenz et al., 1991). As the **membranous labyrinth** enlarges, vacuoles appear in the cartilaginous otic capsule that soon coalesce to form the **perilymphatic space.** The membranous labyrinth is now suspended in **perilymph** (fluid in perilymphatic space). The perilymphatic space related to the cochlear duct develops two divisions, the **scala tympani** and **scala vestibuli** (Fig. 19-18*H* and *I*). The cartilaginous otic capsule later ossifies to form the **bony labyrinth** of the internal ear. The internal ear reaches its adult size and shape by the middle of the fetal period (20 to 22 weeks).

Development of the Middle Ear

Development of the tubotympanic recess (Fig. 19-19*B*) from the first pharyngeal pouch is described in Chapter 10. The proximal part of the tubotympanic

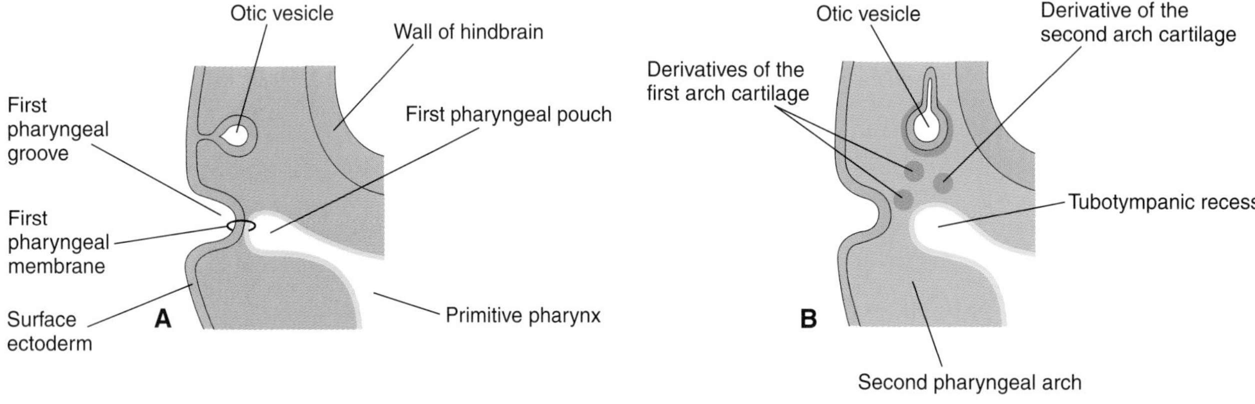

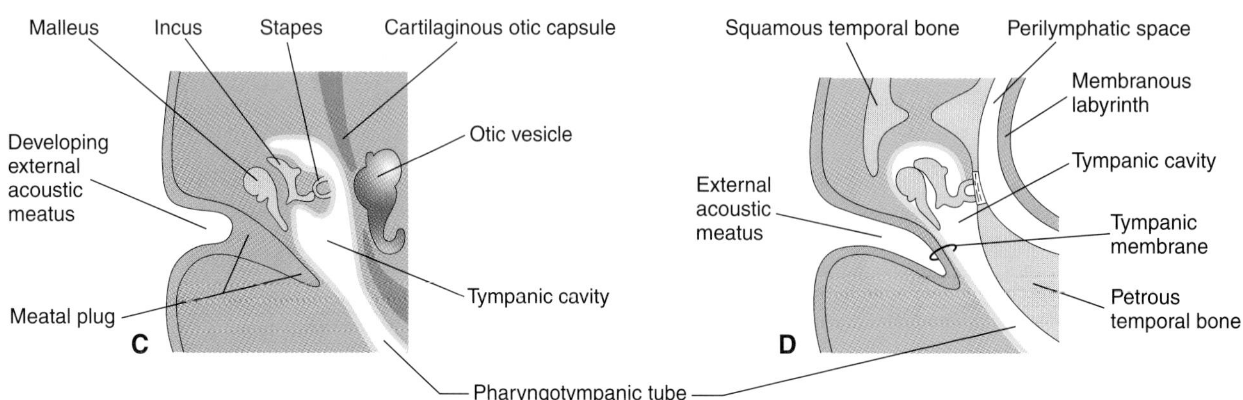

■ **Figure 19-19.** Schematic drawings illustrating development of the external and middle ear. Observe the relationship of these parts of the ear to the otic vesicle, the primordium of the internal ear. *A,* 4 weeks, illustrating the relation of the otic vesicle to the pharyngeal apparatus. *B,* 5 weeks, showing the tubotympanic recess and pharyngeal arch cartilages. *C,* Later stage, showing the tubotympanic recess (future tympanic cavity and mastoid antrum) beginning to envelop the ossicles. *D,* Final stage of ear development, showing the relationship of the middle ear to the perilymphatic space and the external acoustic meatus. Note that the tympanic membrane develops from three germ layers: surface ectoderm, mesoderm, and endoderm of the tubotympanic recess.

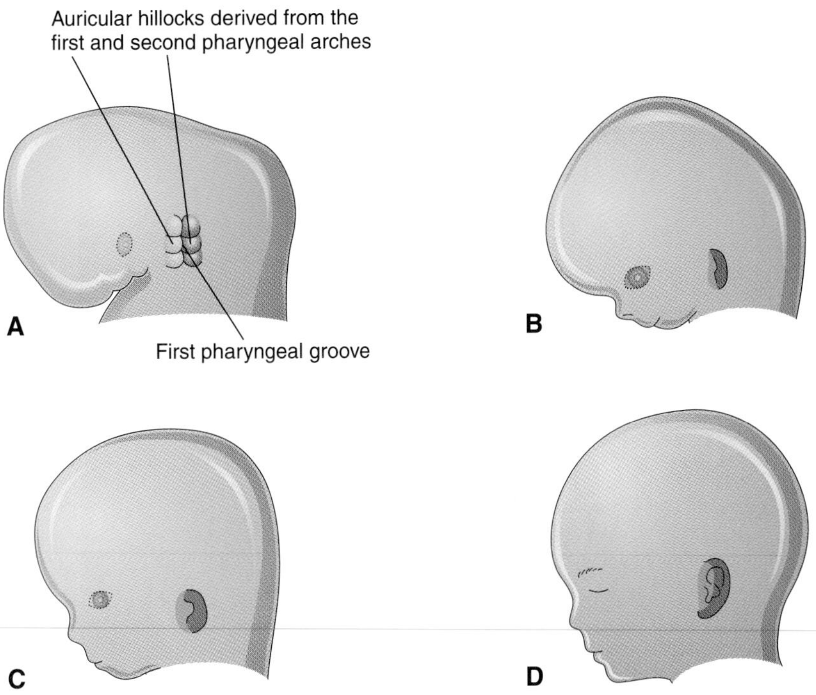

■ **Figure 19–20.** Drawings illustrating development of the auricle. *A*, 6 weeks. Note that three auricular hillocks are located on the first pharyngeal arch and three on the second arch. *B*, 8 weeks. *C*, 10 weeks. *D*, 32 weeks. As the mandible and teeth develop, the auricles move from the neck to the side of the head.

recess forms the **pharyngotympanic tube** (auditory tube). The distal part of the tubotympanic recess expands and becomes the **tympanic cavity** (Fig. 19-19*C*), which gradually envelops the **auditory ossicles** (malleus, incus, and stapes), their tendons and ligaments, and the chorda tympani nerve. All these structures receive a more or less complete epithelial investment. From a study of early human embryos and fetuses, it has been suggested that an epithelial-type organizer located at the tip of the tubotympanic recess probably plays a role in the early development of the middle ear and tympanic membrane (Michaels, 1988).

During the late fetal period, expansion of the tympanic cavity gives rise to the **mastoid antrum,** located in the petromastoid part of the temporal bone (Moore, 1992). The mastoid antrum is almost adult size at birth; however, *no mastoid cells are present in newborn infants.* By 2 years of age the mastoid cells are well developed and produce conical projections of the temporal bones, the **mastoid processes.** The middle ear continues to grow through puberty (Ars, 1989; Behrman et al., 1996). Development of the **auditory ossicles** (middle ear bones) is described in Chapter 10. The *tensor tympani*, the muscle attached to the malleus, is derived from mesenchyme in the first pharyngeal arch and is innervated by CN V, the nerve of this arch. The *stapedius muscle* is derived from the second pharyngeal arch and is supplied by CN VII, the nerve of that arch.

Development of the External Ear

The **external acoustic meatus** develops from the dorsal end of the first pharyngeal groove (cleft). The ectodermal cells at the bottom of this funnel-shaped tube proliferate to form a solid epithelial plate, the **meatal plug** (Fig. 19-19*C*). Late in the fetal period the central cells of this plug degenerate, forming a cavity that becomes the internal part of the external acoustic meatus (Fig. 19-19*D*). This meatus is relatively short at birth; because of this, care must be taken not to injure the tympanic membrane. The external acoustic meatus attains its adult length around the ninth year.

The primordium of the **tympanic membrane** is the first pharyngeal membrane, which separates the first pharyngeal groove from the first pharyngeal pouch (Fig. 19-19*A*). As development proceeds, mesenchyme grows between the two parts of the pharyngeal membrane and differentiates into the collagenic fibers in the tympanic membrane. The external covering (very thin skin) of the tympanic membrane is derived from the surface ectoderm, whereas its internal lining is derived from the endoderm of the tubotympanic recess. To summarize, the tympanic membrane develops from three sources:

- *ectoderm* of the first pharyngeal groove
- *endoderm* of the tubotympanic recess, a derivative of the first pharyngeal pouch
- *mesoderm* of the first and second pharyngeal arches

The **auricle** (pinna) develops from six mesenchymal proliferations in the first and second pharyngeal arches. The prominences—**auricular hillocks**—surround the first pharyngeal groove (Fig. 19-20*A*). As the auricle grows, the contribution by the first arch is reduced (Fig. 19-20*B* to *D*). The lobule (earlobe) is the last part to develop. The auricles begin to develop in the base of the neck (Fig. 19-20*A* and *B*). As the mandible develops, the auricles move to their normal position at the side of the head (Fig. 19-20*D*). The external ears continue to grow through puberty. The parts of the auricle derived from the first pharyngeal arch are supplied by its nerve, the mandibular branch of the trigeminal nerve; the parts derived from the second arch are supplied by cutaneous branches of the **cervical plexus,** especially the lesser occipital and greater auricular nerves. The facial nerve of the second pharyngeal arch has few cutaneous branches; some of its fibers contribute to the sensory innervation of the skin in the mastoid region and probably in small areas on both aspects of the auricle (Moore, 1992).

Congenital Deafness

Because formation of the internal ear is independent of development of the middle and external ears, congenital impairment of hearing may be the result of maldevelopment of the sound-conducting apparatus of the middle and external ears (De la Cruz and Doyle, 1994), or of the neurosensory structures of the internal ear. Most types of congenital deafness are caused by genetic factors. In **deaf-mutism** the ear abnormality is usually perceptive in type. Congenital deafness may be associated with several other head and neck anomalies as a part of the *first arch syndrome* (see Chapter 10). Abnormalities of the malleus and incus are often associated with this syndrome. A **rubella infection** during the critical period of development of the internal ear, particularly the seventh and eighth weeks, can cause maldevelopment of the spiral organ and deafness. Congenital deafness may also be associated with maternal goiter, which may result in fetal hypothyroidism. **Congenital fixation of the stapes** results in conductive deafness in an otherwise normal ear. Failure of differentiation of the *anular ligament,* which attaches the base of the stapes to the fenestra vestibuli (Moore, 1992), results in fixation of the stapes to the bony labyrinth.

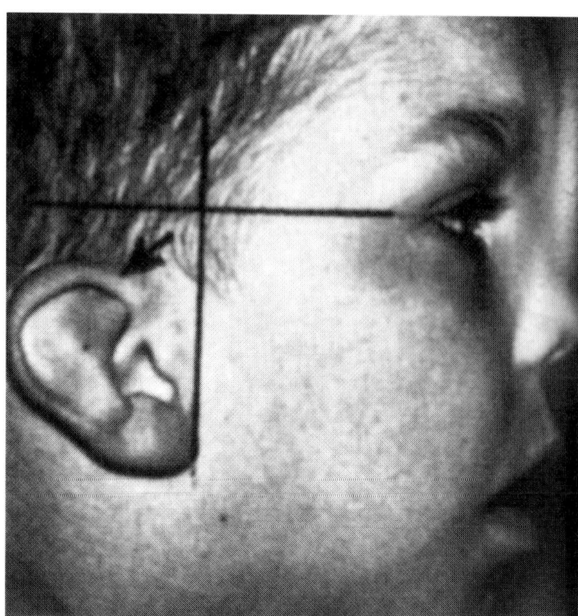

■ **Figure 19–21.** Low-set slanted ear. This designation is made when the margin of the auricle or helix *(arrow)* meets the cranium at a level inferior to the horizontal plane through the corner of the eye. (From Jones KL: *Smith's Recognizable Patterns of Human Malformation,* 5th ed. Philadelphia, WB Saunders, 1996.)

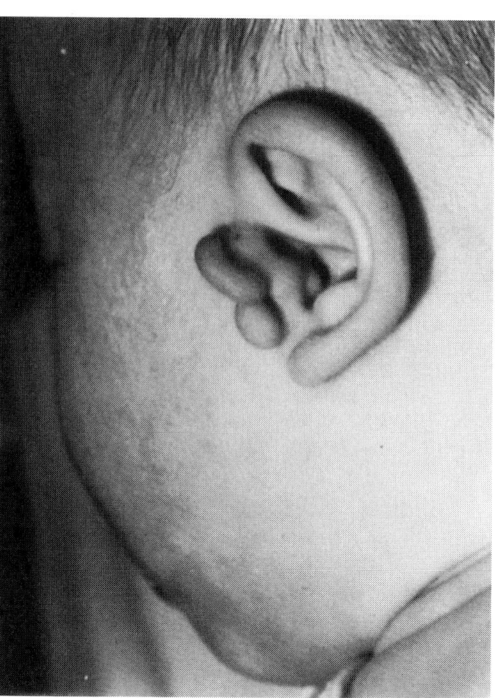

■ **Figure 19–22.** Photograph of a child with two auricular appendages (skin tags), which resulted from the formation of accessory auricular hillocks. (From Swenson O: *Pediatric Surgery,* 1958. Courtesy of Appleton-Century-Crofts.)

Auricular Abnormalities

Severe anomalies of the external ear are rare, but minor deformities are common (Behrman et al., 1996). There is a wide normal variation in the shape of the auricle. Almost any minor auricular defect may occasionally be found as a usual feature in a particular family (Jones, 1997). Minor anomalies of the auricles may serve as indicators of a specific pattern of congenital anomalies. For example, the auricles are often abnormal in shape and low-set in infants with chromosomal syndromes (Fig. 19-21) such as trisomy 18 and in infants affected by maternal ingestion of certain drugs (e.g., trimethadione).

Auricular Appendages

Auricular appendages (skin tags) are common and result from the development of accessory auricular hillocks (Fig. 19-22). The appendages usually appear anterior to the auricle, more often unilaterally than bilaterally. The appendages, often with narrow pedicles, consist of skin but may contain some cartilage.

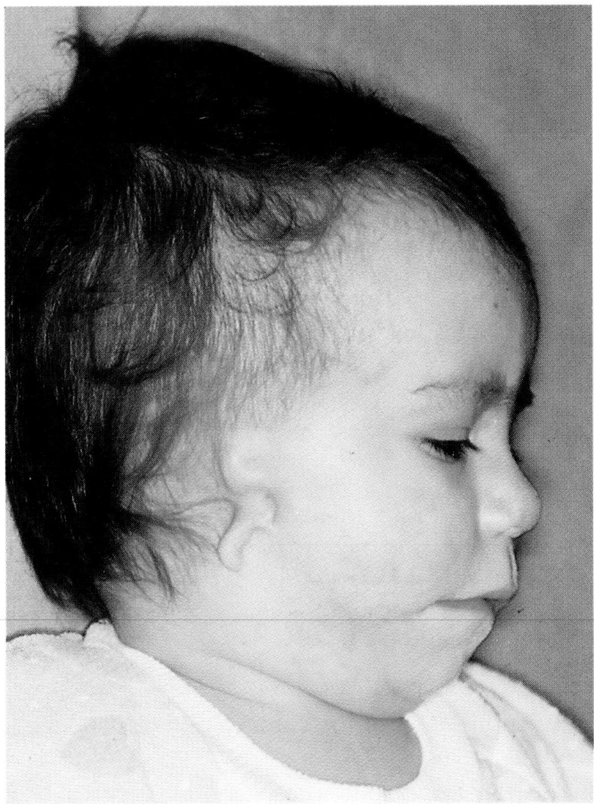

■ **Figure 19–23.** Child with a small rudimentary auricle (microtia). She also had several other congenital anomalies. (Courtesy of Dr. A. E. Chudley, Section of Genetics and Metabolism, Department of Pediatrics and Child Health, Children's Hospital, University of Manitoba, Winnipeg, Manitoba, Canada.)

Absence of the Auricle

Anotia (absence of the auricle) is rare but is commonly associated with the first arch syndrome (see Chapter 10). Anotia results from failure of auricular hillocks to develop.

Microtia

Microtia (small or rudimentary auricle) results from suppressed development of the auricular hillocks (Fig. 19-23). This anomaly often serves as an indicator of associated anomalies, such as an atresia of the external acoustic meatus and middle ear anomalies.

Preauricular Sinuses

Pitlike cutaneous depressions or shallow sinuses are commonly located in a triangular area anterior to the auricle (Fig. 19-24). The sinuses are usually narrow tubes or shallow pits that have pinpoint external openings. Some sinuses contain a vestigial cartilaginous mass. Preauricular sinuses may be associated with internal anomalies, such as deafness and kidney malformations. The embryological basis of auricular sinuses is uncertain but some are related to abnormal development of the auricular hillocks and defective closure of the dorsal part of the first pharyngeal groove. Most of this pharyngeal groove normally disappears as the external auditory meatus forms. Other auricular sinuses appear to represent ectodermal folds that are sequestered during formation of the auricle (Moll, 1991). Preauricular sinuses are familial and frequently bilateral. They are asymptomatic and have only minor cosmetic importance (Raffensperger, 1990); however, they often develop serious infections. *Auricular fistulas* (narrow canals) connecting the preauricular skin with the tympanic cavity or the tonsillar fossa (see Fig. 10-10*F*) are extremely rare.

Atresia of the External Acoustic Meatus

Blockage of this auditory canal results from failure of the meatal plug to canalize (Fig. 19-19*C*). Usually the deep part of the meatus is open, but the superficial part is blocked by bone or fibrous tissue. Most cases are associated with the *first arch syndrome* (see Chapter 10). Often abnormal development of both the first and second pharyngeal arches is involved. The auricle is also usually severely affected and anomalies of the middle and/or internal ear are sometimes present (Parrish and Amedee, 1990). Atresia of the external acoustic meatus can occur bilaterally or unilaterally and usually results from autosomal dominant inheritance.

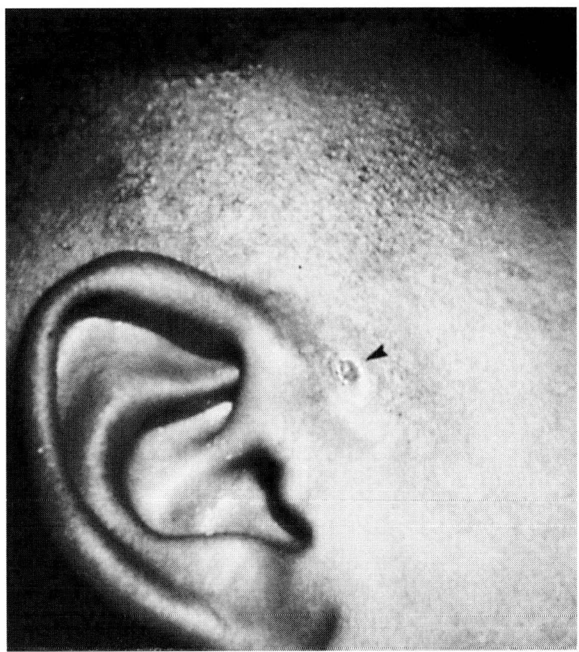

■ **Figure 19–24.** Child with an infected preauricular sinus. There is a small patch of chronic granulation tissue at the external orifice of the sinus. (From Raffensperger JG [ed]: *Swenson's Pediatric Surgery,* 5th ed. Norwalk, CT, Appleton & Lange, 1990.)

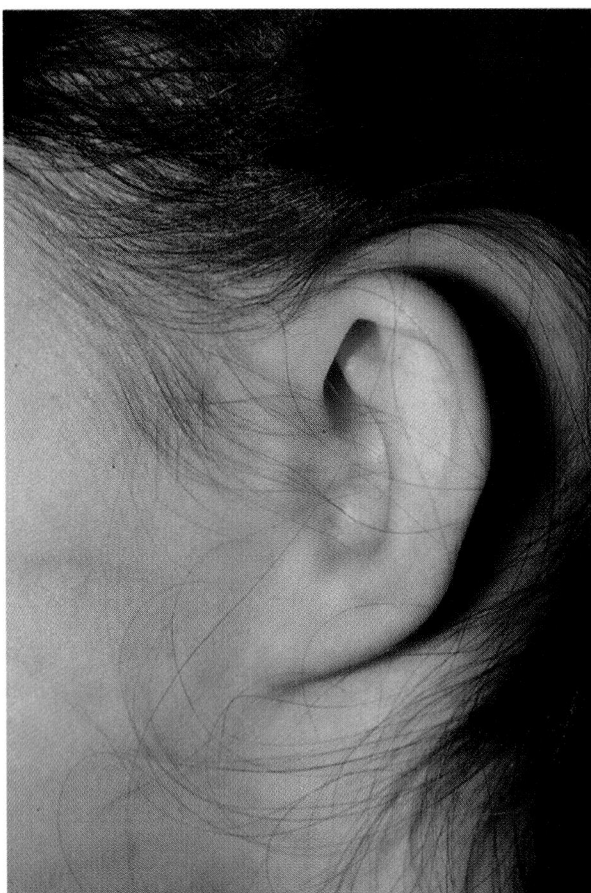

■ **Figure 19–25.** Child with no external acoustic meatus; however, the auricle is normal. A CT scan revealed normal middle and internal ear structures. (Courtesy of Dr. A. E. Chudley, Section of Genetics and Metabolism, Department of Pediatrics and Child Health, Children's Hospital, University of Manitoba, Winnipeg, Manitoba, Canada.)

Absence of the External Acoustic Meatus

Absence of the external acoustic meatus is rare; often the auricle is normal (Fig. 19-25). This anomaly results from failure of inward expansion of the first pharyngeal groove and failure of the meatal plug to disappear (Fig. 19-19*C*).

Congenital Cholesteatoma

This is a rest of epithelial cells (L. *restare*, to remain) that appears as a white cystlike structure medial to or within the tympanic membrane. A rest is a group of cells that are displaced and embedded in tissue of another character. The rest probably consists of cells from the meatal plug that were displaced during its canalization (Fig. 19-19*C*). It has been suggested that congenital cholesteatoma may originate from an epidermoid formation that normally involutes by 33 weeks' gestation.

SUMMARY OF DEVELOPMENT OF THE EYE

The first indication of the eye is the **optic groove,** which forms at the beginning of the fourth week. The groove deepens to form a hollow **optic vesicle** that projects from the forebrain. The optic vesicle contacts the surface ectoderm and induces development of the **lens placode,** the primordium of the lens. As the lens placode invaginates to form a **lens pit** and **lens vesicle,** the optic vesicle invaginates to form an **optic cup.** The retina forms from the two layers of the optic cup.

- The retina, the optic nerve fibers, the muscles of the iris, and the epithelium of the iris and ciliary body are derived from the *neuroectoderm* of the forebrain. The sphincter and dilator muscles of the iris develop from the ectoderm at the rim of the optic cup.
- The *surface ectoderm* gives rise to the lens and the epithelium of the lacrimal glands, eyelids, conjunctiva, and cornea.
- The *mesoderm* gives rise to the eye muscles, except those of the iris, and to all connective and vascular tissues of the cornea, iris, ciliary body, choroid, and sclera.

There are many **ocular anomalies** but most of them are rare. The eye is very sensitive to the teratogenic effects of infectious agents (e.g., cytomegalovirus and rubella virus). The most serious defects result from disturbances of development during the fourth to sixth weeks, but defects of sight may result from infection of tissues and organs by certain microorganisms during the fetal period (e.g., rubella virus and *Treponema pallidum,* the microorganism that causes syphilis). Most ocular anomalies are caused by defective closure of the optic fissure during the sixth week (e.g., coloboma of the iris). *Congenital cataract* and *glaucoma* may result from intrauterine infections (e.g., rubella virus), but most congenital cataracts are inherited.

SUMMARY OF DEVELOPMENT OF THE EAR

The otic vesicle develops from the surface ectoderm during the fourth week. The vesicle develops into the **membranous labyrinth** of the internal ear. The otic vesicle divides into:

- a dorsal utricular part, which gives rise to the utricle, semicircular ducts, and endolymphatic duct
- a ventral saccular part, which gives rise to the saccule and cochlear duct

The cochlear duct gives rise to the **spiral organ** (of Corti). The **bony labyrinth** develops from the mesenchyme adjacent to the membranous labyrinth. The epithelium lining the tympanic cavity, mastoid antrum, and **pharyngotympanic tube** (auditory tube) is derived from the endoderm of the tubotympanic recess, which develops from the first pharyngeal pouch. The **auditory ossicles** (malleus, incus, and stapes) develop from the dorsal ends of the cartilages in the first two pharyngeal arches. The epithelium of the **external acoustic meatus** develops from the ectoderm of the first pharyngeal groove (cleft). The tympanic membrane is derived from three sources:

- endoderm of the first pharyngeal pouch
- ectoderm of the first pharyngeal groove
- mesenchyme between the above layers.

The auricle develops from six **auricular hillocks** which form from mesenchymal prominences around the margins of the first pharyngeal groove. These hillocks fuse to form the auricle.

Congenital deafness may result from abnormal development of the membranous labyrinth and/or bony labyrinth, as well as from abnormalities of the auditory ossicles. *Recessive inheritance is the most common cause of congenital deafness*, but a rubella virus infection near the end of the embryonic period is a major environmental factor known to cause abnormal development of the spiral organ and defective hearing. There are many minor, clinically unimportant anomalies of the auricle; however, they alert the clinician to the possible presence of associated major anomalies (e.g., defects of the middle ear). Low-set, severely malformed ears are often associated with chromosomal abnormalities, particularly trisomy 18 and trisomy 13 (see Chapter 8).

Clinically Oriented Problems

Case 19–1

An infant was born blind and deaf with congenital heart disease. The mother had had a severe viral infection early in her pregnancy.

- Considering the congenital anomalies present, name the virus that was probably involved.
- What is the common congenital cardiovascular lesion found in infants whose mothers have this infection early in pregnancy?
- Is the history of a rash during the first trimester an essential factor in the development of embryonic disease (embryopathy)?

Case 19–2

An infant was born with bilateral ptosis.

- What is the probable embryological basis of this condition?
- Are hereditary factors involved?
- Injury to what nerve could also cause congenital ptosis?

Case 19–3

An infant has small, multiple calcifications in the brain, microcephaly, and microphthalmia. The mother was known to have a fondness for very rare meat.

- What *protozoon* might be involved?
- What is the embryological basis of the infant's congenital anomalies?
- What advice might the doctor give the mother concerning future pregnancies?

Case 19–4

A mentally retarded female infant had low-set, malformed ears, a prominent occiput, and rocker-bottom feet. A chromosomal abnormality was suspected.

- What type of chromosomal aberration was probably present?
- What is the usual cause of this abnormality?
- How long would the infant likely survive?

Case 19–5

An infant was born with partial detachment of the retina in one eye. The eye was microphthalmic, and there was persistence of the distal end of the hyaloid artery.

- What is the embryological basis of congenital detachment of the retina?
- What is the usual fate of the hyaloid artery?

Discussion of problems appears at the back of the book.

REFERENCES AND SUGGESTED READING

Albert DM, Jakobiec FA (eds): *Atlas of Clinical Ophthalmology.* Philadelphia, WB Saunders, 1996.

Ars B: Organogenesis of the middle ear structures. *J Laryngol Otol 103:*16, 1989.

Behrman RE, Kliegman RM, Arvin AM (eds): *Nelson Textbook of Pediatrics,* 15th ed. Philadelphia, WB Saunders, 1996.

Carlson, BM: *Human Embryology and Developmental Biology.* St Louis, Mosby-Year Book, 1994.

Cormack DH: *Essential Histology.* Philadelphia, JB Lippincott, 1993.

Daw NW: *Visual Development.* New York, Plenum, 1995.

De la Cruz A, Doyle KJ: Ossiculoplasty in congenital hearing loss. *Otolaryngol Clin North Am 27:*799, 1994.

Doutreland JJ, Querleu D: Organogenese de l'audition. Developpement de l'oreille. *Rev Fr Gynecol Obstet 83:*23, 1988.

Forrester JV, Dick A, McMenamin PG, Lee WR: *The Eye.* Philadelphia, WB Saunders, 1996.

Frenz DA, Van de Water TR, Galinovic-Schwartz V: Transforming growth factor beta: does it direct otic capsule formation? *Ann Otol Rhinol Laryngol 100:*301, 1991.

Gartner LP, Hiatt JL: *Color Textbook of Histology.* Philadelphia, WB Saunders, 1997.

Gehring WJ: The master control gene for morphogenesis and evolution of the eye. *Genes to Cell 1:*11, 1996.

Gorlin RJ, Toriello HV, Cohen Jr MM: *Hereditary Hearing Loss and its Syndromes.* New York, Oxford University Press, 1995.

Graw J: Genetic aspects of embryonic eye development in vertebrates. *Dev Genet 18:*181, 1996.

Johnson BL, Cheng KP: Congenital aphakia: a clinicopathologic report of three cases. *J Pediatr Ophthalmol Strabismus 34:*35, 1997.

Jones KL: *Smith's Recognizable Patterns of Human Malformation,* 5th ed. Philadelphia, WB Saunders, 1997.

Linberg KA, Fisher SK: A burst of differentiation in the outer posterior retina of the eleven-week human fetus: an ultrastructural study. *Vis Neurosci 5:*43, 1990.

Magnuson T, Har-el G: Middle ear anomalies. *Otolaryngol Head Neck Surg 111:*853, 1994.

Marles SL, Greenberg CR, Persaud TVN, et al: A new familial syndrome of unilateral upper eyelid coloboma, aberrant anterior hairline pattern and anal anomalies in Manitoba Indians. *Am J Med Genet 42:*793, 1992.

Mathers PH, Grinberg A, Mahon KA, Jamrich M: The *Rx* homeobox gene is essential for vertebrate eye development. *Nature 387:*603, 1997.

Michaels L: Evolution of the epidermoid formation and its role in the development of the middle ear and tympanic membrane during the first trimester. *J Otolaryngol 17:*22, 1988.

Michaels L, Soucek S: Development of the stratified squamous epithelium of the human tympanic membrane and external canal: the origin of auditory epithelial migration. *Am J Anat 184:*334, 1989.

Michaels L, Soucek S: Auditory epithelial migration on the human tympanic membrane. II. The existence of two discrete migratory pathways and their embryologic correlates. *Am J Anat 189:*189, 1990.

Moll M: Congenital earpits or auricular sinuses. *Acta Path Microbiol Scand 99:*96, 1991.

Moore KL: *Clinically Oriented Anatomy,* 3rd ed. Baltimore, Williams & Wilkins, 1992.

Moore KL, Agur AMR: *Essential Clinical Anatomy.* Baltimore, Williams & Wilkins, 1995.

Nelson L: Disorders of the eye. *In* Behrman RE, Kliegman RM, Arvin AM (eds): *Nelson Textbook of Pediatrics,* 15th ed. Philadelphia, WB Saunders, 1996.

Noden DM, Van-de-Water TR: Genetic analyses of mammalian ear development. *Trends Neurosci 15:*235, 1992.

Nordquist D, McLoon SC: Morphological patterns in the developing vertebrate retina. *Anat Embryol 184:*433, 1991.

Norlund JJ: The lives of pigment cells. *Clin Geriatr Med 5:*91, 1989.

Ogawa GSH, Gonnering RS: Congenital nasolacrimal duct obstruction. *J Pediatr 119:*12, 1991.

Oguni M, Setogawa T, Otani H, et al: Development of the lens in human embryos; a histochemical and ultrastructural study. *Acta Anat 149:*31, 1994.

Oguni M, Tanaka O, Shinohara H, et al: Ultrastructural study of the retinal pigment epithelium of human embryos, with special reference to the quantitative study on the development of melanin granules. *Acta Anat 140:*335, 1991.

O'Rahilly R: The early development of the otic vesicle in staged human embryos. *J Embryol Exp Morphol 11:*741, 1963.

O'Rahilly R: The prenatal development of the human eye. *Exp Eye Res 21:*93, 1975.

O'Rahilly, Müller F: Interpretation of some median anomalies as illustrated by cyclopia and symmelia. *Teratology 40:*409, 1989.

Otto HD, Gerhardt HJ: Kongenitale Epidermoide des Schlafenbeins. *Teil I: Pathogenese HNO 38:*43, 1990.

Parrish KL, Amedee RG: Atresia of the external auditory canal. *J La State Med Soc 142:*9, 1990.

Penfold PL, Provis JM, Madigan MC, et al: Angiogenesis in normal human retinal development: the involvement of astrocytes and macrophages. *Graefes Arch Clin Exp Ophthalmol 228:*255, 1990.

Raffensperger JG (ed): *Swenson's Pediatric Surgery,* 5th ed. Norwalk, Appleton & Lange, 1990.

Repressa JJ, Moro JA, Gato A, et al: Patterns of epithelial cell death during early development of the human inner ear. *Ann Otol Rhinol Laryngol 99:*482, 1990.

Selland JH: The lens capsule and zonulae. *Acta Ophthalmol (Suppl),* 1992, pp. 7-14.

Sellheyer K: Development of the choroid and related structures. *Eye 4(Pt 2):*255, 1990.

Sellheyer K, Spitznas M: Morphology of the development of choroidal vasculature in the human fetus. *Graefes Arch Clin Exp Ophthalmol 226:*461, 1988.

Sellheyer K, Spitznas M: Differentiation of the ciliary muscle in the human embryo and fetus. *Graefes Arch Clin Exp Ophthalmol 226:*281, 1988.

Sellheyer K, Spitznas M: Licht-und elektronenmikroskopische Untersuchungen zur Entwicklung des menschlichen Ziliakorpers. *Fortschr Ophthalmol 86:*392, 1989.

Sevel D: A reappraisal of the development of the eyelids. *Eye 2(Pt 2):*123, 1988a.

Sevel D: Development of the connective tissue of the extraocular muscles and clinical significance. *Graefes Arch Clin Exp Ophthalmol 226:*246, 1988b.

Sevel D, Isaacs R: A re-evaluation of corneal development. *Trans Am Ophthalmol Soc 86:*178, 1989.

Shah CP, Halperin DS: Congenital deafness. *In* Persaud TVN (ed): *Advances in the Study of Birth Defects, Vol 7. Central Nervous System and Craniofacial Malformations.* New York, Alan R Liss, 1982.

Stromland K, Miller M, Cook C: Ocular teratology. *Surv Ophthalmol 35:*429, 1991.

Takayama S, Yamamoto M, Hashimoto K, Itoh H: Immunohistochemical study in the developing optic nerves in human embryos and fetuses. *Brain Develop 13:*307, 1991.

Tripathi BJ, Tripathi RC, Livingston AM, Borisuth NSC: The role of growth factors in the embryogenesis and differentiation of the eye. *Am J Anat 192:*442, 1991.

Twefik TL, Der Kaloustian VM (eds): *Congenital Anomalies of the Ear, Nose, and Throat.* Oxford, Oxford University Press, 1996.

Waid DK, McLoon SC: Immediate differentiation of ganglion cells following mitosis in the developing retina. *Neuron 14:*117, 1995.

Wilson RS, Char F: Drug-induced ocular malformations. *In* Persaud TVN (ed): *Advances in the Study of Birth Defects, Vol 7. Central Nervous System and Craniofacial Malformations.* New York, Alan R Liss, 1982.

Wright KW: Embryology and eye development. *In* Wright KW (ed): *Textbook of Ophthalmology.* Baltimore, Williams & Wilkins, 1997.

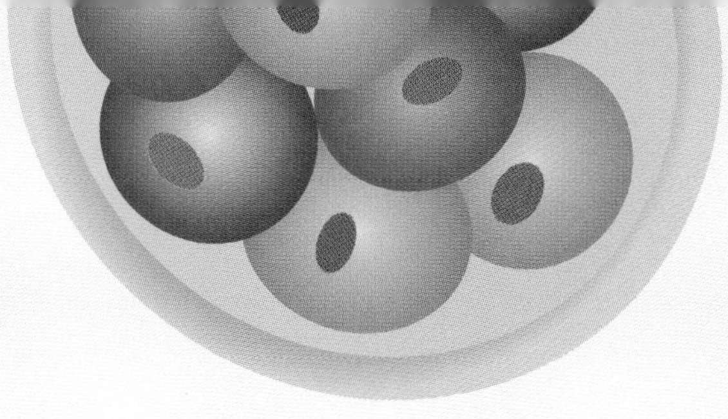

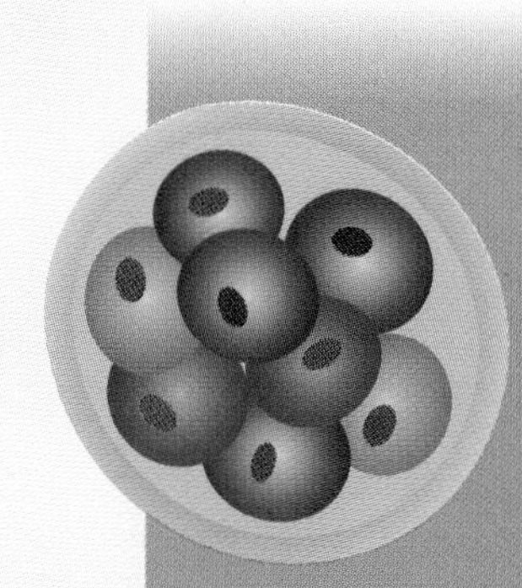

The Integumentary System

20

■ The integumentary system consists of the skin and its derivatives: sweat glands, nails, hair, sebaceous glands, and arrector pili muscles. The system also includes the mammary glands and teeth. At the external orifices, the digestive tract for example, the mucous membrane and integument (L., covering) are continuous.

DEVELOPMENT OF SKIN

The skin—one of the largest structures in the body—is a complex organ system that forms a protective covering for the body. The skin consists of two layers that are derived from two different germ layers (Fig. 20-1): ectoderm and mesoderm.

- The **epidermis** is a superficial epithelial tissue, which is derived from *surface ectoderm.*
- The **dermis** is a deeper layer composed of dense, irregularly arranged connective tissue, which is derived from *mesoderm.* The meshwork of embryonic connective tissue or **mesenchyme** derived from mesoderm forms the connective tissues in the dermis.

Ectodermal (epidermal)/mesenchymal (dermal) interactions involve mutual inductive mechanisms (Collins, 1995). See Haake and Lane (1989) and Nanney et al. (1990) for studies of molecular mechanisms that regulate human skin development. Skin structures vary from one part of the body to another. For example, the skin of the eyelids is thin and soft and has fine hairs; whereas the skin of the eyebrows is thicker and has coarse hairs. The embryonic skin at 4 to 5 weeks consists of a single layer of surface ectoderm overlying the mesenchyme (Fig. 20-1).

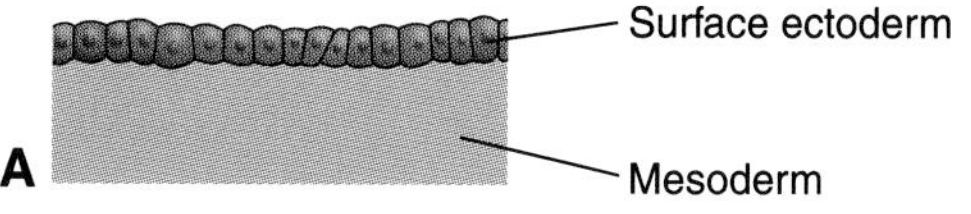

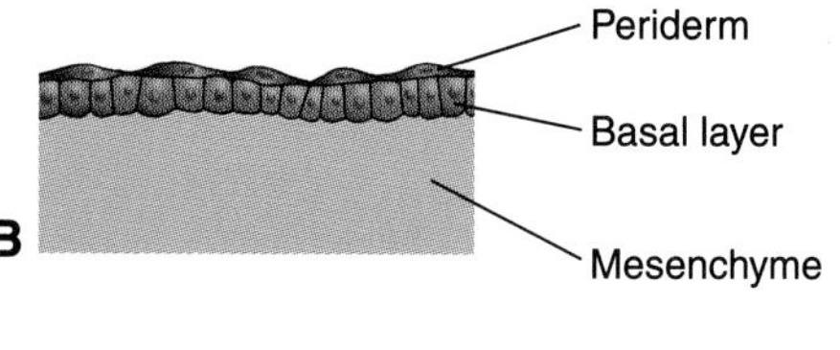

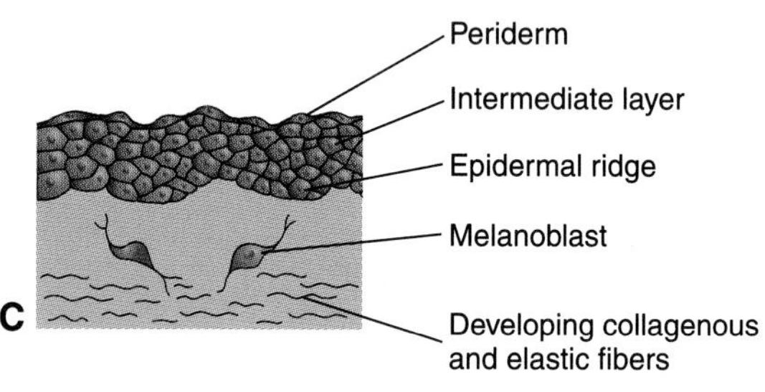

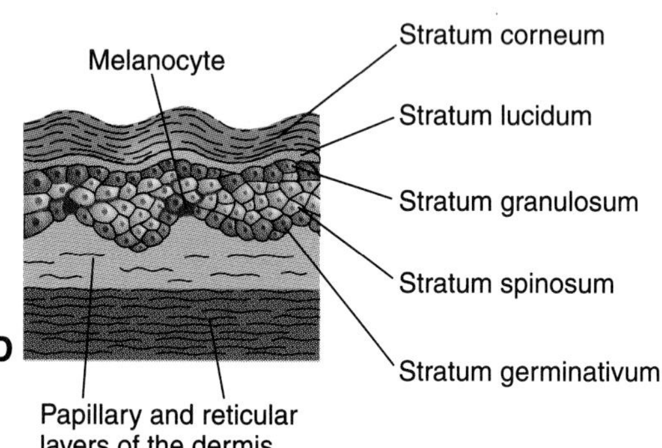

■ **Figure 20-1.** Drawings illustrating successive stages in skin development. *A,* 4 weeks. *B,* 7 weeks. *C,* 11 weeks. The cells of the periderm continually undergo keratinization and desquamation. The exfoliated peridermal cells form part of the vernix caseosa. *D,* Newborn. Note the position of the melanocytes in the basal layer of the epidermis and the way their branching processes extend between the epidermal cells to supply them with melanin.

Epidermis

During the first and second trimesters, epidermal growth occurs in stages, which result in an increase in epidermal thickness (Foster et al., 1988). The primordium of the epidermis is the layer of surface ectodermal cells (Fig. 20-1*A*). These cells proliferate and form a layer of squamous epithelium, the **periderm,** and a basal germinative layer (Fig. 20-1*B*). The cells of the periderm continually undergo keratinization and desquamation and are replaced by cells arising from the **basal layer.** The exfoliated peridermal cells form part of the white greasy substance—the **vernix caseosa**—that covers the fetal skin. Later, the vernix (L., varnish) contains sebum, the secretion from sebaceous glands in the skin. The vernix protects the developing skin from constant exposure to amniotic fluid with its urine content during the fetal period. In addition, the vernix caseosa facilitates birth of the fetus because of its slippery nature.

The basal germinative layer of the epidermis becomes the **stratum germinativum,** which produces new cells that are displaced into the layers superficial to it. By 11 weeks, cells from the stratum germinativum have formed an **intermediate layer** (Fig. 20-1*C*). Replacement of peridermal cells continues until about the twenty-first week; thereafter, the periderm disappears and the **stratum corneum** forms (Fig. 20-1*D*). Proliferation of cells in the stratum germinativum also forms **epidermal ridges,** which extend into the developing dermis (Figs. 20-1*C* and 20-2). These ridges begin to appear in embryos at 10 weeks and are permanently established by the seventeenth week. The epidermal ridges produce grooves on the surface of the palms of the hands and the soles of the feet, including the digits. The type of pattern that develops is determined genetically and constitutes the basis for examining fingerprints in criminal investigations and medical genetics.

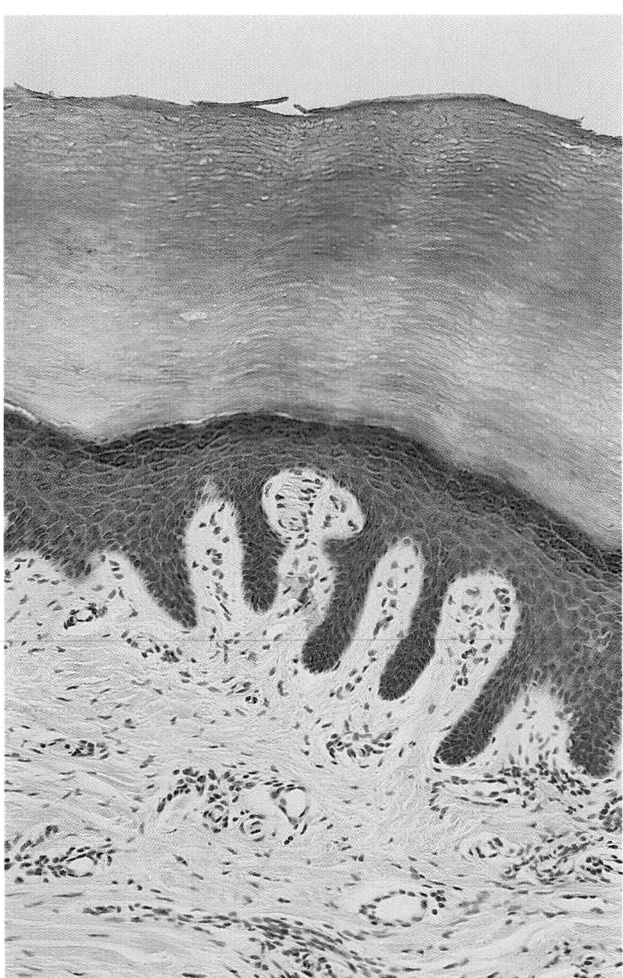

■ **Figure 20–2.** Light micrograph of thick skin (×132). Observe the epidermis and dermis as well as the dermal ridges interdigitating with the epidermal ridges. (From Gartner LP, Hiatt JL: *Color Textbook of Histology.* Philadelphia, WB Saunders, 1997.)

Dermatoglyphics is the study of the patterns of the epidermal ridges of the skin. Abnormal chromosome complements affect the development of ridge patterns; e.g., infants with Down syndrome have distinctive patterns on their hands and feet that are of diagnostic value (see Chapter 8).

Late in the embryonic period, **neural crest cells** migrate into the mesenchyme of the developing dermis and differentiate into **melanoblasts.** Later these cells migrate to the dermoepidermal junction and differentiate into **melanocytes** (Fig. 20 - 1*D*). The differentiation of melanoblasts into melanocytes involves the formation of pigment granules. Recent studies have shown that melanocytes appear in the developing skin at 40 to 50 days, immediately after the migration of neural crest cells (Holbrook et al., 1989). In white races, the cell bodies of melanocytes are usually confined to basal layers of the epidermis; however, their dendritic processes extend between the epidermal cells. Only a few melanin-containing cells are normally present in the dermis (Cormack, 1993). The melanocytes begin producing **melanin** (Gr. *melas,* black) before birth and distribute it to the epidermal cells. Pigment formation can be observed prenatally in the epidermis of dark-skinned races; however, there is little evidence of such activity in light-skinned fetuses. Increased amounts of melanin are produced in response to ultraviolet light. The relative content of melanin in the melanocytes accounts for the different colors of skin.

The transformation of the surface ectoderm into a multilayered epidermis results from continuing inductive interactions with the dermis (Carlson, 1994). Skin is classified as thick or thin based on the thickness of the epidermis (Gartner and Hiatt, 1997).

- **Thick skin** covers the palms and soles; it lacks hair follicles, arrector pili muscles, and sebaceous glands but has sweat glands.
- **Thin skin** covers most of the rest of the body; it contains hair follicles, arrector pili muscles, sebaceous glands, and sweat glands (see Fig. 20 - 3).

Dermis

The dermis develops from mesenchyme, which is derived from the mesoderm underlying the surface ectoderm. Most of the mesenchyme that differentiates into the connective tissue of the dermis originates from the somatic layer of lateral mesoderm; however, some of it is derived from the dermatomes of the somites (see Chapter 15). By 11 weeks, the mesenchymal cells have begun to produce collagenous and elastic connective tissue fibers (Fig. 20 - 1*D*). As the **epidermal ridges** form, the dermis projects into the epidermis forming **dermal ridges** (Fig. 20 - 2). Capillary loops develop in some of these ridges and provide nourishment for the epidermis. Sensory nerve endings form in others. The developing afferent nerve fibers apparently play an important role in the spatial and temporal sequence of dermal (papillary) ridge formation (Moore and Munger, 1989). The development of the *dermatomal pattern of innervation of the skin* is described in Chapter 17.

The blood vessels in the dermis begin as simple, endothelium-lined structures that differentiate from mesenchyme. As the skin grows, new capillaries grow out from the simple vessels. Such simple capillarylike vessels have been observed in the dermis at the end of the fifth week. Some capillaries acquire muscular coats through differentiation of myoblasts developing in the surrounding mesenchyme and become arterioles and arteries. Other capillaries, through which a return flow of blood is established, acquire muscular coats and become venules and veins. As new blood vessels form, some transitory ones normally disappear. By the end of the first trimester, the major vascular organization of the fetal dermis is established (Johnson and Holbrook, 1989).

Glands of the Skin

Two kinds of glands, sebaceous and sweat glands, are derived from the epidermis and grow into the dermis. The mammary glands develop in a similar manner.

SEBACEOUS GLANDS

Most sebaceous glands develop as buds from the sides of developing epithelial root sheaths of hair follicles (Fig. 20-3). The glandular buds grow into the surrounding embryonic connective tissue and branch to form the primordia of several alveoli and their associated ducts. The central cells of the alveoli break down, forming an oily secretion—**sebum**—that is released into the hair follicle and passes to the surface of the skin, where it mixes with desquamated peridermal cells to form **vernix caseosa.** Sebaceous glands independent of hair follicles (e.g., in the glans penis and labia minora) develop in a similar manner to buds from the epidermis.

SWEAT GLANDS

Eccrine sweat glands are located in the skin throughout most of the body. They develop as epidermal downgrowths into the underlying mesenchyme (Fig. 20-3). As the bud elongates, its end coils to form the primordium of the secretory part of the

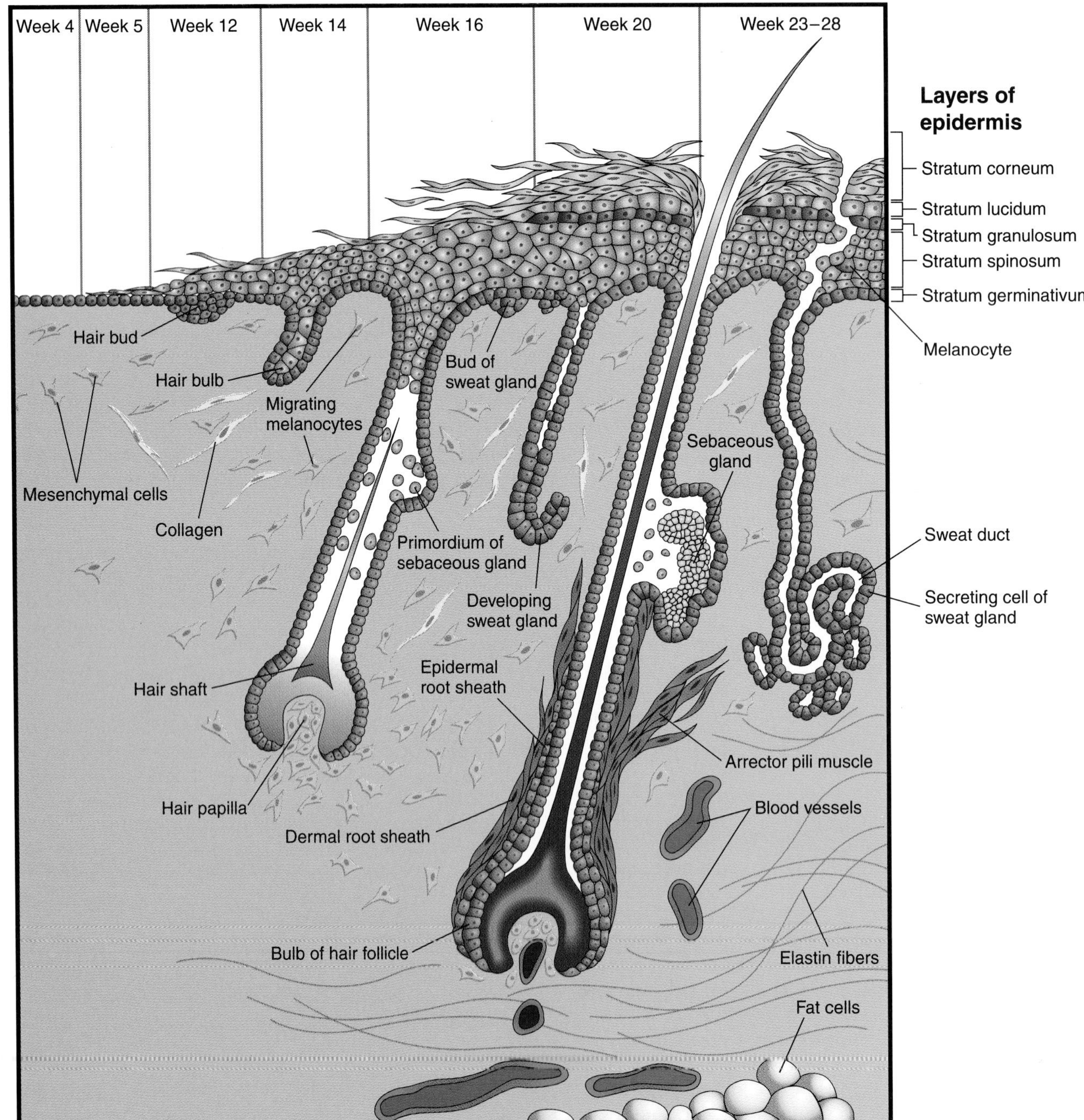

■ **Figure 20-3.** Drawing showing successive stages in the development of a hair and its associated sebaceous gland and arrector pili muscle. Note that the sebaceous gland develops as an outgrowth from the side of the hair follicle.

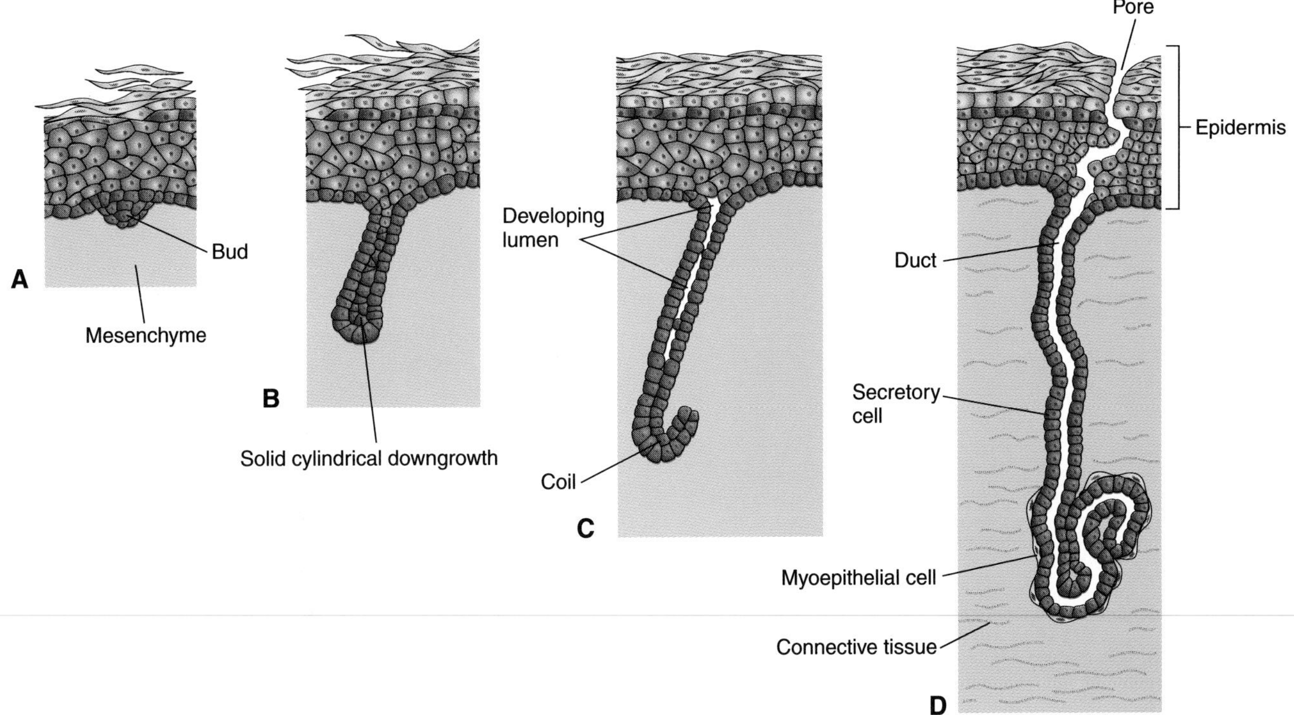

■ **Figure 20–4.** Diagrams illustrating successive stages in the development of a sweat gland. *A* and *B*, The gland develops at about 20 weeks as a solid growth of epidermal cells into the mesenchyme. *C*, Its terminal part coils and forms the body of the gland. The central cells degenerate to form the lumen of the gland. *D*, The peripheral cells differentiate into secretory cells and contractile myoepithelial cells.

gland (Fig. 20-4*A* to *C*). The epithelial attachment of the developing gland to the epidermis forms the primordium of the duct. The central cells of the primordial ducts degenerate, forming a lumen. The peripheral cells of the secretory part of the gland differentiate into myoepithelial and **secretory cells** (Fig. 20-4*D*). The **myoepithelial cells** are thought to be specialized smooth muscle cells that assist in expelling sweat from the glands. Eccrine sweat glands begin to function shortly after birth.

The distribution of the large **apocrine sweat glands** in humans is mostly confined to the axilla, pubic, and perineal regions, and areolae of the nipples. They develop from downgrowths of the stratum germinativum of the epidermis that give rise to hair follicles. As a result the ducts of these glands open, not onto the skin surface as do ordinary sweat glands, but into the upper part of hair follicles superficial to the openings of the sebaceous glands. They secrete only after puberty.

DEVELOPMENT OF HAIR

Hairs begin to develop early in the fetal period (ninth to twelfth week), but they do not become easily recognizable until about the twentieth week (see Chapter 6). Hairs are first recognizable on the eyebrows, upper lip, and chin. A hair follicle begins as a proliferation of the stratum germinativum of the epidermis and extends into the underlying dermis (Fig. 20-3). The **hair bud** soon becomes club-shaped, forming a **hair bulb.** The epithelial cells of the hair bulb constitute the **germinal matrix,** which later produces the hair. The hair bulb (primordium of hair root) is soon invaginated by a small mesenchymal **hair papilla** (Figs. 20-3 and 20-5). The peripheral cells of the developing hair follicle form the **epithelial root sheath,** and the surrounding mesenchymal cells differentiate into the **dermal root sheath.** As cells in the germinal matrix proliferate, they are pushed toward the surface, where they become keratinized to form the **hair shaft.** The hair grows through the epidermis on the eyebrows and upper lip by the end of the twelfth week.

The first hairs that appear—**lanugo hairs** (L. *lana,* wool)—are fine, soft, and lightly pigmented. Lanugo hairs begin to appear toward the end of the twelfth week and are plentiful by 17 to 20 weeks. These hairs help to hold the vernix caseosa on the skin. Lanugo hairs are replaced during the perinatal period by coarser hairs. This hair persists over most of the body, except in the axillary and pubic regions, where it is replaced at puberty by even coarser terminal hairs. In males similar coarse hairs also appear on the face and often on the chest. **Melanoblasts** migrate into the hair bulbs and differentiate into **melanocytes.** The melanin produced by these cells is transferred to the hair-forming cells in the germinal matrix several weeks before birth. The relative content of melanin accounts for different hair colors. **Arrector pili muscles,** small bundles of smooth muscle fibers, differentiate from the mesenchyme surrounding the hair follicle and attach to the dermal root sheath of the hair follicles and the

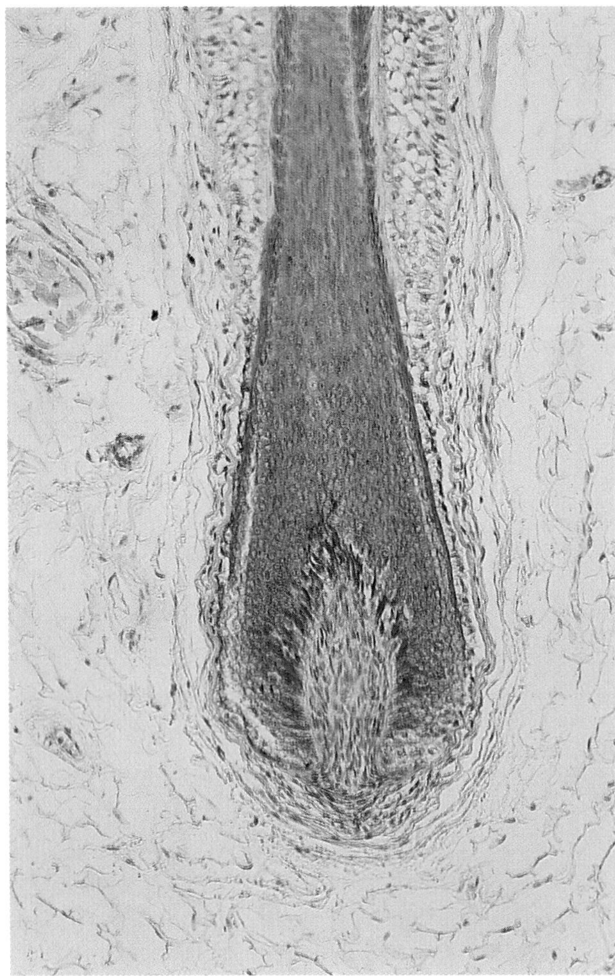

■ **Figure 20–5.** Light micrograph of a longitudinal section of a hair follicle with its hair root and papilla (×132). (From Gartner LP, Hiatt JL: *Color Textbook of Histology.* Philadelphia, WB Saunders, 1997.)

papillary layer of the dermis (Fig. 20-3). Contractions of the arrector pili muscles depress the skin over their attachment and elevate the skin around the hair shafts, forming tiny "goose bumps" on the surface of the skin. The arrector pili muscles are poorly developed in the hairs of the axilla and in certain parts of the face. The hairs forming the eyebrows and the cilia forming the eyelashes have no arrector pili muscles.

Disorders of Keratinization

Ichthyosis (Gr. *ichthys,* fish) is a general term that is applied to a group of disorders resulting from excessive keratinization. The skin is characterized by dryness and fishskin-like scaling, which may involve the entire body surface. A **harlequin fetus** results from a rare keratinizing disorder that is inherited as an autosomal recessive trait (Behrman et al., 1996). The skin is markedly thickened, ridged, and cracked. Affected infants have a grotesque appearance and most of them die during the first week of life. A **collodion baby** is covered at birth by a thick, taut membrane that resembles collodion or parchment. This membrane cracks with the first respiratory efforts and begins to fall off in large sheets. Complete shedding may take several weeks, occasionally leaving normal-appearing skin. **Lamellar ichthyosis** (Fig. 20-6) is an autosomal recessive disorder. A newborn infant with this condition may first appear to be a collodion baby, but the scaling persists. Growth of hair may be curtailed, and development of sweat glands is often impeded. Affected infants often suffer severely in hot weather because of their inability to sweat.

Congenital Ectodermal Dysplasia

This condition represents a group of rare hereditary disorders involving tissues that are ectodermal in origin. The teeth are completely or partially absent. Often the hair, nails, and skin are also severely affected (Buss et al., 1995; Tape and Tye, 1995).

Ectrodactyly-Ectodermal Dysplasia-Clefting Syndrome

Ectrodactyly-ectodermal dysplasia-clefting (EEC) syndrome is a congenital skin condition that is inherited as an autosomal dominant trait. It involves both ectodermal and mesodermal tissues, consisting of **ecto-**

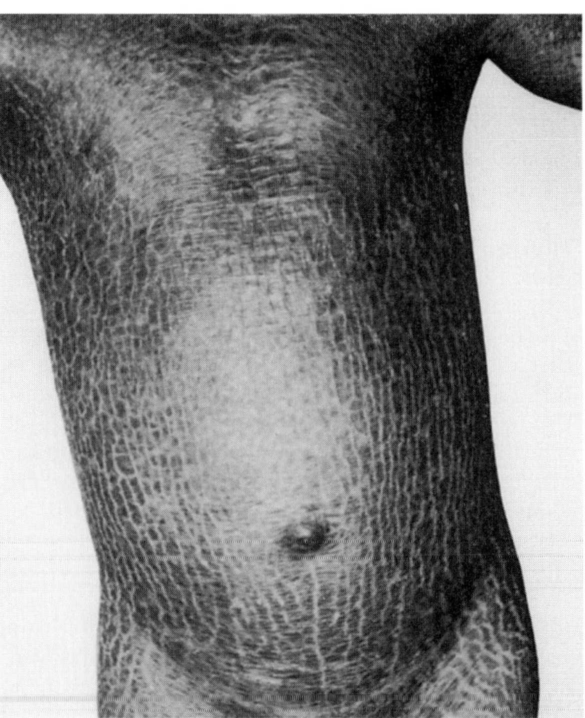

■ **Figure 20–6.** Photograph of an infant with lamellar ichthyosis, a congenital disorder of keratinization of the skin that is characterized by pronounced scaling involving the entire body. (From Behrman RE, Kliegman RM, Arvin AM [eds]: *Nelson Textbook of Pediatrics,* 15th ed. Philadelphia, WB Saunders, 1996.)

dermal dysplasia associated with hypopigmentation of skin and hair, scanty hair and eyebrows, absence of eye lashes, nail dystrophy, hypodontia and microdontia, **ectrodactyly,** and **cleft lip** and **palate** (Buss et al., 1995).

Angiomas of the Skin

These vascular anomalies are developmental defects in which some transitory and/or surplus primitive blood or lymphatic vessels persist. These anomalies are called **angiomas,** even though they may not be true tumors. Those composed of blood vessels may be mainly arterial, venous, or cavernous, but they are often of a mixed type. Angiomas composed of lymphatics are called cystic lymphangiomas or **cystic hygromas** (see Chapter 14). True angiomas are benign tumors of endothelial cells, usually composed of solid or hollow cords; the hollow cords contain blood. Various terms are used to describe angiomatous anomalies ("birthmarks"). **Nevus flammeus** denotes a flat, pink or red, flamelike blotch that often appears on the posterior surface of the neck. A port-wine stain or **hemangioma** is a larger and darker angioma than nevus flammeus and is nearly always anterior or lateral on the face and/or neck. It is sharply demarcated when it is near the median plane, whereas the common angioma (pinkish-red blotch) may cross the median plane. A port-wine stain in the area of distribution of the trigeminal nerve is sometimes associated with a similar type of angioma of the meninges of the brain **(Sturge-Weber syndrome).** A hemangioma is among the most common neoplasms found in infants and children (Behrman et al., 1996).

Albinism

In *generalized albinism,* an autosomal recessive trait, the skin, hair, and retina lack pigment; however, the iris usually shows some pigmentation. Albinism occurs when the melanocytes fail to produce melanin because of the lack of the enzyme tyrosinase. In *localized albinism*—**piebaldism**—an autosomal dominant trait, there is a lack of melanin in patches of skin and/or hair.

Absence of Skin

In rare cases small areas of skin fail to form, giving the appearance of ulcers. The area usually heals by scarring unless a skin graft is performed. Absence of patches of skin is most common in the scalp.

Alopecia

Absence or loss of scalp hair may occur alone or with other abnormalities of the skin and its derivatives. **Congenital alopecia** may be caused by failure of hair follicles to develop, or it may result from follicles producing poor-quality hairs. **Pressure alopecia** results from persistent pressure on the scalp, as may occur in infants lying on their backs.

Hypertrichosis

Excessive hairiness results from the development of supernumerary hair follicles or from the persistence of hairs that normally disappear during the perinatal period. It may be localized (e.g., on the shoulders and back) or diffuse. Localized hypertrichosis is often associated with spina bifida occulta (see Fig. 18-13).

Pili Torti

In this familial disorder the hairs are twisted and bent (L. *tortus,* twisted). Other ectodermal defects (e.g., distorted nails) may be associated with this condition. Pili torti is usually first recognized at 2 to 3 years of age.

DEVELOPMENT OF NAILS

Toenails and fingernails begin to develop at the tips of the digits at about 10 weeks (Fig. 20-7). Development of fingernails precedes that of toenails by about 4 weeks (see Chapter 6). The primordia of nails appear as thickened areas or fields of epidermis at the

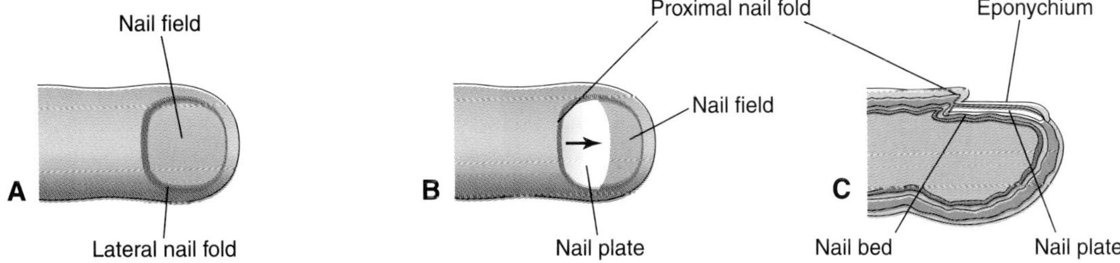

■ **Figure 20-7.** Diagrams illustrating successive stages in the development of a fingernail. *A,* The first indication of a nail is a thickening of the epidermis, the nail field, at the tip of the digit. *B,* As the nail plate develops, it slowly grows toward the tip of the digit. *C,* The fingernail reaches the end of the digit before birth.

tip of each digit. Later these **nail fields** migrate onto the dorsal surface, carrying their innervation from the ventral surface. The nail fields are surrounded laterally and proximally by folds of epidermis, the **nail folds.** Cells from the proximal nail fold grow over the nail field and become keratinized to form the **nail plate** (Fig. 20-7*B*). At first the developing nail is covered by superficial layers of epidermis, the **eponychium.** This later degenerates, exposing the nail, except at its base, where it persists as the **cuticle.** The skin under the free margin of the nail is the **hyponychium.** The fingernails reach the fingertips by about 32 weeks; the toenails reach the toetips by about 36 weeks. Nails that have not reached the tips of the digits at birth indicate prematurity.

Congenital Anonychia

Absence of nails at birth is extremely rare. Anonychia results from failure of the nail fields to form or from failure of the proximal nail folds to form nail plates. The abnormality is permanent. It may be associated with congenital absence or extremely poor development of hair, and with abnormalities of the teeth. Anonychia may be restricted to one or more nails of the digits of the hands and/or feet.

Deformed Nails

This disorder occurs occasionally and may be a manifestation of a generalized skin disease or systemic disease. There are a number of congenital diseases with nail defects (for details, see Behrman et al. [1996]).

DEVELOPMENT OF MAMMARY GLANDS

Mammary glands are a modified and highly specialized type of sweat gland. **Mammary buds** begin to develop during the sixth week as solid downgrowths of the epidermis into the underlying mesenchyme (Fig. 20-8*C*). These changes occur in response to an inductive influence from the mesenchyme (Carlson, 1994). The mammary buds develop as downgrowths from thickened **mammary ridges** (lines), which are thickened strips of ectoderm extending from the axillary to the inguinal regions (Fig. 20-8*A* and *B*). The mammary ridges appear during the fourth week but normally persist in humans only in the pectoral area, where the breasts develop (Fig. 20-8*B*). Each primary bud soon gives rise to several secondary mammary buds that develop into **lactiferous ducts** and their branches (Fig. 20-8*D* and *E*). Canalization of these buds is induced by placental sex hormones entering the fetal circulation. This process continues until late gestation and by term, 15 to 20 lactiferous ducts are formed. The fibrous connective tissue and fat of the mammary gland develop from the surrounding mesenchyme.

During the late fetal period the epidermis at the site of origin of the mammary gland becomes depressed, forming a shallow **mammary pit** (Fig. 20-8*E*). The nipples are poorly formed and depressed in newborn infants. Soon after birth the nipples usually rise from the mammary pits because of proliferation of the surrounding connective tissue of the **areola,** the circular area of skin around the nipple. The smooth muscle fibers of the nipple and areola differentiate from surrounding mesenchymal cells. The rudimentary mammary glands of newborn males and females are identical and are often enlarged. Some secretion, often called **"witch's milk,"** may be produced. These transitory changes are caused by maternal hormones passing through the placental membrane into the fetal circulation.

Only the main lactiferous ducts are formed at birth and the mammary glands remain underdeveloped until puberty. The mammary glands develop similarly and are of the same structure in both sexes. In females the glands enlarge rapidly during puberty (Fig. 20-9), mainly because of fat and other connective tissue development. Growth of the duct system also occurs because of the raised levels of circulating estrogens. Progestogens, prolactin, corticoids, and growth hormone also play a role (Gartner and Hiatt, 1997). If pregnancy occurs, the mammary glands complete their development owing to the raised estrogen levels and the sustained increase in the levels of progesterone. The intralobular ducts undergo rapid development, forming buds that become alveoli. The breasts become hemispherical in shape (Fig. 20-8*D*), largely because of the deposition of fat. Full development occurs at about 20 years (Fig. 20-9*E*).

Gynecomastia

The rudimentary mammary glands in males normally undergo no postnatal development. Gynecomastia (Gr. *gyne,* woman, + *mastos,* breast) refers to excessive development of the male mammary tissue. It occurs in most newborn males because of stimulation of the glandular tissue by maternal sex hormones. This effect disappears in a few weeks (Behrman et al., 1996). During midpuberty about two-thirds of boys develop varying degrees of hyperplasia of the breasts. The subareolar hyperplasia may persist for a few months to 2 years. A decreased ratio of testosterone to estradiol is found in boys with gynecomastia. About 80% of males with Klinefelter syndrome have gynecomastia (see Chapter 8).

Absence of Nipples (Athelia) and Breasts (Amastia)

These rare congenital anomalies may occur bilaterally or unilaterally. They result from failure of development or disappearance of the mammary ridges. These conditions may also result from failure of a mammary bud

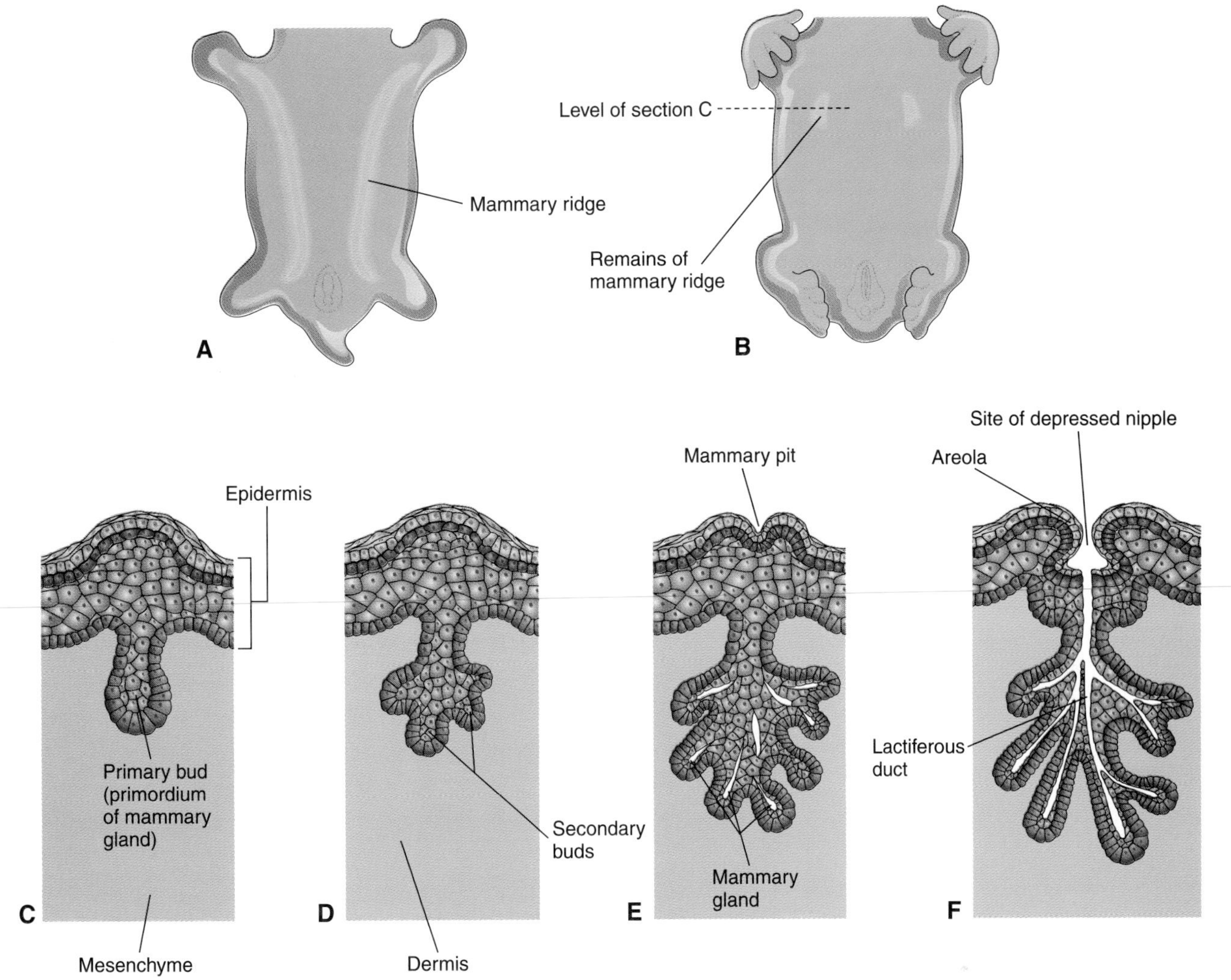

■ **Figure 20–8.** Drawings illustrating the development of mammary glands. *A*, Ventral view of an embryo of about 28 days, showing the mammary ridges. *B*, Similar view at 6 weeks, showing the remains of these ridges. *C*, Transverse section of a mammary ridge at the site of a developing mammary gland. *D*, *E*, and *F*, Similar sections showing successive stages of breast development between the twelfth week and birth.

to form. More common is hypoplasia of the breast, often found in association with gonadal agenesis and Turner syndrome (see Chapter 8).

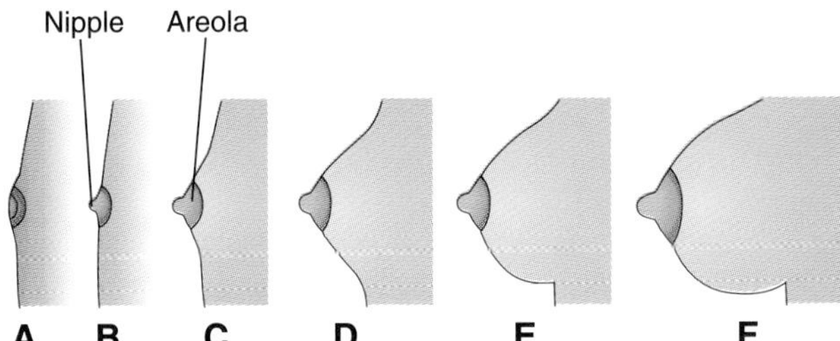

■ **Figure 20–9.** Sketches showing progressive stages in the postnatal development of the breast. *A*, Newborn. *B*, Child. *C*, Early puberty. *D*, Late puberty. *E*, Young adult. *F*, Pregnant female. Note that the nipple is inverted at birth *(A)*. Normally it elevates during childhood to form the usual nipple. Failure of this process to occur gives rise to an inverted nipple. At puberty (12 to 15 years), the breasts enlarge because of development of the mammary glands and the increased deposition of fat.

Aplasia of the Breast

The breasts of a postpubertal female often differ somewhat in size. Marked differences are regarded as anomalies because both glands are exposed to the same hormones at puberty. In these cases there is often associated rudimentary development of muscles, usually the pectoralis major (see Chapter 16).

Supernumerary Breasts and Nipples

An extra breast **(polymastia)** or nipple **(polythelia)** occurs in about 1% of the female population (Fig. 20–10) and is an inheritable condition. An extra breast or nipple usually develops just inferior to the normal breast. **Supernumerary nipples** are also relatively common in males; often they are mistaken for moles (Fig. 20-11). An extra breast or nipple usually develops just inferior to the normal breast. Less commonly, supernumerary breasts or nipples appear in the axillary or abdominal regions. In these positions the nipples or breasts develop from extra mammary buds that develop along the mammary ridges. They usually become obvious in women when pregnancy occurs. About one-third of affected persons have two extra nipples or breasts. Supernumerary mammary tissue very rarely occurs in a location other than along the course of the mammary ridges. It probably develops from tissue that was displaced from these ridges.

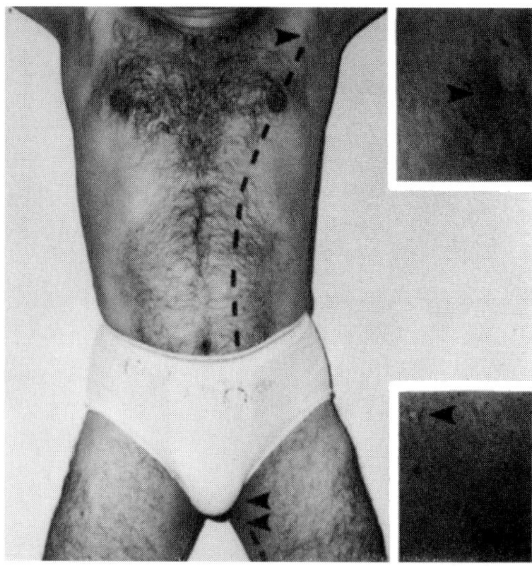

■ **Figure 20-11.** Photograph of a man with nipples in the axillary and thigh regions. The inset photographs are enlargements of the nipples on the left *(arrows)*. The broken line indicates the original position of the left mammary ridge, along which the extra nipples developed. (Courtesy of Dr. Kunwar Bhatnagar, Professor of Anatomy, School of Medicine, University of Louisville, Louisville, Kentucky.)

Inverted Nipples

Sometimes the nipples fail to elevate above the skin surface; i.e., they remain in their newborn location (Figs. 20-8*F* and 20-9*A*). Inverted nipples may make breast feeding of an infant difficult; however, a special exercise can be used to prepare the nipple for feeding an infant.

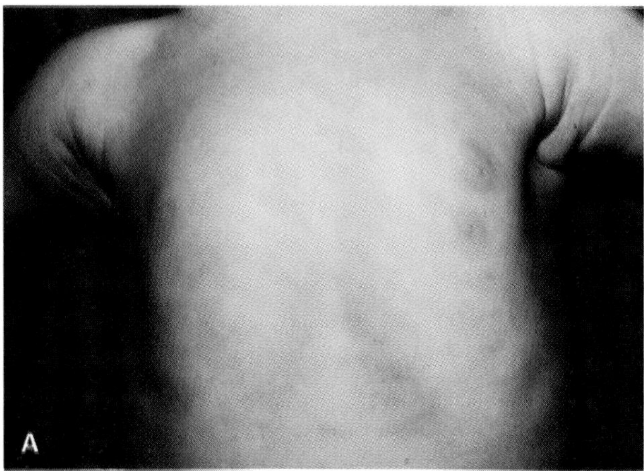

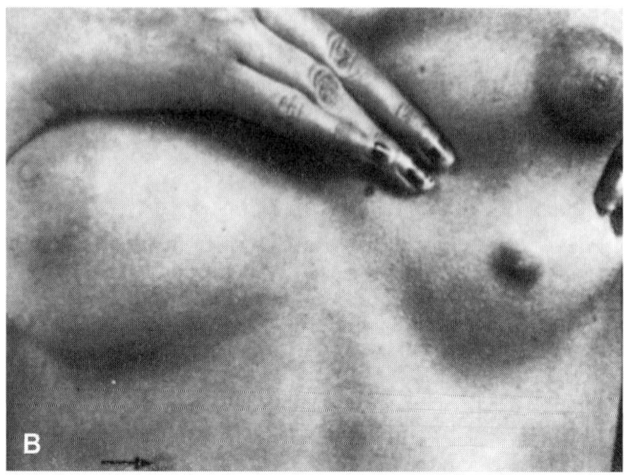

■ **Figure 20-10.** *A*, Female infant with an extra nipple on the left side. *B*, Photograph of a woman with a supernumerary nipple on the right *(arrow)* and a small supernumerary breast inferior to the normal left one. (*A*, Courtesy of Dr. A. E. Chudley, Section of Genetics and Metabolism, Department of Pediatrics and Child Health, Children's Hospital and University of Manitoba, Winnipeg, Manitoba, Canada. *B*, From Haagensen CD: *Diseases of the Breast,* 3rd ed. Philadelphia, WB Saunders, 1986.)

DEVELOPMENT OF TEETH

Two sets of teeth normally develop: the primary dentition or **deciduous teeth** and the secondary dentition or **permanent teeth.** Teeth develop from:

- oral ectoderm
- mesoderm
- neural crest cells

The enamel is derived from ectoderm of the oral cavity; all other tissues differentiate from the surrounding mesenchyme derived from mesoderm and neural crest cells. Experimental evidence suggests that **neural crest cells** are imprinted with morphogenetic information before or shortly after they migrate from the **neural crest** (Carlson, 1994). As the mandible and maxilla grow to accommodate the developing teeth, the shape of the face changes.

Odontogenesis (tooth development) is initiated by the inductive influence of neural crest mesenchyme on the overlying ectoderm (Carlson, 1994). Tooth development is a continuous process; however, it is usually divided into stages for descriptive purposes on the basis of the appearance of the developing tooth. Not all teeth begin to develop at the same time. The first tooth buds appear in the anterior mandibular region; later tooth development occurs in the anterior maxillary region and then progresses posteriorly in both jaws. Tooth development continues for years after birth (Table 20-1). The first indication of tooth devel-

Table 20–1. ■ The Order and Usual Time of Eruption of Teeth and the Time of Shedding of Deciduous Teeth

Tooth	Usual Eruption Time	Shedding Time
Deciduous		
Medial incisor	6–8 mos	6–7 yr
Lateral incisor	8–10 mos	7–8 yr
Canine	16–20 mos	10–12 yr
First molar	12–16 mos	9–11 yr
Second molar	20–24 mos	10–12 yr
Permanent*		
Medial incisor	7–8 yr	
Lateral incisor	8–9 yr	
Canine	10–12 yr	
First premolar	10–11 yr	
Second premolar	11–12 yr	
First molar	6–7 yr	
Second molar	12 yr	
Third molar	13–25 yr	

Modified from Moore KL: *Clinically Oriented Anatomy,* 3rd ed. Baltimore, Williams & Wilkins, 1992.

*The permanent teeth are not shed. If they are not properly cared for, or disease of the gingiva develops, they may have to be extracted.

opment occurs early in the sixth week as a thickening of the oral epithelium, a derivative of the surface ectoderm. These U-shaped bands—**dental laminae**—follow the curves of the primitive jaws (Figs. 20–12*A* and 20–13*A*).

Bud Stage of Tooth Development

Each dental lamina develops ten centers of proliferation from which swellings—**tooth buds**—grow into the underlying mesenchyme (Figs. 20–12*B* and 20–13*B*). These tooth buds develop into the first teeth or **deciduous teeth,** which were given this name because they are shed during childhood (Table 20–1). There are ten tooth buds in each jaw, one for each deciduous tooth. The tooth buds for **permanent teeth** that have deciduous predecessors begin to appear at about 10 weeks from deep continuations of the dental lamina (Fig. 20-13*D*). They develop lingual (toward the tongue) to the deciduous **tooth buds.** The permanent molars that have no deciduous predecessors develop as buds from posterior extensions of the dental laminae. The tooth buds for the permanent teeth appear at different times, mostly during the fetal period. The buds for the second and third permanent molars develop after birth.

Cap Stage of Tooth Development

As each tooth bud is invaginated by mesenchyme—the primordium of the dental papilla—it becomes cap-shaped (Figs. 20–13*C* and 20–14). The ectodermal part of the developing tooth, the **enamel organ** (dental organ), eventually produces enamel. The internal part of each cap-shaped tooth, the **dental papilla,** is the primordium of the dental pulp. Together, the dental papilla and enamel organ form the **tooth germ** (Gartner and Hiatt, 1997). The outer cell layer of the enamel organ is the **outer enamel epithelium,** and the inner cell layer lining the "cap" is the **inner enamel epithelium** (Fig. 20–13*D*). The central core of loosely arranged cells between the layers of enamel epithelium is the **enamel (stellate) reticulum.** As the enamel organ and dental papilla of the tooth develop, the mesenchyme surrounding the developing tooth condenses to form the **dental sac,** a vascularized capsular structure (Fig. 20–13*E*). The dental sac is the primordium of the cementum and periodontal ligament. The **cementum** is the bonelike rigid connective tissue covering the root of the tooth. The **peridontal ligament** is the fibrous connective tissue that surrounds the root of the tooth, separating it from and attaching it to the alveolar bone (Fig. 20–13*G*).

Bell Stage of Tooth Development

As the enamel organ differentiates, the developing tooth assumes the shape of a bell (Figs. 20–13*D* and *E* and 20–14). The mesenchymal cells in the dental papilla adjacent to the inner enamel epithelium differentiate into **odontoblasts,** which produce **predentin** and deposit it adjacent to the epithelium. Later, the predentin calcifies and becomes **dentin.** As the dentin thickens, the odontoblasts regress toward the center

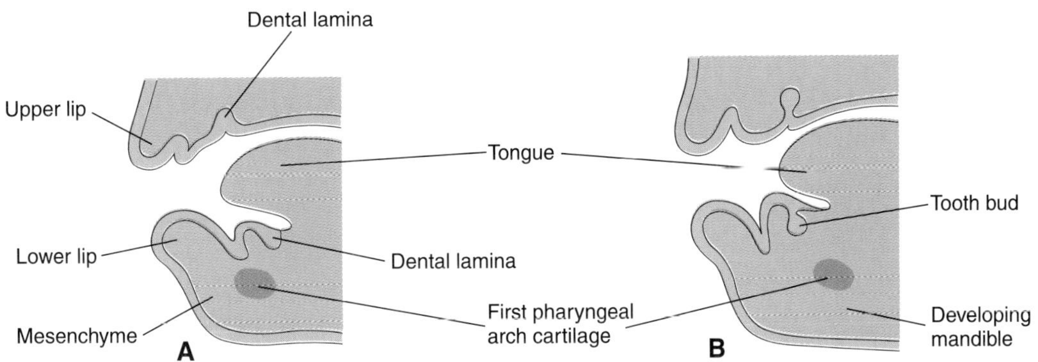

■ **Figure 20–12.** Diagrammatic sketches of sagittal sections through the developing jaws, illustrating early development of the teeth. *A,* Early in the sixth week, showing the dental laminae. *B,* Later in the sixth week, showing tooth buds arising from the dental laminae.

of the dental papilla; however, their fingerlike cytoplasmic processes—**odontoblastic processes** or Tomes processes—remain embedded in the dentin (Fig. 20-13*F* and *I*). The yellowish dentin is the second hardest tissue in the body (Gartner and Hiatt, 1997). It overlies and protects the brittle enamel, the hardest tissue in the body, from being fractured (Fig. 20-15).

Cells of the inner enamel epithelium differentiate into **ameloblasts,** which produce enamel in the form of prisms (rods) over the dentin. As the **enamel** increases, the ameloblasts regress toward the outer enamel epithelium. Enamel and dentin formation begins at the tip (cusp) of the tooth and progresses toward the future root. The **root of the tooth** begins to develop after dentin and enamel formation is well advanced (Fig. 20-16). The inner and outer enamel epithelia come together in the neck region of the tooth, where they form a fold, the **epithelial root sheath** (Fig. 20-13*F*). This sheath grows into the mesenchyme and initiates root formation. The odontoblasts adjacent to the epithelial root sheath form dentin that is continuous with that of the crown. As the dentin increases, it reduces the pulp cavity to a nar-

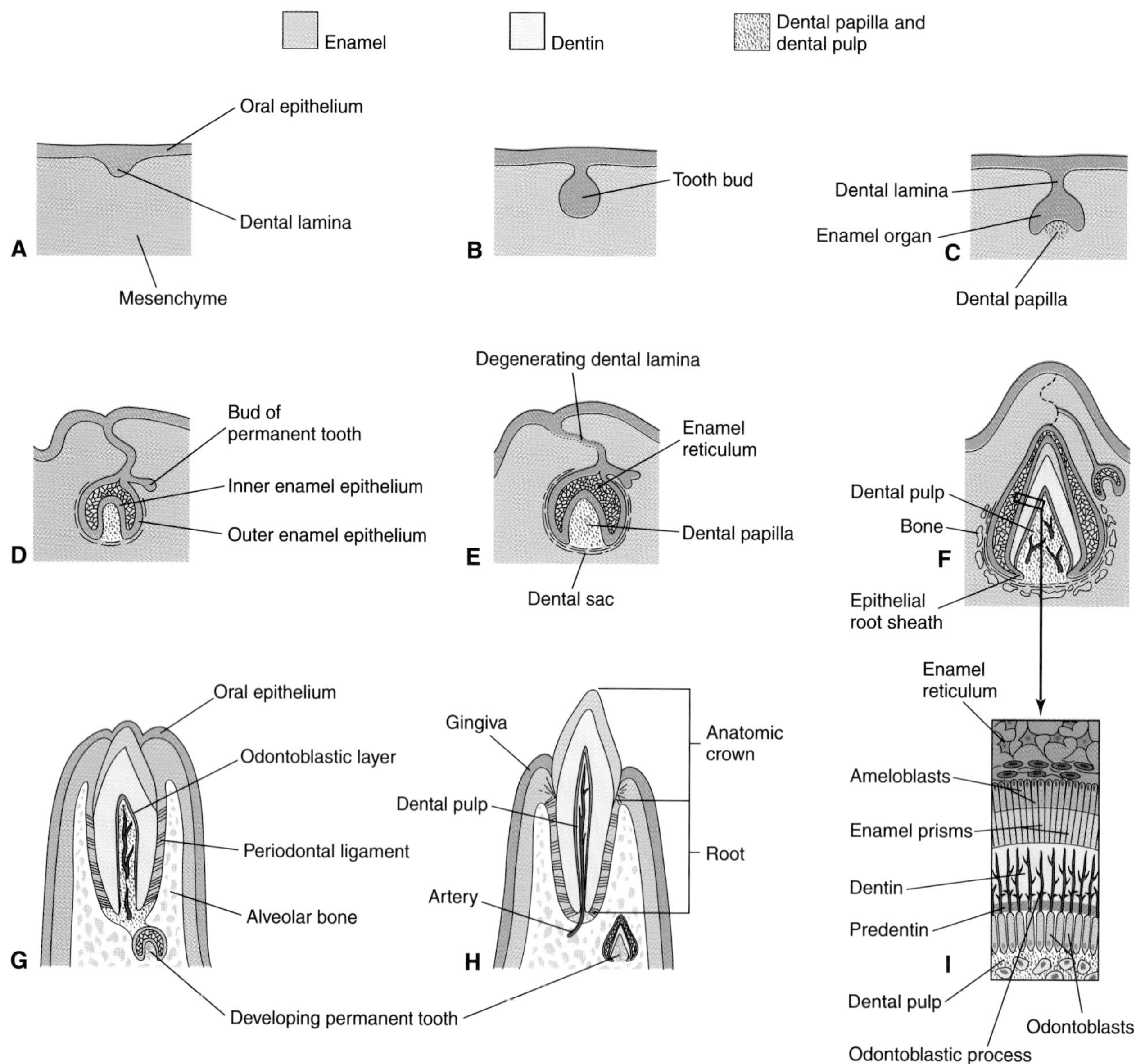

■ **Figure 20-13.** Schematic drawings of sagittal sections illustrating successive stages in the development and eruption of an incisor tooth. *A,* 6 weeks, showing the dental lamina. *B,* 7 weeks, showing the tooth bud developing from the dental lamina. *C,* 8 weeks, showing the cap stage of tooth development. *D,* 10 weeks, showing the early bell stage of a deciduous tooth and the bud stage of a permanent tooth. *E,* 14 weeks, showing the advanced bell stage of tooth development. Note that the connection (dental lamina) of the tooth to the oral epithelium is degenerating. *F,* 28 weeks, showing the enamel and dentin layers. *G,* 6 months postnatal, showing early tooth eruption. *H,* 18 months postnatal, showing a fully erupted deciduous incisor tooth. The permanent incisor tooth now has a well-developed crown. *I,* Section through a developing tooth, showing ameloblasts (enamel producers) and odontoblasts (dentin producers).

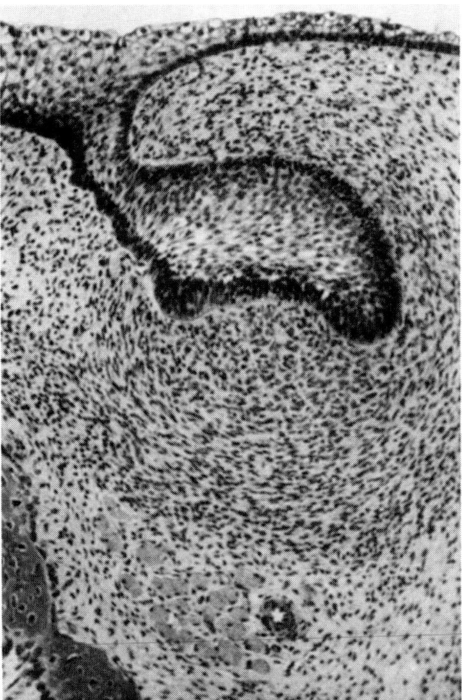

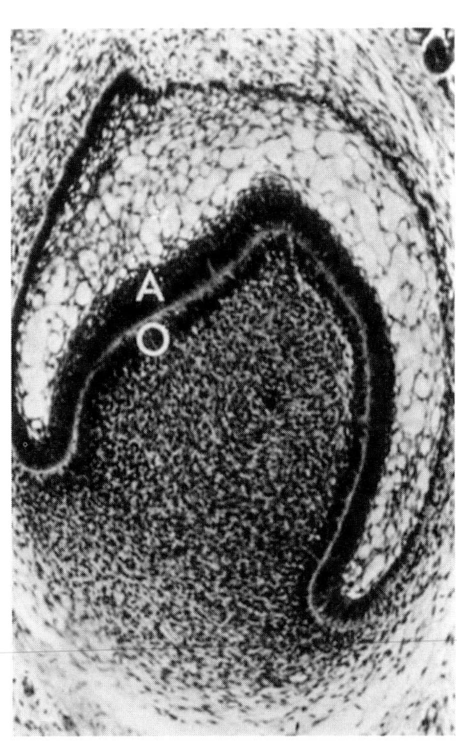

■ **Figure 20-14.** *Left:* Photomicrograph of a developing tooth in the cap stage of development, showing the enamel organ attached to the oral mucosa by the dental lamina (×100). *Right:* Photomicrograph of a developing tooth in the late bell stage with ameloblasts (inner enamel epithelium **[A]**) differentiated and in contact with odontoblasts **(O)**. (From Leeson CR, Leeson TS: *Histology,* 5th ed. Philadelphia, WB Saunders, 1985.)

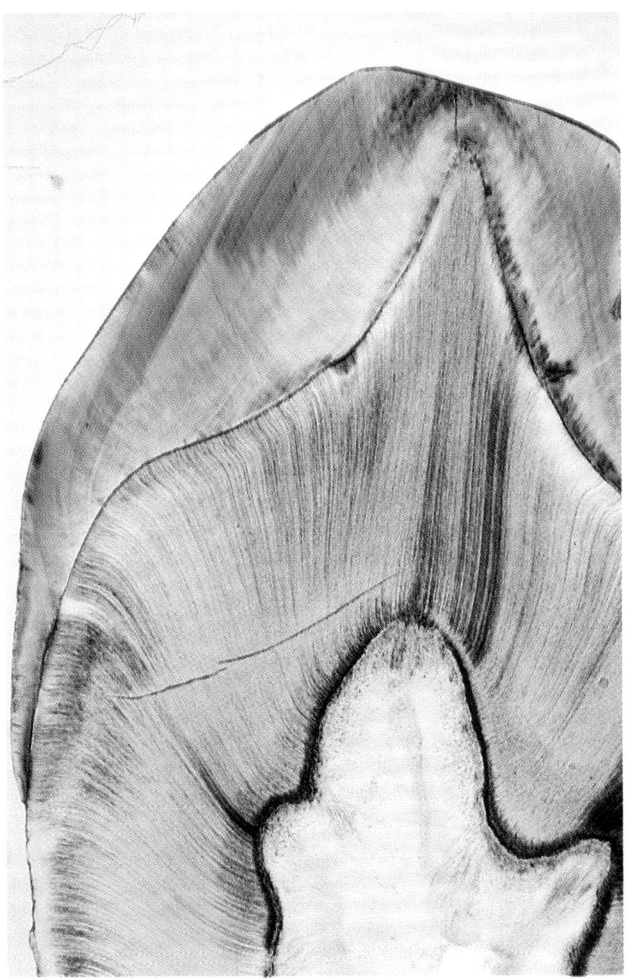

■ **Figure 10-15.** Photomicrograph of the crown and neck of a tooth (×17). (From Gartner LP, Hiatt JL: *Color Textbook of Histology.* Philadelphia, WB Saunders, 1997.)

row **root canal** through which the vessels and nerves pass. The inner cells of the dental sac differentiate into **cementoblasts,** which produce cementum that is restricted to the root. **Cementum** is deposited over the dentin of the root and meets the enamel at the neck of the tooth **(cementoenamel junction).**

As the teeth develop and the jaws ossify, the outer cells of the dental sac also become active in bone formation. Each tooth soon becomes surrounded by bone, except over its crown. The tooth is held in its **alveolus** (bony socket) by the strong **periodontal ligament,** a derivative of the dental sac (Fig. 20-13*G* and *H*). Some fibers of this ligament are embedded in the cementum; other fibers are embedded in the bony wall of the alveolus. The peridontal ligament is located between the cementum of the root and the bony alveolus.

Tooth Eruption

As the teeth develop they begin a continuous slow movement toward the oral cavity (Fig. 20-13*G*). The mandibular teeth usually erupt before the maxillary teeth, and girls' teeth usually erupt sooner than boys' teeth. The child's dentition contains 20 deciduous teeth. The complete adult dentition consists of 32 teeth. As the root of the tooth grows, its crown gradually erupts through the oral epithelium. The part of the oral mucosa around the erupted crown becomes the **gingiva** (gum). Usually eruption of the deciduous teeth occurs between the sixth and twenty-fourth months after birth (Table 20-1). The mandibular medial or **central incisors** usually erupt 6 to 8 months after birth, but this process may not begin until 12 or 13 months in some children. Despite this, all 20 decid-

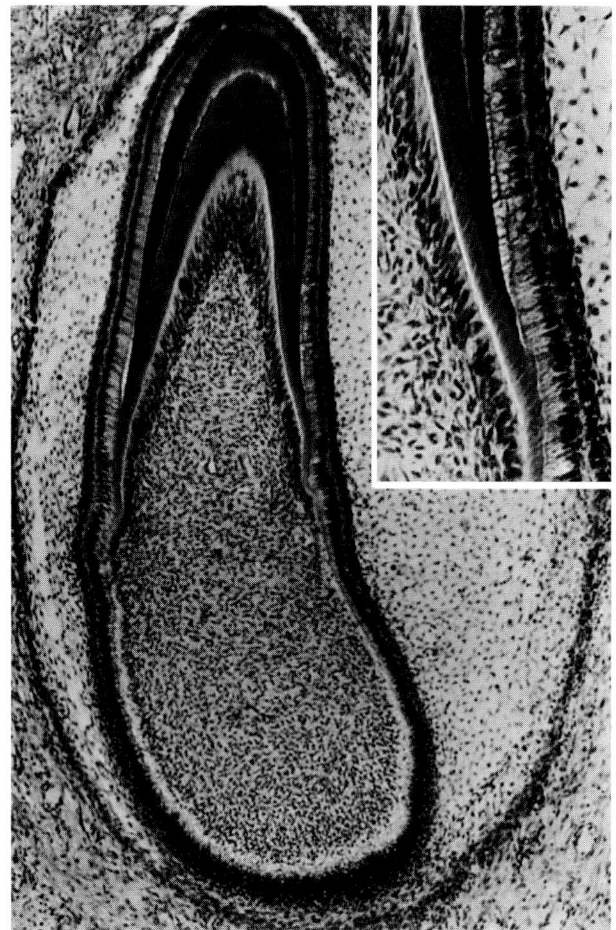

■ **Figure 20–16.** Photomicrograph of a developing tooth at the stage when crown formation is well advanced. Enamel and dentin are present with a thin layer of predentin in relation to the odontoblasts (×75). *Upper right insert:* Higher magnification of part of the tooth showing, from left to right, pulp, odontoblasts, predentin, dentin, enamel (black), ameloblasts, stratum intermedium, and enamel reticulum (×175). (From Leeson CR, Leeson TS, Paparo AA: *Text/Atlas of Histology.* Philadelphia, WB Saunders, 1988.)

uous teeth are usually present by the end of the second year in healthy children. Delayed eruption of all teeth may indicate a systemic or nutritional disturbance such as hypopituitarism or hypothyroidism (Behrman et al., 1996).

The **permanent teeth** develop in a manner similar to that described for deciduous teeth. As a permanent tooth grows, the root of the corresponding deciduous tooth is gradually resorbed by **osteoclasts.** Consequently, when the deciduous tooth is shed, it consists only of the crown and the uppermost part of the root. The permanent teeth usually begin to erupt during the sixth year and continue to appear until early adulthood (Fig. 20-17; Table 20-1). The shape of the face is affected by the development of the paranasal sinuses and the growth of the maxilla and mandible to accommodate the teeth (see Chapter 10). It is the lengthening of the **alveolar processes** (bony sockets supporting the teeth) that results in the increase in the depth of the face during childhood.

Natal Teeth

Natal teeth are erupted at birth (L. *natus,* birth). There are usually two in the position of the mandibular incisors. Natal teeth are observed in about 1 in 2000 newborn infants (Behrman et al., 1996). Natal teeth may produce maternal discomfort during breast-feeding. In addition, the infant's tongue may be lacerated or the teeth may detach and be aspirated; for these reasons natal teeth are sometimes extracted.

Enamel Hypoplasia

Defective enamel formation causes pits and/or fissures in the enamel (Fig. 20-18). These defects result from temporary disturbances of enamel formation. Various factors may injure ameloblasts, the enamel builders (e.g., nutritional deficiency, tetracycline therapy, and infectious diseases such as measles). **Rickets** during the critical period of permanent tooth development is the most common known cause of enamel hypoplasia. Rickets, a disease in children who are deficient in vitamin D, is characterized by disturbance of ossification of the epiphyseal cartilages and disorientation of cells at the metaphysis (see Chapter 15).

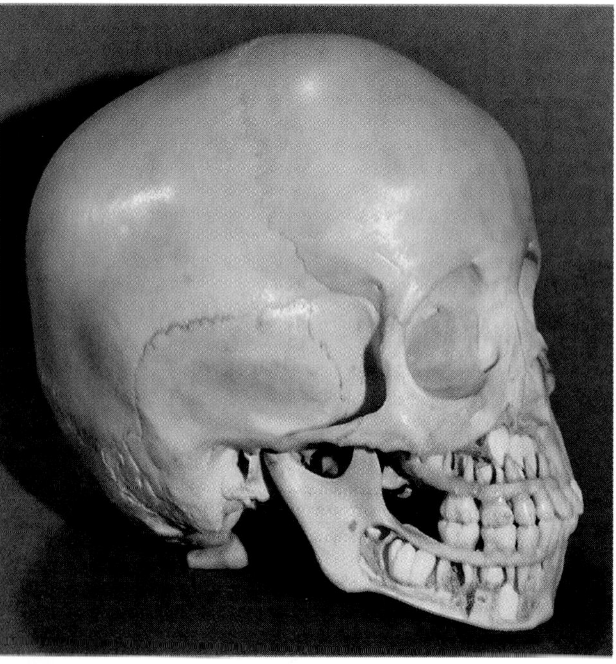

■ **Figure 20–17.** Photograph of a 4-year-old child's skull. Bone has been removed to show the relation of the developing permanent teeth to the erupted deciduous teeth.

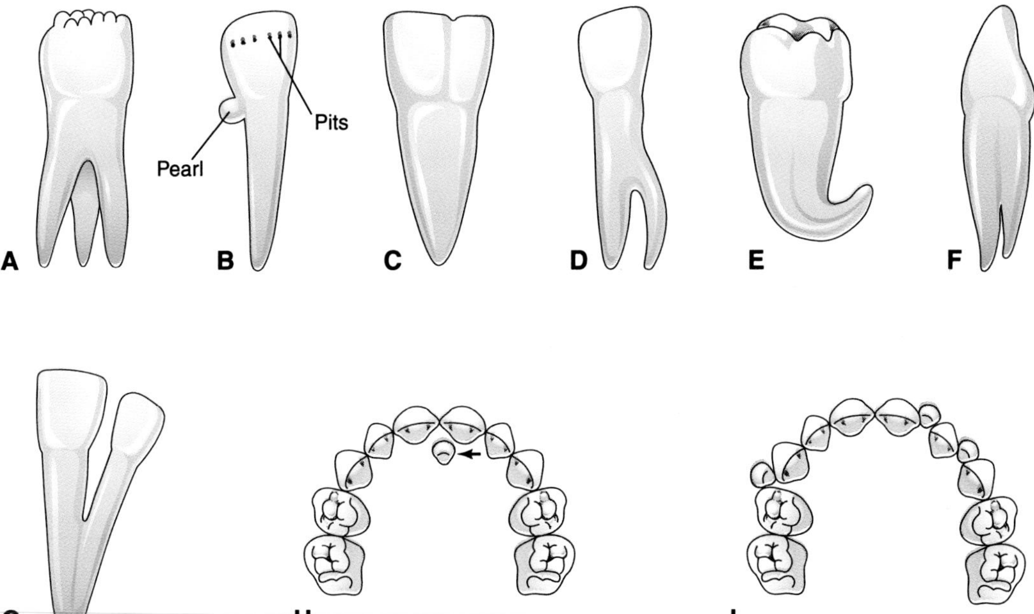

■ Figure 20–18. Drawings illustrating common anomalies of teeth. *A,* Irregular raspberrylike crown. *B,* Enamel pearl and pits. *C,* Incisor tooth with a double crown. *D,* Abnormal division of root. *E,* Distorted root. *F,* Branched root. *G,* Fused roots. *H,* Hyperdontia with a supernumerary incisor tooth in the anterior region of the palate *(arrow). I,* Hyperdontia with 13 deciduous teeth in the maxilla (upper jaw) instead of the normal ten.

Variations of Tooth Shape

Abnormally shaped teeth are relatively common (Fig. 20-18*A* to *G*). Occasionally there are spherical masses of enamel—**enamel pearls**—attached to the tooth. They are formed by aberrant groups of ameloblasts. In other children, the maxillary lateral incisor teeth may have a slender, tapering shape (peg-shaped incisors). **Congenital syphilis** affects the differentiation of the permanent teeth, resulting in screwdriver-shaped incisors, with central notches in their incisive edges.

Numerical Abnormalities

One or more supernumerary teeth may develop, or the normal number of teeth may fail to form (Fig. 20-18*H* and *I*). **Supernumerary teeth** usually develop in the area of the maxillary incisors and disrupt the position and eruption of normal teeth. The extra teeth commonly erupt posterior to the normal ones. In **partial anodontia,** one or more teeth are absent. Congenital absence of one or more teeth is often a familial trait. In **total anodontia,** no teeth develop; this very rare condition is usually associated with *congenital ectodermal dysplasia* (Behrman et al., 1996).

Abnormally Sized Teeth

Disturbances during the differentiation of teeth may result in gross alterations of dental morphology, such as *macrodontia* (large teeth) and *microdontia* (small teeth).

Fused Teeth

Occasionally a tooth bud divides or two buds partially fuse to form fused teeth (Fig. 20-18*C* and *G*). This condition is commonly observed in the mandibular incisors of the primary dentition. "Twinning" of teeth results from division of the tooth bud. In some cases the permanent tooth does not form; this suggests that the deciduous and permanent tooth primordia fused to form the primary tooth.

Dentigerous Cyst

In rare cases a cyst develops in a mandible, maxilla, or maxillary sinus that contains an unerupted tooth. The dentigerous (tooth-bearing) cyst develops because of cystic degeneration of the enamel reticulum of the enamel organ of an unerupted tooth. Most cysts are deeply situated in the jaw and are associated with misplaced or malformed secondary teeth that have failed to erupt.

Amelogenesis Imperfecta

The enamel is soft and friable because of hypocalcification, and the teeth are yellow to brown in color. The teeth are covered with only a thin layer of abnormally formed enamel through which the yellow underlying dentin is visible (Johnsen, 1996). This gives a darkened appearance to the teeth. This autosomal dominant trait affects about 1 in every 20,000 children.

Dentinogenesis Imperfecta

This condition is relatively common in white children (Fig. 20-19). The teeth are brown to gray-blue with an opalescent sheen because the odontoblasts fail to differentiate normally and poorly calcified dentin results (Johnsen, 1996). Both deciduous and permanent teeth are usually involved. The enamel tends to wear down rapidly, exposing the dentin. This anomaly is inherited as an autosomal dominant trait (Thompson et al., 1991).

Discolored Teeth

Foreign substances incorporated into the developing enamel discolor the teeth. The hemolysis (liberation of hemoglobin) associated with erythroblastosis fetalis or hemolytic disease of the newborn (HDN) (see Chapter 7) may produce blue to black discoloration of the teeth. *All tetracyclines are extensively incorporated into the enamel of teeth.* The critical period at risk is from about 14 weeks of fetal life to the tenth postnatal month for primary teeth, and from about 14 weeks of fetal life to 16th postnatal year for permanent teeth (Johnsen, 1996). Tetracyclines produce brownish-yellow discoloration (mottling) and enamel hypoplasia because they interfere with the metabolic processes of the ameloblasts. The enamel is completely formed on all but the third molars by about 8 years of age. For this reason, *tetracyclines should not be administered to pregnant women or children under 8 years of age* (Shepard, 1992).

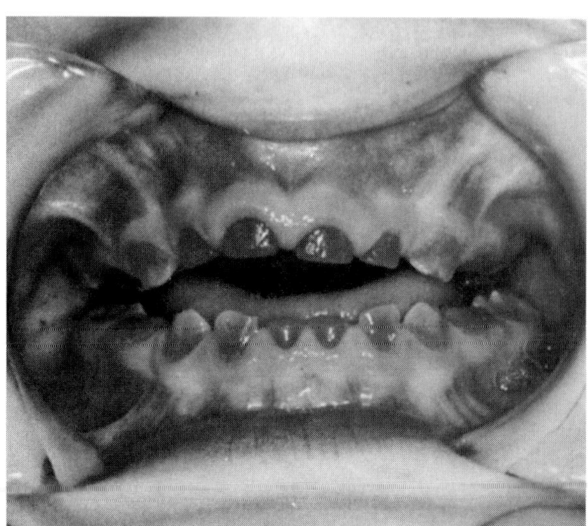

■ **Figure 20-19.** Photograph of the teeth of a child with dentinogenesis imperfecta. (From Thompson MW: *Genetics in Medicine,* 4th ed. Philadelphia, WB Saunders, 1986.)

SUMMARY OF THE INTEGUMENTARY SYSTEM

The skin and its appendages develop from ectoderm, mesoderm, and neural crest cells. The epidermis is derived from surface ectoderm. Melanocytes are derived from **neural crest cells** that migrate into the epidermis. Cast-off cells from the epidermis mix with secretions of sebaceous glands to form the **vernix caseosa,** a whitish, greasy coating for the skin. This fatty substance protects the epidermis, probably making it more waterproof, and facilitates birth because of its slipperiness.

Hairs develop from downgrowths of the epidermis into the dermis. By about 20 weeks the fetus is completely covered with fine, downy hairs—**lanugo hairs.** These hairs are shed by birth or shortly thereafter and are replaced by coarser hairs. Most **sebaceous glands** develop as outgrowths from the sides of hair follicles; however, some glands develop as downgrowths of the epidermis into the dermis. **Sweat glands** also develop from epidermal downgrowths into the dermis. **Mammary glands** develop in a similar manner.

Congenital anomalies of the skin are mainly **disorders of keratinization** (ichthyosis) and pigmentation (albinism). Abnormal blood vessel development results in various types of **angioma.** Nails may be absent or malformed. Hair may be absent or excessive. Absence of mammary glands is rare, but supernumerary breasts (polymastia) or nipples (polythelia) are relatively common.

Teeth develop from ectoderm, mesoderm, and neural crest cells. The enamel is produced by **ameloblasts,** which are derived from the oral ectoderm; all other dental tissues develop from mesenchyme, derived from mesoderm and neural crest cells. The common **congenital anomalies of teeth** are defective formation of enamel and dentin, abnormalities in shape, and variations in number and position. **Tetracyclines** are extensively incorporated into the enamel of developing teeth and produce brownish-yellow discoloration and hypoplasia of the enamel. Consequently, they should not prescribed for pregnant women or children under 8 years of age.

Clinically Oriented Problems

Case 20–1

A newborn infant had two erupted mandibular incisor teeth.

- What are these teeth called?
- How common is this anomaly?
- Are they supernumerary teeth?
- What problems and/or danger might be associated with the presence of teeth at birth?

Case 20–2

The primary dentition of an infant had a brownish-yellow color and some hypoplasia of the enamel. The mother recalled that she had been given antibiotics during the second trimester of her pregnancy.

- What is the probable cause of the infant's tooth discoloration?
- Dysfunction of what cells would cause the enamel hypoplasia?
- Would the secondary dentition be discolored?

Case 20–3

An infant was born with a small, irregularly shaped, light-red blotch on the posterior surface of the neck. It was level with the surrounding skin and blanched when light pressure was applied to it.

- Name this congenital anomaly.
- What do these observations probably indicate?
- Is this condition common?
- Are there other names for this skin anomaly?

Case 20–4

A newborn infant had a tuft of hair in the lumbosacral region of the back.

- What does this tuft of hair probably indicate?
- Is this condition common?
- Is this anomaly clinically important?

Case 20–5

The skin of a newborn infant had a collodion type of covering that fissured and exfoliated shortly after birth. Later, lamellar ichthyosis developed.

- Briefly describe this condition.
- Is it common?
- How is it inherited?

Discussion of these problems appears at the back of the book.

REFERENCES AND SUGGESTED READING

Avery JK: *Essentials of Oral Histology and Embryology.* St Louis, Mosby-Year Book, 1992.

Behrman RE, Kliegman RM, Arvin AM (eds): *Nelson Textbook of Pediatrics,* 15th ed. Philadelphia, WB Saunders, 1996.

Beller F: Development and anatomy of the breast. *In* Mitchell GW Jr, Bassett LW (eds): *The Female Breast and Its Disorders.* Baltimore, Williams & Wilkins, 1990.

Bland KI, Copeland III EM (eds): *The Breast.* Philadelphia, WB Saunders, 1991.

Booth DH, Persaud TVN: Congenital absence of the breast. *Anat Anz 155:*23, 1984.

Buss PW, Hughes HE, Clarke A: Twenty-four cases of the EEC syndrome: clinical presentation and management. *J Med Genet 32:* 716, 1995.

Carlson BM: *Human Embryology and Developmental Biology.* St Louis, Mosby-Year Book, 1994.

Casasco A, Calligaro A, Casasco M, et al: Early stages of ameloblast differentiation as revealed by immunogold detection of enamel matrix proteins. *Proc Roy Micr Soc 30:*113, 1995.

Collins P: Embryology and development. *In* Bannister LH, Berry MM, Collins P, et al (eds): *Gray's Anatomy. The Anatomical Basis of Medicine and Surgery,* 38th ed. New York, Churchill Livingstone, 1995.

Cormack DH: *Essential Histology.* Philadelphia, JB Lippincott, 1993.

Darmstadt GL, Lane AT: The skin. *In* Berhman RE, Kliegman RM, Arvin AM (eds): *Nelson Textbook of Pediatrics,* 15th ed. Philadelphia, WB Saunders, 1996.

Foster CA, Bertram JF, Holbrook KA: Morphometric and statistical analyses describing the *in utero* growth of human epidermis. *Anat Rec 222:*201, 1988.

Gartner LP, Hiatt JL: *Color Textbook of Histology.* Philadelphia, WB Saunders, 1997.

Gilbert-Barness E (ed): *Potter's Pathology of the Fetus and Infant.* 2 vols. St Louis, Mosby-Year Book, 1997.

Haake AR, Lane AT: Retention of differentiated characteristics in human fetal keratinocytes in vitro. *In Vitro Cell Dev Biol 25:*592, 1989.

Holbrook KA, Underwood RA, Vogel AM, et al: The appearance, density and distribution of melanocytes in human embryonic and fetal skin revealed by the anti-melanoma monoclonal antibody. *Anat Embryol 180:*443, 1989.

Horn TD: Developmental defects of the skin. *In* Farmer ER, Hood AF (eds): *Pathology of the Skin.* Norwalk, Appleton & Lange, 1990.

Hunter JAA, Savin JA, Dahl MV: *Clinical Dermatology.* Oxford Blackwell Scientific Publications, 1990.

Johnsen DC: The oral cavity. *In* Behrman RE, Kliegman RM, Arvin AM (eds): *Nelson Textbook of Pediatrics,* 15th ed. Philadelphia, WB Saunders, 1996.

Johnson CL, Holbrook KA: Development of human embryonic and fetal dermal vasculature. *J Invest Dermatol 93(Suppl):*105, 1989.

Mackie RM: *Clinical Dermatology,* 3rd ed. Oxford, Oxford University Press, 1991.

Moore KL: *Clinically Oriented Anatomy,* 3rd ed. Baltimore, Williams & Wilkins, 1992.

Moore SJ, Munger BL: The early ontogeny of the afferent nerves and papillary ridges in human digital glabrous skin. *Dev Brain Res 48:* 119, 1989.

Müller M, Jasmin JR, Monteil RA, Loubiere R: Embryology of the hair follicle. *Early Hum Dev 26:*59, 1991.

Nanney LB, Stoscheck CM, King LE Jr, et al: Immunolocalization of epidermal growth factor receptors in normal developing human skin. *J Invest Dermatol 94:*742, 1990.

Opitz JM: Pathogenetic analysis of certain developmental and genetic ectodermal defects. *Birth Defects 24:*75, 1988.

Osborne MP: Breast development and anatomy. *In* Harris JR, Hellman S, Henderson IC, Kinne DW (eds): *Breast Diseases,* 2nd ed. Philadelphia, JB Lippincott, 1991.

Persaud TVN: *Environmental Causes of Human Birth Defects.* Springfield, IL, Charles C Thomas, 1990.

Shafer WG, Hine MG, Levy BM: *A Textbook of Oral Pathology,* 4th ed. Philadelphia, WB Saunders, 1983.

Shepard TH: *Catalog of Teratogenic Drugs,* 6th ed. Baltimore, The Johns Hopkins University Press, 1992.

Smith DW, Gong BT: Scalp-hair patterning: Its origin and significance relative to early brain and upper facial development. *Teratology 9:* 17, 1974.

Sperber GH: *Craniofacial Embryology,* 4th ed (revised reprint). London, Butterworths, 1993.

Tape MW, Tye E: Ectodermal dysplasia: literature review and a case report. *Compend Contin Educ Dent 16:*524, 1995.

Tavassoli FA: *Pathology of the Breast.* Norwalk, Appleton & Lange, 1995.

Telford IR, Bridgman CF: *Introduction to Functional Histology.* New York, Harper & Row Publishers, 1990.

Ten Cate AR: Development of the tooth. *In* Ten Cate, AR (ed): *Oral Histology. Development, Structure, and Function,* 4th ed. St Louis, Mosby-Year Book, 1994.

Ten Cate AR, Mills C, Solomon G: The development of the periodontium. A transplantation and autoradiographic study. *Anat Rec 170:* 365, 1971.

Termine JD: Development of dental and paradental structures; Enamel. *In* Provenza DV (ed): *Fundamentals of Oral Histology and Embryology,* 2nd ed. Philadelphia, Lea & Febiger, 1988.

Thesleff I: Extracellular matrix and tooth morphogenesis. *In* Pratt RM, Christensen RL (eds): *Current Research Trends in Prenatal Craniofacial Development.* Amsterdam, Elsevier/North Holland, 1980.

Thompson MW, McInnes RR, Willard HF: *Thompson & Thompson Genetics in Medicine,* 5th ed. Philadelphia, WB Saunders, 1991.

Wilflingseder P: Skin hemangiomas; aggressive approach. *In* Huffstadt AJC (ed): *Congenital Malformations.* Amsterdam, Excerpta Medica, 1980.

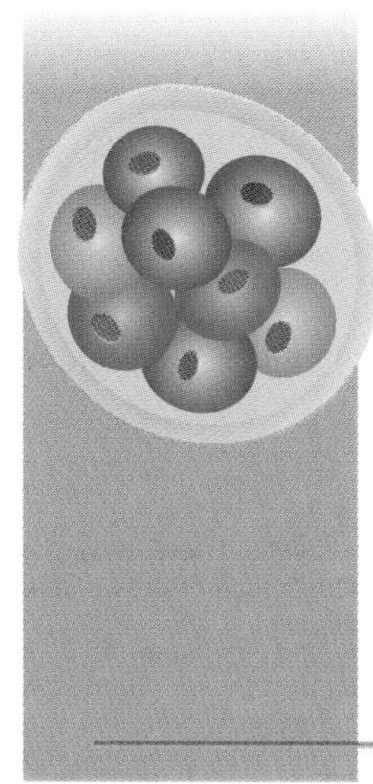

Discussion of Clinically Oriented Problems

Chapter 1

1. *Human development begins with fertilization*, a process during which a sperm unites with an oocyte (ovum). The numbered developmental stages end at 8 weeks; however, development continues during the fetal period and long after birth.

2. At the beginning of its development a human embryo is called a **zygote**. This is an appropriate term because *zygōtus* means united and refers to the union of the oocyte and sperm. The term **conceptus** refers to all structures that develop from a zygote (e.g., the embryo, amnion, and chorionic sac). The terms, therefore, are not synonymous.

3. The term **conceptus** is used when referring to an embryo and its membranes, i.e., the products of conception. The term **abortus** refers to any product or all products of an abortion; that is, the embryo (or part of it) and/or its membranes and placenta (or parts of them). An abortus, therefore, is an aborted conceptus.

4. The development of secondary sexual characteristics occurs, reproductive functions begin, and sexual dimorphism becomes more obvious; consequently, the pubertal changes are not the same in males and females. The ages of presumptive puberty are 12 years in girls and 14 years in boys; however, variations occur.

5. **Embryology** refers to the study of embryonic development; clinically it refers to the study of embryonic and fetal development—*the study of prenatal development*. **Teratology** refers to the study of abnormal embryonic and fetal development. It is the branch of embryology concerned with abnormal development and the factors that cause it. Embryological and teratological studies are applicable to clinical studies because they indicate vulnerable prenatal periods of development.

Chapter 2

1. Numerical changes in chromosomes arise chiefly from **nondisjunction** during a mitotic or meiotic cell division (see Fig. 2-3). Most clinically important abnormalities in chromosome number occur during the first meiotic division. Nondisjunction is the failure of double chromatid chromosomes to dissociate during anaphase of cell division; as a result, both chromosomes pass to the same daughter cell and trisomy results. **Trisomy 21** (Down syndrome) is the most common numerical chromosomal disorder resulting in congenital anomalies (see Fig. 8-6*A* to *D*). It occurs about once in every 700 births; however, it is more common in older mothers.

2. A morula with an extra set of chromosomes in its cells results in **triploidy**. This chromosome abnormality usually results from fertilization of an oocyte by two sperms (*dispermy*). A fetus could develop from a triploid morula and be born alive; however, this is unusual. Most *trisomic fetuses* abort spontaneously or are stillborn, and most *trisomic infants* die shortly after birth.

3. Blockage of the uterine tubes resulting from infection is a major cause of infertility in women. Because occlusion prevents the oocyte from coming into contact with sperms, fertilization cannot occur. Infertility in men usually results from defects in spermatogenesis. Nondescent of the testes is one cause of *aspermatogenesis* (failure of sperm formation); however, normally positioned testes may not produce adequate numbers of actively motile sperms.

4. **Mosaicism** results from nondisjunction of double chromatid chromosomes during early cleavage of a zygote rather than during gametogenesis. As a consequence, the embryo has two cell lines with different chromosome numbers. Persons who develop from these chromosomally abnormal embryos are **mosaics.** About 1% of Down syndrome persons are mosaics. They have relatively mild stigmata of the syndrome and are less retarded than usual. *Mosaicism can be detected before birth* by cytogenetic studies following amniocentesis and chorionic villus sampling (see Chapter 6).

5. *Postcoital birth control pills* ("morning after pills") may be prescribed in an emergency (e.g., following sexual abuse). Ovarian hormones (estrogen) taken in large doses within 72 hours after sexual intercourse usually prevent implantation of the blastocyst, probably by altering tubal motility, interfering with corpus luteum function, or causing abnormal changes in the endometrium. *These hormones prevent implantation, not fertilization.* Consequently, they should not be called contraceptive pills. Conception occurs but the blastocyst does not implant. It would be more appropriate to call them "contraimplantation pills." Because the term *abortion* refers to a premature stoppage of a pregnancy, the term *abortion* could be applied to such an early termination of pregnancy.

Chapter 3

1. Yes, a chest radiograph could be taken because the patient's uterus and ovaries are not directly in the x-ray beam. The only radiation the ovaries receive would be a negligible, scattered amount. Furthermore, this small amount of radiation would be highly unlikely to damage the products of conception if the patient happened to be pregnant. Most physicians, however, would defer the radiographic examination of the thorax if at all possible, because if the woman had an abnormal child she might sue the doctor, claiming that the x-rays produced the abnormality. A jury may not accept the scientific evidence for the nonteratogenicity of low-dose radiation.

2. *Diethylstilbestrol* (DES) appears to affect the endometrium by rendering it unprepared for implantation, a process that is regulated by a delicate balance between estrogen and progesterone. The large doses of estrogen upset this balance. Progesterone makes the endometrium grow thick and succulent so that the blastocyst may become embedded and nourished adequately. DES pills are referred to as "morning after pills" by lay people. When the media refer to the "abortion pill," they are usually referring to RU486. This drug, developed in France, interferes with implantation of the blastocyst by blocking the production of progesterone by the corpus luteum. A pregnancy can be detected at the end of the second week after fertilization using highly sensitive pregnancy tests. Most tests depend on the presence of an *early pregnancy factor* (EPF) in the maternal serum. Early pregnancy can also be detected by ultrasonography.

3. Over 95% of ectopic pregnancies are in the uterine tube, and 60% of them are in the ampulla of the tube. *Endovaginal sonography* is often used to detect ectopic tubal pregnancies. The surgeon would likely perform a *laparotomy* (abdominal section to gain access to the peritoneal cavity) and remove the uterine tube containing the conceptus.

4. No, the surgery could not have produced the anomaly of the brain. Exposure of an embryo during the second week of development to the slight trauma that might be associated with abdominal surgery would not cause a congenital anomaly. Furthermore, the anesthetics used during the operation would not induce an anomaly of the brain. Teratogens present during the first 2 weeks of development are not known to induce congenital anomalies.

5. Women over 40 years of age are more likely to have a baby with congenital anomalies such as Down syndrome; however, women over 40 can have normal children. Prenatal diagnosis (e.g., using chori-

onic villus sampling or amniocentesis) is now available for women over 35 years of age. This procedure will tell whether the embryo has severe chromosomal abnormalities (e.g., trisomy 13) that would cause its death shortly after birth. Ultrasound examination of the embryo in utero may also be carried out for the detection of certain morphological anomalies (e.g., anomalies of the limbs and central nervous system). In most cases the embryo is normal and the pregnancy continues to full term.

Chapter 4

1. The hormones in birth control pills prevent ovulation and development of the secretory stage of the menstrual (uterine) cycle. Severe chromosomal abnormalities may have caused the spontaneous abortion. The incidence of chromosomal abnormalities in early abortions is very high in women who become pregnant shortly after discontinuing the use of birth control pills. A pronounced increase in polyploidy (cells containing three or more times the haploid number of chromosomes) has been observed in embryos expelled during spontaneous abortions when conception occurred within 2 months after discontinuing oral contraception. Polyploidy is fatal to the developing embryo. This information suggests that it is wise to use some other type of contraception for one or two menstrual cycles before attempting pregnancy after discontinuing oral contraceptives. In the present case, the physician probably told the patient that her abortion was a natural screening process, that is, that it was probably the spontaneous expulsion of an embryo that could not have survived because it likely had severe chromosomal abnormalities. Some women have become pregnant 1 month after discontinuing the use of contraceptive pills and have given birth to normal babies.

2. A highly sensitive radioimmune test would likely indicate that the woman was pregnant. The presence of embryonic and/or chorionic tissue in the endometrial remnants would be an absolute sign of pregnancy. By 5 days after the expected menses (about 5 weeks after the last normal menstrual period [LNMP]), the embryo would be in the third week of its development. The blastocyst would be about 2 mm in diameter and can be detected with current transvaginal ultrasound techniques.

3. The central nervous system (brain and spinal cord) begins to develop during the third week. Meroencephaly or anencephaly, in which most of the brain and calvaria are absent, may result from environmental teratogens acting during the third week of development. This severe anomaly of the brain occurs because of failure of the cranial part of the neural tube to develop normally, which usually results from nonclosure of the rostral neuropore.

4. *Sacrococcygeal teratomas* arise from remnants of the primitive streak (see Fig. 4-6). Because cells from the primitive streak are pluripotent, the tumors contain various types of tissue derived from all three germ layers. There is a clear-cut difference in the incidence of these tumors with regard to sex; they are three to four times more frequent in girls than in boys.

5. *Endovaginal sonography* is an important technique for assessing pregnancy during the third week because the conceptus can be visualized. It is, therefore, possible to determine if the embryo is developing normally. A negative pregnancy test in the third week does not rule out an ectopic pregnancy because ectopic pregnancies produce human chorionic gonadotropin (hCG) at a slower rate than intrauterine pregnancies. The hormone hCG is the basis of pregnancy tests.

Chapter 5

1. The physician would likely tell the patient that her embryo was undergoing a critical stage of its development and that it would be safest for her baby if she were to stop smoking and avoid taking any unprescribed medication throughout her pregnancy. The physician would also likely tell her that heavy cigarette smoking is known to cause IUGR and underweight babies, and that the incidence of prematurity increases with the number of cigarettes smoked. The physician would also recommend that she not consume alcohol during her pregnancy because of its known teratogenic effects (see fetal alcohol syndrome in Chapter 8).

2. The embryonic period is the most critical period of development because all the main tissues and organs are forming. It is the time when the embryo is most vulnerable to the injurious effects of environmental agents (e.g., large doses of radiation, drugs, and certain viruses).

3. One cannot predict how a drug will affect the human embryo because human and animal embryos may differ in their response to a drug; for example, thalidomide is extremely teratogenic to human embryos but has very little effect on some experimental animals such as rats and mice. Drugs known to be strong teratogens in animals should not be used during human pregnancy, especially during the embryonic period. The germ layers form during gastrulation. All tissues and organs of the embryo develop from the three germ layers: ectoderm, mesoderm, and endoderm. Formation of the primitive streak and notochord are important events during morphogenesis.

4. Information about the starting date of a pregnancy may be unreliable because it depends upon the patient's remembering an event (last menses) that occurred 2 or 3 months earlier. In addition, she may have had implantation bleeding (breakthrough bleeding) at the time of her last normal menstrual period (LNMP) and may have thought that it was a

light menses. Endovaginal sonography is reliable for estimating the starting date of a pregnancy and embryonic age.

5. No! To cause severe limb defects a known teratogenic drug would have to act during the critical period of limb development (24 to 36 days after fertilization). Teratogens interfere with differentiation of tissues and organs, often disrupting or arresting their development. See Chapter 8 for details.

Chapter 6

1. Physicians cannot always rely on information about the time of the last menstrual period provided by their patients, especially in cases in which determination of gestational age is extremely important, for example, in high-risk pregnancies in which one might wish to induce labor as soon as possible. One can determine with reasonable accuracy the estimated date of confinement (EDC), or expected date of delivery (EDD) using diagnostic ultrasound to estimate the size of the fetal head and abdomen. Normally labor would be induced after 37 weeks, using hormones (e.g., prostaglandins and oxytocin), unless there is a good reason to do so earlier.

2. Chorionic villus sampling (CVS) would likely be performed for study of the fetus's chromosomes. The most common chromosomal disorder detected in fetuses of women over 40 years of age is trisomy 21. If the chromosomes of the fetus were normal but congenital abnormalities of the brain or the limbs were suspected, ultrasonography would likely be performed. These methods allow one to look for morphological abnormalities while scanning the entire fetus. The sex of the fetus could be determined by examining the sex chromosomes in cells obtained by CVS. One can often determine fetal sex using ultrasonography. In persons with technical experience, this method can be used to identify the sex (particularly male) with a certainty that approaches 100% after 30 weeks of gestation.

3. There is considerable danger when uncontrolled drugs (over-the-counter drugs) such as aspirin and cough medicine are consumed excessively or indiscriminately by pregnant women. Withdrawal seizures have been reported in infants born to mothers who are heavy drinkers, and fetal alcohol syndrome (FAS) is present in some of these infants (see Chapter 8). The physician would likely tell the patient not to take any drugs that she does not prescribe. She might also tell her that drugs that are most detrimental to her fetus are under legal control and that she dispenses them with great care.

4. Many factors (fetal, maternal, and environmental) may reduce the rate of fetal growth (intrauterine growth retardation [IUGR]). Examples of such factors are intrauterine infections, multiple pregnancies, and chromosomal abnormalities (see Chapters 7 and 8). Cigarette smoking, narcotic addiction, and consumption of large amounts of alcohol are also well-established causes of IUGR. A mother interested in the growth and general well-being of her fetus consults her doctor frequently, eats a good-quality diet, and does not use narcotics, smoke, or drink alcohol.

5. Amniocentesis is relatively devoid of risk. The chance of inducing an abortion is estimated to be about 0.5%. CVS can also be used for obtaining cells for chromosome study. PUBS refers to percutaneous umbilical cord blood sampling. The needle is inserted into an umbilical vessel with the guidance of ultrasonography. Chromosome and hormone studies can be performed on this blood.

6. *Neural tube defects* are indicated by high levels of alpha-fetoprotein (AFP). Diagnostic studies would be done monitoring the levels of AFP. Further studies would be done using ultrasonography. Low levels of AFP may indicate Down syndrome. Chromosome studies would be done to check the chromosome complement of the fetal cells.

Chapter 7

1. The common method of estimating the expected date of confinement (EDC), or estimated date of delivery (EDD), is to count back 3 months from the first day of the last normal menstrual period (LNMP) and then add 1 year and 7 days (Nägele's rule; see Chapter 6). The biparietal diameter of the fetal head could be measured by ultrasonography in a high-risk obstetrical patient because this measurement correlates well with fetal age. Foot measurements are also very helpful.

2. *Polyhydramnios is the accumulation of an excessive amount of amniotic fluid.* When it occurs over the course of a few days, there is an associated high risk of severe fetal anomalies, especially of the central nervous system (e.g., meroanencephaly and spina bifida cystica). Fetuses with gross brain defects do not drink the usual amounts of amniotic fluid; hence, the amount of liquid increases. *Atresia (blockage) of the esophagus* is almost always accompanied by polyhydramnios because the fetus cannot swallow and absorb amniotic fluid. Twinning is also a predisposing cause of polyhydramnios.

3. There is a tendency for twins to "run in families." It appears unlikely that there is a genetic factor in monozygotic (MZ) twinning, but a disposition to dizygotic (DZ) twinning is genetically determined. The frequency of DZ twinning rises sharply with maternal age up to 35 years and then declines; however, the frequency of MZ twinning is affected very little by the age of the mother. Determination of twin zygosity can usually be made by examining the placenta and fetal membranes. One can later determine zygosity by looking for genetically determined similarities and differences in a twin pair. Differences in genetic markers prove that twins are DZ.

4. A single umbilical artery occurs in about one of every 200 umbilical cords. This abnormality is accompanied by a 15 to 20% incidence of cardiovascular abnormalities (see Fig. 7-20).

5. Two zygotes were fertilized. The resulting blastocysts implanted close together and the placentas fused. The sample of chorionic villi was obtained from the chorionic sac of the female twin. If two chorionic sacs had been observed during ultrasonography, DZ twinning would have been suspected.

6. Amniotic bands form when the amnion tears during pregnancy. The bands surround parts of the embryo's body and produce anomalies such as absence of a hand or deep grooves in a limb (see Fig. 7-24), which constitute the amniotic band syndrome (ABS), or the amniotic band disruption complex (ABDC).

Chapter 8

1. Seven to 10% of congenital anomalies are caused by environmental factors such as drugs and chemicals. It is difficult for clinicians to assign specific defects to specific drugs because:

   - the drug may be administered as therapy for an illness that itself may cause the anomaly.
   - the fetal anomaly may cause maternal symptoms that are treated with a drug.
   - the drug may prevent the spontaneous abortion of an already malformed fetus.
   - the drug may be used with another drug that causes the anomaly.

   Women should know that several drugs, cocaine for instance, cause severe anomalies if taken during pregnancy and that these drugs should be avoided.

2. Women over the age of 35 years are more likely to have a child with Down syndrome (see Fig. 8-6*D*) or some other chromosomal disorder than are younger women (25-30 years). Nevertheless, most women over the age of 35 have normal children. The physician caring for a pregnant, 40-year-old woman would certainly recommend chorionic villus sampling and/or amniocentesis to determine whether the infant had a chromosomal disorder such as trisomy 21 or trisomy 13. A 44-year-old woman can have a normal baby; however, the chances of having a child with Down syndrome are 1 in 25 (Thompson et al., 1991).

3. Penicillin has been widely used during pregnancy for over 25 years without any suggestion of teratogenicity. Small doses of aspirin and other salicylates are ingested by most pregnant women, and, when they are consumed as directed by a physician, the teratogenic risk is very low. Chronic consumption of large doses of aspirin during early pregnancy may be harmful. Alcohol and other social drugs, such as cocaine, should be avoided.

4. The physician would certainly tell the mother that there was no danger that her child would develop cataracts and cardiac defects because she has German measles. He would undoubtedly explain that cataracts often develop in embryos whose mothers contract the disease early in pregnancy and occur because of the damaging effect the rubella virus has on the developing lens (see Fig. 8-23*A* and *B*). The physician might say that it is not necessarily bad for a girl to contract German measles before her childbearing years because this attack would probably confer permanent immunity to rubella.

5. Cats may be infected with the parasite *Toxoplasma gondii*. Oocysts of these parasites appear in the feces of cats and can be ingested if one is careless in handling the cat's litter. If the woman is pregnant, the parasite can cause severe anomalies of the central nervous system (see Fig. 8-25*A* and *B*) such as mental retardation and blindness.

Chapter 9

1. A diagnosis of *congenital diaphragmatic hernia* (CDH) is most likely. The congenital defect in the diaphragm that produces this hernia usually results from the failure of the left pericardioperitoneal canal to close during the sixth week of development; consequently, herniation of abdominal organs into the thorax occurs. This compresses the lungs, especially the left one, and results in respiratory distress. The diagnosis can usually be established by a radiographic or sonographic examination of the chest. The anomaly can also be detected prenatally using ultrasonography. Characteristically, there are air- and/or fluid-filled loops of intestine in the left hemithorax of a newborn infant afflicted with CDH (see Figs. 9-12 and 9-13).

2. In the very rare congenital anomaly *retrosternal hernia*, the intestine may herniate into the pericardial sac, or conversely, the heart may be displaced into the superior part of the peritoneal cavity. Herniation of the intestine through the sternocostal hiatus causes this condition.

3. CDH occurs about once in every 2200 births. A newborn infant in whom a diagnosis of CDH is suspected would immediately be positioned with the head and thorax higher than the abdomen and feet to facilitate the inferior displacement of the abdominal organs in the thorax. After a period of preoperative stabilization, an operation is performed with reduction of the abdominal viscera and closure of the diaphragmatic defect. Mortality rates are about 60%. Newborns with CDH often die because of severe respiratory distress from poor development of the lungs.

4. *Epigastric hernias* occur in the median plane of the epigastric region. This type of hernia is uncommon. The defect through which herniation occurs results

from failure of the lateral body folds to fuse in this region during the fourth week.

Chapter 10

1. The most likely diagnosis is a *branchial sinus* (see Fig. 10-11). When the sinus becomes infected, an intermittent discharge of mucoid material occurs. The material was probably discharged from an *external branchial sinus*, a remnant of the second pharyngeal groove and/or cervical sinus. Normally, this groove and sinus disappear as the neck forms.

2. The position of the inferior parathyroid glands is variable. They develop in close association with the thymus gland and are carried caudally with it during its descent through the neck. If the thymus fails to descend to its usual position in the superior mediastinum, one or both inferior parathyroid glands may be located near the bifurcation of the common carotid artery. If an inferior parathyroid gland does not separate from the thymus, it may be carried into the superior mediastinum with the thymus.

3. The patient very likely has a *thyroglossal duct cyst* that arose from a small remnant of the embryonic thyroglossal duct (see Figs. 10-20 and 10-21). When complete degeneration of this duct does not occur, a cyst may form from it anywhere along the median plane of the neck between the foramen cecum of the tongue and the jugular notch in the manubrium of the sternum. A thyroglossal cyst may be confused with an ectopic thyroid gland, such as one that has not descended to its normal position in the neck.

4. Unilateral cleft lip results from failure of the maxillary prominence on the affected side to fuse with the merged medial nasal prominences (see Fig. 10-41*A* and *B*). Clefting of the maxilla anterior to the incisive fossa results from failure of the lateral palatine process to fuse with the primary palate. About 60 to 80% of persons who have a cleft lip, with or without cleft palate, are males. When both parents are normal and have had one child with a cleft lip, the chance that the next infant will have the same lip anomaly is about 4%.

5. There is substantial evidence that anticonvulsant drugs, such as phenytoin or diphenylhydantoin, when given to epileptic women during pregnancy, increase by two- to threefold the incidence of cleft lip and cleft palate when compared with the general population. Cleft lip with cleft palate is caused by many factors, some genetic and others environmental; therefore, this condition has a multifactorial etiology. In most cases the environmental factor involved is not identifiable.

Chapter 11

1. Inability to pass a catheter through the esophagus into the stomach indicates *esophageal atresia*. Because this anomaly is commonly associated with *tracheoesophageal fistula*, the pediatrician would suspect a fistula. A radiographic or sonographic examination would demonstrate the atresia. The presence of this anomaly would be confirmed by imaging the nasogastric tube arrested in the proximal esophageal pouch. If necessary a small amount (1 to 3 ml) of air would be injected to highlight the image. When certain types of tracheoesophageal fistula are present, there would also be air in the stomach that passed to it from a connection between the esophagus and the trachea (see Fig. 11-5). A combined radiologic, endoscopic, and surgical approach would usually be used to detect and remove a tracheoesophageal fistula.

2. An infant with respiratory distress syndrome (RDS) or hyaline membrane disease tries to overcome the ventilatory problem by increasing the rate and depth of respiration. Intercostal, subcostal, sternal retractions, and nasal flaring are prominent signs of respiratory distress. *Hyaline membrane disease* is a leading cause of RDS and death in liveborn, premature infants. A deficiency of pulmonary surfactant is associated with RDS. *Glucocorticoid treatment* may be given during pregnancy to accelerate fetal lung development and surfactant production.

3. The most common type of tracheoesophageal fistula connects the trachea with the inferior part of the esophagus. This anomaly is associated with *atresia of the esophagus* superior to the fistula. Tracheoesophageal fistula results from incomplete division of the foregut by the tracheoesophageal septum into the esophagus and trachea.

4. In most types of tracheoesophageal fistula, air passes from the trachea through the fistula into the esophagus and stomach. *Pneumonitis* (pneumonia) resulting from aspiration of oral and nasal secretions into the lungs is a serious complication of this anomaly. Giving the baby water or food by mouth is obviously contraindicated in such cases.

Chapter 12

1. Complete absence of a lumen (*duodenal atresia*) usually involves the second (descending) and third (horizontal) parts of the duodenum. The obstruction usually results from incomplete vacuolization of the lumen of the duodenum during the eighth week (see Figs. 12-6*B* and 12-7). The obstruction causes distention of the stomach and proximal duodenum because the fetus swallows amniotic fluid, and the newborn infant swallows air, mucus, and milk. Duodenal atresia is common in infants with Down syndrome, as are other severe congenital anomalies such as annular pancreas, cardiovascular abnormalities, malrotation of the midgut, and anorectal anomalies. *Polyhydramnios* occurs because the duodenal atresia prevents normal absorption of amniotic fluid from the fetal intestine distal to the obstruction. The fetus swallows amniotic fluid before birth; how-

ever, because of duodenal atresia, this fluid cannot pass along the bowel, be absorbed into the fetal circulation, and transferred across the placental membrane into the mother's circulation from which it enters her urine.

2. The yolk stalk normally undergoes complete involution by the tenth week of development, at which time the intestines return to the abdomen. In 2 to 4% of people, a remnant of the yolk stalk persists as a diverticulum of the ileum—a *Meckel diverticulum*—however, only a small number of these anomalies ever become symptomatic (see Figs. 12-21 and 12-22). In the present case, the entire yolk stalk persisted so that the diverticulum was connected to the anterior abdominal wall and umbilicus by a sinus tract. This anomaly is rare, and its external opening may be confused with a granuloma (inflammatory lesion) of the stump of the umbilical cord.

3. The fistula was likely connected to the blind end of the rectum. The anomaly—*imperforate anus with rectovaginal fistula*—results from failure of the urorectal septum to form a complete separation between the anterior and posterior parts of the urogenital sinus. Because the inferior one-third of the vagina forms from the anterior part of the urogenital sinus, it joins the rectum, which forms from the posterior part of the sinus.

4. This anomaly is an omphalocele (exomphalos). A small omphalocele, like the one described here, is sometimes called an *umbilical cord hernia*; however, it should not be confused with an umbilical hernia that occurs after birth and is covered by skin. The thin membrane covering the mass in the present case would be composed of peritoneum and amnion (see Fig. 12-17). The hernia would be composed of small intestinal loops. Omphalocele occurs when the intestinal loops fail to return to the abdominal cavity from the umbilical cord during the tenth week of fetal life. In the present case, because the hernia is relatively small, the intestine may have entered the abdominal cavity and then herniated later when the rectus muscles did not approach each other close enough to occlude the circular defect in the anterior abdominal wall.

5. The ileum was probably obstructed—*ileal atresia*. Congenital atresia of the small bowel involves the ileum most frequently; the next most frequently affected region is the duodenum. The jejunum is involved least often. Some meconium ("fetal feces") is formed from exfoliated fetal epithelium and mucus in the intestinal lumen and is located distal to the obstructed area (atretic segment). At operation the atretic ileum would probably appear as a narrow segment connecting the proximal and distal segments of the small bowel. Atresia of the ileum could result from failure of recanalization of the lumen (see text); more likely, the atresia occurred because of a prenatal interruption of the blood supply to the ileum. Sometimes a loop of small bowel becomes twisted, interrupting its blood supply and causing necrosis (death) of the affected segment. The atretic section of bowel usually becomes a fibrous cord connecting the proximal and distal segments of bowel.

Chapter 13

1. Double renal pelves and ureters result from the formation of two metanephric diverticula, or ureteric buds, on one side of the embryo. Subsequently, the primordia of these structures fuse (see Fig. 13-15). Both ureters usually open into the urinary bladder. Occasionally, the extra ureter opens into the urogenital tract inferior to the bladder. This occurs when the accessory ureter is not incorporated into the base of the bladder with the other ureter; instead, the extra ureter is carried caudally with the mesonephric duct and opens with it into the caudal part of the urogenital sinus. Because this part of the urogenital sinus gives rise to the urethra and the epithelium of the vagina, the ectopic (abnormally placed) ureteric orifice may be located in either of these structures, which accounts for the continual dribbling of urine into the vagina (see Fig. 13-16). An *ectopic ureteral orifice* that opens inferior to the bladder results in urinary incontinence because there is no urinary bladder or urethral sphincter between it and the exterior. Normally, the oblique passage of the ureter through the wall of the bladder allows the contraction of the bladder musculature to act like a sphincter for the ureter, controlling the flow of urine from it.

2. *Accessory (supernumerary) renal arteries are very common* (see Fig. 13-10). About 25% of kidneys receive two or more branches directly from the aorta; however, more than two is exceptional. Supernumerary arteries enter either through the renal sinus or at the poles of the kidney, usually the inferior pole. Accessory renal arteries, more common on the left side, represent persistent, fetal renal arteries that grow out in sequence from the aorta as the kidneys "ascend" from the pelvis to the abdomen. Usually, the inferior vessels degenerate as new ones develop. Supernumerary arteries are about twice as common as supernumerary veins. They usually arise at the level of the kidney. The presence of a supernumerary artery is of clinical importance in other circumstances because it may cross the ureteropelvic junction and hinder urine outflow, leading to dilation of the calices and pelvis on the same side (*hydronephrosis*). Hydronephrotic kidneys frequently become infected (*pyelonephritis*); infection may lead to destruction of the kidneys.

3. *Rudimentary horn pregnancies are very rare*; they are clinically important, however, because it is difficult to distinguish between this type of pregnancy and a tubal pregnancy (see text). In the present

case, the uterine anomaly was the result of retarded growth of the right paramesonephric duct and incomplete fusion of this duct with its partner during development of the uterus (see Fig. 13-44*E*). Most anomalies resulting from incomplete fusion of the paramesonephric ducts do not cause clinical problems; however, a rudimentary horn that does not communicate with the main part of the uterus may cause pain during the menstrual period because of distention of the horn by blood. Because most rudimentary uterine horns are thicker than uterine tubes, a rudimentary horn pregnancy is likely to rupture much later than a tubal pregnancy.

4. *Glandular hypospadias* is the term applied to an anomaly in which the urethral orifice is on the ventral surface of the penis near the glans penis (see Fig. 13-42*A*). The ventral curving of the penis is called *chordee*. Glandular hypospadias results from failure of the urogenital folds on the ventral surface of the developing penis to fuse completely and establish communication with the terminal part of the spongy urethra within the glans penis. Hypospadias may be associated with an inadequate production of androgens by the fetal testes, or there may be resistance to the hormones at the cellular level in the urogenital folds. Hypospadias is thought to have a multifactorial etiology because close relatives of patients with hypospadias are more likely to have the anomaly than persons in the general population. Hypospadias, a common anomaly of the urogenital tract, occurs in about 1 of every 300 male infants.

5. This young woman is female even though she has a 46, XY chromosome complement. She has the *androgen insensitivity syndrome* (see Fig. 13-41). Failure of masculinization to occur in these individuals results from a resistance to the action of testosterone at the cellular level in genitalia.

6. The embryological basis of indirect inguinal hernia is *persistence of the processus vaginalis*, a fetal outpouching of peritoneum. This fingerlike pouch evaginates the anterior abdominal wall and forms the inguinal canal. A persistent processus vaginalis predisposes to indirect inguinal hernia (see Fig. 13-48*B*) by creating a weakness in the anterior abdominal wall and a hernial sac into which abdominal contents may herniate if the intra-abdominal pressure becomes very high (as occurs during straining). The hernial sac would be covered by internal spermatic fascia, cremaster muscle, and cremasteric fascia. For more information about inguinal hernias, see the text.

Chapter 14

1. *Ventricular septal defect* (VSD) is the most common cardiac defect. It occurs in about 25% of children with congenital heart disease. Most patients with a large VSD have a massive left-to-right shunt of blood, which causes cyanosis and congestive heart failure (see Fig. 14-30).

2. *Patent ductus arteriosus* (PDA) is the most common cardiovascular anomaly associated with maternal rubella infection during early pregnancy. When the ductus arteriosus is patent, aortic blood is shunted into the pulmonary artery (see Fig. 14-53*B*). In extreme cases, one-half to two-thirds of the left ventricular output may be shunted through the PDA. This extra work for the heart results in cardiac enlargement.

3. The tetrad of cardiac abnormalities present in the tetralogy of Fallot is: pulmonary stenosis, VSD, overriding aorta, and right ventricular hypertrophy (see Figs. 14-35 and 14-36). Angiocardiography or ultrasonography could be used to reveal the malpositioned aorta (straddling the VSD) and the degree of pulmonary stenosis. Cyanosis occurs because of the shunting of unsaturated blood; however, it may not be present at birth. The main aim of therapy is to improve the oxygenation of the blood in the infant, usually by surgical correction of the pulmonary stenosis and closure of the VSD.

4. *Cardiac catheterization* and ultrasonography would probably be used to confirm the diagnosis of transposition of the great arteries (TGA). If this anomaly were present, a bolus of contrast material injected into the right ventricle would enter the aorta whereas contrast material injected into the left ventricle would enter the pulmonary circulation. The infant was able to survive after birth because the ductus arteriosus remains open in these patients, allowing some mixing of blood between the two circulations. In other cases, there is also an atrial septal defect (ASD) or VSD that permits intermixing of blood. Complete TGA is incompatible with life if there are no associated septal defects or a patent ductus arteriosus.

5. This would probably be a secundum type of ASD. It would be located in the region of the fossa ovalis because this is the most common type of clinically significant ASD (see Fig. 14-27). Large defects, as in the present case, often extend toward the inferior vena cava. The pulmonary artery and its major branches are dilated because of the increased blood flow through the lungs and the increased pressure within the pulmonary circulation. In these cases a considerable shunt of oxygenated blood flows from the left atrium to the right atrium. This blood, along with the normal venous return to the right atrium, enters the right ventricle and is pumped to the lungs. Large ASDs may be tolerated for a long time, as in the present case, but progressive dilation of the right ventricle often leads to heart failure.

Chapter 15

1. The common congenital anomaly of the vertebral column is spina bifida occulta (see text). This defect of the vertebral arch of the first sacral and/or last lumbar vertebra is present in about 10% of people. The defect also occurs in cervical and thoracic ver-

tebrae. The spinal cord and nerves are usually normal, and neurological symptoms are usually absent. Spina bifida occulta does not cause back problems in most people.

2. A rib associated with the seventh cervical vertebra is of clinical importance because it may compress the subclavian artery and/or brachial plexus, producing symptoms of artery and nerve compression. In most cases, cervical ribs produce no symptoms. These ribs develop from the costal processes of the seventh cervical vertebra. Cervical ribs are present in 0.5 to 1% of people (see Fig. 15-11*A*).

3. A hemivertebra can produce a lateral curvature of the vertebral column (*scoliosis*). A hemivertebra is composed of one-half of a body, a pedicle, and a lamina (see Fig. 15-11*B*). This anomaly results when the mesenchymal cells from the sclerotomes on one side fail to form the primordium of half of a vertebra. As a result, there are more growth centers on the one side of the vertebral column; this imbalance causes the vertebral column to bend laterally.

4. *Craniosynostosis* indicates premature closure of one or more of the cranial sutures. This developmental abnormality results in malformations of the skull. *Scaphocephaly*, or a long narrow skull, results from premature closure of the sagittal suture (see Fig. 15-13). This type of craniosynostosis accounts for about 50% of the cases of premature closure of cranial sutures.

5. The features of Klippel-Feil syndrome are short neck, low hair line, and restricted neck movements. In most cases the number of cervical vertebral bodies is less than normal.

Chapter 16

1. Absence of the sternocostal portion of the left pectoralis major muscle is the cause of the abnormal surface features observed (see text). The costal heads of the pectoralis major and pectoralis minor muscles are usually present. Despite its numerous and important actions, absence of all or part of the pectoralis major muscle usually causes no disability; however, the abnormality caused by absence of the anterior axillary fold is striking, as is the inferior location of the nipple. The actions of other muscles associated with the shoulder joint compensate for the absence of part of the pectoralis major.

2. About 13% of people lack a palmaris longus muscle on one or both sides. Its absence causes no disability.

3. It would be the left sternocleidomastoid muscle (SCM) that was prominent when tensed. The left one is the unaffected muscle, and it does not pull the child's head to the right side. It is the short, contracted, right SCM that tethers the right mastoid process to the right clavicle and sternum; hence, continued growth of the left side of the neck results in tilting and rotation of the head. This relatively common condition—*congenital torticollis* (wryneck)—may occur because of injury to the muscle during birth. Tearing of some muscle fibers may have occurred, resulting in bleeding into the muscle. Over several weeks, necrosis of some fibers could have occurred, and the blood was replaced by fibrous tissue. This could result in shortening of the muscle and in pulling of the child's head to the side.

4. Absence of striated musculature in the median plane of the anterior abdominal wall of the embryo is associated with *exstrophy of the urinary bladder*. This severe anomaly is caused by incomplete midline closure of the inferior part of the anterior abdominal wall, and failure of mesenchymal cells to migrate from the somatic mesoderm between the surface ectoderm and the urogenital sinus during the fourth week of development. The absence of mesenchymal cells in the median plane results in failure of striated muscles to develop.

Chapter 17

1. The number of female infants with dislocation of the hip is approximately eight times that of male infants. The hip joint is not usually dislocated at birth; however, the acetabulum is underdeveloped. Dislocation of the hip may not become obvious until the infant attempts to stand up several months after birth. This condition is probably caused by deforming forces acting directly on the hip joint of the fetus.

2. Severe anomalies of the limbs (amelia and meromelia), similar to those produced by thalidomide (see Fig. 8-22), are rare and usually have a genetic basis. The thalidomide syndrome consisted of absence of limbs (amelia), gross defects of the limbs (meromelia) such as the hands and feet attached to the trunk by small, irregularly shaped bones, intestinal atresia, and cardiac defects.

3. The most common type of clubfoot is *talipes equinovarus*, occurring in about one of every 1000 newborn infants (see Fig. 17-18). In this deformation, the soles of the feet are turned medially and the feet are sharply plantarflexed. The feet are fixed in the tiptoe position, resembling the foot of a horse (L. *equinus*, horse).

4. *Syndactyly* (fusion of digits) is the most common type of limb anomaly (see Fig. 17-16). It varies from cutaneous webbing of the digits to synostosis (union of phalanges, the bones of the digits). Syndactyly is more common in the foot than in the hand. This anomaly occurs when separate digital rays fail to form in the fifth week, or the webbing between the developing digits fails to break down between the sixth and eighth weeks. As a consequence, separation of the digits does not occur.

Chapter 18

1. Ultrasound scanning of the fetus can detect absence of the calvaria (acrania) as early as 14 weeks (see Fig. 18-39). Fetuses with *meroanencephaly* (absence of part of brain) do not drink the usual amounts of amniotic fluid, presumably because of impairment of the neuromuscular mechanism that controls swallowing. Inasmuch as fetal urine is excreted into the amniotic fluid at the usual rate, the amount of amniotic fluid increases. Normally, the fetus swallows amniotic fluid, which is absorbed by its intestines and passed to the placenta for elimination through the mother's blood and kidneys. Meroanencephaly, often inaccurately called anencephaly (absence of the brain), can be easily and safely detected by a plain radiograph; however, radiographs of the fetus are not usually taken. Instead, this severe anomaly is usually detected by ultrasonography or amniocentesis. An elevated level of alpha-fetoprotein (AFP) in the amniotic fluid indicates an open neural tube defect, such as acrania with meroanencephaly or spina bifida with myeloschisis.

2. A neurological defect is associated with meningomyelocele because the spinal cord and/or nerve roots are often incorporated into the wall of the protruding sac. This damages the nerves supplying various structures. Paralysis of the lower limbs often occurs, and there may be incontinence of urine and feces resulting from paralysis of the sphincters of the anus and urinary bladder.

3. The condition is called internal or *obstructive hydrocephalus*. The block would most likely be in the cerebral aqueduct of the midbrain. Obstruction at this site (stenosis or atresia) interferes with or prevents passage of ventricular fluid from the lateral and third ventricles to the fourth ventricle. *Hydrocephalus* is sometimes recognized before birth; however, most cases are diagnosed in the first few weeks or months after birth. Hydrocephalus can be recognized using ultrasonography of the mother's abdomen during the last trimester. Surgical treatment of hydrocephalus usually consists of shunting the excess ventricular fluid through a plastic tube to another part of the body (e.g., into the blood stream or peritoneal cavity), from which it will subsequently be excreted by the infant's kidneys.

4. *Hydrocephalus* is not synonymous with a large head because a large brain (*macroencephalon*), a subdural hygroma, or a hematoma can also cause enlargement of the head (see text). Hydrocephalus may or may not enlarge the head. *Hydrocephalus exvacuo* causes enlargement of the ventricles resulting from brain destruction; however, the head is not enlarged. *Microencephaly* (small brain) is usually associated with *microcephaly* (small calvaria). Because growth of the skull is largely dependent upon growth of the brain, arrest of brain development can cause microcephaly. During the fetal period, environmental exposure to agents such as cytomegalovirus, *Toxoplasma gondii*, herpes simplex virus, and high-level radiation is known to induce microencephaly and microcephaly. Severe mental retardation may occur as a result of exposure of the embryo/fetus to high levels of radiation during the 8- to 16-week period of development.

5. *Agenesis of the corpus callosum*, partial or complete, is frequently associated with low intelligence in 70% of cases and seizures in 50% of patients (see text). Some people are asymptomatic and lead normal lives. Agenesis of the corpus callosum may occur as an isolated defect; however, it is often associated with other central nervous system anomalies, such as *holoprosencephalies*—anomalies resulting from failure of cleavage of the prosencephalon (forebrain). As in the present case, a large third ventricle may be associated with agenesis of the corpus callosum. The large ventricle exists because it is able to rise superior to the roofs of the lateral ventricles when the corpus callosum is absent. The lateral ventricles are usually moderately enlarged.

Chapter 19

1. The mother had certainly contracted rubella or German measles during early pregnancy because her infant had the characteristic triad of anomalies resulting from infection of an embryo by the rubella virus (see Fig. 8-23). *Cataract* is common when severe infections occur during the first 6 weeks of pregnancy because the lens vesicle is forming. Congenital cataract is believed to result from invasion of the developing lens by the rubella virus. The most common cardiovascular lesion in infants whose mothers had rubella early in pregnancy is *patent ductus arteriosus*. Although a history of a rash during the first trimester of pregnancy is helpful for diagnosing the congenital rubella syndrome, embryopathy (embryonic disease) can occur after a subclinical maternal rubella infection (i.e., without a rash).

2. *Congenital ptosis* (drooping of upper eyelid) is usually caused by abnormal development or failure of development of the levator palpebrae superioris muscle (see Fig. 19-14). Congenital ptosis is usually transmitted by autosomal dominant inheritance; however, injury to the superior branch of the oculomotor nerve (CN III), which supplies the levator palpebrae superioris muscle, would also cause drooping of the upper eyelid.

3. The protozoon involved was *Toxoplasma gondii*, an intracellular parasite. The congenital anomalies result from invasion of the fetal blood stream and developing organs by toxoplasma parasites (see Figs. 8-24 and 8-25). These parasites disrupt development of the central nervous system, including the eyes, which develop from outgrowths of the brain (optic vesicles). The physician would certainly tell the woman about toxoplasma cysts in meat and advise the woman to cook her meat well, especially

if she decided to have more children. She would tell her that toxoplasma oocysts are often found in cat feces and about the importance of carefully washing her hands after handling a cat or its litter box.

4. The infant had trisomy 18 because the characteristic phenotype is present (see Chapter 8). Low-set, malformed ears associated with severe mental retardation, prominent occiput, congenital heart defect, and failure to thrive are all suggestive of the trisomy 18 syndrome (see Fig. 8-7). This numerical chromosomal abnormality results from nondisjunction of the number 18 chromosome pair during gametogenesis. Its incidence is about 1 in 8000 newborn infants. Probably 94% of trisomy 18 fetuses abort spontaneously. Postnatal survival of these infants is poor, with 30% dying within a month of birth; the mean survival time is only 2 months. Less than 10% of these infants survive more than a year.

5. Detachment of the retina is a separation of the two embryonic retinal layers: the neural pigment epithelium derived from the outer layer of the optic cup and the neural retina derived from the inner layer of the cup. The intraretinal space, representing the cavity of the optic vesicle, normally disappears as the retina forms. The proximal part of the hyaloid artery normally persists as the central artery of the retina; however, the distal part of this vessel normally degenerates.

Chapter 20

1. Natal teeth (L. *natus*, to be born) occur in about 1 in every 2000 newborn infants. There are usually two teeth in the position of the mandibular medial incisors. Natal teeth may be supernumerary ones; however, they are often prematurely erupted primary teeth. If it is established radiologically that they are supernumerary teeth, they would probably be removed so that they would not interfere with the subsequent eruption of the normal primary teeth. Natal teeth may cause maternal discomfort resulting from abrasion or biting of the nipple during nursing. They may also injure the infant's tongue, which, because the mandible is relatively small at birth, lies between the alveolar processes of the jaws.

2. The discoloration of the infant's teeth was likely caused by the administration of tetracycline to the mother during her pregnancy (see text). Tetracyclines become incorporated into the developing enamel of the teeth and cause discoloration. *Dysfunction of ameloblasts* resulting from tetracycline therapy causes hypoplasia of the enamel (e.g., pitting). It is very likely that the secondary dentition would also be affected because enamel formation begins in the permanent teeth before birth (about 20 weeks in the incisors).

3. This is an angiomatous anomaly of the skin—a *capillary angioma* or hemangioma. It is formed by an overgrowth of small blood vessels consisting mostly of capillaries; however, there are also some arterioles and venules in it. The blotch is red because oxygen is not taken from the blood passing through it. This type of angioma is quite common and the mother would be assured that this anomaly is of no significance and requires no treatment. It will fade in a few years. Formerly this type of angioma was called a *nevus flammeus* (flamelike birthmark); however, these names are sometimes applied to other types of angiomas. To avoid confusion, it is better not to use them. Nevus is not a good term because it is derived from a Latin word meaning a mole or birthmark, which may or may not be an angioma.

4. A tuft of hair in the median plane of the lumbosacral region usually indicates the presence of *spina bifida occulta*. This is the most common developmental anomaly of the vertebrae and is present in L5 and/or L1 in about 10% of otherwise normal people. Spina bifida occulta is usually of no clinical significance; however, some infants with this vertebral anomaly also have a developmental defect of the underlying spinal cord and nerve roots.

5. The superficial layers of the epidermis of infants with *lamellar ichthyosis*, resulting from excessive keratinization, consist of fishlike, grayish-brown scales, which are adherent in the center and raised at the edges. Fortunately, the condition is very rare. It is inherited as an autosomal recessive trait.

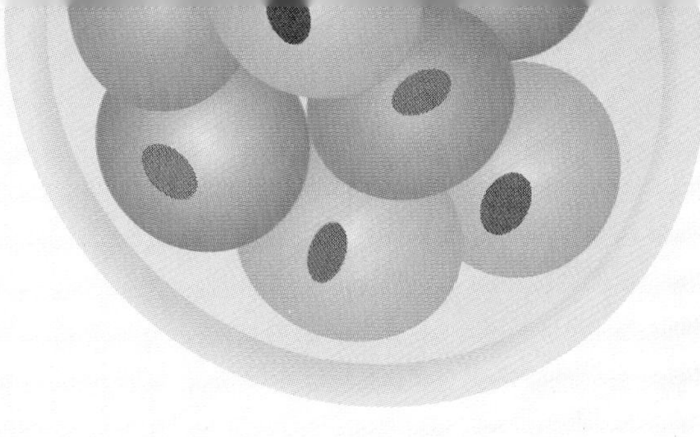

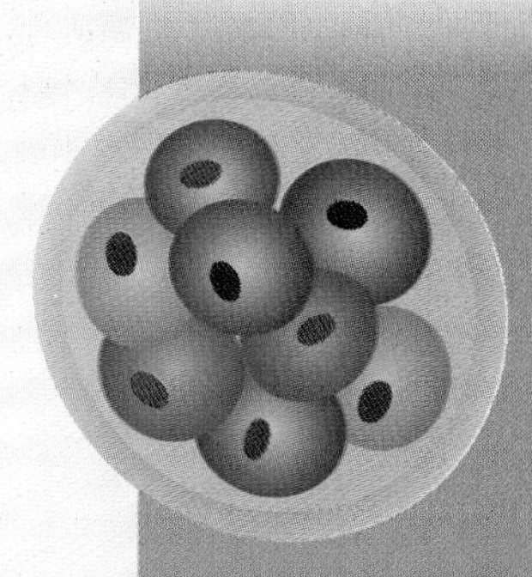

Appendices

Timetable of Human Prenatal Development 1 to 6 weeks

Timetable of Human Prenatal Development 7 to 38 weeks

Critical Periods in Human Development

TIMETABLE OF HUMAN PRENATAL DEVELOPMENT
1 TO 6 WEEKS

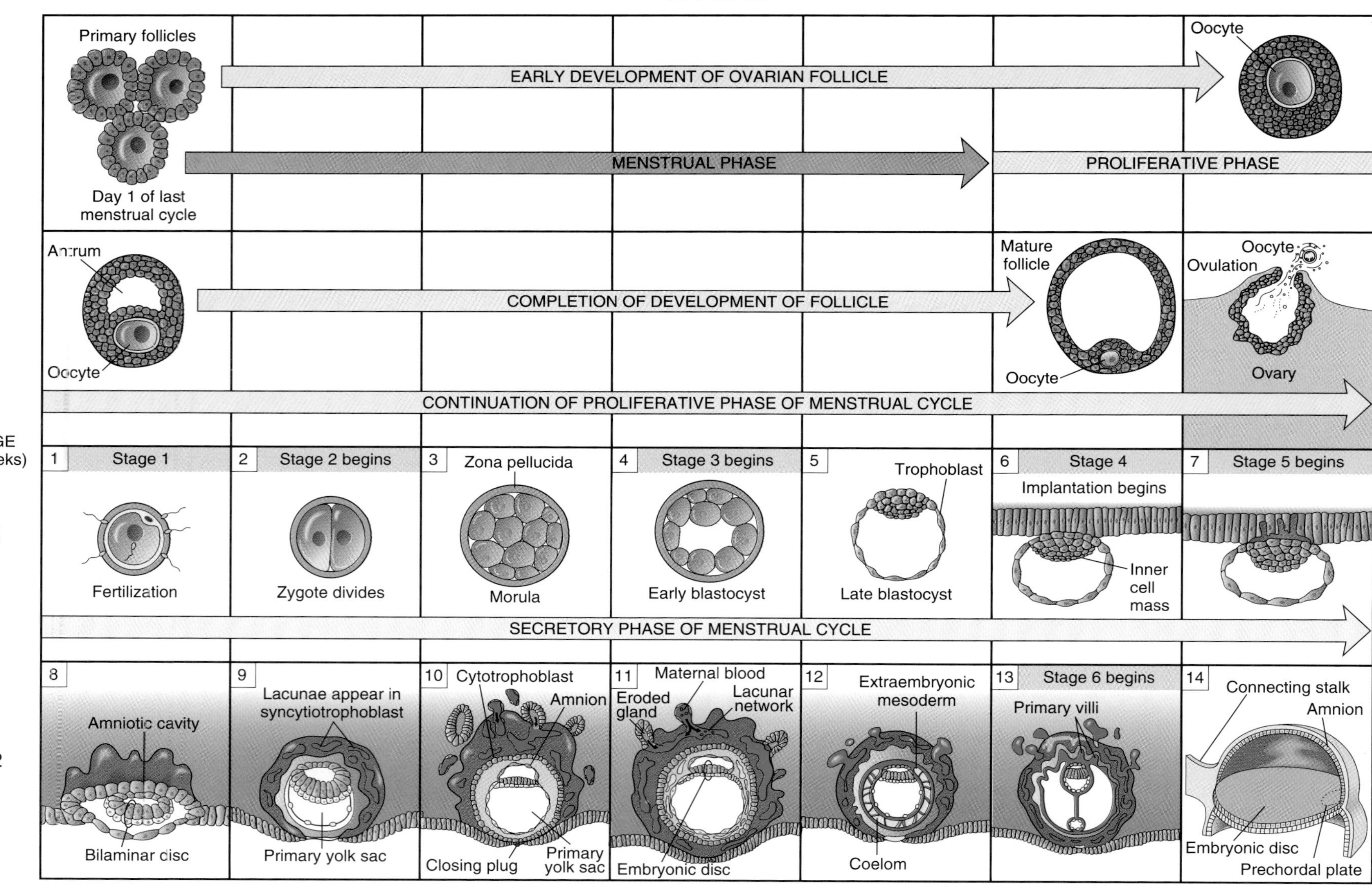

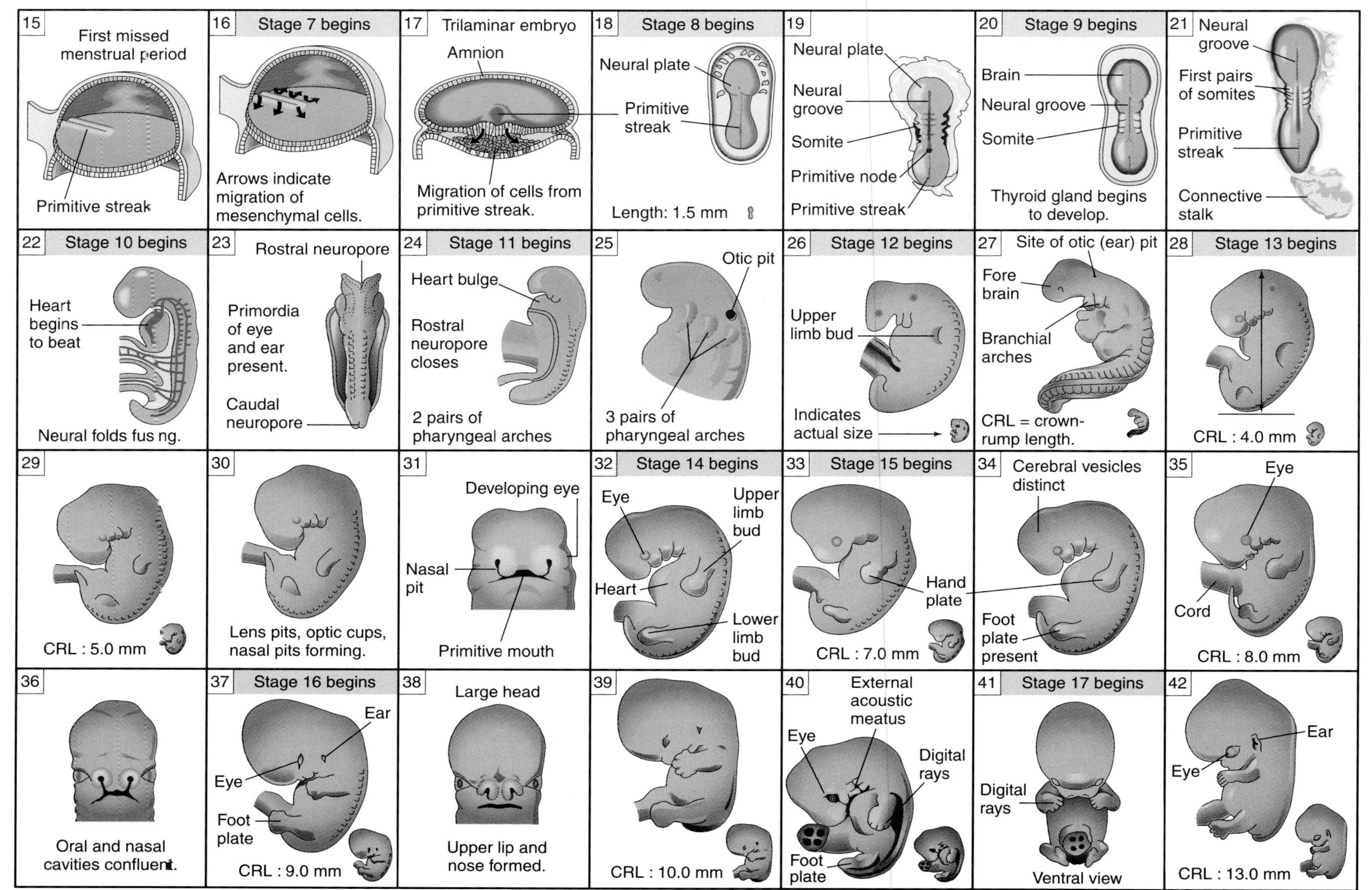

15
First missed menstrual period
Primitive streak
16
Stage 7 begins
Arrows indicate migration of mesenchymal cells.
17
Trilaminar embryo
Amnion
Migration of cells from primitive streak.
18
Stage 8 begins
Neural plate
Primitive streak
Length: 1.5 mm
19
Neural plate
Neural groove
Somite
Primitive node
Primitive streak
20
Stage 9 begins
Brain
Neural groove
Somite
Thyroid gland begins to develop.
21
Neural groove
First pairs of somites
Primitive streak
Connective stalk
22
Stage 10 begins
Heart begins to beat
Neural folds fus ng.
23
Rostral neuropore
Primordia of eye and ear present.
Caudal neuropore
24
Stage 11 begins
Heart bulge
Rostral neuropore closes
2 pairs of pharyngeal arches
25
Otic pit
3 pairs of pharyngeal arches
26
Stage 12 begins
Upper limb bud
Indicates actual size
27
Site of otic (ear) pit
Fore brain
Branchial arches
CRL = crown-rump length.
28
Stage 13 begins
CRL : 4.0 mm
29
CRL : 5.0 mm
30
Lens pits, optic cups, nasal pits forming.
31
Developing eye
Nasal pit
Primitive mouth
32
Stage 14 begins
Eye
Upper limb bud
Heart
Lower limb bud
33
Stage 15 begins
Hand plate
CRL : 7.0 mm
34
Cerebral vesicles distinct
Foot plate present
35
Eye
Cord
CRL : 8.0 mm
36
Oral and nasal cavities confluent.
37
Stage 16 begins
Ear
Eye
Foot plate
CRL : 9.0 mm
38
Large head
Upper lip and nose formed.
39
CRL : 10.0 mm
40
External acoustic meatus
Eye
Digital rays
Foot plate
41
Stage 17 begins
Digital rays
Ventral view
42
Ear
Eye
CRL : 13.0 mm

3

4

5

6

TIMETABLE OF HUMAN PRENATAL DEVELOPMENT
7 to 38 weeks

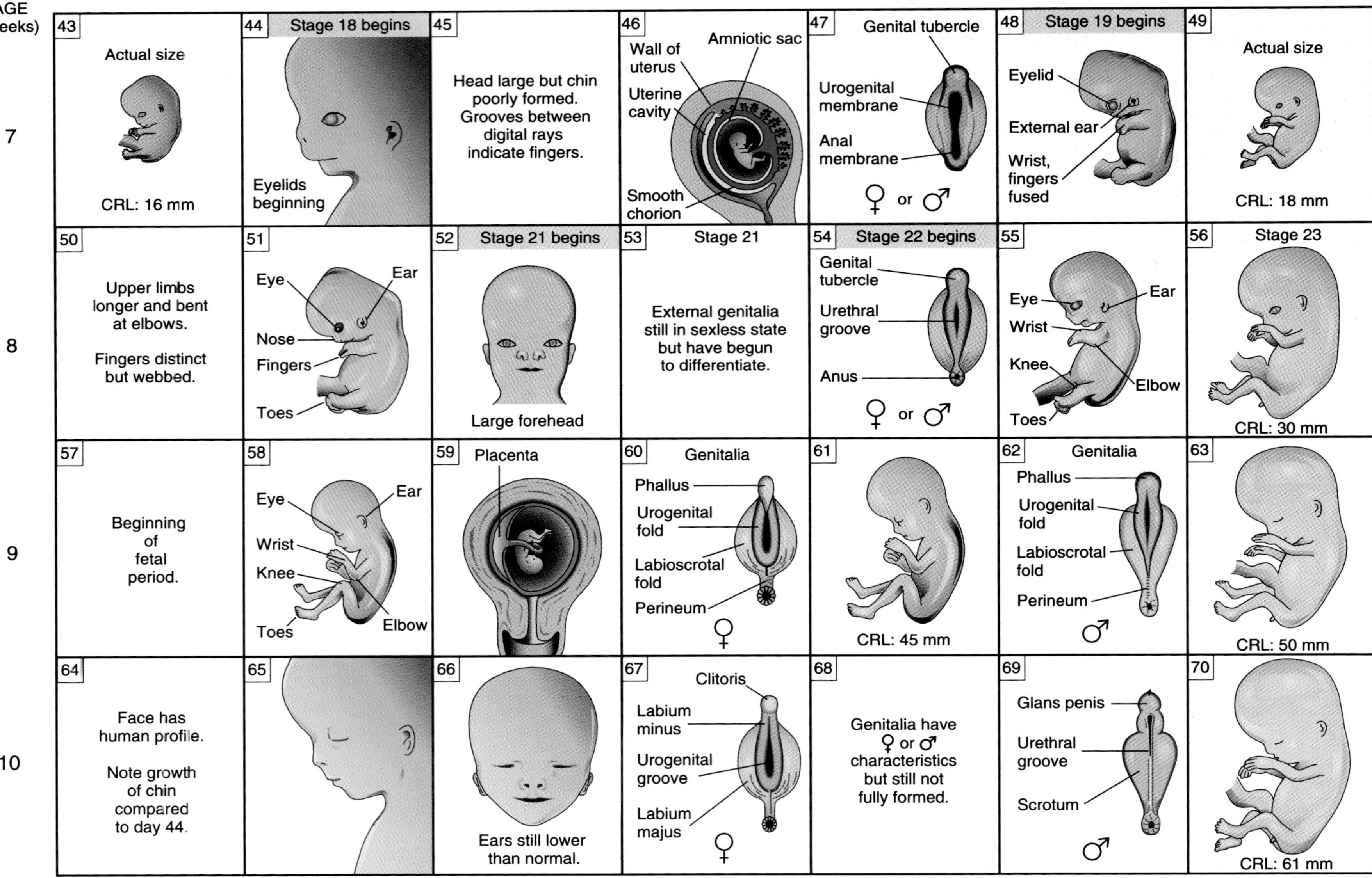

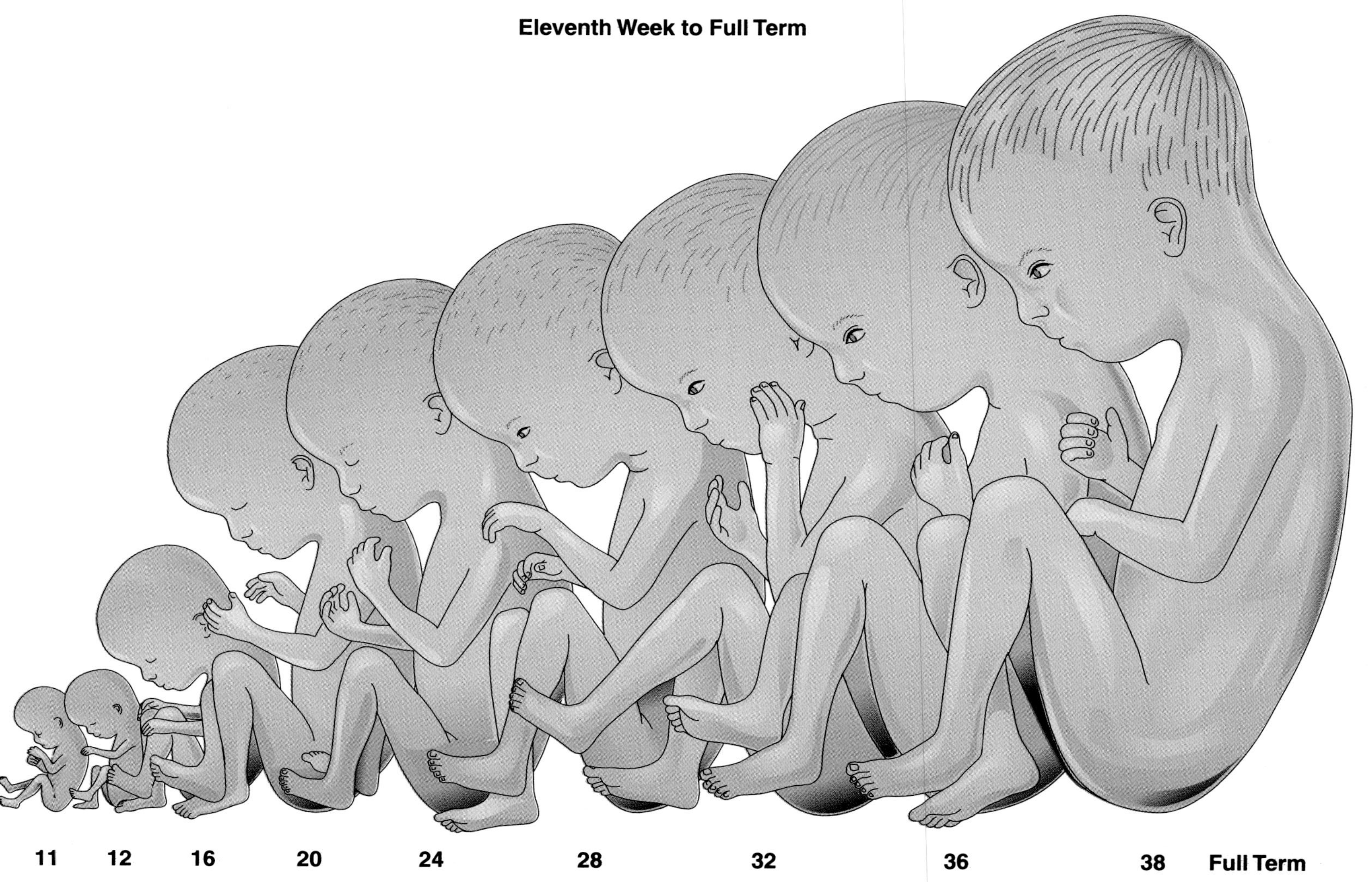
Eleventh Week to Full Term
11
12
16
20
24
28
32
36
38
Full Term

CRITICAL PERIODS IN HUMAN DEVELOPMENT*

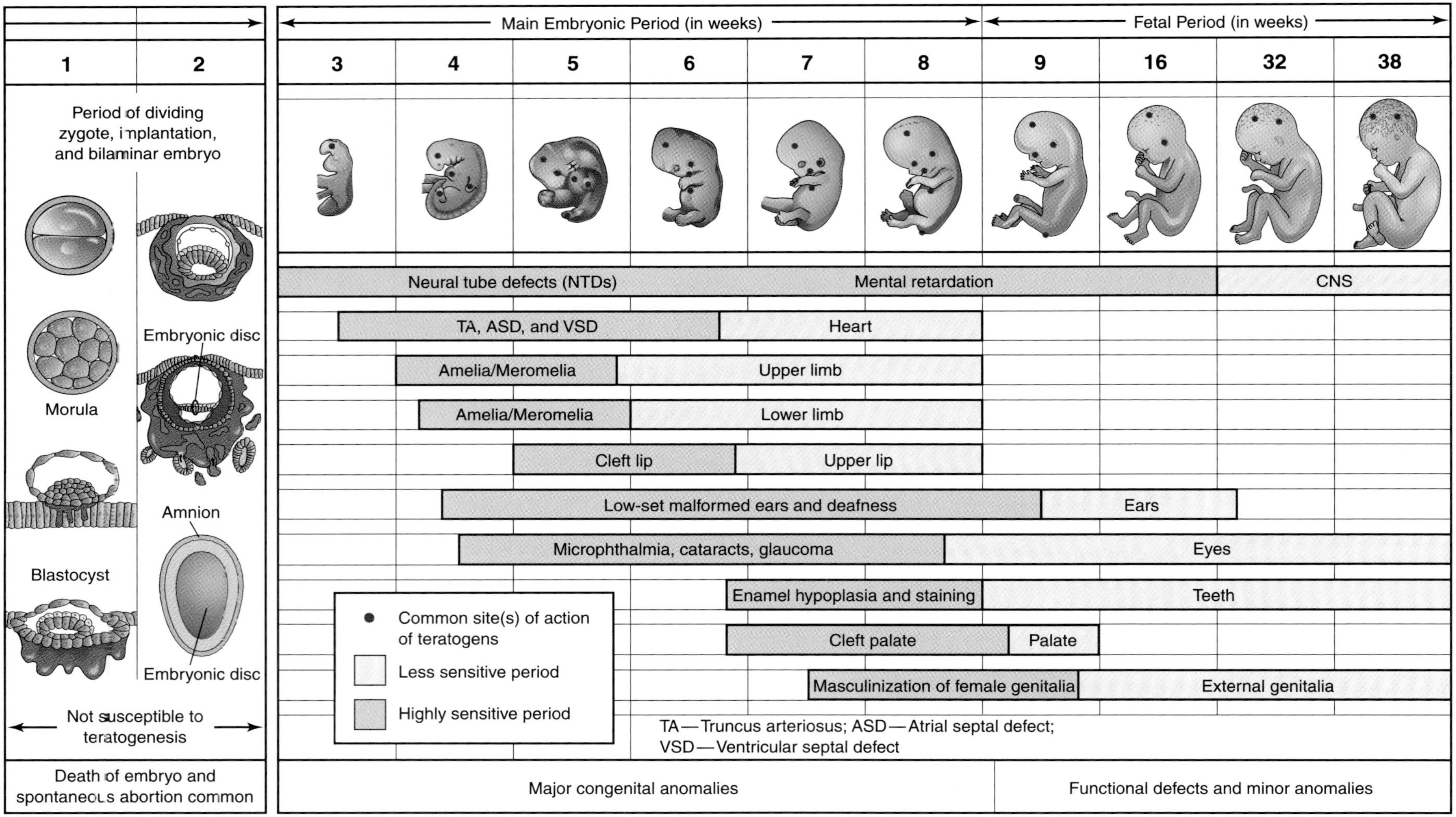

1	2	3	4	5	6	7	8	9	16	32	38

Main Embryonic Period (in weeks) (weeks 3–8)

Fetal Period (in weeks) (weeks 9–38)

Period of dividing zygote, implantation, and bilaminar embryo (weeks 1–2)

Morula

Blastocyst

Embryonic disc

Amnion

Embryonic disc

Not susceptible to teratogenesis

Neural tube defects (NTDs) — Mental retardation — CNS

TA, ASD, and VSD — Heart

Amelia/Meromelia — Upper limb

Amelia/Meromelia — Lower limb

Cleft lip — Upper lip

Low-set malformed ears and deafness — Ears

Microphthalmia, cataracts, glaucoma — Eyes

Enamel hypoplasia and staining — Teeth

Cleft palate — Palate

Masculinization of female genitalia — External genitalia

- ● Common site(s) of action of teratogens
- Less sensitive period
- Highly sensitive period

TA—Truncus arteriosus; ASD—Atrial septal defect;
VSD—Ventricular septal defect

Death of embryo and spontaneous abortion common (weeks 1–2)

Major congenital anomalies (weeks 3–8)

Functional defects and minor anomalies (weeks 9–38)

*Mauve denotes highly sensitive periods when major birth defects may be produced.

Index

Note: Page numbers in *italics* refer to illustrations; page numbers followed by t refer to tables.

B

C

I

N

O

P

T

U